Brief Contents for Volume 2

VOLUME 2

PARAMEDIC PRACTICE TODAY

ABOVE AND BEYOND

VOLUME **2**

PARAMEDIC PRACTICE TODAY ABOVE AND BEYOND

Editor

BARBARA AEHLERT, RN, BSPA

Associate Editor

ROBERT VROMAN, M. Ed, BS, NREMT-P

World Headquarters
Jones & Bartlett Learning
5 Wall Street
Burlington, MA 01803
978-443-5000
info@jblearning.com
www.jblearning.com

Jones & Bartlett Learning books and products are available through most bookstores and online booksellers. To contact Jones & Bartlett Learning directly, call 800-832-0034, fax 978-443-8000, or visit our website, www.jblearning.com.

Substantial discounts on bulk quantities of Jones & Bartlett Learning publications are available to corporations, professional associations, and other qualified organizations. For details and specific discount information, contact the special sales department at Jones & Bartlett Learning via the above contact information or send an email to specialsales@jblearning.com.

The procedures and protocols in this book are based on the most current recommendations of responsible medical sources. The publisher, however, makes no guarantee as to, and assumes no responsibility for, the correctness, sufficiency, or completeness of such information or recommendations. Other or additional safety measures may be required under particular circumstances.

This textbook is intended solely as a guide to the appropriate procedures to be employed when rendering emergency care to the sick and injured. It is not intended as a statement of the standards of care required in any particular situation, because circumstances and the patient's physical condition can vary widely from one emergency to another. Nor is it intended that this textbook shall in any way advise emergency personnel concerning legal authority to perform the activities or procedures discussed. Such local determination should be made only with the aid of legal counsel.

Production Credits
Chief Executive Officer: Ty Field
President: James Homer
SVP, Editor-in-Chief: Michael Johnson
SVP, Chief Marketing Officer: Alison M. Pendergast
Executive Publisher: Kimberly Brophy
Executive Acquisitions Editor—EMS: Christine Emerton
Vice President of Sales, Public Safety Group: Matthew Maniscalco
Director of Sales, Public Safety Group: Patricia Einstein
Production Editor: Tina Chen
Director of Marketing: Alisha Weisman
VP, Manufacturing and Inventory Control: Therese Connell
Director of Photo Research and Permissions: Amy Wrynn
Printing and Binding: Courier Companies
Cover Printing: Courier Companies

ISBN: 978-1-284-03909-2

Library of Congress Cataloging-in-Publication Data
Aehlert, Barbara.
Paramedic practice today : above and beyond / Barbara Aehlert.--lst ed.
p. cm.
Includes bibliographical references and index.
ISBN 978-0-323-08535-9 (vol. 1, hardcover : alk paper)--ISBN 978-0-323-08537-3 (vol. 2, hardcover : alk paper)--ISBN 978-0-323-08539-7 (two volume set, hardcover : alk. paper) 1. Emergency medicine. 2. Emergency medical technicians. I. Title.
RC86.7.A355 2010
616.02'5--dc22

2008041746

6048

Printed in the United States of America
16 15 14 13 10 9 8 7 6 5 4 3 2 1

For our paramedic students and instructors (past, present, and future) who make a personal commitment every shift to provide optimal emergency care to each patient—as if that patient were a member of their own family.

Contributors

Barbara Aehlert, RN, BSPA
Southwest EMS Education, Inc.
Phoenix, Arizona
Pursley, Texas

Imoigele P. Aisiku, MD, MSCR, MBA
Assistant Professor
Department of Anesthesia/Critical Care & Emergency Medicine
Virginia Commonwealth University
Richmond, Virginia

Deanna Aftab Guy, MD
Assistant Professor of Pediatrics
Division of Pediatric Endocrinology
Vanderbilt University Medical Center
Children's Hospital at Vanderbilt
Nashville, Tennessee

David K. Anderson, BS, EMT-P
Director of EMS Education
NW Regional Training Center
Vancouver, Washington

Augie Bamonti III, EMT-P, FF
EMS Training Officer
Chicago Heights Fire Department
Chicago Heights, Illinois

Jeffrey K. Benes, BS, NREMT-P
EMS Coordinator
Aurora Medical Centre
Kenosha, Wisconsin

Scott Bourn, PhD, RN, NREMT-P
National Director of Clinical Programs
American Medical Response National Resource Center
Greatwood Village, Colorado

Jennie A. Buchanan, MD
Chief Resident in Emergency Medicine
Denver Health
Denver, Colorado

Chris Cebollero, NREMT-P
Clinical Services Manager
MedStar
Fort Worth, Texas

Jo Ann Cobble, EdD, NREMT-P, RN
Dean, Division of Health Professions
Oklahoma City Community College
Oklahoma City, Oklahoma

Kevin T. Collopy, BA, NREMT-P, WEMT
Lead Instructor, Wilderness Medical Associates
Bell Ambulance, Inc.
Milwaukee, Wisconsin

Peter Connick, EMT-P, EMT I/C
Captain
Chatham Fire-Rescue
Chatham, Massachusetts
Adjunct Faculty
Cape Cod Community College EMS Program
Emergency Medical Teaching Services Inc
Dennis, Massachusetts

Elizabeth Criss, RN, MEd, CEN, CCRN
Clinical Educator
University Medical Center
Tucson, Arizona

Phil Currance, EMT-P, RHSP
Deputy Commander, National Medical Response Team—Central Task Force
U.S. Department of Homeland Security
Denver, Colorado

Randy D. Danielsen, PhD, PA-C
Dean and Professor
Arizona School of Health Sciences
A.T. Still University
Mesa, Arizona

Roy Danks, DO
Kansas Surgical Consultants
Wichita, Kansas

Thom Dick, BA
Quality Care Coordinator
Platte Valley EMS
Brighton, Colorado

Steven Dralle, LP, BA
Director of Operations
American Medical Response–South Texas
San Antonio, Texas

Marc Eckstein, MD, FACEP
Medical Director
Los Angeles Fire Department
Associate Professor of Emergency Medicine
Keck School of Medicine of the University of Southern California
Director of Prehospital Care
Los Angeles County/University of Southern California Medical Center
Los Angeles, California

Dennis Edgerly, EMT-P
Program Coordinator
HealthONE EMS
Englewood, Colorado

John Elder, EMT-P, CCEMT-P
Forth Worth, Texas

Hunter Elliott, CCEMT-P
Adjunct Faculty
The Center for Emergency Health Services
Williamsburg, Virginia

Jay Fitch, PhD
Fitch & Associates, LLC
Platte City, Missouri

Jeffery S. Force, BA, NREMT-P
EMS Program Director
Pikes Peak Community College
Colorado Springs, Colorado

Greg Frailey, DO
Williamsport Hospital
Williamsport, Pennsylvania

Mark Goldstein, RN, BSN, EMT-P I/C
EMS Coordinator
William Beaumont Hospital–Royal Oak
Royal Oak, Michigan

John B. Gosford, EMT-P
Adjunct Faculty
North Florida Community College
Madison, Florida
CE Broker
Jacksonville, Florida

Keith Griffiths
President
The Red Flash Group
Encinitas, California

Seth C. Hawkins, MD, FACEP
Assistant Medical Director of Special Operations
Burke County EMS
Attending Physician
Blue Ridge HealthCare
Morganton, North Carolina

John C. Hopkins, Paramedic
Retired
Lexington, South Carolina

Davis E. Hill, EMT-P
Program Director
Managing Agricultural Emergencies
The Pennsylvania State University
University Park, Pennsylvania

Lorri Johnston, EMT-P
Owner and Instructor
Emergency Medical Instructor Services
New Carlisle, Indiana
Instructor
LaPorte Hospital
LaPorte, Indiana

Rodger J. Kelley, RN-CEN, EMT-P, I/C
Emergency Department
Ingham Regional Medical Center/Lansing Community College
Lansing, Michigan

Josh Krimston, Firefighter/Paramedic
Director of Operations
EPIC Medics
La Mesa, California

Douglas F. Kupas, MD, EMT-P
Clinical Professor of Emergency Medicine
Department of Emergency Medicine
Geisinger Health System
Danville, Pennsylvania

David T. Lake, BS, MS, EMT-D
Vice President of Academic Affairs
Wichita Area Technical College
Director, State of Kansas Board of EMS, Retired
Wichita, Kansas

Andrea Legamaro, RN
Emergency Room RN
McKinney, Texas

Paul Maxwell, Paramedic
President/Founder
EPIC Medics
San Diego, California

Joanne McCall, RN, MA, CEN, CFN, SANE-A
Senior Education Specialist
St. John Providence Park Hospital
Novi, Michigan

Christine C. McEachin, BSN, CEN, MBA, Paramedic/IC
Clinical Nurse Specialist
Emergency Service Line
William Beaumont Hospital–Troy
Troy, Michigan

Michelle M. McLean, MD, EMT-P
Clinical Faculty
Emergency Medicine Residency
Michigan State University
Covenant Emergency Care Center
Saginaw, Michigan

Michael Meoli, FF/EMTP-TEMS
SEAL Team 17
San Diego Fire Department Special Weapons and Tactics
San Diego Fire Department
San Diego, California

Michael G. Miller, BS, RN, NREMT-P
Coordinator EMS Education
Creighton University EMS Education
Omaha, Nebraska

Joseph B. Mittelman II, BS, NREMTP
Murray City Fire Department
Murray, Utah

Kirk E. Mittelman, BS, NREMTP
Mt. Nebo Training Association
Payson, Utah

Margaret A. Mittelman, BS
Utah Valley State College
Provo, Utah

Ron Moore, Battalion Chief
McKinney Fire Department
McKinney, Texas

Earl H. Neal, BS, EMT-P
Executive Director
Johnson County Ambulance District
Warrensburg, Missouri

Robert G. Nixon, MBA, EMT-P
Manager, Clinical and Educational Services
American Medical Response
New Haven, Connecticutt

William Northington, MD, NREMT-P
Instructor, Department of Emergency Medicine
University of Pittsburgh
Pittsburgh, Pennsylvania

Roger Parvin, Jr, NREMT-P
Field Training Officer
Louisville Metro EMS
Louisville, Kentucky

Mary Jane Pavlick, RN, BA
Program Manager, Emergency Management
Hillcrest Hospital, A Cleveland Clinic Hospital
Mayfield Heights, Ohio

Thomas F. Payton, MD, MBA, EMT-P
Staff Physician, Emergency Medicine
Geisinger Health System
Danville, Pennsylvania

Randall G. Perkins, EMT-P
Paramedic Program Director
Scottsdale Community College
Scottsdale, Arizona

Warren J. Porter, MS, BA, LP, PNCCT
EMS Programs Manager
Garland Fire Department
Garland, Texas

Roy Ramos, NREMT-P
Director Education/Training
Thompson Valley EMS
Loveland, Colorado

William Raynovich, EdD, MPH, NREMTP
Assistant Professor and Director
Creighton University EMS Education
Omaha, Nebraska

Howard Rodenberg, MD, MPH
Director, Division of Health
State Health Officer
Kansas Department of Health and Environment
Topeka, Kansas
Clinical Associate Professor
Department of Preventive Medicine
University of Kansas School of Medicine–Wichita
Wichita, Kansas

Gregory Scott, MBA
EMD QA Instructor
EMD Consultant
Priority Dispatch Corporation
EMD Consultant
National Academies of Emergency Dispatch
Salt Lake City, Utah

Everett Stephens, MD, FAAEM
Assistant Clinical Professor
Department of Emergency Medicine
University of Louisville
Louisville, Kentucky

Rod Thompson, CEP
Deputy Fire Chief
Scottsdale Fire Department
Scottsdale, Arizona

Chris Tilden, PhD
Director, Office of Local and Rural Health
Kansas Department of Health and Environment
Topeka, Kansas
Adjunct Instructor
Department of Health Policy and Management
University of Kansas Medical School
Kansas City, Kansas

Tom Vines
Training Officer
Carbon County Sheriff's Search and Rescue
Red Lodge, Montana

Robert Vroman, M. Ed, BS, NREMT-P
HealthONE EMS
Englewood, Colorado

Richard A. Walker, MD
Associate Professor
Section of Emergency Medicine
University of Nebraska Medical Center
Clinical Director
Nebraska Medical Center Emergency Services
Omaha, Nebraska

Chris Weber, PhD
President
Dr. Hazmat, Inc.
Ann Arbor, Michigan

Elizabeth M. Wertz, RN, BSN, MPM, EMT-P, PHRN, FACMPE
Chief Executive Officer
Pediatric Alliance, PC
Chairperson, EMSC Advisory Committee
Pennsylvania Emergency Health Services Council
Pittsburgh, Pennsylvania

Stephen R. Wirth, JD, BA, MS, EMT-P
Partner, Attorney at Law
Page, Wolfberg & Wirth, LLC
Mechanicsburg, Pennsylvania

Christopher M. Woleben, MD, FAAP
Assistant Professor, Emergency Medicine
Pediatric Division
Virginia Commonwealth University Medical Center
Richmond, Virginia

Douglas M. Wolfberg, JD
Partner, Attorney at Law
Page, Wolfberg & Wirth, LLC
Mechanicsburg, Pennsylvania

Lynn Yancey, MD
Department of Emergency Medicine
University of Colorado Health Sciences Center
Denver, Colorado

Jesse Yarbrough, EMT-P
Operations Paramedic
Louisville Metro EMS
Louisville, Kentucky

Adam M. Yates, MD
Emergency Medicine Attending Physician
Mercy Hospital of Pittsburgh
Pittsburgh, Pennsylvania

Brian S. Zachariah, MD, MBA, FACEP
Associate Professor
Director, Division of Emergency Medicine
University of Texas Medical Branch–Galveston
Galveston, Texas

Reviewers

Michael Armacost, MA, NREMT-P
Owner, Athena Learning Services
Frederick, Colorado
Instructor/Simulation Faculty
Exempla Healthcare
Wheatridge, Colorado

Kathleen A. Ballman, RN, MSN, ACNP, CEN, NREMT-P
Paramedic Training Program
Bethesda North Hospital
Cincinnati, Ohio

Mark Barrier, AAS, NREMT-P, CCEMT-P, EMD
Burke County Emergency Services
Morganton, North Carolina

Rhonda Beck, NREMT-P
Houston Healthcare EMS
Warner Robins, Georgia

Daniel Benard, BS, EMTP-IC
EMS Program Director
Kalamazoo Valley Community College
Kalamazoo, Michigan

Jeffrey K Benes, BS, NREMT-P
EMS Coordinator
Aurora Medical Centre
Kenosha, Wisconsin

Michael Berg, Flight Paramedic
Berklyn Medical Solutions
Gilbert, Arizona

James Blivin, NREMT-P, RRT
F.D. Paramedic/Instructor
Chambersburg, Pennsylvania

Chip Boehm, RN, EMT-P, FF, EMS I/C III
Portland Fire Department
Portland, Maine

Kristen Borchelt, NREMT-P
Cincinnati Children's Hospital
Cincinnati, Ohio

Rob Bozicevich, Paramedic
Instructor
Woodstock, Georgia

Joyce S. Bradley, NREMT-P, AAS, BHCS
Dona Ana Community College
Las Cruces, New Mexico

Bob Breese, CCEMT-P, FP-C
Monroe Community College
Rochester, New York

Brady Breon, AAS, BS, MS, NREMT-P
EMS Operations Chief
Jersey Shore Area EMS
Faculty
Pennsylvania College of Technology
Williamsport, Pennsylvania

Richard Britz, NREMT-P
EMS Captain
Bulverde Spring Branch EMS
Spring Branch, Texas

Rod Brouhard, AA, EMT-P
Former EMS Program Director
Modesto Junior College
Modesto, California

Robert J. Carter, NREMT-P
Flight Paramedic/Instructor
STAT MedEvac
West Mifflin, Pennsylvania
Centre for Emergency Medicine
Pittsburgh, Pennsylvania

Robert Clark, EMT-P, EMSI
Fire Fighter, Paramedic
Warrensville Heights Fire Department
Warrensville Heights, Ohio
Instructor
Cuyahoga Community College
Highland Hill, Ohio

Jo Ann Cobble, EdD, NREMT-P, RN
Dean, Division of Health Professions
Oklahoma City Community College
Oklahoma City, Oklahoma

Kevin T. Collopy, BA, NREMT-P, WEMT
Lead Instructor, Wilderness Medical Associates
Bell Ambulance, Inc.
Milwaukee, Wisconsin

Peter Connick, EMT-P, EMT I/C
Captain
Chatham Fire-Rescue
Chatham, Massachusetts
Adjunct Faculty
Cape Cod Community College EMS Program
Emergency Medical Teaching Services, Inc.
Dennis, Massachusetts

Jon Cooper, NREMT-P
Baltimore City Fire and EMS Academy
Baltimore, Maryland

Ken H. Davis, AS, NREMT-P, CCEMT-P
Eastern New Mexico University
Roswell, New Mexico

John A. DeArmond, NREMT-P
Emergency Management Resources
Half Moon Bay, California

Janice Dorey, RN, BS
EMS Education Coordinator
Advocate Christ Medical Center EMS Academy
Oak Lawn, Illinois

Steven Dralle, LP, BA
Director of Operations
American Medical Response–South Texas
San Antonio, Texas

Kelly J. Drennan, EMT-P
Capital Region EMS
Jefferson City, Missouri

John Dudte, MPA, MICT I/C
Assistant Medical Director
District of Columbia Fire and EMS Department
Washington, D.C.

Cindy Edwards, AAS, NREMT-P, LP
Course Coordinator
Bulverde Spring Branch EMS Training Institute
Spring Branch, Texas

Steven Ernest, NREMT-P
EMS Operations Coordinator/Paramedic Program Coordinator
Kish Health System
Flight Medic
OSF Lifeline Helicopter
DeKalb, Illinois

Thomas E. Ezell III, NREMT-P, CCEMT-P
James City County Fire Department
Williamsburg, Virginia

Mark Fair, BS, NREMT-P, PI, CTM
Director
Fayette Regional Health System School of Paramedic Science
Connersville, Indiana

Joe Ferrell, MS, NREMT-P
EMS Regulation Manager
Iowa Department of Public Health
Des Moines, Iowa

Janet Fitts, RN, BSN, CEN, TNS, EMT-P
Educational Consultant
Prehospital Emergency Medical Education
Pacific, Missouri

Joyce Foresman-Capuzzi, RN, BSN, CEN, CPN, CTRN, PHRN, EMT-P
Business Development Representative
Temple Health System Transport Team, Temple University Health System
Philadelphia, Pennsylvania

Jason Foth, Firefighter/Paramedic
Marshfield Fire and Rescue Department
Marshfield, Wisconsin

Gregory T. Friese, MS, NREMT-P, WEMT
President
Emergency Preparedness Systems, LLC
Plover, Wisconsin

Fidel O. Garcia, EMT-P
President
Professional EMS Education
Mesa State College
Grand Junction, Colorado

Rudy Garrett, AS, NREMT-P, CCEMT-P
Flight Paramedic
Lifenet Kentucky
Lexington, Kentucky

Maylyn Geissler, NREMT-P
Education Coordinator
National EMS Academy
Covington, Louisiana

Lisa Gilmore, MSN/Ed, RN, CEN, CFRN, CC/NREMT-P, FP-C
STC Education Coordinator/Flight Nurse
St. John's Emergency Trauma Center
Springfield, Missouri

Chuck Gipson, AAS, NREMT-P, CCP
Medic, EMS
Des Moines, Iowa

Lynn Goldstein, PharmD
Emergency Medicine Specialist
William Beaumont Hospital–Royal Oak
Royal Oak, Michigan

Mark Goldstein, RN, BSN, EMT-P I/C
EMS Coordinator
William Beaumont Hospital–Royal Oak
Royal Oak, Michigan

James Goss, BS, BA, MHS, MICP
Lead Paramedic Instructor
Northern California Training Institute
Roseville, California
Faculty
Loma Linda University
Loma Linda, California

Thomas G. Gottschalk, Critical Care Paramedic
Educator
Platinum Educational Group, LLC
Jenison, Michigan

Danna S. Hatley, PharmD
Clinical Phramacist
East Alabama Medical Center
Opelika, Alabama

Robert M. Hawkes, MS, PA-C, NREMT-P
EMS Program Director
Southern Maine Community College
South Portland, Maine

Agustin Hernandez, AAS, NREMT-P, I/C
United States Army
Fort Detrick, Maryland

Jon Hibbard, AS, EMT-P, EMS-I
President
Connecticut Medical Training Academy
Windsor Locks, Connecticut

Stephen Hines, BSc, Dip IMC RCS Ed
London Ambulance Service NHS Trust
London, United Kingdom

John C. Hopkins, Paramedic
Retired
Lexington, South Carolina

Mark Hornshuh, BS, EMT-P
Portland Community College
Portland, Oregon

David Hostler, PhD, CSCS
Emergency Responder
Human Performance Lab
Department of Emergency Medicine
University of Pittsburgh
Pittsburgh, Pennsylvania

Eric Howard, NREMT-P, CCEMT-P, FP-C
Senior Flight Crew Member, Flight Paramedic
St. John's Life Line, St. John's Regional Health Center
Springfield, Missouri

Bill Hufford, REMT-P, PI, CTM
Director
Tri-County Training Academy
Connersville, Indiana

Stephen J Huisman, NREMT-P
President/Owner
Great Lakes EMS Academy
Grand Rapids, Michigan

Robert L. Jackson, Jr., EMT-P, CCEMTP, NREMT-P, MAR, MAPS
University of Missouri Health Care
Columbia, Missouri

Captain Thomas Jarman, NREMT-P, AAS
Prince William County Department of Fire and Rescue
Prince William, Virginia

Lorri Johnston, EMT-P
Owner and Instructor
Emergency Medical Instructor Services
New Carlisle, Indiana
Instructor
LaPorte Hospital
LaPorte, Indiana

Scott Jones, MBA, EMT-P
Director, Paramedic Academy
Chairperson, Allied Health
Victor Valley College
Victorville, California

Chad S. Kim, NREMT-P, BA, I/C
Eastern New Mexico University
Roswell, New Mexico

Don Kimlicka, NREMT-P, CCEMT-P
EMS Coordinator
Saint Clare's Hospital
Weston, Wisconsin

Gregory R. LaMay, AS, NREMT-P
Associate Training Specialist
Texas Engineering Extension Service
College Station, Texas

Jane L. LaMay, BSN
Somerville, Texas

Robert W. Lamey, MSIT, NREMT-P
Retired
Baltimore, Maryland

Monica Liebman, RN, MSN, PHRN
Coordinator, Emergency Medical Services
The Children's Hospital of Philadelphia
Philadelphia, Pennsylvania

Lawrence Linder, MA, NREMT-P
Paramedic Faculty
Hillsborough Community College
Tampa, Florida

Shane Lockard, EMT-P, NREMT-P, CCEMT-P
Administrator and Chief
Johnson County Ambulance District
Warrensburg, Missouri

David Lynch, REMT-P, ACLS-I, BLS-I
ALS Coordinator/EMS Training Officer
Mendon Fire Department
Mendon, Massachusetts

Karen F. Marlowe, PharmD
Auburn University Harrison School of Pharmacy
Auburn, Alabama

Dean Martin, EMT-P, AAS
Columbia Missouri Fire Department
Columbia, Missouri

Denise S. Martin, MS, Paramedic I/C
EMS Program Director
Oakland Community College
Auburn Hills, Michigan

John W. McBryde, NREMT-P
Program Director, EMS Department
East Mississippi Community College
Mayhew, Mississippi

Amy C. McCullough, RN, BSN, CEN, NREMT-P
Clayton County Fire Department
Riverdale, Georgia

Captain Gene McDaniel, BS, NREMT-P
Paramedic Education Program Manager
Phoenix Fire Department, EMS Division
Phoenix, Arizona

William McGovern, BS, EMT-P, EMSI, FSI
Quality Assurance Coordinator
Hunter's Ambulance Service
Meriden, Connecticut
Assistant Chief
Yalesville Volunteer Fire Department
Wallingford, Connecticut

Barbara McMahon, RN, BSN, MSN
Nurse Educator
McMahon Consulting
West Palm, Florida

Jeff J. Messerole, Paramedic
Clinical Instructor
Spencer Hospital
Spencer, Iowa

Connie A. Meyer, AAS, MICT
Paramedic Captain
Johnson County Med-Act
Johnson County, Kansas

Joe Middleton, CC/NREMT-P, AAS-P, RN
Deputy Chief of Police
Horse Cave Police, EMS
Horse Cave, Kentucky
Flight Paramedic
Air Evac Lifeteam
Bowling Green, Kentucky
Paramedic
Caverna Hospital Emergency Room, Hart County
Horse Cave, Kentucky

Gregg T. Moriguchi, BS, NREMT-P
Battalion Chief, EMS
Federal Fire Department, CNRH
Pearl Harbor, Hawaii

Greg Mullen, MS, NREMT-P
National EMS Academy
Lafayette, Louisiana

Jad Muntasser
Special Operations Combat Medic
United States Army

Nikhil Natarajan, BPS, NREMT-P, I/C
Strategic National Stockpile Coordinator
New York State Department of Health
Troy, New York

Earl H. Neal, BS, EMT-P
Executive Director
Johnson County Ambulance District
Warrensburg, Missouri

Joshua J. Neumiller, PharmD
College of Pharmacy
Washington State University
Spokane, Washington

Robert G. Nixon, MBA, EMT-P
Manager, Clinical Education
American Medical Response
Springfield, Massachusetts

Chris Parker, MSN/ED, RN, LICP
Office of the Medical Director, Austin County EMS System
Adjunct Faculty
Austin Community College
South Austin Hospital
Austin, Texas

Dennis Parker, MA, EMT-P, I/C
Tennessee Tech University
Cookeville, Tennessee

Richard Patterson, NR/CCEMT-P, MICP, FP-C
Director of Operations, Flight Paramedic, ALS Instructor
Critical Care Concepts, Inc.
Suffolk, Virginia

Captain Tim Peebles, AAS, NREMT-P
EMS Coordinator
Hall County Fire Services
Gainesville, Georgia

Tim Penic, NREMT-P
Field Operations Supervisor
Medstar EMS
Fort Worth, Texas

Warren J. Porter, MS, BA, LP, PNCCT
EMS Programs Manager
Garland Fire Department
Garland, Texas

Merle Potter, NREMT-P
Paramedic/EMS Educator
Wyoming Life Flight
Wyoming Medical Center
Casper, Wyoming

Gregg D. Ramirez, BS, EMT-P
Student Services Director
Northwest Regional Training Center
Vancouver, Washington

Kathleen Rankin, MICT I/C, NREMT-P, AAS
Paramedic, Adjunct Faculty
Johnson County MED-ACT
Johnson County, Kansas

John Rasmussen, REMT-P, PhD
Captain, Support Services
Greenville County EMS
Greenville, South Carolina

David Rathbun, EMT-P, AA
Chairperson
Tactical Emergency Medical Services
LaCanada, California

Kenneth J. Reardon
Flight Paramedic
LifeNet
Valhalla, New York

Lori Reeves, BA, PS/CCP
Program Director
Rural Health Education Partnership, Indiana Hills College
Ottumwa, Iowa

Mark Register, BS, NREMT-P
Lead Paramedic Instructor
Aiken Technical College
Low Country Regional Council EMS
Aiken, South Carolina

William E. Rich, AAS-EMT, EMT-P, CEM
Center for Disease Control and Prevention
Atlanta, Georgia

Larry Richmond, AS, NREMT-P, CCEMT-P
EMS Education Manager
Mountain Plains Health Consortium
Fort Meade, South Dakota

Becky Ridenhour, PharmD
The Medicine Shoppe
Troy, Missouri

Michael W. Robinson, MA, CFO, NREMT-P
Division Chief
Baltimore County Fire Department
Baltimore, Maryland

George Schulp, EMT-P/PI
Director, Education Services
EMS Coordinator
Superior Air-Ground Ambulance Services
Highland, Indiana

Stephen M. Setter, PharmD, CDE, CGP, DVM
Associate Professor of Pharmacotherapy
Washington State University-Spokane
Spokane, Washington

Maureen Shanahan, RN, BSN, MN
EMT Program Coordinator
City College of San Francisco
San Francisco, California

Judson Smith, BSBA, NREMT-P, CCEMT-P
Overland Park Fire Department
Overland Park, Kansas

Derek Sobelman, MPA, NREMT-P
EMS Training Captain
Olathe Fire Department
Olathe, Kansas

Andrew E. Spain, MA, EMT-P
Assistant Manager, Emergency Centers
University of Missouri Health Care
Columbia, Missouri

Randolph Scott Spies, AS, NREMT-P
Emergency Services Program Coordinator
Blue Ridge Community and Technical College
Martinsburg, West Virginia

Robert Spranger, LP
Methodist Dallas Medical Center
Dallas, Texas

David Stamey, CCEMT-P
EMS Training Administrator
District of Columbia Fire and EMS Department
Washington, D.C.

Nerina J. Stepanovsky, PhD, RN, NREMT-P
Chief Flight Nurse
U.S. Air Force Reserve
MacDill Air Force Base, Florida
EMS Program Director
St. Petersburg College
St. Petersburg, Florida

Michael A. Stern, NREMT-P, CCEMT-P
Deputy Chief
Grand County EMS
Granby, Colorado

David L. Sullivan, MA, NREMT-P
EMS/CME Program Director
Critical Care Transport Paramedic and SWAT (Tactical Paramedic)
St. Petersburg College, Pinellas County EMS Sunstar Paramedics
Pinellas Park, Florida
Largo, Florida

Christopher T. Sweeney, NREMT-P, FFI, FFII
Covington Fire Department
Covington, Kentucky

John Tartt, MPH, EMT-P, DHA(c)
Director, Emergency Medical Science
Carolinas College of Health Sciences
Carolinas HealthCare System
Charlotte, North Carolina

Dave M. Tauber, NREMT-P, CCEMT-P, FP-C, I/C
Advanced Life Support Institute
Conway, New Hampshire

Chet Thorne, NREMT-P, I/C, BSN, PALS ACLS
Albuquerque Fire Department
Albuquerque, New Mexico

Donna G. Tidwell, BS, RN, EMT-P
Tennessee Department of Health EMS Division
Nashville, Tennessee

William F. Toon, MeD, NREMT-P
Battalion Chief, Training
Olathe, Kansas

Mark Trueman, BS, NREMT-P
Pennsylvania College of Technology
Williamsport, Pennsylvania

Larry Vandegriff, BS, NREMT-P
Paramedic Instructor, Flight Paramedic
Lifenet Georgia
Griffin, Georgia

Susan Van Egghen, EMT-P
New York State Course Instructor Coordinator and Regional Faculty
Albany, New York

Lisa Vargas, EMT-P, BS
Primary Paramedic Instructor
National College of Technical Instruction
Buellton, California

Jimmy Walker, NREMT-P
Training Coordinator/EMT, EMT-I, Paramedic Instructor
South Carolina Midlands EMS
West Columbia, South Carolina

Laura L. Walker, DM, NREMT-P
Center Director
Weber Simulation Center
Norfolk, Virginia

Michael J. Ward
Assistant Professor of Emergency Medicine
The George Washington University
Washington, D.C.

John J. Watts, MPH, MEP, NREMT-P
Regional Emergency Response and Recovery Coordinator, Region 7
Carolinas HealthCare System
Charlotte, North Carolina

Michael Whitehurst, EMT-P
Albemarle Hospital
Elizabeth City, North Carolina

Marc Yeston, NREMT-P
Canyon District Ranger
National Park Sevice
Grand Canyon, Arizona

Acknowledgments

We would like to thank Jeff Sargent, Cathy Thanner, Roy Ryals, and the employees of Southwest Ambulance for making their staff, facility, vehicles, and equipment available to us for many of the photographs used in this text.

Moulage make-up provided by Graftobian Make-up Company, makers of the EMS Makeup/Severe Trauma Kit. For more information, please visit www.graftobian.com.

Preface

Because being "good enough" isn't good enough for you . . .

Congratulations on your choice to pursue a career in paramedicine. Whether you are just starting out, looking for a refresher, or seeking to perfect your skills, your success in this dynamic field depends on preparation that goes **above and beyond** the standard.

You need the best.

The most clinically comprehensive foundation for practice, **Paramedic Practice Today: Above and Beyond** is designed to help you achieve complete success on the National Registry examination and prepare you for *any* challenge you may encounter in practice.

Paramedic Practice Today: Above and Beyond is more than just a paramedic textbook; it is part of a complete learning system composed of innovative tools that work together to give you the most effective learning experience:

- Textbook
- Companion DVD
- Student Workbook
- Online Resources for Students

HOW TO USE THIS TEXTBOOK

The best possible preparation for the National Registry examination and professional success begins with a solid foundation in the principles and skills of paramedic practice. A conversational, easy-to-read style simplifies topics and helps you master National Standard Curriculum objectives and the National Education Standards. In addition, content corresponding directly to the National Registry of EMTs National EMS Practice Analysis provides unparalleled preparation for the National Registry examination.

Streamlined division and chapter openers help you to navigate each volume with ease and learn more efficiently. *Chapter Objectives* identify learning goals, and the *Chapter Outlines* present a brief overview of each chapter.

DIVISION 8

TRAUMA

CHAPTER 36

Neonatology

Key terms are bolded in each chapter for easy identification. These terms are discussed in the text and are defined for quick reference in the Terminology section at the end of each chapter.

Four-part case scenarios put material into context, enabling you to follow each case from presentation to conclusion. Questions throughout each scenario test your knowledge of each step and are followed by complete answers and expert insight at the end of each scenario.

Forty-nine illustrated, step-by-step skill sequences in this two-volume package guide you through each action to help you review important skills before performing them in class.

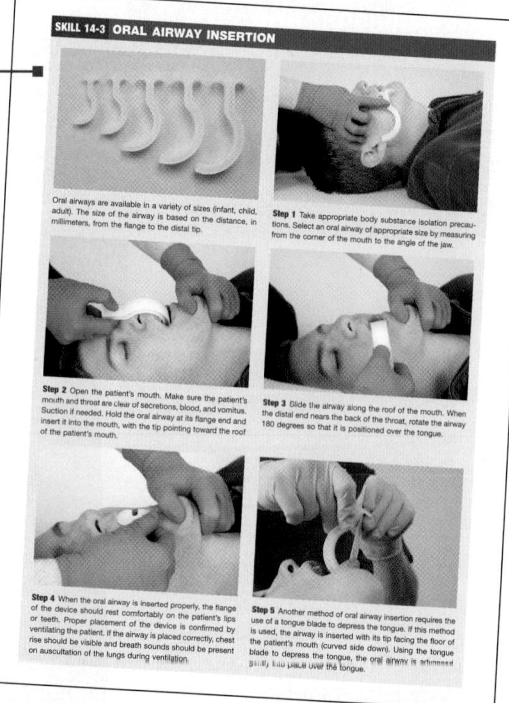
SKILL 14-3 ORAL AIRWAY INSERTION

Oral airways are available in a variety of sizes (infant, child, adult). The size of the airway is based on the distance, in millimeters, from the flange to the distal tip.

Step 1 Take appropriate body substance isolation precautions. Select an oral airway of appropriate size by measuring from the corner of the mouth to the angle of the jaw.

Step 2 Open the patient's mouth. Make sure the patient's mouth and throat are clear of secretions, blood, and vomitus. Suction if needed. Hold the oral airway at its flange end and insert it into the mouth, with the tip pointing toward the roof of the patient's mouth.

Step 3 Slide the airway along the roof of the mouth. When the distal end nears the back of the throat, rotate the airway 180 degrees so that it is positioned over the tongue.

Step 4 When the oral airway is inserted properly, the flange of the device should rest comfortably on the patient's lips or teeth. Proper placement of the device is confirmed by ventilating the patient. If the airway is placed correctly, chest rise should be visible and breath sounds should be present on auscultation of the lungs during ventilation.

Step 5 Another method of oral airway insertion requires the use of a tongue blade to depress the tongue. If this method is used, the airway is inserted with its tip facing the floor of the patient's mouth (curved side down). Using the tongue blade to depress the tongue, the oral airway is advanced gently into place over the tongue.

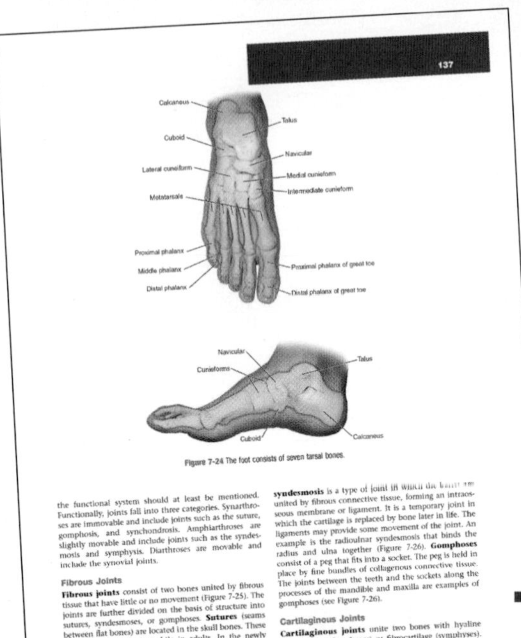
137

Figure 7-24 The foot consists of seven tarsal bones.

the functional system should at least be mentioned. Functionally, joints fall into three categories. Synarthroses are immovable and include joints such as the suture, gomphosis, and synchondrosis. Amphiarthroses are slightly movable and include joints such as the syndesmosis and symphysis. Diarthroses are movable and include the synovial joints.

Fibrous Joints

Fibrous joints consist of two bones united by fibrous tissue that have little or no movement (Figure 7-25). The joints are further divided on the basis of structure into sutures, syndesmoses, or gomphoses. **Sutures** (seams between flat bones) are located in the skull bones. These may be completely immobile in adults. In the newly born, the sutures have gaps called **fontanels.** These gaps allow the skull to expand or contract during birth. They also allow growth of the head during development. A **syndesmosis** is a type of joint in which the bones are united by fibrous connective tissue, forming an intraosseous membrane or ligament. It is a temporary joint in which the cartilage is replaced by bone later in life. The ligaments may provide some movement of the joint. An example is the radioulnar syndesmosis that binds the radius and ulna together (Figure 7-26). **Gomphoses** consist of a peg that fits into a socket. The peg is held in place by fine bundles of collagenous connective tissue. The joints between the teeth and the sockets along the processes of the mandible and maxilla are examples of gomphoses (see Figure 7-26).

Cartilaginous Joints

Cartilaginous joints unite two bones with hyaline cartilage (synchondroses) or fibrocartilage (symphyses). This is a slightly movable joint in which the bones are connected by a fibrocartilage disk or ligaments.

Extensive illustrations clarify key concepts and reinforce your understanding.

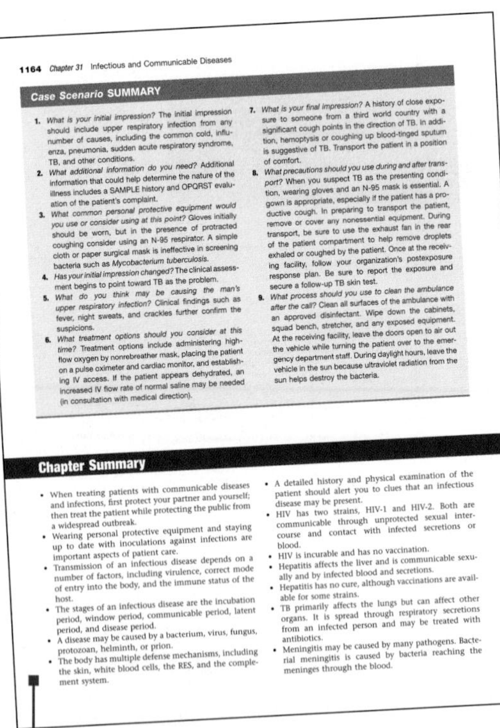
1164 *Chapter 31* Infectious and Communicable Diseases

Case Scenario SUMMARY

1. *What is your initial impression?* The initial impression should include upper respiratory infection from any number of causes, including the common cold, influenza, pneumonia, sudden acute respiratory syndrome, TB, and other conditions.
2. *What additional information do you need?* Additional information that could help determine the nature of the illness includes a SAMPLE history and OPQRST evaluation of the patient's complaint.
3. *What common personal protective equipment would you use or consider using at this point?* Gloves initially should be worn, but in the presence of protracted coughing consider using an N-95 respirator. A simple cloth or paper surgical mask is ineffective in screening bacteria such as *Mycobacterium tuberculosis*.
4. *Has your initial impression changed?* The clinical assessment begins to point toward TB as the problem.
5. *What do you think may be causing the man's upper respiratory infection?* Clinical findings such as fever, night sweats, and crackles further confirm the suspicions.
6. *What treatment options should you consider at this time?* Treatment options include administering high-flow oxygen by nonrebreather mask, placing the patient on a pulse oximeter and cardiac monitor, and establishing IV access. If the patient appears dehydrated, an increased IV flow rate of normal saline may be needed (in consultation with medical direction).
7. *What is your final impression?* A history of close exposure to someone from a third world country with a significant cough points in the direction of TB. In addition, hemoptysis or coughing up blood-tinged sputum is suggestive of TB. Transport the patient in a position of comfort.
8. *What precautions should you use during and after transport?* When you suspect TB as the presenting condition, wearing gloves and an N-95 mask is essential. A gown is appropriate, especially if the patient has a productive cough. In preparing to transport the patient, remove or cover any nonessential equipment. During transport, be sure to use the exhaust fan in the rear of the patient compartment to help remove droplets exhaled or coughed by the patient. Once at the receiving facility, follow your organization's postexposure response plan. Be sure to report the exposure and secure a follow-up TB skin test.
9. *What process should you use to clean the ambulance after the call?* Clean all surfaces of the ambulance with an approved disinfectant. Wipe down the cabinets, squad bench, stretcher, and any exposed equipment. At the receiving facility, leave the doors open to air out the vehicle while turning the patient over to the emergency department staff. During daylight hours, leave the vehicle in the sun because ultraviolet radiation from the sun helps destroy the bacteria.

Chapter Summary

- When treating patients with communicable diseases and infections, first protect your partner and yourself; then treat the patient while protecting the public from a widespread outbreak.
- Wearing personal protective equipment and staying up to date with inoculations against infections are important aspects of patient care.
- Transmission of an infectious disease depends on a number of factors, including virulence, correct mode of entry into the body, and the immune status of the host.
- The stages of an infectious disease are the incubation period, window period, communicable period, latent period, and disease period.
- A disease may be caused by a bacterium, virus, fungus, protozoan, helminth, or prion.
- The body has multiple defense mechanisms, including the skin, white blood cells, the RES, and the complement system.
- A detailed history and physical examination of the patient should alert you to clues that an infectious disease may be present.
- HIV has two strains, HIV-1 and HIV-2. Both are communicable through unprotected sexual intercourse and contact with infected secretions or blood.
- HIV is incurable and has no vaccination.
- Hepatitis affects the liver and is communicable sexually and by infected blood and secretions.
- Hepatitis has no cure, although vaccinations are available for some strains.
- TB primarily affects the lungs but can affect other organs. It is spread through respiratory secretions from an infected person and may be treated with antibiotics.
- Meningitis may be caused by many pathogens. Bacterial meningitis is caused by bacteria reaching the meninges through the blood.

Bulleted summaries at the conclusion of each chapter help you review essential information quickly and easily.

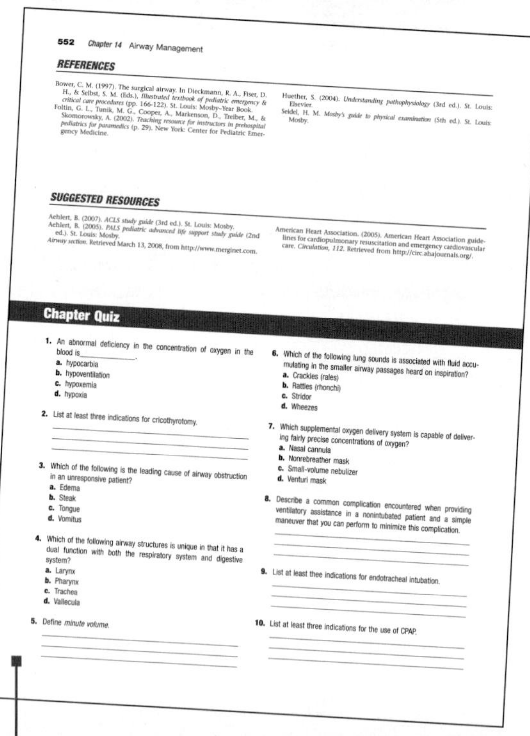
552 *Chapter 14* Airway Management

REFERENCES

Bower, C. M. (1997). The surgical airway. In Dieckmann, R. A., Fiser, D. H., & Selbst, S. M. (Eds.), *Illustrated textbook of pediatric emergency & critical care procedures* (pp. 166-122). St. Louis: Mosby–Year Book.
Foltin, G. L., Tunik, M. G., Cooper, A., Markenson, D., Treiber, M., & Skomorowsky, A. (2002). *Teaching resource for instructors in prehospital pediatrics for paramedics* (p. 29). New York: Center for Pediatric Emergency Medicine.
Huether, S. (2004). *Understanding pathophysiology* (3rd ed.). St. Louis: Elsevier.
Seidel, H. M. *Mosby's guide to physical examination* (5th ed.). St. Louis: Mosby.

SUGGESTED RESOURCES

Aehlert, B. (2007). *ACLS study guide* (3rd ed.). St. Louis: Mosby.
Aehlert, B. (2005). *PALS pediatric advanced life support study guide* (2nd ed.). St. Louis: Mosby.
Airway section. Retrieved March 13, 2008, from http://www.merginet.com.
American Heart Association. (2005). American Heart Association guidelines for cardiopulmonary resuscitation and emergency cardiovascular care. *Circulation, 112.* Retrieved from http://circ.ahajournals.org/.

Chapter Quiz

1. An abnormal deficiency in the concentration of oxygen in the blood is__________.
   a. hypocarbia
   b. hypoventilation
   c. hypoxemia
   d. hypoxia
2. List at least three indications for cricothyrotomy.
3. Which of the following is the leading cause of airway obstruction in an unresponsive patient?
   a. Edema
   b. Steak
   c. Tongue
   d. Vomitus
4. Which of the following airway structures is unique in that it has a dual function with both the respiratory system and digestive system?
   a. Larynx
   b. Pharynx
   c. Trachea
   d. Vallecula
5. Define *minute volume.*
6. Which of the following lung sounds is associated with fluid accumulating in the smaller airway passages heard on inspiration?
   a. Crackles (rales)
   b. Rattles (rhonchi)
   c. Stridor
   d. Wheezes
7. Which supplemental oxygen delivery system is capable of delivering fairly precise concentrations of oxygen?
   a. Nasal cannula
   b. Nonrebreather mask
   c. Small-volume nebulizer
   d. Venturi mask
8. Describe a common complication encountered when providing ventilatory assistance in a nonintubated patient and a simple maneuver that you can perform to minimize this complication.
9. List at least thee indications for endotracheal intubation.
10. List at least three indications for the use of CPAP.

Chapter quizzes included at the end of each chapter test your understanding of chapter content with a variety of multiple-choice, true/false, short-answer, and matching questions. Answers and rationales at the end of each volume provide instant feedback and help you identify areas requiring additional study and review.

***Pediatric Pearl* boxes** identify important distinctions for managing pediatric patients.

PEDIATRIC*Pearl*

Maintaining appropriate temperature is particularly important in the pediatric patient because children have a large body surface area/weight ratio, providing a greater area for heat loss.

***Cultural Considerations* boxes** provide helpful information for interacting with people of various cultures.

CULTURAL*Considerations*

When talking with patients, try to avoid using medical terms. Ask the patient questions and explain what you are going to do to help by using words that are easy to understand. This is important when communicating with any patient, but it is particularly important when speaking with patients for whom English is a second language.

***Geriatric Considerations* boxes** alert you to special considerations for elderly patients.

GERIATRIC*Considerations*

Urinary retention in the elderly may lead to delirium. Carefully question the recent urinary history and bladder habits for any older adult who has a sudden onset of delirium.

***Paramedic Pearl* boxes** highlight important information in the text.

PARAMEDIC*Pearl*

Remember to communicate with the patient throughout your assessment. Make him or her feel a part of your team, not just an object of your work.

A comprehensive, timesaving index presented at the end of each volume spans *both* volumes of the textbook, enabling you to find topics of interest from both volumes in one place.

Drugs and herbal supplements are indexed at the back of the applicable volumes, providing essential dosage information on 50 herbal supplements and approximately 100 drugs.

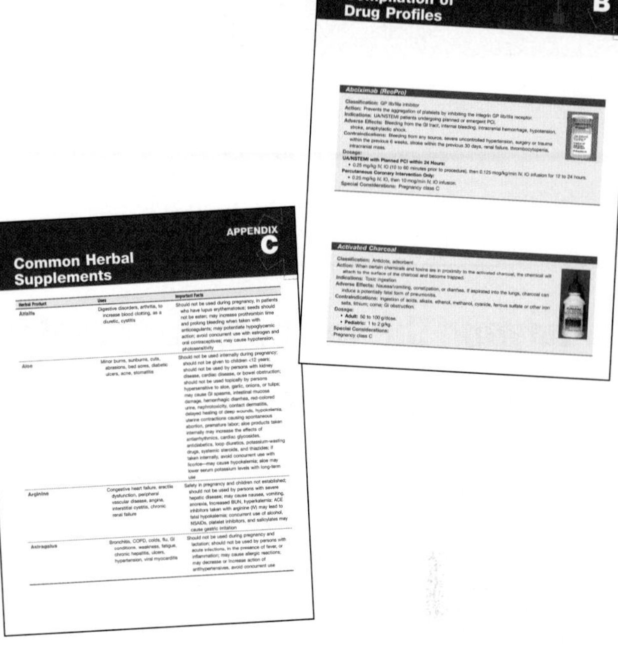

Compilation of Drug Profiles — APPENDIX B

Common Herbal Supplements — APPENDIX C

The comprehensive glossary presented at the end of each volume provides clear definitions for more than 2200 key terms.

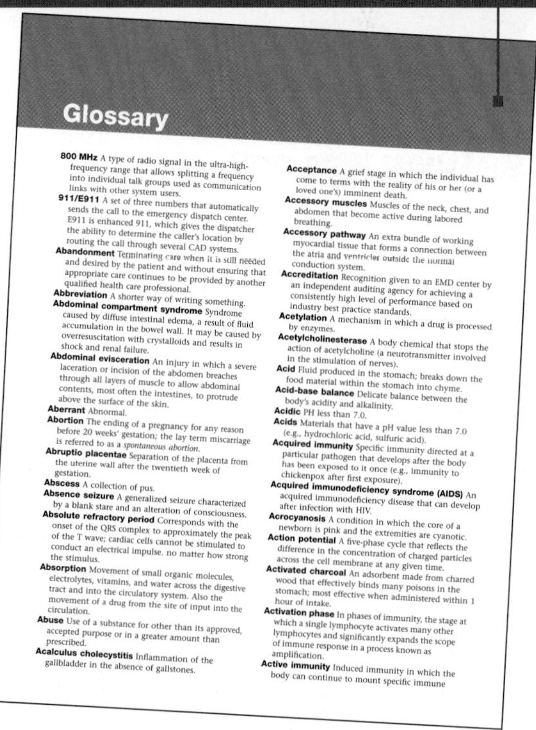

Glossary

800 MHz A type of radio signal in the ultra-high-frequency range that allows splitting a frequency into individual talk groups used as communication links with other system users.

911/E911 A set of three numbers that automatically sends the call to the emergency dispatch center. E911 is enhanced 911, which gives the dispatcher the ability to determine the caller's location by routing the call through several CAD systems.

Abandonment Terminating care when it is still needed and desired by the patient and without ensuring that appropriate care continues to be provided by another qualified health care professional.

Abbreviation A shorter way of writing something.

Abdominal compartment syndrome Syndrome caused by diffuse intestinal edema, a result of fluid accumulation in the bowel wall. It may be caused by overresuscitation with crystalloids and results in shock and renal failure.

Abdominal evisceration An injury in which a severe laceration or incision of the abdomen breaches through all layers of muscle to allow abdominal contents, most often the intestines, to protrude above the surface of the skin.

Aberrant Abnormal.

Abortion The ending of a pregnancy for any reason before 20 weeks' gestation; the lay term miscarriage is referred to as a *spontaneous abortion*.

Abruptio placentae Separation of the placenta from the uterine wall after the twentieth week of gestation.

Abscess A collection of pus.

Absence seizure A generalized seizure characterized by a blank stare and an alteration of consciousness.

Absolute refractory period Corresponds with the onset of the QRS complex to approximately the peak of the T wave; cardiac cells cannot be stimulated to conduct an electrical impulse. no matter how strong the stimulus.

Absorption Movement of small organic molecules, electrolytes, vitamins, and water across the digestive tract and into the circulatory system. Also the movement of a drug from the site of input into the circulation.

Abuse Use of a substance for other than its approved, accepted purpose or in a greater amount than prescribed.

Acalculus cholecystitis Inflammation of the gallbladder in the absence of gallstones.

Acceptance A grief stage in which the individual has come to terms with the reality of his or her (or a loved one's) imminent death.

Accessory muscles Muscles of the neck, chest, and abdomen that become active during labored breathing.

Accessory pathway An extra bundle of working myocardial tissue that forms a connection between the atria and ventricles outside the normal conduction system.

Accreditation Recognition given to an EMD center by an independent auditing agency for achieving a consistently high level of performance based on industry best practice standards.

Acetylation A mechanism in which a drug is processed by enzymes.

Acetylcholinesterase A body chemical that stops the action of acetylcholine (a neurotransmitter involved in the stimulation of nerves).

Acid Fluid produced in the stomach; breaks down the food material within the stomach into chyme.

Acid-base balance Delicate balance between the body's acidity and alkalinity.

Acidic PH less than 7.0.

Acids Materials that have a pH value less than 7.0 (e.g., hydrochloric acid, sulfuric acid).

Acquired immunity Specific immunity directed at a particular pathogen that develops after the body has been exposed to it once (e.g., immunity to chickenpox after first exposure).

Acquired immunodeficiency syndrome (AIDS) An acquired immunodeficiency disease that can develop after infection with HIV.

Acrocyanosis A condition in which the core of a newborn is pink and the extremities are cyanotic.

Action potential A five-phase cycle that reflects the difference in the concentration of charged particles across the cell membrane at any given time.

Activated charcoal An adsorbent made from charred wood that effectively binds many poisons in the stomach; most effective when administered within 1 hour of intake.

Activation phase In phases of immunity, the stage at which a single lymphocyte activates many other lymphocytes and significantly expands the scope of immune response in a process known as amplification.

Active immunity Induced immunity in which the body can continue to mount specific immune

A complete *Pediatric Quick Reference* foldout card, packaged in *Volume 2,* presents key information from *Mosby's Comprehensive Pediatric Emergency Care* in a concise, pocket-sized format for fast reference wherever you go.

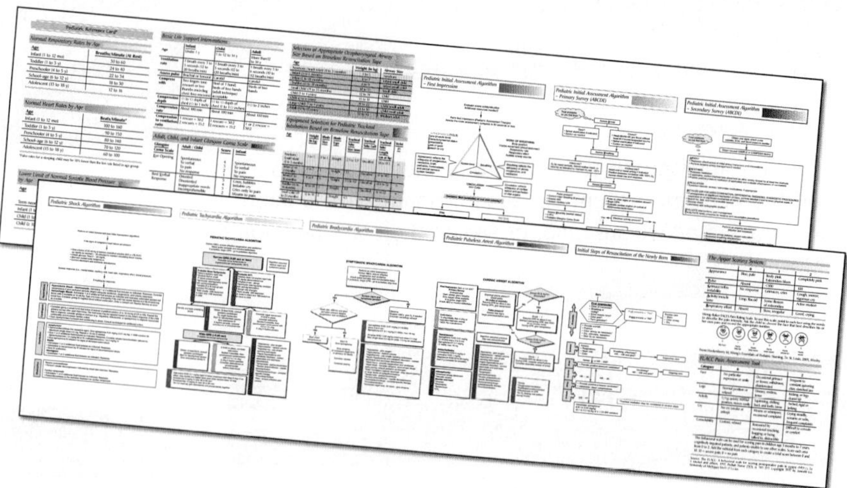

Go *beyond* the textbook for greater understanding . . .

COMPANION DVD-ROM

Load the companion DVD-ROM included with Volume 1 on your computer to access video footage produced exclusively for **Paramedic Practice Today: Above and Beyond.** These detailed videos guide you through the performance of key skills, while lecture videos and other skill clips broaden your understanding of core concepts.

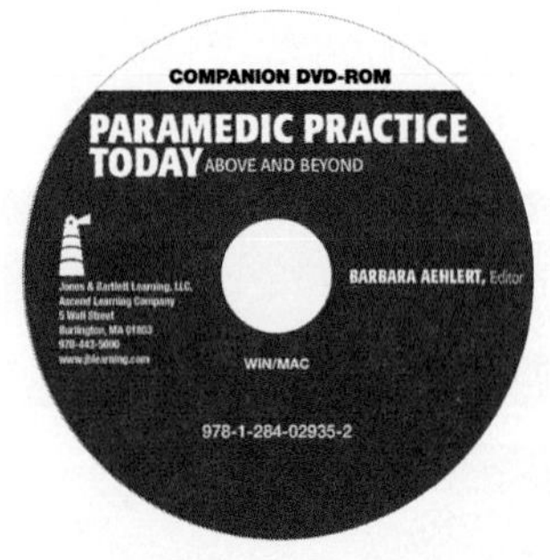

COMPANION WEB SITE

Enhance your knowledge with FREE online access to additional classroom resources, reference materials, and activities on the companion website.
http://EMS.jbpub.com/Aehlert/Paramedic

WORKBOOKS

Practice your skills and prepare for your examinations with detailed, chapter-by-chapter review opportunities in two workbook volumes that correspond directly to the two volumes of the text.
Sold separately.

Volume 1

2009 • Approx. 448 pp., illustd. • ISBN: 978-0-323-04377-9

Volume 2

2009 • Approx. 352 pp., illustd. • ISBN: 978-0-323-04378-6

2-Volume Set

2009 • Approx. 800 pp., illustd. • ISBN: 978-0-323-04390-8

- **Multiple question formats** include matching, short-answer, multiple-choice, true/false, labeling, and case studies to test your knowledge in a variety of different ways.
- **Chapter objectives** identify learning goals and guide you through your review.
- **Chapter summaries** outline the most important points from each corresponding textbook chapter.

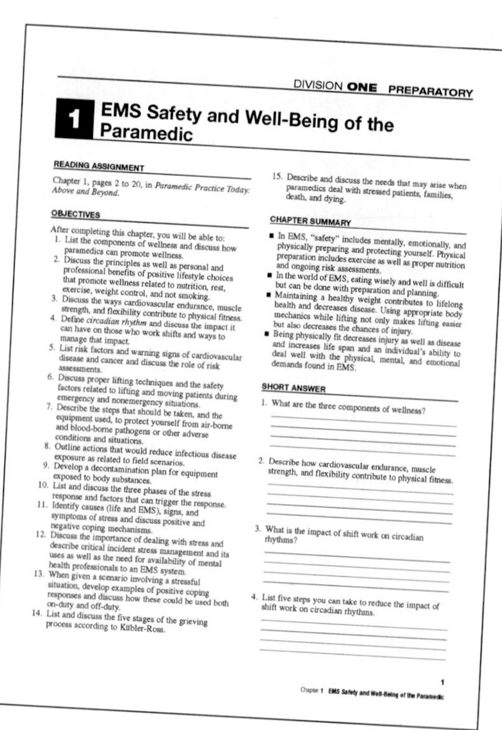

DIVISION **ONE** PREPARATORY

1 EMS Safety and Well-Being of the Paramedic

READING ASSIGNMENT

Chapter 1, pages 2 to 20, in *Paramedic Practice Today: Above and Beyond.*

OBJECTIVES

After completing this chapter, you will be able to:
1. List the components of wellness and discuss how paramedics can promote wellness.
2. Discuss the principles as well as personal and professional benefits of positive lifestyle choices that promote wellness related to nutrition, rest, exercise, weight control, and not smoking.
3. Discuss the ways cardiovascular endurance, muscle strength, and flexibility contribute to physical fitness.
4. Define *circadian rhythm* and discuss the impact it can have on those who work shifts and ways to manage that impact.
5. List risk factors and warning signs of cardiovascular disease and cancer and discuss the role of risk assessments.
6. Discuss proper lifting techniques and the safety factors related to lifting and moving patients during emergency and nonemergency situations.
7. Describe the steps that should be taken, and the equipment used, to protect yourself from air-borne and blood-borne pathogens or other adverse conditions and situations.
8. Outline actions that would reduce infectious disease exposure as related to field scenarios.
9. Develop a decontamination plan for equipment exposed to body substances.
10. List and discuss the three phases of the stress response and factors that can trigger the response.
11. Identify causes (life and EMS), signs, and symptoms of stress and discuss positive and negative coping mechanisms.
12. Discuss the importance of dealing with stress and describe critical incident stress management and its uses as well as the need for availability of mental health professionals to an EMS system.
13. When given a scenario involving a stressful situation, develop examples of positive coping responses and discuss how these could be used both on-duty and off-duty.
14. List and discuss the five stages of the grieving process according to Kübler-Ross.
15. Describe and discuss the needs that may arise when paramedics deal with stressed patients, families, death, and dying.

CHAPTER SUMMARY

- In EMS, "safety" includes mentally, emotionally, and physically preparing and protecting yourself. Physical preparation includes exercise as well as proper nutrition and ongoing risk assessments.
- In the world of EMS, eating wisely and well is difficult but can be done with preparation and planning.
- Maintaining a healthy weight contributes to lifelong health and decreases disease. Using appropriate body mechanics while lifting not only makes lifting easier but also decreases the chances of injury.
- Being physically fit decreases injury as well as disease and increases life span and an individual's ability to deal well with the physical, mental, and emotional demands found in EMS.

SHORT ANSWER

1. What are the three components of wellness?
2. Describe how cardiovascular endurance, muscle strength, and flexibility contribute to physical fitness.
3. What is the impact of shift work on circadian rhythms?
4. List five steps you can take to reduce the impact of shift work on circadian rhythms.

1

Chapter 1 EMS Safety and Well-Being of the Paramedic

RAPID PARAMEDIC

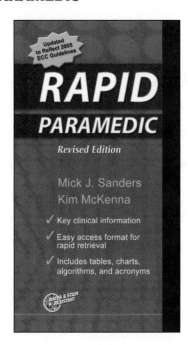

Respond quickly and confidently with this full-color paramedic field guide. Useful both as a classroom resource and as a field reference, **RAPID Paramedic** distills the essentials of paramedic practice into a pocket-sized, spiral-bound, fluid-resistant quick reference to provide the fastest, most convenient access to the information you need in paramedic practice.
Sold separately.
2007 • 172 pp., illustd. • ISBN: 978-0-323-04762-2

Take learning to a new level . . .

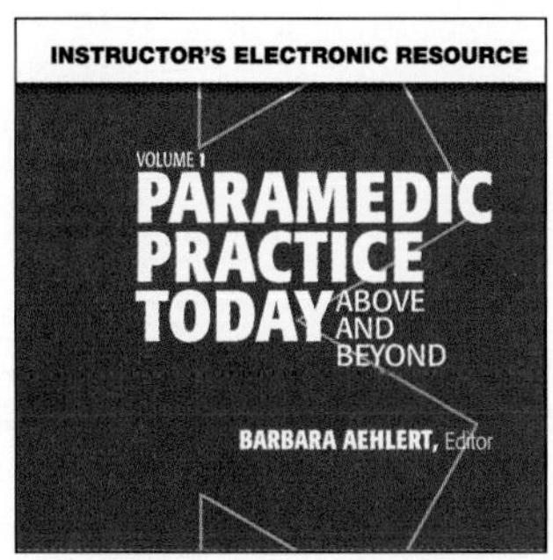

Paramedic Practice Today is supported by extensive **instructor resources** that provide everything needed for easy, efficient class preparation.

The extensive **Instructor's Electronic Resource** includes everything needed to make preparing for class quick and easy: detailed lesson plans, lecture outlines, PowerPoint presentations with *Speaker Notes* and embedded skills video clips, and even tables that correlate content to the National EMS Practice Analysis (on which the National Registry examination is based), NSC objectives, and National Education Standards.

Customizable lesson plans, lecture outlines, and PowerPoint presentations with *Speaker Notes* and embedded skills videos streamline course preparation.

JB Course Manager saves preparation time and helps instructors teach more effectively with online access to all of the instructor electronic resources and valuable course management tools.

Paramedic Practice Today: Above and Beyond is intended to be the most effective paramedic learning resource and provide the best preparation for paramedic practice and the National Registry examination. If you have any questions about the components of this learning system, if you would like to place an order, or if you have suggestions about how **Paramedic Practice Today** could go even further **above and beyond,** please contact Jones & Bartlett Learning at 800-832-0034 or visit www.jblearning.com.

Barbara Aehlert, RN, BSPA

Contents for Volume 1

Contents for Volume 2

DIVISION 7 Special Patient Populations

DIVISION 10 OPERATIONS

63 Vehicle Rescue and Rescue Awareness Operations, 716

64 Response to Hazardous Materials Incidents, 764

65 Tactical EMS, 801

DIVISION 11 DISASTER AND DOMESTIC PREPAREDNESS ISSUES

Appendices

Strategies for Successfully Studying and Taking Examinations

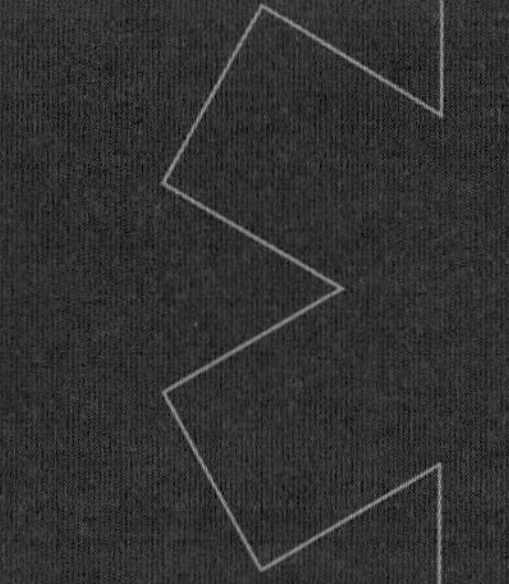

Studying is a skill and, like any skill, it has certain steps or procedures that lead to success. In the academic arena, there are four distinct time frames that require study skills: before class, during class, after class, and while taking examinations. The most successful students have developed study skills in each of these areas. Each of us is an individual; therefore we each have a unique learning style that works best for us. We learn in different ways, and many effective study techniques can be used, based on our learning styles. However, some study techniques are essential and common across all learning styles and will therefore be useful to most students.

STUDYING BEFORE CLASS

Some of the essential and common study techniques that should be used before class are:

- Plan on attending class regularly and being actively involved in classroom activities.
  - Although some subjects may seem boring, simply reading the assignments and taking tests does not promote the best learning. One of the best ways to improve learning is developing knowledge and understanding through classroom discussion and interaction with your instructor. Both listening and participating in class discussions are critical to understanding the subject matter.
- Set a regular time for studying each day.
  - Schedule study time for the time of day you are most alert. For example, if your attention is more focused in the morning, try to schedule your study time for that period.
- Study in a consistent and quiet place.
  - Study produces the best results when distractions are kept to a minimum and the surroundings are familiar. Avoid distractions such as noise, music, television, and radio. Ensure that there is adequate lighting to avoid unnecessary eyestrain. Studying on a bed should be avoided to reduce the possibility of overrelaxation, inattentiveness, and sleepiness.
- Study in half-hour intervals with 10-minute breaks.
  - This format will provide reasonable study time and allow relaxation breaks. The mind will only process so much information without a break. A tired mind is not a good study tool.
- Have everything you need available before you start.
  - This includes textbooks, notebooks, pencils, pens, highlighters, calculators, and anything else that will be required for completion of the assignment.
  - Know how to use your textbook.
  - Learn to use reference materials.
- Read and pay careful attention to assigned materials.
  - This requires reading class assignments and preparing homework assignments before the start of class. Trying to read the assignment while the instructor is presenting the lesson or during classroom discussions causes your hearing and sight to compete for attention, resulting in memory confusion. Plan to read the assignment at least twice. The first reading should be approached as though reading a novel or newspaper (conversational reading). This will allow you to capture the main points in your short-term memory. The second reading should be accomplished while outlining the assignment to allow the prominent points to be recorded into long-term memory.
- Read the assignment again and use outlines to emphasize critical points.
  - Outlining allows you to organize information into useful patterns, which improves recall, application, and problem-solving skills. Use the chapter and section headings as the major points in the outline and then use the following questions to add subpoints.
    - What is the main point of the section?
    - What are the major anatomic, physiologic, and pathophysiologic concepts?
    - Who is most affected by this information or these concepts?
    - When is this important to me, my EMS partner, and/or my patient?
    - Why is this important to me, my EMS partner, and/or my patient?
    - How is this important to me, my EMS partner, and/or my patient?
    - Where will this information be most useful to me?
- Develop your own examples or case studies of information in the assignment.
  - As you develop your own examples and case studies, ask yourself why the author put this information in the reading and what it teaches you about similar situations that you might see in the day-to-day operations as a paramedic. By putting key concepts or illustrations into your own words instead of simply memorizing the words of the author of the assignment, it is easier to understand and remember your own examples

and case studies because they are a product of your learning style and method of processing new information.

STUDYING DURING CLASS

There is no substitute for attending class. Using notes taken by a classmate with a different learning style may not prove beneficial to you.

Some of the essential and common study techniques that should be used during class are:

- Get involved by asking questions on topics that are confusing to you.
  - Remember, your classmates bring a wide variety of perspective and experience to the class discussion and may use a phrase or example that will help your understanding of a concept or principle. In addition, providing your thoughts and insights on topics that you have mastered and actively participating in discussion groups will allow you to hear your own words and explanations of concepts and principles. This may help you to find flaws in your logic or reinforce your understanding of a topic.
- Ask the "stupid" question.
  - Every student at some time has failed to ask a question because he or she thought it might sound stupid or that everybody else already understood the concept being taught. The old adage "the only stupid question is the one that isn't asked" has a lot of validity. You are attending class to learn a topic. If you don't ask, you won't learn.
- Take effective notes.
  - Notes should be focused on critical concepts and principles. Use the outline you developed before class to identify the important points. Write down "additional information" gained during the lecture or classroom discussion that enhances your outline. Take notes in your own words rather than trying to write verbatim what the instructor or classmate said. It is easier to understand and remember your own words, because they are a product of your learning style and method of processing new information.

STUDYING AFTER CLASS

Some of the essential and common study techniques that should be used after class are:

- Study in half-hour intervals with 10-minute breaks.
  - This format will provide reasonable study time and allow relaxation breaks. The mind will only process so much information without a break. A tired mind is not a good study tool.
- Have everything you need available before you start.
  - This includes textbooks, notebooks, pencils, pens, highlighters, calculators, and anything else that will be required for completion of the assignment.
  - Know how to use your textbook.
  - Use additional study materials, such as your workbook, *Virtual Patient Encounters,* and Evolve Resources, to reinforce learning.
  - Learn to use reference materials.
- Develop and use flashcards, acronyms, and memory mnemonics for recall topics.
  - Flashcards and mnemonics are useful for memorizing information at a recall level. They are useful for recall of medical terminology, normal laboratory values, normal age-specific vital signs, rhythm strip recognition, and medication dosages.
- Be selective of the materials to study.
  - There is entirely too much information in any lecture or textbook to be included on an examination or to be added to your memory. While studying, anticipate possible questions that might be included on a test. Use your outline and class notes to highlight areas that have a high potential for inclusion on a test. Concepts and principles that are critical to life and limb or have critical ethical or legal implications are most likely to appear on comprehensive examinations.
- Get involved with study groups.
  - As mentioned earlier, classmates bring a wide variety of perspective and experience to the study groups and may help your understanding of a concept or principle. Remember to take notes in your words so that they match your learning style. Ask the members of the study group to confirm your list of important topics that may appear on a test.
- Set a regular time for studying each day.
  - Schedule study time for the time of day you are most alert. For example, if your attention is more focused in the morning, try to schedule your study time for that period.
- Study in a consistent and quiet place.
  - Study produces the best results when distractions are kept to a minimum and the surroundings a familiar. Avoid distractions such as noise, music, television and radio. Ensure there is adequate lighting to avoid unnecessary eyestrain. Studying on a bed should be avoided to reduce the possibility of overrelaxation, inattentiveness, and sleepiness.
- Study each day for upcoming tests.
  - Consistent study, spread out over a period of time, has been proven to be far more effective in retention of knowledge than "cramming" or massing study the day before class or hours before an examination. Start your study far enough in advance of a class or a test so that you can read and practice the critical information several times over a period of days, not hours.

TAKING EXAMINATIONS

Like studying, there are specific strategies that enhance student success when preparing to take a high-stakes certification examination.

- Course examinations help you determine how well you have managed the topics presented and help you identify whether your study materials and habits are effective.
- There is no substitute for good study habits when preparing for an examination.
  - It is important to remember that using any examination preparation strategy is ineffective if you have not spent time studying effectively. Effective study habits, as outlined earlier, are the single most effective method of improving examination scores. Remember to study consistently over a period of days, not hours. "Cramming" for a test is usually not effective. Focus your study on the critical items most likely to be included on the test. There is too much information in any lecture or textbook to be added to your memory.
- Eat a nutritious meal the night before an examination.
  - Avoid stimulants and depressants.
- Get plenty of rest the night before the examination.
  - Arriving at the examination site well rested will help to reduce anxiety and improve focus and mental acuity necessary for the critical thinking associated with high-stakes certification examinations.
- Take steps to avoid hunger and other physical distraction during the examination.
  - Be sure to eat before arriving at the examination to avoid hunger pains during the examination. Ensure that you empty your bladder before entering the examination room to avoid the distraction of a full bladder during the examination.
- Find out as much information about the test as possible.
  - If you are taking the National Registry of Emergency Medical Technicians test, visit their website at http://www.nremt.org/about/CBT_Home.asp to learn about the examination and take a visual tour of the testing facility. If you are taking a state certification examination, ask your instructor to describe what you should expect when you take the examination. Ensure that you know where and when the examination will be administered and what materials you will need to bring to the examination site.
- Arrive early at the examination site.
  - To reduce any last minute pressure and to allow for unavoidable delays in travel, plan on arriving at the examination site 15 to 20 minutes earlier than the scheduled time.
- Layer clothing to accommodate for variable room temperatures. It is better to be a bit cooler than too warm while taking an examination.
- Expect to experience some stress and anxiety.
  - It is natural to feel stress and anxiety. Do not become focused on the stress or anxiety and do not become overly concerned. A small amount of stress and anxiousness will help you do your best on the examination.
- Stay away from other individuals who are extremely nervous or worried.
  - You have enough stress of your own and do not need to multiply your level of stress by "buying" into others' emotions. Remember, stress is contagious and increasing stress will not help improve test performance.
- Take steps to reduce unproductive stress.
  - Keep a positive and upbeat attitude by deciding to do your best on things you know and understand, and refusing to dwell on those things that you do not know. It is too late to learn new material; simply make sure that you do well on the things that you know and understand.
  - Focus on the task of taking the examination. Answer one question at a time to the best of your ability. Avoid thinking about the remaining questions and do not worry about what others are doing.
  - Try to slow down and focus by taking several deep breaths before reading the first question. If you feel anxiety returning, repeat the deep breathing sequence.

PREPARING FOR EXAMINATIONS

Depending on the developer of the examination, you may be presented with a traditional pen and paper multiple-choice examination or a computer-adaptive multiple-choice examination. Although some of the strategies are similar, it is important to be aware of the type of examination you will be taking and apply the appropriate test-taking strategies to meet the examination format.

Pen and Paper Multiple-Choice Examination

The following are general test-taking strategies for pen and paper examinations that contain multiple-choice questions. Many of these strategies are appropriate for computer-adaptive testing as well.

- Read the examination instructions carefully or listen carefully to the examination proctor if he or she is required to read the instructions to you. If you do not understand any of the instructions or require clarification, ask the proctor for more detailed explanation before you begin reading the examination questions.

- Be sure that you know how much time you have to complete the examination and then plan your time for each part of the test. Allow a few minutes to review your answers before turning in your examination material.
- Read the stem of each question carefully and completely before considering an appropriate response.
- Answer examination items in the order presented and avoid the urge to skip questions. Identify any answer of which you are not completely certain by making a mark in the margin of the answer sheet next to the suspect answer. Once you have completed the test, review the examination question and answers that you marked in the margin. Correct any absolute errors that you identify, but do not change any answers unless you are extremely confident that you have made a mistake.
- Do not stay too long on any single question. If you find a question that appears to be difficult, rule out any answer that does not make sense and then make your best guess among the remaining answer choices. Mark the question for review at the end of the examination and continue with the rest of the examination.
- When confronted with a question that appears to have more than one correct answer, be alert for two or more concepts in the answer phrase. Some test developers will make the first concept of an answer choice correct and the second incorrect. Remember, all parts of the answer must be correct or the entire answer choice is incorrect.
- Reread all questions that contain the words *not, least, except* in the stem. These words have a negative connotation and can be confusing. If they appear on the examination, rereading the stem two or three times will help ensure a better understanding of the question and related answers.
- Be aware of qualifying words in the stem or the answer choices, such as *always, never, all, most, largest, smallest, best,* and *worst.* These words help to identify the correct answer choice, but are easily missed when reading a question. Sometimes test developers use a bold font to make the words more apparent. If you see this on a test, it is a clue that the word has serious implications for understanding the questions and related answers.
- Look for grammar and syntax agreement between the stem of the question and the related answers. Any answer that has a grammatical or syntactical mismatch with the stem of the question must be considered incorrect.

Computer-Adaptive Examination

In addition to the test-taking strategies listed in the previous section, the following are strategies that are unique to computer-adaptive testing:

- If a difficult question is presented to you, use the strategies listed in the section outlining multiple-choice pen and paper examination strategies to select the correct answer.
  - In computer-adaptive testing, you are not permitted to skip questions or review answers as the end of the examination. You are presented only one question at a time and must answer the question before another question is presented to you.
- Avoid random guessing at the correct answer.
  - Random guessing can significantly reduce your overall examination scores. If you are unsure of an answer to a question, ignore any answer choice that is absolutely incorrect, and then use the strategies outlined in the pen and paper multiple-choice examination section to help choose the best answer.
- Expect to get tougher questions.
  - Don't panic—computer-adaptive tests are designed to present you with questions that you will have about a 50/50 probability of answering correctly. This type of test is designed to test you at your maximum ability level; therefore you should not be surprised when you get difficult questions. Once again, don't panic. Take a deep breath and use your test-taking strategies to make the best guess about the correct answer.
- Regardless of the question, always make your best guess at the correct answer.
  - Every examination will contain pilot questions. You will not be able to identify these questions and they may appear anywhere during the examination. You should simply answer every question to the best of your ability even though pilot questions do not count toward your official examination score.

VOLUME **2**

PARAMEDIC PRACTICE TODAY

ABOVE AND BEYOND

DIVISION 7

SPECIAL PATIENT POPULATIONS

CHAPTER 35

Obstetrics and Gynecology

Objectives *After completing this chapter, you will be able to:*

1. Review the anatomic structures and physiology of the female reproductive system.
2. Identify the normal events of the menstrual cycle.
3. Describe how to assess a patient with a gynecologic complaint.
4. Explain how to recognize a gynecologic emergency.
5. Describe the general care for any patient with a gynecologic emergency.
6. Describe the pathophysiology, assessment, and management of specific gynecologic emergencies.
7. Identify the normal events of pregnancy.
8. Describe how to assess an obstetric patient.
9. Describe the procedures for handling complications of pregnancy.
10. Identify the stages of labor and the paramedic's role in each stage.
11. Differentiate normal and abnormal delivery.
12. State indications of an imminent delivery.
13. Identify and describe complications associated with pregnancy and delivery.
14. Explain the use of the contents of an obstetrics kit.
15. Differentiate the management of a patient with predelivery emergencies from a normal delivery.
16. State the steps in the predelivery preparation of the mother.
17. Establish the relation between standard precautions and childbirth.
18. State the steps to assist in the delivery of a newborn.
19. Describe the management of the mother after delivery.
20. Discuss the steps in the delivery of the placenta.
21. Describe how to care for the newborn.
22. Describe how and when to cut the umbilical cord.
23. Summarize neonatal resuscitation procedures.
24. Describe the procedures for handling abnormal deliveries and maternal complications of labor.
25. Describe special considerations of a premature baby.
26. Describe special considerations when meconium is present in amniotic fluid or during delivery.

Chapter Outline

Case Scenario

Dispatch directs you to the home address of a 28-year-old woman who states she is pregnant and having severe vaginal bleeding. The caller states the woman collapsed to the ground, feeling weak. You arrive to find a woman lying on the ground surrounded by a pool of blood. The woman states that she is 18 weeks pregnant. She tells you that she was in an altercation with her boyfriend yesterday, during which he struck her abdomen, chest, and arms. She states that she has been having cramping all day and the bleeding started about 20 minutes ago. She is awake and alert. Approximately 750 mL of blood is on the ground.

Questions

1. *What is your initial impression of this patient?*
2. *What are some important questions about the patient's history?*
3. *Describe the physical examination you will perform.*

Pregnancy and childbirth are a natural part of the human life cycle. As a paramedic, you may be called to assist in a delivery that happens rapidly or unexpectedly, or you may be called to assist a pregnant woman who has been injured or has vaginal bleeding. This chapter introduces you to the anatomy and physiology of the nonpregnant and pregnant patient, the stages of labor and delivery, and postdelivery care of the mother and the newborn. It also introduces you to some of the complications of pregnancy, delivery, and gynecology.

GYNECOLOGY

ANATOMY OF THE FEMALE GENITAL TRACT

[OBJECTIVE 1]

The female reproductive structures include the external female genitalia, uterus, vagina, fallopian tubes, ovaries, and the perineum (Figure 35-1). The **ovaries** are a pair of organs that release eggs, or ova (singular, **ovum**), as well as reproductive hormones. The egg travels down its adjacent **fallopian tube** into the uterus.

The **uterus** is a pear-shaped organ where the **embryo,** or fertilized egg, implants and grows. The upper, convex portion of the uterus is called the **fundus.** Internally the uterus has a **uterine cavity.** The uterine wall consists of a muscular layer, called the **myometrium,** and the **endometrium,** or nutrient-rich inner layer, which is shed during **menstruation.** If the egg is fertilized (which usually occurs within the fallopian tube), it travels to the uterine cavity and implants into the endometrium, where it will grow and mature. The neck of the uterus, called the **cervix,** inserts into the **vagina,** which leads to the outside of the body. Together, the lower part of the uterus, the cervix, and the vagina are referred to as the **birth canal.**

The external female genitalia (Figure 35-2), or **vulv,** includes the **mons pubis,** a hair-covered fat pad overlying the symphysis pubis; the **labia majora,** rounded folds of external adipose tissue; and the **labia minora,** thinner, pinkish-red folds that extend anteriorly to form the **prepuce** and **clitoris,** the region of sexual stimulation. The **urethral meatus** opens into the area between the clitoris and the vagina. Below the urethral meatus lies the **vaginal orifice.** Within the vaginal orifice lies the **hymen,** a thin ring of tissue that partly blocks the orifice. The hymen may be present only as small tags of tissue in the adult woman. The **perineum,** or **perineal body,** refers to the tissue between the vaginal opening and the **anus.**

THE MENSTRUAL CYCLE

[OBJECTIVE 2]

Menstruation occurs approximately every 28 days and is the normal discharge of blood, mucus, and cellular debris from the uterine cavity. **Menarche** is the onset of menstruation during puberty. **Menopause** is the cessation of ovarian function and of the menstrual cycle. The average age at menarche in the United States is 12.5 years, and the average age at menopause is between 51 and 52 years (Stenchever et al., 2001). The menstrual cycle is divided into three phases. The cycle begins with the **proliferative phase,** when the endometrium is stimulated by **estrogen** to grow thicker. **Ovulation** occurs at the end of the proliferative phase when an ovum, or egg, is released from an **ovarian follicle.** This usually occurs 14 days after the start of the previous menstrual period.

After release of the egg, the ovarian follicle begins to secrete **progesterone,** marking the start of the **secretory phase.** During this time, the **ovary** continues to secrete estrogen and the endometrium is maintained by both estrogen and progesterone. In case of fertilization, the endometrium is prepared to receive the fertilized ovum. If the ovum is not fertilized, menstruation ensues with discharge of the endometrial lining. Menstruation lasts 4 to 6 days, with blood loss of approximately 25 to 60 mL.

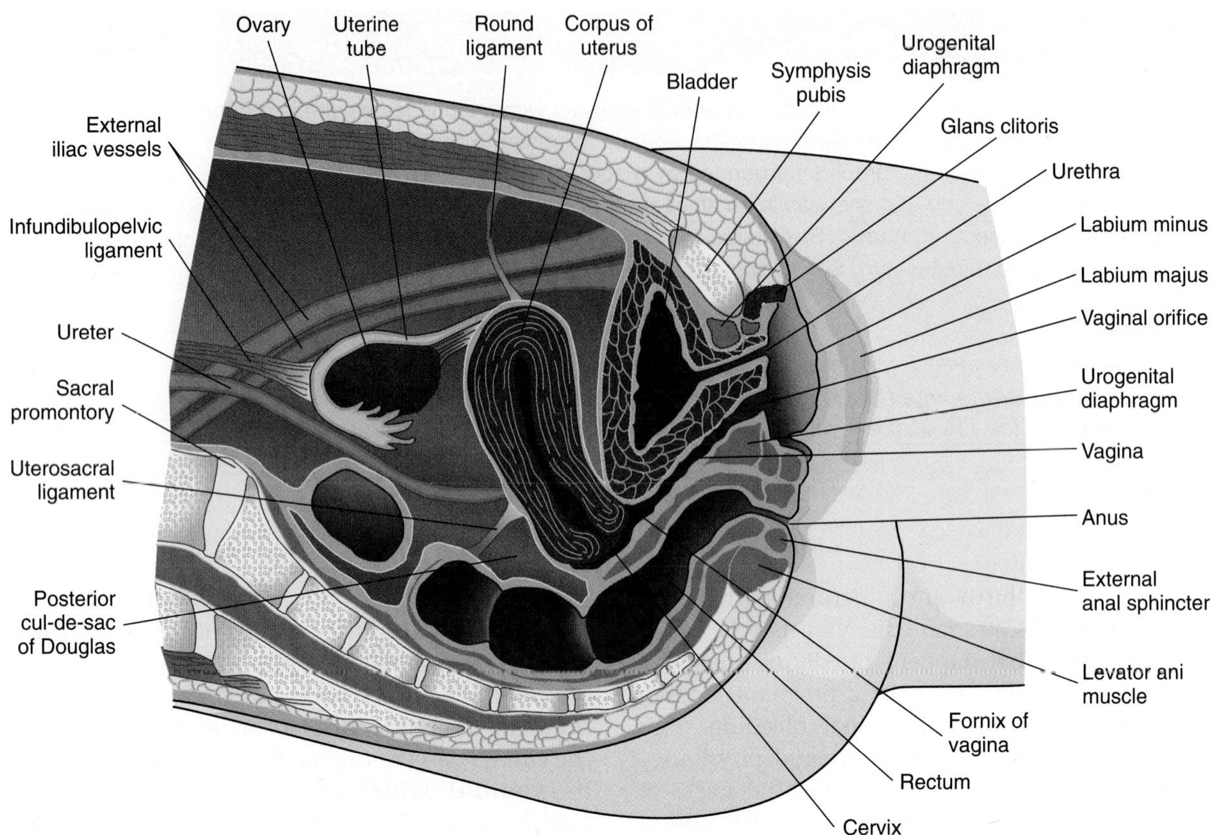

Figure 35-1 Anatomy of the female genital tract.

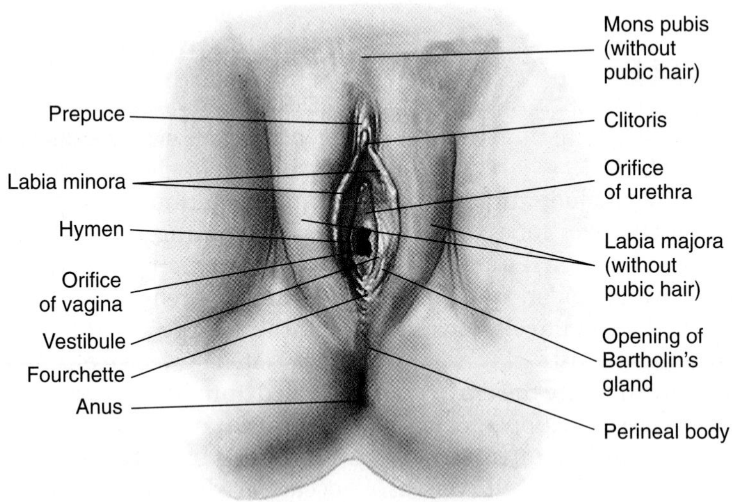

Figure 35-2 Anatomy of the external female genitalia.

GYNECOLOGIC EMERGENCIES

Assessment and Management

[OBJECTIVES 3, 4]

Gynecologic emergencies are usually associated with one or more of the following symptoms: vaginal bleeding, abdominal pain, vomiting, fever, diaphoresis, syncope, changes in stool pattern, **dyspareunia** (pain during intercourse), or urinary symptoms. Signs on physical assessment may include tachycardia, hypotension, fever, abdominal tenderness, and blood from the vagina. A complete gynecologic history should include an exploration of the chief complaint as well as associated symptoms. If vaginal bleeding has occurred, try to quantify this in pads per hour or in comparison with the patient's normal menstrual period. Ask about the date of the last normal menstrual period, regularity of menstrual cycles, whether a current pregnancy exists, number of previous pregnancies, number of pregnancies carried to term, number of miscarriages or abortions, history of prior gynecologic problems or surgeries, current sexual activity, type of birth control, and history of sexually transmitted diseases (Table 35-1).

The maternal history is recorded in one of two formats, either of which is medically acceptable. In the first format the number of pregnancies, births, and abortions, is expressed as **gravida** (pregnancies), **para** (number of births after 20 weeks of **gestation** regardless of outcome), and abortus (spontaneous or induced). For example, a woman who is currently pregnant and has had two prior pregnancies with two living children would be gravida 3, para 2, abortus 0 (G3P2A0). It is important to note that the case of multiple children during one pregnancy (i.e., twins, triplets) still equals one birth. For example, a patient who is pregnant for the second time and has twins from a prior pregnancy would be G2P1A0. In the second format, *gravida* is used in the same manner as described previously, and *para* indicates the number of deliveries regardless of gestational age. Parity is then further clarified in terms of outcome. This is defined using term (deliveries after 37 weeks' gestation), premature (deliveries between 20 and 37 weeks' gestation), abortus (deliveries less than 20 weeks' gestation, spontaneous or induced), and living (currently living children). These clarifications follow the expression of parity and may be identified using the letters *TPAL*, or may simply be expressed as numbers separated by hyphens. For example, suppose a woman who is currently pregnant delivered two children at term, one child at 30 weeks, had a spontaneous abortion (miscarriage) at 16 weeks, and has 3 living children. Her history would be documented as G5P3 [T2P1A1L3] or as G5P3 [2-1-1-3]. As previously stated, multiple children in one pregnancy equals one birth.

When obtaining a sexual and menstrual history, remember that patients sometimes are not reliable in reporting this information. One study demonstrated that, of women with abdominal pain or vaginal bleeding who told hospital personnel there was "no chance" they were pregnant, 11.5% had a positive pregnancy test (Ramouska et al., 1989).

PARAMEDIC*Pearl*

Be careful to maintain your patient's modesty and privacy at all times. Use correct medical and anatomic terms when talking with your patient and your colleagues, never slang. Remember that having to discuss her symptoms and history with a stranger may be distressing to your patient. You are a medical professional—projecting a professional image is reassuring to the patient.

TABLE 35-1 Elements of the Gynecologic and Obstetric History

	Gynecologic History	Obstetric History
Current symptoms: Vaginal bleeding? Amount? Any tissue passed?	x	x
Current symptoms: Abdominal pain? Onset, duration, character, location, radiation, severity?	x	x
Current symptoms: Vaginal discharge? Color, amount, odor, itching?	x	x
Currently pregnant?	x	
Current sexual activity? Birth control?	x	x
Last menstrual period	x	x
Prior pregnancies (gravidity)	x	x
Prior births (parity)	x	x
Prior pregnancy complications or losses?	x	x
Prior cesarean delivery or other abdominal surgery?	x	x
Other past medical history, medications, allergies	x	x
Prior or current sexually transmitted diseases	x	x
Estimated date of confinement (due date)?		x
Prenatal care?		x
Contractions? How long, how far apart?		x
Any bloody show?		x

When evaluating a patient with a gynecologic complaint, assess and treat for shock as you would in any patient. Maintain the ABCs (***a***irway, ***b***reathing, and ***c***irculation), obtain intravenous (IV) access (a second IV line may be needed), and monitor vital signs. Provide analgesia and fluid resuscitation as indicated by the patient's condition. Even if bleeding from the vagina is significant, do not pack any dressings inside the vagina. Make note of the amount, color, and type of discharge or bleeding, including the presence of clots or tissue. Transport these patients to a hospital for further evaluation. If the patient passed any clots or tissue before or during transport, bring these with the patient to the hospital in a clean, sealed container if possible.

PARAMEDIC*Pearl*

Any patient of childbearing years with abdominal pain should be considered to be a gynecologic emergency until proven otherwise.

BOX 35-1 PID: Assessment Findings

- Lower abdominal pain
- Possible fever
- Vaginal discharge
- Dyspareunia
- Patient doubled over when walking
- Abdominal guarding
- Acute onset, typically within 1 week of menstrual period
- Ill appearance

PID, Pelvic inflammatory disease.

BOX 35-2 Ruptured Ovarian Cyst: Assessment Findings

- Possible sudden onset of severe lower abdominal pain
- Typically affects one side, pain may radiate to back
- Possible vaginal bleeding

Specific Gynecologic Emergencies

Nontraumatic Abdominal Pain

[OBJECTIVES 5, 6]

Pelvic Inflammatory Disease. **Pelvic inflammatory disease (PID)** is a sexually transmitted bacterial infection with one or more organisms, most commonly *Chlamydia trachomatis* and *Neisseria gonorrhea*. These infections gain access through the vagina and can ascend to the cervix, uterus, endometrium, fallopian tubes, ovaries, uterine and ovarian support structures, and liver. PID affects approximately 1 million women in the United States each year. If untreated, PID can lead to abscess, sepsis, or scarring of the uterus and tubes, with eventual infertility.

Assessment findings for PID are listed in Box 35-1. Patients often report lower abdominal pain, fever, foul vaginal discharge, and dyspareunia. Rarely, patients may become septic from PID. Assess the patient with abdominal pain and fever for signs of septic shock and manage accordingly (see Chapter 34).

Ovarian Disorders. Ovarian follicles are formed during the proliferative phase of the menstrual cycle. These follicles typically rupture to release an ovum in the midportion of the cycle. Sometimes a follicle may not rupture, but rather continues to grow, forming an ovarian cyst. A cyst can cause pain as it grows or if it eventually ruptures. An ovarian cyst may rupture spontaneously or after mild abdominal injury, intercourse, or exercise. Patients occasionally may have significant internal bleeding, but this is rare. Symptoms often include sudden onset of severe lower quadrant discomfort, which may radiate to the back. Patients also may have a small amount of vaginal bleeding. Typical assessment findings of a ruptured ovarian cyst are shown in Box 35-2.

Ovarian torsion, or twisting of the ovary such that its blood supply is interrupted, must be considered if pain is severe or symptoms worsen. Ovarian torsion is more common in patients with a history of ovarian cysts, as a cyst may make the ovary more prone to twisting on its axis. Torsion is a surgical emergency and can lead to permanent damage to the ovary. The pain associated with this condition is an acute onset of moderate to severe unilateral pain in the lower abdomen that increases over a period of hours. The pain may be intermittent and may radiate to the back, pelvis, or thigh. Nausea and vomiting is common with ovarian torsion; unfortunately, however, this is a nonspecific finding. The affected side will be tender to palpation, and often a mass may be felt. However, the absence of these findings does not rule out the possibility of ovarian torsion. Prehospital treatment involves recognition, quick transport to the emergency department, and treatment of any symptoms.

Bladder Infection. A bladder infection **(cystitis)** is usually caused by bacteria that ascend from the perineum through the genital tract into the urethral opening. Infection is isolated in the bladder. Patients often present with suprapubic pain, cloudy urine, urinary frequency, hematuria, and dysuria (Box 35-3). If untreated, it may lead to **pyelonephritis,** or infection of the kidneys. Pyelonephritis is more serious, and patients may be severely ill, with fevers, chills, and vomiting. Treatment of cystitis and pyelonephritis includes antibiotics and pain relief.

Mittelschmerz. **Mittelschmerz** is pain that can occur with ovulation (Box 35-4). It probably results from a small amount of blood or fluid leaking from the follicle into the peritoneal cavity when the ovum is released. Symptoms usually last a few hours to 1 day and are uni-

BOX 35-3 Cystitis: Assessment Findings

- Suprapubic tenderness
- Frequency of urination
- Painful urination (dysuria)
- Blood in urine (hematuria)
- Cloudy or foul-smelling urine

BOX 35-4 Mittelschmerz: Assessment Findings

- Unilateral lower quadrant abdominal pain
- Low-grade fever
- Symptoms similar to ruptured ovarian cyst

lateral; patients may have a low-grade fever. Mittelschmerz typically is not an immediate life threat, but does require physician evaluation because it can present similarly to a ruptured ovarian cyst.

PARAMEDIC*Pearl*

Mittelschmerz means "middle pain." This information can help you remember when it occurs in the menstrual cycle.

Uterine Disorders. **Endometritis,** or infection of the endometrium, most commonly occurs after childbirth or abortion. Patients often present with lower abdominal pain, fundal tenderness, fever, and vaginal discharge. If untreated, severe infection and sepsis may result.

Endometriosis is the growth of endometrial tissue outside the uterus, usually on the pelvic structures around the uterus such as the ovaries, fallopian tubes, bowel, or rectum. Patients may report pain with intercourse, urination, and bowel movements, with worse pain during menstruation. Although the cause of endometriosis is not entirely clear, the most accepted theory is that menstrual fluid flows backward up through the uterine cavity and out the fallopian tubes to seed in distant sites. An estimated 15% of women have some degree of this disease (Tintinalli et al., 2004). Most women become symptomatic in their late 30s. Generally, endometritis and endometriosis can be managed in an outpatient setting.

Uterine prolapse, or protrusion of part, or all, of the uterus outside the vagina, may happen in an older woman after bearing down or coughing. It also can happen in a younger woman after vaginal delivery. Assessment findings are listed in Box 35-5. If vaginal tissue is visibly prolapsed outside the vaginal orifice, cover it with sterile, moist gauze and transport the patient to the closest appropriate facility for further care.

Vaginal Disorders. **Vaginitis** is an inflammation of the vaginal tissues. **Vulvovaginitis** is an inflammation of the external female genitalia and vagina. Vaginitis and vulvovaginitis often manifest with vaginal discharge, pain, and a foul odor (Box 35-6). If the vulva is involved, patients often report vulvar irritation and pain. This condition often is treated with antibiotics. Vaginitis can spread upward to the cervix, uterus, fallopian tubes, and ovaries to cause PID. Vaginal foreign bodies such as retained tampons, condoms, or other devices may predispose to vaginitis. They are usually removed easily by a physician. Surgery occasionally is required.

BOX 35-5 Uterine Disorders: Assessment Findings

Endometritis

- Lower abdominal pain
- Purulent vaginal discharge

Endometriosis

- Severe pain during and immediately after intercourse and bowel movement

Uterine prolapse

- Protrusion of tissue
- Urinary frequency, urgency
- Urinary incontinence
- Pelvic heaviness or pressure
- Pelvic pain, lower back pain
- Difficulty walking
- Difficulty urinating

BOX 35-6 Vaginal Infection: Assessment Findings

- Vaginal discharge accompanied by a foul odor
- Pain
- Vulvar irritation

Vaginal Bleeding. Although vaginal bleeding is a normal part of the monthly menstrual cycle, it may at times be quite heavy or irregular. It also may be accompanied by severe, cramping pain. Vaginal bleeding in a nonpregnant patient is not usually life threatening. However, a woman may not yet realize she is pregnant if the bleeding occurs early in the pregnancy. An ectopic pregnancy is a life-threatening cause of vaginal bleeding in early pregnancy and is discussed later in this chapter.

Treat these patients as you would any other patient with the potential for hemorrhagic shock (see Chapter 34). Keep the patient warm, give oxygen, obtain IV access, and give IV fluids if indicated. Carefully watch vital signs and give this patient high priority for transport and treatment.

PARAMEDIC*Pearl*

Assume that any woman of childbearing age with vaginal bleeding has a potentially life-threatening condition until proven otherwise.

BOX 35-7 Possible Causes of Traumatic Vaginal Bleeding

- Vigorous intercourse
- Straddle-type injury
- Pelvic fracture
- Direct blow to perineum
- Blunt force to lower abdomen from assault or seat belt
- Foreign body inserted into vagina
- Abortion attempts

Traumatic Abdominal Pain

Vaginal Bleeding. Traumatic vaginal bleeding is not uncommon after vigorous voluntary intercourse, although violent involuntary sexual activity should be considered. Other causes of traumatic vaginal bleeding are shown in Box 35-7. The posterior vaginal wall behind the cervix is most commonly injured, although all pelvic organs can be involved. Complications include bleeding, organ rupture, and hypovolemic shock.

Treat these patients as you would any other patient with the potential for hemorrhagic shock. Keep the patient warm, give oxygen, obtain IV access, and give IV fluids if indicated. Carefully watch vital signs and give this patient high priority for transport and treatment.

Sexual Assault. A sexual assault can be a terrifying and traumatic experience. A person who has been sexually assaulted may respond in a variety of ways. Some patients may be agitated or hysterical; others may react with fear and withdrawal. Anxiety, withdrawal, silence, denial, anger, and fear are all normal behavior patterns. Obtaining a detailed history may not be possible or desirable for a patient who has been sexually assaulted. Be prepared to respond with compassion and patience.

Examine the genitalia only if injury is severe. If the patient is female, you may want to ask whether a female EMS professional is preferred.

A person who is sexually assaulted may sustain physical injuries not limited to the genital tract. Head injuries, abdominal trauma, strangulation injuries, chest trauma, and extremity lacerations or fractures are all reported in the context of sexual assault. Assess and manage these patients as you would any other trauma patient.

Remember that the scene of an alleged assault is a crime scene and law enforcement officials may wish to gather evidence. Ask the patient to not change clothes, eat, bathe, urinate, defecate, or douche because these actions may destroy valuable evidence for later prosecution of the attacker.

PARAMEDIC*Pearl*

Work with law enforcement to preserve the scene whenever possible. However, your primary responsibility is to attend to the physical and emotional needs of your patient.

Intimate Partner Violence. Although the incidence of violence in intimate relationships in this country is higher in women, intimate partner violence is an issue for men as well, in both opposite-sex and same-sex relationships. Statistics from the National Institute of Justice suggest that 25% of women and 8% of men said they were raped and/or physically assaulted by a current or former spouse, cohabiting partner, or date at some time in their lives (Tjaden & Thoennes, 1998). Pregnant women appear to be at increased risk for intimate partner violence (Shah et al., 1998). The abuser is often the father of the child (Poole et al., 1996). The most common injury from domestic violence in a pregnant woman is blunt trauma to the abdomen (Webster et al., 1994). Other common sites of injury are the face, head, and breasts. A woman who has been abused usually does not tell healthcare providers what really happened—at least not initially (Stewart & Cecitto, 1993).

As the first member of the healthcare team to contact the patient outside the hospital or at her home, you may be able to gather valuable information not available to hospital personnel. If you arrive at an uncontrolled scene where you suspect intimate partner violence has occurred, avoid confronting those involved. Your priority is safety—yours and your patient's.

PARAMEDIC*Pearl*

Suspect intimate partner violence in cases in which the patient's injuries do not match the mechanism or the story is confusing or changes over time.

OBSTETRICS

Women have given birth for thousands of years without the assistance of medical professionals. In fact, most childbirths happening on this planet every day occur with little or no medical assistance. The majority of these deliveries happen without complications. However, when complications do occur, they can be terrifying and disastrous for the mother and her infant. In this country, patients who deliver in the prehospital setting are more likely to:

- Have had previous deliveries
- Call for your help because of an unexpected complication, such as premature labor or bleeding
- Have psychosocial issues such as lack of access to medical care, drug and/or alcohol abuse, or domestic violence

Because of this, mothers who deliver infants in the prehospital setting have much higher rates of complications and death than those who deliver in a hospital (Brunette & Sterner, 1989). Common terms used in obstetrics are shown in Table 35-2.

TABLE 35-2 Obstetric Terms

Term	Definition
Antepartum	Before delivery
Gestation (gestational age)	Period of time for intrauterine fetal development
Grand multipara	A woman who has given birth five times or more
Gravida	Number of pregnancies
Multigravida	A woman who has had two or more pregnancies
Multipara	A woman who has given birth at least twice to an infant, live born or not, having a length of gestation of at least 20 weeks or more
Natal	Connected with birth
Nullipara	A woman who has not borne a child
Para	Number of pregnancies carried 20 weeks or more
Parity	Number of times the patient has given birth regardless of outcome
Perinatal	The period from the twenty-eighth week of gestation through the first 7 days after delivery
Postnatal	The period immediately after the birth of a child and lasting for approximately 6 weeks
Postpartum	Pertaining to the mother after delivery
Prenatal	Existing or occurring before birth
Primigravida	A woman pregnant for the first time
Primipara	A woman who has given birth to her first child
Term gestation	Gestation equal to or longer than 37 weeks

ANATOMY AND PHYSIOLOGY OF PREGNANCY

[OBJECTIVE 7]

Pregnancy is a normal event in the life cycle of human beings. However, unique changes in anatomy and physiology take place during pregnancy. Understanding these normal changes will help you better assess and treat the pregnant patient.

Fetal Development

Fertilization usually occurs in the distal third of the fallopian tube. The fertilized egg is referred to as an *embryo* during the first 8 weeks of pregnancy. After that it is called the **fetus.** During its growth in the uterus, the fetus is encased in a protective bag called the **amniotic sac.** Fluid in the sac originates from fetal secretions, primarily urine. The sac can contain approximately 500 to 1000 mL of fluid after 20 weeks. The fetus receives nutrition and oxygen and eliminates waste through the **umbilical cord** (Figure 35-3, *A*). The umbilical cord contains three vessels—two arteries and a vein—and connects the fetus to the **placenta.** The placenta attaches to the wall of the uterus and exchanges nutrients and wastes for the fetus (Box 35-8). Transfer of gases such as carbon dioxide and oxygen; transport of nutrients and electrolytes such as glucose, potassium, sodium, and chloride; and excretion of wastes such as urea, uric acid, and creatinine occur in the placenta. The placenta also acts as an endocrine gland, secreting the hormones estrogen and progesterone, and as a barrier, preventing exposure to harmful substances.

BOX 35-8 Placental Functions

- Transfer of gases
- Transport of nutrients
- Excretion of wastes
- Hormone production
- Protection

The normal length of pregnancy is approximately 40 weeks. For ease of reference, the pregnancy typically is divided into three parts, or trimesters, each lasting approximately 3 months. Fetal gender may be determined by the end of the first trimester. By the twentieth week, fetal heart tones should be detectable by stethoscope. The mother may note fetal movement as early as 18 to 22 weeks.

If born prematurely after the twenty-third week, the fetus may be capable of survival. The fetus is considered term if it has reached the thirty-seventh week. The due date is known as the **estimated date of confinement (EDC)**, or *expected due date* (EDD). This can be calculated easily by the paramedic. This is particularly important when assessing a patient who has not had prenatal care. The most common method used to assess a patient's due date assumes that conception occurred 14 days after the start of the last menstrual period. The approximate date may be obtained by taking the date when the last period began, adding 7 days, then counting back 3 months and adding a whole year. For example, if the first day of the last menstrual period was November 10, 2007, add 7 days and you get November 17, 2007; then count back 3 months and you have August 17; add 1 year and you get the estimated due date: August 17, 2008. Several charts and tables are also available to quickly find the estimated due date.

Maternal Physiology

As early as the first trimester, maternal heart rate increases by 10 to 15 beats/min. Diaphragmatic displacement causes the heart to be rotated slightly and displaced

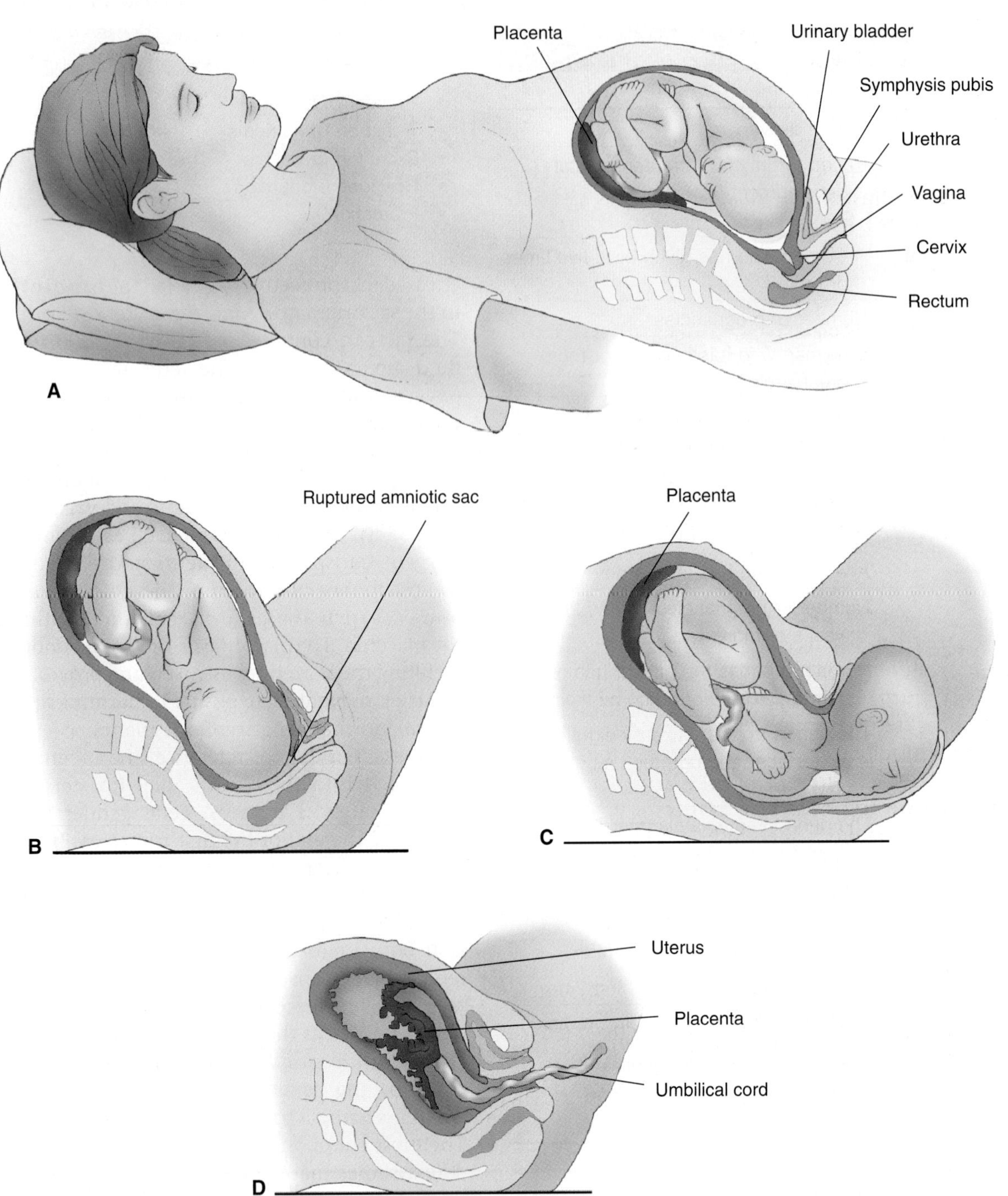

Figure 35-3 **A,** Anatomy of the pregnant woman. **B,** The first stage of labor involves dilation and thinning of the cervix. **C,** The second stage of labor begins when the cervix is fully dilated and ends with the delivery of the infant. **D,** The third stage of labor involves delivery of the placenta.

upward and to the left. This causes slight left axis deviation on the cardiac monitor as well as flattened or negative T waves in lead III. Respiratory rate also increases slightly because of stimulation of the respiratory centers of the brain by the hormone progesterone. Later in pregnancy, as the enlarging uterus pushes up on the diaphragm, breathing often is slightly shallower and faster than in the nonpregnant patient. Because of elevation of the diaphragm, functional residual capacity is reduced. Despite these changes in respirations there is an increase in both tidal volume and minute volume. End-tidal carbon dioxide ($ETCO_2$) decreases because of the increased respiratory rate. Pregnancy hormones also lead to a drop in blood pressure of 10 to 15 mm Hg by the second trimester. The blood pressure gradually returns to the normal range by the end of the third trimester (Morrison, 2002).

A pregnant patient's blood volume, or the total amount of blood circulating in the body, is almost 1.5 times what it was before she became pregnant. Cardiac output increases by 30% by week 34. This increased blood volume helps her body adjust to the blood loss that is a normal part of delivery.

PARAMEDIC*Pearl*

Because a patient's blood volume is increased during pregnancy, in the early setting of trauma, dehydration, or other volume loss the pregnant patient may be able to compensate without a significant change in heart rate and blood pressure. However, her fetus may already be in danger before the mother develops the usual signs and symptoms of shock. As a paramedic, you must be attuned to this and closely monitor all pregnant patients.

During the second half of pregnancy, the uterus is large enough that, when the patient is supine, it can compress the inferior vena cava in the abdomen and impede the return of blood to the heart. This reduces preload and therefore cardiac output. Hypotension can result, with poor blood flow to the uterus, which means poor oxygen delivery to the fetus. This phenomenon is termed **supine hypotensive syndrome** (Cunningham, 2005). To avoid this syndrome, the pregnant patient should be positioned in the left lateral recumbent position whenever possible (Figure 35-4). This position moves the uterus off the large vessels and improves blood return to the heart. Use pillows or blankets to support the patient's hips, back, and abdomen as needed.

During the first trimester, the uterus is still small enough to be entirely protected by the pelvis. After approximately 13 weeks of pregnancy, the uterus begins to rise out of the pelvis and displace the abdominal contents superiorly, laterally, and posteriorly. This displacement has several implications. First, the uterus is now much more susceptible to injury from direct trauma, whereas the other abdominal organs are relatively protected. Second, the enlarging uterus compresses the stomach and contributes to the heartburn common in pregnancy. Third, pressure on the diaphragm from the enlarging abdomen makes breathing deeply more difficult and may contribute to shortness of breath. At term, the fundus of the uterus is near the xiphoid process (Figure 35-5).

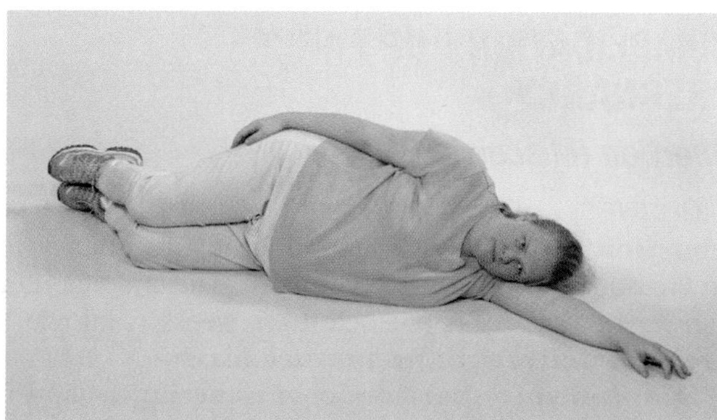

Figure 35-4 Left lateral recumbent position.

Maternal Metabolism and Nutrition

Recommended weight gain during pregnancy varies for underweight, normal-weight, overweight, and obese women but is usually somewhere between 11 and 16 kg (24 to 35 lb). Approximately 2 to 3 lb are from increased fluid volume, 3 to 4 lb from increased blood volume, 1 to 2 lb from breast enlargement, 2 lb from enlargement of the uterus, and 2 lb from amniotic fluid. At term, the infant weighs approximately 6 to 8 lb and the placenta weighs 1 to 2 lb. A 4- to 6-lb increase in maternal stores of fat and protein is important for production of breast milk. Most of this weight gain should occur during the second half of pregnancy (Johnson & Niebyl, 2002).

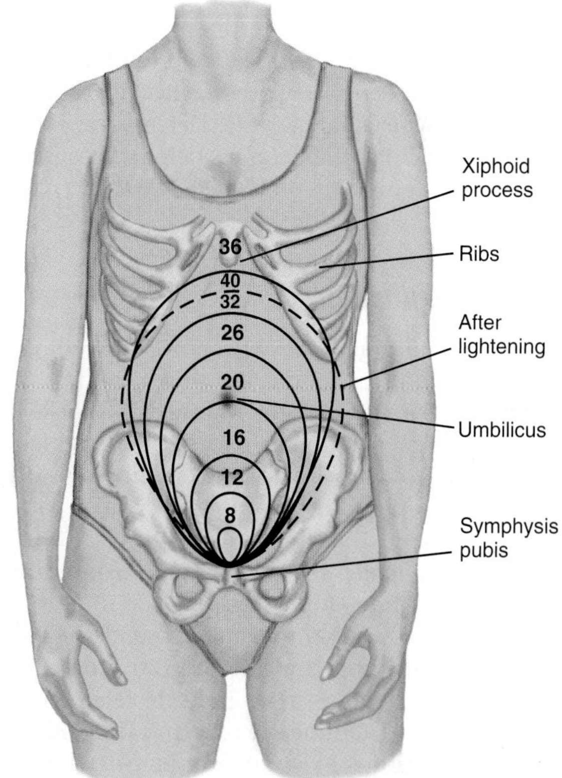

Figure 35-5 Uterine growth during pregnancy.

The average woman retains at least 6.5 L of extra body water during a normal pregnancy. The fetus, placenta, and amniotic fluid account for part of this, and most of the rest is from expanding maternal blood volume.

Pregnancy is also associated with insulin resistance, which increases as pregnancy progresses. This can progress to frank diabetes mellitus during pregnancy, requiring insulin therapy. Although the diabetes may resolve after delivery, women who are diabetic during pregnancy are at increased risk for developing type 2 diabetes later in life (Landon et al., 2002).

ASSESSMENT OF THE PREGNANT PATIENT

[OBJECTIVE 8]

History

An obstetric history should start with the chief complaint and its relation, if any, to the pregnancy. No matter what the chief complaint, ask about the presence of any vaginal bleeding, uterine contractions, or abdominal pain. If the mother is far enough along to have noted fetal movement, ask whether she has felt her baby moving normally during the past few hours. Always establish **gestational age** and EDC as closely as possible. If a woman is unsure of these dates, try to at least establish the last menstrual period. Establish **gravidity** and **parity,** and inquire about any previous pregnancy complications or fetal losses. Pertinent medical history includes diabetes, heart disease, hypertension, seizures, previous cesarean sections, or other gynecologic or obstetric complications (see Box 35-11). Determining whether the woman has had prenatal care is helpful because a lack of care means significant problems may not have been recognized.

Physical Examination

Make sure to note general appearance, including skin color, temperature, and moisture. Assess vital signs, looking for signs of dehydration or shock. If the gestational age is nearing or exceeds 20 weeks, listen for fetal heart tones by placing a stethoscope on the patient's abdomen and moving it in a circular pattern 6 to 8 inches around the umbilicus until heart tones are heard. The paramedic should be sure to monitor the patient's pulse while doing this. If the sounds heard match the patient's pulse, they are those of the mother. Normal fetal heart tones are between 120 and 160 beats/min; rates outside these values indicate fetal distress or maternal hypoxia. Examine the woman's feet and legs for edema. On abdominal examination, palpate the uterine fundus and note its height relative to abdominal landmarks, including the symphysis pubis, umbilicus, and xiphoid process. This can be used as a rough estimate of gestational age (see Figure 35-5). Note any ecchymosis or tenderness.

GENERAL MANAGEMENT OF THE PREGNANT PATIENT

Pregnancy is unique in that assessment and management of the patient (mother) actually involves two patients (mother and baby). In general, your treatment priorities are the same for both patients. In other words, what is best for the pregnant patient also is what is best for her unborn child. The paramedic should assess carefully for the presence of hypoxia and hypovolemia. Oxygen requirements of the pregnant patient increase by 10% to 20%. Because of the previously mentioned changes in blood volume and cardiac output, the pregnant patient can show minimal signs of hypovolemia with up to 35% blood loss. However, because of compensatory mechanisms, blood flow to the uterus will be significantly decreased. Unless you suspect that delivery is imminent, management of the pregnant patient includes only standard diagnostic and treatment modalities. Assess ABCs, and treat these as you would in the nonpregnant patient. Oxygen, IV access, and close monitoring are usually appropriate. Unless a medication is specifically indicated and approved by medical direction, avoiding all medications in pregnancy is best, including pain medications, because they may have adverse effects on the fetus or mask important signs and symptoms of deterioration.

Pregnant patients with respiratory distress or respiratory arrest are at higher risk of vomiting and aspiration of gastric contents into the lungs. Several factors contribute to this. First, the hormones of pregnancy slow gastric emptying. They also cause the lower portion of the esophagus to relax, allowing more reflux of gastric contents. Second, the stomach and intestines are compressed and displaced by the enlarging uterus. Remember to place the patient in a left lateral recumbent position if you anticipate vomiting and have suction ready to clear the airway. The left lateral recumbent position also is important to avoid supine hypotensive syndrome in the second half of pregnancy.

COMPLICATIONS OF EARLY PREGNANCY

Abortion (Miscarriage)

[OBJECTIVE 9]

Abortion is defined as the ending of a pregnancy for any reason before 20 weeks' gestation. The end of a pregnancy after 20 weeks but before 37 weeks is known as **preterm delivery** or **premature birth.**

Spontaneous abortion, or **miscarriage,** happens for many reasons. Often the reason for the miscarriage is never known but is presumed to be that some fatal error occurred in the growth of the embryo or fetus. As many as one in three pregnancies result in early miscarriage, usually before the end of the first trimester (Simpson, 2002; Houry & Abbott, 2002). The most common time is between 8 and 14 weeks' gestation. Sometimes the woman may not even realize she is pregnant yet. **Complete abortion** is passage of all fetal tissue before 20 weeks of gestation. An **incomplete abortion** is failure to pass all fetal tissue. **Threatened abortion** is a pregnancy-related bloody vaginal discharge or frank bleeding during the first half of pregnancy without cervical dilation. A **septic abortion** occurs in the presence of an infection. Planned surgical or medical evacuation of the uterus is a **therapeutic abortion.**

Signs and symptoms of abortion include abdominal cramping, vaginal bleeding, and the passage of tissue or the fetus. The bleeding can be severe and lead to hemorrhagic shock.

Assess any patient with suspected or threatened abortion for signs of hemorrhagic shock and manage accordingly. Assess ABCs. Provide oxygen and treat for shock if necessary, including establishing two large-bore IV lines for fluid resuscitation. Frequently monitor vital signs during transport, particularly if heavy bleeding occurs. If the patient has passed tissue or a fetus, place these in a clean plastic bag or other container and transport them to the hospital with the mother.

Be aware that a miscarriage can be an emotionally traumatic experience for parents, even if it is early in the pregnancy or if the pregnancy was unplanned. Offer compassion and psychological support if needed.

Ectopic Pregnancy

An **ectopic pregnancy** occurs outside the uterus, usually in the fallopian tube. It occurs in approximately 2% of pregnancies in the United States (Houry & Abbott, 2002). Risk factors include anything that may promote scarring or inflammation in the pelvis, such as previous surgical adhesions, PID, tubal ligation, and use of an intrauterine device (IUD) to prevent pregnancy. This is because the IUD prevents pregnancy by interfering with implantation of a fertilized ovum in the uterine cavity. By interfering with implantation in the uterine cavity, the IUD increases the probability of implantation in the fallopian tube.

If the fertilized egg implants in the tube instead of the uterus, it stretches the tube as it grows, causing pain and sometimes vaginal bleeding. Eventually it may cause the tube to rupture, causing severe and even life-threatening bleeding. Symptoms of an ectopic pregnancy usually begin during the fifth to tenth weeks of pregnancy. Usually the woman does not know her pregnancy is ectopic and in fact may not know she is pregnant. Therefore any sudden or severe lower abdominal pain or vaginal bleeding in a woman of child-bearing age should be taken seriously.

An ectopic pregnancy is a potentially life-threatening emergency. Closely monitor the patient for shock and treat it aggressively if suspected. Plan for a second large-bore IV, place the patient in a supine position if shock is impending, and transport the patient to the nearest facility with surgical capabilities.

Hyperemesis Gravidarum

Hyperemesis gravidarum is a more severe form of morning sickness that can persist throughout pregnancy. Patients often present with nausea, vomiting, weight loss, electrolyte imbalance, and dehydration. These patients may require hospitalization, replacement of fluids, electrolytes, and antiemetics. Severe cases occasionally do not respond to antiemetics and may require tube feedings or IV calorie replacement. Other, more serious causes of vomiting must be ruled out, including pancreatitis, cholecystitis, hepatitis, and thyroid disease.

Case Scenario—continued

You begin your primary survey. The patient is awake and alert. She has an open airway and is breathing regularly at 24 breaths/min. Her pulse rate is 90 beats/min and her blood pressure is 118/96 mm Hg. She states she was working around the house when she felt lower abdominal cramping. She states that she began bleeding approximately 1 hour after the cramping. She denies any passage of tissue. She tells you that this is her first pregnancy and that she receives routine obstetric care at a local clinic. The patient denies any previous medical or surgical history. She also denies smoking or using alcohol or drugs. On secondary examination, the patient appears in mild distress. She has clear heart and lung sounds. Her abdomen is firm but tender to palpation. The patient has some recent bruises on her arms.

Questions

4. *Discuss domestic violence in pregnant patients.*
5. *What is the significance of the blood pressure?*
6. *What are important treatment considerations?*
7. *Describe possible differential diagnoses for this patient.*

COMPLICATIONS OF LATE PREGNANCY

[OBJECTIVE 9]

Placental Abruption

Abruptio placentae, or **placental abruption,** is defined as separation of part of the placenta from its normal attachment to the inner wall of the uterus. This leads to bleeding from the site of separation. Placental abruption occurs in approximately 2% of pregnancies, 1 in 200 deliveries, and 1 in 400 fetal deaths (American College of Obstetricians and Gynecologists, 2004).

A number of studies have shown abruption to be correlated with certain conditions, including abdominal trauma, high blood pressure, maternal cocaine and tobacco use, poor nutrition, advanced maternal age, and infection of the uterus or placenta. The most common causes of abdominal trauma in pregnancy are motor vehicle accidents and domestic violence (Simpson, 2002).

Abruption is usually accompanied by painful uterine contractions and vaginal bleeding that is dark in color. However, it may not always be an obvious diagnosis, as blood loss may be minimal. Although significant separation of the placenta often results in vaginal bleeding, the bleeding also may be contained between the uterine wall and the placenta. In addition, the signs and symptoms normally associated with blood loss may not be obvious because the normal increase in blood volume during pregnancy initially protects the mother from developing obvious shock. Also, in the case of abruption from abdominal trauma, little or no external bruising or injury may be present and yet the abruption may be significant.

Abruption may be a life-threatening event for both mother and fetus. Some studies have shown mortality rates as high as 25% to 30% in fetuses and newborns with placental abruption (Simpson, 2002). If a woman has vaginal bleeding and abdominal pain in the third trimester, always consider this diagnosis. The uterus can become tender and boardlike if blood is retained. Patients may present in shock with minimal vaginal bleeding. Ask about risk factors for abruption, be aggressive about treating shock, position in the left lateral recumbent position, and transfer the patient to a surgically capable facility because cesarean section often is the treatment of choice.

Placenta Previa

Placenta previa is the abnormal placement of the placenta such that it partly or completely covers the cervical opening. It occurs in 1 in 300 pregnancies and accounts for 20% of bleeding episodes in the second half of pregnancy (Houry & Abbott, 2002). Risk factors include previous cesarean sections, multiparity, increasing age, and preterm births. When the cervix begins to dilate during labor, the placenta separates at the edge of the cervix and causes painless bright-red vaginal bleeding with little or no contractions. Consider the diagnosis of placenta previa in any woman with third-trimester bleeding. Differentiating placenta previa from abruption may be difficult. Placental insufficiency may cause fetal hypoxia. As with any vaginal bleeding in pregnancy, closely monitor the mother for shock and transport to a facility with obstetric capabilities.

Preeclampsia and Eclampsia

Preeclampsia, also known as *pregnancy-induced hypertension,* is a potentially life-threatening condition that occurs in approximately 5% to 7% of pregnancies (Wagner, 2004). Although the causes are not fully understood, it appears to be related to abnormal blood vessel constriction, leading to multiple complications after 20 weeks of pregnancy. Risk factors are listed in Box 35-9.

Symptoms of this disorder can include headache; severe swelling of the hands, feet, and face; right upper quadrant and epigastric pain; nausea and vomiting; and visual disturbances. Proteinuria is usually present in patients with preeclampsia. In severe cases symptoms can progress to include seizures. The condition is then known as **eclampsia.** Seizures increase the incidence of placental abruption. Severe preeclampsia or eclampsia can lead to stroke, clotting or bleeding problems, kidney or liver failure, and death.

Remember that blood pressure in pregnancy should be normal or slightly lower than normal. A blood pressure of 140/90 mm Hg or an acute systolic rise more than 20 mm Hg or diastolic rise more than 10 mm Hg, which might be considered normal in a nonpregnant patient, may indicate preeclampsia. A woman with signs and symptoms of preeclampsia should be transported on her left side to a hospital with obstetric capabilities.

Assume that seizures in pregnancy indicate eclampsia until proven otherwise. Treatment in the field is the same as for any other seizure (see Chapter 23). Manage the patient's airway, provide oxygen, transport her on her left side, obtain IV access, and transport her to a medical facility with obstetric capabilities. IV magnesium sulfate diluted in 50 to 100 mL of 5% dextrose in water is the treatment of

BOX 35-9 Preeclampsia: Risk Factors

- Primigravidity
- Twin or multiple gestation
- Prior pregnancies with different fathers
- Hypertension
- Excessive amniotic fluid
- Diabetes
- Renal disease
- Obesity
- Maternal age >35 years
- History of preeclampsia

choice for seizures caused by eclampsia. Magnesium sulfate can cause respiratory depression in high doses. Monitor deep tendon reflexes that are lost at magnesium levels of 10 mg/dL. Respiratory depression occurs at levels of 12 mg/dL. The effects of hypermagnesemia can be reversed with calcium gluconate administered slowly IV. Be sure to have calcium gluconate readily available when giving magnesium. IV benzodiazepines may be required if seizures are refractory to magnesium. The ultimate treatment of eclampsia is delivery by cesarean section.

Infection

Infectious diseases are one of the most common causes of pregnancy-related complications worldwide. Many infections present unique risks to the fetus and mother when acquired during gestation. Some infections, including those of the vagina and lower urinary tract, primarily affect the mother and have little effect on the fetus. Other infections, such as rubella (measles) or cytomegalovirus, may have relatively little effect on the mother but cause devastating birth defects for the infant if the mother acquires the infection during pregnancy. Still other infections, such as varicella (chickenpox), gonorrhea, syphilis, human immunodeficiency virus, and group B streptococcal infection can cause significant illness for both mother and baby.

Pyelonephritis, or kidney infection, is more common during pregnancy because of stasis of urine in the ureters and kidneys. This is caused in part by progesterone, which reduces the normal peristaltic action of the ureters, and in part by the enlarging uterus, which compresses the ureters, creating additional stasis. This stasis facilitates migration of bacteria from the bladder into the ureters and kidneys. Symptoms include fever, chills, flank pain and tenderness, frequency, urgency, hematuria, and dysuria. Patients also may have signs of preterm labor, septic shock, and respiratory distress. Assess and treat for septic shock if present and transport the patient to a hospital for antibiotic therapy.

Chorioamnionitis, or infection of the amniotic sac and its contents, most commonly arises when normal bacterial organisms ascend from the vagina into the uterus. Risk factors for chorioamnionitis include young age, low socioeconomic status, nulliparity, extended duration of labor and ruptured membranes, multiple vaginal examinations, and preexisting infections of the lower genital tract (Duff, 2002). The most common bacteria are group B streptococci and *Escherichia coli.* Chorioamnionitis predisposes a woman to preterm labor. Infection with these organisms can cause pneumonia or sepsis in a newborn.

Premature Rupture of Membranes

Rupture of the amniotic sac before labor is called *premature rupture of membranes* (PROM) even if the baby is at term. Preterm PROM occurs before 37 weeks' gestation. Patients usually present with a gush of fluid from the vagina with persistent leakage. Their course often is complicated by chorioamnionitis. Other risks to the fetus from PROM include cord prolapse, cesarean delivery, and placental abruption. PROM is usually treated with antibiotics and steroids.

Diabetes

Diabetes may complicate pregnancy and often can become unstable during pregnancy. Diabetes complicates approximately 2% to 3% of all pregnancies (Tintinalli et al., 2004). These patients are at higher risk for poor fetal outcomes, including stillbirth and fetal distress. Pregnant women with diabetes are more susceptible to hypertensive diseases, preterm labor, spontaneous abortion, pyelonephritis, diabetic ketoacidosis, cerebral hemorrhage, cardiac failure, and renal failure. In particular, they are prone to having large babies and are at risk for shoulder dystocia at delivery. The mother is at higher risk of mental status changes from either high or low blood sugar.

NORMAL CHILDBIRTH

[OBJECTIVES 10, 11]

Labor

Labor is defined as the onset of regular, coordinated **contractions** of the uterus, combined with opening **(dilation)** and effacement of the cervix, which ultimately lead to delivery of the infant and the placenta. The time course of labor varies greatly, lasting from a few hours to more than 1 day. Labor tends to be longer with the first pregnancy and shorter with subsequent pregnancies.

Braxton-Hicks contractions, also called *false labor,* are a normal occurrence during the second half of pregnancy. They help prepare the uterus for the work of delivery. These typically are mild, irregular contractions that do not increase in duration over time. They are also not associated with dilation of the cervix. They occur more frequently when the patient walks and are primarily located in the lower abdomen and groin rather than in the upper abdomen and back. They are not associated with the vaginal discharge (described later) that occurs in the first stage of labor. However, in the field Braxton-Hicks contractions cannot be distinguished from early labor. Assume any patient with contractions may be in labor and treat accordingly.

First Stage

Normally labor is divided into three stages (see Figure 35-3; Box 35-10). The first stage begins with the onset of contractions and ends when the cervix is fully dilated and effaced (thinned out). This stage usually takes 12.5 hours in a **primiparous** and 7 hours in a **multipa-**

BOX 35-10 Stages of Labor

Stage I (dilation stage): Onset of regular uterine contractions to complete cervical dilation
Stage II (expulsion stage): Full dilation of the cervix to the delivery of the newborn
Stage III (placental stage): Immediately after delivery of the baby until expulsion of the placenta

rous patient. Contractions usually start out shorter in duration and farther apart. They become longer, stronger in intensity, and closer together as labor progresses. Contractions of true labor are usually painful. Measuring the **contraction time** (length of each contraction) and the **contraction interval** (time from the beginning of one contraction to the beginning of the next) can help determine whether delivery is imminent. Contractions that last longer than 1 minute or are closer than every 2 to 3 minutes may indicate that birth is very near.

Another clue to the first stage of labor may be the presence of **bloody show.** This is the passage of a small amount of mucus and blood from the vagina. It indicates that the protective mucous plug that normally seals off the cervix has been released as the cervix dilates. Bloody show consists of only a small amount of blood. Any significant or persistent bleeding is abnormal and may indicate a serious complication.

Second Stage

The *second stage* of labor is defined as the time from complete dilation and effacement of the cervix until the delivery of the infant (see Figure 35-3, *C*). During this time the infant is moving out of the uterus and down into the birth canal. This causes a strong pressure sensation in the perineal area. The mother usually has an overwhelming urge to bear down or push. Contractions are intense and close together, sometimes with a contraction interval of less than 1 minute. The amniotic sac usually ruptures but may not in some situations: the amniotic sac may be the first thing to present, or it may present covering the child during crowning. In these cases the sac should be ruptured. As the baby moves down the birth canal, the **presenting part** becomes visible at the vaginal opening. The presenting part, or the first part of the baby's body to come into view, is usually the head. When the head is visible at the perineum, the infant is said to be **crowning.** The second stage usually lasts an average of 80 minutes for a primipara and 30 minutes for a multipara.

Third Stage

The third stage of labor begins after the infant is delivered and ends with delivery of the placenta (see Figure 35-3, *D*). Do not delay transport for placental delivery. This stage usually lasts less than 20 minutes but can last as long as 30 to 45 minutes. Do not attempt to hasten the delivery of the placenta by pulling on the umbilical cord. This can lead to incomplete separation of the placenta from the uterine wall, or a uterine inversion. Traction on the umbilical cord can also lead to separation of the cord from the placenta. This is particularly true if there is a velamentous insertion of the umbilical cord. In this situation, the arteries and vein of the umbilical cord leave the Wharton's jelly and "branch out" before connecting with the placenta. If the placenta does deliver in the prehospital setting, inspect it for missing pieces and place it in a container for transport. The hospital must be notified of the delivery of an incomplete placenta, as this can cause significant maternal hemorrhage. Normal hemorrhage following delivery of the placenta presents as a rush of blood that slows to a trickle.

Delivery

Decision to Transport versus Delivery in the Field

[OBJECTIVES 12, 13]

Transporting the mother to the hospital before delivery is obviously preferable if time allows. However, in some instances delivery is imminent and likely will occur before you can safely transport the mother. When deciding whether to transport a patient immediately or deliver an infant in the prehospital setting, some considerations include estimated transport time to the closest hospital and whether the mother's condition is complicated by other immediate life threats, such as active vaginal bleeding, hypotension, diabetes, seizures, or trauma.

If the mother states that she has an urge to bear down, strongly consider visually inspecting the perineum. To do this, find or create a private area for the mother to remove her pants or undergarments. Have her lie on her back with her knees flexed and spread apart to allow inspection. If you see crowning or bulging present, prepare for delivery.

Box 35-11 contains some questions to help determine if delivery is imminent. Table 35-3 lists additional factors to consider when deciding to transport the patient or deliver in the field.

Preparation for Delivery

[OBJECTIVE 14]

Preparation for delivery includes preparing the mother, yourself, and your surroundings. Begin by finding a private, protected place for the delivery to occur if possible. If you cannot move the patient to the ambulance and no private area exists where you are, consider creating some privacy by draping sheets and blankets to create visual barriers.

As always, use standard precautions, including gloves, a mask, a gown, and eye protection. If you have a commercially prepared obstetric kit, these items are probably included. If you do not have a kit, you will need to prepare the following supplies (Figure 35-6):

BOX 35-11 Questions to Determine Whether Delivery Is Imminent

Start with identifying urgent signs and symptoms:

- *Do you feel like you need to push or have a bowel movement?*
  - Women often feel the sensation of needing to push when the baby's head has moved into the birth canal. They also may describe this as an urge to have a bowel movement or as intense pressure in the vaginal area.
- *Are you bleeding or having any vaginal discharge?*
  - Bloody show may indicate the start of labor. Significant bleeding in labor is not normal and should prompt immediate stabilization and transport.
- *Has your water broken?*
  - The amniotic sac usually ruptures at some point during labor. If it has already ruptured, delivery may be imminent.

Other important pieces of history include:

- *Is this your first pregnancy?*
  - Labor and delivery are usually more rapid with each successive pregnancy. If the woman has had babies before, ask how long her previous labors lasted.
- *How long have you been having contractions?*
  - Contractions become more forceful and last longer as labor progresses.
- *How far apart are your contractions?*
  - As a woman gets closer to delivery, the contractions come closer together.
- *What is your due date?*
  - Delivery more than 3 weeks before the due date is considered preterm or premature. Knowing this is important in anticipating the needs of the infant after birth.
- *Is there any chance you are having more than one baby?*
  - A woman who has had regular prenatal care during the pregnancy will likely know this. If more than one infant is expected, you may need to call for additional resources.

- Gown, gloves, mask, and protective eyewear
- Clean towels and blankets
- 1 bulb syringe
- 2 plastic umbilical cord clamps
- Gauze sponges
- 1 pair of scissors or scalpel
- Sanitary napkin
- Container for the placenta

Next, help the mother position herself for delivery (Figure 35-7). Have her remove her underwear if she has not already done so.

The easiest position for delivery is to have her lie on her back with her knees flexed and her feet flat on the

TABLE 35-3 Considerations Regarding Transport versus Delivery in the Field

History and Assessment Findings	Significance
Factors Related to the Imminence of Delivery	
Number of pregnancies	Labor is shortened with multiparity
Frequency of contractions	2 minutes apart may signal imminent delivery
Maternal urge to push	Desire to push signals imminent delivery
Crowning of the presenting part	Imminent delivery
Factors Related to the Presence of Complications	
Abnormal presentations Fetal distress Multiple births	Increased risk of complications

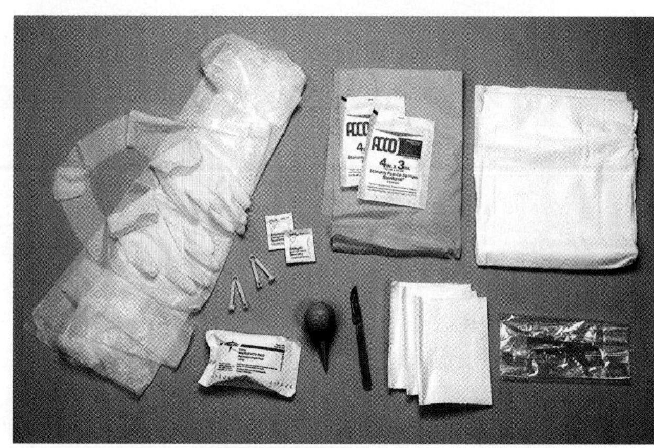

Figure 35-6 Supplies in a typical delivery kit.

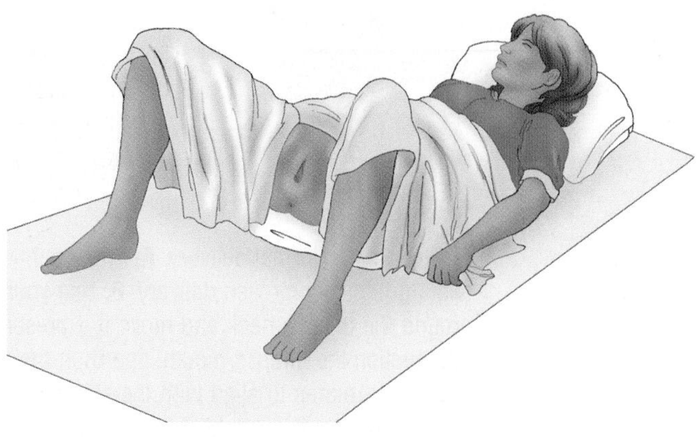

Figure 35-7 Position for delivery.

stretcher or other surface. You may want to place a clean sheet or towel under her buttocks to elevate her hips slightly. You can drape a sheet over her lower abdomen and upper legs for modesty's sake if time permits, but make sure it is not in your way for the actual delivery.

If the mother feels the urge to push, encourage her to keep her chin down and her knees flexed. She can push more effectively if her head and back are elevated to a partial sitting position. Encourage her to push for approximately 10 seconds, then rest and breathe for 10 seconds. Long, sustained (more than 10 seconds) pushing can rupture blood vessels and tear the perineum.

Delivery Procedure

[OBJECTIVES 15, 16, 17, 18]

Once the baby's head is crowning, follow these steps to help deliver the infant (Figure 35-8):

- Allow the head to deliver in a controlled, gradual manner. This allows the mother's perineum to stretch more and therefore tear less. To do this, put one hand on the baby's head and the other hand, holding a towel or piece of gauze, on the perineum. Exert gentle pressure with your hands to avoid an explosive delivery. The head will most commonly be facing downward at this point.
- Once the head has delivered, use the bulb syringe to suction the baby's mouth and nose. First squeeze all the air out of the syringe. Then, with the syringe still compressed, place the tip into the infant's mouth and release the compression to suction out any fluids. Move the syringe away from the baby's face and squeeze it several times to expel the contents. Repeat this procedure one or two times for the mouth and then each nostril. If you do not have a bulb syringe, use a gauze pad to wipe any fluid from the mouth and nose area.
- Check around the neck for a loop of umbilical cord. If one is present, gently hook your finger under the loop and pull it over the baby's head. You may have to repeat this procedure if more than one loop is

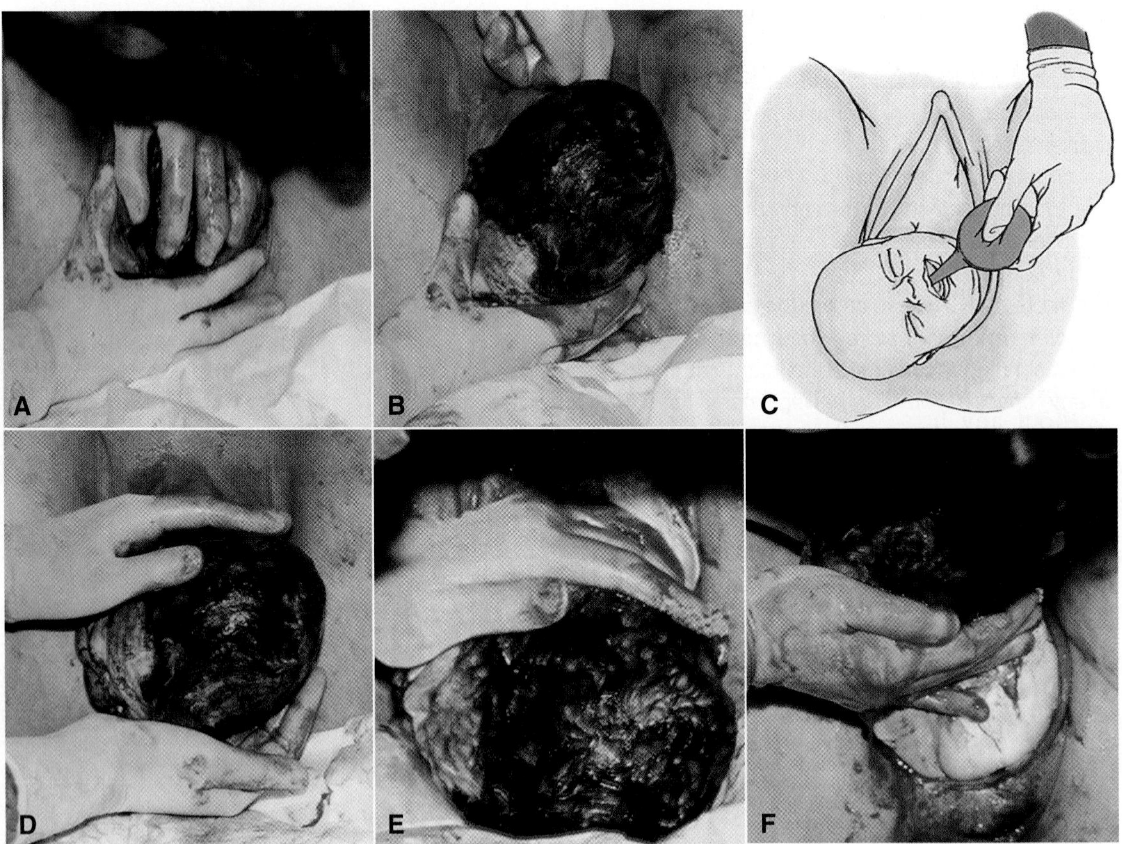

Figure 35-8 Normal delivery. **A,** Apply gentle pressure to the infant's head during crowning to allow gradual, controlled delivery. **B,** Use your index finger to feel for a loop of umbilical cord around the infant's neck and move it if present. **C,** After the head is delivered, support the head and suction the infant's mouth, and then the nose, with a bulb syringe. **D,** Support the infant's head as it rotates to align with the shoulders. **E,** Gently guide the infant's head downward to deliver the anterior shoulder. **F,** Guide the infant's head upward to deliver the posterior shoulder and the rest of the body.

around the newborn's neck. If you are unable to free the cord, clamp the cord in two places and cut the cord between the clamps.
- During the previous steps, the baby's head will probably have started to turn toward one side or the other. Gently direct the head downward to allow the anterior shoulder to slip out from under the pubic bone. Once the anterior shoulder is delivered, the rest of the baby's body will usually appear quickly. Remember that the baby will be slippery. Be careful not to drop the baby!
- Keep the infant at about the level of the vagina while you use a gauze pad to wipe away any remaining secretions around the mouth and nose.
- Dry the infant to reduce body heat loss and stimulate the infant to breathe. The easiest way to do this is to place the infant on a firm surface and rub the infant dry with a towel. If needed, you can also stimulate the baby by flicking the soles of the feet.
- Cut the umbilical cord. Place the two plastic cord clamps on the umbilical cord several inches away from the baby's abdomen (4 and 6 inches, respectively) and cut *between* the clamps.
- Wrap the infant in clean towels or blankets. This step is important to prevent hypothermia.
- Note the time of delivery.
- If you expect multiple births, prepare for the next delivery.
- Watch for the placenta to deliver spontaneously. This can take up to 30 to 45 minutes.
- If the placenta delivers, place it in a clean container and transport it to the hospital with the mother and infant.

Remember, normal childbirth usually happens spontaneously without any intervention or assistance. The actual delivery of the infant's body from the birth canal usually happens in a matter of 1 to 2 minutes. Be prepared, but do not panic. Box 35-12 summarizes some paramedic pearls regarding vaginal delivery.

BOX 35-12 Paramedic Pearls: Do's and Dont's of Delivery

- **DO** . . . dry, cover, and warm the baby as soon as possible after delivery. Newborns lack the ability to regulate their body temperature as effectively as adults. On top of this, the newborn comes out wet into a cooler environment than the womb. These factors predispose a newborn to hypothermia.
- **DO** . . . clamp each umbilical cord separately when there are multiple births. More than one placenta may deliver after the babies are born. If so, preserve and transport all to the hospital.
- **DO** . . . begin cardiopulmonary resuscitation on a baby that appears to be very premature or stillborn unless signs of death are obvious. Loss of a baby at any stage of pregnancy can be emotionally devastating to the parents. Even if your efforts are unsuccessful, it may be one of the kindest things you can do for the survivors.
- **DON'T** . . . put the mother's legs together in an effort to delay the birth. This will not stop the delivery and is extremely dangerous to both mother and baby.
- **DON'T** . . . pull hard on the infant's head or extremities during the delivery process. You can break bones or cause permanent damage to the spinal cord and nerves.
- **DON'T** . . . drop the baby! Remember, the baby will be wet and slippery. One maneuver is to let the infant deliver into your hands and immediately tuck it under your arm (like a football) as you wipe off the face and body.
- **DON'T** . . . pull on the umbilical cord while waiting for the placenta to deliver. Doing so could cause the cord to tear or the uterus to invert. If the placenta has not delivered by the time you arrive at the hospital, simply note this in your report to the hospital care providers.

POSTDELIVERY CARE OF THE MOTHER

[OBJECTIVES 19, 20]

After delivery, the mother will likely feel weak and tired. Women occasionally experience involuntary trembling in the legs or entire body after the infant is born. This will resolve naturally in a few minutes. During this time, continue regular monitoring of blood pressure and heart rate. Keep the mother warm and watch for signs of shock.

The average volume of blood lost with a vaginal delivery is approximately 500 mL. Because of the increased blood volume that occurs in pregnancy, most women can tolerate this blood loss without any symptoms. Monitor the amount of blood loss; if needed, provide clean pads or bedding. If blood loss continues or seems excessive, massage the uterus to promote uterine contraction and reduce bleeding (Figure 35-9). Place your fingers flat on the mother's abdomen, just above the pubic bone, and massage in a circular fashion. You probably will feel the enlarged uterus through the abdominal wall under your fingers. The mother will experience a cramping sensation; this is a sign of effective massage. If mother and baby are able, you also can encourage the mother to breastfeed her newborn to promote uterine contraction and slow the bleeding. Breastfeeding stimulates the release of oxytocin, a hormone that causes the uterus to contract.

Remember that delivery of the placenta can take 30 to 45 minutes. Do not delay transport to await delivery of the placenta.

POSTDELIVERY CARE OF THE INFANT

[OBJECTIVES 21, 23]

Newborns are usually blue or purplish immediately after delivery. A pink core and cyanotic extremities are referred to as **acrocyanosis;** this is also a normal finding at delivery. As newborns begin to breathe, they normally "pink up" within several minutes. If the mother is frightened by this, reassure her that the color change is normal. Your priorities in caring for a newborn are the same as any other patient: manage ABCs.

Airway

You should already have cleared the baby's airway immediately after the head delivered. Check again to ensure no more mucus or other material is blocking the airway. Repeat bulb suctioning if necessary and position the baby on his or her side. During this time, also dry and cover the infant with a clean, dry blanket to prevent heat loss.

Breathing

Clearing the airway and drying procedures usually stimulate the baby to begin breathing. If not, stimulate the baby by either rubbing his or her back vigorously or flicking the feet with your fingers. If the infant is still not breathing after these maneuvers, make sure the airway is open. Use a chin lift or jaw thrust to open the airway if needed. Provide bag-mask breaths for approximately 30 seconds at a rate of 40 to 60 per minute and reevaluate.

If the infant is breathing, ensure the respiratory rate is at least 30 breaths/min (normal rate for a newborn is approximately 40 breaths/min). If the baby is not breathing at least 30 times/min or is having trouble breathing, assist breathing with a bag-mask device.

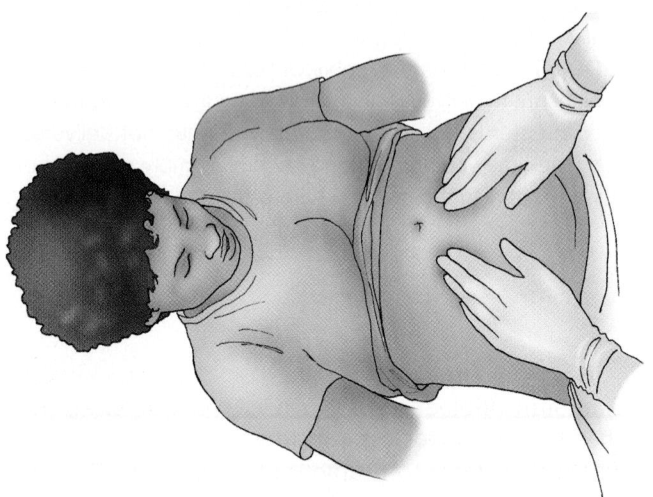

Figure 35-9 Uterine massage to control postdelivery bleeding.

Circulation

Check for a pulse either in the umbilical cord or in the brachial artery. If no pulse is present or if it is less than 60 beats/min, begin chest compressions. Neonatal resuscitation is discussed in more detail in Chapter 36.

Apgar Scores

Apgar scores are commonly assigned to newborns according to the infant's appearance and activity 1 and 5 minutes after delivery. The scoring system is based on assigning a score of 0 to 2 for five areas (Table 35-4). Scores average 8 to 10. Do not delay resuscitation of an infant to assign Apgar scores.

COMPLICATIONS OF CHILDBIRTH

Preterm Delivery

[OBJECTIVES 24, 25]

Preterm or **premature delivery** is defined as any delivery between the twentieth and thirty-seventh weeks of pregnancy. Only approximately 10% of babies are born preterm, but 80% of newborn deaths are related to prematurity (Gianopoulos, 1994). Risk factors include physiologic abnormalities, uterine or cervical abnormalities, PROM, multiple gestations, and intrauterine infection. Be sure to ask the mother how far along she is in her pregnancy and whether she has noticed fluid leakage that might indicate her amniotic sac has broken. Treatment includes rapid transport to an appropriate facility, rest, fluids, and administration of a **tocolytic** to slow contractions. The uterus is made of smooth muscle. As a result, the administration of $beta_2$ agonists or smooth muscle

TABLE 35-4 Apgar Scoring System

Sign	0	1	2
Appearance (skin color)	Blue or pale	Blue extremities, pink torso	Completely pink
Pulse	Absent	Slow (<100)	>100
Grimace (reflex irritability)	No response	Grimace	Cough, sneeze, cry
Activity (muscle tone)	Limp	Some flexion	Active motion
Respiratory effort	Absent	Slow, irregular	Good, crying

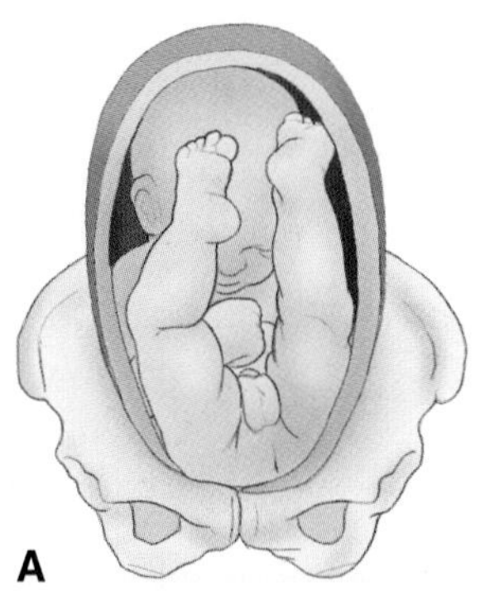

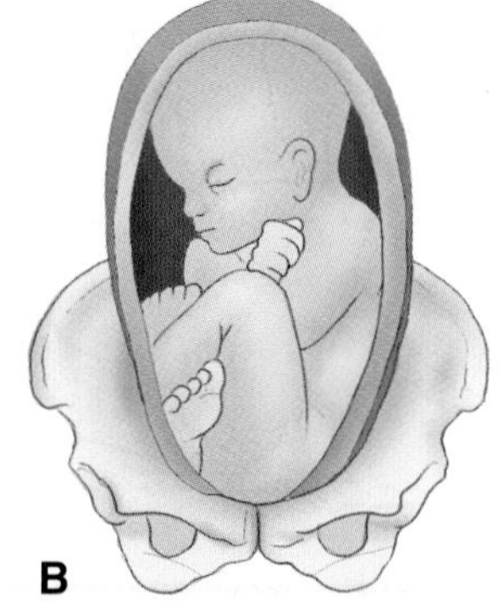

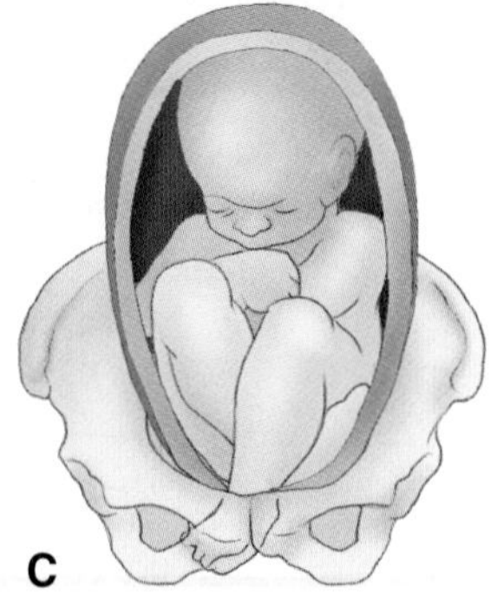

Figure 35-10 Breech delivery. **A,** Frank breech. **B,** Complete breech. **C,** Footling breech.

relaxants reduces labor by causing the relaxation of smooth muscles. Magnesium sulfate, ritodrine, and terbutaline are examples of tocolytic agents.

If you must deliver a preterm infant in the field, expect that the baby may need more aggressive resuscitation. Provide humidified blow-by oxygen. Ventilatory assistance with a bag-mask device is likely, and be more careful than usual to keep the infant warm.

The age at which a fetus is generally considered old enough to survive is approximately 24 weeks. However, unless the baby is clearly dead, begin resuscitative measures even if you think the infant is likely too small to survive. A mother may be unsure or incorrect regarding how far along her pregnancy is. Besides, making every attempt to save the baby may help the family cope with the loss.

Breech Delivery

A **breech presentation** means that either the baby's buttocks or lower extremities are the first part of the body to enter the birth canal. This occurs in approximately 4% of deliveries (Cunningham, 2005) and is the most common abnormal presentation. Breech presentation has three presentations: frank breech, complete breech, and footling breech (Figure 35-10). Often the baby will deliver on its own, although the process may be slower because the head, which is the largest part, is the last to be delivered. For a breech delivery, assist as follows:

- As the infant's body delivers, support the legs and pelvis with your gloved hands. Do not grasp the infant around the abdomen because this can lead to damage of the internal organs. Instead, gently grasp the infant over the bony part of the pelvis to help guide the body out or support the baby's body on your forearm. Do not pull on the body.
- Gently rotate the torso such that the shoulders are oriented anteriorly to posteriorly.
- Guide the infant's body upward to allow the posterior shoulder to deliver, then downward to deliver the anterior shoulder.

At this point, the infant's head may spontaneously deliver. If it does not deliver shortly, assist as follows:

- Support the baby's body on your forearm.
- Place the mother in a knee-chest position (Figure 35-11). This position creates the widest possible diameter of the mother's pelvis and allows more room for the baby's head to pass.
- Use your fingers to create an airway for the baby (Figure 35-12). Do this by placing two fingers inside the vagina, one on either side of the baby's nose. Bend your fingers slightly to push the birth canal away from the baby's face and create a breathing space.
- With the next contraction, lift the baby's body slightly upward to create a better angle for the head to deliver.
- Provide blow-by oxygen to the area near the baby's nose to increase the oxygen concentration. You also can provide oxygen to the mother if you have not already done so.
- If the head does not deliver on its own, maintain the airway with your fingers as described above and transport rapidly to the nearest hospital.

Shoulder Dystocia

Shoulder dystocia occurs when the head has delivered but the shoulder is trapped under the mother's pelvic bone and the infant's body does not easily slide out. It is the second most common abnormal presentation and is more likely with a very large infant or a mother whose pelvis is very small. Often this presents with "turtle sign," in which the head will appear with a contraction and retract during relaxation.

If the baby's body does not slide out easily with limited traction on the head, do *not* pull hard to deliver the shoulder. This makes the shoulder impaction worse and may cause serious and permanent brachial plexus damage to the baby. Instead, place the mother in the knee-chest position as for breech presentation. You can also press downward with your fingers on the baby's shoulder through the mother's abdominal wall just above the pubic bone. Together these maneuvers often dislodge the wedged shoulder and allow the baby to deliver.

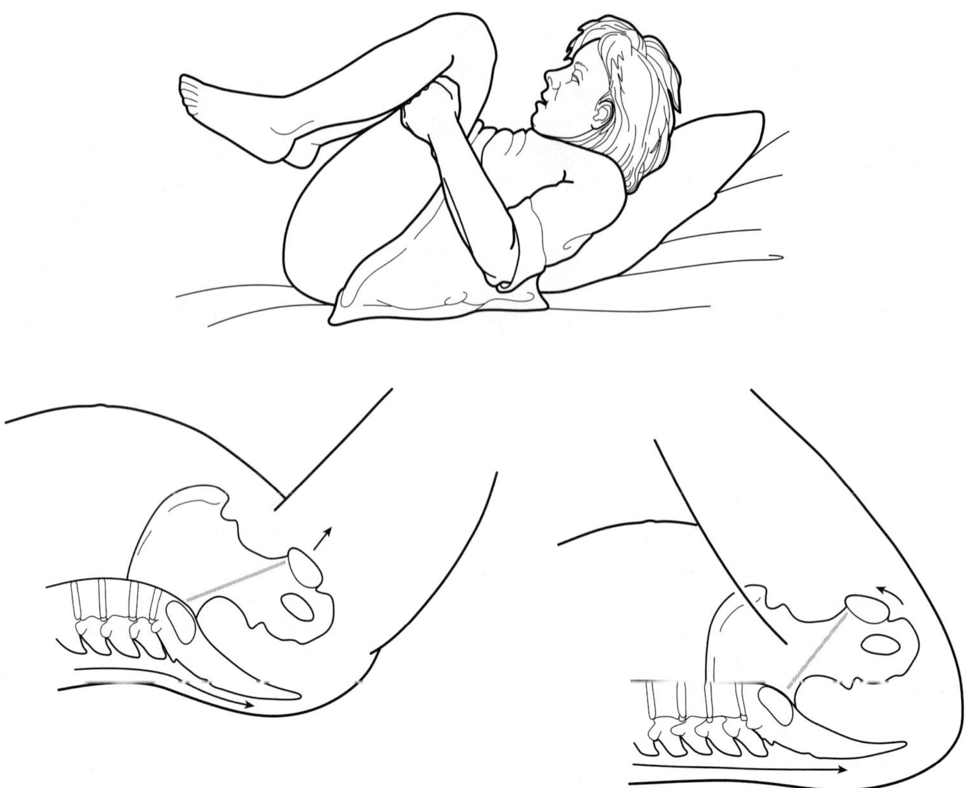

Figure 35-11 Knee-chest position for shoulder dystocia, breech delivery, prolapsed umbilical cord, and limb presentation.

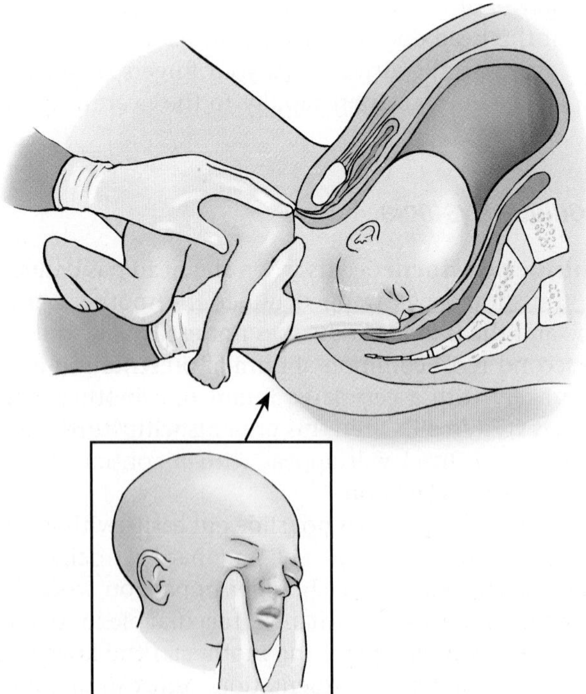

Figure 35-12 Creating an airway for the infant during a breech delivery.

If these maneuvers are unsuccessful, remain calm and keep the mother calm. Transport her immediately and call ahead to let hospital personnel know of your arrival.

Cephalopelvic Disproportion

Cephalopelvic disproportion results when the head of the baby is too large for the maternal pelvic opening. In this situation the child cannot be delivered vaginally and a cesarean section is required. Often these patients have strong and frequent contractions that may lead to exhaustion and possibly uterine rupture. Prehospital care is limited to recognition, treatment of presenting symptoms, and transport to the hospital.

Prolapsed Umbilical Cord

Umbilical cord prolapse refers to a situation in which the umbilical cord is in front of the presenting part and becomes compressed, cutting off blood supply and oxygen to the baby (Figure 35-13). This is more likely to happen when the presenting part is something other than the head, such as in breech or limb presentations. This is a rare but potentially catastrophic event in which the baby will quickly die without intervention.

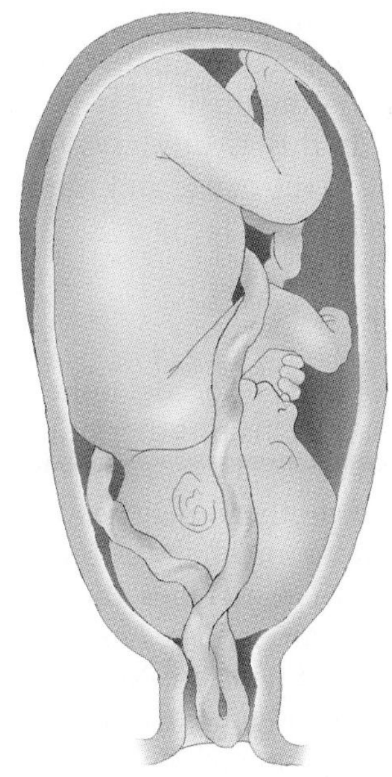

Figure 35-13 Prolapsed umbilical cord.

If you see the umbilical cord protruding from the vagina before the baby has delivered, immediately place the mother in a knee-chest position. If possible, place the bed in Trendelenburg position. Both these maneuvers reduce pressure on the cord. Place your gloved hand inside the vagina and push upward on the presenting part to further reduce pressure on the cord. Keep pressure on the presenting part during transport. Cover the cord with wet dressings but avoid manipulating it.

Umbilical cord prolapse often requires emergency cesarean section to save the infant's life. The infant's survival is directly related to the time from prolapse to surgical intervention (Cunningham, 2005). Your top priority is to transport the mother immediately. Notify hospital personnel of the prolapsed cord during transport so that they can prepare for immediate surgery.

Compound Presentation

A **compound presentation** refers to the presentation of an extremity alongside or in front of the major presenting fetal part. The combination of an upper extremity and the head is the most common compound presentation. Compound presentations are seen most commonly in preterm babies and in twin delivery, specifically delivery of the second twin. Fortunately this occurrence is rare. In this case, specialized intervention is necessary for delivery and the baby is unlikely to be born outside the hospital. If an extremity is visible in the birth canal, do not pull on the extremity to try to help deliver the infant. Remember that umbilical cord prolapse is more likely to occur in any kind of abnormal presentation, so check to see if the cord is visible or palpable in the vagina. If it is, manage as discussed above for umbilical cord prolapse. Place the mother in the knee-chest position, give her oxygen, and prepare to transport her immediately. Stay calm and try to keep the mother calm.

Multiple Births

Most mothers who are expecting more than one baby know this before delivery and will tell you during evaluation. However, if the mother has not had prenatal care, she may not realize she is carrying multiple fetuses. If a woman still has a markedly enlarged abdomen after delivery and has had no prenatal care, consider the possibility of multiple births. Try to auscultate for fetal heart sounds over the abdomen with a stethoscope.

The procedures for delivering multiple infants are the same as for a single baby. Keep in mind that infants of multiple births are more likely to be born prematurely and often are smaller than a single term infant. This means they are at higher risk for breathing difficulties and hypothermia. Be ready to resuscitate them and continue close observation and assessment during transport.

Vaginal Bleeding

Bleeding during and after delivery is a normal part of childbirth. Remember that the mother's blood volume is increased during pregnancy, which allows her body to compensate for the expected blood loss. Up to 500 mL of blood loss is considered normal, but more than 500 mL is considered excessive. Excessive bleeding may be caused by a lack of uterine tone, vaginal or cervical tears, incomplete passage of the placenta, or clotting disorders. Do not be alarmed by the normal bleeding that occurs, but do watch for signs of excess bleeding. If bleeding is brisk and does not slow within several minutes of delivery, take appropriate steps. Excessive vaginal bleeding is the most common complication of labor and delivery (Mallon & Henderson, 2002).

To help slow vaginal bleeding and reduce the risk of excess bleeding, massage the abdomen over the uterus as described previously. You also can encourage the mother to breastfeed if she is able and apply direct pressure to obvious external bleeding sources. Watch for signs and symptoms of shock and treat as for hemorrhagic shock. Provide oxygen, keep the mother warm, consider two large-bore IVs with normal saline or lactated Ringer's solution, and rapidly transport the patient to the closest appropriate facility.

Meconium

[OBJECTIVE 26]

Meconium is a yellow to dark-green substance that constitutes a newborn's first bowel movement. It occurs in approximately 8% to 30% of deliveries. Normally a newborn does not pass stool until after delivery. However, an infant occasionally will pass meconium while still in the uterus. This is important to recognize for two reasons. First, meconium passage in utero means that the baby may already be in some distress from a lack of oxygen, infection, or other causes. Second, the infant may aspirate meconium into the lungs when taking the first breath. Meconium aspiration syndrome can result in pneumonia and lung damage.

If the infant has passed meconium in the uterus, you or the mother may note a greenish tint to the amniotic fluid. You also may see a thick, dark-greenish substance coming from the vagina or covering the baby as the head emerges.

If you suspect that the baby has passed meconium, special delivery procedures are required. Closely monitor after delivery for breathing difficulties, provide oxygen, and be prepared to intubate if needed. Be sure to inform hospital personnel of your suspicions on arrival. Care of the newborn is discussed in more detail in Chapter 36.

Fetal Death

Loss of a child is probably one of the most significant traumas human beings can experience. Although an indication that something was wrong may have been noted ahead of time, it also may be an unexpected tragedy, especially in the case of trauma.

Unless signs of death are obvious, err on the side of performing cardiopulmonary resuscitation. The family may better cope with the loss if they believe that "everything possible was done." Be ready to offer emotional support to the parents and be prepared for a range of responses from the family.

Uterine Inversion

Uterine inversion is uncommon but can be life threatening. In this condition the uterus is turned inside out. Inversion complicates approximately 1 in 2000 deliveries. It is usually associated with a placenta that is attached to the fundus, coughing or sneezing, or aggressive umbilical cord traction and improper massage. On examination, the uterine fundus may be visibly protruding from the cervix. Treatment includes fluid and restoration of the normal position of the uterus. This should be accomplished with sterile gloves and without removing the placenta. The exact restoration of anatomic position should be discussed under the direction of a physician. Administer oxygen and IV fluids to the patient. One attempt at replacing the uterus may be made in the prehospital setting. If this is unsuccessful, cover exposed tissue with moist sterile gauze and transport the patient immediately to a medical facility.

Uterine Rupture

Uterine rupture is rare but occurs more often in patients with prior cesarean births or other prior uterine surgery. It also may be seen when delivery is mechanically blocked, such as when the mother's pelvis is too small to allow expulsion of the fetus, or when the fetus has some physical malformation that stretches the uterus or impedes delivery. Mortality rate is lower in an inpatient setting when the mother and fetus are continuously monitored. Unfortunately, fetal and maternal death is far more likely to occur in the prehospital setting, such as when a woman has been laboring at home. Uterine rupture is extremely difficult to diagnose in the field. Patients may report severe shooting pain during contractions, but pain actually can improve with complete rupture. The mother may note decreased fetal movement. Rapid shock may ensue, although external bleeding often is minimal. Any woman suspected of uterine rupture should be treated for shock and immediately transported to a hospital.

Pulmonary Embolism

Pulmonary embolism is one of the leading causes of maternal death, complicating approximately 17% of pregnancies. Pregnancy increases the risk of pulmonary embolism fivefold in the perinatal and postpartum period when compared with age-matched, nonpregnant patients (Whitty & Dombrowski, 2002). Pulmonary embolism is commonly seen with cesarean section and often results from a clot in the pelvic circulation. Amniotic fluid may also cause a pulmonary embolism. Patients often present with dyspnea, tachypnea, cough, pleuritic chest pain, tachycardia, hemoptysis, and diaphoresis. Management includes oxygenation, ventilation, placement in a comfortable position, cardiac monitoring, and emergency transport.

Case Scenario CONCLUSION

After initial stabilization, you prepare for transport to the receiving facility. The patient continues to complain of cramping and states she feels she is bleeding more heavily. After asking permission to inspect the vaginal area, you notice that she is passing some tissue and blood clots. The patient is awake and conversant throughout transport. She asks if she is having a miscarriage.

Questions

8. *What are your critical concerns regarding treatment and care of this patient?*
9. *What information should be relayed to the receiving facility?*
10. *What comfort measures can be provided for this patient?*

TRAUMA IN PREGNANCY

Trauma is the leading cause of death among pregnant women in the United States (Fildes et al., 1992). Motor vehicle crashes account for the majority of injuries and injury-related deaths in pregnant women. In motor vehicle crashes, the most common cause of death in the fetus is death of the mother. Intimate partner violence also should be considered as a possible cause of injury. In addition, pregnant women are more prone to accidents because of the weight gain and body changes of pregnancy. They may experience loosening of the joints and be more likely to fall because of their changing center of gravity. They also may be more prone to syncopal episodes.

Trauma in pregnancy means you have two patients—the mother and her unborn infant. Although remembering this axiom is important, you also must remember that, in general, the best treatment for the fetus is to take care of the mother. Therefore treatment priorities will be the same in pregnant and nonpregnant trauma victims (Van Hook, 2002).

Immediately assess ABCs in a pregnant patient just as you would any other patient. Supplemental oxygen is especially important because the mother's enlarged uterus makes deep breathing more difficult. She therefore is more prone to becoming hypoxic. In addition, the developing fetus is particularly sensitive to hypoxia.

Position the mother on her left side if possible after the twenty-fourth week. If a pregnant patient has injuries that require a cervical collar and backboard, immobilize her just as you would the nonpregnant patient. Remember that placing a pregnant woman flat on her back reduces blood flow to the uterus and blood return to the mother (supine hypotensive syndrome). Avoid this problem by tilting the backboard 15 degrees to the left. To do this, place linens or other items under the right side of the backboard (Figure 35-14). You also may need to place a pillow or blanket under the mother's abdomen for her comfort.

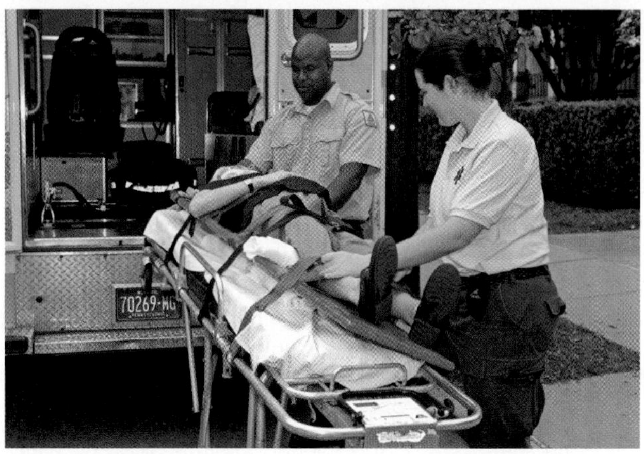

Figure 35-14 A pregnant woman who requires spinal motion restriction should be placed on a backboard that is tilted 15 degrees to the left.

Even relatively minor trauma to the abdomen can cause injury to the placenta and uterus. Placental abruption can be life threatening for the mother and baby. Transport any pregnant patient with possible abdominal or chest trauma, no matter how trivial, to the hospital for further evaluation and fetal monitoring.

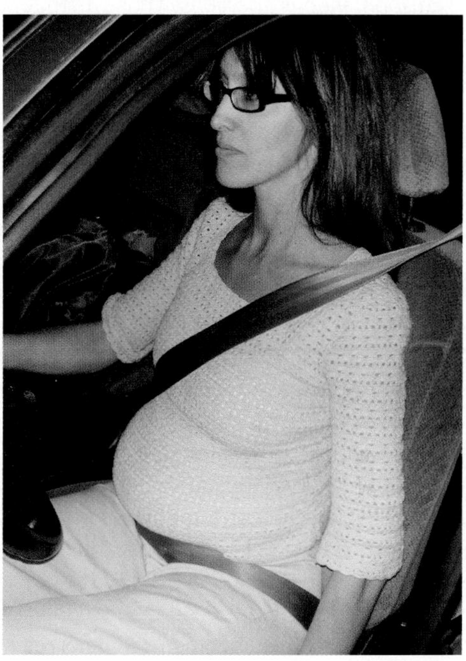

Figure 35-15 Proper seat belt use in pregnancy. The lap belt is positioned over the pelvis and under the abdomen, and the shoulder harness is between the breasts.

Seat Belt Use in Pregnancy

Motor vehicle crashes account for the majority of injuries and injury-related deaths in pregnant women in the United States. As many as one third to half of all pregnant women do not use seat belts or do not use them properly. Yet the evidence is clear: maternal injuries from car crashes can be effectively reduced or prevented by three-point restraints (American College of Obstetricians and Gynecologists, 1991). No evidence shows that properly worn restraints increase the chance of fetal injury. Proper positioning includes placing the lap belt snugly and comfortably under the abdomen and across the thighs, with the shoulder belt positioned between the breasts (Figure 35-15).

Women who receive information on seat belt use during pregnancy from a healthcare professional are more likely to use seat belts and use them properly (Pearlman & Phillips, 1996). As a healthcare professional, you should emphasize the use of three-point restraints for all passengers, including pregnant women.

Case Scenario SUMMARY

1. *What is your initial impression of this patient?* This patient has vaginal bleeding. On your arrival, you notice a moderate amount of blood near the victim. This can indicate a serious condition and possible shock. The history provided indicates the patient is pregnant and she was struck in the abdomen, chest, and arms yesterday by her boyfriend. Possible conditions to consider include chest, abdominal, and/or fetal trauma, possible miscarriage, or preterm delivery.
2. *What are some important questions about the patient's medical history?* You should obtain a SAMPLE history and OPQRST. Also ask questions regarding trauma, abuse, last menstrual period, EDC, prenatal care, social history, and specific questions regarding her pain. The patient reports a pregnancy dated at 18 weeks. The duration of the pregnancy is important. Pregnancies that spontaneously terminate before 20 weeks are called *spontaneous abortions*. Those after 20 weeks are considered *preterm deliveries*.
3. *Describe the physical examination you will perform.* The physical examination should begin with the primary survey. Immediately treat any life-threatening findings. Reassessment is essential. The secondary physical examination should include a head-to-toe examination. Although this patient appears to have significant vaginal bleeding, be sure to look for additional medical conditions, including cardiac, pulmonary, and hematologic complaints. Signs of pulmonary edema, murmur, and bruising are important to investigate. After a thorough secondary examination, perform ongoing assessments until the patient's care is transferred to staff at the receiving facility.
4. *Discuss domestic violence in pregnant patients.* Pregnant women are at increased risk for intimate partner violence (Shah et al., 1998). The abuser is often the father of the child (Poole et al., 1996). The most common injury from domestic violence in a pregnant woman is blunt trauma to the abdomen (Webster et al., 1994). Other common sites of injury are the face, head, and breasts. A patient who is the victim of domestic violence may not report the event. Be sure to ask the patient whether abuse has occurred. This should be done in all cases, but with particular attention in patients who have additional injuries such as bruising, burns, or broken bones.
5. *What is the significance of the blood pressure?* The patient's blood pressure, although appearing normal, suggests the compensatory phase of shock. This is indicated by a pulse pressure (difference between systolic and diastolic pressures) of less than 30 mm Hg. If bleeding is controlled, the risk of the shock progressing is decreased. However, if bleeding continues, hypotension, tachycardia, and other forms of shock will develop. Constant monitoring of this patient is essential.
6. *What are important treatment considerations?* This patient should be placed on high-flow supplemental oxygen. She is losing a large amount of blood and should be treated for shock. Place the patient on the cardiac monitor and establish IV access with two large-bore catheters. Administer fluids per protocol. If the patient continues to bleed, place a pad underneath her. This will help quantify the blood loss. Any tissue that passes also should be kept and delivered to the receiving facility.
7. Describe possible differential diagnoses for this patient. This patient appears to be having a spontaneous abortion. However, you need to consider other causes of second-trimester vaginal bleeding, including placenta previa, abruptio placenta, and (possibly) uterine rupture.
8. *What is critical regarding treatment and care of this patient?* This patient likely is having a miscarriage with significant bleeding. Prompt care and transport are essential. Place the patient in a left lateral recumbent position, administer oxygen, establish IV access, and transport her to the nearest appropriate facility for stabilization.
9. *What information should be relayed to the receiving facility?* Relay the patient's age, duration of pregnancy, history, and physical examination findings and treatment provided to the receiving facility. Other important information includes previous problems with pregnancy, comorbid medical problems, and other traumatic injuries. If abuse is suspected, this also should be conveyed in your report. Law enforcement personnel also should be notified.
10. *What can be done to comfort this patient?* The patient should be made as comfortable as possible in a left lateral recumbent position during transport. Consider pain medication for this patient because it will alleviate her pain and perhaps her anxiety. However, the patient's blood pressure suggests compensatory shock, so this should be critically evaluated. Consult medical direction for assistance regarding this decision. The patient also asks if she is having a miscarriage. The patient should not be told that "everything will be okay." An appropriate response is to state that you are unsure of the cause of her bleeding but a miscarriage is a concern. The exact diagnosis should be made by a specialist after appropriate evaluation and diagnostic testing.

Chapter Summary

- The major female reproductive structures include the uterus, ovaries, fallopian tubes, and vagina. During the menstrual cycle, the endometrium is prepared by the hormones estrogen and progesterone to receive a fertilized egg. If the egg is not fertilized, the lining is shed as menstruation.
- Assessment and management of the patient with a gynecologic emergency should include a history that focuses on the chief complaint and specifically addresses vaginal bleeding, abdominal pain, and the possibility of pregnancy. These may be sensitive issues for the patient and you should maintain a caring, professional attitude at all times.
- Most gynecologic problems are not life threatening; however, ectopic pregnancy can kill otherwise healthy women. Any woman with vaginal bleeding and abdominal pain who might be pregnant should be monitored for shock and transported for further evaluation.
- Domestic violence and sexual assault are terrifying for the patient. Your primary responsibility is to keep your patient and yourself safe from further violence. Try to cooperate with law enforcement authorities in collecting evidence whenever possible.
- Pregnancy is a normal event in the human life cycle. When an egg is fertilized, it travels down the fallopian tube and implants in the lining of the uterus. The egg develops into an embryo, which is attached by the umbilical cord to the placenta. The placenta is the organ that exchanges nutrition and toxins for the embryo. After 8 weeks the embryo is called a *fetus*. The normal duration of pregnancy is 38 to 40 weeks.
- The enlarging uterus causes physiologic changes unique to pregnancy. Heart rate and respiratory rate increase slightly, and blood pressure decreases slightly. Blood volume is significantly increased. The enlarging uterus can compress major blood vessels in the abdomen to cause supine hypotension syndrome. To avoid this, transport a woman on her left side during the second half of pregnancy.
- An obstetric history should start with the chief complaint and its relation, if any, to the pregnancy. Always ask about the presence of vaginal bleeding, contractions, or abdominal pain. Try to establish the EDC, gravidity, and parity of the patient. If the mother is at least 20 weeks pregnant, listen for fetal heart tones on physical examination of the abdomen.
- Vaginal bleeding and abdominal pain in the first trimester of pregnancy may be signs of a miscarriage or an ectopic pregnancy. Both conditions may cause life-threatening bleeding. Closely monitor these patients for shock and transport them as soon as possible.
- Placental abruption and placenta previa are complications of late pregnancy that may cause vaginal bleeding. Previa often is associated with painless, bright-red bleeding, whereas abruption may be associated with abdominal pain and a tender uterus. Significant vaginal bleeding is not normal before delivery and should prompt careful monitoring for shock and rapid transport.
- Preeclampsia is a disorder of the second half of pregnancy that may include signs such as hypertension, severe swelling of the extremities, and vomiting and symptoms such as abdominal pain and headaches. The most serious complication of preeclampsia is seizures. Assume that any seizure in pregnancy is caused by preeclampsia and treat with careful airway management, supplemental oxygen, IV access, and prompt transport. The drug of choice for eclamptic seizures is magnesium sulfate.
- Like pregnancy, childbirth is a normal event in the human life cycle and usually progresses without difficulty no matter where it happens. In this country most deliveries occur in hospitals or birthing centers with medical professionals in attendance. If you are called to help with a delivery, reassure the mother, prepare for delivery, assist with the birth, and then monitor the mother and baby closely after delivery. The ABCs apply here, as they do in any patient.
- Labor is divided into three stages. The first stage begins with the onset of contractions and ends when the cervix is fully dilated. The second stage is the time from complete dilation of the cervix until the delivery of the infant. The third stage begins after the infant is delivered and ends with delivery of the placenta.
- Some indicators that delivery may be imminent include the sensation of needing to push, rupture of membranes, and contractions longer than 1 minute and closer than 2 to 3 minutes apart. If you suspect that delivery is imminent, examine the mother for crowning or perineal bulging.
- If you must deliver the infant outside the hospital, try to find a private and protected place. Remember to use standard precautions, including wearing a gown, gloves, mask, and protective eyewear.
- Supplies for delivery include clean linens, a bulb syringe, umbilical cord clamps, gauze, sponges, scissors, and a container for the placenta.
- Allow the head to deliver in a gradual, controlled manner. Check for the umbilical cord wrapped around the baby's neck and, if present, pull the cord over the baby's head. Immediately suction the infant's nose and mouth before the body delivers. If meconium is present, suction the mouth and nose thoroughly, provide oxygen, and watch for breathing difficulties.
- After the body delivers, dry the baby and clamp and cut the umbilical cord. Assess the baby's ABCs. Stimu-

Chapter Summary—continued

late the infant to breathe if necessary and provide oxygen as needed.
- If the placenta delivers, place it in a clean container and transport it to the hospital with mother and infant.
- It is easy to focus on only one of your patients after delivery. Continue to reassess ABCs in both mother and baby and provide support as needed.
- Up to 500 mL of blood loss after delivery is normal and should be expected. If the mother continues to have brisk bleeding, massage the uterus through the abdominal wall and encourage her to breastfeed if possible to slow the bleeding.
- *Preterm delivery* is defined as delivery before the thirty-seventh week of pregnancy. Preterm infants may need more aggressive resuscitation than term infants and are more prone to hypoxia, respiratory distress, and hypothermia. Keep the infant warm and provide ventilatory assistance as needed.
- Abnormal presentations include breech presentation, shoulder dystocia, limb presentation, and cord prolapse. In all these situations placing the mother in a knee-chest position provides the widest possible diameter of the pelvis and may expedite delivery. In the case of cord prolapse, it will help reduce pressure on the cord.
- Fetal demise is a horrific event for the mother. A gentle, supportive demeanor should be maintained at all times. Err on the side of doing everything to aid in the infant's survival.
- Uterine complications of delivery can include inversion or rupture. Both are life-threatening events that require prompt recognition and treatment for shock.
- Pregnant women are at increased risk of pulmonary embolism. Suspect this diagnosis if a woman is short of breath, reports pleuritic chest pain, and coughs up blood.
- Trauma is the leading cause of death among pregnant women in the United States. The best care for the fetus is good care for the mother. Treat her aggressively, as you would any other trauma victim. Always position a pregnant woman in the left lateral recumbent position when possible. If she requires a backboard, it can be tilted to the left to reduce the risk of supine hypotensive syndrome.

REFERENCES

American College of Obstetricians and Gynecologists. (1991). Trauma during pregnancy. *ACOG Technical Bulletin*, 161.

American College of Obstetricians and Gynecologists. (2004). Placental abruption. *ACOG Technical Bulletin*, 58, 10.

Brunette, D. D., & Sterner, S. P. (1989). Prehospital and emergency department delivery: A review of eight years experience, *Annals of Emergency Medicine*, *18*(10), 1116-1118.

Cunningham, F. G. (2005). *Williams' obstetrics* (22nd ed.). New York: McGraw-Hill.

Duff, P. (2002). Maternal and perinatal infection. In S. G. Gabbe, J. R. Niebyl, & J. L. Simpson (Eds.), *Obstetrics: Normal and problem pregnancies* (4th ed.). New York: Churchill Livingstone.

Fildes, J., Reed, L., Jones, N., Martin, M., & Barrett, J. (1992). Trauma: The leading cause of maternal death. *Journal of Trauma*, *32*(5), 643-645.

Gianopoulos, J. G. (1994). Emergency complications of labor and delivery. *Emergency Medicine Clinics of North America*, *12*(1), 201-217.

Houry, D., & Abbott, J. T. (2002). Acute complications of pregnancy. In J. M. Marx (Ed.), *Rosen's emergency medicine: Concepts and clinical practice* (5th ed.). St. Louis: Mosby.

Johnson, T. R., & Niebyl, J. R. (2002). Preconception and prenatal care: Part of the continuum. In S. G. Gabbe, J. R. Niebyl, & J. L. Simpson (Eds.). *Obstetrics: Normal and problem pregnancies* (4th ed.). New York: Churchill Livingstone.

Landon, M. B., Catalano, P. M., & Gabbe, S. G. (2002). Diabetes mellitus. In S. G. Gabbe, J. R. Niebyl, & J. L. Simpson (Eds.), *Obstetrics: Normal and problem pregnancies* (4th ed.). New York: Churchill Livingstone.

Mallon, W. K., & Henderson, S. (2002). Labor and delivery. In J. M. Marx (Ed.), *Rosen's emergency medicine: Concepts and clinical practice* (5th ed.). St. Louis: Mosby.

Morrison, L. J. (2002). General approach to the pregnant patient. In J. M. Marx (Ed.), *Rosen's emergency medicine: Concepts and clinical practice* (5th ed.). St. Louis: Mosby.

Pearlman, M. D., & Phillips, M. E. (1996). Safety belt use during pregnancy. *Obstetrics and Gynecology*, *88*, 1026-1029.

Poole, G. V., Martin, J. N. Jr., Perry, K. G. Jr., Griswold, J. A., Lambert, C. J., & Rhodes, R. S. (1996). Trauma in pregnancy: The role of interpersonal violence. *American Journal of Obstetrics and Gynecology*, *174*(6), 1873-1877.

Ramouska, E., Sachetti, A. D., & Nepp, M. (1989). Reliability of patient history in determining the possibility of pregnancy. *Annals of Emergency Medicine*, *18*(10), 48.

Shah, K. H., Simons, R. K., Holbrook, T., Fortlage, D., Winchell, R. J., & Hoyt, D. B. (1998). Trauma in pregnancy: Maternal and fetal outcomes. *Journal of Trauma*, *45*(1), 83-86.

Simpson, J. L. (2002). Fetal wastage. In S. G. Gabbe, J. R. Niebyl, & J. L. Simpson (Eds.), *Obstetrics: Normal and problem pregnancies* (4th ed.). New York: Churchill Livingstone.

Stenchever, M. A., Droegemueller, W., Herbst, A. L., & Mishell, D. R. (2001). *Comprehensive gynecology* (4th ed.). St. Louis: Mosby.

Stewart, D. E., & Cecitto, A. (1993). Physical abuse in pregnancy. *Canadian Medical Association Journal*, *149*, 1257-1263.

Tintinalli, J. E., Kelen, G. D., & Stapczynski, J. S. (2004). *Emergency medicine: A comprehensive study guide* (6th ed.) (pp. 657, 670). New York: McGraw-Hill.

Tjaden, P., & Thoennes, N. (1998). *Prevalence, incidence, and consequences of violence against women: Findings from the national violence against women survey* (pp. 1-15). Washington, DC: U.S. Department of Justice.

Van Hook, J. W. (2002). Trauma in pregnancy. *Clinical Obstetrics and Gynecology*, *45*(2), 414-424.

Wagner, L. K. (2004). Diagnosis and management of preeclampsia. *American Family Physician*, *70*(12), 2317-2324.

Webster, J., Sweett, S., & Stolz, T. A. (1994). Domestic violence in pregnancy: A prevalence study. *Medical Journal of Australia*, *161*(8), 466-470.

Whitty, J. E., & Dombrowski, M. P. (2002). Respiratory diseases in pregnancy. In S. G. Gabbe, J. R. Niebyl, & J. L. Simpson (Eds.), *Obstetrics: Normal and problem pregnancies* (4th ed.). New York: Churchill Livingstone.

SUGGESTED RESOURCES

Abbott, J. (1998). Obstetric and gynecologic emergencies. In P. T. Pons & V. J. Markovchick (Eds.), *Prehospital emergency care secrets*. Philadelphia: Hanley and Belfus.

Abbott, J., & Gifford, M. J. (1996). *Prehospital emergency care: A guide for paramedics* (3rd ed.). New York: Parthenon Publishing Group.

American College of Obstetricians and Gynecologists. (2004). *2004 Compendium of selected publications from the American College of Obstetricians and Gynecologists*. Washington, DC: American College of Obstetricians and Gynecologists.

Doan-Wiggins, L. (2004). Emergency childbirth. In J. R. Roberts & J. R. Hedges (Eds.), *Clinical procedures in emergency medicine* (4th ed.). Philadelphia: Elsevier.

Gordon, J. D., Rydfors, J. T., Druzin, M. L., & Tadir, Y. (2001). *Obstetrics, gynecology and infertility*. Arlington, VA: Scrub Hill Press.

Pons, P. T. (1994). Prehospital considerations in the pregnant patient. *Emergency Medical Clinics of North America, 12*(1), 1-7.

Chapter Quiz

1. What is an ectopic pregnancy and why is it a life threat?

____

____

2. Describe the management of seizures in pregnancy.

____

____

3. What is the difference between placenta previa and abruption?

____

____

4. List three interventions in the face of excessive vaginal bleeding after delivery.

____

____

____

5. Define the three stages of labor.

____

____

____

6. Describe the contents of an obstetric kit.

____

____

7. What is the left lateral recumbent position and why is it important?

____

____

8. Describe the steps you would take while delivering a breech presentation.

____

____

9. Describe cervical spine precautions in the pregnant patient.

____

____

Terminology

Abortion The ending of a pregnancy for any reason before 20 weeks' gestation; the lay term *miscarriage* is referred to as *a spontaneous abortion*.

Acrocyanosis A condition in which the core of a newborn is pink and the extremities are cyanotic.

Amniotic sac (bag of waters) The fluid-filled protective sac that surrounds the fetus inside the uterus.

Antepartum The period before childbirth.

Anus The end of the anal canal.

Apgar score A scoring system applied to an infant after delivery; key components include appearance, pulse, grimace, activity, and respiration.

Birth canal Part of the female reproductive tract through which the fetus is delivered; includes the lower part of the uterus, the cervix, and the vagina.

Bloody show Passage of the protective blood and mucus plug from the cervix; often an early sign of labor.

Braxton-Hicks contractions (false labor) Benign and painless contractions that usually occur after the third month of pregnancy.

Breech presentation Presentation of the buttocks or feet of the fetus as the first part of the infant's body to enter the birth canal.

Cervix The inferior portion of the uterus; it connects to the vagina as part of the birth canal.

Chorioamnionitis Infection of the amniotic sac and its contents.

Clitoris Small, erectile structure superior to the entrance to the vagina.

Complete abortion Passage of all fetal tissue before 20 weeks of gestation.

Terminology—continued

Compound presentation Presentation of an extremity beside the major presenting fetal part.

Contraction Rhythmic tightening of the muscular uterine wall that occurs during normal labor and leads to expulsion of the fetus and placenta from the uterus.

Contraction interval The time from the beginning of one contraction to the beginning of the next contraction.

Contraction time The time from the beginning to the end of a single uterine contraction.

Crowning The appearance of the first part of the infant at the vaginal opening during delivery.

Cystitis Infection isolated in the bladder.

Dilation Spontaneous opening of the cervix that occurs as part of labor.

Dyspareunia Pain during sexual intercourse.

Eclampsia A life-threatening condition of pregnancy and the postpartum period characterized by hypertension, edema, and seizures.

Ectopic pregnancy A pregnancy that implants outside the uterus, usually in the fallopian tube.

Embryo The developing egg from fertilization until approximately 8 weeks of pregnancy.

Endometriosis Growth of endometrial tissue outside the uterus, often causing pain.

Endometritis Infection of the endometrium.

Endometrium Innermost tissue lining of the uterus that is shed during menstruation.

Estrogen A female hormone produced mainly by the ovaries from puberty to menopause that is responsible for the development of secondary sexual characteristics and cyclic changes in the thickness of the uterine lining during the first half of the menstrual cycle.

Estimated date of confinement (EDC) The due date of the fetus.

Fallopian tube Paired structures extending from each side of the uterus to each ovary; they provide a way for the egg to reach the uterus.

Fetus The term used for an infant from approximately 8 weeks of pregnancy until birth.

Fundus The superior aspect of the uterus.

Gestation or gestational age The number of completed weeks of pregnancy from the last menstrual period.

Gravida Number of pregnancies.

Gravidity The number of times a patient has been pregnant.

Hymen Thin layer of tissue that may cover the vaginal orifice in women who have not had sexual intercourse.

Incomplete abortion An abortion in which the uterus retains part of the products of the pregnancy.

Labia majora Rounded folds of external adipose tissue of the external female genitalia.

Labia minora Thinner, pinkish folds of skin that extend anteriorly to form the prepuce of the external female genitalia.

Labor The process by which the fetus and placenta are expelled from the uterus; usually divided into three stages, starting with the first contraction and ending with delivery of the placenta.

Meconium A dark-green substance that constitutes the infant's first bowel movement.

Menarche The onset of menstrual cycles.

Menopause Cessation of ovarian function and menstrual activity.

Menstruation Cyclical shedding of endometrial lining.

Miscarriage (spontaneous abortion) Loss of the products of conception before the fetus can survive on its own.

Mittelschmerz Pain occurring at time of ovulation.

Mons pubis A hair-covered fat pad overlying the symphysis pubis.

Multipara A woman who has given birth multiple times.

Myometrium Muscular region of the uterus.

Natal Connected with birth.

Nullipara A woman who has not borne a child.

Ovarian follicle The ovum and its surrounding cells.

Ovarian torsion Twisting of an ovary on its axis such that the venous flow to the ovary is interrupted.

Ovary A paired organ that releases eggs and hormones in a female.

Ovulation Mid-cycle release of an ovum during the menstrual cycle.

Ovum (oocyte) A human egg that, when fertilized, implants in the lining of the uterus and results in pregnancy.

Para The number of pregnancies carried to 20 weeks or more.

Parity The number of pregnancies that have resulted in birth.

Pelvic inflammatory disease (PID) An infection of a woman's reproductive organs, usually from a bacterial infection, that spreads from the vagina to the upper parts of the reproductive tract.

Perinatal From the twenty-eighth week of gestation through the first 7 days after delivery.

Perineal body See *Perineum*.

Perineum The tissue between the mother's vaginal and rectal openings; may be torn during delivery.

Placenta (afterbirth) The organ inside the uterus that exchanges nutrition and waste between mother and fetus.

Placental abruption (abruptio placenta) Separation of part of the placenta away from the wall of the uterus.

Placenta previa Placement of the placenta such that it partially or completely covers the cervix.

Postnatal The period immediately after the birth of a child and lasting for approximately 6 weeks.

Postpartum Pertaining to the mother after delivery.

Preeclampsia A complication of pregnancy that includes hypertension, swelling of the extremities, and, in its most severe form, seizures (see Eclampsia).

Premature birth Delivery between the twentieth and thirty-seventh weeks of pregnancy.

Prenatal Preceding birth.

Prepuce A fold formed by the union of the labia minora over the clitoris.

Presenting part The first part of the infant to appear at the vaginal opening, usually the head.

Preterm delivery Delivery between the twentieth and thirty-seventh week of pregnancy.

Primigravida A woman who is pregnant for the first time.

Primipara A woman who has given birth to her first child.

Progesterone A female hormone secreted after ovulation has occurred that causes changes in the lining of the uterus necessary for successful implantation of a fertilized egg.

Proliferative phase Portion of the menstrual cycle in which the endometrial lining grows under the influence of estrogen.

Pyelonephritis Infection of the kidney.

Secretory phase Portion of the menstrual cycle in which the corpus luteum secretes progesterone to maintain the endometrial lining in case of fertilization.

Septic abortion An abortion associated with intrauterine infection.

Shoulder dystocia Impaction of the baby's anterior shoulder underneath the mother's pubic bone, slowing or preventing delivery.

Spontaneous abortion See *Miscarriage*.

Supine hypotensive syndrome A physiologic phenomenon in which the enlarged uterus compresses the major blood vessels in the abdomen and impedes the return of blood to the heart when a pregnant woman lies in a supine position.

Term gestation A gestation equal to or longer than 37 weeks.

Therapeutic abortion Planned surgical or medical evacuation of the uterus.

Threatened abortion Vaginal bleeding or uterine cramping during the first half of pregnancy without cervical dilation.

Tocolytic A medication used to slow uterine contractions.

Umbilical cord The cord, containing two arteries and a vein, that connects the fetus to the placenta.

Umbilical cord prolapse Appearance of the umbilical cord in front of the presenting part, usually with compression of the cord and interruption of blood supply to the fetus.

Urethral meatus Opening of the urethra between the clitoris and vagina.

Uterine cavity Innermost region of the uterus.

Uterine prolapse Protrusion of part or all of the uterus out of the vagina.

Uterus (womb) The muscular organ where the fetus develops.

Vagina The lower part of the birth canal extending from the uterus to the outside of the body.

Vaginal orifice Opening of the vagina.

Vaginitis An inflammation of the vaginal tissues.

Vulva The region of the external genital organs of the female, including the labia majora, labia minora, mons pubis, clitoris, and vagina.

Vulvovaginitis Inflammation of the external female genitalia and vagina.

CHAPTER 36

Neonatology

Objectives

After completing this chapter, you will be able to:

1. Define the terms *newly born, neonate,* and *newborn.*
2. Discuss antepartum and intrapartum factors associated with an increased risk for neonatal resuscitation.
3. Identify the factors that lead to premature birth and low birth weight newborns.
4. Discuss the assessment findings associated with primary and secondary apnea in the neonate.
5. Discuss pulmonary perfusion and asphyxia.
6. Describe the etiology, epidemiology, history, and physical findings for the following congenital anomalies:
   - Tracheoesophageal fistula
   - Diaphragmatic hernia
   - Choanal atresia
   - Pierre Robin sequence
   - Meningomyelocele
   - Cleft lip and palate
   - Omphalocele
7. With the patient history and physical examination findings, develop a treatment plan for newborns with the following conditions:
   - Tracheoesophageal fistula
   - Diaphragmatic hernia
   - Choanal atresia
   - Pierre Robin sequence
   - Meningomyelocele
   - Cleft lip and palate
   - Omphalocele
8. Discuss the indications, necessary equipment, technique, and assessment of the newborn's response for the following interventions:
   - Blow-by oxygen delivery
   - Ventilatory assistance
   - Orogastric tube insertion
   - Chest compressions
   - Tracheal intubation
   - Vascular access
   - Needle chest decompression
9. Identify the primary signs used for evaluating a newborn during resuscitation.
10. Discuss the initial steps in and formulate a treatment plan for providing initial care to a newborn, including transport guidelines.
11. Identify the appropriate use of the Apgar score in caring for a newborn.
12. Calculate the Apgar score for various newborn situations.
13. Describe the etiology, epidemiology, history, and physical findings for newborn cardiac arrest.
14. Develop a treatment plan for a newborn in cardiac arrest.
15. Discuss the signs of hypovolemia in a newborn.
16. Discuss the treatment plan to stabilize the neonate after cardiac arrest.
17. Describe the etiology, epidemiology, history, and physical findings for the following conditions:
   - Meconium aspiration
   - Apnea
   - Bradycardia
   - Prematurity
   - Respiratory distress or cyanosis
   - Seizures
   - Fever
   - Hypothermia
   - Hypoglycemia
   - Vomiting
   - Diarrhea
   - Birth injury
18. With the patient history and physical examination findings, develop a treatment plan (including transport destination) for newborns with the following conditions:
   - Meconium aspiration
   - Apnea
   - Bradycardia
   - Prematurity
   - Respiratory distress or cyanosis
   - Seizures
   - Fever
   - Hypothermia
   - Hypoglycemia
   - Vomiting
   - Diarrhea
   - Birth injury
19. Discuss the effects of maternal narcotic use on the newborn and formulate a treatment plan for the newborn with narcotic depression.

CHAPTER OUTLINE

Case Scenario

You are called to the scene of a 32-year-old woman who is 38 weeks pregnant with her first child. She is experiencing cramping and thinks she is having the baby. She states that her prenatal visits have indicated that the baby is healthy, and she has no health problems of her own. You begin assessing the patient.

Questions

1. *What are the important questions to ask the patient?*
2. *What is important in preparation for delivery?*
3. *What are the signs of a problematic delivery?*

[OBJECTIVE 1]

Calls involving babies and children are among the most stressful for EMS professionals. A **newly born** refers to a baby in the first minutes to hours after birth. A **neonate** (also called a **newborn** infant) is a baby from the time of birth through the first 28 days of life. This chapter focuses on the assessment and emergency care of the newly born outside of the delivery room.

PRINCIPLES OF RESUSCITATION OF THE NEWLY BORN

Transitional Physiology (Adjustments to Extrauterine Life)

In utero, all the oxygen and nutrients used by the fetus, as well as waste products produced by the fetus, diffuse across the placenta from the mother's blood to the baby's blood (Figure 36-1). Because of this, fetal circulation has several intrauterine adaptations that must be adjusted to allow extrauterine life soon after delivery. In addition to physical differences in the cardiovascular system, the fetal blood has chemical alterations allowing intrauterine survival. The hemoglobin concentration is approximately 50% greater than maternal blood and has a greater affinity for oxygen than maternal blood. This allows it to carry 20% to 30% more oxygen than an equal amount of maternal blood. The fetal circulation interacts with the placenta via the umbilical cord. This structure contains two arteries that carry deoxygenated blood and one vein that carries oxygenated blood. Once entering the fetus, oxygenated blood is directed toward the liver. Because the normal functions of filtration are performed by maternal circulation, approximately one half of the blood entering the fetus enters portal circulation to go through the liver. The other half (40% to 60%) bypasses the liver through a vessel called the *ductus venosus* and enters the inferior vena cava.

Once entering the inferior vena cava, the blood from the ductus venosus is joined by the blood from portal circulation as well as deoxygenated blood returning from the lower extremities. As in extrauterine circulation, the inferior vena cava terminates at the right ventricle. Because fetal oxygenation is a function of maternal oxygenation, the fetal lungs are nonfunctional and blood flow to the lungs for purposes of oxygenation is not required. As a result only a minimal amount of blood follows the standard path of the right atrium to the right ventricle to the lungs. Blood that does follow this path still may not reach the lungs, as it is shunted from the pulmonary artery directly to the descending aortic arch through a vascular connection called the *ductus arteriosus*. The majority of the blood in the right atrium passes directly into the left atrium through an opening in the atrial septum called the foramen ovale. Blood flow from the left atrium to the right atrium through the foramen ovale is prevented because the pressures in the right atrium are higher than the left; in addition a valve called the *septum primum* in the left atrium prevents blood flow from left to right. Blood from the left atrium follows the standard path to the left ventricle and to the aorta, where it is distributed primarily to the heart, brain, and upper extremities. The blood that enters the descending aortic arch from the ductus arteriosus is distributed to the remainder of the body and to the umbilical arteries to be returned to the placenta (Figure 36-2).

The alveoli of the fetus are open and filled with fetal lung liquid instead of air, and the pulmonary blood vessels are constricted. Before labor, the production of fetal lung fluid decreases dramatically, decreasing the volume by approximately one third. During vaginal delivery, the newborn's chest is squeezed, further reducing the volume of fetal lung fluid by approximately one third.

At birth the newborn must adjust from intrauterine to extrauterine function. This includes the need to obtain nutrients, perform digestion, eliminate waste products, and regulate temperature, all independent of maternal circulation. The most important extrauterine activity is respiration so that hypoxia and hypercapnea are avoided. With the first breath, the newborn must pull air into his or her fluid-filled airways and alveoli. This requires sufficient negative pressure (approximately 22 to 30 mm Hg, or 30 to 40 cm H_2O) as the newborn's lungs

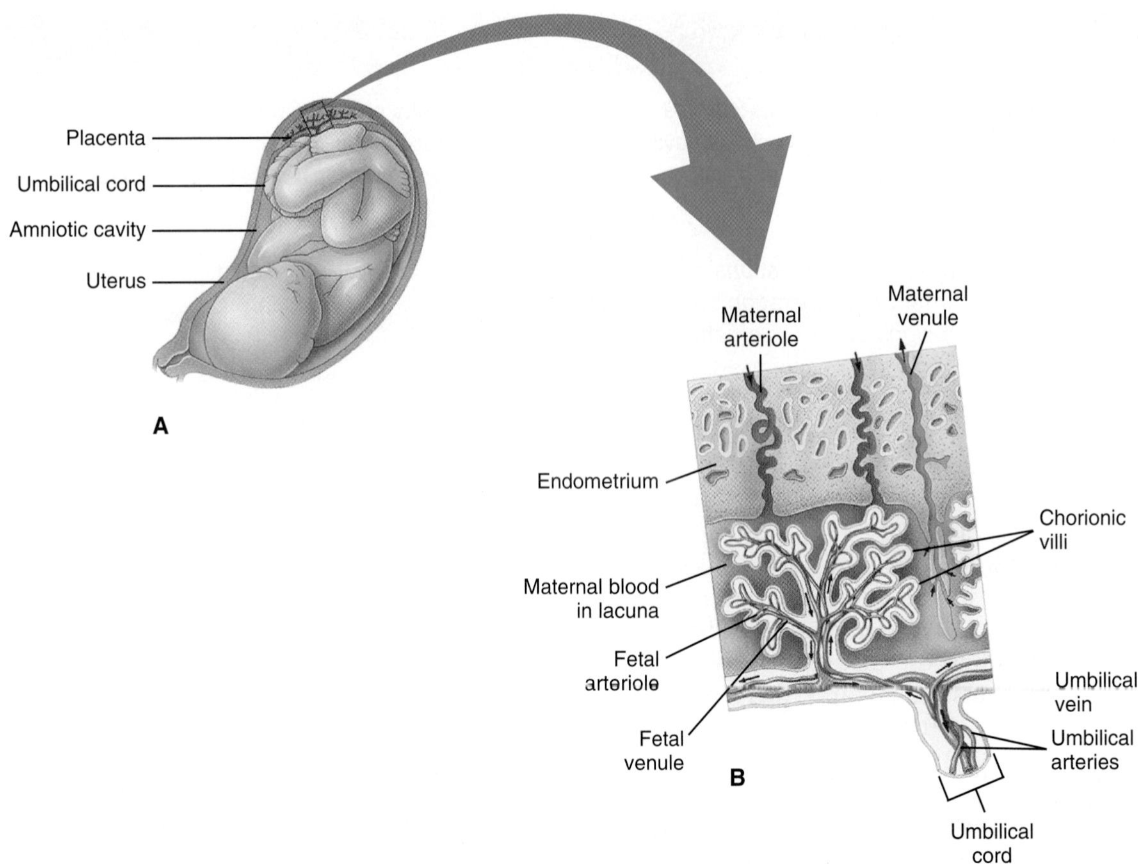

Figure 36-1 The placenta: interface between maternal and fetal circulation. **A,** Relation of uterus, developing infant, and placenta. **B,** The close placement of the fetal blood supply and the maternal blood in the placenta permits diffusion of nutrients and other substances.

are collapsed and the airways are small, all leading to significant resistance to airflow. When the alveoli begin to fill with air for the first time, surfactant helps them remain partially open and keeps the walls of the alveoli from sticking together when the newborn exhales. Surfactant production occurs at approximately 28 to 32 weeks of gestation. Recall from prior chapters that this fluid is a mixture of lipids and proteins that is produced by alveolar type II cells. The fluid creates a hydrophobic film on the insides of the alveoli at the alveolar–air interface. This prevents the moist alveoli from collapsing and sticking together secondary to their surface tension. Those born at less than 32 weeks' gestation are likely to be surfactant deficient and suffer from respiratory distress syndrome. These patients require the administration of synthetic surfactant at birth.

The newborn's initial cries and deep breaths help move the fetal lung fluid out of the airways. As air enters the lungs, pressure drives the remaining fetal lung fluid into the interstitium. In the interstitium, half of the fetal lung fluid is absorbed by pulmonary lymph vessels. The other half is absorbed by the interstitium and is then carried away by the pulmonary blood vessels. Breathing becomes easier and easier as the air sacs fill and then remain full of air. Unless the lungs are immature, absorption of fetal lung liquid is usually complete within 24 hours of birth.

As the lungs fill with air, the pulmonary blood vessels relax. This significantly increases blood flow to the lungs. As a result, pressures in the vena cava, pulmonary arteries, right atrium, and right ventricle are reduced. At approximately the same time, the umbilical arteries and vein constrict, increasing systemic blood pressure. Blood flow through the umbilical vein, ductus arteriosus, and ductus venosus decreases. The reduction in pressure in the right side of the heart and the increase in pressure in the left side of the heart result in closure of the foramen ovale and a transition to "normal" cardiac circulation. The newborn's skin turns from gray-blue to pink as oxygen-enriched blood enters the systemic circulation. Possible problems that may disrupt the newborn's transition to life outside the uterus are shown in Table 36-1.

The structures that are unique to fetal circulation eventually disappear, leaving only remnants after their closure. Blood in the umbilical vein begins to clot after birth, and the vein is completely occluded between the second and fifth day of life. Over a period of months the umbilical vein transitions into the ligamentum teres hepatis. This ligament can cause significant injury to the liver in

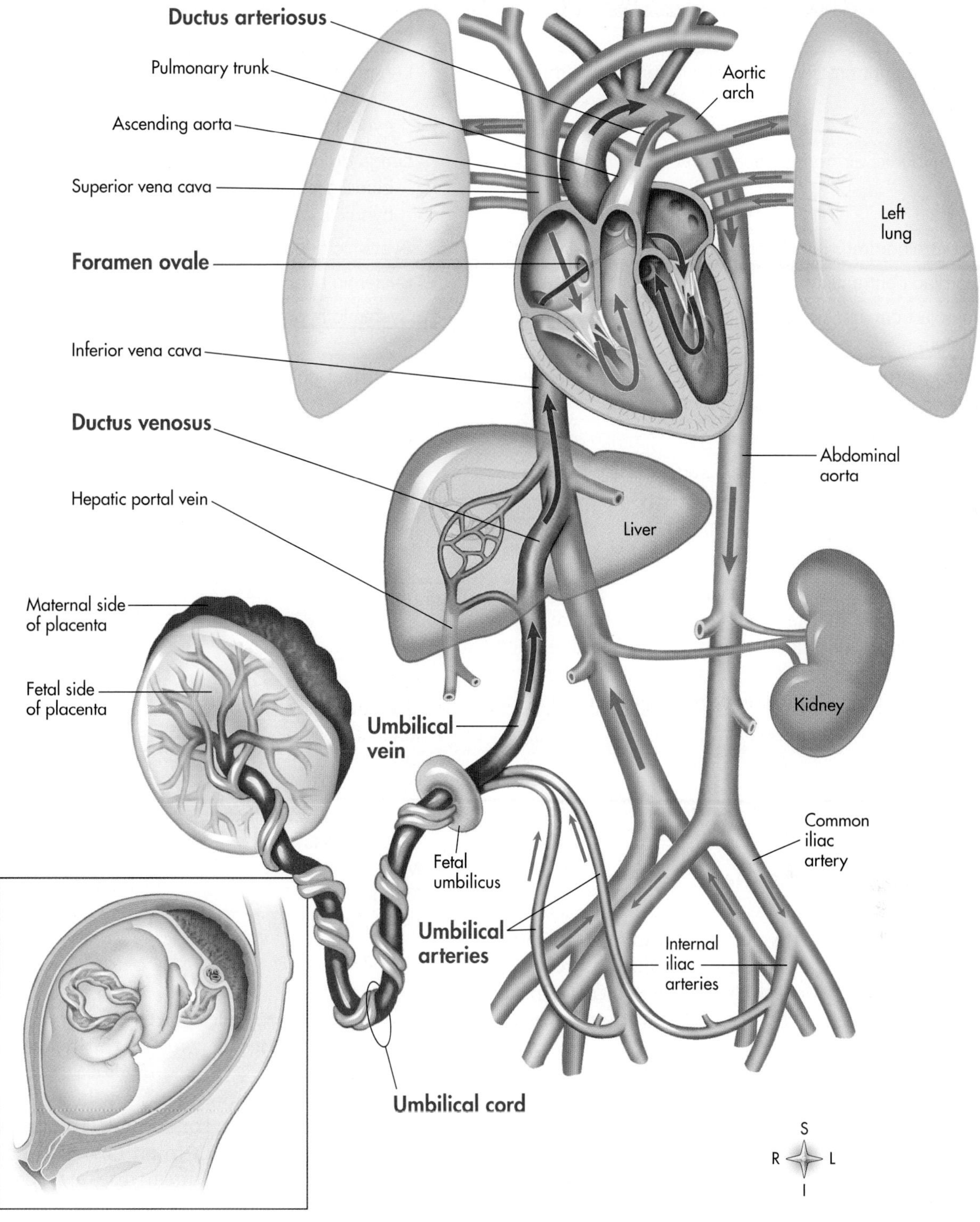

Figure 36-2 Fetal circulation.

the setting of trauma, as will be discussed in Chapter 50. The ligamentum arteriosum, which firmly attaches the descending aorta to the spine, develops from the closure of the ductus arteriosus. This structure plays a critical role in the development of traumatic aortic aneurysms and dissections, as will be described in Chapter 49. The cause of closure of the ductus venosus is not completely understood, but it may be related to the decrease in pressure within the hepatic portal system. Closure starts immediately after birth and is completed between the fifteenth and twentieth day of life. The resulting structure is the ligamentum venosum. The septum primum causes an almost immediate cessation of blood flow through the foramen ovale. However, anatomic closure is not com-

TABLE 36-1 Problems That May Disrupt Normal Transition to Extrauterine Life

Problem	Possible Result
Newborn does not breathe sufficiently to force fluid from alveoli	Lungs do not fill with air; oxygen is not available to blood circulating through the lungs, leading to hypoxia, cyanosis
Meconium blocks air from entering alveoli	Lungs do not fill with air; oxygen is not available to blood circulating through the lungs, leading to hypoxia, cyanosis
Insufficient blood return from placenta before or during birth	Systemic hypotension hypoxia
Poor cardiac contractility	Systemic hypotension hypoxia
Bradycardia from insufficient delivery of oxygen to heart or brainstem	Systemic hypotension
Lack of oxygen or failure to distend lungs with air may result in sustained constriction of pulmonary arterioles	Persistent pulmonary hypertension
Insufficient oxygen delivery to brain	Depressed respiratory drive
Insufficient oxygen delivery to brain and muscles	Poor muscle tone

plete until approximately 1 year of age. This leaves an oval depression in the atrial septum called the *fossa ovalis*. In some individuals the foramen ovale does not completely close, resulting in a condition called *patent foramen ovale*. This will be discussed in greater detail in Chapter 37.

Factors Associated with Increased Risk for Neonatal Resuscitation

Low Birth Weight and Preterm Birth

[OBJECTIVES 2, 3]

An estimated 99% of births occur in hospitals. It is estimated that about 5% to 10% of newborns require some form of active resuscitation at birth (Zideman & Hazinski, 2008). The rate of complications increases as birth weight decreases.

Neonatal deaths occur most often during the first 24 hours of life and overall account for 65% of all infant deaths (i.e., deaths before 1 year of age) (Stoll & Kliegman, 2004b). A preterm infant is a neonate who is delivered before 37 completed weeks of gestation. Preterm infants can be further classified according to their birth weight. A low birth weight (LBW) infant weighs less than 2500 g (5.5 lb) at birth. A very low birth weight (VLBW) rate infant weighs 1500 g (3.3 lb) or less at birth. An extremely low birth weight (ELBW) infant has a birth weight less than 1000 g.

LBW may be a result of an infant born early, restricted growth within the uterus, or both. The leading cause of LBW in the United States is **preterm birth.** The shorter the duration of the pregnancy, the smaller the infant and the higher the risk of death or disability. The causes of preterm birth are complex and not completely understood. Possible causes of preterm birth are shown in Box 36-1.

BOX 36-1 Possible Causes of Preterm Birth

- Severe preeclampsia
- Premature rupture of membranes
- Uterine abnormalities
- Placental bleeding (abruptio, previa)
- Multiple gestation
- Drug misuse
- Maternal chronic illnesses
- Fetal distress
- Maternal infection
- Trauma
- Unknown cause

The mother's nutrition, diet, and lifestyle affect fetal growth and development. For example, the use of alcohol, tobacco, or drugs can result in an LBW child. The duration of the pregnancy, exposure to diseases such as human immunodeficiency virus, or complications of conditions such as high blood pressure also can affect fetal growth and development.

PEDIATRIC*Pearl*

According to the World Health Organization, infants who weigh less than 2500 g are approximately 20 times more likely to die than heavier babies (United Nations Children's Fund and World Health Organization, 2004).

Depending on gestational age, a **premature** newborn may not have sufficient lung development for survival and is at higher risk of needing resuscitative efforts because of the following factors:

- The lungs may lack sufficient surfactant and be more difficult to ventilate.
- The brain substance is soft, gelatinous, and easily torn and has fragile capillaries that may bleed during stress.
- Premature newborns are more likely to be born with an infection.
- Premature newborns are predisposed to problems with temperature regulation because of their thin skin, large surface area/body mass ratio, and lack of subcutaneous fat.

Successful resuscitation of the newly born presents a challenge that requires the following:

- An understanding of the adjustments the newborn must make to life outside the uterus
- The ability to anticipate high-risk situations in which the newborn may require resuscitation
- Adequate training with appropriate equipment and medications for newborn resuscitation
- The ability to begin resuscitative efforts in a timely and effective manner

Although relatively few newborns require emergency care, *always* be prepared for newborn resuscitation when assisting with a delivery. Some conditions increase the likelihood that resuscitation will be necessary (Box 36-2). The presence of these conditions can result in a depressed newborn and the need for neonatal resuscitation. Because asking the mother-to-be too many questions is impractical when delivery is about to happen in the field, answers to the questions in Table 36-2 may be helpful in preparing for the birth. Use the information you find out to prepare appropriate equipment and transport the patient to the most appropriate facility.

PEDIATRIC*Pearl*

Less than 10% of newborns require emergency care to establish a vigorous cry or regular breathing, maintain a heart rate greater than 100 beats/min, and achieve good color and tone.

Newborn Asphyxia

[OBJECTIVES 4, 5]

Newborn asphyxia is the inability of a newborn to begin and continue breathing at birth. Cerebral palsy, mental retardation, and speaking, hearing, visual, and learning disabilities are examples of conditions that may occur in newborns who survive asphyxia at birth.

When deprived of oxygen, a newborn's responses follow a predictable pattern. The child initially responds by breathing faster. This is the newborn's attempt to maintain perfusion and oxygen delivery to vital organs. Because of hypoxia the heart rate drops abruptly. Skin color typically becomes progressively blue and then blotchy. These changes occur because of vasoconstriction in an effort to maintain systemic blood pressure (blood pressure increases slightly). If oxygen levels do not improve, breathing efforts slow and eventually stop. This is called **primary apnea.** In animal studies, this initial period of apnea typically lasts 30 to 60 seconds. If stimulated by drying or gently rubbing the back during this period, the newborn responds by resuming spontaneous breathing.

PEDIATRIC*Pearl*

Ventilations are the first vital sign to stop when a newborn is deprived of oxygen.

With ongoing asphyxia, the newborn takes several gasping ventilations. Oxygen saturation falls, the skin turns blue, heart rate slows further, and blood pressure falls. Gasping ventilations become weaker and slower and then stop. This is called **secondary apnea.** During secondary apnea, the newborn does not respond to stimulation. More vigorous and prolonged resuscitation is needed to restore adequate breathing and circulation. Death will follow unless resuscitation begins *immediately.* Emergency care includes bag-mask ventilation and chest compressions if necessary. The first sign of recovery after positive-pressure ventilation is an increase in heart rate. The blood pressure then rises and the skin becomes pink. Gasping occurs and is followed by rhythmic breathing. Because no definitive method differentiates primary apnea from secondary apnea, assume that any newborn who does not immediately respond to gentle stimulation and blow-by oxygen has secondary apnea. Immediately provide positive-pressure ventilation (Box 36-3). It is imperative the paramedic realize that newborns are extremely sensitive to hypoxia. Bradycardia is almost always secondary to hypoxia, as are changes in mental status. Additionally hypoxia can quickly lead to permanent brain damage.

PEDIATRIC*Pearl*

Unlike adults, who develop tachycardia in response to hypoxia, the newly born initially responds with a reflex bradycardia.

BOX 36-2 Factors Associated with Increased Risk for Neonatal Resuscitation

Antepartum Risk Factors

- Maternal age older than 35 y or younger than 16 y
- Maternal preeclampsia, diabetes
- Maternal bleeding in second or third trimester
- Maternal drug therapy (magnesium, adrenergic-blocking drugs, CNS depressants, alcohol, lithium carbonate)
- Maternal substance abuse (heroin, methadone)
- Chronic or pregnancy-induced hypertension
- Chronic maternal illness (cardiovascular, thyroid, neurologic, pulmonary, renal)
- Maternal anemia or infection
- Premature rupture of membranes
- Previous fetal or neonatal death
- Postterm gestation
- Multiple gestation
- Size/date discrepancy
- Inadequate or no prenatal care
- Diminished fetal activity
- Fetal malformation

Intrapartum Risk Factors

- Abruptio placentae
- Placenta previa
- Premature labor
- Precipitous labor
- Prolonged rupture of membranes (more than 18 hours before delivery)
- Prolonged labor (longer than 24 hours)
- Prolonged second stage of labor (longer than 2 hours)
- Uterine tetany
- Narcotics administered to mother within 4 hours of delivery
- Breech or other abnormal presentation
- Fetal bradycardia
- Prolapsed cord
- Meconium-stained amniotic fluid
- Bleeding

CNS, Central nervous system.

TABLE 36-2 Focused Maternal History

Risk Factor	Question	Possible Risk	Preparation or Action
Estimate gestational age	When is your baby due?	Prematurity	Assisted ventilation Ensure availability of size-appropriate equipment
Multiple gestation	How many babies are there?	If more than one, newborns at greater risk for prematurity	Additional personnel and equipment needed
Meconium in amniotic fluid	Did your bag of water rupture? What was the color of the water?	Respiratory distress Hypoxemia Aspiration pneumonia	Immediate suction Possible tracheal intubation
Maternal medications	Have you taken any medications or drugs?	Narcotic use within 4 hours of delivery may result in neonatal respiratory depression	Assisted ventilation
Maternal diabetes	Do you have high blood sugar or diabetes?	Neonatal hypoglycemia Congenital anomalies Large for gestational age	Assisted ventilation Vascular access
Breech position	Has your doctor told you if the baby is coming head first or feet first?	Birth trauma Prematurity Umbilical cord prolapse	Assisted ventilation Additional personnel and equipment needed
Vaginal bleeding	Have you experienced any vaginal bleeding? How long ago? Did you have any pain with the bleeding?	Maternal/placental hemorrhage Increased likelihood of hypovolemic shock and respiratory distress in neonate	Vascular access Fluid/blood administration
Fetal movement	When was the last time you felt the baby move?	Fetal distress	Assisted ventilation

Congenital Anomalies

[OBJECTIVES 6, 7]

Congenital anomalies (birth defects) are structural abnormalities present at or before birth. Anomalies occur in 3% to 4% of births and are a major cause of stillbirths and neonatal deaths. Some anomalies are obvious at birth. Others may not be recognized until later in childhood. Birth defects may affect one organ system or one local area, such as a congenital hip dislocation or cleft lip. In some cases a congenital anomaly may be part of a multiple malformation syndrome. The probability of an infant having a major anomaly increases with the number of minor anomalies found.

A minor anomaly poses no significant problems to the patient's health. Examples of minor birth defects include birthmarks, skin tags, and extra fingers or toes (Figure 36-3). A major anomaly has significant medical and social or cosmetic consequences for the patient (Figure 36-4). Examples of major birth defects include tracheoesophageal fistula, diaphragmatic hernia, and choanal atresia. These major birth defects require immediate medical and/or surgical care.

Congenital anomalies may be caused by genetic factors. Down syndrome is one of the most common birth defects caused by chromosomal abnormalities. Environmental toxins, radiation, diet, drugs, infection, and metabolic disorders also may cause anomalies. For example, birth defects may occur if the mother is exposed to rubella during the first trimester of pregnancy, which is a critical period of fetal development.

Most babies who need resuscitation at birth do not require deviations from recommended resuscitation guidelines. However, some babies who have congenital anomalies require special care because of their altered anatomy.

BOX 36-3 Oxygen in Neonatal Resuscitation

For more than 5 years, neonatologists and researchers have discussed and debated the use of room air or 100% oxygen during neonatal resuscitation. Most guidelines recommend the use of 100% oxygen, but some studies have shown that room air is adequate (Vento et al., 2003). At this time the optimal concentration of oxygen for newborn resuscitation is unknown. Be sure to check local protocols to find out about oxygen use in these situations.

Esophageal Atresia and Tracheoesophageal Fistula

Description and Definition. **Esophageal atresia** (EA) is failure of the esophagus to develop as a continuous passage. Instead the section of the esophagus from the mouth and the section of the esophagus from the stomach end as a blind pouch without connecting to each other. A **tracheoesophageal fistula** (TEF) is an abnormal opening between the trachea and esophagus.

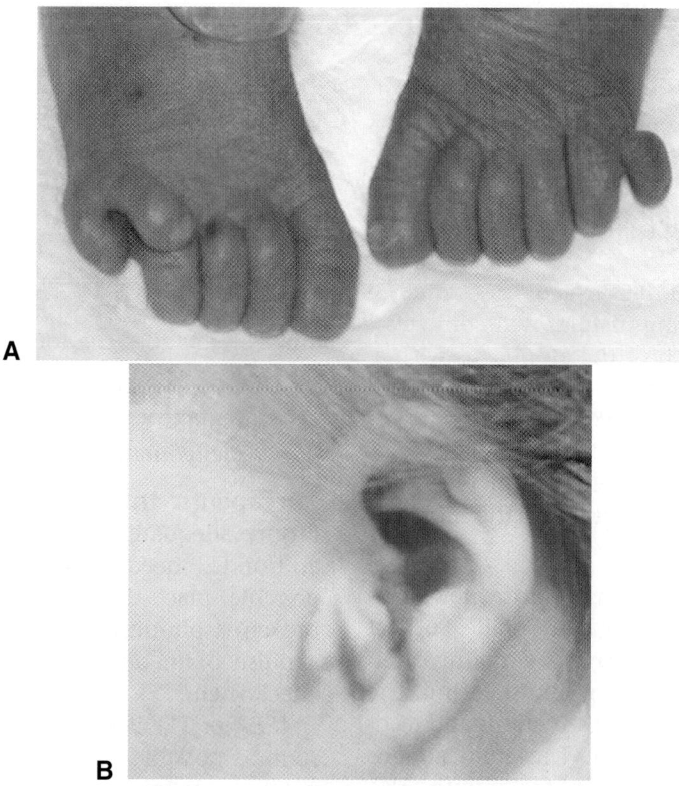

Figure 36-3 Examples of minor congenital anomalies. **A,** Polydactyly (duplication of digits) of the fifth toe. **B,** Skin tags of the ear.

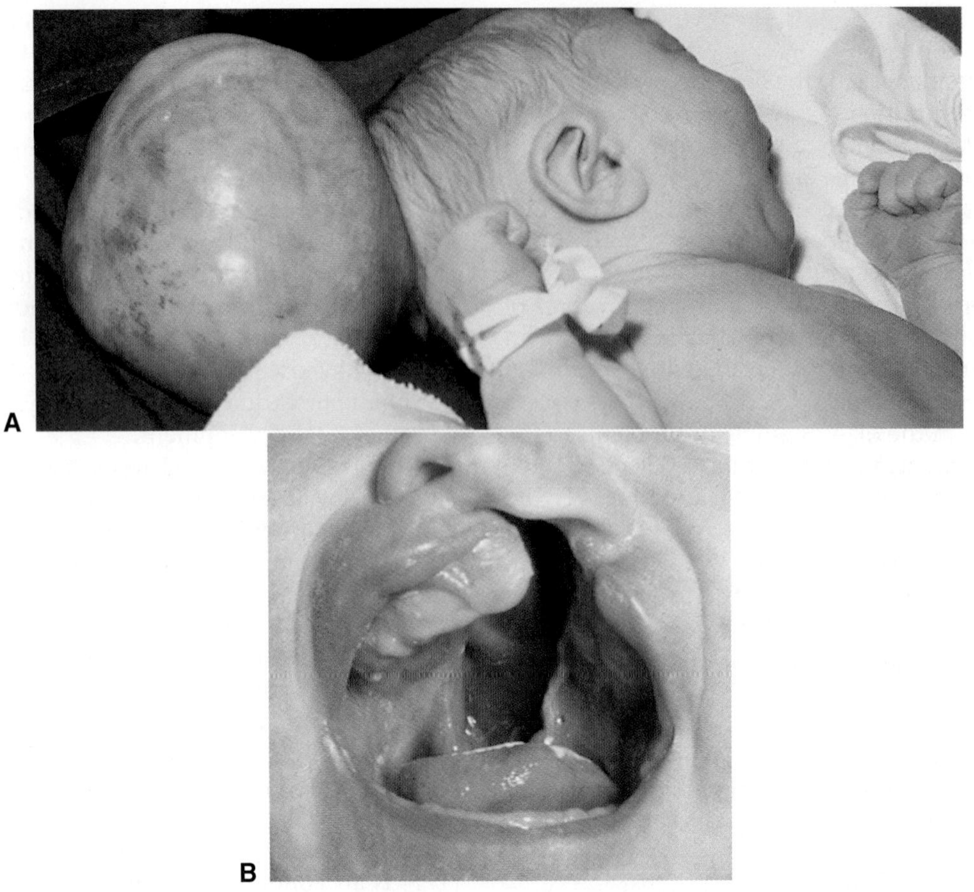

Figure 36-4 Examples of major congenital anomalies. **A,** Encephalocele. **B,** Cleft palate and lip.

Etiology. The etiologies of EA and TEF are not known.

Epidemiology and Demographics. Statistics regarding EA and TEF include the following:

- Approximately 1 in 4000 babies has one or both of these problems.
- EA rarely occurs by itself. It is usually associated with an abnormal opening (fistula) that connects the lower or upper pouch of the esophagus with a bronchus or the trachea (TEF). Sometimes an infant has EA with no TEF, but TEF without atresia is uncommon.
- Associated anomalies are present in 50% to 70% of patients. Cardiac abnormalities are the most common.

History and Physical Findings. Most newborns show symptoms of EA in the first few hours of life. Suspect EA in a newborn who drools excessively. Drooling often is accompanied by choking, coughing, and sneezing. The newborn swallows normally, but oral secretions and feedings pool in the esophageal pouch. The child coughs when the fluid returns through the nose and mouth. Also suspect EA if you are unable to advance an orogastric tube or nasogastric tube into the stomach.

If TEF exists, fluid from the esophageal pouch or gastrointestinal secretions spill over into the trachea. This results in cyanosis, wheezing, tachypnea, and chemical pneumonitis. Babies who have TEF without EA may not have obvious symptoms at birth. These babies may have chronic respiratory problems and/or repeated episodes of pneumonia associated with feeding.

Differential Diagnosis. Differential diagnosis of EA and TEF includes the following:

- Gastroesophageal reflux disease
- Premature lungs
- Tracheomalacia

Therapeutic Interventions

Ensure adequate oxygenation. A newborn who has EA and/or TEF needs constant monitoring of the airway. If possible, place the child in an upright position to help prevent aspiration of secretions. Suction as needed. Apply a pulse oximeter and cardiac monitor and constantly check them.

If EA or TEF is suspected, consult medical direction as soon as possible. Transport the child to the closest perinatal center for further care.

Patient and Family Education. Provide emotional support and reassurance to the parents. Explain what is being done for the newborn. A newborn who has EA needs surgery to connect the esophagus to the stomach. If TEF is present, the opening between the esophagus and trachea must be surgically closed. After surgery, many patients have long-term gastroesophageal reflux problems. All children with these conditions need regular follow-up after discharge from the hospital.

Diaphragmatic Hernia

Description and Definition. A **diaphragmatic hernia** is a protrusion of the abdominal contents into the chest cavity through an opening in the diaphragm.

Etiology. During early pregnancy a very small hole is normally present in the diaphragm of the fetus. The hole usually closes by the end of the first trimester. In cases of diaphragmatic hernia, the diaphragm has a defect, which can vary from a small slit to the complete absence of the diaphragm on the affected side. This defect allows some of the stomach, small intestine, or even the spleen to invade the chest cavity. The lungs of newborns with this condition are small because they had to share the space with abdominal contents in the chest cavity during fetal development.

The lung on the side of the defect is more severely affected. The number of alveoli and bronchial branches also is decreased. The presence of other anomalies is reported to be as high as 50%.

Epidemiology and Demographics. Statistics regarding diaphragmatic hernia include the following:

- Reports of the incidence of diaphragmatic hernia vary from 1 in 3000 live births to 1 in 5000 live births.
- Approximately 85% to 90% of hernias are left sided and 5% are bilateral.
- Survival for a newborn whose symptoms are noted within the first 8 hours of life is approximately 50%. If the newborn has no respiratory distress within the first 24 hours of life, survival approaches 100%.

History and Physical Findings. The newborn may present with little to severe respiratory distress. Breath sounds are decreased. Bowel sounds can be heard in the chest. Because most hernias occur on the left, heart sounds may be displaced to the right side of the chest. Cyanosis may be present that does not improve despite ventilation. The abdomen is usually scaphoid (flat).

Differential Diagnosis. The differential diagnosis for diaphragmatic hernia is pneumothorax.

Therapeutic Interventions. Ensure that the newborn is adequately oxygenated. A newborn with a diaphragmatic hernia is at high risk for developing a pneumothorax if positive-pressure ventilation is needed. To avoid this complication, perform tracheal intubation first if positive-pressure ventilation is required. Positive-pressure ventilation will distend the abdominal organs within the chest cavity and worsen respiratory distress. Place an orogastric tube to deflate the stomach and/or intestines and minimize distention. Apply a pulse oximeter and cardiac monitor and constantly check them.

If diaphragmatic hernia is suspected, consult medical direction as soon as possible. Transport the newborn to the closest perinatal center for further care.

Patient and Family Education. Provide emotional support and reassurance to the parents. Explain what is being done for the child. After the newborn is stabilized at the hospital, the hole in the diaphragm is surgically closed. After the operation, a significant number of infants have long-term gastroesophageal reflux and intestinal motility problems. Regular follow-up care is essential.

Choanal Atresia

Description and Definition. In **choanal atresia,** one or both nares is narrowed or blocked by membranous or bony tissue. If the obstruction is limited to one side, unilateral atresia is present (Figure 36-5). If the obstruction affects both sides, bilateral atresia is present.

Etiology. Although several theories exist, the etiology of choanal atresia is unknown.

Epidemiology and Demographics. Statistics regarding choanal atresia include the following:

- The incidence of choanal atresia is 1 in every 7000 to 8000 births.
- Unilateral atresia occurs twice as often as bilateral atresia, usually on the right side.
- Approximately 50% of babies with choanal atresia have associated anomalies.
- 90% of nasal obstructions involve bone; 10% are membranous.
- 47% of cases have other congenital defects.

History and Physical Findings. Bilateral choanal atresia is usually recognized at birth. Remember that

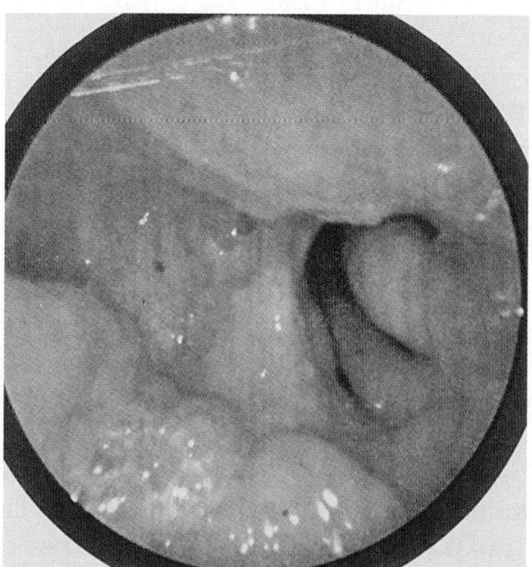

Figure 36-5 Unilateral choanal atresia. The left nasal passage *(right)* is open. The right nasal passage *(left)* is clearly blocked.

babies are obligatory nose breathers until approximately 6 months of age. Complete or partial obstruction of the nose often results in respiratory distress. In bilateral choanal atresia, both sides of the nose are blocked. When the child's mouth is closed, he or she has gasping ventilations and becomes cyanotic. Cyanosis disappears when the infant cries and returns with rest (paradoxic cyanosis). The infant is unable to feed and breathe at same time. Retractions may be seen unless the infant is breathing through the mouth or crying.

A few newborns who have unilateral choanal atresia may have signs of respiratory distress at birth. However, many patients do not have symptoms for months or years until the nasal obstruction is complicated by infection. The patient often has a foul-smelling discharge of mucus from the affected side of the nose. The patient's caregiver often reports that the infant or child is susceptible to upper respiratory infections.

Differential Diagnosis. Differential diagnosis of choanal atresia includes the following:

- Deformity of the nasal septum
- Nasal foreign body
- Nasal polyp

Therapeutic Interventions. An infant who has bilateral choanal atresia needs close airway monitoring. Open the newborn's airway and then size and insert an oral airway. This will help relieve respiratory distress and ensure adequate oxygenation. It also will help teach the newborn how to breathe through the mouth. The use of an oral airway is temporary because the newborn will not be able to feed through it. The oral airway is replaced at the hospital with a McGovern nipple, a large nipple with its end cut off. Ties are attached to secure it in place. The nipple allows the child to feed and acts as an oral airway until the defect is surgically corrected. Endotracheal (ET) intubation is usually unnecessary. Apply a pulse oximeter and cardiac monitor and continuously watch them.

If choanal atresia is suspected, consult medical direction as soon as possible. Transport the newborn to the closest perinatal center for further care.

Patient and Family Education. Provide emotional support and reassurance to the parents. Explain what is being done for the newborn.

Pierre Robin Sequence

Description and Definition. Pierre Robin sequence is a congenital anomaly characterized by three conditions: a small lower jaw (micrognathia), a tongue that tends to fall back and downward (glossoptosis), and cleft palate.

Etiology. During weeks 7 to 11 of fetal development, the mandible does not develop normally. The exact cause is unknown. One theory suggests that the head of the fetus is flexed with the chin resting on the chest in utero. This prevents appropriate growth of the mandible.

Epidemiology and Demographics. Statistics of Pierre Robin sequence include the following:

- Pierre Robin sequence occurs in 1 in 2000 live births.
- The mortality rate ranges from 19% to 65%. In most cases the cause of death is respiratory failure from airway obstruction.
- Pierre Robin sequence does not tend to run in families.

History and Physical Findings. A newborn with Pierre Robin sequence is prone to airway obstruction (Figure 36-6). The lower jaw is very small. Although the tongue is of normal size, it is large relative to the jaw. The tongue tends to ball up at the back of the mouth and fall back toward the throat, further decreasing airflow. These factors narrow the space in the nasopharynx and lead to an increase in airway resistance. To overcome the increase in airway resistance, the newborn uses accessory muscles to breathe. Retractions often are seen.

Therapeutic Interventions. A newborn with Pierre Robin sequence may have an airway obstruction. Verify that the newborn's airway is open. If it is not open, size and insert an oral airway. If you are able to insert the airway, continuously reassess the airway to make sure it remains open. If the airway is not open and you are unable to insert an oral airway, insert an orogastric tube. This will prevent the tongue from making a tight seal with the wall of the throat. It also will help prevent the newborn from developing large negative pressures in the pharynx and sucking the tongue into the pharynx (Gregory, 2005). Place the patient on a pulse oximeter and cardiac monitor. Intubating a patient with Pierre Robin sequence is very difficult. This procedure is best performed by an anesthesiologist.

If Pierre Robin sequence is suspected, consult medical direction as soon as possible. Transport the child to the closest perinatal center for further care.

Patient and Family Education. Provide emotional support and reassurance to the parents. Explain what

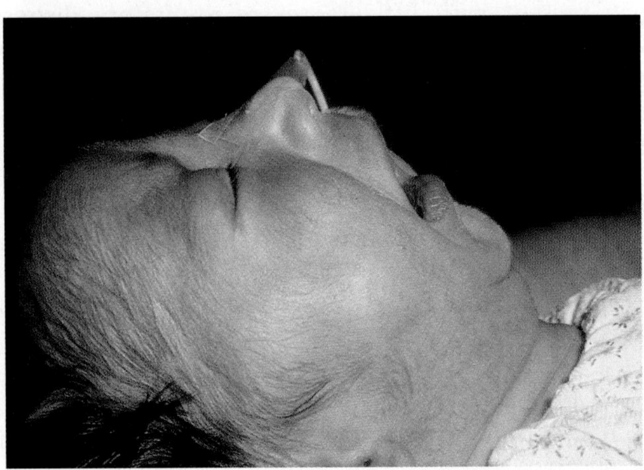

Figure 36-6 Pierre Robin sequence. Note the small lower jaw and recessed chin.

is being done for the child. Newborns with Pierre Robin sequence often have feeding problems and frequent ear infections. Because the infant expends so much energy to breathe, he or she often is too exhausted to eat. Caregivers may be instructed to nurse in a prone position. This allows the tongue to fall forward and keeps the airway open. As the infant's jaw grows (allowing more room for the tongue), breathing and feeding problems usually decrease. Surgery will be needed to correct the infant's cleft palate. Regular follow-up care is essential.

Meningomyelocele

Description and Definition. **Neural tube defects** are congenital anomalies that involve incomplete development of the brain, spinal cord, and/or their protective coverings. **Spina bifida (SB)** is a neural tube defect. The three most common types of SB are spina bifida occulta, meningocele, and meningomyelocele.

Spina bifida occulta is the mildest form of SB. In this type of SB, the spinal cord is intact but one or more vertebrae fail to close in the lumbosacral area. This type of SB is not usually visible and neurologic deficits are not typically present. External findings of this type of SB, if present, are limited to a small dimple in the lumbsacral area that is often associated with a tuft of hair.

Meningocele is a more severe form of SB. In this type of SB, the spinal cord develops normally but a saclike cyst that contains the meninges and cerebrospinal fluid (CSF) protrudes from an opening in the spine, usually in the lumbosacral area. The sac is usually covered by a thin layer of skin. The spinal cord is not involved and neurologic deficits are not usually present.

Meningomyelocele (also called *myelomeningocele*) is the severest form of SB. In this type of SB, the meninges, CSF, and a portion of the spinal cord protrude from an opening in the spine. They are encased in a sac that is covered by a thin membrane (Figure 36-7). The membrane is prone to leakage or rupture. Neurologic deficits are present. **Hydrocephalus,** an abnormal buildup of CSF in the brain, is common.

Etiology. SB results when the spine does not close properly during the first month of fetal development. The specific etiology of SB is unknown. Genetics, maternal hyperthermia, environmental factors, and maternal nutrition are factors in neural tube defects. Folic acid is an important vitamin in fetal development. A deficiency of folic acid, also called *folate,* is believed to play a significant role in neural tube defects. Certain medications such as the anticonvulsants carbamazepine (Tegretol), phenytoin (Dilantin), and phenobarbital antagonize folic acid, increasing the risk of meningomyelocele. Ingestion of the anticonvulsant valproic acid (Depakene) by the mother has been associated with an increased risk of neural tube defects.

Epidemiology and Demographics. Statistics regarding SB include the following:

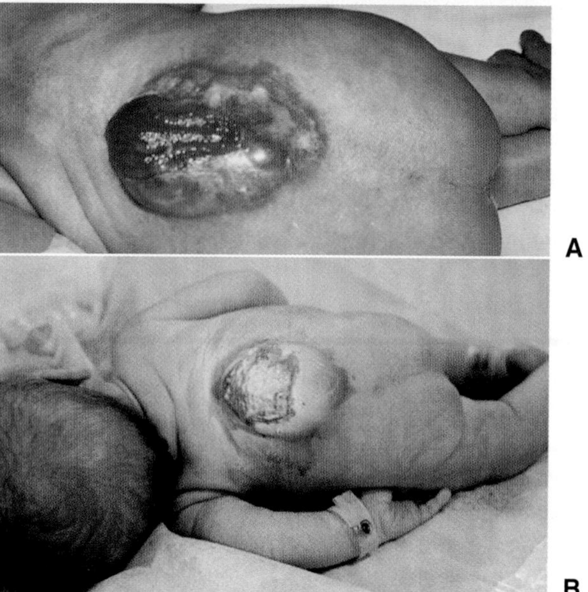

Figure 36-7 **A,** Meningomyelocele. **B,** Another example of a meningomyelocele.

- The incidence of meningomyelocele is approximately 1 in every 4000 live births.
- Females are more often affected than males.
- The areas most often affected are the lumbar and lumbosacral areas of the spine. The cervical and thoracic areas of the spine are the least commonly affected.
- A woman who has SB or already has a child with SB is at greater risk of having another child with SB or another neural tube defect.

History and Physical Findings. Meningomyelocele is associated with varying degrees of dysfunction depending on the part of the spinal cord involved. The higher the defect occurs on the back, the greater the amount of nerve damage and loss of muscle function and sensation (National Institute of Neurological Disorders and Stroke, 2005).

A newborn with a meningomyelocele has a visible spinal defect. Flaccid paralysis of the legs and altered bladder and bowel function may be obvious. The child may not respond to touch and pain in the areas below the defect. Clubfeet and hip dislocations may be present.

Differential Diagnosis. Differential diagnosis of SB meningomyelocele includes the following:

- SB meningocele
- SB occulta

Therapeutic Interventions. Priorities in the care for a newborn with meningomyelocele include preventing infection through the exposed spinal defect and protecting the exposed area from trauma. To reduce the risk of rupturing the thin membranous sac, an infant with a meningomyelocele should not be placed on his or her back. Position the infant on the side and handle gently. Apply a pulse oximeter and cardiac monitor and constantly check them. Watch for early signs of increased intracranial pressure, as hydrocephalus is commonly associated with this condition. Cover the spinal defect with sterile gauze pads soaked in warm sterile normal saline. Keep the gauze pads moist at all times and make sure that the child is kept warm. The area may also be covered with plastic to decrease the loss of water and heat.

If meningomyelocele is present, consult medical direction as soon as possible. Transport the child to the closest perinatal center for further care.

PARAMEDIC*Pearl*

Because up to 50% of patients with meningomyelocele may be latex sensitive, be sure to use latex precautions when caring for these patients.

Patient and Family Education. Explain the care you are providing for the patient. A visible anomaly such as a meningomyelocele often is traumatic for the family. Provide emotional support. The newborn will need surgery to correct the spinal defect. If the infant has hydrocephalus, a shunt may need to be inserted to drain the excess CSF. At the hospital, a pediatrician will coordinate the child's care with surgeons, physicians, nurses, and therapists. Hospital personnel will teach the parents about the infant's condition and discuss various procedures and treatment plans.

Cleft Lip and Cleft Palate

Description and Definition. Cleft lip and cleft palate are among the more common congenital anomalies. A **cleft lip** is incomplete closure of the upper lip. A **cleft palate** is incomplete closure of the hard and/or soft palate of the mouth. These anomalies may occur separately or together.

Etiology. In most cases, the etiology of cleft lip and cleft palate is unknown. Possible causes include maternal drug exposure, exposure to radiation, exposure to the rubella virus, or genetic factors. In Pierre Robin sequence, cleft palate occurs because the infant's tongue prevents the two sides of the palate from joining in the midline.

Epidemiology and Demographics. Cleft lip occurs in 1 in 1000 live births in the United States. Cleft palate occurs in approximately 1 in 2000 live births in the United States. Cleft lip occurs most often in Native Americans (3.6 of 1000 live births), Asians (2.1 of 1000), and whites (1 in 1000). It occurs with the lowest incidence among African Americans (0.41 in 1000) (Dyleski et al., 2001). Cleft lip is more common in males, and cleft palate is more common in females. Both conditions often occur with other congenital anomalies such as SB.

History and Physical Examination. Cleft lip and palate are usually recognized at birth. A cleft lip may occur on one or both sides. It may vary from a slight notch to complete separation from the floor of the nose. Cleft palate may occur in the midline and involve only the uvula, involve only one side, or extend into or through the soft and hard palates, exposing one or both of the nasal cavities (Figure 36-8).

Differential Diagnosis. Cleft lip or cleft palate must be differentiated from Pierre Robin sequence.

Therapeutic Interventions. When an infant is born with a cleft, you must be concerned about the possible risk of aspiration and airway obstruction. A risk of aspiration exists because of communication between the oral and nasal cavities. Airway obstruction may occur if a cleft exists as part of the Pierre Robin sequence. Positioning the newborn on his or her side can help alleviate this problem. If positive-pressure ventilation is required a good face-to-mask seal may be difficult if the child has a cleft lip. If suctioning is required, be careful when inserting the catheter into the mouth. Apply a pulse oximeter and cardiac monitor and frequently check them.

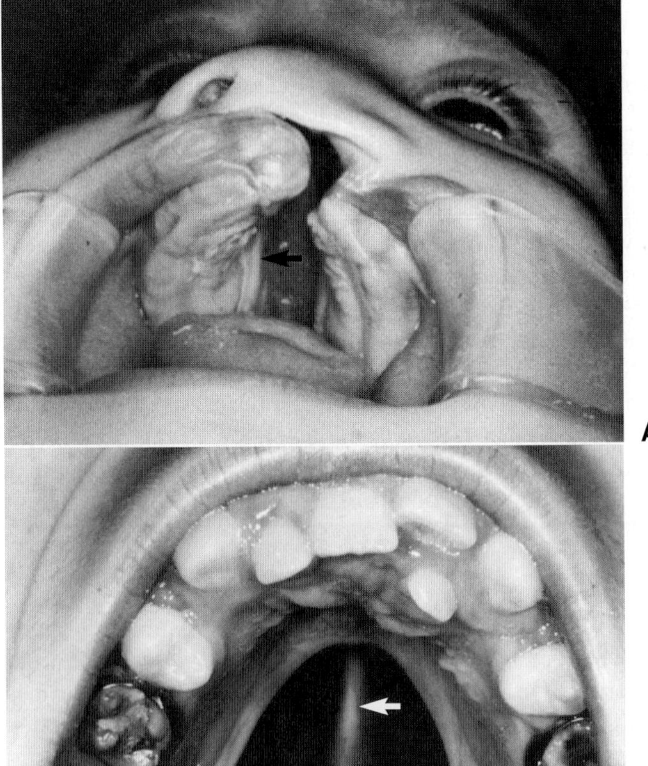

Figure 36-8 Cleft lip and palate. **A,** A patient with complete unilateral cleft of lip and palate. The *arrow* points to the junction of the nasal septum with the noncleft side of the palate. **B,** A patient with bilateral complete cleft palate. The *arrow* points to the nasal septum.

If a cleft lip and/or palate is present, consult medical direction as soon as possible. Transport the patient to the closest perinatal center for further care.

Patient and Family Education. The birth of an infant with cleft lip and/or palate often is traumatic to the family. Be prepared for their emotional reactions and provide emotional support. Explain all procedures you are performing as you provide care.

Cleft lip and cleft palate anomalies can cause feeding difficulties, problems with speech development, and ear infections. An infant with a cleft lip requires surgery to correct the anomaly. An infant with a cleft palate requires ongoing care from a team of specialists, including nurses; a cosmetic surgeon; an ear, nose, and throat surgeon; a speech language therapist; a dentist; and an orthodontist. Soft, elongated nipples and compressible bottles often are used for feeding. In some cases, an artificial device is fitted over the palate for feeding until surgery can be performed. Regular follow-up care is essential.

Omphalocele

Description and Definition. An **omphalocele** is protrusion of abdominal organs into the umbilicalcord. The defect is usually covered by a sac of peritoneum. The umbilical vessels are usually present within the sac.

Etiology. The origin of an omphalocele is not known. It may occur because the anterior wall of the abdomen does not completely close during fetal development.

Epidemiology and Demographics. Statistics regarding omphalocele include the following:

- The incidence of omphalocele varies between 1 in 5000 to 1 in 6000 live births.
- Approximately 15% to 25% of newborns with an omphalocele have cardiac defects. Neurologic, genitourinary, chromosomal, and skeletal anomalies also may be present.

History and Physical Examination. An omphalocele is visible at birth, and the size varies (Figure 36-9). An umbilical cord that looks unusually fat should be examined before clamping to make sure it is not a small omphalocele. Large omphaloceles may include the stomach, intestines, liver, and spleen. Rupture of an omphalocele may occur immediately before or during delivery. This exposes the abdominal organs to amniotic fluid. Exposure to amniotic fluid results in intense inflammation.

Differential Diagnosis. Omphalocele should be differentiated from gastroschisis (an abdominal wall defect through which the internal organs push outside of the infants body).

Therapeutic Interventions. Priorities in the care for a newborn with an omphalocele include preventing infection through the exposed bowel and protecting the exposed area from trauma. Position the newborn on his or her side and handle the newborn gently. Apply a pulse oximeter and cardiac monitor and constantly check them. Cover the exposed bowel with sterile gauze pads soaked in warm sterile normal saline. Keep the gauze pads moist at all times and make sure the patient is kept warm. The area may also be covered with plastic to decrease the loss of water and heat.

If an omphalocele is present, consult medical direction as soon as possible. Transport the patient to the closest perinatal center for further care.

Patient and Family Education. Explain the care you are providing for the child. A visible anomaly such as an omphalocele often is traumatic for the family. Provide emotional support. Surgery is needed to correct the defect. At the hospital, a pediatrician will coordinate care with surgeons, physicians, nurses, and therapists. Hospital personnel will teach the parents about the infant's condition and discuss various procedures and treatment plans.

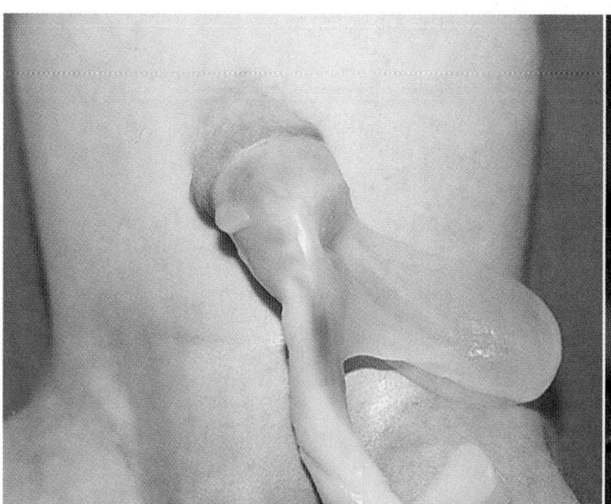

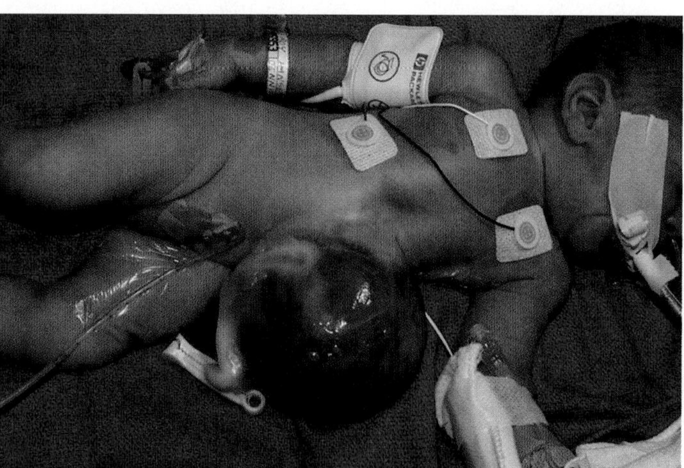

Figure 36-9 Omphalocele. **A,** A small omphalocele. **B,** A giant omphalocele that contains the intestines, stomach, and liver.

PARAMEDIC*Pearl*

In some areas specialized neonatal teams are available to transport high-risk newborns. Neonatal transport teams consist of skilled personnel and specialized equipment. Modes of transport include ground ambulance, helicopter, or fixed-wing aircraft. Neonatal team configurations vary but may include paramedics, nurses, respiratory therapists, nurse practitioners, and physicians. The most common configuration is a nurse and paramedic. Check with your instructor to find out about the availability and use of neonatal transport services in your area.

INITIAL STEPS OF RESUSCITATION OF THE NEWLY BORN

Before delivery, prepare the environment and equipment. If two paramedics are available, one paramedic should assume care of the mother by organizing the obstetric kit and creating a sterile field around the vaginal opening with sterile towels or sterile packaged paper drapes. The other paramedic should assume care of the newborn and prepare blankets, suctioning equipment, and other items. Box 36-4 lists suggested supplies, medications, and equipment that should be readily available during delivery of a newborn. The availability of properly sized equipment is

BOX 36-4 Prehospital Equipment List for Newborn Delivery

Obstetric Kit

- Sterile gloves
- Scalpel or surgical scissors
- 2 hemostats or cord clamps
- Bulb syringe
- 4 or more clean, dry towels
- Gauze sponges
- 2 or more baby blankets
- Sanitary napkins

Suction Equipment

- Bulb syringe
- Suction source and tubing
- 8F feeding tube and 20-mL syringe
- Suction catheters in sizes 5F or 6F, 8F, and 10F or 12F
- Meconium aspirator

Bag-Mask Equipment

- Oxygen source and tubing
- Bag-mask (200 to 750 mL) with pressure-release valve; must have oxygen reservoir
- Transparent face mask with soft, inflatable rim (sizes for preterm and term babies)

ET Intubation Equipment

- Pediatric laryngoscope handle with extra batteries
- Straight laryngoscope blades in sizes 0 (preterm) and 1 (term) with extra bulbs
- Uncuffed ET tubes in sizes 2.5, 3.0, 3.5, and 4.0 mm
- ET tube stylets (small)
- Tape or securing device for tracheal tube
- End-tidal CO_2 detector (optional)
- Laryngeal mask airway (optional)
- Stethoscope

Intraosseous Equipment

- 18-gauge intraosseous needle and syringe
- Normal saline

Umbilical Vessel Catheterization Equipment

- Povidone-iodine solution
- Scalpel with blade
- Sterile gauze sponges, 5 cm^2 or 10 cm^2
- Size 3.5F and 5F umbilical catheters
- Three-way stopcock
- Mosquito clamp
- Fine forceps without teeth
- Umbilical tape

Medications

- Epinephrine 1:10,000
- Sodium bicarbonate 4.2%
- Naloxone 0.4 mg/mL
- Dextrose 10%, 250 mL
- Normal saline for flushes and sterile water if dilution of bicarbonate or hypertonic glucose solutions is necessary
- Normal saline for volume expansion

Gastric Decompression Equipment

- 8F gastric or feeding catheter
- 20-mL syringe

Additional Supplies

- Personal protective equipment
- Oropharyngeal airways (0, 00, and 000 sizes)
- Cardiac monitor and electrodes (optional)
- Clock or watch
- Tape ($\frac{1}{2}$ or $\frac{3}{4}$ inch)
- 1-, 3-, 5-, 10-, 20-, and 50-mL syringes
- Pulse oximeter and probe (optional)
- 18,- 21-, and 25-gauge needles or puncture device for needleless systems

Modified from Aehlert, B. (2005). *Mosby's comprehensive pediatric emergency care.* St. Louis: Elsevier.
ET, Endotrachial.

essential, particularly equipment used for airway management and ventilation, which is most likely to be used.

During delivery, suction the mouth and nose as the head delivers. As the torso and full body are born, support the newborn with both hands. As the feet are born, grasp the feet. Wipe blood and mucus from the newborn's mouth and nose with sterile gauze. Suction the mouth and nose again with a bulb syringe as necessary. Note the time of delivery. When time permits, write the last name of the infant's mother on a gauze pad. Secure the gauze pad to one of the child's limbs with tape. Make sure the tape is not wrapped too tightly around the limb and that the adhesive of the tape is not in direct contact with the newborn's skin.

Be sure to position the newborn at the same level as the mother's vaginal opening until the cord has been clamped because blood can continue to flow between the newborn and the placenta.

General Impression

Ask yourself three questions at the time of birth:

- Is the infant full term?
- Is the newborn breathing or crying?
- Does the newborn have good muscle tone?

These questions can be answered by simply looking at the newborn. If the answer to all these questions is "yes," proceed with routine newborn care (provide warmth, clear the airway, dry). If the answer to any question is "no," continue to the initial steps of resuscitation (Figure 36-10).

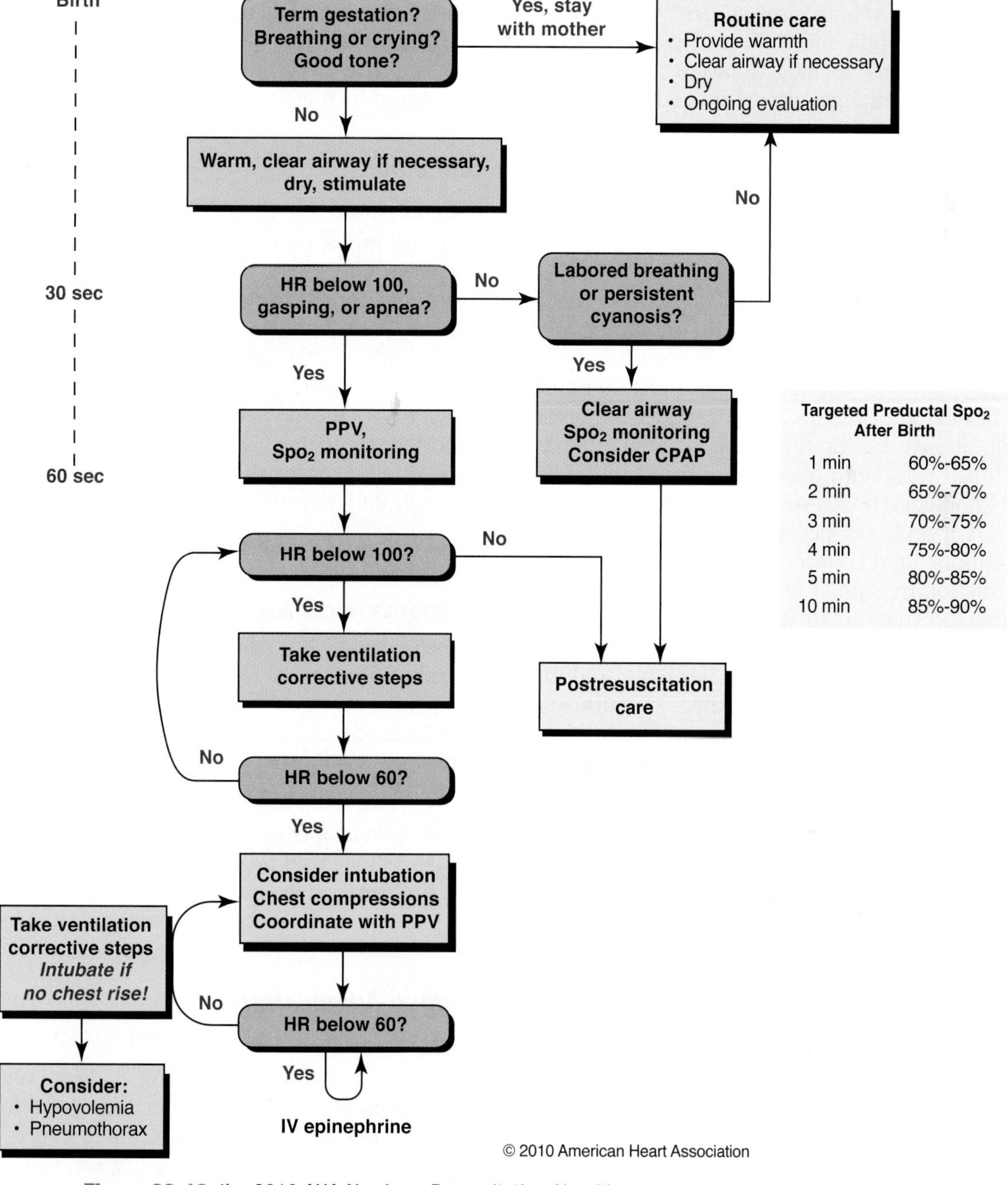

Figure 36-10 the 2010 AHA Newborn Resuscitation Algorithm.

Provide Warmth

Take care to maintain the newborn's body temperature. Preventing heat loss in the newborn is important because cold stress can lead to increased oxygen consumption, metabolic acidosis, hypoglycemia, and apnea. It is important to realize that newborns lack the ability to shiver to generate heat when cold. Therefore early signs of heat loss can be missed, allowing the development of the more serious conditions listed previously.

Increased oxygen consumption in a poorly oxygenated newborn can cause aerobic metabolism to cease, leaving only anaerobic metabolism for the production of energy. This change may lead to tissue hypoxia and acidosis because of the buildup of metabolic byproducts, such as lactate.

Hypoglycemia may develop in response to cold stress because the newborn rapidly uses glucose and glycogen reserves during anaerobic metabolism. Signs and symptoms of hypoglycemia include apnea, color changes, respiratory distress, lethargy, jitteriness, and seizures.

Whenever possible, deliver the newborn in a warm, draft-free area. Methods to minimize heat loss are shown in Box 36-5.

Position and Suction

Quickly dry the newborn. Place the infant supine with the head in a sniffing position. The newborn has a relatively large occiput and anterior airway; therefore hyperextension or flexion of the neck may produce an airway obstruction. Proper positioning may be facilitated by placing a rolled washcloth, blanket, or towel under the newborn's shoulders. If excessive secretions are present, place the infant on his or her side.

If the amniotic fluid is clear of meconium and signs of infection, suctioning should be reserved for babies who have obvious obstruction to spontaneous breathing or who require positive-pressure ventilation (Kattwinkel et al., 2010). If suctioning is necessary, keep in mind that newborns are primarily nose breathers. Suction the mouth first to ensure the newborn does not aspirate if he or she gasps when the nose is suctioned. When using a bulb syringe, squeeze the bulb of the syringe before inserting it into the newborn's mouth or nose. Gentle suctioning is usually adequate to remove secretions. Be careful not to insert the bulb syringe or suction catheter too far. Stimulation of the back of the throat can cause severe reflex bradycardia or apnea when performed within the first few minutes of delivery.

If meconium-stained fluid is present but the newborn is vigorous (strong ventilatory effort, good muscle tone, heart rate above 100 beats/min), proceed with routine newborn care (i.e., provide warmth, clear the airway, dry). If the newborn is depressed (poor ventilatory effort, decreased muscle tone, and/or a heart rate slower than 100 beats/min), insert a tracheal tube into the trachea and attach the tracheal tube to suction. Apply suction as the tube is slowly withdrawn. Repeat intubation and suctioning until little additional meconium is obtained or until the newborn's heart rate indicates that resuscitation must proceed immediately. If the newborn's heart rate or breathing is severely depressed, positive-pressure ventilation may be necessary despite the presence of some meconium in the airway.

BOX 36-5 Methods to Minimize Heat Loss

- Rapidly dry the infant's skin.
- Immediately remove wet linens from the newborn.
- Wrap the newborn in blankets, towels, or insulating film blankets.
- Cover the newborn's body and top of the head.
- Place the dried newborn against the mother's chest (skin-to-skin contact).
- Increase room temperature.

Stimulate

In most cases the stimulation received during drying, warming, and suctioning is enough to cause the newborn to breathe effectively. These may be the only resuscitative measures needed. However, if adequate breathing is not present, provide additional stimulation by rubbing the back, trunk, or extremities or tapping or flicking the soles of the feet (Figure 36-11). These methods may be tried for 5 to 10 seconds to stimulate breathing. If a brief period of stimulation is not effective in initiating ventilations, the newborn is in secondary apnea. Positive-pressure ventilation with a bag-mask device is required.

PEDIATRIC*Pearl*

When stimulating a newborn, avoid methods that are too vigorous because they will not help initiate respirations and may harm the newborn. Examples of methods that should *not* be used include the following:

- Slapping the back
- Forcing the thighs onto the abdomen
- Using hot or cold compresses
- Blowing cold oxygen onto the face or body
- Squeezing the rib cage

Oxygen Administration

[OBJECTIVE 8]

Studies have revealed conflicting evidence regarding the use of room air versus supplemental oxygen during resuscitation. Tissue damage may occur because of oxygen deprivation during and after asphyxia. Conversely, cell

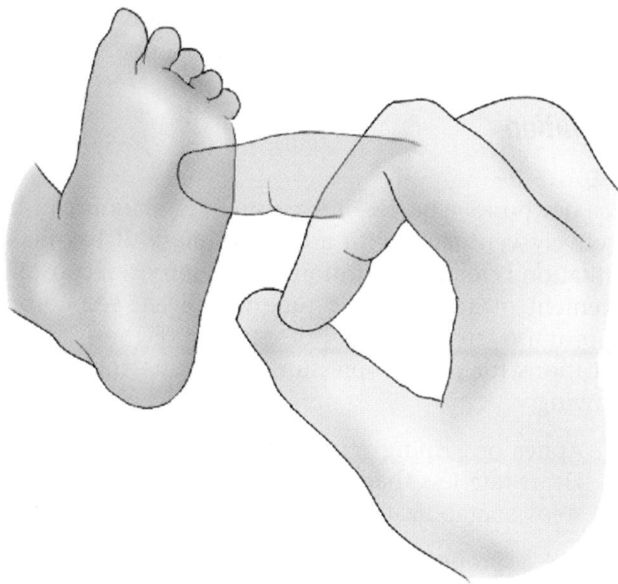

Figure 36-11 If adequate ventilations are not present, provide additional stimulation by rubbing the newborn's back, trunk, or extremities or tapping or flicking the soles of the feet.

and tissue injury may increase if hypoxic tissue is exposed to high concentrations of oxygen. Supplemental oxygen should be available for use if resuscitation is begun with room air and there no appreciable improvement within 90 seconds after birth. If the infant's heart rate is slower than 60 beats per minute after 90 seconds of resuscitation with a lower concentration of oxygen, increase the oxygen concentration to 100% until recovery of a normal heart rate (Kattwinkel et al., 2010).

Blow-by oxygen is the delivery of oxygen over the newborn's nose to improve breathing of oxygen-enriched air. Blow-by oxygen can be delivered by a simple face mask held firmly (but not too tightly) to the newborn's face or by a hand cupped around oxygen tubing. The oxygen source should be set to deliver at least 5 L/min and held close to the face to maximize oxygen flow to the newborn's nose and mouth. Do not administer oxygen at high flow rates (more than 10 L/min) if it is unheated and dehumidified, because convective heat loss can become a problem.

PARAMEDIC*Pearl*

Many bag-mask devices will not passively deliver sufficient oxygen flow (i.e., when not being squeezed) for effective use in blow-by oxygen administration.

Assess Ventilations and Heart Rate

[OBJECTIVES 9, 10]

Assessment of the newborn begins immediately after birth (Figure 36-12). Assessment of the newborn's ventilatory effort and heart rate is necessary to determine if resuscitative efforts beyond the initial steps of stabilization (providing warmth, clearing the airway, drying, and stimulating) are required.

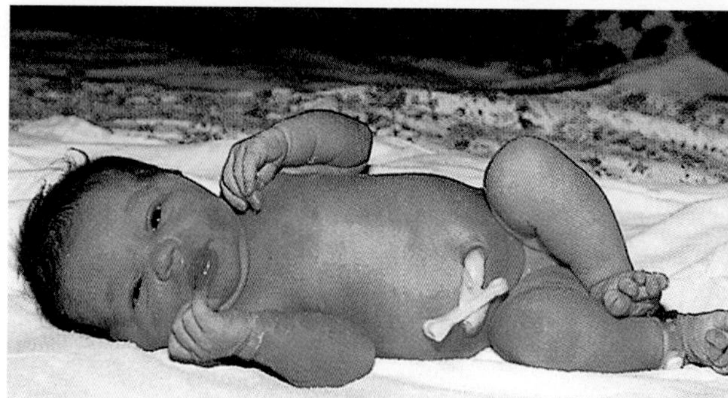

Figure 36-12 Assessment of the newborn begins immediately after birth.

Ventilations

Assess the newborn's ventilatory rate and effort (e.g., apnea, gasping, or labored or unlabored breathing). The term newborn's ventilatory rate is normally between 40 and 60 breaths/min in the first 12 hours of life. Apply a pulse oximeter to an upper extremity and continuously monitor oxygen saturation. Correct gasping ventilations or apnea with positive-pressure ventilation.

Heart Rate

The term newborn's heart rate normally is 100 to 180 beats/min during the first 12 hours of life. Heart rate may be evaluated by listening to the apical beat with a stethoscope or feeling the pulse by lightly grasping the base of the umbilical cord. Pulse oximetry and cardiac monitoring are other methods that may be used to monitor heart rate. However, if using pulse oximetry or the cardiac monitor, the paramedic should feel the pulse to make sure it correlates with these devices. Feeling the umbilical pulse allows assessment of the newborn's heart rate without affecting ventilation to listen to heart sounds. If pulsations cannot be felt at the base of the cord, auscultate the apical pulse. Because the rate is rapid, tapping out the heart rate as you count it may be helpful.

In general, a spontaneously breathing newborn with effective ventilations, pink color, and a heart rate greater than 100 beats/min will need no further emergency care. If the heart rate is less than 100 beats/min, begin positive-pressure ventilation. A heart rate less than 60 beats/min indicates that additional resuscitative measures are needed. Cardiac output in the newborn is almost exclusively dependent on heart rate. In fact, these patients have a cardiac output requirement of 500 mL per minute, yet only physically have 300 mL of blood. The only way to meet this requirement is to circulate it very fast. For this reason, newborns have minimal cardiac reserves. Essentially their normal heart rate is already so fast that they are unable to further increase it to compensate for decreases in cardiac output.

PEDIATRIC*Pearl*

In an uncompromised newborn, the heart rate should be consistently more than 100 beats/min. An increase or decrease in heart rate can provide clues about improvement or worsening of the infant's condition.

Studies have shown that clinical assessment of skin color is a very poor indicator of oxyhemoglobin saturation during the immediate neonatal period and that lack of cyanosis appears to be a very poor indicator of the state of oxygenation of an uncompromised newborn following birth. It is normal for the oxygen saturation level to remain in the 70% to 80% range for several minutes following birth with the appearance of cyanosis during this period (Kattwinkel et al., 2010). **Acrocyanosis** (cyanosis of the extremities) is a common finding immediately after delivery. It is not a reliable indicator of hypoxemia. Acrocyanosis may be an indicator of cold stress. Pallor may indicate decreased cardiac output, severe anemia, hypothermia, acidosis, or hypovolemia.

Apgar Scoring System

[OBJECTIVES 11, 12]

The Apgar scoring system is a numerical method of rating five specific signs pertaining to the newborn's condition after birth. Each sign is assigned a value of 0, 1, or 2 and added for a total Apgar score. Components of the Apgar scoring system are shown in Table 36-3. In general, the higher the score, the better the condition of the newborn.

Do not delay resuscitative efforts to obtain an Apgar score. Although the Apgar score is an important tool used in the assessment of a newborn, it is not recorded until 1 and 5 minutes after birth. If resuscitation of the newborn is needed, waiting until the first Apgar score is obtained could be disastrous. The decision to begin resuscitative efforts and the newborn's response to resuscitation can be more accurately determined by assessing the newborn's ventilatory effort and heart rate.

Ventilation

[OBJECTIVE 10]

Most newborns who require assisted ventilation can be effectively ventilated with a bag and mask. If bag-mask ventilation is required for more than 2 minutes, consider placement of an orogastric tube to prevent respiratory compromise from gastric distention (Figure 36-13). Indications for positive-pressure ventilation include the following:

- Apnea or gasping ventilations
- Heart rate less than 100 beats/min despite initial steps of stabilization

Select a properly sized face mask. Face masks are available in a variety of sizes and shapes. Use a mask equipped with a cushioned rim that is anatomically shaped. A mask of the proper size avoids the eyes and covers the nose, mouth, and tip of the chin. Masks fitting preterm, term, and large newborns should be available. A mask that is too large will not seal well and may damage the newborn's eyes. Ocular pressure also induces bradycardia. A mask that is too small will not cover the mouth and nose and may block the nose.

For a term newborn, select a resuscitation bag with a minimum volume of 450 to 500 mL and a maximum volume of 750 mL. A term newborn requires approximately 15 to 25 mL with each ventilation (5 to 8 mL/kg). A preterm newborn requires even less volume; some require as little as 5 to 10 mL per ventilation. Using a 750-mL (or larger) bag makes providing such small tidal volumes difficult and increases the risk of complications (e.g., hyperinflation). If the bag-mask has a pop-off valve, it should release at approximately 30 to 35 cm H_2O pressure. It should also have an override feature to permit delivery of higher pressures if necessary to achieve good chest expansion. To open the alveoli in a newborn, pressures of 30 to 40 cm H_2O may be needed during the first few breaths. This may necessitate temporary disabling of the pop-off valve.

TABLE 36-3 Apgar Scoring System

	0	1	2
Appearance	Blue, pale	Body pink Extremities blue	Completely pink
Pulse	Absent	Slower than 100 beats/min	100 beats/min or faster
Grimace/reflex irritability	No response	Grimaces, cries	Cough, sneeze, vigorous cry
Activity/muscle tone	Limp, flaccid	Some flexion of extremities	Active motion
Respiratory effort	Absent	Slow, irregular	Good, crying

Reprinted from Aehlert, B. (2005). *Mosby's comprehensive pediatric emergency care.* St. Louis: Elsevier.

PARAMEDIC*Pearl*

Two methods are used to express pressure. Pressures expressed in mm Hg represent the pressure needed to elevate a column of mercury the stated number of millimeters, whereas pressures expressed in cm H_2O represent the pressure needed to elevate a column of water the stated number of centimeters. Because both methods are commonly used in medicine, the paramedic may need to convert pressures between these two measurements. Conversion from cm H_2O to mm Hg is done with the formula cm $H_2O \div 1.36 =$ mm Hg. Conversion from mm Hg to cm H_2O is done with the formula mm Hg $\times$ 1.36 = cm H_2O.

Ventilate the newborn's lungs at a rate of 40 to 60 breaths/min to achieve or maintain a heart rate of at least 100 beats/min. Signs of adequate assisted ventilation are shown in Box 36-6.

A poor response to ventilation efforts may be the result of the following:

- *A poor seal between the newborn's face and the mask.* Corrective action: Reapply the mask to the face. Check the seal when you reapply the mask, particularly between the cheek and the bridge of the nose.
- *Poor alignment of the head and neck.* Corrective action: Reposition the head.
- *Insufficient ventilation pressure.* Corrective action: Increased inflation pressure may be required. If adequate chest rise is still not achieved, tracheal intubation may be required.
- *Improper tracheal tube position (if intubated).* Corrective action: Reassess tube placement; remove if the tube is improperly positioned or position is uncertain.
- *Blocked airway.* Corrective action: Reposition the head, suction as needed, and ventilate with the mouth slightly open.
- *Gastric distention.* Corrective action: Insert an orogastric tube and leave the end open to air. Periodically aspirate the tube with a syringe.

Once adequate ventilation with oxygen has been established for 30 seconds, recheck the heart rate and

BOX 36-6 Signs of Adequate Positive-Pressure Ventilation

- Gentle chest rise
- Presence of bilateral breath sounds
- Improvement in color and heart rate

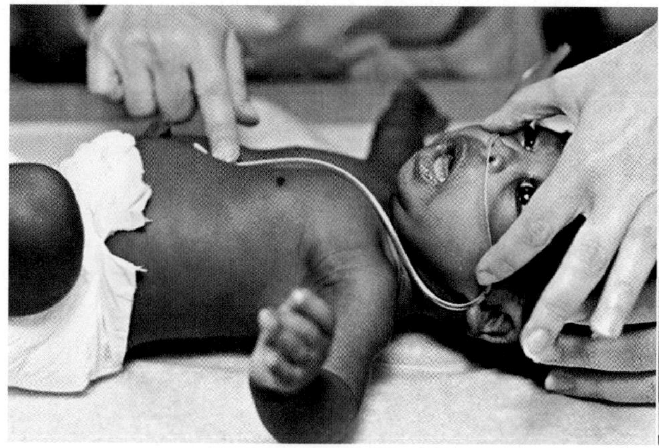

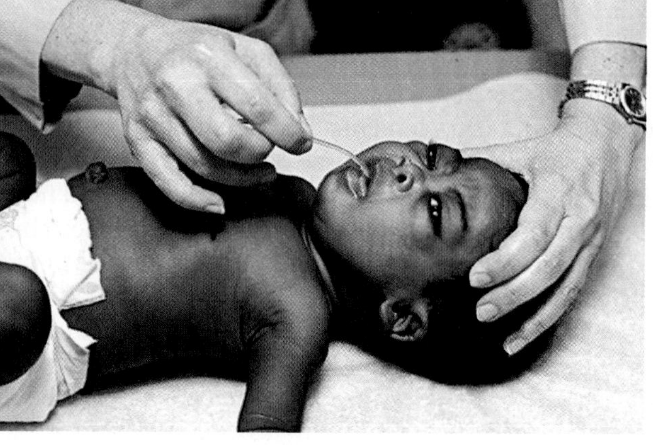

Figure 36-13 Placement of an orogastric tube. **A,** Take appropriate standard precautions. Assemble the necessary equipment. Select an orogastric tube of proper size as indicated on a length-based resuscitation tape. To determine the correct insertion depth, use the tube to measure the distance from the lips to the earlobe. Add the distance from the earlobe to the xiphoid process. Lubricate the end of the tube with a water-soluble lubricant. **B,** Grasp the tube and gently insert it into the patient's mouth over the tongue. Use a tongue blade if necessary. Gently advance the tube to the premeasured length. *Do not force the tube.* If the infant begins coughing as the tube is advanced, it may have entered the trachea. Remove the tube. Ventilate the patient for 30 seconds and then try to reinsert the tube. Once the tube is in position, attach an air-filled syringe to the end of the tube near the patient's mouth. Auscultate over the patient's stomach as you push the plunger on the syringe. Gurgling or the sound of rushing air suggests that the tube is in proper position. After air has been aspirated from the stomach, remove the syringe from the catheter. Reapply the face mask to the patient and continue positive-pressure ventilation. Additional air will be vented through the open catheter as assisted ventilation continues. Secure the tube in place.

ventilatory effort. If the newborn is spontaneously breathing and the heart rate is greater than 100 beats/min, positive-pressure ventilation may be gradually discontinued. Closely watch for signs of adequate spontaneous breathing before stopping ventilation. Gently stimulating the infant may help maintain spontaneous breathing. If spontaneous breathing is adequate, administer blow-by oxygen.

If spontaneous breathing is inadequate, continue assisted ventilation. If the newborn is unresponsive to positive-pressure ventilation and the heart rate is less than 60 beats/min, continue positive-pressure ventilation and begin chest compressions. Consider tracheal intubation.

Chest Compressions

[OBJECTIVES 13, 14]

Cardiac arrest in newborns is primarily related to hypoxia. The outcome is poor if care is not begun quickly. The longer the delay in beginning care, the greater the likelihood of brain and organ damage. Risk factors for cardiac arrest in the newborn are shown in Box 36-7. Causes of newborn cardiac arrest include the following:

- Primary apnea
- Secondary apnea
- Bradycardia
- Persistent fetal circulation
- Pulmonary hypertension

Chest compressions are indicated if the newborn's heart rate is less than 60 beats/min despite adequate ventilation with supplemental oxygen for 30 seconds (Kattwinkel et al., 2010). Because chest compressions may diminish the effectiveness of ventilation, they should not be initiated until adequate ventilation has been established. Two compression techniques can be used, both of which should be delivered on the lower third of the sternum to a depth of approximately one third of the anteriorposterior diameter of the chest.

Thumb Technique

To use the thumb technique, place your thumbs side by side on the lower third of the sternum unless the infant is small (or the rescuer's hands are extremely large), in which case the thumbs may be placed one over the other (Figure 36-14). The fingers encircle the chest and support the back. This technique may be used in newly born infants and older infants whose size permits its use. The two thumb-encircling hands technique is preferred for performing chest compressions in the newly born because studies suggest that this technique may generate higher peak systolic and coronary perfusion pressure than the two-finger method.

Two-Finger Method

Two fingers of one hand are placed on the lower third of the sternum (Figure 36-15). The other hand should support the newborn or infant's back.

Compression-to-Ventilation Ratio

Compressions and ventilations must be coordinated to avoid simultaneous delivery. Deliver compressions smoothly. Compress approximately one third of the anteriorposterior diameter of the chest. The compression to ventilation ratio is 3:1. Three chest compressions should be followed by a brief pause to deliver one ventilation. Allow the newborn's chest to fully recoil during relaxation while keeping your fingers or thumbs (depending on the technique used) in contact with the chest.

Unlike adults, newborns have no or minimally established functional residual capacity. Resuscitation efforts attempt to replenish oxygen with effective ventilation and deliver proportionally more ventilations over a specific period in relation to chest compressions. The 3 to 1

BOX 36-7 Risk Factors for Cardiac Arrest in the Newborn

- Intrauterine asphyxia
- Prematurity
- Drugs administered to or taken by the mother
- Congenital neuromuscular diseases
- Congenital malformations
- Intrapartum hypoxemia

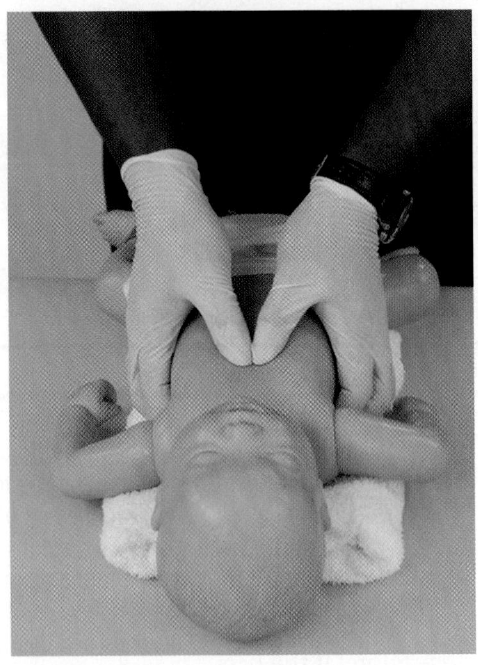

Figure 36-14 Newborn chest compressions with the two thumb-encircling hands technique. The thumbs are placed side by side on the lower third of the sternum unless the infant is small (or the rescuer's hands are extremely large), in which case the thumbs may be placed one over the other. The fingers encircle the chest and support the back.

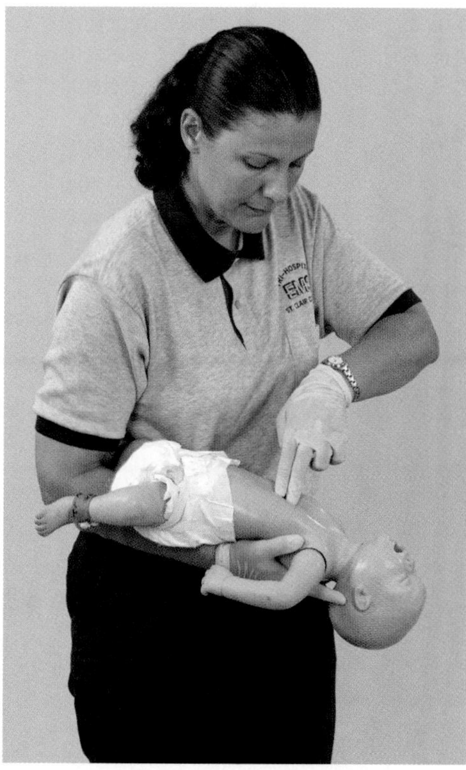

Figure 36-15 Two-finger method of chest compressions. Two fingers of one hand are placed on the lower third of the sternum. The other hand should support the infant's back.

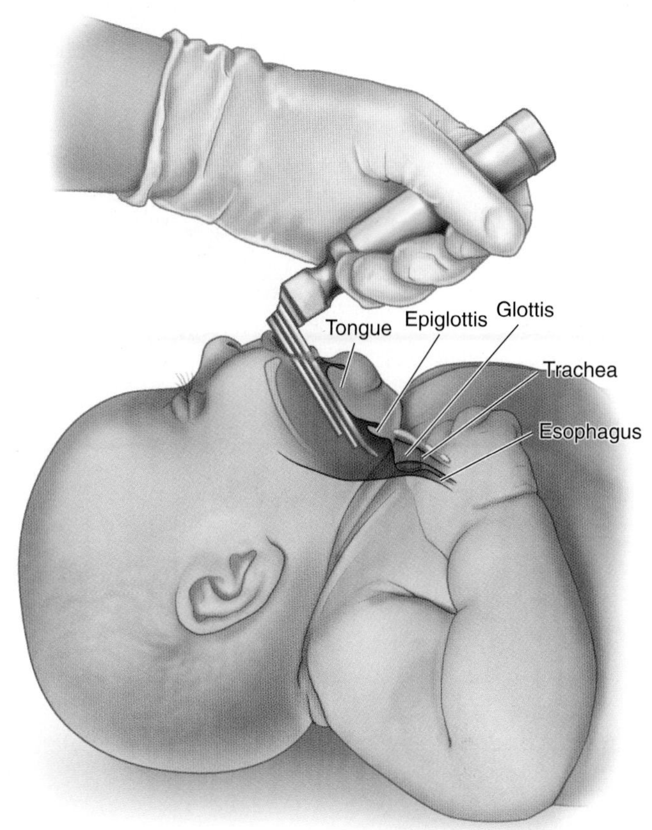

Figure 36-16 Using a straight blade for tracheal intubation of a newborn.

ratio is a consensus opinion of experts that is based on the likelihood that newborns who require cardiac compressions are asphyxiated and that newborns have higher ventilatory rates than adults and older children even when not asphyxiated. Consider using a compression to ventilation ratio of 15:2 if the arrest is believed to be of cardiac origin (Kattwinkel et al., 2010).

Periodically reassess oxygenation, ventilation, and heart rate. Myocardial blood flow is dependent on coronary perfusion pressure, which is generated when performing external chest compressions. Because it takes time to build up cerebral and coronary perfusion pressures, interrupting chest compressions causes cerebral and coronary perfusion pressures to fall quickly and dramatically, reducing blood flow to the brain and heart. Even after compressions are resumed, several chest compressions are needed to restore coronary perfusion pressure. Therefore, it is important to minimize interruptions in chest compressions during resuscitation. Discontinue chest compressions when the heart rate reaches 60 beats per minute or more. If the heart rate remains slower than 60 beats per minute, continue compressions.

Tracheal Intubation

Tracheal intubation may be indicated at the following points during neonatal resuscitation:

- When tracheal suctioning for meconium is required
- If bag-mask ventilation is ineffective (inadequate chest expansion, persistent low heart rate) or prolonged
- When chest compressions are performed
- Special resuscitation circumstances, such as diaphragmatic hernia or extremely LBW

If tracheal intubation is required, use a size 0 blade for a preterm and size 1 for a term newborn for intubation (Figure 36-16). Tracheal tube sizes are generally 2.5 for preterm and 3.0 to 3.5 for term newborns. Most tracheal tubes intended for newborn use have a vocal cord guide (a black line) near the distal tip of the tube (Figure 36-17). Insert the tip of the tracheal tube until the vocal cord guide is at the level of the cords. In this position, the tip of the tube should be between the vocal cords and carina. Intubation attempts should be limited to 20 seconds to minimize the risk of hypoxia.

After placement of the tube, check the centimeter marking on the tube at the newborn's upper lip (Table 36-4). The tube should be located 7 cm at the lip for a 1000-g infant, 8 cm for a 2000-g infant, and 9 cm for a 3000-g infant. Keep in mind that changes in head position will change the depth of insertion. This can result

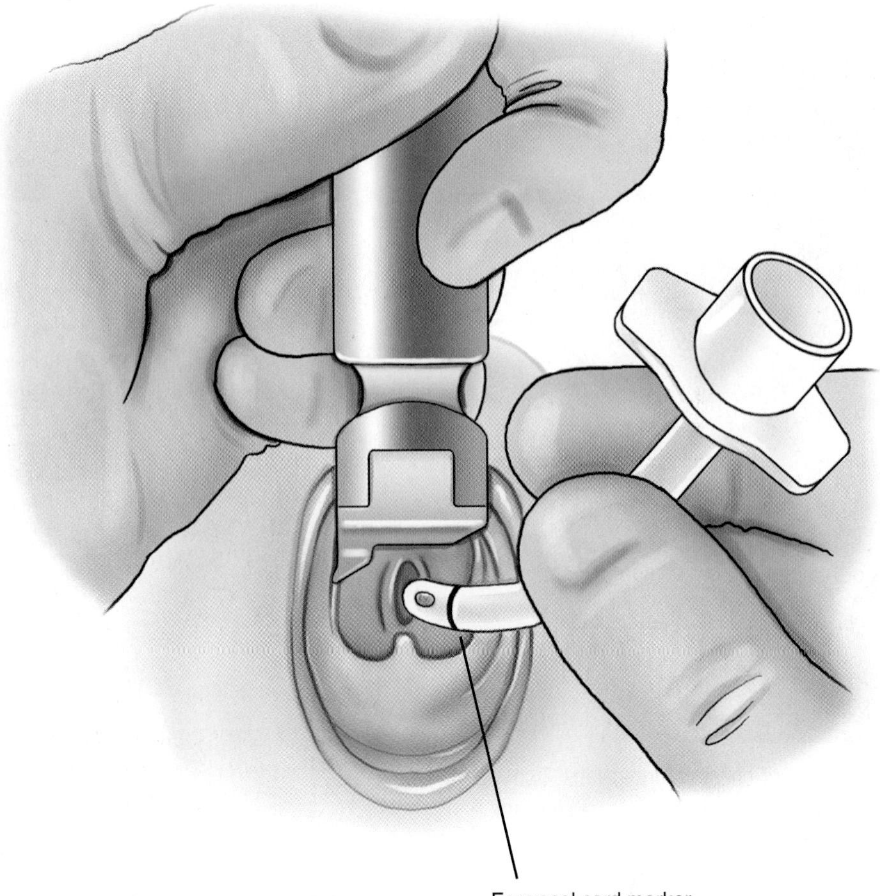

Figure 36-17 Most tracheal tubes intended for newborn use have a vocal cord guide near the distal tip. The tip of the tracheal tube should be inserted until the vocal cord guide is at the level of the cords.

TABLE 36-4 Estimation of Laryngoscope Blade and ET Tube Size Based on Infant Gestational Age and Weight

Weight (g)	Gestational Age (weeks)	Laryngoscope Blade Size	Laryngoscope Blade Type	Et Tube Size (mm)	Depth of ET Tube Insertion from Upper Lip (cm)
<1000	<28	0	Straight	2.5	6.5 to 7.0
1000-2000	28-34	0	Straight	2.5 to 3.0	7.0 to 8.0
2000-3000	34-38	0 to 1	Straight	3.0 to 3.5	8.0 to 9.0
>3000	>38	1	Straight	3.5 to 4.0	>9.0

Modified from Aehlert, B. (2005). *Mosby's comprehensive pediatric emergency care*. St. Louis: Elsevier.
ET, Endotracheal.

in unintentional extubation or right primary bronchus intubation. After proper tube position is confirmed, document and maintain this depth of insertion.

PEDIATRIC*Pearl*

A guide to determining proper distance for insertion of the tracheal tube is the "tip to lip" measurement: 6 cm + weight in kg = distance (in cm) from the tracheal tube tip to the infant's lips.

Exhaled carbon dioxide monitoring is the preferred method for confirming tracheal tube position. These devices are most useful if a perfusing rhythm is present and the newborn weighs more than 2 kg. False-negative results (i.e., no carbon dioxide detected despite tube placement in the trachea) may occur in newborns with poor or absent pulmonary blood flow (Kattwinkel et al., 2010).

In addition to exhaled carbon dioxide detection, the following actions can confirm the position of the tube:

- Watch for symmetric rise and fall of the chest
- Listen high in the axillae for equal breath sounds and for an absence of sounds over the stomach
- Confirm absence of gastric distention with ventilation
- Watch for improvement in the infant's color, heart rate, and activity

Sudden worsening of the patient's condition (bradycardia, decreased oxygen saturation) after intubation suggests one of the following problems (the mnemonic *DOPE*):

- ***D***islodgement: the tube is no longer in the trachea (right primary bronchus or esophagus).
- ***O***bstruction: secretions are obstructing airflow through the tube; suspect obstruction of the tube when there is resistance to bagging and no chest wall movement.
- ***P***neumothorax: decreased or absent breath sounds on the side of the affected lung.
- ***E***quipment: oxygen is not being delivered to the patient (check equipment).

PEDIATRIC*Pearl*

Possible causes for a newborn's failure to respond to intubation and ventilation include mechanical difficulties, profound asphyxia with myocardial depression, or an inadequate circulating blood volume. If the patient's condition suddenly worsens after intubation, quickly check your equipment. If no explanation is obvious, remove the tracheal tube and ventilate the patient with a bag-mask device. If the patient is bradycardic, do not waste time adjusting or suctioning the tracheal tube.

Medications and Fluids

Medications are rarely needed for resuscitation of a newborn. Bradycardia in the newborn is usually secondary to inadequate lung inflation and hypoxia, so ensuring adequate ventilation is an essential step in correcting a low heart rate. However, epinephrine administration or volume expansion, or both, may be necessary if the heart rate remains slower than 60 beats per minute despite adequate ventilation with 100% oxygen and chest compressions.

PEDIATRIC*Pearl*

The Broselow-Luten tape is a length-based resuscitation tape. The tape may be used to determine appropriate medication dosages and equipment on any child younger than 12 years. If a child is longer than the tape, use adult doses and equipment.

Routes of Medication Administration

The IV route is the preferred method for medication administration during newborn resuscitation. In the past, it was recommended that the tracheal route be used for epinephrine administration because this route was often the most rapidly accessible route for during newborn resuscitation. Studies have shown that epinephrine has no effect when it is administered tracheally using the currently recommended IV dose (0.01 to 0.03 mg/kg of 1:10,000 solution) (Kattwinkel et al., 2010). Current resuscitation guidelines recommend that epinephrine be administered IV as soon as venous access is available. Administration of tracheal epinephrine can be considered while attempting to obtain venous access but the safety and efficacy of this practice have not been evaluated (Kattwinkel et al., 2010).

Although rarely used as a means of vascular access outside the delivery room, the umbilical vein is the preferred means of vascular access during resuscitation of the newly born because it is easily located and easily cannulated. An umbilical catheter is inserted into the umbilical vein until the tip of the catheter is just below the skin and a good blood return is present. Umbilical vein catheterization may be attempted *only* by those specially trained in this technique, usually after attempts at IV and intraosseous access prove unsuccessful. Complications of umbilical vein cannulation include infection, hemorrhage, vessel perforation, and catheter tip embolism. A fatal air embolus can result if air enters the umbilical catheter. Advancing the catheter too far into the umbilical vein may cause infusion of medications directly into the liver with the potential for liver damage. Complications of umbilical vein cannulation are summarized in Box 36-8.

Veins of the scalp and extremities are acceptable routes for administration of fluids and medications but are difficult to access during resuscitation. Many EMS agency protocols advise the use of the intraosseous route as the primary means of vascular access during cardiac arrest. Keep in mind that the newborn's bones are small and fragile and the intraosseous space is small in a preterm infant. The technique for intraosseous access is discussed in Chapter 37.

Volume Expanders

[OBJECTIVE 15]

Volume expanders should be considered when acute blood loss is known or suspected with signs of hypovolemia:

BOX 36-8 Complications of Umbilical Vein Cannulation

- Infection
- Hemorrhage
- Air embolism
- Liver damage
- Catheter tip embolism
- Vessel perforation

SKILL 36-1 Umbilical Vein Cannulation

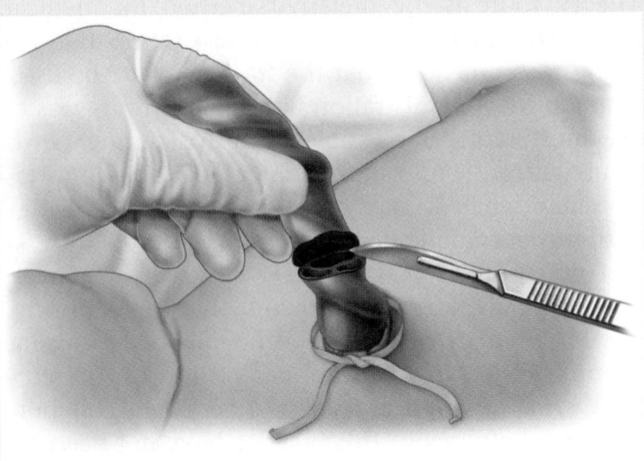

Step 1 Trim the umbilical cord down to ½ to 1 inch from the abdomen. The umbilical cord has two arteries and one vein. The vein is a thin-walled vessel. The arteries are thicker walled, paired, and often constricted. Identify the umbilical vein.

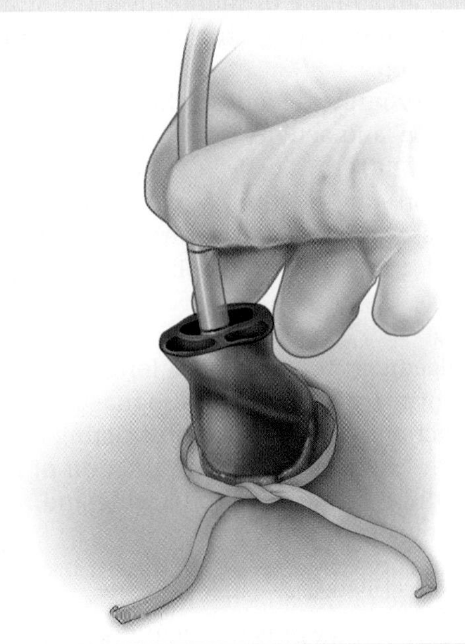

Step 2 Insert the umbilical catheter into the vein. Gently advance the catheter while watching for a free flow of blood. Advance the catheter only about to ¾ inch (1 to 2 cm) beyond the point at which the flashback of blood is seen. This usually is only 1½ to 2 inches (4 to 5 cm) in a term infant.

Slowly and gently pull back on the syringe to confirm a lack of resistance. If no flashback of blood is seen, the catheter may be inserted too far. Withdraw the catheter slightly. Check again for blood flow. If blood flow is present, inject normal saline.

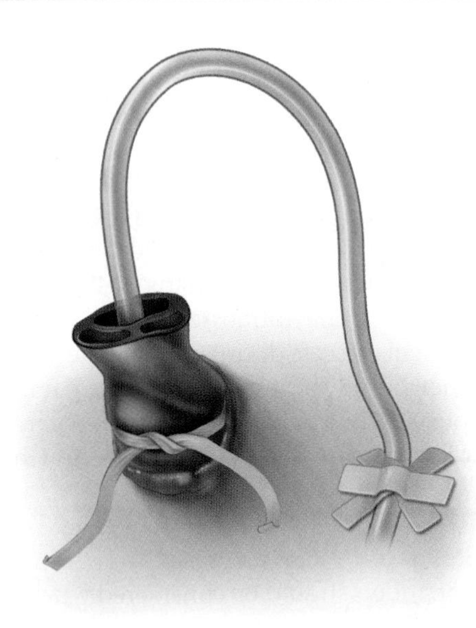

Step 3 Tighten the umbilical tape around the base of the cord. Secure the catheter in place.

- Pallor that persists despite oxygenation
- Poor perfusion
- Weak pulses with a heart rate faster than 100 beats per minute
- Poor response to resuscitative efforts, including effective ventilation

The fluid of choice for volume expansion is an isotonic crystalloid solution, such as normal saline or Ringer's lactate. Initially 10 mL/kg of IV fluid is usually given slow IV push over a 5- to 10-minute period. Boluses may be repeated several times, as guided by patient assessment. Because portions of a preterm infant's brain are at risk of bleeding when subjected to rapid changes in vascular pressure and osmolarity, seek guidance from medical direction when giving medications to a preterm newborn.

Medications

Table 36-5 lists medications that may be used during newborn resuscitation. Table 36-6 lists other medications that may be given to newborns.

Postresuscitation Care

[OBJECTIVE 16]

Continued monitoring and supportive care are essential for any newborn. Postresuscitation monitoring should include the following:

- Monitoring of heart rate, ventilatory rate, blood pressure, temperature, and oxygen saturation

TABLE 36-5 Medications Used in Neonatal Resuscitation

Drug	Indications	Mechanism of Action	Route	Notes
Epinephrine	Asystole or when the heart rate remains less than 60 beats per minute despite adequate ventilation with 100% oxygen and chest compressions	Vasoconstriction increases perfusion pressure during chest compressions, increasing oxygen delivery to the heart and brain; also improves myocardial contractility and increases heart rate	IV, IO	May be repeated every 3 to 5 minutes as needed Give rapidly

Modified from Aehlert, B. (2005). *Mosby's comprehensive pediatric emergency care*. St. Louis: Elsevier.
IV, Intravenous; *IO*, intraosseous; *IM*, intramuscular.

TABLE 36-6 Other Medications Given to Newborns

Drug	Indications	Mechanism of Action	Route	Notes
Glucose	Documented and symptomatic hypoglycemia	Rapidly increases serum glucose concentration; reverses central nervous system effects of hypoglycemia	IV, IO	There are currently no neonatal studies that have addressed the question of whether early supplemental glucose during and/or following delivery room resuscitation can or will improve outcome (Kattwinkel et al., 2010).
Naloxone	Reversal of respiratory depression	Competes with opioid receptor sites in the central nervous system, displacing previously administered narcotic analgesics	IV, IO, IM	Current resuscitation guidelines do not recommend administration of naloxone as part of the initial resuscitative efforts for newborns with respiratory depression. Support of ventilation should be the primary means used to restore oxygenation and heart rate. (Kattwinkel et al., 2010)

Modified from Aehlert, B. (2005). *Mosby's comprehensive pediatric emergency care*. St. Louis: Elsevier.
IV, Intravenous; *IO*, intraosseous; *IM*, intramuscular.

- Maintaining normal body temperature
- Rechecking blood sugar level
- Frequently assessing ventilatory effort and placement of tubes and catheters
- Detecting possible complications of resuscitation, such as pneumothorax
- Treating hypotension with volume expanders, vasopressors, or both
- Treating seizures, if present
- Establishing vascular access and appropriate fluid therapy
- Documenting your observations and actions
- Transporting the patient to the closest, most appropriate facility for further care

Case Scenario—continued

You set up all your equipment, and the mother is in a supine position. She states that she needs to push. You inspect the perineal area and notice that the head is crowning.

Questions

4. *What are the steps of delivering the head?*
5. *What are important steps with clearing the airway?*
6. *What should be done to assist with delivery of the body?*
7. *What are the steps immediately after delivery?*

SPECIFIC NEWBORN SITUATIONS

[OBJECTIVES 17, 18]

Because of the number of newborn situations presented, the epidemiology, history, physical findings, and therapeutic interventions are briefly discussed with each condition.

Meconium Aspiration

Meconium is material that collects in the digestive tract of a fetus and forms the first stools of a newborn. Meconium is thick, sticky, and usually greenish to black in color. It contains swallowed amniotic fluid, mucus, fine hair, blood, bile, and other byproducts of growth.

The presence of meconium in the amniotic fluid is an indication of possible fetal distress. If the fetus experiences hypoxia during birth, it may have a bowel movement and pass meconium into the amniotic fluid. Conditions that may cause hypoxia include compression of the umbilical cord, abruptio placenta, maternal hypertension, preeclampsia, or maternal shock.

Amniotic fluid is normally colorless. Amniotic fluid containing meconium may be thin and watery or thick and may be brownish-yellow or green in color. Meconium-stained amniotic fluid usually occurs in term or postterm infants and newborns who are small for gestational age. Meconium aspiration can occur in utero or immediately after delivery when the infant takes his or her first breaths. If inhaled, meconium may cause severe inflammation of the lungs, hypoxemia, aspiration pneumonia, pneumothorax, or pulmonary hypertension in the newborn.

Aspiration of meconium-stained amniotic fluid irritates the airways, causing a chemical pneumonitis. Pneumonia may begin within a few hours of aspiration. Substances within meconium strip surfactant from the surface of the alveoli. Meconium aspiration also results in a complete or partial airway obstruction. A complete airway obstruction results in atelectasis. Partial obstruction of some airways with thick, particulate meconium causes air trapping and distention of the alveoli. Hyperinflation of the lung may lead to pneumothorax. Needle decompression may be required if signs of a tension pneumothorax are present (Figure 36-18).

In the past, tracheal intubation and direct tracheal suctioning was recommended for all meconium-stained newborns. Today, the decision to perform tracheal intubation with tracheal suctioning after delivery of a meconium-stained newborn is based on the vigor of the infant (not the consistency of the meconium). For example, an infant born through meconium who has a strong ventilatory effort, good muscle tone, and a heart rate faster than 100 beats/min may require suctioning of the mouth and nose as you would for a newborn born through clear fluid but would not require tracheal intubation and suctioning. In contrast, an infant born through meconium may show signs of significant distress, including rapid breathing, absent or depressed breathing, retractions, grunting, nasal flaring, cyanosis, poor muscle tone, and possible bradycardia. Current resuscitation guidelines maintain that there is insufficient evidence to recommend a change in the current practice of performing tracheal suctioning of nonvigorous meconium-stained newborns. If intubation is prolonged and unsuccessful, consider bag-mask ventilation – particularly if persistent bradycardia is present (Kattwinkel et al., 2010).

While providing care for the patient, be sure to explain to the parents what is being done. Do not discuss chances of survival with the newborn's family. Transport

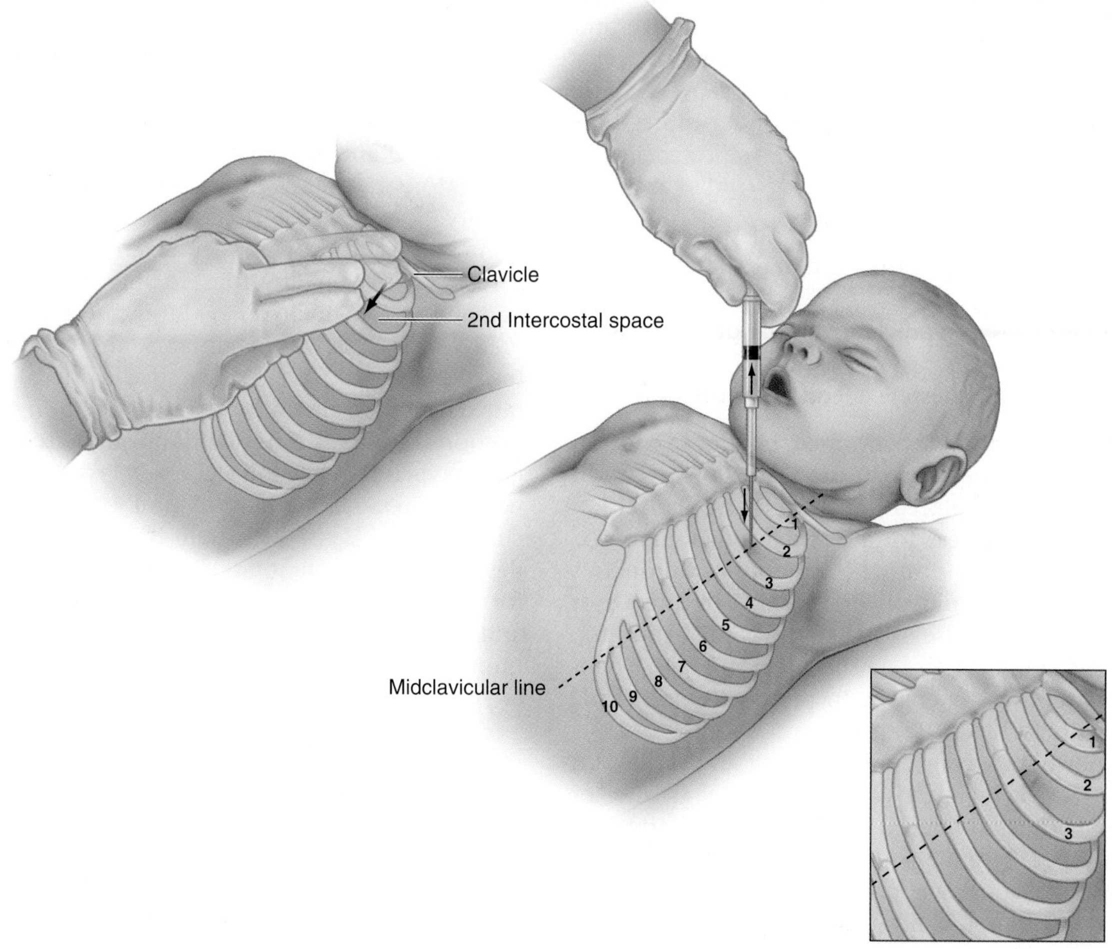

Figure 36-18 Needle chest decompression. Place the patient in a supine position. Find the second intercostal space at the midclavicular line. Cleanse the site. With an 18-gauge over-the-needle catheter, hold the catheter at a 90-degree angle to the chest wall and insert the needle through the skin. Slowly advance the needle over the superior border of the rib until the pleural space is entered. Entry into the pleural space is evidenced by a popping sound or giving-way sensation, a sudden rush of air, or the ability to aspirate air into a syringe (if used). Remove the needle from the catheter, leaving the catheter in place. Connect the catheter to a one-way valve if required by local protocol. Secure the catheter to the patient's chest wall to prevent dislodgement. Assess the patient's response to the procedure.

the infant to a facility capable of handling high-risk newborns.

Apnea

[OBJECTIVE 19]

Apnea is a common finding in preterm infants. If prolonged, apnea can lead to hypoxemia and bradycardia. **Serious apnea** is defined as cessation of breathing for longer than 20 seconds or any duration if accompanied by cyanosis and sinus bradycardia (Stoll & Kliegman, 2004c). Risk factors for apnea include prematurity, drug exposure, and prolonged or difficult labor and delivery.

Apnea in a newborn is usually caused by hypoxia or hypothermia. Apnea also may be caused by ventilation defects, disturbances in oxygen delivery, or disorders that depress the central nervous system's control of respiration (Stoll & Kliegman, 2004c). Ventilation defects include pneumonia, respiratory distress syndrome, or airway and respiratory muscle weakness. Disturbances in oxygen delivery include anemia, sepsis, and shock. Central nervous system depression may be caused by hypoglycemia, meningitis, hemorrhage, seizures, or drugs such as narcotics or central nervous system depressants.

Assessment may reveal a newborn that does not breathe on his or her own after stimulation, or the infant may have respiratory pauses that last more than 20 seconds. If apnea is present, bradycardia usually follows within 1 to 2 seconds.

Emergency care of an apneic newborn should begin with stimulating the infant to breathe. Flick the soles of the feet and/or rub the back. If the patient does not begin breathing, assist breathing with a bag-mask device and oxygen. Disable the pop-off valve on the bag-mask device and ventilate with just enough pressure to cause a gentle chest rise. Suction as needed. Perform chest compressions if needed. Tracheal intubation may be indicated in the following situations:

- Heart rate less than 60 beats/min despite adequate bag-mask ventilation and chest compressions
- Prolonged positive-pressure ventilation
- Prolonged apnea
- Central cyanosis despite adequate ventilation

If tracheal intubation is performed, be sure to confirm placement of the tube using an exhaled CO_2 detector. If the tube is correctly placed and the infant's condition suddenly worsens, assess for a possible pneumothorax, displacement of the tube into the right primary bronchus or esophagus, or obstruction of the tube by mucus or meconium. Apply a pulse oximeter and cardiac monitor. Continuously monitor the newborn's heart rate. Maintain normal body temperature to prevent hypothermia while providing care.

If the newborn's condition does not improve, gain circulatory access by means of a peripheral IV line or intraosseous infusion. Check the glucose level and give dextrose if hypoglycemia is present and you are permitted to do so per your local protocols.

Newborns with apnea have a relatively good outcome if they are treated early and aggressively. While providing care be sure to explain to the parents what is being done. Transport the patient to a facility capable of handling high-risk newborns.

Bradycardia

Bradycardia is present if the heart rate is slower than the lower limit of normal for the patient's age. Bradycardia can be classified as either primary or secondary. A primary bradycardia is usually caused by structural heart disease. A secondary bradycardia is a slow heart rate from a noncardiac cause. Causes of secondary bradycardia include increased vagal (parasympathetic) tone (vomiting, increased intracranial pressure, suctioning, or tracheal intubation procedure), hypothermia, hypothyroidism, acidosis, and hyperkalemia. Bradycardia in a newborn is most often caused by hypoxia. Risk to the newborn is minimal if hypoxia is quickly corrected.

Remember: Cardiac output = Stroke volume × Heart rate. Therefore a decrease in either stroke volume or heart rate may result in a decrease in cardiac output. Bradycardia can produce significant symptoms unless stroke volume increases to compensate for the decrease in heart rate. However, as discussed earlier, newborns do not have the ability to increase stroke volume to compensate for decreased heart rates. Unless corrected promptly, decreasing cardiac output eventually produces hemodynamic compromise.

Search for the cause of the bradycardia. Assess for signs of an upper airway obstruction. Check for secretions or the presence of a foreign body. Check the position of the tongue and soft tissues of the airway. Assess the ventilatory rate and effort. Assess the pulse rate and quality.

As you begin providing emergency care, do not be in a rush to give medications to increase the heart rate. Remember that hypoxia is the most common cause of bradycardia in newborns, infants, and children. Correcting the hypoxia (if present) should increase the heart rate. Ensure the airway is open and breathing is adequate. Suction the airway if needed. Apply a pulse oximeter and give oxygen if needed. If necessary, assist breathing with positive-pressure ventilation and oxygen. Begin chest compressions if the heart rate is less than 60 beats/min despite adequate ventilation with supplemental oxygen for 30 seconds. You may need to establish vascular access and give epinephrine if the infant's condition does not improve despite suctioning, positioning, and adequate oxygenation and ventilation.

Explain to the parents what is being done while caring for the infant. Maintain normal temperature while transporting the patient to the closest appropriate facility.

PARAMEDIC*Pearl*

Before suctioning any patient, note the patient's heart rate, oxygen saturation, and color. Monitor the patient's heart rate and appearance during suctioning. Bradycardia may result from stimulation of the back of the throat, larynx, or trachea. If bradycardia occurs or the patient's appearance deteriorates, interrupt suctioning and ventilate with oxygen until the patient's heart rate returns to normal.

Prematurity

A preterm infant weighs 0.6 to 2.2 kg (1.3 to 4.5 lb) or is born before the thirty-seventh completed week of gestation. Healthy preterm infants weighing more than 1700 g (3.7 lb) have a survivability and outcome similar to that of term infants. Mortality rate decreases weekly with gestation beyond the age of fetal viability (currently approximately 23 to 24 weeks of gestation).

Preterm babies are at increased risk of respiratory suppression, hypoglycemia, hypothermia, and infection as well as head or brain injuries caused by hypoxemia, changes in blood pressure, intraventricular hemorrhage, or fluctuations in serum osmolarity. They often require resuscitation.

Although retinopathy of prematurity (damage to the retina of the eye) may result from long-term oxygen use, hypoxemia causes irreparable brain damage. The use of oxygen should not be a factor in the short-term management of a preterm infant.

The degree of immaturity determines the physical characteristics of a preterm infant. Preterm infants generally have a large trunk and short extremities. Their skin is transparent and has less wrinkles and subcutaneous fat than a term newborn (Figure 36-19).

Attempt resuscitation if the newborn has any sign of life. Ensure the airway is open and breathing is adequate. Suction as needed. If breathing is inadequate, assist breathing with a bag-mask device and oxygen. Perform chest compressions if needed. Maintain body temperature to prevent hypothermia. Apply a pulse oximeter and cardiac monitor. Establish vascular access and give epinephrine if indicated per instructions from medical direction.

Explain to the parents what is being done while caring for the infant. Transport the patient to a facility with special services for LBW newborns.

Respiratory Distress and Cyanosis

Prematurity is the single most common factor causing newborn respiratory distress and cyanosis. Preterm infants have an immature central respiratory control center. They are easily affected by environmental or metabolic changes. Respiratory distress occurs most often in newborns who weigh less than 1200 g (approximately 2.6 lb) and are less than 30 weeks' gestation. Multiple gestations or prenatal maternal complications increase the risk of respiratory distress and cyanosis. Respiratory distress in the newborn may be caused by pulmonary, cardiovascular, or noncardiopulmonary conditions. Examples of these conditions are shown in Box 36-9.

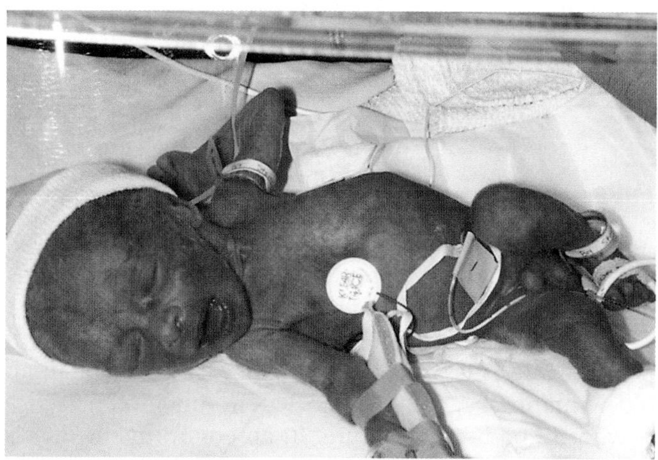

Figure 36-19 Retractions can be seen in this preterm infant.

Assessment of the newborn in respiratory distress may reveal the following:

- Tachypnea
- Paradoxic breathing
- Periodic breathing
- Intercostal retractions
- Nasal flaring
- Expiratory grunt

For a newborn in respiratory distress, maintaining an airway takes priority over any other procedures. Suction the airway as needed. Apply a pulse oximeter and give oxygen if indicated. Keep the oxygen saturation level above 95%. Assist breathing with a bag-mask device if needed. Consider tracheal intubation if prolonged assisted ventilation will be needed. Perform chest compressions if indicated. Check the glucose level and give dextrose if the infant is hypoglycemic and you are permitted to do so according to your local protocols. Maintain normal body temperature. Explain to the parents what is being done while caring for the patient, and transport the patient to the closest appropriate facility.

Seizures

Seizures occur in a small percentage of all newborns. However, they are relative medical emergencies because they are usually a sign of an underlying abnormality. Prolonged and frequent multiple seizures may result in metabolic changes and cardiopulmonary difficulties. Causes of neonatal seizures are shown in Box 36-10.

BOX 36-9 Causes of Respiratory Distress in the Newborn

CARDIOVASCULAR	PULMONARY	NONCARDIOPULMONARY
Transposition of great vessels	Diaphragmatic hernia	Metabolic acidosis
Shock, hemorrhage	Choanal atresia	Hypoglycemia
Coarctation of the aorta	Meconium aspiration	Hypothermia or hyperthermia
	Pneumonia	Phrenic nerve injury
	Lung immaturity	Drug withdrawal
	Pneumothorax	Skeletal abnormalities
	Asphyxia	Central nervous system disorders
	Amniotic fluid aspiration	Sepsis
	Spontaneous pneumothorax	Neuromuscular disease
	Primary pulmonary hypertension	
	Mucous obstruction of nasal passages	

BOX 36-10 Causes of Neonatal Seizures

- Hypoxic-ischemic encephalopathy (most common cause)
- Intracranial bleeding (intraventricular hemorrhage, subdural or subarachnoid bleeds, stroke; second most common cause)
- Central nervous system infection, such as meningitis
- Central nervous system malformation
- Metabolic disturbances (hypoglycemia, hypocalcemia, hypomagnesemia, pyridoxine deficiency)
- Drug withdrawal
- Developmental abnormalities
- Disorders of amino and organic acid metabolism
- No cause found (10% of cases)

Seizures in a newborn may be difficult to recognize because only slight changes may be seen. Types of seizures in neonates include the following:

- *Subtle seizure.* A subtle seizure is recognized by eye deviation, blinking, sucking, swimming movements of the arms, pedaling movements of the legs, and apnea.
- *Tonic seizure.* A tonic seizure is recognized by stiffening and extension of the limbs. Less commonly, flexion of the upper extremities and extension of the lower extremities occurs. A tonic seizure is more common in preterm infants, especially in those with intraventricular hemorrhage.
- *Clonic seizure.* Clonic seizures are characterized by rhythmic contractions (one to three jerks per second) alternating with relaxation of muscle groups. In focal clonic seizures, jerking or twitching movements involve localized muscle groups. Focal clonic seizures may occur in both term and preterm infants. Multifocal clonic seizures involve jerking or twitching movements of multiple muscle groups that randomly migrate to another area of the body. Multifocal seizures occur primarily in term infants.
- *Myoclonic seizure.* Myoclonus is a shocklike contraction of a muscle. A myoclonic seizure is characterized by sudden but short contractions of either single muscles or muscle groups. Contractions may occur singly or in a series of repetitive jerks. A myoclonic seizure is distinguished from a clonic seizure by the more rapid speed with which jerking occurs and the tendency to involve flexor muscle groups of the upper or lower extremities.

Assessment of a newborn having a seizure will reveal an altered level of responsiveness and seizure activity. Emergency care focuses on maintaining an open airway and adequate oxygen saturation. Suction the airway as needed. Avoid stimulation of the back of the throat during suctioning because this may stimulate vomiting. Give oxygen and assisted ventilation if necessary. Provide positive-pressure ventilation with oxygen if the seizure is prolonged or if the infant is cyanotic, has shallow chest rise with slow breathing, or has an oxygen saturation reading below 90% despite supplemental oxygen. Assess the adequacy of the ventilations delivered. ECG monitoring generally is indicated for any patient who has an abnormal ventilatory rate or effort, heart rate, perfusion, blood pressure, or mental status. However, do not delay lifesaving interventions to set up a monitor.

Check the glucose level and give dextrose if the infant is hypoglycemic and you are permitted to do so according to your local protocols. Benzodiazepines (diazepam, lorazepam, or midazolam) may be required to stop persistent or repetitive seizures. After the seizure has stopped, place the newborn on his or her side to aid drainage of secretions. Maintain normal body temperature and transport the patient to the closest appropriate facility.

Seeing a seizure for the first time can be frightening for the parents. Be considerate of their emotional reactions. Explain what is being done for the infant as you provide emergency care.

Fever

A newborn's average normal temperature is 37.5° C (99.5° F). A fever is present if the rectal temperature is 38.0° C (100.4° F) or higher.

A newborn has a limited ability to control body temperature and is less able to dissipate excess heat than an older infant is. A warm or hot environment can raise a newborn's body temperature. In an environment that is too warm the primary means of heat loss is through dilation of the vessels in the skin and sweating. Term infants who have a fever will have beads of sweat on the brow but usually not over the rest of the body. Preterm infants will have no visible sweat.

A prolonged fever can seriously weaken a newborn because of exhausted energy stores and increased work of breathing. To maintain normal body temperature the newborn uses more glucose. When glucose is depleted, anaerobic metabolism results. Increased metabolism places the infant at risk for dehydration because of evaporative heat loss and a reduction in feeding. Newborns can quickly become dehydrated because they rapidly lose large amounts of fluid in proportion to their body weight.

Infants in the first 3 months of life have an immature immune system and are more susceptible to severe infections and infections by unusual organisms than are older infants or children. Some of the causes of fever in

BOX 36-11 Causes of Fever in Newborns

- Upper respiratory infection
- Lower respiratory infection (pneumonia, bronchiolitis)
- Sepsis
- Meningitis
- Urinary tract infection
- Ear infection (otitis media)
- Gastroenteritis
- Undetermined cause

newborns are listed in Box 36-11. Excessive clothing or overbundling and excessive room temperature also may contribute to an elevated body temperature.

A newborn who has a fever may show mental status changes ranging from irritability to somnolence. The skin may appear pink, mottled, ashen, or pale and feel warm. Look at the skin for signs of a rash or petechiae. Check for signs of dehydration such as dry mucous membranes and decreased skin turgor. Sweating may be present in term infants.

Treatment for a feverish newborn is primarily supportive. Ensure the airway is open and breathing is adequate. Perform chest compressions if indicated. Giving an antipyretic agent to a newborn is of questionable value in the prehospital setting. Do not use ice or cold water baths to reduce fever. These methods cause shivering and constriction of the peripheral blood vessels, which then increases the core temperature. If signs of dehydration or shock are present, establish vascular access and give fluids.

Explain to the parents what is being done for the infant as you provide emergency care, and transport the patient to the closest appropriate facility.

Case Scenario CONCLUSION

You have delivered the newborn and suctioned the airway. You notice a greenish-brown fluid on the body and near his mouth and nose. His body is pink and extremities are blue. The heart rate is faster than 100 beats/min. He grimaces, his extremities have active motion, and he is crying very loudly as you dry him.

Looking back

8. *What is the significance of the greenish-brown fluid on the newborn?*
9. *What is the Apgar score?*
10. *When is it appropriate to start resuscitation on a newborn?*

Hypothermia

Hypothermia (a core body temperature below 35° C [95° F]) may result from a decrease in heat production, an increase in heat loss, or a combination of these factors. A newborn is at risk for heat loss because of its relatively large surface area to body mass ratio, wet amniotic fluid covering, and exposure to a relatively cool environment, especially in contrast to the temperature within the uterus. Furthermore, the newly born cannot generate heat by shivering and has less tissue insulation because of less subcutaneous fat. Hypothermia can be a sign of sepsis. The increased metabolic demand can cause metabolic acidosis, pulmonary hypertension, and hypoxemia.

Because the increased surface area/volume ratio makes newborns extremely sensitive to environmental conditions (especially when they are wet after delivery), control the four methods of heat loss: evaporation, conduction, convection, and radiation. Signs and symptoms of hypothermia include the following:

- Pale color
- Cool skin, particularly of the extremities
- Acrocyanosis
- Slow and shallow ventilatory effort, possible apnea
- Bradycardia
- Central cyanosis
- Irritability initially, lethargy in later stages

Emergency care for hypothermia includes making sure the airway is open and breathing is adequate. Assist ventilations if needed. Perform chest compressions if indicated. Warm your hands before touching the patient. Dry the newborn's skin and wrap the patient with warm blankets. If the torso must be exposed for frequent assessments, increase the temperature in the patient compartment of the ambulance to 24° to 26.5° C (75° to 80° F). Check the glucose level and give dextrose if the infant is hypoglycemic and you are permitted to do so according to your local protocols. Warm IV fluids may also be considered. To do this, give the IV fluids through an IV heater designed for this purpose.

Explain to the parents what is being done while caring for the newborn. Transport the patient rapidly to the closest appropriate facility.

PEDIATRIC*Pearl*

Infants may die of cold exposure at temperatures that adults find comfortable.

Hypoglycemia

The level of glucose in the blood must remain fairly constant to ensure proper functioning of the brain and body cells. Hypoglycemia in a newborn is a blood glucose level of less than 40 mg/dL. Prolonged low blood glucose levels can lead to irreversible brain damage. Hypoglycemia may be caused by inadequate glucose intake or increased use of glucose.

A newborn's glycogen stores are adequate to meet glucose requirements for only 8 to 12 hours. In the healthy newborn, the glucose level falls over the first 1 to 2 hours after birth and then stabilizes at a minimum of approximately 40 mg/dL. By 3 hours of life, the glucose level rises to 50 to 80 mg/dL (Rosenberg, 2002). Hypoglycemia may occur in a much shorter period if conditions exist that increase the newborn's need for glucose. Risk factors for newborn hypoglycemia are shown in Box 36-12.

To overcome hypoglycemia, the body releases counterregulatory hormones, including glucagon, epinephrine, cortisol, and growth hormone. These hormones may cause symptoms of hyperglycemia that last for several hours. However, preterm babies are less able to respond to hypoglycemia with counterregulatory hormones than term newborns are. Hypoglycemia may occur as early as 30 to 60 minutes after birth in children of diabetic mothers. Hypoglycemia may begin 2 to 6 hours after birth in preterm infants and those who are small for gestational age (Rosenberg, 2002).

Check blood glucose levels in all sick babies and those at risk for hypoglycemia. Signs and symptoms of hypoglycemia are shown in Box 36-13.

Emergency care starts with ensuring the newborn has an open airway and is breathing adequately. Perform chest compressions if indicated. Maintain normal body temperature. Establish vascular access, check the glucose level, and give dextrose if the infant is hypoglycemic and you are permitted to do so according to your local protocols. Explain to the parents what is being done while caring for the newborn. Transport the patient to the closest appropriate facility.

Vomiting

Vomiting in the first 24 hours of life suggests obstruction in the upper digestive tract, pyloric stenosis, or increased intracranial pressure. Vomiting also may occur because of a duodenal ulcer, stress ulcer, overfeeding, ineffective burping, or an allergy to milk. Persistent vomiting is a warning sign. Vomiting mucus that may occasionally be blood streaked in the first few hours of life is not uncommon. Vomitus containing dark blood is usually a sign of a serious illness but can be caused by swallowed maternal blood. Aspiration of vomitus can cause respiratory insufficiency or obstruction of the airway.

Vomiting of non–bile-stained fluid suggests an anatomic or functional obstruction at or above the first portion of the duodenum or gastroesophageal reflux. Vomiting of bile-stained fluid suggests an obstruction below the opening of the bile duct.

Assessment findings may reveal a distended stomach, signs of infection, increased intracranial pressure, or drug withdrawal.

When caring for a newborn who is vomiting, maintain an open airway. Suction or clear vomitus from the airway and ensure adequate breathing. Apply a pulse oximeter and give oxygen if needed. If necessary, assist breathing with positive-pressure ventilation and oxygen. After the airway is cleared, place the newborn on his or her side. This will help drain fluid from the mouth. Because vomiting may cause bradycardia, apply a cardiac monitor and watch the heart rate closely. You may need to establish vascular access and give IV fluids if there are signs and symptoms of hypovolemia.

Explain to the parents what is being done while caring for the infant. Maintain normal temperature while transporting the newborn to the closest appropriate facility.

BOX 36-12 Risk Factors for Newborn Hypoglycemia

- Maternal diabetes
- Preterm birth
- Hypoxia, asphyxia
- Hypothermia
- Small for gestational age infant
- Sepsis
- Toxemia
- Smaller twin
- Central nervous system hemorrhage
- Respiratory distress

BOX 36-13 Signs and Symptoms of Hypoglycemia

- Jitteriness
- Twitching or seizures
- Cyanosis
- Respiratory distress
- Limpness
- Eye rolling
- Lethargy
- High-pitched cry
- Apnea
- Irregular respirations

Diarrhea

A breastfed newborn can have five to six stools per day. Diarrhea is present when the normal pattern of stools changes, with an increase in their frequency or volume and a change in stool consistency. Severe cases of diarrhea can cause dehydration and electrolyte imbalances.

Diarrhea in a newborn may be caused by overfeeding or may be a sign of a serious illness. It may occur as an isolated symptom or in conjunction with other symptoms, such as vomiting and fever. Causes of diarrhea in a newborn are shown in Box 36-14.

Neonatal abstinence syndrome is a disorder that occurs in newborns born to narcotic-addicted mothers. If the mother is addicted to narcotics, the newborn also will be addicted. After birth the supply of narcotics is suddenly cut off, which results in symptoms of narcotic withdrawal called *neonatal abstinence syndrome.* Withdrawal symptoms usually begin within 48 to 72 hours after birth but may be delayed up to 2 weeks. Signs of withdrawal include irritability, jitters, tremors, rapid breathing, mottling of the skin, tachycardia, respiratory distress, wheezing, vomiting, diarrhea, and dehydration. Seizures may also result.

Phototherapy and thyrotoxicosis also may cause diarrhea in a newborn. Phototherapy is exposure to sunlight or artificial light. In newborns, phototherapy is used to treat jaundice (hyperbilirubinemia). Phototherapy uses radiant energy to change bilirubin to a soluble form that can be excreted by the kidneys and digestive tract. Phototherapy can result in diarrhea, producing bilirubin stools. **Thyrotoxicosis** (hyperthyroidism) results when the thyroid gland produces too much thyroid hormone. The infant usually has diarrhea, tremors, and tachycardia and is very hungry.

Take appropriate standard precautions when caring for a newborn with diarrhea. A newborn with diarrhea will have loose stools and may have decreased urinary output. Look for signs of dehydration, including delayed capillary refill, poor skin turgor, dry mucous membranes, and lethargy.

Maintain an open airway and make sure breathing is adequate. Apply a pulse oximeter and give oxygen if needed. Perform chest compressions if indicated. Because diarrhea may cause electrolyte disturbances, apply a cardiac monitor and closely watch the newborn's heart rate. You may need to establish vascular access and give IV fluids.

Explain to the parents what is being done while caring for the newborn. Maintain normal temperature while transporting the patient to the closest appropriate facility.

BOX 36-14 Causes of Diarrhea in a Newborn

- Overfeeding
- Bacterial or viral infection
- Gastroenteritis
- Lactose intolerance
- Phototherapy treatment
- Neonatal abstinence syndrome
- Thyrotoxicosis
- Malabsorption
- Cystic fibrosis

Birth Injuries

Birth injuries are defined as occurring during labor and delivery. Birth injuries are estimated to occur in 2 to 7 of every 1000 live births. Five to 8 in every 100,000 newborns die of birth trauma. Twenty-five in every 100,000 die of anoxic injuries. Such injuries account for 2% to 3% of infant deaths. Risk factors predisposing to birth injury include the following:

- Cephalopelvic disproportion
- Shoulder dystocia
- Postmaturity
- Prolonged or difficult labor
- Explosive delivery
- Abnormal presentations (including breech)

Soft tissue injuries such as lacerations, abrasions, and bruising are the most common birth injuries. Cranial injuries may include the following:

- Molding of the head and overriding of the parietal bones
- Redness, abrasions, bruising, and subcutaneous fat necrosis
- Subconjunctival and retinal hemorrhage
- Subperiosteal hemorrhage
- Skull fracture

Intracranial hemorrhage, including subdural and subarachnoid bleeds, may result from trauma or asphyxia. Injuries to the spine and spinal cord may occur if strong traction is exerted when the spine is hyperextended or there is a lateral pull. Peripheral nerve injury, such as brachial plexus injury, can occur when nerve roots are stretched during delivery (Figure 36-20). This can occur when shoulder dystocia is present. Facial palsy may be caused by pressure from the sacral bones as the fetus passes through the birth canal. Fractures of the clavicle may result from shoulder dystocia or breech birth. Fractures of the extremities also may occur. The humerus is the most commonly fractured long bone. Other birth injuries include rupture of the spleen, liver injury, adrenal hemorrhage, and hypoxic ischemia.

Assessment of the newborn with a birth injury may reveal the following:

- Diffuse, sometimes ecchymotic, swelling of the soft tissues of the scalp
- Paralysis below the level of spinal cord injury
- Paralysis of the upper arm with or without paralysis of the forearm
- Paralysis of the diaphragm

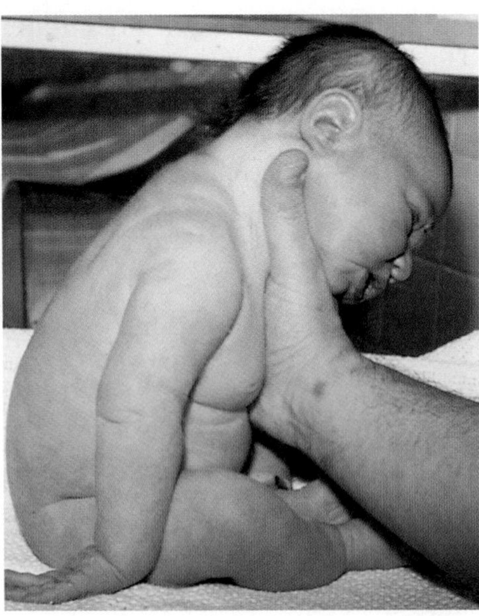

Figure 36-20 Brachial plexus injury.

- Movement on only one side of the face when the newborn cries
- Lack of free arm movement on side of fractured clavicle
- Lack of spontaneous movement of the affected extremity
- Hypoxia
- Shock

Emergency care includes ensuring adequate oxygenation and ventilation. Perform chest compressions if indicated. Maintain normal body temperature. Medical direction may instruct you to establish vascular access and administer medications depending on the type and severity of the birth injury. Consult medical direction to determine the most appropriate facility to which the infant should be transported. Explain to the parents what is being done while caring for the newborn.

Case Scenario SUMMARY

1. *What are the important questions to ask the patient?* Questions that are helpful include the following:
   - Do you feel like you need to push or have a bowel movement?
   - How long have you been having contractions? How far apart are they?
   - When is your baby due?
   - How many babies are there?
   - Did your bag of water rupture? What was the color of the water?
   - Have you taken any medications or drugs?
   - Do you have high blood sugar or diabetes?
   - Has your doctor told you if the baby is coming head first or feet first? Did your physician mention any need for a cesarean section?
   - Have you experienced any vaginal bleeding? How long ago?

   If the patient states she feels the need to push or that the baby is coming out, proceed directly to delivery.
2. *What is important in preparation for delivery?* First locate the obstetric kit. If delivery is imminent, open the kit and put the patient in position for delivery. The easiest position for you to assist her with the delivery is to have her lie down on her back with her knees flexed and feet flat on the stretcher or other surface. Place the blue pads or sheets from the obstetric kit under her hips. Because exposure to body fluids is possible and likely during a delivery, you should have on a sterile gown, gloves, goggles, and a mask. All the necessary equipment should be set out and easy to reach. This includes a bulb syringe, blankets, towels, hemostats/clips for the cord, and scissors. If time permits, place the mother on the cardiac monitor and establish IV access.
3. *What are the signs of a problematic delivery?* Problematic deliveries, although rare, can occur. Twin deliveries can be difficult. Patients who have diabetes may have large children because of their hyperglycemia. Abnormal presenting parts also can cause a difficult or impossible field delivery. When looking at the perineal area, note the presenting part. If the presenting part is the cord, this condition is very serious. Breech deliveries can be accomplished in the field but can be difficult. A limb as the presenting part requires emergent transport. When preparing for delivery, two EMS providers may need to assist.
4. *What are the steps of delivering the head?* Support the perineal tissue to prevent an explosive delivery and tearing of the tissue. As the head begins to come out of the vaginal canal, support it with gentle pressure. As the head delivers, instruct the mother not to push. Once the head has delivered, use the bulb syringe to suction out the mouth and then the nose. Do not pull on the neck while the newborn is exiting the vaginal canal.

Continued

Case Scenario SUMMARY—continued

5. *What are important steps with clearing the airway?* A bulb syringe often is effective in clearing the airway and typically is a standard part of the obstetric kit. Begin by squeezing all the air out of the syringe. Then, with the syringe still compressed, place the tip into the mouth and release the compression to suction out any fluids. Move the syringe away from the newborn's face and squeeze it several times to expel the contents. Eject the secretions onto a towel. Repeat this procedure one or two times for the mouth and then each nostril.
6. *What should be done to assist with delivery of the body?* The shoulder-to-shoulder distance is the widest diameter of the newborn's body. Delivering the child with the mother supine, legs bent at the knees, and knees to her chest is typically the easiest position. This provides the widest opening of the pelvic outlet. Gently direct the head downward to allow the anterior shoulder to slip out from under the pubic bone. Once the anterior shoulder is delivered, the rest of the body usually will be born quickly.
7. *What are the steps immediately after delivery?* Dry the newborn to reduce body heat loss and stimulate breathing. The easiest way to do this is to place the child on a firm surface and rub him or her dry with a towel. If needed, you also can stimulate the newborn by flicking the soles of the feet. Calculate an Apgar score at 1 and 5 minutes after delivery. Do not delay resuscitation of an infant to assign Apgar scores. Assess breathing and heart rate. Begin resuscitation if necessary and keep the newborn warm.
8. *What is the significance of the greenish-brown fluid on the newborn?* Meconium staining can occur if a newborn has the first bowel movement in utero. If fluid is meconium stained but the newborn is vigorous, suctioning may be done with the bulb syringe. Give blow-by oxygen throughout the suctioning procedure. If the newborn is depressed with poor ventilatory effort, decreased muscle tone, and/or a heart rate less than 100 beats/min, quickly examine the back of the throat with a laryngoscope. Suction any residual meconium with a 12F or 14F suction catheter. Suction while withdrawing the catheter. Insert a tracheal tube into the trachea and attach the tube to suction. Apply suction as the tube is slowly withdrawn. Repeat intubation and suctioning until little additional meconium is obtained or until the newborn's heart rate indicates that resuscitation must proceed immediately. If the newborn's heart rate or breathing is severely depressed, positive-pressure ventilation may be necessary despite the presence of some meconium in the airway.
9. *What is the Apgar score?* The Apgar scoring system assigns a score of 0 to 2 for five elements: color (0, blue/pale; 1, pink; 2, completely pink), pulse (0, absent; 1, slow; 2, over 100 beats/min), grimace (0, no response; 1, grimace; 2, cry), activity (0, limp; 1, some extremity flexion; 2, active movement), and respiration (0, absent; 1, slow; 2, good, strong cry). This infant receives a 1 for appearance because the body is pink but the extremities are blue. He receives a 2 for pulse because his heart rate is greater than 100 beats/min. He receives a 2 for grimace and irritability because he is grimacing and crying loudly. He receives a 2 for activity and a 2 for respirations. The total Apgar score is 8. Document this and provide it in your radio report to the receiving facility.
10. *When is it appropriate to start resuscitation on a newborn?* Resuscitation should occur if the newborn is not responding appropriately. A newborn may require some stimulation to begin breathing effectively. However, if you do not see some effort at breathing, coughing, or sneezing within 15 seconds, start blow-by oxygen. If the infant is still not responding, positive-pressure ventilation may be required. Definite indications for positive-pressure ventilation include apnea, gasping ventilations, or a heart rate less than 100 beats/min after providing the initial steps of stabilization. Adequate ventilation is primarily determined by a prompt improvement in heart rate. If the newborn is spontaneously breathing and the heart rate is greater than 100 beats/min, positive-pressure ventilation may be gradually discontinued.

The newborn needs to be closely watched for signs of deterioration. Periodic gentle stimulation may help maintain spontaneous breathing. Blow-by oxygen may be used if the patient maintains adequate ventilations. If spontaneous breathing is inadequate, continue assisted ventilation. Begin chest compressions if the newborn's heart rate is less than 60 beats/min despite adequate ventilation with supplemental oxygen for 30 seconds.

Chapter Summary

- Although fewer than 10% of newborns require emergency care, you must always be prepared for newborn resuscitation when assisting with a delivery.
- Some conditions increase the likelihood that resuscitation will be necessary.
- In most cases, drying, warming, and suctioning are sufficient to cause a newborn to breathe effectively and may be the only resuscitative measures needed. If additional care is required, you must know how to manage a newborn's airway, assist ventilations, perform chest compressions, establish vascular access, and give medications.
- You must be aware of the capabilities of the hospitals in your area to determine the most appropriate destination for healthy and high-risk newborns.
- Although your care will be focused on the newborn, remember to explain what you are doing to family members as you provide care.

REFERENCES

Dyleski, R. A., Crockett, D. M., & Seibert, R. W. (2001). Cleft lip and palate. In B. J. Bailey (Ed.), *Head and neck surgery—otolaryngology* (3rd ed.) (p. 961). Philadelphia: Lippincott, Williams & Wilkins.

Gregory, G. A. (2005). Resuscitation of the newborn. In R. D. Miller (Ed.), *Miller's anesthesia* (6th ed.) (pp. 2345-2355). Philadelphia: Elsevier.

Kattwinkel, J., Perlman, J. M., Aziz, K., et al. (2010). Part 15: neonatal resuscitation: 2010 American Heart Association Guidelines for Cardiopulmonary Resuscitation and Emergency Cardiovascular Care. *Circulation 122*(suppl 3), S909-S919.

National Institute of Neurological Disorders and Stroke. (2005). *Spina bifida fact sheet.* Retrieved July 1, 2008, from www.ninds.nih.gov.

Rosenberg, A. A. (2002). The neonate. In S. G. Gabbe, J. R. Niebyl, & J. L. Simpson (Eds.), *Obstetrics: Normal and problem pregnancies* (4th ed.) (pp. 653-692). New York: Churchill Livingstone.

Stoll, B. J., & Kliegman, R. M. (2004a). Delivery room emergencies. In R. E. Behrman, R. M. Kliegman, & H. B. Jenson (Eds.), *Nelson textbook of pediatrics* (17th ed.) (pp. 570-573). Philadelphia: W.B. Saunders.

Stoll, B. J., & Kliegman, R. M. (2004b). Overview of mortality and morbidity. In R. E. Behrman, R. M. Kliegman, & H. B. Jenson (Eds.), *Nelson textbook of pediatrics* (17th ed.) (pp. 519-522). Philadelphia: W.B. Saunders.

Stoll, B. J., & Kliegman, R. M. (2004c). Respiratory tract disorders. In R. E. Behrman, R. M. Kliegman, & H. B. Jenson (Eds.), *Nelson textbook of pediatrics* (17th ed.) (pp. 574-588). Philadelphia: W.B. Saunders.

United Nations Children's Fund and World Health Organization. (2004). *Low birthweight: Country, regional and global estimates,* New York: UNICEF.

Vento, M., Asensi, M., Sastre, J., Lloret, A., Garcia-Sala, F., & Vina, J. (2003). Oxidative stress in asphyxiated term infants resuscitated with 100% oxygen. *Journal of Pediatrics, 142,* 240-246.

Zideman, D. A., Hazinski, M. F. (2008). Background and epidemiology of pediatric cardiac arrest. *Pediatr Clin North Am* Aug;55(4):847-59, ix. Review.

Chapter Quiz

1. Which of the following signs are associated with secondary apnea?
a. Pink skin, increasing heart rate, normal blood pressure
b. Cyanotic skin, falling heart rate, falling blood pressure
c. Pink skin, falling heart rate, falling blood pressure
d. Cyanotic skin, increasing heart rate, normal blood pressure

2. Which of the following signs are the *most* important when determining if additional resuscitative efforts are needed in the newly born?
a. Heart rate, muscle tone, and color
b. Absence of meconium, muscle tone, and color
c. Heart rate and ventilatory effort
d. Ventilatory effort and absence of meconium

3. The heart rate of the newly born should be assessed by palpating
a. the carotid pulse.
b. the femoral pulse.
c. the umbilical pulse.
d. the brachial pulse.

4. When delivering positive-pressure ventilations with a bag-mask device to a newborn, the assisted ventilation rate should be ____ breaths/min and ______ breaths/min when chest compressions also are being delivered.
a. 10 to 20; 30
b. 20 to 40; 20
c. 30 to 40; 40
d. 40 to 60; 30

5. Assessment of a newly born infant 1 minute after delivery reveals the infant is crying vigorously on light tapping of the foot. Her heart rate is 130 beats/min and some flexion of the extremities is noted. Ventilations are regular at approximately 40 breaths/min. Her body is pink and extremities are blue. You would assign an Apgar score of
a. 7
b. 8
c. 9
d. 10

Chapter Quiz—continued

6. Which of the following most appropriately defines *newly born*?
   a. The first week of life
   b. The first month of life
   c. From 1 month to 1 year of life
   d. From the first minutes to hours of life
7. You are working with a newly born infant who experienced an explosive delivery and is now vomiting. Which of the following should you *most* likely suspect?
   a. Gastric ulcer
   b. Gastrointestinal infection
   c. Increased intracranial pressure
   d. Obstructed upper gastrointestinal tract
8. The protrusion of abdominal organs into the umbilical cord is known as which of the following?
   a. Fistula
   b. Omphocele
   c. Meningocele
   d. Choanal atresia

Terminology

Acrocyanosis Cyanosis of the extremities.

Atresia Absence of a normal opening.

Choanal atresia Narrowing or blockage of one or both nares by membranous or bony tissue.

Cleft lip Incomplete closure of the upper lip.

Cleft palate Incomplete closure of the hard and/or soft palate of the mouth.

Congenital Present at or before birth.

Diaphragmatic hernia Protrusion of the abdominal contents into the chest cavity through an opening in the diaphragm.

Esophageal atresia (EA) A condition in which the section of the esophagus from the mouth and the section of the esophagus from the stomach end as a blind pouch without connecting to each other.

Fistula An abnormal passage from a body organ to the body surface or between two internal body organs.

Hydrocephalus An abnormal buildup of cerebrospinal fluid in the brain.

Meningocele A type of SB in which the spinal cord develops normally but a saclike cyst that contains the meninges and cerebrospinal fluid protrudes from an opening in the spine, usually in the lumbosacral area.

Meningomyelocele The severest form of SB in which the meninges, cerebrospinal fluid, and a portion of the spinal cord protrude from an opening in the spine and are encased in a sac covered by a thin membrane; also called *myelomeningocele.*

Neonatal abstinence syndrome Withdrawal symptoms that occur in newborns born to opioid-addicted mothers.

Neonate An infant from birth to 1 month of age; also called *newborn.*

Neural tube defects Congenital anomalies that involve incomplete development of the brain, spinal cord, and/or their protective coverings.

Newborn asphyxia The inability of a newborn to begin and continue breathing at birth.

Newly born An infant in the first minutes to hours after birth.

Omphalocele Protrusion of abdominal organs into the umbilical cord.

Pierre Robin sequence A congenital anomaly characterized by a very small lower jaw (micrognathia), a tongue that tends to fall back and downward (glossoptosis), and cleft palate.

Premature or preterm infant Infant born before 37 completed weeks of gestation.

Preterm birth Birth before 37 completed weeks of gestation.

Primary apnea The newly born's initial response to hypoxemia consisting of initial tachypnea, then apnea, bradycardia, and a slight increase in blood pressure; if stimulated, responds with resumption of breathing.

Secondary apnea When asphyxia is prolonged, a period of deep, gasping respirations with a simultaneous fall in blood pressure and heart rate; gasping becomes weaker and slower and then ceases.

Serious apnea Cessation of breathing for longer than 20 seconds or any duration if accompanied by cyanosis and sinus bradycardia.

Spina bifida (SB) A neural tube defect that affects the back portion of the vertebrae, which fail to close, usually in the area of the lower back; meninges, the spinal cord, or both may protrude through this opening.

Spina bifida occulta Mildest form of SB in which the spinal cord is intact but one or more vertebrae fail to close in the lumbosacral area.

Thyrotoxicosis A condition in which the thyroid gland produces excess thyroid hormone; also called *hyperthyroidism* or *Graves' disease.*

Tracheoesophageal fistula (TEF) An abnormal opening between the trachea and the esophagus.

Vomiting Forceful ejection of stomach contents through the mouth.

CHAPTER 37

Pediatrics

Objectives *After completing this chapter, you will be able to:*

1. Describe Emergency Medical Services for Children and discuss how an integrated system can affect patient outcome.
2. Identify methods and mechanisms that prevent injuries and discuss the paramedic's role in the reduction of infant and childhood morbidity and mortality from acute illness and injury.
3. Describe techniques for successful assessment and treatment of infants and children.
4. Identify typical age-related vital signs and the appropriate equipment used to obtain pediatric vital signs.
5. Identify common responses of families to acute illness and injury of an infant or child and techniques for successful interaction.
6. Determine appropriate airway adjuncts and ventilation devices for infants and children and complications of improper use of these devices.
7. Discuss appropriate tracheal intubation equipment for infants and children.
8. Identify complications of an improper tracheal intubation procedure in infants and children.
9. List the indications for gastric decompression for infants and children.
10. Discuss age-appropriate vascular access sites and necessary equipment for infants and children.
11. Identify complications of vascular access for infants and children.
12. Discuss appropriate transport guidelines for infants and children.
13. Discuss appropriate receiving facilities for low- and high-risk infants and children.
14. Differentiate upper airway obstruction from lower airway disease.
15. Define respiratory distress, failure, and arrest and describe the general approach to the treatment of a child with each of these conditions.
16. Describe the etiology, epidemiology, history, and physical findings of croup, epiglottitis, and bacterial tracheitis.
17. By using the patient history and physical examination findings, develop a treatment plan for a patient who has croup, epiglottitis, or bacterial tracheitis.
18. Describe the etiology, epidemiology, history, and physical findings of asthma, bronchiolitis, and pneumonia.
19. By using the patient history and physical examination findings, develop a treatment plan for a patient who has asthma, bronchiolitis, or pneumonia.
20. Describe the etiology, epidemiology, history, and physical findings of shock in infants and children.
21. By using the patient history and physical examination findings, develop a treatment plan for a patient in shock.
22. Identify the major classifications of pediatric cardiac rhythms.
23. Describe the etiology, epidemiology, history, and physical findings of cardiac dysrhythmias in infants and children.
24. By using the patient history and physical examination findings, develop a treatment plan for a patient who has a cardiac dysrhythmia.
25. Discuss the primary causes of cardiopulmonary arrest in infants and children.
26. Describe the primary causes of altered mental status in infants and children.
27. Describe the etiology, epidemiology, history, and physical findings of neurologic emergencies in infants and children.
28. By using the patient history and physical examination findings, develop a treatment plan for a patient who has a neurologic emergency.
29. Identify common lethal mechanisms of injury in infants and children.
30. Discuss anatomic features of children that predispose or protect them from certain injuries.
31. Describe the pathophysiology, assessment, and treatment of infants and children with trauma.
32. Describe aspects of infant and child airway management affected by potential cervical spine injury.
33. Identify infant and child trauma patients who require spinal immobilization.
34. Discuss fluid management and shock treatment for infant and child trauma patients.
35. Determine when pain management and sedation are appropriate for infants and children.
36. Define *child abuse* and *child neglect*.
37. Define *sudden infant death syndrome* and describe its etiology, epidemiology, history, and physical findings.
38. Discuss the parent and caregiver responses to the death of an infant or child.
39. Identify appropriate parameters for performing infant and child cardiopulmonary resuscitation.
40. Define *children with special healthcare needs* and *technology assistance*.
41. Discuss the unique assessment and treatment considerations for a child with special healthcare needs.

Chapter Outline

Case Scenario

You are called to a private residence for a 4-year-old boy who is having difficulty breathing. His mother states that he has a history of asthma. She says that he feels warm, his breathing has gotten worse, he has developed a barky cough, and his appetite has been decreased today.

You find the child to be resting comfortably. His heart rate is 110 beats/min, blood pressure is 90/68 mm Hg, and ventilations are 34 breaths/min and slightly labored. Pulse oximetry is 93% on room air. His skin is warm and dry. Capillary refill is less than 2 seconds. His oral temperature measures 103° F.

Questions

1. *What is your impression of the patient?*
2. *What is the appropriate initial therapy?*
3. *Describe how you would perform the complete physical examination.*

You have an important role in treating infants and children during prehospital care (primary transport) and interfacility transfer (secondary transport). To give appropriate care, you must be familiar with the differences in body size, development, and conditions pertinent to infants and children. Make it a priority to maintain and improve your pediatric knowledge, assessment, and emergency care skills. Use textbooks, journals, continuing education programs, and clinical environments such as a pediatric emergency department, clinic, or pediatrician's office to help you meet this important goal.

EMERGENCY MEDICAL SERVICES FOR CHILDREN

History and Legislation

[OBJECTIVE 1]

Early EMS systems (mid- to late 1960s and early 1970s) focused on providing rapid intervention for sudden cardiac arrest in adults and rapid transport for motor vehicle crash victims. Because these systems focused on adult care, outcomes for adults in emergencies improved dramatically, but the specialized needs of children experiencing a medical emergency went largely unrecognized. As a result the equipment, training, experience, and expertise of prehospital personnel often were less developed to meet the needs of children.

In the mid-1970s this weakness in the EMS system began to be recognized. Healthcare professionals worked to make sure that the unique needs of children were included in the EMS system. Their efforts remained unfunded until the U.S. Congress enacted legislation in 1984 (Public Law 98-555) authorizing the use of federal funds for Emergency Medical Services for Children (EMSC).

EMSC efforts have improved the availability of child-size equipment in emergency vehicles and emergency departments. EMSC has initiated hundreds of programs to prevent injuries and has provided thousands of hours of training to EMTs, paramedics, and other emergency medical care providers.

Purpose

Following are the EMSC program's aims:

- Ensure state-of-the-art emergency medical care for the ill or injured child and adolescent.
- Ensure that pediatric service is well integrated into an EMS system backed by optimal resources.
- Ensure that the entire spectrum of emergency services, including primary prevention of illness and injury, acute care, and rehabilitation, is provided to children and adolescents as well as adults.

PARAMEDIC*Pearl*

Use of the term *accident,* which implies an unpredictable or unavoidable event, is being replaced with the term *injury* to reflect the nature of the problem more accurately.

ILLNESS AND INJURY PREVENTION

[OBJECTIVE 2]

Children are at high risk for many injuries that can lead to death or disability. In fact, one in every five U.S. children requires medical care for an injury each year (Dowd & Bull, 2003). Traumatic injury is the leading cause of death in children after infancy (Dowd et al., 2002).

Two criteria by which the significance of childhood injuries can be measured are death and **morbidity.** Although death is the worst possible outcome, injuries cause widespread morbidity, which results in the need for medical care and an inability to perform normal daily activities. The leading causes of childhood injury deaths are shown in Table 37-1.

Most injuries are predictable and preventable. Predictable injuries stem from a dangerous situation or risky behavior. To prevent injuries, think about them in terms of cause and effect. If we can identify how, when, and where injuries typically occur, we can identify who may be at higher risk for injuries. Efforts can then be targeted at prevention of specific types of injuries.

In addition to age, the type, number, and severity of pediatric injuries in a given area partly depend on the following regional characteristics:

- Geography (type of terrain, average response times for emergency care)
- Climate and weather conditions (temperature extremes, violent storms)
- Population density (crime rates, 9-1-1 coverage, availability of medical services)
- Population traits (economic resources, ethnic backgrounds, education levels)

You play an important role in injury prevention. *Primary prevention* involves measures that can be applied in advance to reduce the likelihood that an injury will occur, such as installing a pedestrian overpass at a dangerous intersection. *Secondary prevention* includes interventions that help prevent or minimize an injury when it happens, such as the use of bicycle helmets. Although you may not realize it, you participate in primary and secondary injury prevention every time you fill out a prehospital care report. These reports provide information that helps determine injury rates and pattern and form a basis for effective injury prevention efforts.

Traditionally, the prehospital professional's role in injury management has focused on emergency care of victims *after* injuries occur. This is called *tertiary prevention.* Tertiary prevention measures lessen the severity of an injury and improve the patient's outcome after an injury, such as advanced trauma care and rehabilitation. Tertiary prevention cannot change the fact that the victim is injured, and it cannot help those whose injuries are too severe for them to be saved.

PARAMEDIC*Pearl*

Injury prevention activities have high visibility within a community. This helps improve relationships between community members and emergency personnel. Increase your involvement in primary and secondary prevention by educating children and families about safety issues and participating in organized injury prevention projects in your community.

TABLE 37-1 Leading Causes of Deaths from Unintentional Injuries in the United States by Age, 2005

Rank	1-4 Years	5-9 Years	10-14 Years
1	Drowning	Motor vehicle traffic	Motor vehicle traffic
2	Motor vehicle traffic	Fire or burn	Drowning
3	Fire or burn	Drowning	Fire or burn
4	Other pedestrian	Other land transport	Other land transport
5	Suffocation	Suffocation	Suffocation

Data from National Center for Health Statistics, National Vital Statistics System. Retrieved August 5, 2008, from http://webappacdc.gov/sasweb/ncipc/leadcaus10.html.

Pediatric Chain of Survival

In adults, sudden, nontraumatic cardiopulmonary arrests are usually the result of underlying respiratory or cardiac disease. Some of the causes of nontraumatic cardiopulmonary arrest in children are shown in Box 37-1.

BOX 37-1 Some Causes of Nontraumatic Cardiopulmonary Arrest in Children

- Bronchospasm
- Congenital cardiac abnormalities
- Dysrhythmias
- FBAO
- Gastroenteritis
- Seizures
- Sepsis
- Drowning
- SIDS
- Upper and lower respiratory tract infection

FBAO, Foreign body airway obstruction; *SIDS,* sudden infant death syndrome.

The pediatric chain of survival represents a sequential series of events to assess, support, or restore effective ventilation and circulation to the infant or child in respiratory or cardiopulmonary arrest. The sequence consists of the following five important steps:

- Prevention of illness or injury
- Early cardiopulmonary resuscitation (CPR)
- Early EMS activation
- Rapid advanced life support (ALS)
- Integration of post-cardiac arrest care

The importance of prevention is reflected by the links of the chain. Note that activating EMS is delayed until after a trial of early CPR. This is based on the higher likelihood of respiratory conditions and lower likelihood of ventricular fibrillation as the cause of cardiopulmonary arrest in the pediatric patient.

ASSESSMENT OF THE ILL OR INJURED CHILD

[OBJECTIVES 3, 4]

Scene Size-Up

When you are called to care for an ill or injured child, survey the scene before approaching the patient. Take appropriate infection control precautions. Note any hazards or potential hazards and any visible mechanism of injury or illness. For example, the presence of pills, medicine bottles, or household chemicals may indicate a possible toxic ingestion. An injury and history that do not match the mechanism of injury may indicate child abuse.

Watch the interaction between the caregiver and the child. Does the interaction demonstrate concern or anger and indifference? Other important assessments that can be made during the scene survey include the following:

- Orderliness, cleanliness, and safety of the home
- General appearance of other children in the family
- Presence of any medical devices used for the child (such as a home ventilator)
- Indications of parental substance abuse

Determine whether additional resources are necessary, including law enforcement, fire equipment, extrication equipment, special rescue services, additional medical personnel, or special transport services (e.g., aeromedical transport).

Initial Assessment

General Impression

When you are called to assist an older child or adolescent, begin your assessment as you would with an adult by asking, "Are you all right?" Because they are often frightened by the presence of strangers, a different approach is needed for younger children and infants. Pause a short distance from the patient and use your senses of sight and hearing (look and listen) to find out whether a life-threatening problem exists. If you find a child unresponsive or observe severe trauma, immediately approach (after assessing for scene safety) and begin necessary care. However, if you find the child alert and responsive, you can proceed at a more moderate pace, assessing the child's condition through observation and background information gathered from the parents.

The pediatric assessment triangle (PAT) summarizes the major points for the general impression assessment. It is a useful tool for quickly determining whether a child is "sick" or "not sick" (Figure 37-1). Three main areas are assessed by the PAT: appearance, (work of) breathing, and circulation. *Appearance* refers to the child's mental status, muscle tone, and body position. *Breathing* includes the presence or absence of visible movement at the chest or abdomen and signs of breathing effort. *Circulation* refers to the child's skin color. With practice you will be able to perform these assessments almost simultaneously.

If the child is bundled, ask the child's caregiver to remove enough of the coverings briefly so that you can see the child's skin color and find out if the child is breathing. Because children quickly lose body heat, remove coverings only as needed to perform assessments and give emergency care, then replace them promptly. Always protect the patient's modesty.

> **PEDIATRIC*Pearl***
>
> Because approaching an ill or injured child can increase agitation, possibly worsening the child's condition, the PAT is performed *before* approaching or touching the child (across the room survey).

Appearance. TICLS (pronounced "tickles") is a memory aid that can help you recall the areas to be assessed relevant to the child's appearance (Table 37-2). If the child is alert, his or her condition is nonurgent. If the child's appearance is anything other than alert, his or her condi-

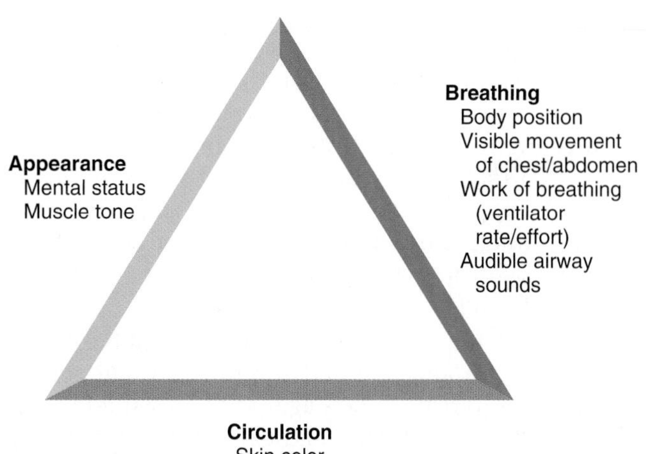

Figure 37-1 The pediatric assessment triangle.

TABLE 37-2 TICLS Assessment Tool

***T**one*	Is the child moving vigorously, or is the child limp, listless, or flaccid?
***I**nteractivity*	Is the child alert and attentive to his or her surroundings or uninterested and apathetic?
Consolability	Can the child be comforted by you or the caregiver?
Look or gaze	Do the child's eyes follow your movement, or is a vacant stare present?
Speech or cry	Is the child's speech or cry strong, or is it weak or hoarse?

Modified from the American Academy of Pediatrics. (2000). *Textbook of pediatric education for prehospital professionals*. Sudbury, MA: Jones & Bartlett.

BOX 37-2 Appearance: Abnormal Findings

- Agitation
- Marked irritability
- Reduced responsiveness
- Drooling (beyond infancy)
- Limp or rigid muscle tone
- Inconsolable crying
- Failure to recognize caregiver
- Paradoxic irritability (irritable when held and lethargic when left alone)

tion is urgent. Begin immediate care as needed. Normal findings include normal muscle tone, response to name (if more than 6 to 8 months of age), equal movement of all extremities, eyes open, and normal speech or cry. Abnormal findings are shown in Box 37-2. If the child exhibits abnormal findings, proceed immediately to the ABCDE assessment.

(Work of) Breathing. Watch the chest and abdomen for movement to tell if the child is breathing and if breathing requires extra effort. Visible movement of the chest or abdomen without obvious sounds or effort indicates a nonurgent situation. If no movement is visible or the child is struggling to breathe, his or her condition is urgent. Begin immediate airway and breathing interventions as needed. With practice, you may learn to spot very fast or slow breathing rates during your general impression. However, this is less critical than the presence or absence of breathing and the degree of effort involved.

Normal findings include quiet, nonlabored breathing; equal chest rise and fall; and a ventilatory rate within normal range for the child's age. Abnormal findings are shown in Box 37-3. If the child exhibits abnormal findings, proceed immediately to the ABCDE assessment.

BOX 37-3 Breathing: Abnormal Findings

- Abnormal body position (sniffing position, **tripod position**, **head bobbing**)
- **Nasal flaring**
- **Retractions**
- Muffled or hoarse speech
- Stridor, **grunting,** gasping, **gurgling,** wheezing
- Ventilatory rate outside normal range
- **Accessory muscle** use

BOX 37-4 Circulation: Abnormal Findings

- Bleeding
- Pallor
- Mottling
- Cyanosis

Circulation. To assess the child's circulation, note the skin color. The child's skin color should appear normal for his or her ethnic group. To assess skin color in a child with darker skin tones, look at the lips and tongue or ask the parents to uncover the child's palms or soles of the feet. A pink skin color indicates a nonurgent condition. If the child's skin is pale, bluish, or mottled, his or her condition is urgent (Box 37-4). Begin immediate care as needed.

Based on your general impression, decide whether the child is sick (unstable) or not sick (stable). If the child's condition is urgent, immediately proceed with rapid assessment of airway, breathing, and circulation. If a problem is identified, give necessary care: "treat as you find." If the child's condition appears nonurgent, proceed with a full assessment of airway, breathing, circulation, and mental status. Then obtain a focused history and perform a detailed physical examination. This may be performed on the scene or during transport. As long as the patient's condition does not change, continue to work at a moderate pace. Remember to take the time to explain what you are doing.

PEDIATRIC*Pearl*

Never let the initial appearance of a child fool you. Both infants and children compensate to maintain homeostasis extremely well. By the time children look seriously ill they often are about to begin a rapid deterioration. Too often EMS professionals do not obtain accurate vital signs to back up the patient's appearance. Although children who look sick are sick, do not assume that a healthy appearance means they are otherwise healthy. Because children are able to compensate longer than adults, they also can deteriorate much more quickly.

ABCDE Assessment

The primary survey is also called the ABCDE assessment. During the ABCDE assessment, assessment and manage-

BOX 37-5 Components: ABCDE Assessment

- *A*irway, level of responsiveness, and cervical spine protection
- *B*reathing (ventilation)
- *C*irculation (perfusion)
- *D*isability mini-neurologic exam
- *E*xpose/environment

ment occur at the same time (Box 37-5). The purpose of the assessment is to find and treat any life-threatening conditions. It usually requires less than 60 seconds to complete the assessment, but may take longer if interventions are needed at any point. Periodically repeat the assessment, particularly if you note a change in the patient's condition.

Airway. At this stage of your patient assessment, simultaneously establish the patient's mental status and his ability to maintain an open airway. Determine level of responsiveness using AVPU:

- A = **A**lert
- V = **R**esponds to verbal stimuli
- P = **R**esponds to painful stimuli
- U = **U**nresponsive

If cervical spine injury is suspected (by examination, history, or mechanism of injury), ask your partner to stabilize the head and neck manually in a neutral, in-line position. Smaller children (who have larger heads and occipital regions) must have their torsos elevated to keep the airway in a neutral position. Not padding under the torso results in the occipital area pushing the head forward, flexing the neck and constricting the airway. If the child is responsive and the airway is open, assess breathing. If the child is responsive but cannot talk, cry, or forcefully cough, assess for possible airway obstruction. If the child is unresponsive, quickly check to see if he is breathing. If normal breathing is present, continue the primary survey. If the child is not breathing (or only gasping), check for a pulse for up to 10 seconds. If there is no pulse or you are unsure if there is a pulse, begin chest compressions.

If the child is unresponsive and a pulse is present, use manual maneuvers such as a head tilt-chin lift or jaw thrust without head tilt to open the airway. If trauma is suspected, use the jaw-thrust without head tilt maneuver to open the airway. If the airway is not patent (clear of debris and obstruction), assess for sounds of airway compromise (snoring, gurgling, or stridor). Gurgling is an indication for immediate suctioning. Look in the mouth for blood, broken teeth, gastric contents, and foreign objects (e.g., loose teeth, gum, small toys). If present, position the patient to facilitate drainage and suction the mouth. If solid material is visualized, remove it with a gloved finger covered in gauze. If a foreign body obstruction is suspected but not visualized, clear the obstruction by performing abdominal thrusts (if the patient is 1 year of age or older) or chest thrusts (if the patient is younger than 1 year of age).

PEDIATRIC*Pearl*

The responsive child may have assumed a position to maximize his or her ability to maintain an open airway. Allow the child to maintain this position as you continue your assessment.

Emergency Care during Airway Assessment. If the child shows little or no sign of air movement, immediately begin to establish an airway. In a child with a complete airway obstruction, open and maintain the airway. Use airway adjuncts if needed. If attempts to open the airway are unsuccessful, begin airway clearing maneuvers, suction visible secretions, and attempt assisted ventilation with a bag-mask device and supplemental oxygen. In a child with a partial airway obstruction, give supplemental oxygen and help the child maintain a position of comfort.

Breathing. The assessment sequence described here assumes the patient is responsive or that a pulse is present if he is unresponsive. If the patient is unresponsive and not breathing (or only gasping), current cardiopulmonary resuscitation guidelines recommend a change in the assessment sequence to Circulation-Airway-Breathing (C-A-B). Confirm that the child is breathing and note significant abnormalities in the work of breathing. In the responsive patient (and in an unresponsive patient with a pulse), look, listen, feel – inspect, auscultate, palpate. In these patient situations, evaluation of breathing during the primary survey should take no more than 10 seconds. If the child is breathing, determine if breathing is adequate or inadequate. If breathing is adequate, move on to assessment of circulation.

Count the ventilatory rate, assess the depth and pattern of the child's breathing, check the color of the lips and tongue, and look for chest trauma. A child with breathing difficulty often has a ventilatory rate outside the normal limits for his or her age (Table 37-3).

If the child's condition is urgent, quickly proceed through the following steps. Look for the following signs, which indicate an increased work of breathing (ventilatory effort):

- Anxious appearance, concentration on breathing
- Use of **accessory muscles**
- Leaning forward to inhale
- Nasal flaring (Figure 37-2)
- Retractions (Figure 37-3)

TABLE 37-3 Normal Respiratory Rates by Age

Age	Breaths/min (at Rest)
Infant (1-12 months)	30-60
Toddler (1-3 years)	24-40
Preschooler (4-5 years)	22-34
School-age (6-12 years)	18-30
Adolescent (13-18 years)	12-20

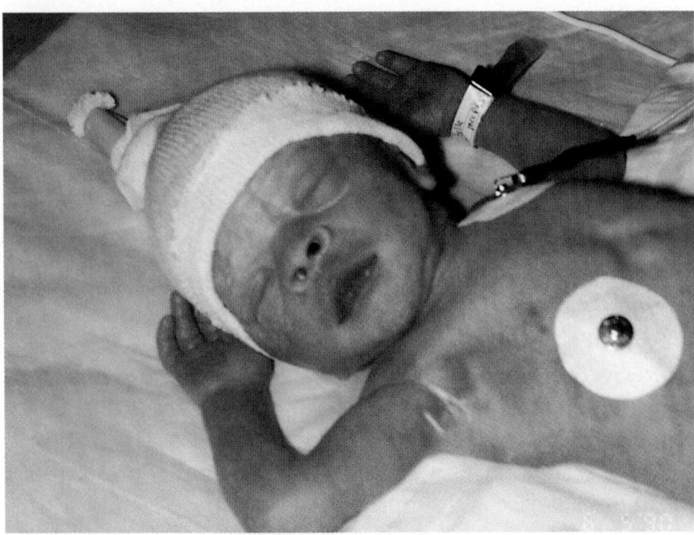

Figure 37-2 Nasal flaring. Widening of the nares may be seen in infants with respiratory distress.

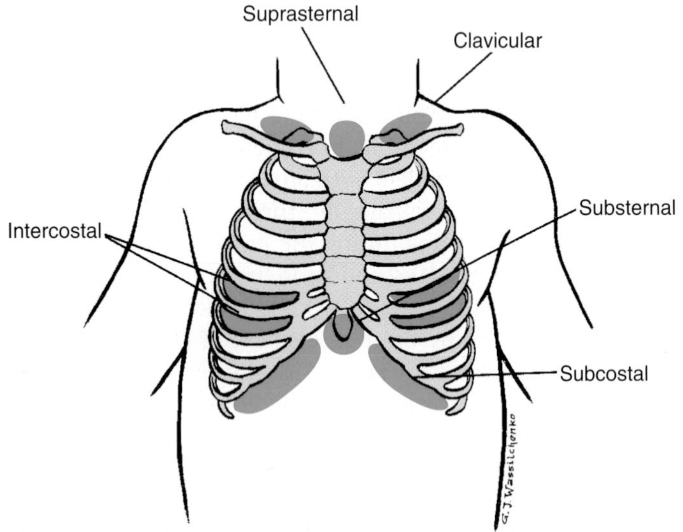

Figure 37-3 Location of retractions.

- Seesaw (chest/abdominal) movement. Increased ventilatory effort draws in the chest while thrusting out the abdomen. This is a sign of severe respiratory distress.

Note the rhythm of breathing (regular, irregular, or periodic). Prolonged inspiration suggests an upper airway obstruction. Prolonged expiration suggests a lower airway obstruction.

Listen for air movement at the nose and mouth. Note whether ventilations are quiet, absent, or noisy (e.g., stridor, wheezing, snoring, crowing, grunting). Wheezing may be heard throughout the lungs or, in the case of a foreign body obstruction, may be localized.

Breath sounds are normally quiet. Because the chest of a child is small and the chest wall is thin, breath sounds are easily transmitted from one side of the chest to the other. As a result, breath sounds may be heard despite the presence of a pneumothorax, hemothorax, or atelectasis. To minimize the possibility of sound transmission from one side of the chest to the other, listen under each armpit (axillary region) and in the midclavicular line under each clavicle. Alternate from side to side and compare the findings.

Feel for air movement from the nose or mouth against your chin, face, or palm. Palpate the chest for tenderness, instability, and crepitation.

PARAMEDIC*Pearl*

If the chest wall does not rise during positive-pressure ventilation, ventilation is inadequate or the airway is obstructed.

Emergency Care during Breathing Assessment. If the child has signs of mild to moderate respiratory distress, help the child into a position of comfort. Do not increase the patient's oxygen demand by forcing the child to wear the oxygen mask. The child may be most comfortable sitting upright in a caregiver's arms. If breathing is difficult and the rate is too slow or too fast, give supplemental oxygen and positive-pressure ventilation if indicated. If breathing is absent, insert an airway adjunct (if not previously done) and deliver two breaths with a pocket mask or bag-mask device with

Case Scenario—continued

While examining the child, you note that he has a seal-like barking cough. He is able to sit up. No evidence of drooling is present. He does have subcostal retractions. Wheezes are present in all lung fields. His abdomen is soft.

Questions

4. *What pharmacologic treatment would be appropriate?*
5. *What is the most likely cause of his symptoms?*
6. *What physical examination findings would warrant immediate transport?*

supplemental oxygen. Give each breath over 1 second. Make sure the child's chest wall rises with each ventilation. If the child is unresponsive but breathing adequately and no signs of trauma are present, place the patient in the recovery position and administer oxygen.

If is the patient has an open pneumothorax, cover it with an occlusive dressing taped on three sides. If the child shows signs of respiratory failure and has diminished or absent breath sounds on one side of the chest, a tension pneumothorax may be present. To release pressure, a needle must be placed between the ribs and into the air pocket.

Circulation. Look for visible external bleeding and control major bleeding if present by applying direct pressure over the bleeding site. Consider possible areas of major internal bleeding. Significant internal bleeding may occur in the chest, abdomen, pelvis, retroperitoneum, and femoral areas. Pain or swelling in any of these areas may signal possible internal bleeding.

Determine whether the patient's heart rate is within normal limits for the child's age. Normal heart rates by age are listed in Table 37-4. Compare the strength and quality of central and peripheral pulses. The location for assessment of a central pulse varies according to the age of the child. In the newly born, assess the strength and quality of a central pulse by palpating the base of the umbilical cord between your thumb and index finger. In an infant, assess the brachial pulse. Assess the carotid pulse in any child older than 1 year.

Assess a peripheral pulse while keeping one hand on the central pulse location. For example, if you are assessing a central pulse by the brachial artery, keep one hand on the brachial pulse and use your other hand to assess the peripheral (radial) pulse in the same extremity. Compare the strength and quality of the central and peripheral pulses. Although a peripheral pulse is not quite as strong as a central pulse, the rate should be the same.

A weak central pulse may indicate **decompensated shock.** A peripheral pulse that is difficult to find, weak, or irregular suggests poor peripheral perfusion and may be a sign of shock or hemorrhage.

Assess the child's skin color, temperature, and moisture. Decreased skin perfusion is an early sign of shock. Skin color is most reliably evaluated in the sclera, conjunctiva, nail beds, tongue, oral mucosa, palms, and soles. A child's hands and feet are normally warm, dry, and pink. A newborn often has acrocyanosis (cyanotic hands and feet while the rest of the body is pink). Pale skin may be observed in shock or respiratory failure. Cool, pale extremities are associated with decreased cardiac output, as seen in shock and hypothermia. Blue (cyanosis) skin suggests **hypoxemia** or inadequate perfusion. In patients with darker skin, cyanosis may be observed as ashen gray lips and tongue. Mottled skin suggests decreased cardiac output, ischemia, and **hypoxia** but can be normal in an infant exposed to a cool environment.

The skin surface is normally warm and equal bilaterally. Use the dorsal surfaces of your hands and fingers to assess skin temperature. As cardiac output decreases, coolness will begin in the hands and feet and rise toward the trunk. The skin is normally dry with a minimum of perspiration. Use the dorsal surfaces of your hands and fingers to assess the moisture of the skin.

Assess skin turgor (elasticity) by grasping the skin on the abdomen between your thumb and index finger (Figure 37-4). Pull the skin taut and then quickly release it. Note how quickly the skin returns to its original shape when released. The skin should resume its shape immediately with no tenting or wrinkling. Good skin turgor indicates adequate hydration. Poor skin turgor (a sign of dehydration and/or malnutrition) is present when the skin is released but remains pinched (tented) and then slowly returns to its normal shape. Never assume a child is well hydrated on the basis of good skin turgor. Other signs of dehydration include a dry mouth, sunken eyes, an absence of tears when crying, and sunken or depressed fontanelles. A dehydrated child may be at risk for shock.

Assess capillary refill by firmly pressing the skin over the warmest point on the child's body and release. Observe the time required for the blanched tissue to

TABLE 37-4 Normal Heart Rate by Age

Age	Beats/min*
Infant (1-12 months)	100-160
Toddler (1-3 years)	90-150
Preschooler (4-5 years)	80-140
School-age (6-12 years)	70-120
Adolescent (13-18 years)	60-100

Reprinted from Aehlert, B. (2005). Comprehensive pediatric emergency care. St. Louis: Mosby.

*Pulse rates for a sleeping child may be 10% lower than the low rate listed in age group.

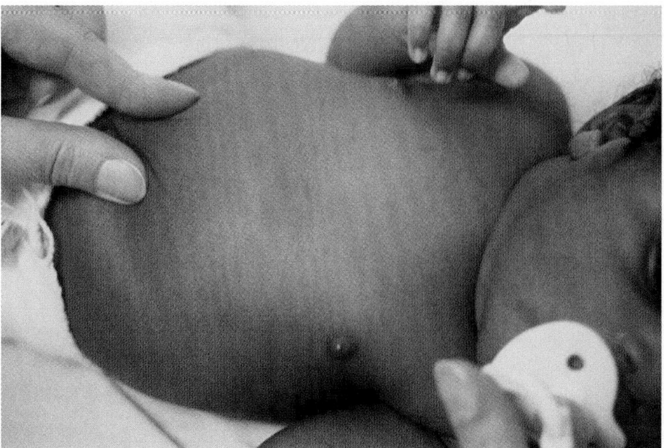

Figure 37-4 Assessing skin turgor (elasticity) in an infant.

return to its original color. If the ambient temperature is warm, color should return within 2 seconds. Capillary refill time of 3 to 5 seconds is delayed and may indicate poor perfusion or exposure to cool ambient temperatures. Capillary refill time greater than 5 seconds is markedly delayed and suggests shock. If capillary refill is initially assessed in the hand or fingers and it is delayed, recheck it in a more central location, such as the chest. Never assume a child is well perfused on the basis of a good capillary refill time.

Emergency Care during Circulation Assessment. Because children can maintain a normal blood pressure and strong central pulse well into early (compensated) shock, take the following steps for any child who is at risk for shock, particularly if the child shows signs of poor perfusion (weak pulses, delayed capillary refill rate, or cool, blue, or mottled skin):

- Place the child in a supine position.
- Administer oxygen if indicated.
- Control external bleeding.
- Conserve body heat.
- Begin chest compressions if no pulse is present or if the heart rate is less than 60 beats/min with signs of poor perfusion.
- Transport the patient promptly to definitive care.

Disability (Mental Status). Question the caregiver about the child's normal mood, activity level, attention span, and willingness and ability to cooperate.

During this phase of the primary survey, use the Glasgow Coma Scale (GCS) modified for pediatric use (Table 37-5). The pediatric GCS may be used to establish a baseline and for comparison in later, serial assessments.

Emergency Care during Mental Status Assessment. If the child responds only to voice, perform further assessment and give supplemental oxygen. If the child responds only to pain or is unresponsive, you also may need to provide assisted ventilations. Rapid interventions (such as correcting hypoxia or hypoglycemia) are indicated for any child who is not alert or is not easily awakened by a verbal stimulus. Begin transport before starting the detailed physical examination for any child who is not alert.

Expose/Environment. Undress the patient as needed for examination, but be sure to replace clothing promptly after assessing each body area. Keeping the head of an infant covered is especially important. Maintaining appropriate temperature is particularly important in the pediatric patient because children have a large body surface area/weight ratio, providing a greater area for heat loss.

Vital Signs

See Tables 37-3 and 37-4 for normal values for ventilatory rates and heart rates by age. Blood pressure (BP) should be measured only after the rest of the circulatory assessment has been completed. In children aged 3 years or younger, a strong central pulse is a good sign of an adequate blood pressure. For children older than 3 years, blood pressure can be measured if time allows. Be aware that getting an accurate BP reading in a young child is a time-consuming procedure that may not be worth the time invested. Children often become agitated and tearful during this procedure, which raises their pulse and ventilatory rate. To decrease the child's anxiety about BP measurements, state you are going to give his arm "a

TABLE 37-5 Adult, Child, and Infant Glasgow Coma Scale

Area Assessed	Adult/child	Score	Infant
***E**ye Opening*	Spontaneous	4	Spontaneous
	To verbal	3	To verbal
	To pain	2	To pain
	No response	1	No response
Best ***V**erbal* Response	Oriented	5	Coos, babbles
	Disoriented	4	Irritable cry
	Inappropriate words	3	Cries only to pain
	Incomprehensible sounds	2	Moans to pain
	No response	1	No response
Best ***M**otor* Response	Obeys commands	6	Spontaneous
	Localizes pain	5	Withdraws from touch
	Withdraws from pain	4	Withdraws from pain
	Abnormal flexion (decorticate)	3	Abnormal flexion (decorticate)
	Abnormal extension (decerebrate)	2	Abnormal extension (decerebrate)
	No response	1	No response
	Total = E + V + M	3 to 15	

hug." Because children have lower BPs than adults, inflating the cuff to high pressures is not necessary.

To obtain an accurate measurement, the bladder of the BP cuff should completely encircle the upper portion of the extremity. The width of the cuff should cover one half to two thirds of the length of the upper arm or thigh. The cuff should be at heart level and the arm should be fully supported by the rescuer. Use the upper extremity to get the most accurate reading and follow the same technique used in adults. If a child's condition is urgent, do not delay transport to obtain a BP reading. Table 37-6 shows the lower limit of normal systolic BP by age.

PEDIATRIC*Pearl*

To determine the *minimum* systolic BP for a child 1 to 10 years of age, the following formula may be used: 70 + (2 × age in years). For example, the minimum systolic BP for a 5-year-old child would be 70 + (2 × 5), or 80 mm Hg.

If necessary, obtain the child's temperature by an appropriate route (oral, axillary, tympanic, or rectal in infants) considering the child's age and clinical condition. Note that a rectal temperature is considered the most accurate reflection of core body temperature. However, rectal temperature is not typically taken in the field. Keep in mind that temperature varies with exercise, crying, stress, and clothing. Common signs of increased body temperature include flushed face and skin, malaise, low energy level, increased ventilatory and heart rates, and a glassy look to the eyes.

CUPS Assessment

After you have completed the initial assessment and given appropriate care for life-threatening emergencies, determine the child's CUPS status. The CUPS assessment scale classifies patients as:

- ***C***ritical
- ***U***nstable
- ***P***otentially unstable
- ***S***table

TABLE 37-6 Lower Limit of Normal Systolic BP by Age

Age	Lower Limit of Normal Systolic BP
Term neonate (0-28 days)	More than 60 mm Hg or strong central pulse
Infant (1-12 months)	More than 70 mm Hg or strong central pulse
Child 1-10 years	More than 70 + (2 × age in years)
Child 10 years or older	More than 90 mm Hg

Reprinted from Aehlert, B. (2005). *Comprehensive pediatric emergency care.* St. Louis: Mosby.
BP, Blood pressure.

The CUPS assessment also can be used to help determine the speed of transport and the facility to which the child should be transported if a choice is available. If the child's CUPS status is critical or unstable, perform initial emergency care and immediately transport. Management of airway and breathing is a priority during transport. Further assessments and interventions may be performed if time allows. Completing the focused history and detailed physical examination may not be possible during a brief transport.

For children who are potentially unstable, complete the initial assessment and emergency care, then transport them promptly because these children may worsen rapidly. The focused history and detailed physical examination may be completed during transport.

For children with a stable CUPS status, you may want to complete the focused history and detailed physical examination with appropriate emergency care before transport. Revise the CUPS assessment as needed on the basis of your findings.

Focused History

When treating a child whose condition is urgent, your priority is to provide initial emergency care and promptly transport the child. If time allows, try to get important background information from the child's caregiver during transport. However, do not delay treatment or transport to obtain a complete medical history.

In nonurgent cases, you can take more time to focus on the child's medical history. Although much of the information will probably come from the caregiver, any child who is old enough to speak and understand simple phrases should be included in the process as much as possible.

A good starting point for the focused history is the SAMPLE history. After noting findings from the SAMPLE history, cover any of the following areas that apply to the specific situation. If any of the findings listed below is positive, upgrade the child's CUPS assessment and reevaluate management actions.

Mental Status. If the child's caregiver is available, ask whether the child's behavior appears unusual. When did the patient's symptoms begin? Was the onset of symptoms gradual or sudden? What was the child doing when the symptoms started? How rapidly have the patient's symptoms progressed? Any history of a similar episode?

Is there any history of head trauma, diabetes, seizures, poisoning, infection with fever (suggesting sepsis), meningitis, or brain tumor? Is there any history of toxic exposure to alcohol, sedatives, or hypnotic agents? Is there any history of exposure to extremes of temperature (hot or cold)? What medications (including vitamin supplements and herbal remedies) does the child currently take? Dosages? Is the child compliant with medications?

Emergency care for positive findings includes reassessing the child's mental status during examination and transport.

Airway and Breathing. Consider the following questions when obtaining a history for a condition affecting the respiratory system. This list requires modification based on the patient's age and chief complaint.

- Is the child having any trouble breathing? When did it start or occur (time, sudden, gradual)? What was the child doing when it began? How long did it last? Does it come and go? Is it still present?
- Does the child have a cough? If yes, what does the cough sound like? When does it occur? Does the cough bring up any sputum? What does the sputum look like? Does the child have a history of a similar episode? If yes, what was the diagnosis?
- Does anything make the symptoms better or worse (e.g., cool air, tripod position, use of inhaler)?
- Does the child have any allergies to medications, foods, pets, dust, perfume, pollen, or cigarette smoke? If yes, how does the child's allergy affect his or her breathing?
- Does the child have a history of asthma or reactive airway disease? Has the child ever been hospitalized or intubated for this condition?
- What medications does the child take (e.g., prescription, over-the-counter, recreational)? When was the last dose?
- Does the child depend on a machine to assist breathing, such as a home ventilator?
- Has the child recently had a cold, flu, earache, pneumonia, or other infection? What about recent injuries or accidents (e.g., chest trauma, submersion incident)? Is there a possibility of foreign body aspiration?
- Will the child drink? Has he been drooling? Has the child had a fever? For how long? Has the child's voice changed? Are siblings sick?
- What treatments have you already provided for the child?

Emergency care for positive findings includes monitoring the child's breathing during assessment and transport.

Circulation. If any external bleeding is present, ask the parents how much blood they think the child has lost in tablespoons or cups (but remember that their estimate may not be accurate). If the child has had vomiting or diarrhea, ask how often and for how long it has occurred. Make a note if the child is not drinking fluids. Try to determine when the child last urinated. Ask about the volume, color, and odor of the urine.

Emergency care for positive findings includes carefully reassessing the child for signs of poor circulation and shock.

Neurologic and Developmental History. Ask the following questions if the child has had a seizure:

- What was the child doing at the time of the seizure?
- Did the child cry out or attract your attention in any way?
- What did the seizure look like? When did the seizure start? How long did it last?
- Did the seizure begin in one area of the body and progress to others?
- Did the child lose bowel or bladder control?
- When the child awoke, did he or she show any change in speech or ability to move the arms or legs?
- Did the child hit his or her head or fall?
- Has the child recently had a fever, headache, or stiff neck?
- Does the child have a history of seizures? Was this seizure different from past seizures?

Ask about the child's normal behavior and abilities. How well does the child generally move, sit, and talk? Have any changes occurred in the child's behavior or abilities?

Emergency care for positive findings includes monitoring the child's airway and breathing.

Fever. Ask the following questions regarding an elevated temperature:

- When did the fever begin and how high was it? Record the temperature reading and the method used to measure it (e.g., rectal, oral, axillary, tympanic). If the child has a fever (rectal temperature of 100.5° F or higher), ask whether any changes in mental status, breathing, muscle tone, or coordination have occurred.
- What remedies have been used to reduce the fever (e.g., sponging with tepid water, giving acetaminophen or ibuprofen)? If medication was given, how much was given? When was the last dose? What was the child's response to the measures taken?
- Has the child had recent immunizations? What about exposure to other ill children or adults?
- Does the child have any associated symptoms such as chills, headache, malaise, earache, sore throat, cough, flank pain, painful or frequent urination, poor feeding, irritability, vomiting, diarrhea, altered mental status, bulging or sunken fontanelles, rash, or stiff neck?
- Does the child have any risk factors for serious infections such as sickle cell disease, human immunodeficiency infection, recent cancer therapy, or respiratory, cardiac, or renal disease?
- Has the child's physician mentioned any reason the child might need special care during a fever?

All children with fever should be evaluated by a physician if possible. Fever and any other risk factor give additional cause to transport. Reassess for changes in mental status and ABCs during transport. If a child shows signs of heat stroke and altered mental status, work quickly to lower the child's temperature (see Chapter 52).

Poisoning. If **poisoning** is suspected, determine the following:

- What is the **poison**? Determine the exact name of the product if possible. Obtain histories from different family members to help confirm the type and dose of exposure. Do any pill bottles, commercial products, or plants support the history?
- How was the poison taken (ingested, inhaled, absorbed, or injected)?
- When was it taken?
- Where was the child found? How long was the child alone? Did anyone witness the event? Were any other children around?
- How much was taken?
  - Number of pills, amount of liquid
  - What was the available amount before ingestion?
  - How much is now in the container?
- Where is the substance stored?
- What is the child's age and weight?
- Has the child had any seizures, abdominal pain, rashes, or changes in behavior? Has the child vomited? How many times?
- What home remedies have been attempted (ask specifically about herbal or folk remedies)?
- Has a poison control center been contacted? If so, what instructions were received? What treatment has already been given?
- Has the child been depressed or experienced recent emotional stress?

Immediately contact a poison control center or medical direction for instructions. Instructions offered by poison control may or may not be able to be followed depending on local protocol. *Always* ask for the container the poison was in and take it to the hospital if possible. If the child took pills but which kind is unclear, take all the pill bottles in the home. Make sure receiving personnel know if the incident may have been a suicide attempt. Transport all children who have been poisoned.

Trauma and Burns

Mechanism of Injury

- How did the injury occur? When?
  - Circumstances of the incident: Does the explanation for how the trauma occurred fit the injury and the child's abilities?

Fall Injury

- What was the height of the fall?
- On what type of surface did the child land?

Motor Vehicle Crash

- What was the site of impact (lateral, frontal)? What was the estimated speed of the vehicle? What was struck (a moving or stationary object)? What is the amount of damage to the vehicle?
- Where was the child located in the vehicle? Was the child restrained? Was the child's safety seat properly secured?
- Was the vehicle equipped with an air bag? If so, did the air bag deploy?
- Was the child ejected from the vehicle? Was prolonged extrication required? Did anyone die on the scene?

Pedestrian Injury

- If the child was struck by a car and thrown while walking, roller skating, or bicycling, was he or she wearing a helmet? If so, is it still in place or was it knocked off the head on impact? Was the helmet damaged?
- How fast was the car traveling?
- Where was the child struck?
- How far was the child thrown? On what type of surface did the child land?

Bicycle Injury

- If struck by a motor vehicle, was the vehicle moving or stationary? If moving, what was the estimated speed?
- Was the child wearing a helmet? If so, is it still in place or was it knocked off the head on impact? Was the helmet damaged?

Penetrating Trauma

- Where is the wound(s) located?
- What are the type, caliber, and velocity of the weapon?
- From what distance was the child shot (close range or long range) or stabbed?
- Are powder burns surrounding the wounds?
- How many shots or stab wounds are present?
- What was the estimated blood loss at the scene?

Burns

- Where is the burn located?
- What caused the burn (e.g., fire, scalding, electrical shock, chemicals)?
- How long ago did the injury occur?
- What treatment has been given?

Chronology

- What was the initial GCS score?
- What was the child's behavior like immediately after the incident (e.g., crying, stunned, seizure, unconscious)?

- Did the child lose consciousness immediately or shortly after the incident? Duration?
- Did the child have any breathing problems after the injury?

Watch the child for changes involving responsiveness, breathing, or circulation. Make a note regarding the possibility of child abuse if the caregiver's explanation for how the trauma occurred does not seem to fit the injury and the child's abilities. Do not delay transport or confront the caregiver about it.

Children with burns from a fire in an enclosed space are at high risk for respiratory problems caused by breathing smoke and hot gases. Monitor airway and breathing, give oxygen, and transport to a pediatric critical care center, if available.

Drowning. In situations involving a drowning victim, you should determine how long the victim was submersed, the fluid in which the victim was submersed, and the events surrounding the incident. Questions to consider include the following:

- When was the child last seen? What is the estimated length of submersion?
- How much time elapsed before CPR was started?
- Did the child lose consciousness?
- Could any trauma be possible (e.g., diving injury)?
- What was the approximate water temperature (e.g., warm, tepid, cold, icy)?
- Did the child use alcohol or other drugs before the incident?
- Was the water clean or contaminated, salt or fresh?
- Does the patient have any medical history that may have contributed to the incident (e.g., seizures, asthma)?
- Were barriers present around the body of water (e.g., pool fence)?
- Was the child using a flotation device? What type? Did it fit properly?
- What was the child's appearance when pulled from the water (e.g., limp, blue, apneic, pulseless)?

Emergency care for positive findings includes beginning efforts to restore oxygenation, ventilation, and perfusion as quickly as possible.

History for a Newborn. If you are called to assist in a field delivery, ask whether the mother is expecting more than one baby. Find out whether labor is occurring more than 4 weeks before the expected due date. If the mother's bag of waters has broken, ask whether the fluid was brownish or greenish. If possible, determine whether the mother has a recent history of substance abuse, especially heroin or methadone. If multiple births are expected, call for additional help.

Physical Examination

In patients with urgent problems, provide initial care for life-threatening conditions and begin rapid transport without delay. Begin the physical examination during transport if time allows and does not interfere with ongoing assessment and management of ABCDE. Do not be concerned if you do not have time to complete the examination before reaching the hospital. For patients whose condition is nonurgent, begin the physical examination on the scene. If possible, try to examine whatever the caregiver is most worried about first and whatever is most painful last. If something hurts, avoid moving it.

The assessment procedure outlined appears as a head-to-toe sequence; however, the sequence should be reversed (toe to head) in infants and young children. By beginning with the extremities and then moving toward the head, you reduce the likelihood of frightening an infant or young child. Try to gain the child's trust as you provide care by being calm, friendly, and reassuring.

The purpose of the physical examination is to detect non–life-threatening conditions and provide care for those conditions and injuries. A detailed physical examination is presented here for completeness. A focused physical examination may be more appropriate depending on the patient's presentation and chief complaint.

Inspect and palpate each of the major body areas for DCAP-BLS-TIC (***d***eformities, ***c***ontusions, ***a***brasions, ***p***enetrations/punctures, ***b***urns, ***l***acerations, ***s***welling/edema, ***t***enderness, ***i***nstability, ***c***repitus). Auscultate breath and heart sounds.

Head and Face

- *Scalp and skull.* Look for DCAP-BLS. Feel for DCAP-BLS-TIC, depressions, and protrusions. In a child younger than 14 months, gently palpate the anterior and posterior fontanelles on the top of the head with the child in a sitting position (if no trauma is suspected). A bulging anterior fontanel may be caused by crying, coughing, vomiting, or increased intracranial pressure from a head injury, meningitis, or hydrocephalus. A depressed anterior fontanelle is seen in dehydrated or malnourished infants. If the fontanels are bulging or sunken, reassess the child's mental status and airway.
- *Ears.* Look for DCAP-BLS, ecchymosis behind the ears (Battle's sign), and blood or clear fluid in the ears. Feel for DCAP-BLS-TIC, including tenderness or pain. If drainage is coming from the ears, consider the child's condition urgent and reassess for breathing problems and changes in mental status.
- *Face.* Look for DCAP-BLS, singed facial hair, and symmetry of facial expression. Feel the orbital rims, zygoma, maxilla, and mandible for DCAP-BLS-TIC, neurovascular impairment, muscle spasm, false motion, or motor impairment.

- *Eyes*. Look for DCAP-BLS, foreign body, blood in the anterior chamber of the eye (hyphema), presence of eyeglasses or contact lenses, raccoon eyes, color of sclera and conjunctiva, periorbital edema, pupils (size, shape, equality, reactivity to light), and eye movement (dysconjugate gaze, ocular muscle function). Determine the pediatric GCS score.
- *Nose*. Look for DCAP-BLS, blood or fluid from the nose, singed nasal hairs, and nares for flaring. Feel for DCAP-BLS-TIC.
- *Mouth, throat, and pharynx*. Look for DCAP-BLS, blood, absent or broken teeth, gastric contents, and foreign objects (e.g., loose teeth, gum, small toys) as well as an injured or swollen tongue, color of the mucous membranes of the mouth, presence and character of fluids, vomitus, sputum color, amount, and consistency. Listen for hoarseness or inability to talk. Note any unusual odors (e.g., alcohol, acetone).

Neck

Look for DCAP-BLS, neck veins (flat or distended), use of accessory muscles, presence of a stoma, and presence of a medical identification device. Assessing distended neck veins in infants and young children is difficult. Feel for DCAP-BLS-TIC, subcutaneous emphysema, and tracheal position. If you find neck stiffness in an infant or child who appears sick, particularly with a history of fever, watch for altered mental status, breathing problems, and shock.

Chest

- *Look:* Work of breathing, symmetry of movement, use of accessory muscles, retractions, abnormal breathing patterns, DCAP-BLS, vascular access devices.
- *Listen:* Equality of breath sounds; abnormal breath sounds **(crackles, wheezes);** and heart sounds for rate, rhythm, murmurs, and muffled heart tones. If breath sounds seem louder on one side than the other, reassess for breathing problems and obtain further history information.
- Feel for DCAP-BLS-TIC, including chest wall tenderness, symmetry of chest wall expansion, and subcutaneous emphysema.

Abdomen

- Look for DCAP-BLS, distention, scars from healed or recent surgical incisions, penetrating wounds, feeding tubes, use of abdominal muscles during respiration, signs of injury, and discoloration.
- Although not always possible (or feasible), consider auscultating to determine the presence or absence of bowel sounds in all quadrants.
- Feel all four quadrants for DCAP-BLS for guarding, distention, rigidity, or masses.
- If guarding and tenderness are present, reassess the child's circulatory status for signs of shock. If the abdomen appears distended and the child has been crying, watch for breathing problems. The child may have swallowed a lot of air from crying. The swallowed air can press against the diaphragm, making the child's breathing difficult to hear.

Pelvis and Genitalia

- If the child reports pain, injury, or other problems in the genital area, look for DCAP-BLS, discharge or drainage from the meatus, priapism (spinal cord injury, sickle cell disease), and scrotal bleeding or swelling.
- Feel for DCAP-BLS-TIC. Assess strength and quality of femoral pulses. Grating sounds suggest a pelvic fracture. In such cases look for signs of internal bleeding and shock.

Extremities

In an alert child, begin your assessment of the extremities by evaluating the lower extremities first. In an injured extremity, be sure to assess distal pulses and neurovascular integrity distal to the injury. Compare an injured extremity with an uninjured extremity and document your findings.

- Look for DCAP-BLS, vascular access devices, **purpura, petechiae,** presence of congenital anomalies (e.g., finger clubbing, clubfoot), abnormal extremity position, and medical identification bracelet.
- Feel for DCAP-BLS-TIC. Assess skin temperature, moisture, and capillary refill in each extremity. Assess the strength and quality of pulses, motor function, and sensory function in each extremity.

If any area shows swelling, deformity, tenderness, or ecchymoses, immobilize the area. If movement in the extremities is unequal, stabilize the spine and immobilize the affected extremity. If an injured arm or leg has poor capillary refill and lacks a pulse or sensation, consider it to be at risk, especially if, after gentle straightening or splinting, these signs are noticeably different from the other arm or leg. Consider the child's condition urgent and prepare for rapid transport.

Posterior Body

If trauma is suspected, make sure that manual in-line stabilization of the head and spine is maintained during the examination. If a child requires stabilization on a spine board, quickly assess for injuries to the child's back before placing the child on the board.

- Look for DCAP-BLS, purpura, petechiae, rashes, and edema.
- Auscultate the posterior chest.
- Feel the posterior trunk for DCAP-BLS.

Reassessment

Continually monitor the following:

- Ventilatory effort
- Color
- Mental status
- Pulse oximetry
- Vital signs

CAREGIVER'S RESPONSE TO EMERGENCIES

[OBJECTIVE 5]

Situations involving an ill or injured child are stressful for the patient and the child's family. Therefore when treating a child, you also must remember to treat the family.

Expect a grief reaction. Initially the caregiver may show guilt, fear, anger, denial, shock, or a loss of control. Remain calm and professional. This behavior is likely to change during the course of the emergency. Accept their fears and concerns and reassure them that their feelings are legitimate. Do not condescend to them or ignore their concerns.

Remember that infants, toddlers, preschool, and school-age patients do not like to be separated from their caregiver. Use the child's caregiver to help make the infant or child more comfortable. For example, have the caregiver locate the child's favorite toy or blanket. Enlist the caregiver's help to calm the child during painful procedures. Keep the caregiver informed about what you are doing as you assess and care for the child.

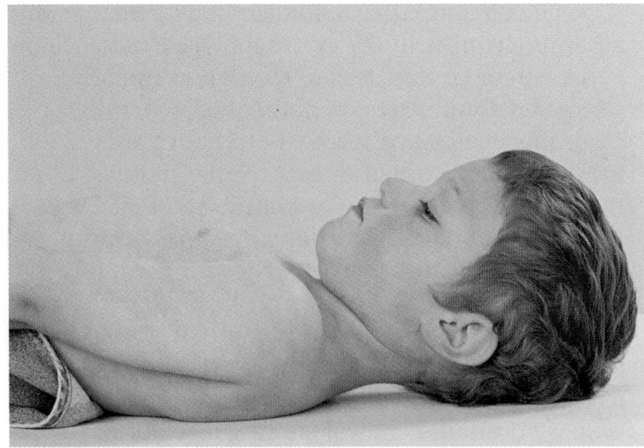

Figure 37-5 The prominent occiput of an infant or young child often causes passive flexion of the neck when the child is placed in a supine position on a flat surface.

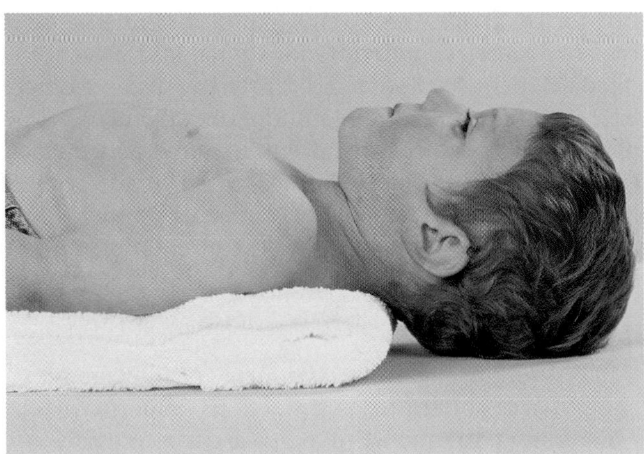

Figure 37-6 To maintain the head and cervical spine in a neutral position, place padding under the torso of an infant or young child. The padding should be of appropriate thickness so that the child's shoulders are in horizontal alignment with the ear canal.

GENERAL MANAGEMENT OF INFANTS AND CHILDREN

Airway and Breathing Support

[OBJECTIVES 6, 7, 8, 9]

Allow an ill child to assume a position of comfort. The prominent occiput of infants and young children often causes flexion of the neck when the child is placed in a supine position on a flat surface (Figure 37-5). Flexion of the neck may compromise air exchange or aggravate an existing spinal cord injury. An injured child younger than 3 years usually needs padding under the torso. The padding should be firm, evenly shaped, and extend from the shoulders to the pelvis (Figure 37-6). It should be of appropriate thickness so that the child's shoulders are in horizontal alignment with the ear canal.

A foreign body airway obstruction should be cleared according to current resuscitation guidelines. Use back slaps and chest thrusts for infants. Use abdominal thrusts for children.

Apply a pulse oximeter and administer oxygen as necessary to maintain an oxygen saturation of at least 94%. When suctioning, avoid hypoxia and upper airway stimulation. If the child will not tolerate a nonrebreather mask, use blow-by oxygen. Direct the oxygen tubing or mask near the child's nose and mouth. Consider attaching the oxygen tubing to a toy and encourage the child to hold the toy near the face or try placing the tubing in a paper cup, then ask the child to drink from the cup. When possible, allow the child's caregiver to give blow-by oxygen.

To determine the proper size oral airway for an infant or child, hold the device against the side of the patient's face. Select an airway that extends from the corner of the mouth to the angle of the jaw. The preferred technique for oral airway insertion in an infant or child requires the use of a tongue blade to depress the tongue.

To determine the proper size of nasal airway, hold the device against the side of the patient's face and select an airway that extends from the tip of the nose to the angle of the jaw or the tip of the ear. In general, nasal airways are not useful in infants and small children. The small internal size of an airway that will fit these patients does not allow adequate airflow.

Bag-mask devices are available in various sizes. Be sure to select a device with sufficient volume for the patient's size. Use a 450- to 500-mL (pediatric) bag for term newborns, infants, and children. Use a 1200-mL (adult) bag for larger children and adolescents. Do not use a 250-mL (neonatal) bag because this size does not provide sufficient volume for term newborns.

Gastric distention is a complication of positive-pressure ventilation that can lead to vomiting and aspiration. Gastric distention also restricts movement of the diaphragm, impeding ventilation. Consider insertion of a gastric tube to decrease gastric distention when the patient requires bag-mask ventilation.

You may need to attempt endotracheal intubation around a foreign body or use direct laryngoscopy with Magill forceps to remove a foreign body airway obstruction. If a complete upper airway obstruction is present, consider needle cricothyroidotomy only as a last resort and in consultation with medical direction. If endotracheal intubation is necessary in an infant or child, determine the correct size of equipment with a length-based resuscitation tape. Reassess and confirm the position of the tracheal tube at the following times:

- Immediately after tube insertion
- Whenever the patient is moved or repositioned
- Whenever a procedure is performed (suctioning)
- When the patient's clinical status changes
- During transport

The procedure for endotracheal intubation and complications of this procedure are discussed in Chapter 14.

Circulatory Support

Peripheral Venous Access

[OBJECTIVES 10, 11]

If peripheral intravenous (IV) access is needed, scalp veins may be used in infants. Scalp veins are very small veins found close to the surface and are more easily seen than extremity veins. However, they are rarely useful during resuscitation efforts. They may be useful for fluid and medication administration after patient stabilization. In infants and children, forearm veins and dorsal hand veins may be used (Figure 37-7). Forearm veins may be hard to locate in chubby infants.

Lower extremity veins such as the saphenous and dorsal venous arch also may be used (Figure 37-8).

Intraosseous Infusion

Intraosseous infusion is the process of infusing medications, fluids, and blood products into the bone marrow cavity. Because the marrow cavity is continuous with the venous circulation, fluids and medications administered by the intraosseous (IO) route subsequently are delivered to the venous circulation. In the presence of cardiac arrest or decompensated shock, an IO infusion should be established in any patient when IV access cannot be rapidly obtained. Venous access often is easier to obtain after initial fluid and medication resuscitation by the IO route.

Indications. Indications for the IO route of administration include the following circumstances:

- Cardiopulmonary arrest or decompensated shock in which vascular access is essential and venous access is not readily achieved
- Multisystem trauma with associated shock and/or severe hypovolemia
- Unresponsive patient in need of immediate medications or fluid resuscitation (e.g., burns, sepsis, drowning, anaphylaxis, status epilepticus)
- Presence of burns or a traumatic injury preventing access to the venous system at another site

Procedure. The preferred site for IO infusion is the anteromedial surface of the proximal tibia because of the broad flat surface of the bone, the thin layer of skin that covers it, and the ease of palpation of this bony landmark. Use of the proximal tibia does not interfere with airway management and CPR.

To perform this procedure, begin by assembling all necessary equipment and taking infection control precautions. Place the infant or child in a supine position. Place a towel roll or small sandbag in the popliteal fossa to provide support, optimize positioning, and minimize the risk of fractures (Figure 37-9).

Identify the landmarks for needle insertion. Palpate the tibial tuberosity. The site for IO insertion lies 1 to 3 cm (1 finger width) below this tuberosity on the medial flat surface of the anterior tibia. Cleanse the intended insertion site. Stabilize the patient's leg. With the needle angled away from the joint, insert the needle with firm pressure. Advance the needle by using a twisting motion at an angle of 60 to 90 degrees away from the epiphyseal plate (i.e., toward the toes). Advance the needle until a sudden decrease in resistance or a "pop" is felt as the needle enters the marrow cavity. Unscrew the cap, remove the stylet from the needle, attach a 10-mL saline-filled syringe to the needle, and attempt to aspirate bone marrow into the syringe. If aspiration is successful, slowly inject 10 to 20 mL of saline to clear the needle of marrow, bone fragments, and/or tissue. Observe for any swelling at the site. If aspiration is unsuccessful, consider the following indicators of correct needle position:

- The needle stands firmly without support.
- A sudden loss of resistance occurred on entering the marrow cavity (this is less obvious in infants than in older children because infants have soft bones).

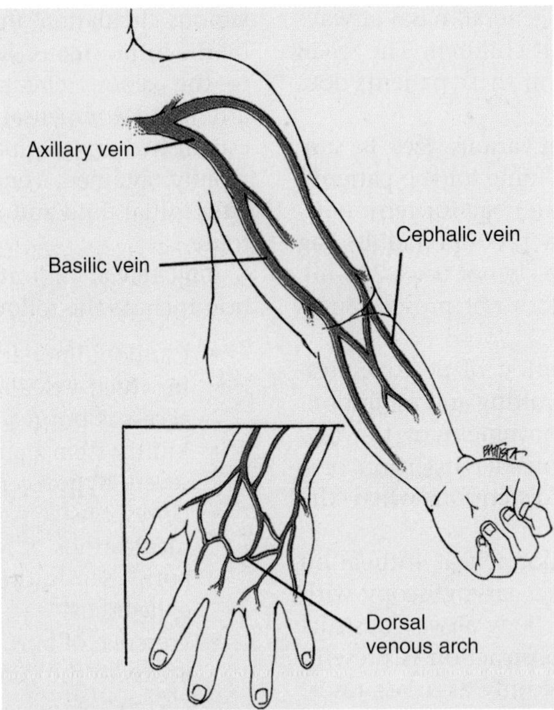

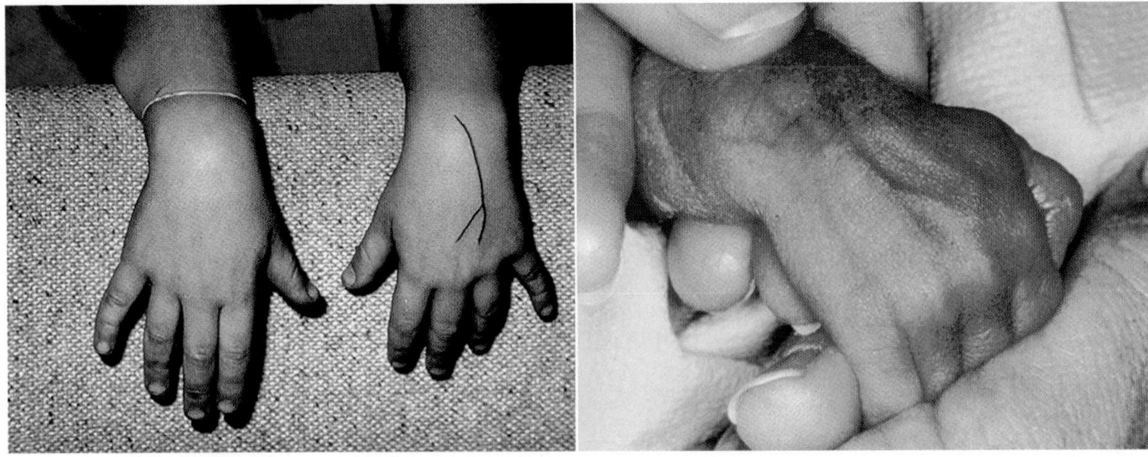

Figure 37-7 Veins of the forearm and hand.

- Fluid flows freely through the needle without signs of significant swelling of the subcutaneous tissue.

If signs of infiltration are present, remove the IO needle and attempt the procedure at another site. If no signs of infiltration are present, attach standard IV tubing. A syringe, pressure infuser, or IV infusion pump may be needed to infuse fluids. Secure the needle and tubing in place with a sterile dressing and tape. Check the site every 5 to 10 minutes for the duration of the infusion. Watch for signs of infiltration and assess distal pulses. Document the procedure.

Contraindications

- Femoral fracture on the same side as the proposed insertion site
- Fracture at or above the insertion site
- Severe burn overlying the insertion site (unless this is the only available site)
- Infection at insertion site (unless this is the only available site)
- Use of the same bone in which an unsuccessful IO attempt was made
- Congenital bone disorders (osteopetrosis, osteogenesis imperfecta [high fracture potential])

Possible Problems Encountered with Intraosseous Infusion. Possible complications of IO infusion include the following:

- Incomplete penetration of the bony cortex
- Penetration of the posterior cortex
- Fluid or medications escaping around the needle through the puncture site

- Fluid leaking through a nearby previous cortical puncture site
- Fracture of the tibia
- Local abscess or cellulitis
- Lower extremity compartment syndrome
- Osteomyelitis
- Loss of vascular access site because of needle obstruction by marrow, bone fragments, or tissue

Transport Considerations

[OBJECTIVES 12, 13]

The goal in the emergency treatment of children is to stabilize the patient for transport to an appropriate facility that can provide definitive care. Depending on the situation, this may be a pediatric emergency department, pediatric trauma center, burn center, or other specialty center (if available in your area). Decide if the patient's condition requires transport by ground ambulance, with or without lights and sirens, or air ambulance.

En route to the hospital, remember to use age-appropriate words and phrases when talking to the child. Keep the child warm and allow him or her to have his favorite toy or blanket if possible.

Do not delay transport to perform procedures that can be done en route. Be sure that appropriate basic life support care is performed before advanced life support care. If you must perform ongoing care that requires a flat surface, such as bag-mask ventilation or CPR, place the child on a spine board or stretcher. For children with less serious conditions that do not require spine board stabilization and ongoing care, transport them with a restraint device (e.g., a child safety seat) appropriate for their size and age. Properly secure safety seats in the ambulance. Parents riding along with the patient should use seat belts or other restraints.

During transport, relay your initial assessment findings, vital signs, care you have provided, and any other critical information to the receiving facility so that hospital staff will be prepared with appropriate personnel and equipment.

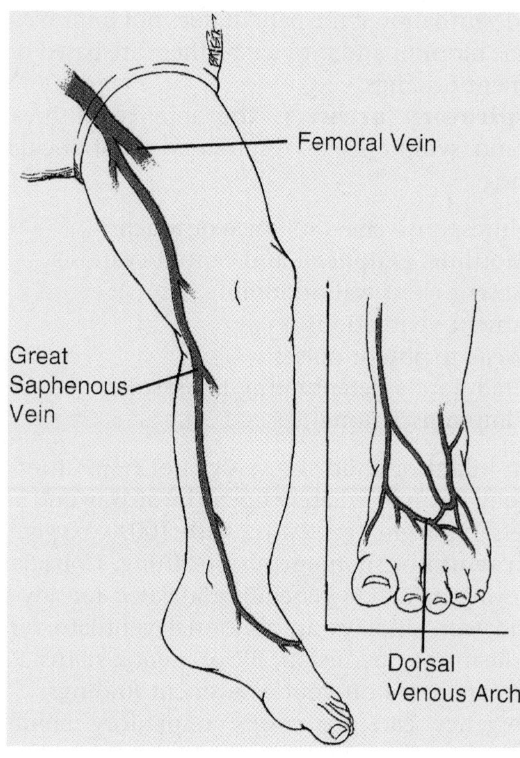

Figure 37-8 Lower extremity veins.

SPECIFIC PATHOPHYSIOLOGY, ASSESSMENT, AND MANAGEMENT

Respiratory Compromise

[OBJECTIVES 14, 15]

Respiratory illnesses can cause respiratory compromise in the upper and lower airways. Categories of respiratory compromise include upper airway obstruction and lower airway disease. A foreign body may block the upper or lower airways. Conditions that may cause upper airway obstruction include croup, epiglottitis, and bacterial tracheitis. Conditions that may cause lower airway disease include asthma, bronchiolitis, and pneumonia.

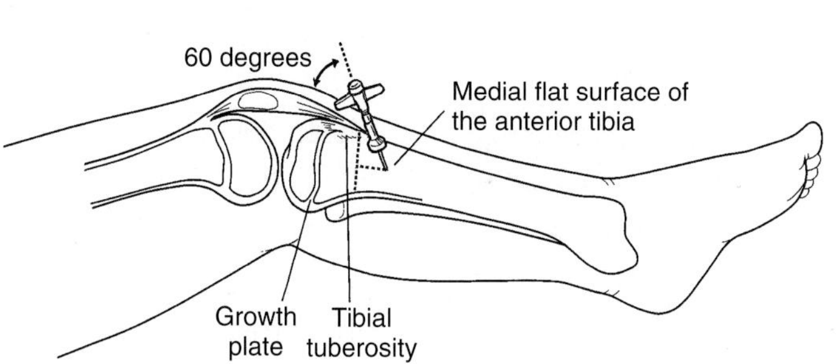

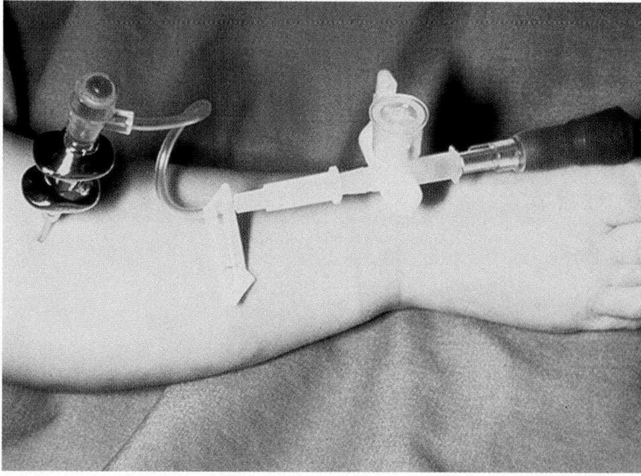

Figure 37-9 Anterior tibial approach for intraosseous infusion.

Respiratory compromise can be classified according to severity: respiratory distress (least severe), respiratory failure, and respiratory arrest (most severe). The severity of respiratory compromise depends on the extent of respiratory illness. Your treatment plan for a child with a respiratory problem depends on the severity of respiratory compromise.

Respiratory distress is increased work of breathing (ventilatory effort). As the child's breathing rate increases, arterial carbon dioxide levels in the blood initially decrease. With continued respiratory distress, the child will begin to tire and arterial carbon dioxide levels will increase. If uncorrected, respiratory distress leads to respiratory failure.

Respiratory distress may result from a problem in the tracheobronchial tree, lungs, pleura, or chest wall. Causes of respiratory distress are shown in Box 37-6.

Signs and symptoms of respiratory distress include the following:

- Irritability, anxiety, restlessness
- Stridor, grunting, gurgling
- Audible wheezing
- Retractions
- Ventilatory rate faster than normal for age (tachypnea)
- Increased depth of breathing **(hyperpnea)**
- See-saw breathing (abdominal breathing)
- Nasal flaring
- Neck muscle use
- Central cyanosis that resolves with oxygen
- Mild tachycardia

Approach a child in respiratory distress promptly, but work at a moderate pace. Permit the child to assume a position of comfort. Correct hypoxia by giving oxygen without causing agitation. Apply a cardiac monitor and provide further care based on your assessment findings.

Respiratory failure is a clinical condition in which blood oxygenation and/or ventilation is inadequate to meet the metabolic demands of body tissues. Respiratory failure is the most common cause of cardiopulmonary arrest in children. It often is preceded by respiratory distress in which the child's work of breathing is increased in an attempt to compensate for hypoxia. Possible causes of respiratory failure are listed in Box 37-7.

BOX 37-6 Respiratory Distress: Possible Causes

- Asthma or reactive airway disease
- Aspiration
- Foreign body
- Congenital heart disease
- Infection, such as pneumonia, croup, epiglottitis, or bronchiolitis
- Medication or **toxin** exposure
- Trauma

Signs and symptoms of respiratory failure include the following:

- Sleepiness, intermittent combativeness or agitation
- Normal or decreased muscle tone
- Central cyanosis despite giving oxygen; mottling
- Decreased level of responsiveness or response to pain
- Inadequate ventilatory rate, effort, or chest excursion
- Tachypnea with periods of bradypnea, slowing to bradypnea or agonal breathing

If an infant or child shows signs of respiratory failure, move quickly. Open the airway and suction if necessary. Correct hypoxia by giving supplemental oxygen. Begin assisted ventilation if the patient does not improve. Apply a cardiac monitor and provide further care based on your assessment findings.

Respiratory arrest is the absence of breathing. Signs and symptoms of respiratory arrest include the following:

- Unresponsiveness to voice or touch
- Mottling; peripheral and central cyanosis
- Absent chest wall motion
- Absent ventilations
- Weak to absent pulses
- Bradycardia deteriorating to asystole
- Limp muscle tone

If an infant or child shows signs of respiratory arrest, move quickly. Immediately open the airway and suction if necessary. Begin ventilating with 100% oxygen. Reassess for return of spontaneous breathing. Consider ECG monitoring, which is generally indicated for any infant or child who displays an abnormal ventilatory rate or effort, heart rate, perfusion, BP, or mental status. Provide further care based on your assessment findings.

Emergency care for severe respiratory failure and respiratory arrest includes ventilation with a bag-mask

BOX 37-7 Respiratory Failure: Possible Causes

- Infection such as croup, epiglottitis, bronchiolitis, pneumonia
- Foreign body
- Asthma or reactive airway disease
- Smoke inhalation
- Submersion syndrome
- Pneumothorax, hemothorax
- Congenital abnormalities
- Neuromuscular disease
- Medication or toxin exposure
- Trauma
- Heart failure
- Metabolic disease with acidosis

device with 100% oxygen. Endotracheal intubation may be needed if positive-pressure ventilation does not rapidly improve the child's condition. Consider gastric decompression if abdominal distention is impeding ventilation. Consider needle decompression per medical direction if a tension pneumothorax is present. Consider cricothyroidotomy per medical direction only as a last resort if complete upper airway obstruction is present. Indicators of improvement in the child's condition include improvement in level of responsiveness, color, oxygen saturation, and pulse rate.

Foreign Body Airway Obstruction

Definition and Description. Foreign body airway obstruction (FBAO) may be seen at any age, but children younger than 5 years are especially vulnerable. Suspect FBAO in any previously well, afebrile child with a sudden onset of respiratory distress and associated coughing, choking, stridor, or wheezing.

Etiology. Common causes of FBAO in children are given in Box 37-8. Hot dogs and bread are two of the most common causes of fatal aspiration. Because they absorb moisture, dried foods (such as beans and peas) may cause progressive airway obstruction. Peanut butter is particularly hard to remove by coughing or with the use of instruments such as Magill forceps.

Epidemiology and Demographics. Children younger than 3 years of age account for 73% of cases of FBAO. In adults, FBAO most often occurs during eating. In infants and children, most episodes of choking occur during eating or play. Poor supervision by adults or older siblings occasionally is a contributing factor.

History. Fewer than 50% of children will have a history of witnessed or suspected foreign body aspiration or a choking spell. The child is frequently examined after a sudden episode of coughing or choking while eating, with subsequent wheezing, coughing, or stridor.

PARAMEDIC*Pearl*

The symptoms, physical findings, and complications produced by a foreign body depend on the following:

- The size and composition of the material aspirated (inert, caustic, organic)
- The location of the foreign body (esophagus, larynx, trachea, bronchus)
- The degree and duration of obstruction

Physical Examination. Signs and symptoms of FBAO include a sudden onset of respiratory distress; abnormal respiratory sounds, including wheezing, inspiratory stridor, or decreased breath sounds; coughing or gagging; agitation; and/or cyanosis.

Therapeutic Interventions. Emergency care for FBAO depends on whether the patient is an infant or a child and conscious or unconscious. Procedures to remove an FBAO are discussed in Chapter 14.

BOX 37-8 Common Causes of FBAO in Children

- Nuts
- Raisins
- Sunflower seeds
- Popcorn
- Peanut butter
- Beans, peas
- Bread
- Improperly chewed pieces of meat, grapes, hot dogs, raw carrots, sausages
- Fruit-flavored gel snacks
- Balloons
- Disc batteries
- Pins
- Rings
- Nails
- Buttons
- Coins
- Plastic or metal toy objects
- Marbles

FBAO, Foreign body airway obstruction.

Patient and Family Education. Give the family tips about how to childproof the home. Check all toys for loose, chipped, or broken parts. Check the clothing of an infant or small child for loose snaps or buttons and mend if needed. Check pacifiers and bottle nipples for cracks. Cracked ones should be thrown away. Because toddlers often pick up items such as pins and small bits of food off the floor, vacuum floors often. Discourage school-age children from placing the cap of a pen, rubber band, or paper clip in their mouth.

Croup

[OBJECTIVES 16, 17]

Description and Definition. Croup (laryngotracheobronchitis) is a viral respiratory infection that affects the upper respiratory tract. The area below the glottis is most commonly affected, resulting in swollen, inflamed mucosa with associated hoarseness, inspiratory stridor, and a barking cough. The diagnosis is usually based on history and physical findings.

Etiology. Croup is caused by a respiratory virus. Parainfluenza types 1, 2, and 3 are the most common cause in up to 80% of cases (Sobal & Zapata, 2008), but it may also result from adenovirus, respiratory syncytial virus (RSV) (most common in patients younger than 5 years), varicella, herpes simplex virus measles, enteroviruses, *Mycoplasma pneumoniae*, and influenza viruses A and B.

Epidemiology and Demographics

- Croup is the most common infectious cause of acute upper airway obstruction in pediatrics.

- It primarily affects children aged 6 months to 3 years, peaking at age 2 years.
- The three parainfluenza viruses most often are seen in the fall. RSV has a midwinter peak and can be found in increasing numbers in the spring.
- Croup spreads by person-to-person contact or large droplets and contaminated nasopharyngeal secretions.
- Incubation period is 2 to 4 days.

History. The child's typical history of symptoms includes upper respiratory infection for 1 to 2 days, but it may be spasmodic (usually wakes from a nap or sleep). Croup is usually worse at night or when the child is agitated.

Physical Examination. Signs and symptoms of respiratory distress or failure depend on severity (Table 37-7) and include the following:

- Vital signs: increased ventilatory rate, increased heart rate, low-grade fever (usually less than 102.2° F)
- Loud stridor with hoarse voice and barking (seal-like) cough; stridor diminishes as muscles fatigue
- Nasal flaring
- Retractions (Figure 37-10)

Differential Diagnosis. Differential diagnosis includes the following conditions:

- Viral croup versus spasmodic croup
- Epiglottitis
- Bacterial tracheitis
- FBAO
- Asthma
- Anaphylaxis

Therapeutic Interventions. Keep the child as calm and as comfortable as possible, usually in the arms of the caregiver. Assess for FBAO *by history;* do not examine the oropharynx. This may agitate the child and worsen respiratory distress. Initiate pulse oximetry. Maintain an oxygen saturation of 94% or higher. It is important to note that the use of pulse oximetry in croup can be inaccurate. This is because a large degree of upper airway obstruction is required to produce hypoxia in an otherwise previously healthy child (Wright et al., 2002). If breathing is adequate and the child shows signs of respiratory distress, give oxygen in a way that does not agitate the child. If the child has mild croup, medical direction may instruct you to give nebulized saline. Nebulized racemic or levo-epinephrine may be ordered for moderate or severe croup. For many years, the use of cool, humidified air was thought to improve airflow through the edematous subglottis by decreasing the viscosity of secretions however, despite this common practice, studies have failed to demonstrate the benefit of cool mist in the outcome of moderate and severe croup. If signs of respiratory failure or respiratory arrest are present, assist breathing with a bag-mask device and 100% oxygen and apply a cardiac monitor.

Patient and Family Education. Tell the family to call 9-1-1 right away if the child starts drooling or has difficulty swallowing.

TABLE 37-7 Croup Severity

Severity	Signs and Symptoms
Mild croup	Normal color, normal mental status, air entry with stridor audible only with stethoscope, no retractions
Moderate croup	Normal color, audible stridor, mild to moderate retractions, slightly diminished air entry in an anxious child
Severe croup	Cyanosis, loud stridor, significant decrease in air entry, marked retractions in a highly anxious child

Epiglottitis

Description and Definition. Epiglottitis is a bacterial infection of the upper airway. It may progress to complete airway obstruction and death within hours unless adequate treatment is provided (Figure 37-11). Diagnosis often is based on history and observation of the child from a distance.

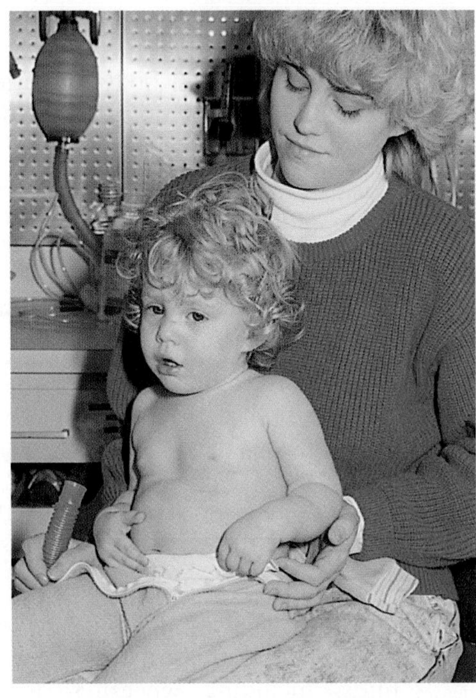

Figure 37-10 Croup. This toddler with moderate upper airway obstruction caused by croup had suprasternal and subcostal retractions. Her anxious expression was the result of mild hypoxia confirmed by pulse oximetry.

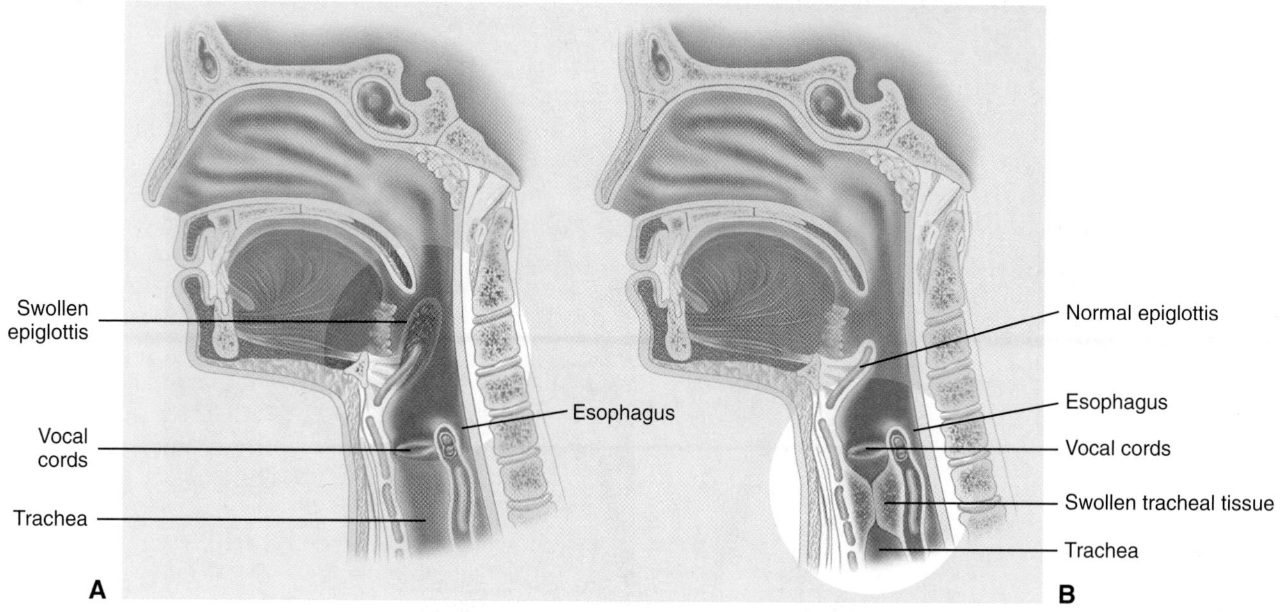

Figure 37-11 **A,** Acute epiglottitis. **B,** Laryngotracheobronchitis (croup).

Etiology. In the past, *Haemophilus influenzae* type B (HiB) was the most commonly identified cause of acute epiglottitis. Because of the widespread use of the HiB vaccine in the United States, the incidence of epiglottitis due to HiB in children has been greatly reduced. *Streptococcus pyogenes, Streptococcus pneumoniae,* and *Staphylococcus aureus* now represent a larger proportion of pediatric cases of epiglottitis.

Epidemiology and Demographics. Facts about epiglottitis include the following:

- Can occur at any age but typically affects children 2 to 7 years old
- Incidence is decreased in children because of widespread use of *H. influenzae* vaccine; prevalence is increasing in adolescents and adults
- No seasonal preference has been detected

History. The history of the patient with epiglottitis usually includes the following:

- Typically no previous history but a rapid onset of symptoms (6 to 8 hours)
- Can quickly progress to respiratory arrest
- Quiet, wet stridor; a muffled voice; difficulty swallowing; and a preference for sitting upright are characteristic of supraglottic disorders; absence of a cough is an important diagnostic clue
- Sudden onset of high fever
- Typically no other family members are ill with an acute upper respiratory illness

Physical Examination. Signs and symptoms of respiratory distress or failure depend on severity but may include the following:

- Acutely ill appearance
- Preference for sitting up and leaning forward (tripod position) with the mouth open (Figure 37-12)
- The "three Ds" (drooling, dysphagia, and distress) are considered the classic clinical findings of acute epiglottitis
- Muffled voice
- Shallow breathing
- Stridor is a *late* finding and suggests near-complete airway obstruction
- Vital signs: increased ventilatory rate, increased heart rate, and elevated temperature, usually 102° to 104° F

PEDIATRIC*Pearl*

Never force a child with respiratory distress to lie down. This may compromise the airway and cause immediate obstruction.

Differential Diagnosis. Differential diagnosis for epiglottitis includes the following:

- Croup
- Laryngitis
- Bacterial tracheitis
- FBAO
- Anaphylaxis

Therapeutic Interventions. Close observation and frequent reassessment are critical. Help the child into a position of comfort. Keep the child as calm and comfortable as possible, usually in the arms of the caregiver. *Do not examine the oropharynx* (this may agitate the child and worsen respiratory distress). Do not administer

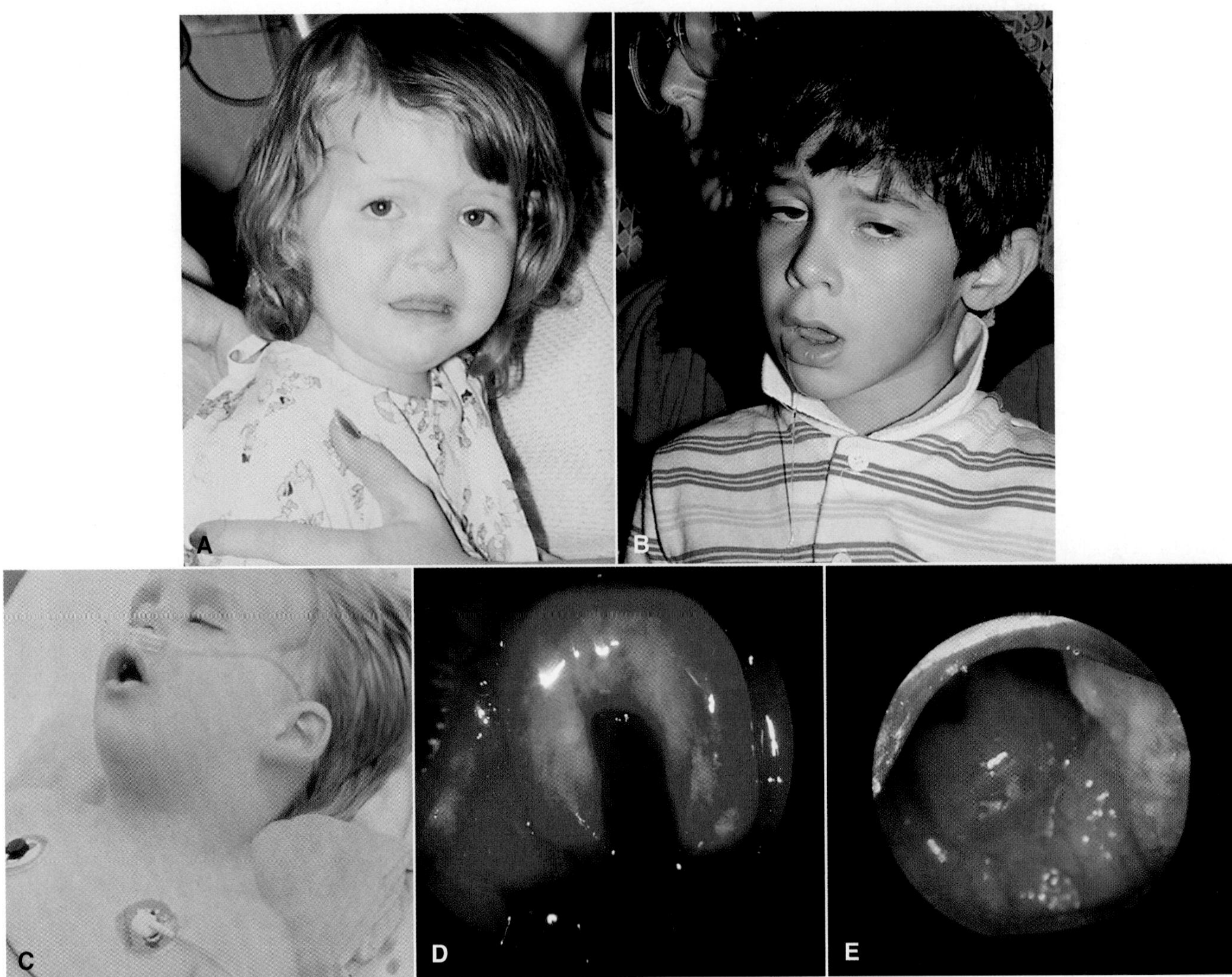

Figure 37-12 Epiglottitis. These three patients with acute epiglottitis demonstrate the varying degrees of distress that may be seen depending on age and time of presentation. **A,** This 3-year-old seen a few hours after the onset of symptoms was anxious and still, but had no positional preference or drooling. **B,** This 5-year-old, who had been symptomatic for several hours, holds his neck extended with the head held forward, is mouth breathing and drooling, and shows signs of tiring. **C,** This 2-year-old was in severe distress and was too exhausted to hold his head up. **D** and **E,** In the operating room, the epiglottis was visualized and appears intensely red and swollen. It may retain its omega shape or resemble a cherry.

anything by mouth. If breathing is adequate and the patient exhibits signs of respiratory distress, administer supplemental oxygen in a manner that does not agitate the child. Maintain an oxygen saturation of 94% or higher. If signs of respiratory failure or respiratory arrest are present, assist breathing with a bag-mask device with 100% oxygen.

Patient and Family Education. The incidence of epiglottitis caused by HiB can be decreased with a vaccine that is recommended for infants and children beginning at 2 months of age. At this time, epiglottitis caused by other organisms cannot be prevented.

Bacterial Tracheitis

Description and Definition. Bacterial **tracheitis** is an acute bacterial infection of the subglottic area of the upper airway. Bacterial tracheitis is complicated by copious thick, pus-filled secretions. The diagnosis is based on signs of bacterial upper airway disease, high fever, pus-like airway secretions, and an absence of the classic findings of epiglottitis. The child may worsen quickly because of airway obstruction from a pus-filled membrane that has loosened.

Etiology. Bacterial tracheitis is most often caused by *Staphylococcus aureus* and *Streptococcus pyogenes* (Sobal & Zapata, 2008).

Epidemiology and Demographics. Facts about bacterial tracheitis include the following:

- This life-threatening illness is now more common than epiglottitis (Roosevelt, 2004).
- Bacterial tracheitis can occur at any age and in any season.
- No clear gender differences are seen in incidence or severity.
- Controversy exists regarding whether bacterial tracheitis exists alone or whether it is a bacterial complication of a preexistent viral respiratory infection (e.g., croup).
- Fifty percent of children with bacterial tracheitis have an associated pneumonia.

History. The patient with bacterial tracheitis frequently has a several-day history of viral upper respiratory symptoms, such as fever, cough, and stridor, similar to croup. This may be followed by a rapid onset of high fever, respiratory distress, and a toxic appearance. Drooling is usually absent.

Physical Examination. Signs and symptoms of respiratory distress or failure may be present depending on severity in addition to the following:

- Inspiratory stridor with or without expiratory stridor
- Barking or brassy cough
- Hoarseness
- Typically no drooling
- Variable degrees of respiratory distress: retractions, dyspnea, nasal flaring, cyanosis
- Sore throat (minimal)
- Worsening or abruptly occurring stridor or respiratory distress

Differential Diagnosis. Differential diagnosis of bacterial tracheitis includes the following:

- Croup
- Epiglottitis
- FBAO

Therapeutic Interventions. Keep the child as calm and comfortable as possible, usually in the arms of the caregiver. Apply a pulse oximeter. If breathing is adequate and the patient exhibits signs of respiratory distress, administer oxygen in a manner that does not agitate the child.

Maintain an oxygen saturation of 94% or higher. If signs of respiratory failure or respiratory arrest are present, assist ventilation using a bag-mask device with supplemental oxygen.

If required, endotracheal intubation should be performed with an endotracheal tube 0.5 to 1 mm smaller than that calculated for age because of tracheal swelling and inflammation. Frequent suctioning often is necessary to maintain the patency of the tube. Apply a cardiac monitor and provide additional care based on your assessment findings.

Patient and Family Education. Bacterial tracheitis frequently follows a viral upper respiratory infection and is not preventable.

Asthma and Reactive Airway Disease

[OBJECTIVES 18, 19]

Definition and Description. **Asthma** (see Chapter 21) is a reversible obstructive airway disease characterized by chronic inflammation, hyperreactive airways, and episodes of bronchospasm.

Etiology. Asthma may be triggered by a stimulus such as an allergen, air pollution, exercise, cold air, or infection. The resulting swelling of the bronchial mucosa, bronchospasm, and mucus plugging vary in severity depending on the age of the child, the size and anatomy of the airways, the type of irritant that precipitates the obstruction, and the duration and severity of the asthma attack (Huether & McCance, 2000).

In most children both larger and smaller airways are obstructed. Ineffective ventilation results in hypoxemia. As the obstruction becomes more severe, air trapping, inadequate ventilation, more severe hypoxemia, and hypercapnia (hypoventilation) with respiratory acidosis occur. Respiratory failure becomes imminent.

Epidemiology and Demographics. Asthma is the most common pediatric chronic disease, affecting nearly 5 million children younger than 18 years in the United States. Although allergens play an important role in asthma, 20% to 40% of children with asthma have no evidence of allergic disease (Hueckel & Wilson, 2007). Factors influencing asthma development and factors that trigger asthma symptoms (some do both) include the following:

- Personal or family history of asthma or allergy
- Viral respiratory infections
- Indoor allergens (domestic mites, furred animals, cockroach allergen, fungi, molds, yeasts)
- Outdoor allergens (pollens, fungi, molds, yeasts)
- Occupational sensitizers
- Tobacco smoke
- Air pollution
- Diet

History. History of asthma typically includes recurrent respiratory symptoms (cough, wheeze, difficulty breathing, chest tightness) that often are worse at night. Wheezing, chest tightness, or cough may occur after exposure to airborne allergens or pollutants. Symptoms occur or worsen in the presence of exercise, viral infections, animals with fur (dogs, cats, mice), house dust mites, molds, smoke (tobacco, wood), pollen, changes in weather, and strong emotional depression.

Physical Examination. Signs and symptoms of respiratory distress or failure depend on severity and include the following:

- Wheezing (most common symptom)
- Dry cough

- Chest tightness
- Shortness of breath with exertion
- Retractions
- Tachypnea
- Poor air entry
- Prolonged expiratory phase

PEDIATRIC*Pearl*

- Assess the child's ability to complete a sentence (age dependent), presence of a cough, breathlessness, and chest tightness. Close monitoring is *essential*.
- Wheezing is an unreliable sign when evaluating the degree of distress in an asthmatic patient. An absence of wheezing may represent severe obstruction. With improvement, wheezing may become more prominent.
- In infants, breathlessness severe enough to prevent feeding is an important symptom of impending respiratory failure.

Differential Diagnosis. Differential diagnosis of asthma includes the following:

- Bronchiolitis
- Obstruction by foreign body or tumor
- Bronchospasm
- Congestive heart failure
- Epiglottitis
- Croup
- Anaphylaxis
- Inhalation injury

Therapeutic Interventions. Help the child into a position of comfort. If ventilation is adequate and the patient shows signs of respiratory distress, administer supplemental oxygen (if necessary) in a manner that does not agitate the child. Keep the oxygen saturation above 94%. If signs of respiratory failure or respiratory arrest are present, assist breathing with a bag-mask device with supplemental oxygen. Place the child on a cardiac monitor. If the child shows signs of respiratory distress or respiratory failure with evidence of bronchospasm or a history of asthma, give aerosolized bronchodilators as ordered by medical direction. Watch for tachycardia and vomiting. Endotracheal intubation may be needed for respiratory failure or arrest with prolonged bag-mask ventilation or an inadequate response to bag-mask ventilation.

Patient and Family Education. Patients and their families frequently do not understand asthma causes, treatment, and symptom prevention. Many children with asthma have frequent and/or severe symptoms, but the child's caregiver tends to underestimate the frequency of the child's symptoms. Frequent follow-up visits with the child's physician are important until symptoms are controlled. Ensure that the child and the family know how to use inhaled medications, including the use of a spacer. Stress the importance of making sure the child's asthma medications are readily available and promptly refilled when they run out. The child's pediatrician will develop an asthma action plan that outlines what to do when the child has asthma symptoms. Review environmental control measures to limit the child's exposure to potential asthma triggers. For example, smoking should not be permitted in the home. Heating and cooling system filters should be changed regularly. If the child wheezes after contact, limit the child's exposure to animals, grass, weeds, and dust.

Bronchiolitis

Description and Definition. Bronchiolitis is an inflammation of the smaller bronchioles caused by a virus. It is characterized by thick mucus. Inflammation and swelling make the small air passages in infants particularly vulnerable to obstruction.

Etiology. In bronchiolitis, airway obstruction is usually gradual and is caused by inflammation, secretions, and swelling of varying degrees in the small bronchi and bronchioles.

RSV is the primary cause of bronchiolitis and pneumonia in children younger than 1 year. Parainfluenza viruses are the second most common cause. An RSV infection can affect any part of the respiratory tract. RSV is highly contagious and is spread from respiratory secretions through close contact (less than 6 feet) with infected persons or contact with contaminated surfaces or objects. Infection can occur when infectious material comes in contact with mucous membranes of the eyes, mouth, or nose and possibly through the inhalation of droplets generated by a sneeze or cough. In the health care setting, RSV often is spread from child to child on the hands of caregivers. The incubation period from exposure to first symptoms is approximately 4 days.

Epidemiology and Demographics. RSV occurs in yearly epidemics. In mild climates, these epidemics occur each winter and last 4 to 5 months.

RSV is most common in infants younger than 1 year of age. Fifty percent of all infants will be infected with RSV by the end of the first year of life. Infants 1 to 4 months of age are at particular risk of severe infection and hospitalization.

History. History of bronchiolitis typically includes the following:

- Upper respiratory infection with runny nose and cough for several days
  - Low-grade fever
  - Increasingly productive cough
  - Increasing respiratory distress
  - Caregiver often reports wheezing at home
- Ear infection (otitis media)
- Contact with older siblings or children at daycare who have viral respiratory symptoms
- Family history of asthma or allergies

PEDIATRIC*Pearl*

Because asthma and bronchiolitis present similarly, determining the difference between these conditions may be difficult.

Physical Examination. Signs and symptoms of respiratory distress or failure depend on severity. RSV begins with signs and symptoms limited to an upper respiratory tract infection, such as a runny nose and sore throat. Within 1 to 3 days, a cough usually appears and may be accompanied by sneezing and a low-grade fever (temperature less than 101° F). Wheezing develops soon after the cough appears and may be detectable without a stethoscope. Auscultation often reveals diffuse rhonchi, fine rales or crackles, and wheezes. Mild cases of RSV may not progress beyond this stage.

If RSV progresses, coughing and wheezing increase and air hunger follows. These signs and symptoms are accompanied by an increased respiratory rate, retractions, peripheral cyanosis, and restlessness. Tachypnea and tachycardia often are present. Signs of dehydration may be present because of decreased fluid intake and increased fluid losses from fever and tachypnea.

Signs of severe, life-threatening illness include nasal flaring, retractions, central cyanosis, tachypnea of more than 70 breaths/min, listlessness, and apnea spells. The chest may be hyperexpanded and almost silent on auscultation because of poor air exchange.

Differential Diagnosis. Differential diagnosis of bronchiolitis includes the following:

- Asthma
- Cystic fibrosis
- Bronchopulmonary dysplasia
- Pneumonia

Therapeutic Interventions. Keep the child as calm and as comfortable as possible, usually in the arms of the caregiver. If breathing is adequate and the child shows signs of respiratory distress, administer supplemental oxygen (if necessary) in a way that does not agitate the child. Keep the oxygen saturation above 94%. If signs of respiratory failure or respiratory arrest are present, assist breathing with a bag-mask device with supplemental oxygen. The use of epinephrine and beta2-agonist bronchodilators is controversial because studies have demonstrated no convincing evidence of their effectiveness. Endotracheal intubation may be needed for respiratory failure or arrest with prolonged bag-mask ventilation or an inadequate response to ventilation.

Patient and Family Education. Teach the family the importance of handwashing to decrease the spread of RSV. Because eating is tiring for a patient with a respiratory illness, advise the family to feed the child smaller amounts than usual but at more frequent intervals. The child should not be exposed to cigarette smoke because it can trigger coughing. Because dry air tends to make coughs worse, recommend the use of a humidifier in the child's bedroom. Steam vaporizers should be avoided because they can cause burns.

Pneumonia

Description and Definition. **Pneumonia** is an inflammation and infection of the lower airway and lungs caused by a viral, bacterial, parasitic, or fungal organism. Pneumonia may occur as a primary infection or secondary to another illness or infection. It is often classified by anatomic location as follows:

- Lobar pneumonia: localized to one or more lobes of the lung
- Bronchopneumonia: inflammation around medium-sized airways, which causes patchy consolidation of parts of the lobes
- Interstitial pneumonia: inflammation of lung tissue between air sacs, usually generalized, often viral symptoms

Etiology. The organism responsible for pneumonia varies with the age of the child. The most common causes are RSV in infants, respiratory viruses (RSV, parainfluenza viruses, influenza viruses, adenoviruses) in children younger than 5 years, and *M. pneumoniae* and *S. pneumoniae* in children older than 5 years (Jenson & Baltimore, 2006).

Epidemiology and Demographics. Pneumonia usually occurs in infants, toddlers, and preschoolers but can occur at any age. Children who are immunocompromised or who have underlying lung disease are at greater risk for significant pneumonia. It is most prevalent in the winter months.

History. Pneumonia is often preceded by symptoms of an upper respiratory infection. Signs and symptoms may include fever, malaise, anorexia, and chest pain.

Physical Findings. Signs and symptoms of respiratory distress or failure depend on severity. Other symptoms include the following:

- Fever (less prominent in viral pneumonia, high in bacterial pneumonia)
- Chills
- Malaise
- Headache
- Lethargy
- Anorexia or poor feeding in infants
- Grunting
- Tachypnea
- Tachycardia
- Crackles may be present over affected lobes (other lobes normal) in lobar pneumonia; scattered crackles in bronchopneumonia; scattered crackles and wheezes in interstitial pneumonia
- Retractions
- Pleuritic chest pain
- Apnea spells

Differential Diagnosis. Differential diagnosis of pneumonia includes the following:

- Heart failure
- Asthma
- Bronchopulmonary dysplasia
- Cystic fibrosis

Therapeutic Interventions. Keep the child as calm and comfortable as possible, usually in the arms of the caregiver. If breathing is adequate and the child shows signs of respiratory distress, administer supplemental oxygen (if necessary) in a way that does not agitate the child. Keep the oxygen saturation above 94%. If signs of respiratory failure or respiratory arrest are present, assist breathing with a bag-mask device with supplemental oxygen.

Patient and Family Education. The child, family, daycare personnel, and teachers should be taught the importance of handwashing and other measures to reduce the spread of respiratory illnesses. Unless specifically contraindicated, the child should receive the usual childhood vaccines as recommended by the child's pediatrician.

Case Scenario—continued

You provide the patient nebulized albuterol per local protocol. He continues to wheeze and his oxygen saturation remains in the low 90s. His parents are concerned because he typically responds well to his breathing treatments.

Questions

7. *What is the appropriate transport decision for this patient?*
8. *What are other treatment options for this patient?*
9. *What are important findings to document in the written and oral report?*

Shock

[OBJECTIVES 20, 21]

Perfusion is the circulation of blood through an organ or a part of the body. Perfusion delivers oxygen and other nutrients to the cells of all organ systems and removes waste products. **Shock (hypoperfusion)** is the inadequate circulation of blood through an organ or a part of the body. Shock is described in detail in Chapter 34. This chapter focuses on the signs, symptoms, and treatment of shock in an infant or child.

Shock Severity

The initial signs of shock may be subtle in an infant or child. The effectiveness of compensatory mechanisms largely depends on the child's previous cardiac and pulmonary health. The presence of hypotension differentiates compensated shock from decompensated shock. Hypotension is a *late* sign of cardiovascular compromise in an infant or child. In the pediatric patient, the progression from compensated to decompensated shock occurs suddenly and rapidly. When decompensation occurs, cardiopulmonary arrest may be imminent. Signs and symptoms of compensated and decompensated shock are given in Box 37-9.

Although the amount and type of information gathered will vary depending on the child's condition, obtain a history as soon as possible from the caregiver. The information obtained may help identify the type of shock

BOX 37-9 Signs and Symptoms of Shock

Compensated Shock

- Irritability or anxiety
- Tachycardia
- Tachypnea
- Weak peripheral pulses, full (normal or adequate) central pulses
- Delayed capillary refill
- Cool, pale extremities
- Systolic BP within normal limits
- Decreased urinary output

Decompensated Shock

- Lethargy or altered mental status (V, P, or U on AVPU scale)
- Marked tachycardia or bradycardia
- Marked tachypnea or bradypnea
- Absent peripheral pulses, weak central pulses
- Markedly delayed capillary refill
- Cool, pale, dusky, mottled extremities
- Hypotension
- Markedly decreased urinary output

BP, blood pressure.

present, ascertain the child's previous health, and determine the onset and duration of symptoms.

Hypovolemic Shock

Hypovolemia and sepsis are the most common causes of shock in children (Frankel & Kache, 2007). In children, the average circulating blood volume is approximately 80 mL/kg. Although the circulating blood volume is proportionately larger in infants and children than in adults, their *total* blood volume is smaller than in adults. As a result, a small volume loss can result in hemodynamic compromise.

Hypovolemic shock may be caused by a loss of blood, plasma, fluids, and electrolytes or by endocrine disorders. Causes of major blood loss are listed in Box 37-10. Plasma loss may be caused by burns or third spacing (as in pancreatitis or peritonitis). Fluid and electrolyte loss may be from a kidney disorder, excessive sweating (cystic fibrosis), diarrhea, vomiting, or dehydration. Shock also may be caused by endocrine disorders such as diabetes mellitus or hypothyroidism. The response of an infant or child to fluid and blood loss is shown in Table 37-8.

Signs and symptoms of compensated or decompensated shock may be present depending on severity. Other signs that may be present include internal or external bleeding, poor skin turgor, decreased saliva and/or tears, or a sunken fontanelle (in infants).

BOX 37-10 Causes of Major Blood Loss

- Vascular injury
- Ruptured liver or spleen
- Hemothorax
- Scalp lacerations
- Intracranial hemorrhage (newborn or infant)
- Fractured femur with vascular laceration

TABLE 37-8 Response to Fluid and Blood Loss in the Pediatric Patient

		Stage of Shock		
Assessment	**Class I**	**Class II Compensated**	**Class III Decompensated**	**Class IV Irreversible**
% Blood volume loss	Up to 15%	15%-30%	30%-45%	>45%
Mental status	Slightly anxious	Mildly anxious; restless	Altered; lethargic; apathetic; decreased pain response	Extremely lethargic; unresponsive
Muscle tone	Normal	Normal	Normal to decreased	Limp
Ventilatory rate/effort	Normal	Mild tachypnea	Moderate tachypnea	Severe tachypnea to agonal (preterminal event)
Skin color (extremities)	Pink	Pale, mottled	Pale, mottled, mild peripheral cyanosis	Pale, mottled, central and peripheral cyanosis
Skin turgor	Normal	Poor; sunken eyes and fontanelles in infant or young child	Poor; sunken eyes and fontanelles in infant or young child	Tenting
Skin temperature	Cool	Cool	Cool to cold	Cold
Capillary refill	Normal	Poor (>2 sec)	Delayed (>3 sec)	Prolonged (>5 sec)
Heart rate	Usually normal if gradual volume loss; increased if sudden loss of volume	Mild tachycardia	Significant tachycardia; possible dysrhythmias; peripheral pulse weak, thready, or absent	Marked tachycardia to bradycardia (preterminal event)
BP	Normal	Lower range of normal	Decreased	Severe hypotension
Pulse pressure	Normal or increased	Narrowed	Decreased	Decreased
Urine output	Normal; concentrated	Decreased	Minimal	Minimal to absent

Reprinted from Aehlert, B. (2005). *Comprehensive pediatric emergency care.* St. Louis: Mosby.
BP, Blood pressure.

Therapeutic Interventions. If trauma is suspected, maintain cervical spine stabilization and open the airway with a jaw thrust without head tilt maneuver if necessary. Administer supplemental oxygen if indicated and ensure oxygenation and breathing are effective. Apply a pulse oximeter and maintain oxygen saturation at greater than 94%. If a pulse or other signs of circulation are absent, or if the heart rate is less than 60 beats/min with signs of poor perfusion, begin chest compressions. Attach a cardiac monitor. If immediate vascular access is needed, attempt IV access with two large peripheral IV lines. If unsuccessful, attempt IO access. Venous access may be difficult to obtain in an infant or child in shock. When decompensated shock is present, the most readily available vascular access site is preferred. If immediate vascular access is needed and reliable venous access cannot be rapidly achieved, establish IO access. If decompensated shock is present, immediate IO access is appropriate. If CPR is in progress, attempt vascular access by the route most readily available that will not require interruption of CPR.

Signs of shock should be treated with a bolus of 20 mL/kg of isotonic crystalloid (normal saline or lactated Ringer's solution) even if the blood pressure is normal (Kleinman et al., 2010). Assess the child's response by checking mental status, capillary refill, heart rate, ventilatory effort, and BP. If no improvement occurs, give additional fluid boluses as ordered by medical direction. Assess the child's response after each bolus. Check the child's glucose level. Some children in shock are hypoglycemic because of rapidly depleted carbohydrate stores. If the serum glucose is less than 60 mg/dL, administer IV dextrose (per medical direction). Maintain normal body temperature.

Distributive Shock. Distributive shock may be caused by a severe infection (septic shock), severe allergic reaction (anaphylactic shock), spinal cord injury (neurogenic shock), or certain overdoses (e.g., sedatives, narcotics). Signs and symptoms of distributive shock that are unusual in the presence of hypovolemic shock include warm, flushed skin (especially in dependent areas) and, in neurogenic shock, a normal or slow pulse rate (relative bradycardia).

Septic Shock. Suspect septic shock when a child with fever, tachycardia, and vasodilation experiences a change in mental status. This may be evidenced by inconsolable irritability, lack of interaction with parents, or an inability to be aroused.

Septic shock occurs in two clinical stages. In the early stage, peripheral vasodilation (warm shock) is present. The late (decompensated) stage is characterized by cool extremities (cold shock). Late septic shock is usually indistinguishable from other types of shock.

Administer supplemental oxygen if indicated and ensure oxygenation and breathing are effective. Apply a pulse oximeter and maintain oxygen saturation at greater than 94%. If a pulse or other signs of circulation are absent, or if the heart rate is less than 60 beats/min with signs of poor perfusion, begin chest compressions. Attach a cardiac monitor. Establish vascular access and give fluid boluses as ordered by medical direction. Most patients in decompensated septic shock require aggressive fluid administration. Carefully monitor the patient for crackles and increased work of breathing when giving fluids. If the child's condition does not improve with fluids, medical direction may order a dopamine or epinephrine IV infusion. IV antibiotics will be given at the hospital.

Anaphylactic Shock. Anaphylaxis occurs when an individual is exposed to a substance to which the patient has been previously sensitized. On reexposure to the same substance, histamine and other chemical mediators are released, which produce the signs and symptoms of anaphylaxis (Box 37-11). Common causes of anaphylaxis include insect stings, medications (e.g., penicillin, sulfa), and some foods (e.g., shellfish, nuts, strawberries).

Treatment is directed at removing or discontinuing the causative substance. Administer supplemental oxygen if indicated and ensure oxygenation and breathing are effective. Apply a pulse oximeter and maintain oxygen saturation at greater than 94%. If a pulse or other signs of circulation are absent, or if the heart rate is less than 60 beats/min with signs of poor perfusion, begin chest compressions. Attach a cardiac monitor. Medical direction will usually order epinephrine intramuscularly (site of choice is the lateral aspect of the thigh). Other medications that may be ordered include bronchodilator therapy (e.g., albuterol), an antihistamine (e.g., diphenhydramine), and a steroid (e.g., methylprednisolone). If signs of decompensated shock are present, establish vascular access. Medical direction may order IV epinephrine and fluid boluses of normal saline or Ringer's lactate. Monitor closely for increased work of breathing and the development of crackles. Check the child's glucose level. Administer IV dextrose if the serum glucose is less than 60 mg/dL, per medical direction.

Neurogenic Shock. Neurogenic shock is caused by a severe injury to the head or spinal cord that results in a loss of sympathetic vascular tone below the level of the spinal cord injury. The loss of peripheral vascular tone results in widespread vasodilation below the level of the injury. The total blood volume remains the same, but vessel capacity is increased (relative hypovolemia). Situations in which spinal cord damage may occur include high-speed motor vehicle crashes in which the child is a pedestrian, an unrestrained or improperly restrained

BOX 37-11 Possible Signs and Symptoms of Anaphylaxis

- Stridor, wheezing, coughing, hoarseness, intercostal and suprasternal retractions
- Tachycardia, hypotension, dysrhythmias
- Vomiting, diarrhea
- Anxiety, restlessness
- Facial swelling and angioedema
- Urticaria (hives)
- Abdominal pain, cramping
- Pruritus (itching)

passenger, falls from extreme heights, and diving accidents.

If trauma is suspected, maintain cervical spine stabilization and open the airway with a jaw thrust without head tilt maneuver if necessary. Administer supplemental oxygen if indicated and ensure oxygenation and breathing are effective. Apply a pulse oximeter and maintain oxygen saturation at greater than 94%. If a pulse or other signs of circulation are absent, or if the heart rate is less than 60 beats/min with signs of poor perfusion, begin chest compressions. Attach a cardiac monitor. Obtain vascular access. If IV access cannot be rapidly established, place an IO needle. Give a 20-mL/kg isotonic crystalloid solution (normal saline or Ringer's lactate) fluid bolus as ordered by medical direction. If the child's condition does not improve, repeat fluid boluses may be ordered. Assess the child's response after each fluid bolus. Monitor closely for increased work of breathing and the development of crackles. Maintain normal body temperature. In neurogenic shock, widespread vasodilation may result in a loss of body heat. Be aware of possible hypothermia. Check the child's glucose level. If the serum glucose is less than 60 mg/dL, administer IV dextrose if approved by medical direction. Medical direction may order vasopressors if poor perfusion persists despite adequate ventilation, oxygenation, and volume expansion.

Obstructive Shock

Shock that develops from cardiac tamponade, tension pneumothorax, or a massive pulmonary embolism is called *obstructive shock* because the common pathophysiology in these conditions is obstruction to blood flow from the heart. Cardiac tamponade and tension pneumothorax present with clear lung sounds; however, lung sounds are unequal in a tension pneumothorax.

Treatment of obstructive shock depends on the cause. If trauma is suspected, maintain cervical spine stabilization and open the airway with a jaw thrust without head tilt maneuver if necessary. Administer supplemental oxygen if indicated and ensure oxygenation and breathing are effective. Apply a pulse oximeter and maintain oxygen saturation at greater than 94%. If a pulse or other signs of circulation are absent, or if the heart rate is less than 60 beats/min with signs of poor perfusion, begin chest compressions. Attach the cardiac monitor. Obtain vascular access. If immediate vascular access is needed, attempt IV access. If unsuccessful, attempt IO access. Medical direction may order fluid boluses of normal saline or Ringer's lactate. Assess the child's response after each bolus. If signs and symptoms of a tension pneumothorax are present, perform needle decompression on the affected side (if permitted by medical direction). Reassess the child's response.

Cardiogenic Shock

Respiratory failure associated with decompensated shock leads to inadequate oxygenation, ventilation, and perfusion, resulting in cardiopulmonary failure. Cardiopulmonary failure is a clinical condition identified by deficits in oxygenation, ventilation, and perfusion. Without prompt recognition and management, cardiopulmonary failure will deteriorate to cardiopulmonary arrest. Signs of cardiopulmonary failure are shown in Box 37-12.

Cardiogenic shock occurs because of impaired cardiac muscle function that leads to decreased cardiac output. Cardiogenic shock may occur as a primary event in patients who have congenital heart disease or as a complication of shock of any cause. Possible causes of cardiogenic shock are listed in Box 37-13. Congenital heart disease and cardiomyopathy are discussed in Chapter 22.

In cardiogenic shock, signs and symptoms of compensated or decompensated shock are present depending on severity in addition to crackles, jugular venous distention, and peripheral edema. Jugular venous distention is difficult to assess in infants and young children.

The treatment of cardiogenic shock is generally based on increasing contractility, altering preload and afterload, and controlling dysrhythmias if they are present and contributing to shock.

Dysrhythmias

[OBJECTIVE 22]

In the pediatric patient, dysrhythmias are divided into four broad categories based on heart rate: (1) normal for age, (2) slower than normal for age (bradycardia), (3) faster than normal for age (tachycardia), or (4) absent or pulseless (cardiac arrest).

In children, dysrhythmias are treated only if they compromise cardiac output or have the potential for

BOX 37-12 Signs of Cardiopulmonary Failure

- Bradypnea with irregular, ineffective respirations
- Decreasing work of breathing (tiring)
- Delayed capillary refill time (longer than 5 seconds)
- Bradycardia
- Weak central pulses and absent peripheral pulses
- Cool extremities
- Mottled or cyanotic skin
- Diminished level of responsiveness

BOX 37-13 Possible Causes of Cardiogenic Shock

- Cardiomyopathy
- Severe congenital heart disease
- Myocardial dysfunction after cardiac surgery
- Myocardial trauma
- Heart failure
- Hypothermia
- Drug intoxication
- Severe electrolyte or acid-base imbalances
- Cardiac dysrhythmias

deteriorating into a lethal rhythm. Although disorders of heart rate and rhythm are uncommon in infants and children, when they do occur they most often are because of hypoxia secondary to respiratory arrest and asphyxia.

Tachydysrhythmias: Too-Fast Rhythms

[OBJECTIVES 23, 24]

In infants and children, tachycardia is present if the heart rate is faster than the upper limit of normal for the patient's age. Tachycardia may represent either a normal compensatory response to the need for increased cardiac output or oxygen delivery or an unstable dysrhythmia.

Three types of tachycardia are generally seen in children: sinus tachycardia, supraventricular tachycardia (SVT), and ventricular tachycardia (VT) with a pulse. Sinus tachycardia is the most common of these rhythms. SVT and VT can produce ventricular rates so rapid that ventricular filling time is reduced, stroke volume decreases, and cardiac output falls.

Sinus tachycardia is a normal compensatory response to the need for increased cardiac output or oxygen delivery. In sinus tachycardia, the heart rate is usually less than 220 beats/min in infants or 180 beats/min in children. Onset of the rhythm occurs gradually. The history given typically explains the rapid heart rate (e.g., pain, fever, volume loss from trauma, vomiting, or diarrhea). Treatment is directed at the underlying cause that precipitated the rhythm, such as administering medications to relieve pain or fluids to correct hypovolemia from diarrhea.

SVT is the most common tachydysrhythmia that requires treatment in the pediatric patient. The most frequent age of presentation is in the first 3 months of life, with secondary peaks occurring at 8 to 10 years of age and again during adolescence (Park & Beerman, 2002). Unlike sinus tachycardia, SVT is not a normal compensatory response to physiologic stress. In SVT, the heart rate is usually more than 220 beats/min in infants or 180 beats/min in children. Onset of the rhythm occurs abruptly. The electrocardiogram (ECG) shows a regular, narrow QRS complex rhythm that does not vary in response to activity or stimulation. P waves often are indiscernible because of the rapid rate and may be lost in the T wave of the preceding beat (Figure 37-13). If P waves are visible, they differ in appearance from P waves that originate in the sinoatrial node. In the absence of known congenital heart disease, the history obtained is usually nonspecific. In other words, the history does not explain the rapid heart rate. Use Table 37-9 to help differentiate sinus tachycardia from SVT.

A child with normal cardiovascular function may tolerate a rapid ventricular rate for several hours before signs

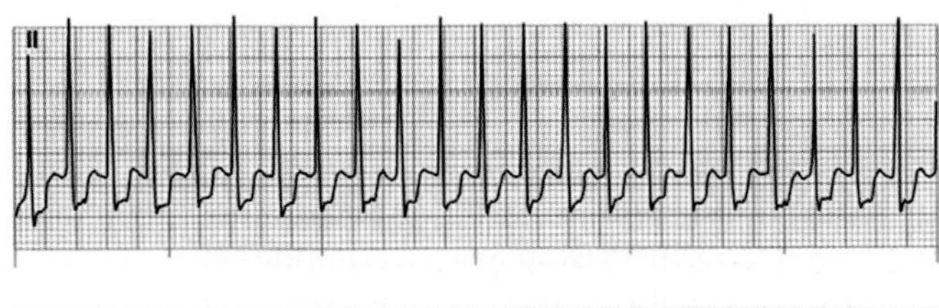

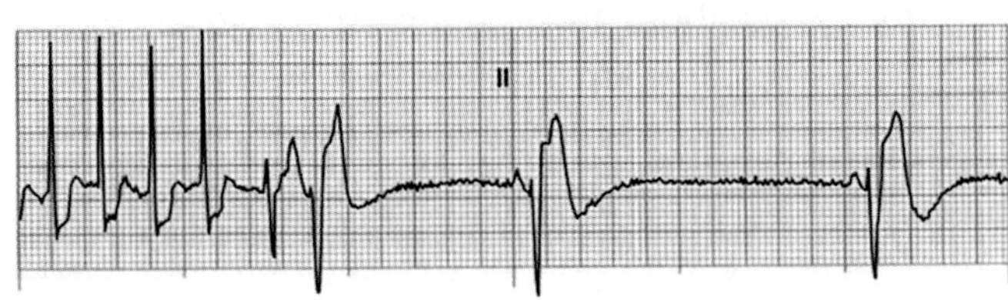

Figure 37-13 A, Supraventricular tachycardia (SVT) in a child complaining of chest pain. **B,** The same child after one intravenous (IV) dose of adenosine.

TABLE 37-9 Differentiation of Sinus Tachycardia and Supraventricular Tachycardia

Characteristic	Sinus Tachycardia	Supraventricular Tachycardia
Rate	Usually <220 beats/min in infants and <180 beats/min in children	Usually 220 beats/min or more in infants and 180 beats/min or more in children
Ventricular rate and regularity	Varies with activity or stimulation	Constant with activity or stimulation
Onset and end	Gradual	Abrupt
P waves	Visible; normal appearance	Often indiscernible; if visible, differ in appearance from sinoatrial node P waves
History	History given explains rapid heart rate; pain, fever, volume loss from trauma, vomiting, or diarrhea	In the absence of known congenital heart disease, history usually is nonspecific (i.e., history given does not explain rapid heart rate)
Physical examination	May be consistent with volume loss (blood, diarrhea, vomiting), possible fever, clear lungs, liver of normal size	Signs of poor perfusion, including diminished peripheral pulses, delayed capillary refill, pallor, increased work of breathing, possible crackles, enlarged liver

Reprinted from Aehlert, B. (2005). *Comprehensive pediatric emergency care,* St. Louis: Mosby.

of heart failure or shock develop. Infants may tolerate the rapid ventricular rate associated with SVT for hours or days before developing signs of poor cardiac output, heart failure, and cardiogenic shock.

VT is uncommon in infants and children unless an underlying cardiovascular disorder exists. This dysrhythmia may be seen in children who have had open-heart surgical repair for tetralogy of Fallot or other anomalies or who have cardiomyopathy, myocarditis, or a myocardial tumor. VT may occur in an infant or child with a preexisting conduction abnormality and may be seen in the end stages of acidosis, hypoxemia, hypovolemia, or hypothermia. Secondary causes of VT include electrolyte imbalance (as seen in hyperkalemia or hypomagnesemia) and ingestion of certain toxins (e.g., tricyclic anti-depressants).

Rapid ventricular rates may be associated with lightheadedness, syncope, dyspnea, weakness, nervousness, and reports of palpitations, chest pain, or pressure in the older child. Signs of shock may be evident depending on the duration and rate of the tachycardia and the presence of primary cardiac disease. Be sure to obtain ECG tracings before, during, and after interventions for any patient with a cardiac dysrhythmia. Recommended treatment for symptomatic tachycardias is shown in the pediatric tachycardia algorithm (Figure 37-14).

PEDIATRIC*Pearl*

The initial emergency management of pediatric dysrhythmias requires a response to four important questions:

1. Are a pulse and other signs of circulation present?
2. Is the rate within normal limits for age, too fast, too slow, or absent?
3. Is the QRS wide (ventricular in origin) or narrow (supraventricular in origin)?
4. Is the patient sick (unstable) or not sick (stable)?

Bradydysrhythmias: Too-Slow Rhythms. In infants and children, bradycardia is present if the heart rate is slower than the lower limit of normal for the patient's age. Bradycardia can be classified as either primary or secondary. Primary bradycardia is usually caused by structural heart disease. An infant or child with structural cardiac disease may develop bradycardia because of atrioventricular block or sinus node dysfunction. Physical examination of these children may reveal a midline sternal scar, and they may have an implanted pacemaker to treat the bradycardia.

Secondary bradycardia is a slow heart rate from a noncardiac cause. Causes of secondary bradycardia include increased vagal tone (e.g., vomiting, increased intracranial pressure, vagal maneuvers, suctioning, endotracheal intubation procedure), hypothermia, hyperkalemia, and ingestion of medications such as calcium channel blockers (verapamil, diltiazem), digoxin, and beta-blockers (propranolol).

A bradycardia can produce significant symptoms unless stroke volume increases to compensate for the decrease in heart rate. Unless promptly corrected, decreasing cardiac output eventually produces hemodynamic compromise.

Treatment for a slow rhythm is unnecessary if the patient is asymptomatic. For example, adolescent athletes at rest or children who are sleeping may show no symptoms with a slow heart rate. If an infant or child is symptomatic because of bradycardia, initial treatment is directed at assessment of the airway and breathing rather than giving epinephrine, atropine, or other drugs. Problems with adequate oxygenation and ventilation are more common in children than are cardiac causes of bradycardia (Figure 37-15).

PEDIATRIC*Pearl*

In the pediatric patient, most slow rhythms occur because of hypoxia and acidosis.

Absent or Pulseless Rhythms

[OBJECTIVE 25]

In adults, sudden, nontraumatic cardiac arrests are usually the result of underlying cardiac disease. In children, cardiac arrests are usually the result of respiratory failure (asphyxia precipitated by acute hypoxia or hypercarbia) or circulatory shock (ischemia from hypovolemia, sepsis, or myocardial dysfunction [cardiogenic shock]) (Berg et al., 2008). The cause of cardiac arrest in the pediatric patient also varies with age, the underlying health of the child, and the location of the event.

Absent or pulseless rhythms include pulseless VT, ventricular fibrillation, asystole, or pulseless electrical activity (see Chapter 22). When these rhythms are seen, they usually signify serious myocardial disease or dysfunction from congenital heart disease, cardiomyopathy, or an acute inflammatory injury to the heart (e.g., myocarditis). Recommended treatment for absent/pulseless rhythms is shown in the pediatric pulseless arrest algorithm (Figure 37-16).

Seizures

Description and Definition

[OBJECTIVES 26, 27, 28]

Many conditions can interfere with brain activity and result in abnormal mental status, including metabolic problems, infectious diseases, intracranial structural abnormalities, trauma, hypoxia, and poisonings. Possible causes of altered mental status are listed in Table 37-10.

A child with altered mental status displays changes in personality, behavior, or responsiveness inappropriate for age. The child may appear agitated, combative, sleepy, withdrawn, slow to respond, or completely unresponsive. The most common causes of altered mental status in the pediatric patient are hypoxia, head trauma, seizures, infection, hypoglycemia, and drug or alcohol ingestion.

General impression findings that indicate altered mental status include unusual agitation, irritability, or confusion; reduced responsiveness; and moaning or a

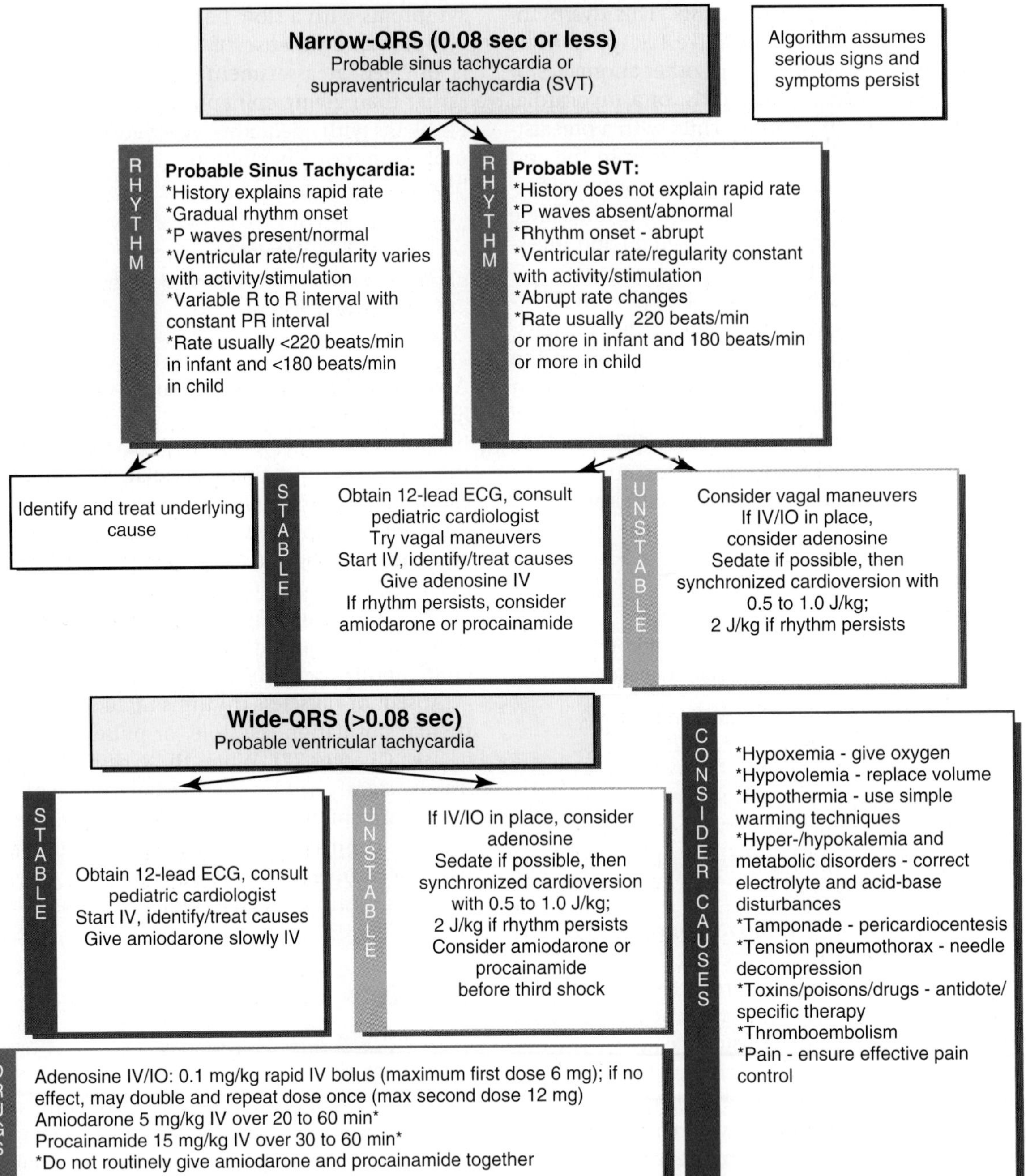

THE 2010 AHA PEDIATRIC TACHYCARDIA ALGORITHM
Assess ABCs, ensure effective oxygenation and ventilation
Attach pulse oximeter and monitor/defibrillator
If pulseless, begin CPR—go to pulseless algorithm
Narrow-QRS (0.08 sec or less)
Probable sinus tachycardia or supraventricular tachycardia (SVT)
Algorithm assumes serious signs and symptoms persist
RHYTHM
Probable Sinus Tachycardia:
*History explains rapid rate
*Gradual rhythm onset
*P waves present/normal
*Ventricular rate/regularity varies with activity/stimulation
*Variable R to R interval with constant PR interval
*Rate usually <220 beats/min in infant and <180 beats/min in child
RHYTHM
Probable SVT:
*History does not explain rapid rate
*P waves absent/abnormal
*Rhythm onset - abrupt
*Ventricular rate/regularity constant with activity/stimulation
*Abrupt rate changes
*Rate usually 220 beats/min or more in infant and 180 beats/min or more in child
Identify and treat underlying cause
STABLE
Obtain 12-lead ECG, consult pediatric cardiologist
Try vagal maneuvers
Start IV, identify/treat causes
Give adenosine IV
If rhythm persists, consider amiodarone or procainamide
UNSTABLE
Consider vagal maneuvers
If IV/IO in place, consider adenosine
Sedate if possible, then synchronized cardioversion with 0.5 to 1.0 J/kg;
2 J/kg if rhythm persists
Wide-QRS (>0.08 sec)
Probable ventricular tachycardia
STABLE
Obtain 12-lead ECG, consult pediatric cardiologist
Start IV, identify/treat causes
Give amiodarone slowly IV
UNSTABLE
If IV/IO in place, consider adenosine
Sedate if possible, then synchronized cardioversion with 0.5 to 1.0 J/kg;
2 J/kg if rhythm persists
Consider amiodarone or procainamide before third shock
CONSIDER CAUSES
*Hypoxemia - give oxygen
*Hypovolemia - replace volume
*Hypothermia - use simple warming techniques
*Hyper-/hypokalemia and metabolic disorders - correct electrolyte and acid-base disturbances
*Tamponade - pericardiocentesis
*Tension pneumothorax - needle decompression
*Toxins/poisons/drugs - antidote/specific therapy
*Thromboembolism
*Pain - ensure effective pain control
DRUGS
Adenosine IV/IO: 0.1 mg/kg rapid IV bolus (maximum first dose 6 mg); if no effect, may double and repeat dose once (max second dose 12 mg)
Amiodarone 5 mg/kg IV over 20 to 60 min*
Procainamide 15 mg/kg IV over 30 to 60 min*
*Do not routinely give amiodarone and procainamide together

Figure 37-14 Pediatric tachycardia algorithm. *ABC,* Airway, breathing, and circulation; *CPR,* cardiopulmonary resuscitation; *SVT,* supraventricular tachycardia; *VT,* ventricular tachycardia; *IV,* intravenous; *IO,* intraosseous; *ECG,* electrocardiogram.

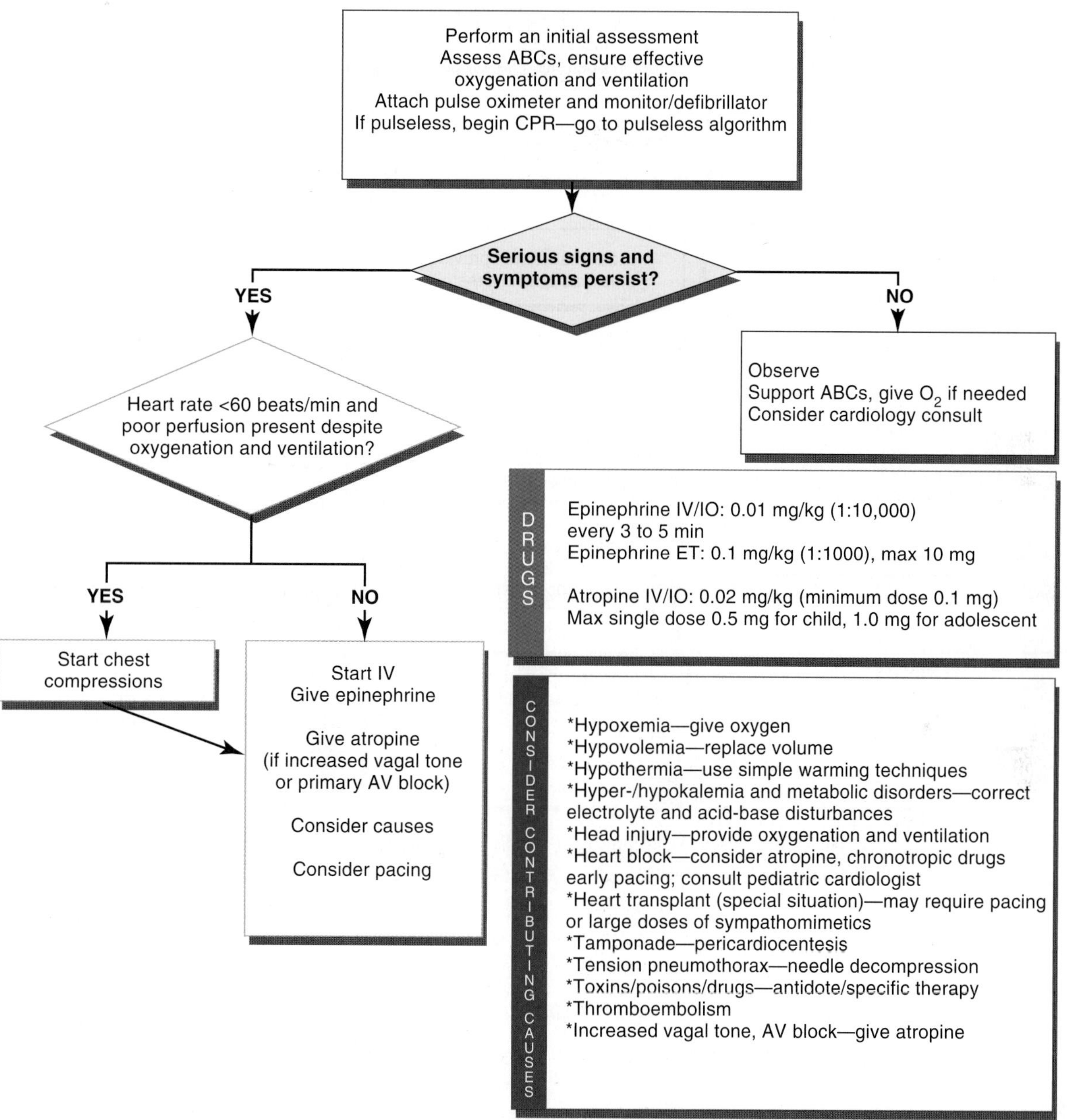

Figure 37-15 Symptomatic bradycardia algorithm. *ABCs,* Airway, breathing, and circulation; *CPR,* cardiopulmonary resuscitation; *IV,* intravenous; *IO,* intraosseous; *ET,* endotracheal, *AV,* atrioventricular.

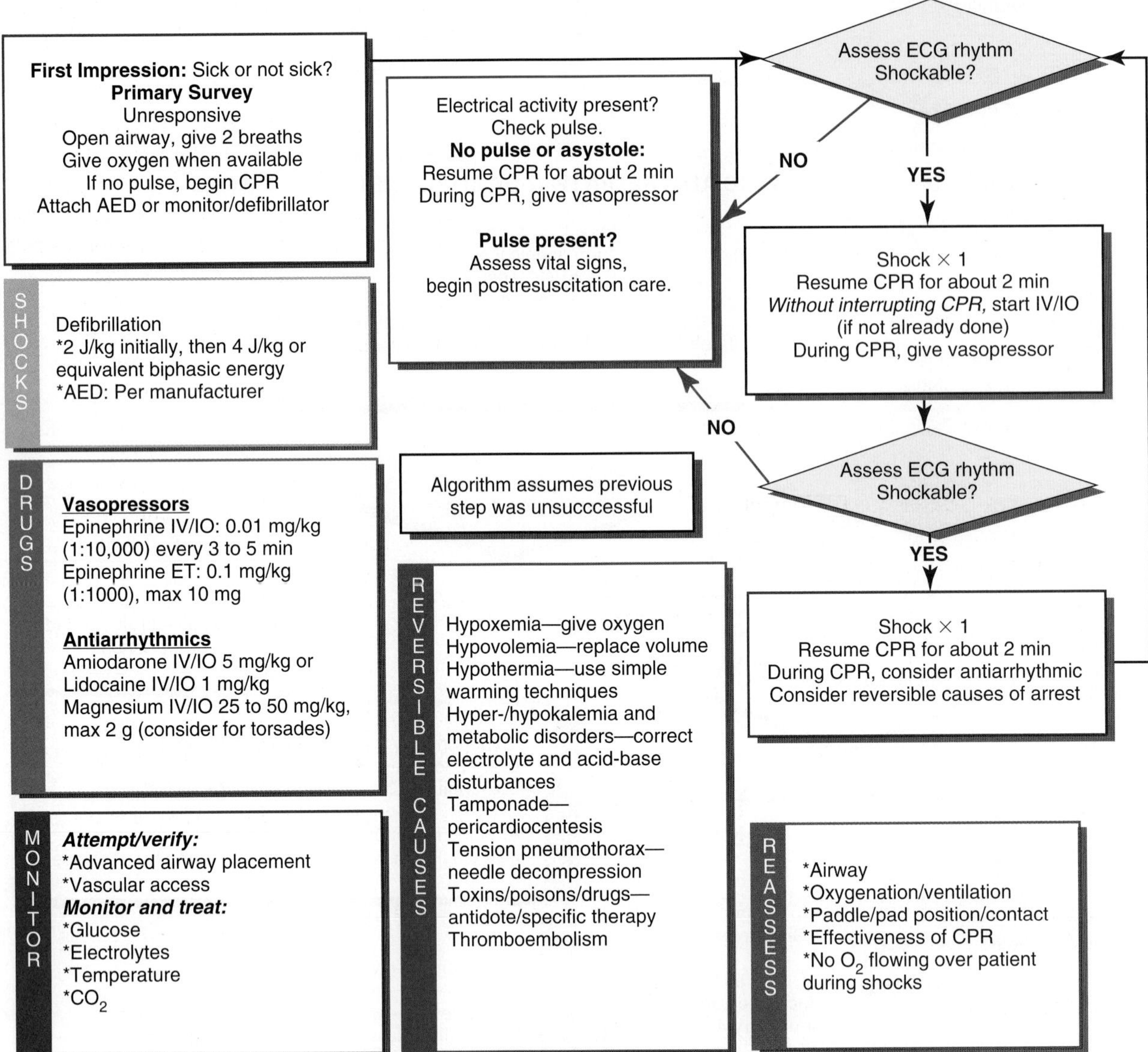

Figure 37-16 Cardiac arrest algorithm. *CPR,* Cardiopulmonary resuscitation; *AED,* automated external difibrillator; *ET,* endotracheal; *ECG,* electrocardiogram; *IV,* intravenous; *IO,* intraosseous.

TABLE 37-10	Possible Causes of Altered Mental Status
A	***A**lcohol, **A**buse*
E	***E**pilepsy, **E**lectrolyte disorders, **E**ncephalopathy, **E**ndocrine*
I	***I**nsulin, **I**ntussusception, **I**ntoxication*
O	**O**verdose (opiates, lead, sedatives, aspirin, carbon monoxide)
U	**U**remia (kidney failure) and other metabolic causes, **U**nderdosage
T	***T**rauma, **T**emperature, **T**umor*
I	***I**nfection (encephalitis, meningitis, Reye's syndrome, sepsis)*
P	**P**sychological (fake, hysterical, or pseudoseizures)
P	**P**oisoning
S	**S**hock, **S**ickle cell disease, **S**ubarachnoid hemorrhage, **S**pace-occupying lesion, **S**hunt-related problems

Reprinted from Aehlert, B. (2005). *Comprehensive pediatric emergency care.* St. Louis: Mosby.

weak cry. Other general impression findings associated with altered mental status include abnormal muscle tone or body position for the child's age, abnormal work of breathing, and pallor.

A **seizure** is a temporary change in behavior or consciousness caused by abnormal electrical activity of one or more groups of neurons in the brain. The two categories of seizures are partial and generalized. **Partial seizures** may be simple or complex. Simple partial seizures also are called *focal* or *focal motor seizures* (Table 37-11). Complex partial seizures are the most common type of seizure in children and adults. This type of seizure often includes automatisms (purposeless repetitive movements such as picking at clothes, lip smacking, chewing, eye blinking, rubbing or caressing objects). Automatisms are not remembered by the child.

Generalized seizures begin suddenly and involve an alteration of consciousness. Absence seizures (petit mal) and tonic-clonic seizures (also called *generalized motor seizures* or *grand mal seizures*) are types of generalized seizures. Tonic-clonic seizures are quite common.

Status epilepticus is any prolonged series of similar seizures without return to full consciousness between them. Status epilepticus is potentially life threatening and requires immediate treatment.

A febrile seizure is a generalized seizure that occurs with fever in childhood between the ages of 3 months and 5 years (most occur between ages 6 and 18 months). A simple febrile seizure is associated with a core body

TABLE 37-11	Characteristics of Partial and Generalized Seizures
Partial Seizures	
Simple partial seizure	Lasts an average of 10 to 20 seconds Patient remains conscious May verbalize during the seizure No postictal event after the seizure Characterized by motor or sensory symptoms without impairment of consciousness Motor: forceful turning of the head and eyes to one side, clonic movements on one side of the body beginning in the face or extremities Sensory: paresthesias or pain localized to a specific area
Complex partial seizure	Consciousness is always impaired May begin as a simple partial seizure and progress or may begin as a complex seizure Lasts an average of 1 to 2 minutes Often preceded by a sensory aura Postictal confusion or sleep may follow the seizure
Generalized Seizures	
Absence (petit mal) seizure	Transient loss of awareness of surroundings without loss of motor tone May have automatisms Uncommon before age 5 years; more prevalent in girls Never associated with an aura Rarely last longer than 30 seconds No postictal state
Tonic-clonic (grand mal) seizure	Typical phases: aura, loss of consciousness, tonic phase, clonic phase, postictal phase

BOX 37-14 Possible Causes of Seizures in Children

- Head trauma
- Toxins, including alcohol and pharmacologic agents
- Hypoxia
- Fever
- Hypoglycemia
- Infection
- Metabolic disorders
- Brain tumor or abscess
- Vascular disorders
- Cardiac dysrhythmias
- Genetic and hereditary factors

temperature that increases rapidly to 38.8° C (101.8° F) or greater. The seizure is usually tonic-clonic and lasts a few seconds to 15 minutes. It is followed by a brief post-ictal period of drowsiness. A complicated (also known as *atypical*) febrile seizure lasts longer than 15 minutes. The child may have repeated seizures within the same day.

Etiology

Seizures are common in children. Possible causes are listed in Box 37-14. Other events, such as breath-holding spells and gastroesophageal reflux, can cause events that mimic seizures (Johnston, 2007).

Epidemiology and Demographics

An estimated 10% of the population will experience at least one seizure during their lifetimes. Peak incidences of seizures are in the neonatal period, between 5 and 10 years, and adolescence. Febrile seizures occur in 2% to 4% of children with most occurring between 1 and 2 years of age (Lewis, 2010).

Epilepsy is considered present when two or more unprovoked seizures occur at an interval greater than 24 hours apart.

History

The history is the most important diagnostic tool in evaluating seizures in children. If possible, obtain a history from the patient and someone who witnessed the seizure. Interestingly, the physical portrayal of the seizure by the caregiver often is surprisingly similar to the actual seizure and is much more accurate than the verbal description (Johnston, 2007).

Physical Findings

If the child is actively seizing, note pertinent findings, including a tongue laceration, head wound, and/or incontinence. If the child is stable and the seizure has stopped, look for clues to the cause, such as the following:

- Check for a medical identification device.
- Look for evidence of burns or suspicious substances that might indicate poisoning or toxic exposure.
- Look for any signs of recent trauma.

Differential Diagnosis

Differential diagnosis of seizure should include the following:

- Hypoglycemia
- Syncope
- Dysrhythmias
- Tetralogy spells
- Breath-holding spells
- Acute intoxication
- Pseudoseizures

Therapeutic Interventions

Protect the child from injury and aspiration of vomitus. Do *not* insert your fingers, an oral airway, a padded tongue blade, or bite block into the child's mouth during an active seizure. Do not try to restrain body movements during the seizure. Provide positive-pressure ventilation with supplemental oxygen if the seizure is prolonged or if the child is cyanotic, has shallow chest rise with bradypnea, or has an oxygen saturation reading less than 90% despite oxygen administration. Consider ECG monitoring, which is generally indicated for any infant or child who displays an abnormal ventilatory rate or effort, heart rate, perfusion, BP, or mental status. However, do not delay lifesaving interventions to set up a monitor. Treat hypoglycemia if present.

Most physicians delay treatment with medications until a second seizure occurs unless the first episode was status epilepticus. All patients with status epilepticus require treatment. If the child has persistent or repetitive tonic-clonic seizures, medical direction usually orders a benzodiazepine (e.g., diazepam, lorazepam, midazolam) to stop the seizures. These medications are effective for immediate control of prolonged tonic-clonic seizures in most children.

After the seizure, place the patient in the recovery (lateral recumbent) position to aid drainage of secretions if cervical spine injury is not an issue. If the patient's spine has been stabilized because of suspected trauma and the patient vomits, turn the patient and backboard as a unit and clear the airway with suctioning.

Patient and Family Education

First-time seizures in any patient require further evaluation by a physician. Factors that may trigger seizures in susceptible patients include fever, lack of sleep, video games, and flashing (strobe) lights. Some pediatricians recommend early administration of acetaminophen or ibuprofen when a child has an illness accompanied by a fever greater than 39° C (102° F).

If the child has a seizure history and is prescribed anticonvulsant medication, make sure the patient and family understand the importance of taking the medication as ordered. The child's family, daycare personnel, and teachers should be taught first aid for seizures, including moving objects away from the child during the seizure and loosening clothing around the neck. The child should wear medical identification that says he or she has a seizure history and avoid activities that would be unsafe if he or she suddenly had a seizure. For example, the child should not swim or bathe unless someone else is nearby.

Hypoglycemia

Description and Definition

Hypoglycemia (low blood sugar) may occur in diabetic patients, often because of treatment with insulin or oral hypoglycemic agents. Hypoglycemia is common in metabolically stressed children because a child is unable to store large quantities of glucose and mobilize what they can store. Prolonged hypoglycemia can lead to irreversible brain damage. In children, alcohol intoxication increases susceptibility to hypoglycemia and altered mental status because alcohol suppresses the ability of the liver to make glucose.

Etiology

The blood sugar level may become too low if the diabetic patient has taken too much insulin, not eaten enough food, overexercised and burned off sugar faster than normal, or experienced significant physical or emotional stress.

Physical Examination

Signs and symptoms of hypoglycemia are nonspecific (Table 37-12). Early signs include headache, hunger, nausea, weakness, irritability, and agitation. Later signs include cool, pale, clammy skin; tachycardia; tachypnea; abdominal pain (stomachache); dizziness; sweating; pallor; confusion; tremors; seizures; and coma. Signs and symptoms of hypoglycemia in a neonate include poor muscle tone, tremors, jitteriness, increased work of breathing, apnea, lethargy, seizures, acidosis, and coma.

Differential Diagnosis

Consider other causes of altered mental status, including alcohol, electrolyte disorders, overdose, infection, and poisoning.

Therapeutic Interventions

In addition to appropriate care to ensure an open airway, adequate breathing, and effective circulation, consider the following actions if the patient shows signs of hypoglycemia. Give normal saline or Ringer's lactate at a to-keep-open rate unless signs of shock are present. If signs of shock are observed or if the child is dehydrated, give a fluid bolus of normal saline at 20 mL/kg as instructed by medical direction. Reassess the child's response.

Determine the child's blood glucose level. If the glucose level is low, treat with dextrose or glucagon as instructed by medical direction. Give oral glucose gel only if the patient can swallow, has a gag reflex, and is alert or can be roused to alertness. If the child has

TABLE 37-12 Assessment and Treatment of Pediatric Diabetic Emergencies

Assessment	Hypoglycemia	Hyperglycemia
General Impression	Normal or decreased responsiveness; pale, diaphoretic	Normal or decreased responsiveness; face flushed
Breathing	Normal to increased rate	Initial ventilations deep, rapid Late: Kussmaul breathing
Circulation	Tachycardia; normal or delayed capillary refill; normal or cool, pale, clammy skin	Normal heart rate or tachycardia; skin dry, warm, flushed
History	Rapid onset (minutes to hours); took too much insulin; ate less food than usual; increased exercise; headache, dizziness, seizures	Gradual onset (hours to days); excessive food intake containing sugar; insufficient insulin dosage; polyuria, polydipsia, polyphagia
Physical Examination	Normal breath odor; tremors, staring, inability to concentrate, incoordination, irritability	Possible fruity breath odor; abdominal pain; signs of dehydration; nausea and/or vomiting
Initial Management	ABCs, O_2, IV, dextrose orally or IV (depending on mental status) or glucagon intramuscularly	ABCs, O_2, IV, fluid challenge for signs of dehydration or shock

Modified from Aehlert, B. (2005). *Comprehensive pediatric emergency care.* St. Louis: Mosby.
ABCs, Airway, breathing, circulation; *IV,* intravenous.

an altered mental status and blood glucose level is less than 60 mg/dL, establish IV access and administer dextrose as ordered by medical direction. The dextrose concentration and dosage are age dependent. If IV access cannot be established, medical direction may order glucagon intramuscularly. If glucagon is given, place the child on his or her side after administration (unless contraindicated) because glucagon may cause nausea. Closely assess the child's response. Recheck and document vital signs often. Recheck the blood glucose level within 10 minutes and frequently thereafter until the level stabilizes.

Patient and Family Education

The diabetic child and family must be taught about diabetes, including signs and symptoms of low blood sugar, checking blood glucose levels, urine ketone monitoring, meal planning, and insulin adjustment. They also should be made aware of the availability of support groups through the American Diabetes Association and Juvenile Diabetes Foundation.

Hyperglycemia

Description and Definition

Excess glucose in the blood is called *hyperglycemia.* Hyperglycemia leads to dehydration and ketoacidosis.

Etiology

The blood sugar level may become too high when the diabetic patient has not taken insulin, has eaten too much food that contains or produces sugar, or experiences physical (e.g., infection, surgery) or emotional stress.

History

The hyperglycemic patient's history commonly includes the following:

- Excessive food intake containing sugar
- Insufficient insulin dosage
- Infection, surgery, or emotional stress

Common presenting symptoms of new-onset or worsening diabetes include **polydipsia** (excessive thirst), **polyuria** (frequent urination), and/or **polyphagia** (excessive eating).

Physical Examination

A slight increase in ventilatory rate is seen early in diabetic ketoacidosis. Kussmaul breathing may develop later. Tachycardia is common in hypoglycemic patients and those with diabetic ketoacidosis. BP may be decreased as a result of dehydration. Poor skin turgor, dry mucous membranes, and/or a sunken fontanel may be evident because of dehydration. Assessment of the abdomen may reveal nonspecific pain, tenderness, or distention.

Differential Diagnosis

Consider other causes of dehydration, including vomiting and diarrhea, and other causes of altered mental status, including alcohol intoxication, electrolyte disorders, overdose, infection, and poisoning.

Therapeutic Interventions

Maintain an open airway, suction as necessary, and administer oxygen. Place the child on a cardiac monitor and pulse oximeter. Check the child's blood glucose level. If signs of dehydration or shock are present, establish IV access and administer a 20-mL/kg fluid bolus of normal saline if ordered by medical direction. Reassess. Do not give dextrose-containing solutions. Multiple boluses may be needed to restore adequate circulation in the severely ill child. Closely monitor the child's response. Electrolyte imbalances (particularly of potassium) may lead to ECG abnormalities and dysrhythmias. Closely monitor the ECG.

Patient and Family Education

The child must be taught the importance of carrying medical identification that says the child has diabetes. The diabetic patient and family must be taught how to monitor the child's blood glucose level and urine ketones. They also need to learn how to adjust the child's dose of insulin according to the advice of the child's physician.

Meningitis

Description and Definition

Meningitis is an inflammation of the meninges, which are the membranes covering the brain and spinal cord. Viral meningitis (also called *aseptic meningitis*) is the most common type. Meningitis also can be caused by infections with several types of bacteria or fungi. Because the meninges are continuous around the central nervous system (CNS) and cerebrospinal fluid (CSF) flows in the arachnoid space, infection spreads quickly through the coverings of the brain. The inflammatory response causes the brain to become swollen and covered with a layer of pus.

In newborns, bacterial meningitis is usually acquired by contact and aspiration of maternal intestinal and genital tract secretions shortly before or during delivery. In older infants and children, the infection that causes meningitis is usually secondary to another bacterial infection, such as an upper respiratory infection, ear infection, pneumonia, or sinusitis. Bacterial meningitis also may occur because of direct invasion of the CNS by bacteria. Examples of situations in which this may occur include skull fracture (CSF leak) or penetrating injuries of the skull (e.g., by toys, teeth).

Etiology

Many viruses are responsible for viral meningitis. Before the 1990s, most cases of bacterial meningitis among children younger than 5 years were from HiB. Vaccines now given to children as part of their routine immunizations (beginning at approximately 2 months of age) have reduced the occurrence of HiB meningitis. *S. pneumoniae* and *Neisseria meningitidis* are now the leading causes of bacterial meningitis.

Epidemiology and Demographics

Enteroviruses, the most common cause of viral meningitis, most often are spread through the fecal-oral and less commonly by the respiratory route (direct contact with respiratory secretions of an infected person). The incubation period for enteroviruses is usually between 3 and 7 days.

Meningitis caused by *S. pneumoniae* (also called *pneumococcal meningitis*) most commonly occurs in infants younger than 8 months and after head injury. Meningitis caused by *N. meningitidis* (also called *meningococcal meningitis*) most often occurs in children younger than 5 years.

History

The onset of acute meningitis has one of the following predominant patterns (Prober, 2004):

- *Sudden onset* (less common presentation): rapidly progressive manifestations of shock, purpura, disseminated intravascular coagulopathy, and reduced levels of responsiveness, frequently resulting in death within 24 hours.
- *Gradual onset* (more common presentation): preceded by several days of fever accompanied by upper respiratory tract or gastrointestinal symptoms, followed by nonspecific signs of CNS infection such as increasing lethargy and irritability.

The child usually has a history of the following:

- Recent ear or upper respiratory infection
- Fever (may not be present in the neonate)
- Apnea, respiratory distress in neonates
- Vomiting, headache, poor feeding, photophobia
- Altered mental status
- Excessive lethargy or irritability in infants (does not quiet when comforted by caregiver)

Physical Examination

Signs and symptoms vary depending on the child's age, underlying medical condition, and the causative organism (Table 37-13). Common signs and symptoms of infection in an infant or child are shown in Box 37-15.

High fever, headache, and stiff neck (nuchal rigidity) are common symptoms of meningitis in patients older than 2 years. Symptoms can develop over several hours, or they may take 1 to 2 days to develop.

In newborns and infants younger than 2 to 3 months, fever, headache, and neck stiffness may be absent or hard to detect. Newborns and young infants initially may have subtle signs such as poor feeding, decreased activity, and irritability. A bulging fontanel or high-pitched cry may be evident.

Signs of meningeal irritation are usually present in older children, but may not be present (or present late in the course of the disease) in infants.

As the disease progresses, patients of any age may have seizures. Rash (petechiae and/or purpura) may or may not be present in meningococcal meningitis (Figure 37-17).

Differential Diagnosis

Differential diagnosis of meningitis includes the following:

- Pneumonia
- Hantavirus
- Drug reaction
- Blood disorder
- Kawasaki disease

TABLE 37-13 Bacterial Meningitis: Presentation by Age

Assessment Findings	Younger Than 2-3 Months	2-3 Months to 2 Years	Older Than 2 Years
Apnea/Cyanosis	Common	Rare	Rare
Fever	Common	Common	Common
Hypothermia	Common	Rare	Rare
Altered Mental Status	Common	Common	Common
Headache	Rare	Rare	Common
Seizures	Early finding	Early finding	Late finding
Ataxia	Rare	Variable	Early finding
Jitteriness	Common	Common	Rare
Vomiting	Common	Common	Variable
Stiff Neck	Rare	Late finding	Common
Bulging Fontanel	Common	Common	Closed

Modified from Barkin, R. M., Marx, J. A., & Rosen, P. (1999). Neurologic disorders. In R. M. Barkin & P. Rosen (Eds.), *Emergency pediatrics: A guide to ambulatory care* (5th ed.). St. Louis: Mosby.

BOX 37-15 Signs and Symptoms of Infection in an Infant or Child

- Fever
- Chills
- Tachycardia
- Cough
- Sore throat
- Nasal congestion
- Malaise
- Tachypnea
- Cool or clammy skin
- Petechiae
- Respiratory distress
- Poor feeding
- Vomiting
- Diarrhea
- Dehydration
- Shock
- Purpura
- Seizures
- Severe headache
- Irritability
- Stiff neck
- Bulging fontanel (infant)

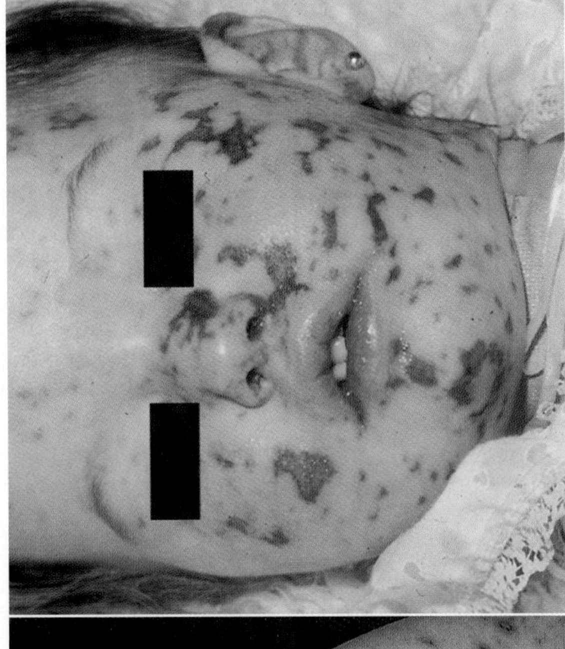

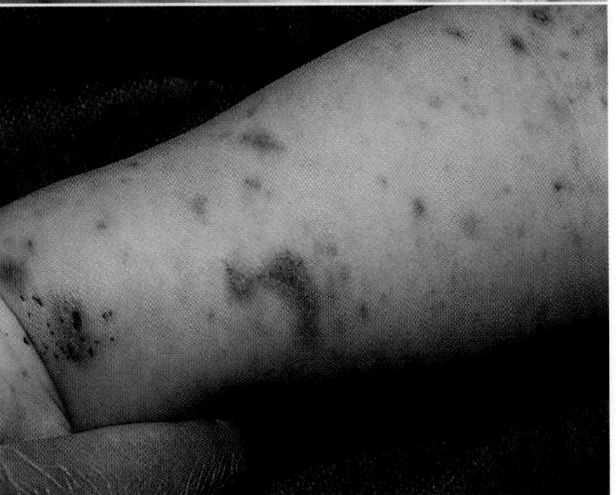

Figure 37-17 Meningococcemia. **A,** The purpuric and petechial rash characteristic of acute meningococcemia. **B,** Petechiae in an infant.

Therapeutic Interventions

Take appropriate infection control precautions. Provide care to ensure an open airway, adequate breathing, and effective circulation. Emergency care for meningitis is mainly supportive. Monitor the child for seizures. If signs of decompensated shock or dehydration are present, administer oxygen and place the child on a cardiac monitor and pulse oximeter. Medical direction may instruct you to give an IV fluid bolus of normal saline or Ringer's lactate. Reassess the child.

Patient and Family Education

If the child has bacterial meningitis, persons in the same household or daycare center and all individuals with direct contact with a patient's oral secretions are at increased risk of acquiring the infection. Close contacts should receive antibiotic therapy.

Poisoning and Toxic Exposure

Description and Definition

Children are at risk for toxic exposures because of their developmental and environmental characteristics. Developmental characteristics of children include the following:

- Curious by nature
- Mobile
- Explore their environment by putting most things in their mouths
- Imitate the behavior of others
- Inability to discriminate a toxic substance from a nontoxic one
- Drawn to attractive packaging and smell of many products found around the home

Environmental characteristics include the following:

- Toxic substances (such as household cleaning agents, gardening chemicals, plants) are often accessible to a child (improper storage, availability of substances in their immediate environment)
- Inattentiveness of caregiver or inadequate supervision

Etiology

Most cases of pediatric toxic exposure are unintentional, occur in the home, and involve only a single substance. Substances most frequently involved in pediatric exposures (children younger than 6 years) are listed in Table 37-14.

Epidemiology and Demographics

Children younger than 6 years are at the greatest risk for unintentional poisoning. Poisonings in older children and adolescents usually represent manipulative behavior, chemical or drug abuse, or genuine suicide attempts (Dart & Rumack, 2003).

Many poisonings take place during mealtime or when the family routine is disrupted. Death from unintentional poisoning in young children is uncommon for the following reasons:

- Increased product safety measures (e.g., child-resistant packaging)
- Increased poison prevention education
- Early recognition of exposure
- Improvements in medical management

History

Critical questions to ask in a toxic exposure situation include what, when, where, why, and how.

TABLE 37-14 Substances Most Frequently Involved in Pediatric Exposures (Children <6 Years)

Substance	Number Affected (%)*
Cosmetics and personal care products	13.3
Cleaning substances	10.3
Analgesics	7.4
Foreign bodies	7.1
Topicals	7.0
Plants	5.1
Cough and cold preparations	5.1
Pesticides	4.1
Vitamins	3.7
Gastrointestinal preparations	3.2
Antimicrobials	2.8
Antihistamines	2.6
Arts, crafts, or office supplies	2.6
Hormones and hormone antagonists	2.3
Hydrocarbons	1.8

Data source: Watson, W. A., Litovitz, T. L., Rodgers, G. C., Jr., et al. (2002). 2002 Annual report of the American Association of Poison Control Centers Toxic Exposure Surveillance System. *American Journal of Emergency Medicine, 21*, 353-421.

*Percentages are based on total number of exposures in children younger than 6 years (1,227,381) rather than the total number of substances.

Physical Examination

Many toxins can produce changes in mental status, skin temperature and moisture, pupils, BP, heart rate, and respiratory rate. These changes may provide a collection of physical findings that are typical of a specific toxin. Frequent reassessment is important to note any trends or changes in the patient's condition.

As you assess the patient's airway, note the presence of any odors that may help pinpoint the cause of the patient's condition. Your physical examination findings may provide the only clues to the presence of a toxin if the patient is unresponsive.

Therapeutic Interventions

The effects of toxins may result in altered mental status, vomiting, or seizures, increasing the child's risk of airway obstruction, aspiration, and lung damage. Be alert to potential airway problems and make sure suction is readily available. If breathing is inadequate, assist breathing with a bag-mask device with supplemental oxygen. Severe upper airway injury after a caustic ingestion may prevent advanced airway insertion. Because many toxins affect heart rate, place the child on a cardiac monitor. Consult with a poison control center as needed for specific treatment to prevent further absorption of the toxin (or to determine antidote). Safely obtain any substance or substance container of a suspected poison and transport it with the patient.

Patient and Family Education

Give the child's caregiver the nationwide Poison Control Center hotline number: 800-222-1222. Talk to the caregiver about how to childproof the home. This should include keeping medications, cosmetics, cleaning solutions, and pesticides up and out of reach of children.

PEDIATRIC TRAUMA

[OBJECTIVES 29, 30 31]

The most common factor in acute traumatic injuries is kinetic energy (the energy of motion), and the dissipation of that energy. A child's small size and shape permit distribution of intense force over a smaller area. Blunt trauma is the most common mechanism of serious injury in the pediatric patient.

Penetrating trauma is less common in young children but is becoming an increasing problem in adolescents, particularly in urban areas. When assessing a patient who has a penetrating injury, bear in mind that you cannot assess the extent of internal injuries by simply looking at the external injury. For example, the severity of a knife wound depends on the length of the blade, angle of penetration, the area of the body pierced with the knife, and the motion applied to the blade. The severity of a firearm injury is related to the size or caliber of the bullet, alteration in the trajectory of the bullet within the body, the bullet's velocity, and the distance of the victim from the weapon.

Mechanism of Injury

Falls

Falls are the single most common cause of injury in children. Important factors to consider in a fall are shown in Box 37-16. In general, the greater the height from which the child falls, the more severe the injury. However, the type of surface onto which the child falls (concrete and trash are the most common) and the degree to which the fall is broken on the way down affect the type and severity of injuries.

Motor Vehicle Crashes

The injuries that result from a motor vehicle crash (MVC) depend on the following:

- The type of collision
- The position of the occupant inside the vehicle
- The use or nonuse of active or passive restraint systems

Child safety seats are available in several shapes and sizes to adapt to the different stages of physical development, including infant carriers, toddler seats, and booster seats. Safety seats use a combination of lap belts, shoulder belts, full-body harnesses, and harness and shield apparatuses to protect the child during MVCs. When used properly, the restraints transfer the force of the impact from the patient's body to the restraint belts and restraint system.

An improperly worn restraint may not protect against injury in the event of a crash and may even cause injury. For example, if an infant is properly restrained in a car seat but the car seat is not properly secured to the vehicle, the infant may be ejected from the vehicle or strike various parts of the vehicle during a crash. Predictable injuries that may occur even with proper use of a child safety seat include blunt abdominal trauma, change-of-speed injuries from deceleration forces, and neck and spinal injury.

Motor Vehicle and Pedestrian Crashes

Pedestrian injuries are a common cause of traumatic death for children 5 to 9 years of age in the United States. Most pedestrian injuries occur during the day, peaking in the after-school period. It has been estimated that about 30% of pedestrian injuries occur while the child is in a marked crosswalk (Rivara & Grossman, 2007). Pedestrian injuries are a frequent cause of serious lower extremity fractures, particularly in the school-aged child (Rivara & Grossman, 2007).

Adults typically turn away if they are about to be struck by an oncoming vehicle, resulting in lateral or posterior injuries. In contrast, a child usually faces an oncoming vehicle, resulting in anterior injuries. Factors affecting the severity of injury are shown in Box 37-17.

Pedestrian versus motor vehicle crashes have three separate phases, each with its own injury pattern. Because a child is usually shorter, the initial impact of the automobile occurs higher on the body than in adults. The bumper typically strikes the child's pelvis or legs (above the knees) and the fender strikes the abdomen. Predictable injuries from the initial impact include injuries to the chest, abdomen, pelvis, or femur. The second impact occurs as the front of the vehicle's hood continues forward and strikes the child's thorax. The child is thrown backward, forcing the head and neck to flex forward. Depending on the position of the child in relation to the vehicle, the child's head and face may strike the front or top of the vehicle's hood. An impression from the child's head may be left on the hood or windshield. Primary and contrecoup injuries to the head are common in this situation. Predictable injuries from the second impact include facial, abdominopelvic, and thoracic trauma and head and neck injury. The third impact occurs as the child is thrown to the ground. Because of the child's smaller size and weight, the child may fall in the following ways:

- Under the vehicle and become trapped and dragged for some distance
- To the side of the vehicle, causing the child's lower limbs to be run over by a front wheel
- Backward, ending up completely under the vehicle (in this situation, almost any injury can occur, such as being run over by a wheel or being dragged)

Bicycle Injuries

Most severe and fatal bicycle injuries involve head trauma. Other injuries associated with bicycle crashes include

BOX 37-16 Factors to Consider in a Fall

- The height from which the child fell
- The mass of the child
- The surface on which the child landed
- The part of the child's body that struck first
- Protective equipment (e.g., helmet, knee pads)

BOX 37-17 Pedestrian versus Motor Vehicle Crashes: Factors Affecting the Severity of Injury

- Speed of the vehicle
- Point of initial impact
- Additional points of impact
- Height and weight of the child
- Surface on which the child lands

facial and extremity trauma and abdominal injuries (from striking the handlebars).

All young children should wear a bicycle helmet, whether they are riding a bicycle, a tricycle, roller skates, or skateboards or are a passenger on a parent's bicycle. The use of helmets can reduce the risk of head injury. A helmet absorbs some of the energy and dissipates the blow over a larger area for a slightly longer time.

PEDIATRIC*Pearl*

- The only wheeled vehicle a child does not need a helmet to ride is a wheelchair.
- If a helmet is damaged, it must be replaced.

Specific Injuries

Traumatic Brain Injury

The skull of infants and children is thin and pliable and more likely to transfer force to the brain beneath it instead of fracturing and absorbing some of the force along the fracture line. A linear skull fracture is the most common type of skull fracture in a child. Most linear fractures have an overlying hematoma or soft tissue swelling, although the swelling may not be detectable if the child is assessed soon after the trauma or if the swelling is under the patient's hair.

The disproportionately large size and weight of a child's head add to the momentum of acceleration-deceleration forces and account for the fact that infants and children tend to lead with their heads when falling or when thrown (whether bodily or ejected from a motor vehicle). The larger relative mass of the head and lack of neck muscle strength also add greater stress to the cervical spine region.

In adults, an epidural hematoma is usually from an arterial tear, typically the middle meningeal artery. A pediatric epidural hematoma occasionally may be the result of *venous* bleeding. This predisposes the infant or child to more subtle signs and symptoms that occur over days (Cantor & Leaming, 2002).

In children, subdural hematomas most commonly occur in patients younger than 2 years, with 93% of cases involving children younger than 1 year (Cantor & Leaming, 2002). A subdural hematoma may be acute or chronic. Chronic subdural hematomas are most often seen in patients who have been subjected to shaken baby syndrome. An acute subdural hematoma is the most common cause of death in sports-related head injuries because it also is associated with cerebral contusion and edema (Cantor & Leaming, 2002). A newborn or infant often presents with focal seizures, decreased level of consciousness, bulging fontanelle, weak cry, pallor, and vomiting. Retinal hemorrhages, which may occur as a result of the primary injury, are common. In children older than 2 to 3 years, signs and symptoms often include pupillary changes, hemiparesis, restlessness, focal neurologic signs, and altered mental status.

In the field, determining which type of hematoma is present may be impossible. Recognizing the presence of a brain injury and signs of increasing intracranial pressure is more important. Signs and symptoms of increasing intracranial pressure are shown in Box 37-18. Because of open fontanelles and sutures, infants up to an average age of 16 months may be more tolerant of an increase in intracranial pressure and can have delayed signs. As intracranial pressure increases, a portion of the brain may herniate through the foramen magnum. Signs of herniation include asymmetric pupils, decorticate posturing, and decerebrate posturing.

General Management. Suspect cervical spine injury and take cervical spine precautions (see the discussion of spinal stabilization). Stabilize the cervical spine in a neutral, not sniffing, position. Hypoxia must be prevented to avoid secondary injury to brain tissue. If you need to open the airway, use the jaw thrust without head tilt maneuver. Suction as needed. Administer supplemental oxygen if indicated. Be prepared to assist inadequate breathing.

Endotracheal intubation often is necessary for the severely head-injured child. If permitted by medical direction and local protocol, consider rapid sequence intubation and the use of IV or endotracheal lidocaine before the procedure. Lidocaine is given to blunt the rise in intracranial pressure that often is associated with the procedure. Make sure suction is readily available (within reach).

Control external bleeding if present. Significant blood loss can occur through scalp lacerations and should be immediately controlled. Spontaneous vomiting in the first 30 to 60 minutes after a head injury is common in children. Consider placement of an orogastric tube. Elevate the head of the stretcher or backboard 30 degrees unless contraindicated. Start an IV of isotonic fluid

BOX 37-18 Signs and Symptoms of Increasing Intracranial Pressure

- Headache that becomes increasingly severe (early sign)
- Vomiting (early sign)
- Confusion, changes in consciousness (early sign)
- Bulging fontanelle in infants (late sign)
- Comatose (late sign)
- Pupil changes (late sign)
- Pulse slows or becomes irregular (late sign)
- Respirations become irregular (late sign)
- Posturing (late sign)
- Seizures (late sign)

(normal saline or Ringer's lactate). Consult medical direction to determine the appropriate rate at which fluids should be infused. If hypotension is present, look for signs of internal bleeding.

Treat seizures if present. Perform frequent neurologic checks, including vital signs, arousability, size and reactivity of the pupils to light, and extent and symmetry of motor responses. Repeated assessments are crucial to detect signs of increasing intracranial pressure. Use the modified GCS for ongoing comparisons. The initial GCS score often influences treatment and transport decisions. A GCS score that falls 2 points suggests significant deterioration. Urgent patient reassessment is needed. Transport the patient rapidly to the closest appropriate facility.

Spinal Trauma

Children can have spinal nerve injury without damage to the vertebrae, a condition called *spinal cord injury without radiographic abnormality* (SCIWORA). SCIWORA is thought to be caused by the increased mobility of a child's spine because of the relatively large size of the child's head, weakness of the soft tissues of the neck, incomplete development of the bony spine, and frequency with which ligamentous injuries occur without cervical spine injury.

Spinal cord and spinal column injuries are uncommon in the pediatric patient. Children younger than 8 years tend to sustain injury to the upper (C1 and C2) cervical spine region. Nearly 80% of spine injuries in children younger than 2 years affect the upper cervical spine region. Adults and older children tend to have cervical spine injuries in the lower cervical spine area (between C5 and C6 and between C6 and C7). As a child approaches 8 to 10 years of age, the spinal anatomy and injury pattern more closely resemble those of adult injuries. Half of all children with spinal cord injury die immediately or within the first hour of injury, and another 20% of survivors succumb to complications within 3 months (Dickman & Rekate, 1993). Signs and symptoms of possible spinal trauma are shown in Box 37-19.

BOX 37-19 Signs and Symptoms of Possible Spinal Trauma

- Pain to the neck or back
- Pain on movement of the neck or back
- Pain on palpation of the posterior neck or midline of the back
- Deformity of the spinal column
- Guarding or splinting of the muscles of the neck or back
- Priapism
- Signs and symptoms of neurogenic shock (peripheral vasodilation, bradycardia, and hypotension)
- Paralysis, paresis, numbness, or tingling in the arms or legs at any time after the incident
- Diaphragmatic breathing

General Management. Give appropriate care to ensure an open airway, adequate breathing, and effective circulation. Stabilization of the spine begins in the initial assessment and continues until the child's spine is completely immobilized on a long backboard or evidence of spinal injury has been definitively ruled out by a physician. Spinal stabilization indications include the following:

- Mechanisms of injury involving blunt or penetrating trauma directly to the spine or forces applied to the spine involving flexion, extension, or rotation of the head and neck (e.g., sports injuries, falls from heights)
- Mechanism of injury that may have resulted in rapid, forceful head movement
- Any child with an altered mental status and no history available, found in setting of possible trauma, or drowning with history or probability of diving
- Neurologic deficit in the arms or legs
- Significant helmet damage
- Local tenderness or deformity in the cervical, thoracic, or lumbar region

Possible contraindications for spinal stabilization include a combative child. Efforts to immobilize forcefully a combative child with a possible head or spinal injury may result in further manipulation of the spine and worsen the injury. If the risks of agitation and increased spinal movement from full spinal stabilization are greater than the benefits, defer the stabilization procedure and consider other stabilization options. For example, enlist the help of the child's caregiver to hold the child in a position the child can tolerate that has a neutral effect on the spine and minimizes movement. Other contraindications include the following (Carruthers, 1997):

- Penetrating foreign body to the neck with hemorrhage
- Massive cervical swelling
- Presence of a tracheal stoma essential to the management of the patient's airway
- Requirement for any maneuver to ensure adequate oxygenation and ventilation

Manual stabilization should be used in these situations. If full spinal stabilization is indicated but not performed, be sure to consult medical direction and clearly document the circumstances in your prehospital care report.

If spinal stabilization is indicated, begin by manually stabilizing the child's head and neck in a neutral in-line position. Use pediatric immobilization equipment of appropriate size. Apply a properly sized rigid cervical collar (Figure 37-18, *A*). If a properly sized device is not available, use towels, washcloths, or other material to stabilize the head as best as possible. Avoid the use of IV bags or sand bags. Their weight may push the cervical spine out of alignment. Logroll the child onto a rigid board. Secure the child to the board with straps around the chest, pelvis, and legs to restrict patient movement from side to side and prevent the child from sliding up and down on the backboard. Secure the torso to the board first and the head to the board last (Figure 37-18, *B*). Manual stabilization can be discontinued after the head has been secured to the board. Additional padding may be necessary along the torso and between the legs. Secure the board to the stretcher and reassess the patient.

If the child's condition is stable, a child safety seat can be used for stabilization. Because car seat manufacturers do not recommend using a child safety seat after a crash, some transport services have inflatable car seats that are used to transport a stable child. Manually stabilize the child's head and neck (Figure 37-19, *A*). If the seat includes a protection plate over the child's chest, remove it to enable easy visualization and assessment of the child's chest. If a chest plate is not present, use the chest straps to secure the child in place whenever possible. Additional padding and/or cravats between the straps and the child or tightening of the straps may be needed. If a properly fitting rigid cervical collar is available, apply it and use towel rolls to limit movement. If a rigid cervical collar of appropriate size is not available, use towels, washcloths, or small blankets (depending on the child's size) and adhesive tape across the forehead to immobilize the head (Figure 37-19, *B*). Use a cravat or similar material around the head to prevent forward movement (Figure 37-19, *C*). Use small blankets, towels, or similar materials to pad all open areas (voids) around the child's body so that the child does not move. Once adequately stabilized, transfer the patient and seat to the ambulance. Carefully secure the seat to the stretcher or captain's seat so that it is not mobile during transport (Figure 37-19, *D*).

If a child is critically injured or the child's condition has the potential to worsen, a child safety seat should *not* be used for stabilization. Instead, the child should be removed from the seat and placed on a rigid board. To remove the child from the child safety seat safely, place the seat on its back onto a long backboard. Slide the child out of the seat as a unit. Unstrap the child and slide him or her onto the long backboard with a padded board splint to keep the child's spine in a neutral, in-line position (Figure 37-20, *A*). Do *not* pull on the child's head or neck. Slide the child along the backboard and remove the safety seat (Figure 37-20, *B*). Stabilize the child to the backboard. Transport the patient rapidly to the closest appropriate facility.

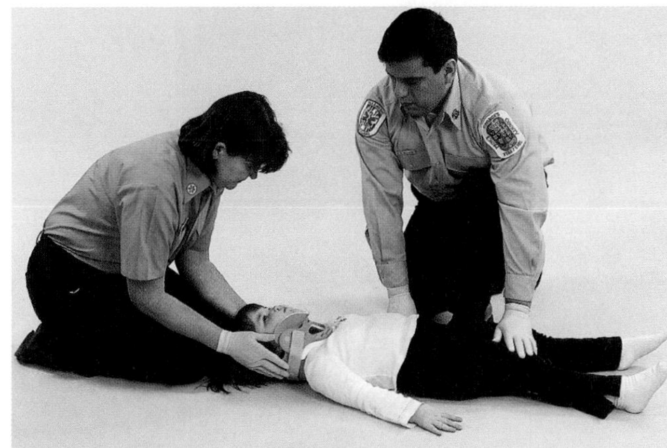

A

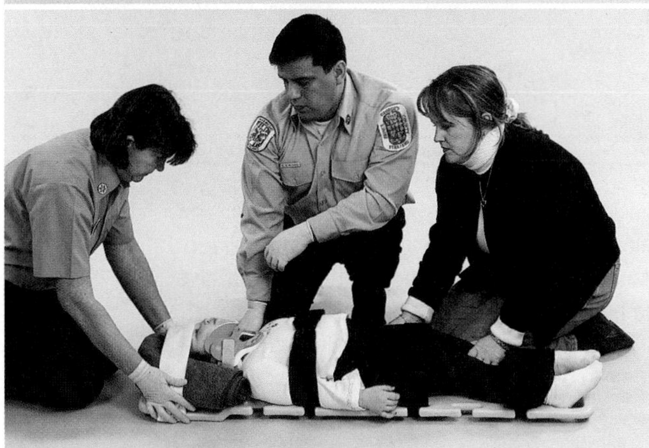

B

Figure 37-18 Immobilizing a pediatric patient on a backboard. **A,** Apply a properly sized rigid cervical collar. **B,** Secure the child to the board with straps around the chest, pelvis, and legs. Secure the head to the board last.

Chest Trauma

In children, chest trauma is associated with a high mortality rate. The greater elasticity and flexibility of the chest wall in children make rib and sternum fractures less common than in adults; however, force is more easily transmitted to the underlying lung tissues, resulting in pulmonary contusion, pneumothorax, or hemothorax. The most common chest injuries seen in children are given in Box 37-20.

Children are less likely to sustain rib fractures than adults are because a child's chest wall is more flexible than that of an adult. The presence of a rib fracture suggests significant force caused the injury. Rib fractures are most often caused by blunt trauma. They may be associated with injury to the underlying lung (pulmonary contusion) or the heart (myocardial contusion). The seriousness of the injury increases with age, the number of fractures, and the location of the fractures. A left lower rib injury is associated with injury to the spleen. A right lower rib injury is associated with injury to the liver.

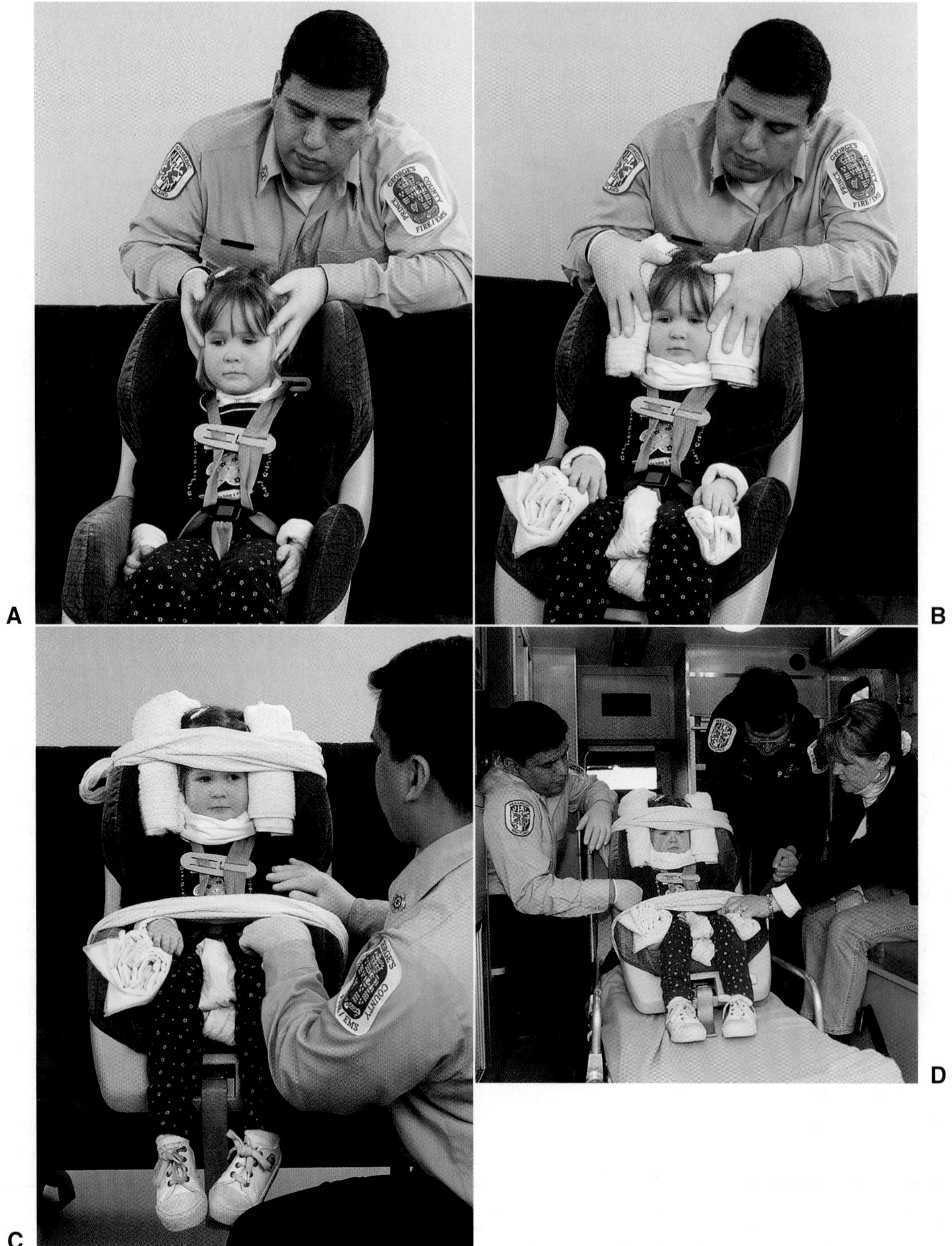

Figure 37-19 **A,** Manually stabilize the child's head and neck. Use the safety seat's chest straps to secure the child in place whenever possible. **B,** If a properly fitting rigid cervical collar is not available, use towels, washcloths, or small blankets (depending on the child's size) and adhesive tape across the forehead to immobilize the head. **C,** Use a cravat or similar material around the head to prevent forward movement. Use small blankets, towels, or similar materials to pad all open areas around the child's body so the child does not move. **D,** Secure the safety seat in place for transport.

Multiple rib fractures may result in inadequate breathing and pneumonia.

Flail chest is a life-threatening injury. It most commonly occurs from an MVC but also may occur from falls from a height, assault, and birth trauma. Because a child's ribs are flexible, flail chest is uncommon in children. When a flail chest is seen without a significant mechanism of injury, suspect child abuse.

A pulmonary contusion is one of the most frequently observed chest injuries in children. It is a potentially

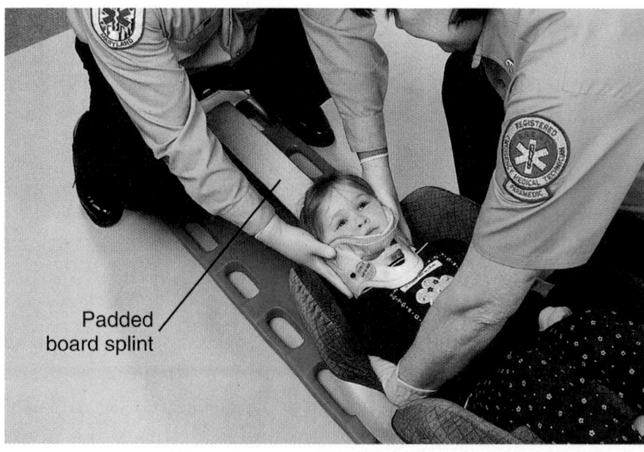

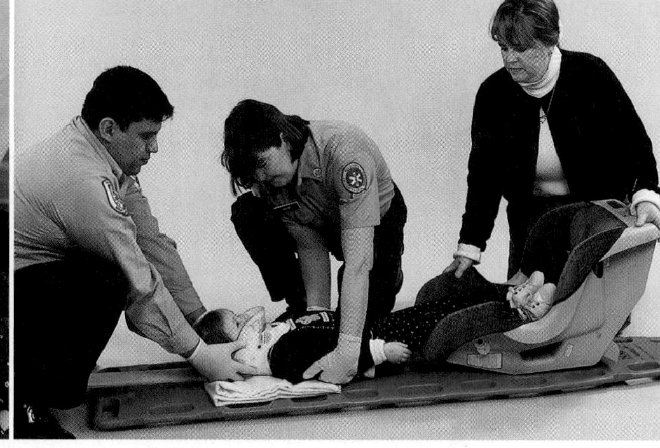

Figure 37-20 **A,** Place the seat on its back onto a long backboard. Unstrap the child and slide her onto the long backboard with a padded board splint to keep the child's spine in a neutral, in-line position. **B,** Slide the child along the board and remove the safety seat. Immobilize the child to the backboard.

BOX 37-20 Common Pediatric Chest Injuries

- Pneumothorax
- Hemothorax
- Pulmonary contusion
- Rib or sternal fractures
- Major blood vessel injury
- Cardiac injury, diaphragm injury

Reprinted from Jarjossa, J. L. (2008). Trauma, Burns, and Common Critical Care Emergencies in Johns Hopkins. In J. W. Custer, R. E. Rau (Eds.), *The Harriet Lane handbook: A manual for pediatric house officers* (18th ed.), St. Louis: Mosby.

life-threatening injury and often is missed because of the presence of other associated injuries. Tension pneumothorax is poorly tolerated and is an immediate threat to life. A massive hemothorax indicates great vessel or cardiac injury. It produces both respiratory failure and circulatory collapse. Massive hemothorax is rare in children. It is usually associated with a high-speed MVC, fall from a great height, or a high-powered or close-range gunshot wound. Many children with cardiac tamponade have no physical signs of tamponade other than hypotension. If profound hypovolemia is present, jugular venous distention is absent. If bradycardia occurs, the child is about to arrest.

General Management. Give oxygen and assist breathing with a bag-mask device if needed. Evaluate the need for endotracheal intubation and analgesics. Closely monitor the child for development of a tension pneumothorax. If the child has an open pneumothorax, promptly close the chest wall defect with an airtight (occlusive) dressing. Tape the dressing on three sides. After taping, if the child develops signs of a tension pneumothorax, remove the dressing over the wound for a few seconds. If the wound in the chest wall has not sealed under the dressing, air will rush out of the wound. Reseal the wound with the airtight dressing once the pressure has been released. You may need to repeat this procedure periodically if pressure again builds up in the chest. If this procedure does not relieve the signs of a tension pneumothorax, perform needle decompression. Treat hypovolemia and shock with IV fluids. Do not delay transport to establish an IV on the scene. Transport rapidly to the closest appropriate facility.

Abdominal and Pelvic Trauma

Abdominal trauma is the third leading cause of traumatic death after head and thoracic injuries. It is the most common cause of unrecognized fatal injury in children. The abdominal organs of an infant or child are susceptible to injury for several reasons. The abdominal wall is thin, so the organs are closer to the surface of the abdomen. Children have proportionally larger solid organs, less subcutaneous fat, and less protective abdominal musculature than adults do. The liver and spleen of a small child are lower in the abdomen and are less protected by the rib cage.

Blunt abdominal trauma in an infant or child is primarily caused by motor vehicle collisions (poorly placed seat belts or improperly sized child seat), motorcycle collisions, falls, sports-related injuries, pedestrian crashes, and child abuse. Blunt trauma related to MVCs is the cause of most abdominal injuries in children and is the most lethal.

The spleen is the most frequently injured abdominal organ during blunt trauma such as MVCs, sudden-deceleration injuries, and contact sports–related injuries. The spleen is completely protected by the rib cage in adolescents and adults, but in infants and small children the rib cage does not extend down far enough to provide adequate protection. The rib cage of the infant and small child also is quite pliable and does not provide the same degree of protection as the rib cage of an adult. An injury to the spleen often is associated with other intraabdominal injuries.

The liver is the second most commonly injured solid organ in the pediatric patient with blunt abdominal trauma but the most common cause of lethal hemorrhage. Injuries may be the result of blunt or penetrating trauma. A firm blow to the right upper quadrant or right-sided rib fractures may cause liver injury. The pancreas may be injured as a result of falling from a bicycle with injury caused by the handlebars, pedestrian traffic collisions, MVCs, and child abuse.

Kidney injury is usually caused by blunt trauma, such as deceleration forces, and is rarely caused by penetrating trauma. Children are more susceptible to kidney injuries because of the following facts:

- The kidneys are large in proportion to the abdomen.
- The lower ribs do not shield the kidneys from injury.
- Underdevelopment of abdominal wall muscles and a lack of extensive fat around the kidneys provide less protection for the kidneys.
- Their kidneys are mobile; they may be bruised or torn by ribs or spinal transverse process.

Fractures of the pelvis in children are uncommon. Associated soft tissue injuries may be severe and require emergency care. Many pelvic fractures occur in children struck by moving vehicles.

General Management. Give appropriate care to ensure an open airway, adequate breathing, and effective circulation. Because of the small size of the abdomen, be certain to palpate only one quadrant at a time. Any child who is hemodynamically unstable without evidence of an obvious source of blood loss should be considered to have an abdominal injury until proven otherwise. Treat hypovolemia and shock with IV fluids. Do not delay transport to establish an IV on the scene.

Because the pelvis contains major blood vessels, the patient with a pelvic fracture is at significant risk for serious hemorrhage. In some EMS systems, the pneumatic antishock garment is applied when a child has an unstable pelvis and shows signs of shock. Follow local protocol. Transport the patient rapidly to the closest appropriate facility.

Extremity Trauma

Extremity trauma is relatively more common in children than in adults. A child's skeletal system is dynamically more flexible than that of adults. Clean fractures are uncommon. Instead, when an infant and child's bones break, they typically demonstrate a **greenstick fracture.** Think of a small, green branch on a tree. When you bend it, it can flex quite far before beginning to break. When the branch breaks, it splinters into many pieces but also remains connected to itself. The same phenomenon occurs in the bones of small children.

The muscles of children are smaller than an adult's, offering less protection to the body's organ systems and the neurovascular bundles in extremities. This leads to an increased risk of underlying structure damage when infants and children are involved in traumatic events.

Fractures are among the most often missed injuries in children with multiple trauma. Growth plate injuries are common. Bilateral femur fractures can cause significant blood loss, resulting in hypovolemic shock. Be alert for evidence of possible child abuse under the following circumstances:

- Fractures of differing ages
- Discrepancy between history and injury
- Prolonged and/or unexplained delay in treatment
- Different stories at different times
- Poor health and hygiene

General Management. Give appropriate care to ensure an open airway, adequate breathing, and effective circulation. Control any sites of active bleeding. Splint to prevent further injury and blood loss. Immobilize the joint above and below the injury. Assess and document pulses, motor function, and sensation in the affected extremity before and after splinting. Consider the need for applying extra padding and protection when preparing the patient for transport. Treat hypovolemia and shock with IV fluids. Transport the patient to the closest appropriate facility.

Burns

In children, chemical burns usually involve household products. Minor electrical burns usually occur as a result of an infant or toddler biting on an extension cord, resulting in localized burns to the mouth that usually involve the upper and lower lip in contact with the extension cord. High-tension electrical wire burns may occur at high-voltage installations, such as electric power stations. The child may touch an electric box or accidentally touch a high-tension electric wire such as flying a kite into overhead wires. Electrical burns require hospital admission for observation regardless of the extent of the surface area burn because the extent of damage may not be initially apparent.

General Management. Prompt management of the airway is required because swelling can rapidly develop. If intubation is required, a tracheal tube up to two sizes smaller than what would normally be used may be required. Assess for associated injuries or shock. Assess for dysrhythmias with a cardiac monitor. Be sure to assess the child's back for burn injury. Keep burned extremities elevated above the level of the heart. Do not place ice or wet sheets on the burn; if burns are more than 10% of the body surface area, apply clean, dry towels to the burn to avoid hypothermia. Check local protocol. Maintain normal body temperature. Establish vascular access. Most burn centers prefer the use of lactated Ringer's solution. Check local protocol. Monitor vital signs *at least* every 15 min-utes. Give analgesics as ordered by medical direction.

Suspect musculoskeletal injuries if the child has an electrical burn and perform spinal immobilization. If the child has a chemical burn, contact a poison control center for advice before treating the patient, particularly if the substance was ingested. While you wear protective clothing, brush dry chemicals from the child's skin by using towels, sheets, or gloved hands. Remove any of the child's clothing that has come in contact with the chemical. Do *not* waste time trying to obtain specific neutralizing chemicals.

Drowning

Drowning is the process of experiencing respiratory impairment from immersion or submersion in a liquid. Immersion refers to covering of the face and airway in water or other fluid. In a submersion incident, the victim's entire body, including his airway, is under the water or other fluid. Delayed drowning refers to survival, at least temporarily, after an immersion or submersion episode.

Drowning is the second most common cause of death by unintentional injury among children. Drowning may occur in lakes, rivers, streams, swimming pools, hot tubs, bathtubs, toilets, buckets, and washing machines. Toddlers most commonly drown in pools and bathtubs and occasionally toilets or buckets of water. Adolescents most commonly drown in larger bodies of water, such as a lake, river, or ocean, and frequently have diving-related spine injuries. The major physiologic consequences of submersion are hypoxia, acidosis, and pulmonary edema. Of these, hypoxia is the most important. Factors affecting patient outcome include water temperature, duration and degree of hypothermia, the diving reflex, the victim's age, water contamination, duration of cardiac arrest, the promptness and effectiveness of initial treatment, and cerebral resuscitation (Feldhaus, 2002). The child's prognosis is poor if he or she is comatose or CPR is in progress on arrival in the emergency department.

Depending on the type and duration of water-related incident, the child's signs and symptoms may vary from no symptoms to cardiac arrest. All drowning victims should be transported to the hospital for evaluation and observation, even those who appear to have recovered fully because signs of pulmonary infection may appear many hours after the event.

General Management. Begin efforts to restore oxygenation, ventilation, and perfusion as quickly as possible. Start rescue breathing as soon as the victim's airway can be opened and the rescuer's safety can be ensured (usually when the victim is in shallow water or out of the water). Cervical spine stabilization is unnecessary unless the incident included diving, use of a water slide, signs of injury, or signs of alcohol intoxication (American Heart Association, 2005). If the incident was not witnessed, assume cervical spine injury and provide in-line stabilization.

If possible, open the child's airway as soon as the head is above water. According to current resuscitation guidelines, clearing the airway of aspirated water is not necessary; however, debris, gastric contents, or other foreign material may need to be removed. Routine use of abdominal thrusts or the Heimlich maneuver is not recommended. These procedures can cause injury, vomiting, and aspiration and delay CPR. Administer supplemental oxygen if indicated. If the child is apneic, intubate and give positive-pressure ventilation. Medical direction may instruct you to provide positive end-expiratory pressure if the patient has increased resistance to ventilation, crackles on auscultation of the lungs, or continuing hypoxia despite assisted ventilation. Use pulse oximetry to monitor oxygenation. Decompress the stomach with an orogastric or nasogastric tube if significant distention is present from swallowed water or air.

Drowning victims are at risk from immersion hypothermia. Remove wet clothing, dry the patient, and apply blankets to reduce further heat loss and hypothermia. Monitor the patient's cardiac rhythm. Begin CPR immediately if no pulse is present or if the heart rate is below 60 beats per minute with signs of hypoperfusion. Keep in mind that detecting a pulse may be difficult because of peripheral vasoconstriction and decreased cardiac output. Attach an automated external defibrillator and attempt defibrillation if a shockable rhythm is identified. Treat dysrhythmias according to resuscitation guidelines. Establish IV access with normal saline or Ringer's lactate. In patients with signs of shock, give a bolus of normal saline or lactated Ringer's solution at 20 mL/kg (or the amount ordered by medical direction), then reassess circulation. Shivering and vigorous struggling can lower blood glucose levels. After the initial assessment and warming, check the child's blood glucose level. Assess for hypoglycemia and give dextrose if indicated. Transport the patient to the closest appropriate facility for physician evaluation.

PARAMEDIC*Pearl*

- When providing emergency care for a drowning victim, always remember personal safety.
- If *any* type of resuscitation is required for a drowning victim, the patient should be transported to the hospital for evaluation.

Special Considerations

[OBJECTIVES 32, 33, 34]

Airway Control

In general, perform the following actions in regard to airway control:

- Maintain in-line stabilization in a neutral, not sniffing, position.
- Give supplemental oxygen if indicated.
- Maintain an open airway by suctioning and jaw thrust without head tilt maneuver.
- Be prepared to assist ineffective breathing.
- Perform intubation when the airway remains inadequate.
- Place a gastric tube after intubation.
- Needle cricothyroidotomy is rarely indicated for traumatic upper airway obstruction.

Immobilization

Use appropriately sized equipment for pediatric immobilization, including the following:

- Rigid cervical collar
- Towel or blanket roll
- Child safety seat
- Vest-type device or short wooden backboard
- Pediatric immobilization device
- Long backboard
- Straps and cravats
- Tape
- Padding

Because the high cervical region is the most likely area of spinal injury in a pediatric patient, placing a child's neck in a flexed position is particularly dangerous. Proper stabilization of infants, toddlers, and preschoolers requires either a special board with a recess for the back of the head, allowing the head to rest in line with the body, or placement of padding under the shoulders to the hips.

Fluid Management

Management of the airway and breathing takes priority over management of circulation because circulatory compromise is less common in children than adults. When establishing vascular access, insert a large-bore IV catheter into a large peripheral vein. Do not delay transport to gain vascular access. If an IV cannot be established, attempt IO access. In consultation with medical direction, give an initial fluid bolus of 20 mL/kg of Ringer's lactate or normal saline (usually 10 mL/kg for a newborn). Reassess vital signs. Give another bolus of 20 mL/kg if no improvement. If improvement does not occur after the second bolus, significant blood loss and the need for rapid surgical intervention are likely. *Do not wait for the second fluid bolus to finish before deciding how or where to transport the patient.* The patient needs rapid transport to the closest appropriate facility.

ANALGESIA AND SEDATION

[OBJECTIVE 35]

Pain should be assessed in *all* patients. Adequate pain management requires ongoing assessment of the presence and severity of pain and the child's response to treatment. The answers a patient provides in response to questions about pain is called a *self-report*. The patient's self-report is considered the most reliable method for assessing pain (in patients who can communicate verbally) because it is the child's verbal statement and description of pain. Self-reporting is appropriate for most children 3 years and older.

The methods for assessing pain in the pediatric patient vary according to the age of the child. Use an age-appropriate pain rating scale. The same scale should be used consistently by all persons caring for the child. A good assessment tool to use is the Wong-Baker Faces pain rating scale. This scale combines three scales in one: facial expressions, numbers, and words. The scale consists of six cartoon faces ranging from a smiling face depicting "no hurt" to a tearful, sad face illustrating "worst hurt" (Figure 37-21). This scale is best used for children aged 3 years or older.

Pain relief is important for all patients. Fractures of long bones and burns are examples of situations in which an analgesic should be given as long as no contraindications are present (e.g., hypotension). Consult medical direction before giving an analgesic. In some situations a sedative is more appropriate. For example, sedation should be considered before procedures such as cardio-

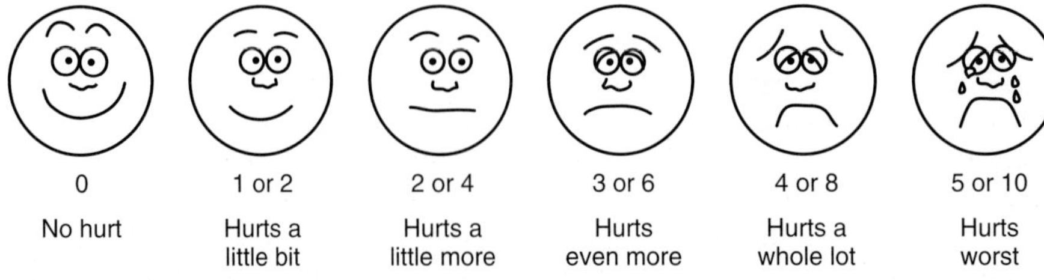

Figure 37-21 Wong-Baker Faces pain rating scale. To use this scale, point to each face and use the words to describe the pain intensity. Ask the child to choose the face that best describes his or her own pain. Document the appropriate number.

version. Keep in mind that analgesics used to manage severe pain usually cause sedation, but most sedatives do not provide analgesia.

CHILD ABUSE

[OBJECTIVE 36]

Terminology

Child maltreatment includes intentional physical abuse or neglect, emotional abuse or neglect, and sexual abuse of children, usually by adults. The Child Welfare Information Gateway has established definitions of the various types of abuse. State law defines specific acts that constitute the various forms of abuse, and they vary from state to state.

Neglect is the failure of a parent or other person with responsibility for the child to provide needed food, clothing, shelter, medical care, or supervision such that the child's health, safety, and well-being are threatened with harm. Neglect can be physical, educational, or emotional. Physical neglect can include not providing adequate food or clothing, appropriate medical care, supervision, or proper weather protection (heat or coats). Educational neglect includes failure to provide appropriate schooling or special educational needs or allowing excessive truancies. Emotional neglect includes the lack of any emotional support and love, chronic inattention to the child, exposure to spouse abuse, or drug and alcohol abuse.

Physical abuse is the inflicting of a nonaccidental physical injury upon a child. This may include burning, hitting, punching, shaking, kicking, beating, or otherwise harming a child. It may, however, have been the result of overdiscipline or physical punishment that is inappropriate to the child's age. Sexual abuse is inappropriate adolescent or adult sexual behavior with a child.

Emotional abuse is a pattern of caregiver behavior or extreme incidents that convey to a child that he or she is worthless, flawed, unloved, unwanted, endangered, or only of value to meeting another's needs. This can include parents or caretakers using extreme or bizarre forms of punishment or threatening or terrorizing a child. Abuse and assault are covered in more detail in Chapter 39.

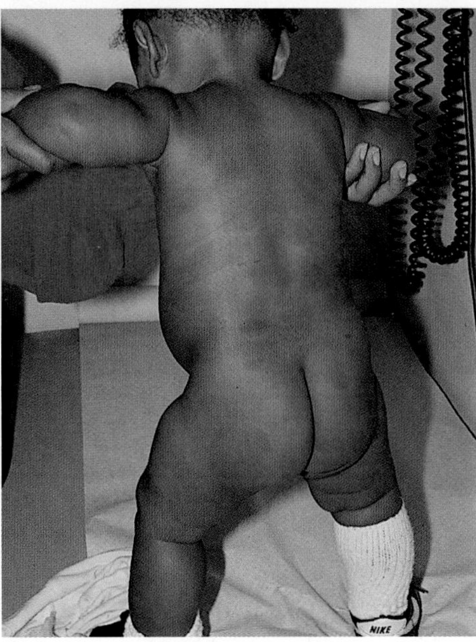

Figure 37-22 This toddler was referred from a daycare center because of "multiple bruises," but actually had an unusual number of Mongolian spots.

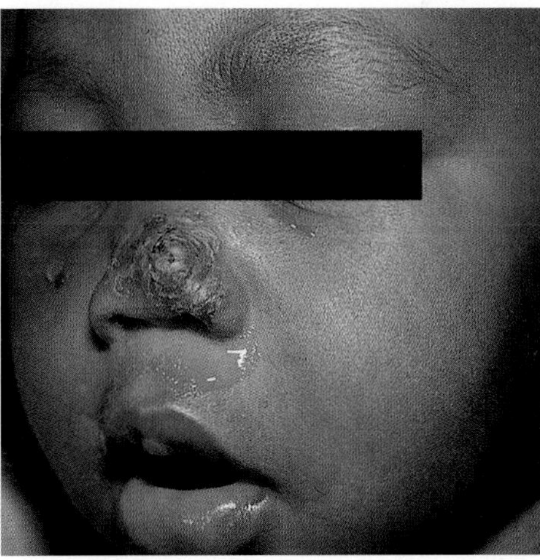

Figure 37-23 This infant was initially suspected of having a cigar burn. Close inspection by a physician and the presence of another lesion on the cheek enabled the correct diagnosis of impetigo.

Accidental versus Inflicted Injury

Children often are injured, but not all children with injuries are abused. Child abuse is unlikely if the child's story is volunteered without hesitation and matches that of the caregiver. Determining the difference between an intentional injury and an accident is often difficult.

Some medical conditions and folk medicine practices may be mistaken for child abuse. For example, Mongolian spots are benign and not associated with any conditions or illnesses (Figure 37-22). Ehlers-Danlos syndrome is a condition associated with cuts, bruises, and scars attributable to the fragility of the child's skin. Blood disorders such as hemophilia, von Willebrand disease, and leukemia also can cause skin changes such as those seen in child abuse situations. For example, bruises at various stages of healing may appear on different parts of the body. Impetigo, a contagious bacterial skin infection, may resemble a burn (Figure 37-23). Chickenpox may resemble cigarette burns. Burns caused by hot areas of a child safety seat may be mistaken for an abusive injury.

Cao Gio, also known as *coining* or *coin rubbing,* is a folk remedy used by Southeast Asians to treat conditions such as fever, chills, and headaches. A balm or ointment is spread over the back, neck, head, shoulder, or chest. A coin is then pressed on the skin and drawn a short distance in one direction without breaking the skin. The

TABLE 37-15 Suspected Child Abuse: Documentation Recommendations

Description of the scene	General appearance of the home and other children Appearance of the room where the injury occurred Any unusual, unsafe, or unsanitary conditions Behavior of those present at the scene
History of the injury or illness	Document the when, where, and how regarding the injury Document who was present Indicate any discrepancies in statements in the report Document statements made by the caregivers exactly as stated and noted in quotation marks
Findings from the physical examination	Objectively document physical examination findings, including the type, number, size, and location of injuries Document any pattern of injury, if observed
Emergency care	Document the emergency care provided and the patient's response to that care

procedure is repeated until blood appears under the skin, producing dark red welts. Coining is said to release excess "wind" or energy considered responsible for illness. Cupping is practiced by Russians, Chinese, and Latin Americans. A heated cup is applied to a part of the body to treat illness. This practice results in circular first-degree burns, usually of the chest, back, or abdomen.

Reporting Requirements and Documentation

Each state and U.S. territory designates individuals, typically by professional group, who are mandated by law to report child maltreatment. Any person, however, may report incidents of abuse or neglect. Individuals typically designated as mandatory reporters have frequent contact with children. Such individuals include healthcare workers, school personnel, childcare providers, social workers, law enforcement officers, and mental health professionals.

Remember that no matter how difficult the situation, you must maintain a professional and nonjudgmental attitude. Do not confront or accuse the child's caregivers in cases of suspected abuse. Objectively document all pertinent physical examination findings and the emergency care given. Information that should be contained in your report is shown in Table 37-15. Notify the receiving facility staff (preferably a physician or charge nurse) of your suspicions.

SUDDEN INFANT DEATH SYNDROME

Description and Definition

[OBJECTIVES 37, 38, 39]

Significant controversy revolves around the cause(s) of sudden infant death syndrome (SIDS). It has been suggested that that SIDS is the final common pathway of three coinciding factors: (1) an infant must first have an underlying vulnerability, (2) the infant is then stressed by an outside source (such as sleeping in a prone position), and (3) the stress must occur during a critical developmental period, as in the first year of life (Willinger et al., 1991).

Etiology

Current SIDS research topics include defects in normal arousal mechanisms, gene mutations affecting autonomic nervous system development, prenatal and postnatal exposure to cigarette smoke and the effects of nicotine on the developing brain, and ion channel disorders, such as those that cause QT interval prolongation. Risk factors for SIDS are shown in Box 37-21.

Epidemiology and Demographics

SIDS is the third leading cause of infant death in the United States and the most common cause of postneonatal infant death (1 month to 1 year of age) (Hunt & Hauck, 2004). The majority of SIDS deaths occur during the first 6 months of life, most between the ages of 2 and 4 months. Most of these infants die at home, usually during the night after a period of sleep.

SIDS occurs more often in infant boys than in girls (approximately a 3:2 male:female ratio). African American and Native American infants are two to three times more likely to die from SIDS than other infants. A lower incidence is seen among Hispanic and Asian infants.

The SIDS rate has declined by 42% since 1992, when the recommendation was issued to have infants sleep on their backs and sides rather than their stomachs.

Interventions

From a distance, form your first impression of the patient. Evaluate the child's appearance, work of breathing, and circulation to determine the severity of the child's illness

BOX 37-21 Risk Factors for SIDS

Maternal Risk Factors

- Smoking during pregnancy
- Drug use (cocaine, opiates)
- Alcohol use
- Late or no prenatal care
- Low socioeconomic status
- Single parent status
- Nutritional deficiency
- Young age (less than 20 y)
- Shorter interpregnancy interval

Infant Risk Factors

- Male gender
- Prematurity
- Native American or African American ancestry
- Low Apgar scores
- Overheating
- Prenatal and postnatal smoking exposure
- Prone or side sleep position
- Soft sleeping surface, soft bedding
- Recent febrile illness
- Infant/caregiver bed sharing

SIDS, Sudden infant death syndrome.

BOX 37-22 SIDS History and Documentation

Questions

- What is the baby's name?
- What happened?
- What is baby's* age?
- What does baby weigh?
- What time was baby put to bed?
- When did baby fall asleep?
- Who last saw baby alive?
- Who found baby? What did that person do?
- What position was baby in when he/she was found?
- Was CPR attempted?
- Did baby share a bed with anyone else?
- What was the general health of baby?
- Had baby been ill recently?
- Was baby taking any medications?

Observations of the Scene

- Position and location of the infant on arrival
- General appearance of the home and other children, appearance of the room where the death occurred, condition and characteristics of the crib or sleep area
- Bedding (e.g., pillows, sheets, blankets), any objects in the crib (toys or bottles), or any unusual or dangerous items that could cause choking or suffocation
- Medications
- Electrical and mechanical devices in use in the room including vaporizers, space heaters, fans, and infant electronic monitors (apnea monitor or heart rate monitor)
- Behavior of those present at the scene

CPR, Cardiopulmonary resuscitation; *SIDS*, sudden infant death syndrome.

*When asking these questions, substitute the infant's name for "baby."

or injury and the urgency for care. Perform an initial assessment and determine the need for CPR.

You must obtain a focused history and carefully document the call whether or not resuscitation efforts are initiated. Find the answers to the information you need as tactfully as possible. Begin by asking the infant's name. After obtaining this information, use the baby's name when asking questions about the incident. Do not refer to the infant as "the baby" or "it" or use other nonspecific words. If time permits, obtain the information in Box 37-22.

Begin resuscitation with standard resuscitation guidelines if your assessment does not clearly indicate death, as in cases in which the infant is still warm and flexible. Rigor mortis is an obvious sign of death. Dependent lividity is considered an obvious sign of death only when extensive areas of reddish-purple discoloration of the skin are present on dependent areas of an unresponsive, breathless, and pulseless patient. In some EMS systems both lividity and rigor mortis must be present to be considered signs of obvious death.

If resuscitation is provided, calmly explain what you are doing. Explain the roles of each member of the crew to the caregiver. If sufficient personnel are on the scene, assign one EMS professional to remain with the caregiver and provide comfort during the resuscitation effort. While keeping your explanations simple, provide frequent updates about what is happening and the infant's status, even if no change. Allow the caregivers to remain within sight of the infant. If possible, allow a caregiver to accompany the infant during transport to the emergency department.

If the physical examination clearly indicates death or if the infant's response to resuscitation efforts was unsuccessful, follow local protocols regarding resuscitation and transport. Do not express your own opinion about the cause of an infant's death in front of caregivers. Objectively document your findings. Some service areas have an obvious death, field termination, death in the field, or similar protocol applicable to this type of situation. In some service areas you may be required to leave the body at the scene pending the arrival of the medical examiner. In others you may be asked to transport the body to a hospital or morgue.

If the body must remain at the scene, tell the caregivers in a sensitive manner and explain why. Explain that the infant is dead. Do not use words or phrases such as "expired" or "passed away." Preface the bad news by saying, "This is hard to tell you, but . . . " Assume nothing regarding how the news is going to be received. The caregiver's reaction to the news may be anger, shock, withdrawal, disbelief, extreme agitation, guilt, or sorrow. In some cases the person may show no response, or the response may seem inappropriate. Allow time for the shock to be absorbed and as much time as necessary for questions. Questions frequently asked include, "Was I to blame?" and "Did my baby suffer?" Emphasize to the grieving caregivers that they were not responsible for the infant's death and the death could not be prevented. You may need to repeat your answers or explanations to ensure they are understood.

Begin grief support for the family as soon as possible. Remain with the family until law enforcement personnel assume responsibility for the body and grief support personnel are on the scene to assist the family. While awaiting the arrival of grief support, law enforcement personnel, or the medical examiner, find out the names of neighbors, relatives, or friends that you can contact to help care for other children in the home.

If you are asked to transport the body to a hospital, encourage the caregivers to hold or touch the infant while you are on the scene. This enables the caregivers to focus on the reality of the death and provides an opportunity for them to say goodbye. Tell the caregivers the name and address of the hospital, and then take the time to write down the information for them. If the caregivers cannot accompany you to the hospital, contact a family member or close friend who can arrive quickly and drive them to the hospital.

PEDIATRIC*Pearl*

Although difficult for the family, the death of an infant or child also is emotionally difficult for healthcare professionals and law enforcement personnel. You may find that meeting with a co-worker to discuss the feelings that normally follow a pediatric death may be helpful.

Prevention

The prevention of SIDS includes the following:

- Place an infant supine for sleep. The infant should sleep in the same room as his or her parents, but in his or her own crib or bassinette.
- The American Academy of Pediatrics recommends offering a pacifier at bedtime and naptime. The pacifier should be used when placing the infant down for sleep and not be reinserted once it falls out. For breast-fed infants, delay introduction of the pacifier until breast-feeding is well established (i.e., after one month of age).
- Place an infant on a firm surface for sleep. Avoid placing the infant on soft or padded sleep surfaces (e.g., pillows, sheepskins, sofas, soft mattresses, waterbeds, beanbag cushions, quilts, comforters).
- Avoid the use of soft materials in the infant's sleep environment (over, under, or near the infant). This includes pillows, comforters, quilts, sheepskins, and stuffed toys. Blankets, if used, should be tucked in around the crib mattress.
- Do not overheat the infant (keep the room temperature comfortable, do not overdress the infant, use a light blanket).
- Avoid exposure to cigarette smoke.
- Do not sleep with a baby on a sofa or armchair. Parents who smoke, are obese or especially tired, or have taken medicines, drugs, or alcohol that impairs their responsiveness should not share a bed with their infant.

CHILDREN WITH SPECIAL HEALTHCARE NEEDS

Overview

[OBJECTIVES 40, 41]

Children with special healthcare needs have or are at risk for chronic physical, developmental, behavioral, or emotional conditions that require use of health and related services of a type and amount not usually required by typically developing children (Box 37-23). Infants and children with special needs can include many different types of children. Examples of children who may have special healthcare needs include preterm babies and babies with lung disease, heart disease, neurologic disease,

BOX 37-23 Children with Special Healthcare Needs

A child with special healthcare needs who has any of the following conditions should be considered unstable or critical:

- Partial or total airway obstruction in children with tracheostomies
- Respiratory difficulties in ventilator-dependent children
- Bradycardia, irregular pulses, or signs of compensated shock in children with pacemakers
- Fever, nausea, vomiting, headache, or a change in mental status in children with CSF shunts
- Signs of worsening illness despite appropriate home therapy in any child with a chronic health problem

Because ventilator-dependent children always require assisted ventilation, critical status applies only if one or more additional signs are present.

Reprinted from Foltin, G. L., Tunik, M. G., Cooper, A., et al. (2002). *Teaching resource for instructors in prehospital pediatrics for paramedics*. New York: Center for Pediatric Emergency Medicine.
CSF, Cerebrospinal fluid.

chronic disease, or altered functions from birth. Children who use assistive technology are a subgroup of children with special healthcare needs that depend on medical devices for their survival. Equipment failure may result in a medical emergency.

The number of children with special healthcare needs is increasing. Children with gastrostomy tubes, indwelling central lines, tracheostomies, pacemakers, and home ventilators often are encountered by healthcare professionals. These children are particularly susceptible to medical problems involving the airway, breathing, and circulation.

A child with special healthcare needs may be small for his or her age. Baseline vital signs may fall outside the typical range for the child's age. He or she may require equipment sizes that differ from those estimated by age. Physical and mental abilities may not be the same as those for other children of similar age.

The child's caregiver often is the best resource regarding the child's special healthcare needs. The caregiver can usually tell you what is normal for the child regarding mental status, vital signs, normal assessment findings and level of activity, ongoing health problems, medications, and medical devices currently in use. Ask the child's caregiver if an Emergency Information Form (EIF) is available (Figure 37-24). The American Academy of Pediatrics and the American College of Emergency Physicians encourage the use of this form for children with special healthcare needs. Medic Alert also participates in the project and stores the information if the child has a Medic Alert bracelet or necklace.

The document is completed and updated by the child's primary care physician. It is then given to the parents, daycare provider, school nurse, or anyone with whom the child spends a part of his or her day. During an emergency, this form relays pertinent information that may affect treatment.

Cerebrospinal Fluid Shunts

Cerebrospinal fluid is produced in the choroid plexus located in the ventricles of the brain. CSF circulates through the ventricular system and around the spinal cord. It is then reabsorbed by vessels in the brain.

Hydrocephalus (water on the brain) develops when this normal circulation is interrupted because of an increase in CSF production, obstruction of CSF flow, or a decrease in CSF absorption. To drain excess CSF and reduce intracranial pressure, a shunting system is surgically implanted into the brain to drain (shunt) CSF from the ventricular system into another part of the body (Figure 37-25). A typical shunting system consists of a proximal catheter, a one-way valve system, and a distal catheter. The proximal catheter is usually inserted into one of ventricles of the brain and exits the skull through a surgically created hole (burr hole). The one-way valve usually contains a reservoir used to withdraw CSF or administer medications. The distal catheter is placed into a body cavity to allow drainage and absorption of CSF. On-off valves, antisiphon devices, and reservoirs also may be attached. The on-off valve is used for intermittent shunting and can be used to assess shunt function.

BOX 37-24 Causes of CSF Shunt Malfunction

- ***D***isplacement (catheter migration), disconnection of shunt components, drainage (overdrainage or inadequate drainage)
- ***O***bstructed or fractured catheter, kinking of distal catheter
- ***P***erforated abdominal viscus, peritonitis, pseudocyst
- ***E***rosion of the equipment through the skin

CSF, Cerebrospinal fluid.

Complications

When a shunt malfunctions (Box 37-24), the child may have symptoms of irritability, headache, neck pain, vomiting, a bulging or full fontanelle in infants, new seizures or a change in the child's seizure pattern, behavioral changes, or reports of "just not acting right." These are signs of increased intracranial pressure caused by fluid buildup within the brain. The child's caregiver is usually most familiar with the child's condition and can tell you if the shunt is the problem.

An infection may occur in the first few months after surgery. If infection is present, you may see redness, edema, or tenderness along the path of the shunt tubing (Figure 37-26). A child with a shunt infection usually, but not always, has a fever. Abdominal pain may be present. This occurs because infected CSF drains into the peritoneal cavity, causing peritoneal inflammation. Perforation of the stomach or intestinal wall may result in peritonitis with signs and symptoms of shock.

Emergency Care

A child with signs of increasing intracranial pressure may vomit, increasing the risk of aspiration. Make sure suction equipment is readily available. Administer oxygen, assist breathing as necessary, and be prepared to intubate. If the child shows signs of shock or if hypotension is present, contact medical direction about volume resuscitation with normal saline or Ringer's lactate. Check the child's blood sugar and give IV dextrose if indicated and ordered by medical direction. Treat seizures if indicated.

At the hospital, a CSF shunt infection is usually treated with antibiotics. Tapping the reservoir of the CSF shunt and removing fluid to lower intracranial pressure temporarily may be necessary. This procedure is only performed by qualified and experienced healthcare professionals. Additional patient conditions and equipment you are likely to encounter in the home care setting are covered in Chapter 42.

Emergency Information Form for Children With Special Needs

American College of Emergency Physicians* | American Academy of Pediatrics

Date form completed By Whom | Revised | Initials | Revised | Initials

Last name:

Name: Birth date: Nickname:

Home Address: Home/Work Phone:

Parent/Guardian: Emergency Contact Names & Relationship:

Signature/Consent*:

Primary Language: Phone Number(s):

Physicians:

Primary care physician: Emergency Phone: Fax:

Current Specialty physician: Specialty: Emergency Phone: Fax:

Current Specialty physician: Specialty: Emergency Phone: Fax:

Anticipated Primary ED: Pharmacy:

Anticipated Tertiary Care Center:

Diagnoses/Past Procedures/Physical Exam:

1. Baseline physical findings:

2.

3. Baseline vital signs:

4.

Synopsis:

Baseline neurological status:

*Consent for release of this form to health care providers

Last name:

Diagnoses/Past Procedures/Physical Exam continued:

Medications:

1.
2.
3.
4.
5.
6.

Significant baseline ancillary findings (lab, x-ray, ECG):

Prostheses/Appliances/Advanced Technology Devices:

Management Data:

Allergies: Medications/Foods to be avoided **and why:**

1.
2.
3.

Procedures to be avoided **and why:**

1.
2.
3.

Immunizations

Dates					
DPT					
OPV					
MMR					
HIB					

Dates					
Hep B					
Varicella					
TB status					
Other					

Antibiotic prophylaxis: Indication: Medication and dose:

Common Presenting Problems/Findings With Specific Suggested Managements

Problem	Suggested Diagnostic Studies	Treatment Considerations

Comments on child, family, or other specific medical issues:

Physician/Provider Signature: **Print Name:**

Figure 37-24 Emergency Identification Form (EIF) for children with special healthcare needs.

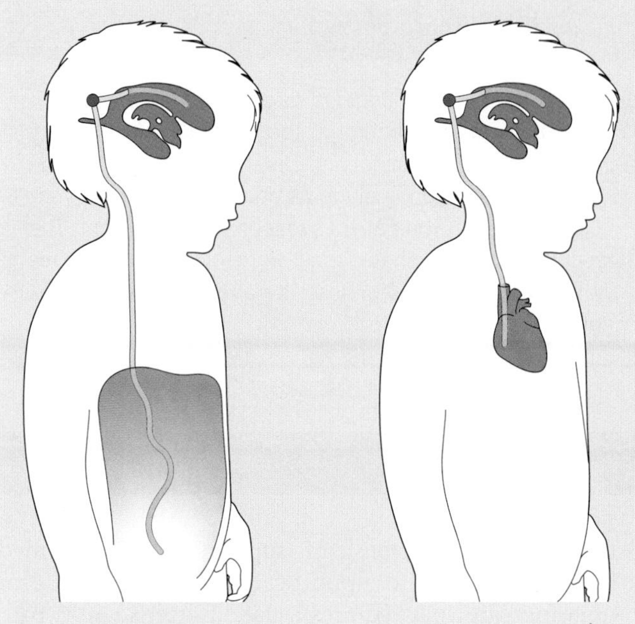

Figure 37-25 Routes of drainage of ventriculoperitoneal *(VP)* and ventriculoatrial *(VA)* shunts. VP shunts drain CSF from the cerebral ventricles to the peritoneal cavity by catheter tubing implanted superficially over the rib cage. The lower end of the peritoneal catheter lies free in the abdomen. VA shunts drain CSF by a convenient neck vein such as the jugular and the superior vena cava to the right atrium.

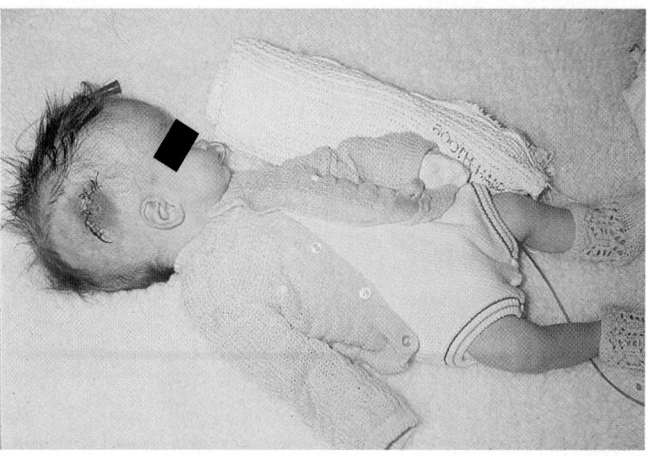

Figure 37-26 External shunt infection in a premature infant with poor nutritional status.

Case Scenario SUMMARY

1. *What is your impression of the patient?* This patient has a history of asthma and is presently having difficulty breathing as evidenced by his increased respiratory rate and labored breathing. Although he is having difficulty breathing, his pulse and BP are currently within normal limits. He does not require immediate intubation but does require further monitoring.
2. *What is the appropriate initial therapy?* The patient should receive supplemental oxygen and a beta$_2$ agonist medication per protocol. Albuterol (Ventolin) is an example of a commonly used beta$_2$ agonist. Ipratropium bromide is an anticholinergic medication that also may be used per protocol.
3. *Describe how you would perform the complete physical examination.* With children, it is often helpful if the child's caregiver holds the patient during the examination. Starting from the feet and working toward the head may help alleviate the child's fear. The examination should focus on head, ears, eyes, nose, and throat; lungs; heart; and abdomen.
4. *What pharmacologic treatment would be appropriate?* Nebulized treatments should be repeated per protocol. They are typically repeated every 15 minutes. Methylprednisolone (SoluMedrol) is often given to children with reactive airway disease and should be administered per protocol or medical direction. Fever control with acetaminophen or ibuprofen also may be part of your protocol. These are weight-based doses (in kilograms), so be sure to ask the caregiver for the child's most recent weight. Supplemental oxygen, respiratory treatments, and fever control will provide patient comfort.
5. *What is the most likely cause of his symptoms?* This child could have a number of conditions. Pneumonia, viral respiratory infection, exacerbation of asthma, and acute laryngotracheobronchitis (croup) are all possibilities. The seal-like, barking cough is consistent with croup.
6. *What physical examination findings would warrant immediate transport?* If the patient was in a tripod position, unable to manage his airway secretions, or if respiratory failure was a concern, transport should not be delayed. The child's airway should be closely watched. If respiratory failure occurs, administer oxygen and implement positive-pressure ventilation.
7. *What is the appropriate transport decision for this patient?* Administer bronchodilators and place the patient on a cardiac monitor. Because the patient's oxygen saturation is in the low 90s, transport the patient

Continued

Case Scenario SUMMARY—continued

for further evaluation and definitive treatment. Allow the child to assume a position of comfort during transport if possible.

8. *What are other treatment options for this patient?* For refractory croup, racemic epinephrine often is used. This is a nebulized form of epinephrine. It also is important to monitor the patient continually after these interventions are begun.

9. *What are important findings to document in the written and oral report?* Document the patient's initial history and physical examination. Note any change in the patient's condition. Include all pharmacologic interventions as well as the patient's response to treatment. The receiving facility should be aware of the patient, his chief complaint, and the therapeutic interventions provided.

Chapter Summary

- The EMSC program works to make sure that the entire spectrum of emergency services, including primary prevention of illness and injury, acute care, and rehabilitation, is provided to children and adolescents as well as adults.
- Children are at high risk for many injuries that can lead to death or disability. Predictable injuries stem from a dangerous situation or risky behavior.
- The pediatric chain of survival represents a sequential series of events to assess, support, or restore effective ventilation and circulation to the infant or child in respiratory or cardiopulmonary arrest. The sequence consists of five important steps: prevention of illness or injury, early CPR, early EMS activation, rapid advanced life support, and post-cardiac arrest care. The importance of prevention is reflected in the links of the chain.
- The PAT is a useful tool for quickly determining whether a child is "sick" or "not sick." Three main areas are assessed: appearance, (work of) breathing, and circulation.
- Determine a child's CUPS status after completing the initial assessment and giving appropriate care for life-threatening emergencies. The CUPS assessment scale classifies patients as ***c***ritical, ***u***nstable, ***p***otentially unstable, or ***s***table. The CUPS assessment also can be used to help determine the speed of transport and the facility to which the child should be transported if a choice is available.
- Allow an ill child to assume a position of comfort. When suctioning, avoid hypoxia and upper airway stimulation. Monitor oxygenation using pulse oximetry. Keep the oxygen saturation above 94%. If a child requires transport to the hospital, decide if the patient requires transport by ground ambulance with or without lights and sirens or air ambulance. Do not delay transport to perform procedures that can be done en route.
- Use age-appropriate words and phrases when talking to a child. Keep the child warm and allow him or her to have a favorite toy or blanket if possible.
- Be sure appropriate basic life support care is performed before advanced life support care. If you must perform ongoing care that requires a flat surface, such as bag-mask ventilation or CPR, place the child on a spine board or stretcher. Transport children with less serious conditions who do not require spine board stabilization and ongoing care with a restraint device (such as a child safety seat) appropriate for size and age. Properly secure safety seats in the ambulance. Parents riding along with the patient should use seat belts or other restraints.
- Categories of respiratory compromise include upper airway obstruction and lower airway disease. A foreign body may block the upper or lower airways. Conditions that may cause upper airway obstruction include croup, epiglottitis, and bacterial tracheitis. Conditions that may cause lower airway disease include asthma, bronchiolitis, and pneumonia.
- Perfusion is the circulation of blood through an organ or a part of the body. Perfusion delivers oxygen and other nutrients to the cells of all organ systems and removes waste products. Shock (hypoperfusion) is the inadequate circulation of blood through an organ or a part of the body. The initial signs of shock may be subtle in an infant or child. The effectiveness of compensatory mechanisms largely depends on the child's previous cardiac and pulmonary health. The presence of hypotension differentiates compensated shock from decompensated shock. Hypotension is a late sign of cardiovascular compromise in an infant or child. In the pediatric patient, the progression from compensated to decompensated shock occurs suddenly and rapidly. When decompensation occurs, cardiopulmonary arrest may be imminent.
- In the pediatric patient, dysrhythmias are divided into four broad categories based on heart rate: normal for age, slower than normal for age (bradycardia), faster than normal for age (tachycardia), or absent or pulseless (cardiac arrest). In children, dysrhythmias are

treated only if they compromise cardiac output or have the potential to deteriorate into a lethal rhythm. Although disorders of heart rate and rhythm are uncommon in infants and children, when they do occur they most often are because of hypoxia secondary to respiratory arrest and asphyxia.

- In infants and children, tachycardia is present if the heart rate is faster than the upper limit of normal for the patient's age. Tachycardia may represent either a normal compensatory response to the need for increased cardiac output or oxygen delivery or an unstable dysrhythmia. If an infant or child is symptomatic because of bradycardia, initial treatment is directed at assessment of the airway and breathing rather than giving epinephrine, atropine, or other drugs. This is because problems with adequate oxygenation and ventilation are more common in children than cardiac causes of bradycardia.
- In adults, sudden, nontraumatic cardiac arrests are usually the result of underlying cardiac disease. In children, cardiac arrests are usually the result of respiratory failure (asphyxia precipitated by acute hypoxia or hypercarbia) or circulatory shock (ischemia from hypovolemia, sepsis, or myocardial dysfunction [cardiogenic shock]).
- A child with altered mental status displays changes in personality, behavior, or responsiveness inappropriate for age. The child may appear agitated, combative, sleepy, withdrawn, slow to respond, or completely unresponsive. The most common causes of altered mental status in the pediatric patient are hypoxia, head trauma, seizures, infection, hypoglycemia, and drug or alcohol ingestion.
- Most pediatric seizures are provoked by disorders that begin outside the brain, such as high fever, infection, syncope, head trauma, hypoxia, toxins, or dysrhythmias. A febrile seizure is a generalized seizure that occurs with fever in childhood between the ages of 3 months to 5 years (most occur between ages 6 and 18 months).
- Meningitis is an inflammation of the meninges, the membranes covering the brain and spinal cord. Viral meningitis (also called *aseptic meningitis*) is the most common type. Meningitis also can be caused by infections with several types of bacteria or fungi.
- Most cases of pediatric toxic exposure are unintentional, occur in the home, and involve only a single substance. Children younger than 6 years are at the greatest risk for unintentional poisoning.
- Blunt trauma is the most common mechanism of serious injury in the pediatric patient. Penetrating trauma is less common in young children but is becoming an increasing problem in adolescents, particularly in urban areas.
- Children can have spinal nerve injury without damage to the vertebrae (SCIWORA). Although spinal cord and spinal column injuries are uncommon in the pediatric patient, children younger than 8 years tend to sustain injury to the upper (C1 and C2) cervical spine region.
- In children, chest trauma is associated with a high mortality rate. The greater elasticity and flexibility of the chest wall in children makes rib and sternum fractures less common than in adults; however, force is more easily transmitted to the underlying lung tissues, resulting in pulmonary contusion, pneumothorax, or hemothorax.
- In children, abdominal trauma is the third leading cause of traumatic death after head and thoracic injuries. It is the most common cause of unrecognized fatal injury in children. The spleen is the most frequently injured abdominal organ during blunt trauma. The liver is the second most commonly injured solid organ in the pediatric patient with blunt abdominal trauma but the most common cause of lethal hemorrhage.
- In a submersion incident, a child's signs and symptoms may vary from no symptoms to cardiac arrest depending on the type and duration of submersion. All submersion victims should be transported to the hospital for evaluation and observation, even those who appear to have recovered fully.
- Methods for assessing pain in the pediatric patient vary according to the age of the child. Use an age-appropriate pain rating scale. The same scale should be used consistently by all persons caring for the child. A good assessment tool to use is the Wong-Baker Faces pain rating scale. This scale combines three scales in one: facial expressions, numbers, and words. The scale consists of six cartoon faces ranging from a smiling face depicting "no hurt" to a tearful, sad face illustrating "worst hurt."
- Child maltreatment includes intentional physical abuse or neglect, emotional abuse or neglect, and sexual abuse of children, usually by adults. Child abuse is unlikely if the child's story is volunteered without hesitation and matches that of the caregiver. Determining the difference between an intentional injury and an accident often is difficult.
- SIDS is the sudden and unexpected death of an infant that remains unexplained after a thorough case investigation, including performance of a complete autopsy, examination of the death scene, and review of the clinical history. Most SIDS deaths occur during the first 6 months of life, most between the ages of 2 and 4 months.
- Children with special healthcare needs are those who have or are at risk for chronic physical, developmental, behavioral, or emotional conditions that require use of health and related services of a type and amount not usually required by typically developing children. Children reliant on technology are a subgroup of children with special healthcare needs that depend on medical devices for their survival. Equipment failure may result in a medical emergency.

REFERENCES

American Heart Association. (2005). 2005 American Heart Association Guidelines for cardiopulmonary resuscitation and emergency cardiovascular care, part 10.3: Drowning. *Circulation, 112*(suppl IV), IV-133.

Barkin, R. M., & Marx, J. A. (1999). Abdominal trauma. In R. M. Barkin, J. A. Marx, & P. Rosen (Eds.), *Emergency pediatrics: A guide to ambulatory care* (5th ed.) (pp. 476-487). St. Louis: Mosby.

Berg, M. D., Nadkarni, V. M., Zuercher, M., Berg, R. A. (2008). In-hospital pediatric cardiac arrest. *Pediatric Clinics of North Amarica 55*(3), 589-604, x. Review.

Cantor, R. M., & Leaming, J. M. (2002). Pediatric trauma. In J. A. Marx, R. S. Hockberger, & R. M. Walls (Eds.), *Rosen's emergency medicine: Concepts and clinical practice* (5th ed.) (pp. 267-281). St. Louis: Mosby.

Carruthers, G. N. (1997). Spinal immobilization. In R. A. Dieckmann, D. H. Fiser, & S. M. Selbst (Eds.), *Illustrated textbook of pediatric emergency & critical care procedures*. St. Louis: Mosby–Year Book.

Dart, R. C., & Rumack, B. H. (2003). Poisoning. In W. W. Hay, Jr., A. R. Hayward, M. J. Levin, et al. (Eds.), *Current pediatric diagnosis and treatment* (15th ed.). New York: McGraw-Hill/Appleton & Lange.

Dickman, C. A., & Rekate, H. L. (1993). Spinal trauma. In M. R. Eichelberger (Ed.), *Pediatric trauma: Prevention, acute care, rehabilitation* (pp. 362-377). St. Louis: Mosby–Year Book.

Dowd, M. D., & Bull, M. (2003). Emergency medicine and injury prevention: Meeting at the intersection. *Clinical Pediatric Emergency Medicine, 4*(2), 83-89.

Dowd, M. D., Keenan, H. T., & Bratton, S. L. (2002). Epidemiology and prevention of childhood injuries. *Critical Care Medicine, 30*(11 suppl), S385-S392.

Feldhaus, K. M. (2002). Submersion. In J. A. Marx, R. S. Hockberger, & R. M. Walls (Eds.), *Rosen's emergency medicine: Concepts and clinical practice* (5th ed.) (pp. 2051-2052). St. Louis: Mosby.

Frankel, L. R., Kache, S. Shock. (2007). In R. M. Kliegman, R. E. Behrman, H. B. Jenson, B. F. Stanton (Eds.), *Nelson textbook of pediatrics* (18th ed.). Philadelphia: WB Saunders.

Hueckel, R., Wilson, D. (2007). The child with respiratory dysfunction. In M. H. Hockenberry, D. Wilson (Eds.), *Wong's Nursing Care of Infants and Children* (8th ed.). Canada: Mosby.

Huether, S. E., & McCance, K. L. (2000). Alterations of pulmonary function in children. In Huether, S. E., & McCance, K. L. (Eds.), *Understanding pathophysiology* (2nd ed.) (pp. 775-788). St. Louis: Mosby.

Hunt, C. E., & Hauck, F. R. (2004). Sudden infant death syndrome. In R. E. Behrman, R. M. Kliegman, & H. B. Jenson (Eds.), *Nelson textbook of pediatrics* (17th ed.) (pp.1380-1385). Philadelphia: W.B. Saunders.

Idris, A. H., Berg, R. A., Bierens, J., Bossaert, L., Branche, C. M., Gabrielli, A., et al. (2003). Recommended guidelines for uniform reporting of data from drowning: the "Utstein style." *Resuscitation, 59*, 45-57.

Jenson, H. B., Baltimore, R. S. Pneumonia. (2006). In R. M. Kliegman, K. J. Marcdante, H. B. Jenson, R. E. Behrman (Eds.), *Nelson Essentials of Pediatrics* (5th ed.). Philadelphia: Elsevier.

Johnston, M. V. (2007). Seizures in Childhood. In R. M. Kliegman, R. E. Behrman, H. B. Jenson, B. F. Stanton (Eds.), *Nelson textbook of pediatrics* (18th ed.). Philadelphia: WB Saunders, .

Kleinman, M. E., Chameides, L., Schexnayder, S.M., et al. (2010). Part 14: pediatric advanced life support: 2010 American Heart Association Guidelines for Cardiopulmonary Resuscitation and Emergency Cardiovascular Care. *Circulation, 122*(suppl 3), S876-S908.

Lasley, M. V. Asthma. (2006) In R. M. Kliegman, K. J. Marcdante, H. B. Jenson, R. E. Behrman (Eds.). *Nelson Essentials of Pediatrics* (5th ed.). Philadelphia: Elsevier.

Lewis, D. W. (2010). Seizures (Paroxysmal Disorders). In K. J. Marcdante, R. B. Kliegman, H. B. Jenson, R. E. Behrman, (Eds.). *Nelson essentials of pediatrics* (6th ed.). Philadelphia: WB Saunders.

Park, S. C., & Beerman, L. B. (2002). Cardiology. In B. J. Zitelli, & H. W. Davis (Eds.), *Atlas of pediatric physical diagnosis* (4th ed.) (pp. 141-143). St. Louis: Mosby.

Poets, C. F., & Southhall, D. P. (1999). Sudden infant death syndrome and apparent life-threatening events. In L. M. Taussig, L. I. Landau (Eds.), *Pediatric respiratory medicine* (pp. 1079-1099). Philadelphia: Mosby.

Lasley, M. V. Asthma. (2006). In R. M. Kliegman, K. J. Marcdante, H. B. Jenson, R. E. Behrman (Eds.). *Nelson Essentials of Pediatrics* (5th ed.). Philadelphia: Elsevier, .

Prober, C. J. (2004). Central nervous system infections. In R. E. Behrman, R. M. Kliegman, & H. B. Jenson (Eds.), *Nelson textbook of pediatrics* (17th ed.) (pp. 2039-2047). Philadelphia: W.B. Saunders.

Rivara, F. P., Grossman, D. (2007). Injury control. In R. M. Kliegman, R. E. Behrman, H. B. Jenson, B. F. Stanton, (Eds.). *Nelson textbook of pediatrics* (18th ed.). Philadelphia: WB Saunders.

Roosevelt, G. E. (2004). Acute inflammatory upper airway obstruction. In R. E. Behrman, R. M. Kliegman, & H. B. Jenson (Eds.), *Nelson textbook of pediatrics* (17th ed.) (pp. 1405-1409). Philadelphia: W.B. Saunders.

Soar, J., Deakin, C. D., Nolan, J. P., Abbas, G., Alfonzo, A., Handley, A. J., et al. (2005). European Resuscitation Council guidelines for resuscitation 2005. Section 7. Cardiac arrest in special circumstances. *Resuscitation, 67*(suppl 1), S135-S1370.

Sobol, S. E., Zapata, S. (2008). Epiglottitis and Croup. *Otolaryngol Clinis of North America 41*(3), 551-566, ix. Review.

Willinger, M., James, L. S., & Catz, C. (1991). Defining the sudden infant death syndrome (SIDS): Deliberations of an expert panel convened by the National Institute of Health and Human Development. *Pediatric Pathology, 11*, 677-684.

Wright, R. B., Pomerantz, W. J., Joseph, W., Luria, J. W. (2002). New approaches to respiratory infections in children: bronchiolitis and croup. *Emergency Medicine Clinics of North Ameria 20*, 93–114.

SUGGESTED RESOURCES

Aehlert, B. (2005). *Comprehensive pediatric emergency care*. St. Louis: MosbyJems.

American Academy of Pediatrics: http://www.aap.org.

The State of Asthma in America: http://www.asthmainamerica.com.

Centers for Disease Control and Prevention: http://www.cdc.gov.

Children's Safety Network: http://www.childrenssafetynetwork.org.

Emergency Medical Services for Children: http://bolivia.hrsa.gov/emsc.

Injury Control Resource Information Network: http://www.injurycontrol.com/icrin.

Injury Free Coalition for Kids: http://www.injuryfree.org.

Jarvis, C. (1996). *Pocket companion for physical examination and health assessment* (2nd ed.). Philadelphia: W.B. Saunders.

National Association of EMS Physicians: http://www.naemsp.org.

Chapter Quiz

1. Which of the following correctly reflects the sequential steps in the pediatric chain of survival?
   - **a.** Early ALS, early EMS activation, early CPR, prevention of illness or injury, post-cardiac arrest care
   - **b.** Early CPR, prevention of illness or injury, early ALS, early EMS activation
   - **c.** Early EMS activation, early ALS, prevention of illness or injury, early CPR
   - **d.** Prevention of illness or injury, early CPR, early EMS activation, rapid ALS, post-cardiac arrest care

2. Complete the following table.

	Croup	Epiglottitis	Bacterial Tracheitis
Age			
Cause			
Seasonal preference			
Onset			
Fever			
Appearance			
Posture			
Sore throat			
Cry			

3. List the four broad categories of pediatric dysrhythmias.

   ____

   ____

   ____

   ____

4. What are the two most commonly injured abdominal organs in the pediatric patient?

   ____

   ____

5. What is the single most common cause of injury in children?

   ____

6. Bradycardia that causes severe cardiopulmonary compromise in an infant or child is initially treated with
   - **a.** effective oxygenation and ventilation.
   - **b.** transcutaneous pacing.
   - **c.** synchronized cardioversion.
   - **d.** administration of atropine.

7. The most common types of shock in the pediatric patient are
   - **a.** anaphylactic and septic.
   - **b.** cardiogenic and neurogenic.
   - **c.** hypovolemic and septic.
   - **d.** septic and neurogenic.

8. A 9-month-old infant has a history of poor feeding. You note that the infant appears pale and limp in her mother's arms. Intercostal retractions are present. She does not respond when her mother speaks her name. From the information provided, complete the following documentation regarding the PAT.

   Appearance: ________________________

   Breathing: ________________________

   Circulation: ________________________

9. Which of the following are conditions that affect the upper airway?
   - **a.** Asthma, bronchiolitis, and pneumonia
   - **b.** Bacterial tracheitis, epiglottitis, and bronchiolitis
   - **c.** Bronchiolitis, croup, and asthma
   - **d.** Croup, epiglottitis, and bacterial tracheitis

10. For each of the following, record the estimated values for a 3-year-old child.
    - **a.** Ventilatory rate:
    - **b.** Heart rate:
    - **c.** BP:

Terminology

Accessory muscles Muscles of the neck, chest, and abdomen that become active during labored breathing.

Asthma A reversible obstructive airway disease characterized by chronic inflammation, hyperreactive airways, and episodes of bronchospasm.

Cognitive disability An impairment that affects an individual's awareness and memory as well as ability to learn, process information, communicate, and make decisions.

Crackles High-pitched breath sounds (formerly referred to as *rales*) that indicate lower airway pathology, such as pneumonia or asthma.

Croup A viral infection of the upper airway; respiratory distress caused by narrowing below the glottis characterized by hoarseness, inspiratory stridor, and a barking cough.

Decompensated shock A clinical state of tissue perfusion that is inadequate to meet the body's metabolic demands; accompanied by hypotension; also called *progressive* or *late shock*.

Drowning The process of experiencing respiratory impairment from immersion or submersion in a liquid.

Epiglottitis A bacterial infection of the epiglottis and supraglottic structures; also called *acute supraglottitis*.

Terminology—continued

Greenstick fracture The incomplete fracturing of an immature bone.

Grunting A short, low-pitched sound heard at the end of exhalation that represents an attempt to generate positive end-expiratory pressure by exhaling against a closed glottis, prolonging the period of oxygen and carbon dioxide exchange across the alveolar-capillary membrane; a compensatory mechanism to help maintain patency of small airways and prevent atelectasis.

Gurgling Abnormal respiratory sound associated with collection of liquid or semisolid material in the patient's upper airway.

Head bobbing Indicator of increased work of breathing in infants; the head falls forward with exhalation and comes up with expansion of the chest on inhalation.

Hyperpnea Increased respiratory rate or deeper than normal breathing.

Hypoperfusion The inadequate circulation of blood through an organ or a part of the body; shock.

Hypoxemia Insufficient oxygenation of the blood; a decrease in the arterial blood oxygen tension; in adults, children, and infants older than 28 days, hypoxemia is defined as an arterial oxygen tension (PaO_2) of less than 60 mm Hg or arterial oxygen saturation (SaO_2) of less than 90% in an individual breathing room air or with a PaO_2 and/or SaO_2 below the desirable range for a specific clinical situation.

Hypoxia A deficiency of oxygen reaching the tissues of the body.

Intraosseous infusion The infusion of fluids, medications, or blood directly into the bone marrow cavity.

Laryngotracheobronchitis Croup.

Morbidity Nonfatal injury rates; state of being diseased; the propensity to cause disease or illness.

Nasal flaring Widening of the nostrils on inhalation; an attempt to increase the size of the airway and increase the amount of available oxygen.

Neglect The failure of a parent or other person with responsibility for the child to provide needed food, clothing, shelter, medical care, or supervision such that the child's health, safety, and well-being are threatened with harm; can be physical, educational, or emotional.

Partial seizure A seizure confined to one area of the brain.

Penetrating trauma Any mechanism of injury that causes a cut or piercing of skin.

Perfusion The circulation of blood through an organ or a part of the body.

Petechiae A tiny pinpoint rash on the upper area of the neck and the face; may indicate near strangulation or suffocation; caused by an occlusion of venous return from the head while arterial pressure remains normal; may be present in mothers after childbirth; reddish-purple, nonblanchable discolorations in the skin less than 0.5 cm in diameter.

Pneumonia An inflammation and infection of the lower airway and lungs caused by a viral, bacterial, parasitic, or fungal organism.

Poison A substance that, on ingestion, inhalation, absorption, application, injection, or development within the body in relatively small amounts, may cause structural damage or functional disturbance.

Poisoning Exposure to a substance that is harmful in any dosage.

Polydipsia Excessive thirst.

Polyphagia Excessive eating.

Polyuria Frequent urination.

Purpura Reddish-purple, nonblanchable discolorations greater than 0.5 cm in diameter; large purpura are called *ecchymoses*.

Respiratory arrest Absence of breathing.

Respiratory distress Increased work of breathing (ventilatory effort).

Respiratory failure A clinical condition of inadequate blood oxygenation and/or ventilation to meet the metabolic demands of body tissues.

Retractions Use of accessory muscles of respiration to assist in ventilation during times of distress; sinking in of the soft tissues above the sternum or clavicle or between or below the ribs during inhalation.

Seizure A temporary change in behavior or consciousness caused by abnormal electrical activity of one or more groups of neurons in the brain.

Shock Inadequate tissue perfusion resulting from the failure of the cardiovascular system to deliver sufficient oxygen and nutrients to sustain vital organ function.

Status epilepticus Any prolonged series of similar seizures without return to full consciousness between them.

Toxin A poisonous substance of plant or animal origin.

Tracheitis Inflammation of the mucous membranes of the trachea.

Tripod position Position used to maintain airway patency; sitting upright and leaning forward with the neck slightly extended, chin projected, and mouth open and supported by the arms.

Wheezes High-pitched whistling sounds produced by air moving through narrowed airway passages.

CHAPTER 38

Geriatrics

Objectives *After completing this chapter, you will be able to:*

1. Discuss population demographics demonstrating the rise in the elderly population in the United States.
2. Discuss societal issues concerning the elderly.
3. Discuss society's view of aging and the social, financial, and ethical issues facing the elderly.
4. Assess the various living environments of elderly patients.
5. Describe the local resources available to assist the elderly and create strategies to refer at-risk patients to appropriate community services.
6. Discuss common emotional and psychological reactions to aging, including causes and manifestations.
7. Compare pharmacokinetics in elderly patients versus younger adults.
8. Discuss drug distribution, metabolism, and excretion in the elderly patient.
9. Discuss the impact of polypharmacy and medication noncompliance on patient assessment and management.
10. Discuss medication issues pertinent to the elderly, including polypharmacy, dosing errors, and increased drug sensitivity.
11. Discuss the problems with mobility in the elderly and develop strategies to prevent falls.
12. Discuss how problems with sensation affect communication and patient assessment.
13. Discuss problems with continence and elimination and develop communication strategies to provide psychological support.
14. Apply the pathophysiology of multisystem failure to the assessment and management of medical conditions in the elderly patient.
15. Discuss factors that may complicate assessment of the elderly patient.
16. Describe principles to use when assessing and communicating with an elderly patient.
17. Compare the assessment of an elderly patient versus a younger patient.
18. Discuss common complaints of the elderly.
19. Discuss the normal and abnormal age-related changes of the pulmonary system.
20. Describe the epidemiology of pulmonary diseases in the elderly, including incidence, morbidity and mortality rates, risk factors, and prevention strategies for patients with pneumonia, chronic obstructive pulmonary disease, and pulmonary embolism.
21. Compare the pathophysiology of pulmonary diseases in the elderly versus younger adults, including pneumonia, chronic obstructive pulmonary disease, and pulmonary embolism.
22. Discuss the assessment of the elderly patient with pulmonary complaints, including pneumonia, chronic obstructive pulmonary disease, and pulmonary embolism.
23. Identify the need for intervention and transport of the elderly patient with pulmonary complaints.
24. Develop a treatment and management plan for the elderly patient with pulmonary complaints, including pneumonia, chronic obstructive pulmonary disease, and pulmonary embolism.
25. Discuss the normal and abnormal cardiovascular system changes with age.
26. Describe the epidemiology of cardiovascular diseases in the elderly, including incidence, morbidity and mortality rates, risk factors, and prevention strategies for patients with myocardial infarction, heart failure, dysrhythmias, aneurysm, and hypertension.
27. Compare the pathophysiology of cardiovascular diseases in the elderly versus younger adults, including myocardial infarction, heart failure, dysrhythmias, aneurysm, and hypertension.
28. Discuss assessment of the elderly patient with complaints related to the cardiovascular system, including myocardial infarction, heart failure, dysrhythmias, aneurism, and hypertension.
29. Identify the need for intervention and transportation of the elderly patient with cardiovascular complaints.
30. Develop a treatment and management plan for the elderly patient with cardiovascular complaints, including myocardial infarction, heart failure, dysrhythmias, aneurism, and hypertension.
31. Discuss the normal and abnormal age-related changes of the nervous system.
32. Describe the epidemiology of nervous system diseases in the elderly, including incidence, morbidity and mortality rates, risk factors, and prevention strategies for patients with cerebral vascular disease, delirium, dementia, Alzheimer's disease, and Parkinson's disease.
33. Compare the pathophysiology of nervous system diseases in the elderly versus younger adults, including cerebral vascular disease, delirium, dementia, Alzheimer's disease, and Parkinson's disease.
34. Discuss the assessment of the elderly patient with complaints related to the nervous system, including cerebral vascular disease, delirium, dementia, Alzheimer's disease, and Parkinson's disease.
35. Identify the need for intervention and transportation of the patient with complaints related to the nervous system.

Objectives—continued

36. Develop a treatment and management plan for the elderly patient with complaints related to the nervous system, including cerebral vascular disease, delirium, dementia, Alzheimer's disease, and Parkinson's disease.
37. Discuss the normal and abnormal age-related changes of the endocrine system.
38. Describe the epidemiology of endocrine diseases in the elderly, including incidence, morbidity and mortality rates, risk factors, and prevention strategies for patients with diabetes and thyroid diseases.
39. Compare the pathophysiology of diabetes and thyroid diseases in the elderly versus younger adults.
40. Discuss the assessment of the elderly patient with complaints related to the endocrine system, including diabetes and thyroid diseases.
41. Identify the need for intervention and transportation of the patient with endocrine problems.
42. Develop a treatment and management plan for the elderly patient with endocrine problems, including diabetes and thyroid diseases.
43. Discuss the normal and abnormal age-related changes of the gastrointestinal system.
44. Discuss assessment of the elderly patient with complaints related to the gastrointestinal system.
45. Identify the need for intervention and transportation of the patient with gastrointestinal complaints.
46. Develop and execute a treatment and management plan for the elderly patient with gastrointestinal problems.
47. Discuss the assessment and management of an elderly patient with gastrointestinal hemorrhage and bowel obstruction.
48. Compare the pathophysiology of gastrointestinal hemorrhage and bowel obstruction in the elderly versus younger adults.
49. Discuss the normal and abnormal age-related psychiatric changes.
50. Describe the epidemiology of depression and suicide in the elderly, including incidence, morbidity and mortality rates, risk factors, and prevention strategies.
51. Compare the psychiatry of depression and suicide in the elderly versus younger adults.
52. Discuss the assessment of the elderly patient with psychiatric complaints, including depression and suicide.
53. Identify the need for intervention and transport of the elderly psychiatric patient.
54. Develop a treatment and management plan for the elderly psychiatric patient pertinent to depression and suicide.
55. Discuss the normal and abnormal age-related changes of the integumentary system.
56. Describe the epidemiology of pressure ulcers in the elderly, including incidence, morbidity and mortality rates, risk factors, and prevention strategies.
57. Compare the pathophysiology of pressure ulcers in the elderly versus younger adults.
58. Discuss the assessment of the elderly patient with complaints related to the integumentary system, including pressure ulcers.
59. Identify the need for intervention and transportation of the patient with complaints related to the integumentary system.
60. Develop a treatment and management plan for the elderly patient with complaints related to the integumentary system, including pressure ulcers.
61. Discuss the normal and abnormal age-related changes of the musculoskeletal system.
62. Describe the epidemiology of osteoarthritis and osteoporosis, including incidence, morbidity and mortality rates, risk factors, and prevention strategies.
63. Compare the pathophysiology of osteoarthritis and osteoporosis in the elderly versus younger adults.
64. Discuss the assessment of the elderly patient with complaints related to the musculoskeletal system, including osteoarthritis and osteoporosis.
65. Identify the need for intervention and transportation of the patient with musculoskeletal complaints.
66. Develop a treatment and management plan for the elderly patient with musculoskeletal complaints, including osteoarthritis and osteoporosis.
67. Discuss the normal and abnormal age-related changes relevant to toxicology.
68. Discuss the assessment of the elderly patient with complaints related to toxicology.
69. Identify the need for intervention and transportation of the patient with toxicologic problems.
70. Develop and execute a treatment and management plan for the elderly patient with toxicologic problems.
71. Describe the epidemiology of drug toxicology in the elderly, including the incidence, morbidity and mortality rates, risk factors, and prevention strategies.
72. Compare the pathophysiology of drug toxicity in the elderly versus younger adults.
73. Discuss the use and effects of commonly prescribed drugs in the elderly patient.
74. Discuss the assessment findings common in elderly patients with drug toxicity.
75. Discuss the management and considerations when treating an elderly patient with drug toxicity.
76. Describe the epidemiology of drug and alcohol abuse in the elderly, including incidence, morbidity and mortality rates, risk factors, and prevention strategies.
77. Compare the pathophysiology of drug and alcohol abuse in the elderly versus younger adults.
78. Discuss the assessment findings common in elderly patients with drug and alcohol abuse.
79. Discuss the management and considerations when treating an elderly patient with drug and alcohol abuse.
80. Discuss the normal and abnormal age-related changes of thermoregulation.
81. Discuss the assessment of the elderly patient with complaints related to thermoregulation.

82. Identify the need for intervention and transportation of the patient with environmental considerations.
83. Develop and execute a treatment and management plan for the elderly patient with environmental considerations.
84. Compare the pathophysiology of hypothermia and hyperthermia in the elderly versus younger adults.
85. Discuss the assessment findings and management plan for elderly patients with hypothermia or hyperthermia.
86. Describe the epidemiology of trauma in the elderly, including incidence, morbidity and mortality rates, risk factors, and prevention strategies for patients with orthopedic injuries, burns, and head injuries.
87. Compare the pathophysiology of trauma in the elderly versus younger adults, including orthopedic injuries, burns, and head injuries.
88. Discuss the assessment findings common in elderly patients with traumatic injuries, including orthopedic injuries, burns, and head injuries.
89. Discuss the management and considerations when treating an elderly patient with traumatic injuries, including orthopedic injuries, burns, and head injuries.
90. Identify the need for intervention and transport of the elderly patient with trauma.

Chapter Outline

Case Scenario

You are called to the scene of a 77-year-old woman who has fallen. Her daughter arrived shortly before your crew. The patient states she fell and cannot remember what happened. You notice she is lying on the ground. She reports pain in her right hip. You notice that she also has a large contusion above her right eye. Her blood pressure is 108/76 mm Hg, pulse is 77 beats/min, and respirations 16 breaths/min and nonlabored.

Questions

1. *What is your impression of this patient?*
2. *What are important questions regarding the chief complaint and history?*
3. *What should be the focus of the physical examination?*

[OBJECTIVES 1, 2]

The geriatric population deserves special attention. Elderly patients often have much more subtle presentations of life-threatening disease processes and require adept clinical skills to diagnose and treat potentially serious conditions. You should understand the normal physiologic changes accompanying the aging process, the different disease processes commonly presenting in the geriatric population, the side effects and interactions of the medications often prescribed to elderly patients, social issues directly affecting the aged population, and how to proficiently interact and elicit a history and physical examination.

GERIATRIC POPULATION

An estimated 34% of all EMS calls are for older patients (American Geriatrics Society, 2003). As the baby-boomer generation ages, a significantly larger proportion of the population is becoming elderly (age 65 years and older). According to the 2000 U.S. Census, 12.4% of the U.S. population at that time was older than 65 years, with more than 9 million individuals older than 80 years. During that same period the baby-boomer generation comprised 22% of the population (U.S. Census Bureau, 2000). As this generation begins to turn 65 years old in 2011, demands on the healthcare system, including EMS, will significantly increase. A study from 1998 showed that 15.7% of visits to emergency departments (EDs) were by the elderly, and nearly 40% of all patients transported to an ED were older than 65 years (Strange & Chen, 1998).

SOCIAL ISSUES FACING THE AGED

[OBJECTIVE 3]

Unfortunately, **ageism** exists in today's society. Many believe that the older population is frail and less capable compared with their younger counterparts. However, most elderly lead healthy, productive, and active lives. Although the elderly population does have more medical problems than younger generations simply because of the process of aging, this cannot be applied on an individual basis. Many octogenarians are much healthier than those half their age. Thanks to the work of several advocacy groups such as the Gray Panthers, the National Council of Senior Citizens, and the American Association of Retired Persons, federal legislation such as the Older Americans Act of 1965 and the Age Discrimination in Employment of 1967 have been passed that aim to eliminate ageism in America (Administration on Aging, 2004).

Social activity remains an important issue in the lives of the elderly. Many satisfy the need for social companionship with their spouses. According to the 2000 Census, more than 85% of all individuals older than 65 years have been married, with 62% of those aged 65 to 74 years currently married and living with their spouses (Kreider & Simmons, 2003). Yet those who are widowed or without a spouse often lead active and healthy lives. Those without access to a suitable social venue often become isolated. The cause of this isolation is multifactorial. Financial constraints and detrimental health conditions often force elders to give up their cars and driving privileges—an important means of transportation. Chronic health problems also may make venturing outside the house for extended periods more difficult. As the population ages, many retire and decide to move to a different location to be closer to family members or to move to a location they always wanted to live. After the age of 30 years, the mortality rate begins to increase with each subsequent decade (Kochanek et al., 2004). This means that as human beings age, we are more likely to have those in our peer group die (including spouses). As an elder slowly loses friends from his or her peer group, remaining active enough to mingle in social settings is imperative to maintain and establish new relationships and avoid isolation.

BOX 38-1 Support and Assistance Resources for the Geriatric Patient

- Adult day service centers
- Area agencies on aging
- Counseling
- Employment services
- Energy assistance
- Religious or faith organizations
- Handyman, chore, and housekeeping services
- Home healthcare assistance
- Home-delivered meals and nutrition programs
- Legal assistance
- Protective services
- Respite care
- Senior centers and living facilities
- Transportation assistance

Living Situation

[OBJECTIVES 4, 5, 6]

The ability to live independently and care for oneself is an important facet of life that many take for granted. Most seniors are able to live independently, but when the decision is made to change to a dependent living situation, it is life altering. Several programs at the local, state, and national level ensure that the elderly receive the assistance they need in their appropriate living environment (Box 38-1).

Independent Living

More than 85% of all individuals older than 65 years are married or widowed and have had the social companionship and support that a spouse offers (Kreider & Simmons, 2003). Most persons, when they turn 65 years, are living independently with a spouse. With the support of a spouse, the married couple helps care for each other and lives independently for several years. Often an elderly couple (or widowed elder) may elect to move in with other family members to have more support to continue independent living. For those who do not wish to move in with or do not have family members who can accommodate them, a visiting nurse or caregiver is another viable option. A visiting caregiver tends to an individual or couple who are mostly independent and able to complete most activities of daily living without assistance. The caregiver often runs errands outside the house, such as shopping for groceries, helping with household chores, and providing transportation. A visiting nurse, on the other hand, is a healthcare professional who tends to the specific health needs of an individual. A visiting nurse often administers and supervises medications, obtains samples for laboratory testing, and monitors medical conditions on a daily to weekly basis in an attempt to avoid frequent visits to the physician's office, inpatient hospital care, or placement in a nursing home or other dependent living situation.

Special attention should be given to those family members who elect to care for an older relative in their home. Although spending time with this relative, as illness sets in also, the cared-for individual may become quite impaired and require more intense care. This higher level of required care often takes a physical and emotional toll on the caregiver. The caregiver is frequently faced with the dilemma of placing the loved one in a dependent living facility to provide better care and alleviate some of increased stressful difficulties that the caregiver may be experiencing.

Dependent Living

As disease processes progress or after an acute event (e.g., stroke) occurs, an individual often may no longer be able to care for himself or herself and perform the activities of daily living. If no other persons the individual can depend on to help provide care, other options may need to be explored. An expensive option that allows the individual to remain in the home is live-in nursing care. This form of nursing care most often entails the employment of a single nurse who moves into the home with the patient to provide care. This option provides the individual the luxury of remaining in the home while still receiving needed care.

Unfortunately, live-in nursing care is costly and far exceeds the financial budget of most seniors. More commonly, seniors who require a higher level of care and a dependent living condition must move from their homes into assisted living communities or nursing homes. Assisted living communities most often are composed of several private apartments for which tenants are responsible. The advantages of assisted living are that meals are provided, property maintenance is not required, and it is a social environment. Some facilities offer other basic services such as providing transportation and ensuring that patients have all needed prescriptions filled.

Nursing homes provide a higher level of care and are staffed by licensed nurses who are permitted to dispense medications. Residents often are unable to care for themselves or require close monitoring and nursing care. Nurses at the nursing home are in close contact with physicians and can execute the orders that a doctor may give—in person or over the phone. The level of care provided in nursing homes often is regarded as a step below that provided in the hospital.

Financial Situation

Between 1960 and 1995, the poverty rate of those aged 65 years and older has fallen dramatically from 35% to 10% (National Bureau of Economic Research, 2004). Social Security, private pension plans, Medicare, and the Older Americans Act have all been cited as helping the elderly stay financially secure. When reaching retirement, income often becomes fixed and is derived from Social Security, a pension check, and personal savings. Those who did not adequately plan for retirement savings often find the income from Social Security to be limiting. Although the elder poverty rate is relatively low, the financial future for this population is uncertain. With longer life expectancy, escalating medical costs, and the possible need for long-term care, the limited income of an elder can quickly dwindle.

End-of-Life Decisions

Over the past several years advanced directives have become much more commonplace. Two types of advanced directives are typical: a durable power of attorney for health care and a living will. A **durable power of attorney for healthcare** (also called a *healthcare proxy*) allows an individual to appoint someone to make healthcare decisions for him or her if the person loses the ability to make these decisions or communicate wishes. A **living will** provides specific instructions to healthcare providers about the individual's wishes regarding what types of healthcare measures or treatments should be undertaken to prolong life. Advanced directives allow an individual to guide medical care and decision making concerning end-of-life care or life-prolonging measures when that individual can no longer communicate his or her wishes.

Policies concerning advanced directives vary from state to state. Local guidelines must be followed. As a prehospital professional, if no written proof that an advanced directive exists, each patient must be treated as if he or she would want comprehensive medical care and treatment—including endotracheal intubation and chest compressions. At the other end of the spectrum, a patient may have an advanced directive stating that the patient has a **do not resuscitate (DNR)** order in place. DNR orders may be individualized for each patient about what medical interventions should and should not be done in the event of a cardiac arrest. Remember that DNR orders do not mean "do not treat." These patients deserve the same assessment as all other patients, and all appropriate treatment should be taken as allowed by the DNR order. Keep in mind that a living will may be changed at any time. If any doubt exists regarding the status of a living will, treat the patient.

PATHOPHYSIOLOGY OF AGING

As it ages, the body goes through many natural changes that cause altered function of most body systems. Different people age at different rates, so the timing of specific effects of aging occur varies from person to person. However, certain organ systems demonstrate predictable declines in function in all people with advancing age (Figure 38-1).

Pharmacology in the Elderly

Although the elderly population constitutes 12.4% of the total U.S. population, the group accounts for 30% of all prescription medications (American Association of Retired Persons, 1999). In fact, 61% of the elderly who see a physician are taking at least one prescription medication, with the majority of these individuals taking between three and five (Rathore et al., 1998). An estimated 11% of ED visits by the elderly are related to adverse drug reactions (Hohl et al., 2001). The most frequent adverse drug reactions include confusion, sedation, loss of balance or falls, change in bowel or urinary patterns, nausea, and electrolyte abnormalities (Table 38-1).

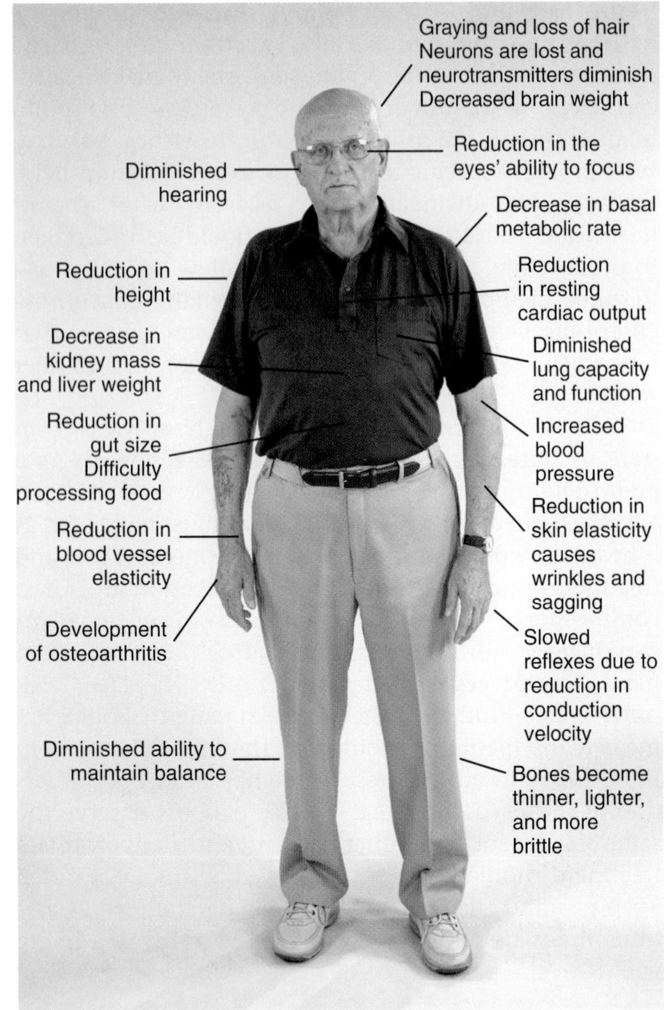

Figure 38-1 The changes of aging.

Pharmacokinetics

[OBJECTIVES 7, 8]

To gain a better appreciation for some age-related changes regarding medications, a brief review of pharmacokinetics is helpful. Pharmacokinetics includes the absorption, distribution, metabolism, and excretion of medications.

Absorption, the amount of medication taken up in the bloodstream, may be slower in the elderly but is otherwise the least affected of the four processes.

Distribution most often is related to body weight and composition. The normal aging process is accompanied by an increase in body fat, decrease in lean muscle mass, and decrease in total body water volume; because of these changes, older individuals often require different doses of medication to obtain the same effect as younger individuals.

Drug metabolism most often occurs in the liver. Liver metabolism is quite variable and depends on age and hepatic blood flow and the presence of hepatic diseases.

Finally, excretion of drugs is primarily carried out by the kidneys and is associated with creatinine clearance, which declines approximately 50% between the ages of 25 and 85 years. This means that the elderly are more likely to have a medication circulating in their bodies for a longer period and experience a prolonged period of the drug's effects.

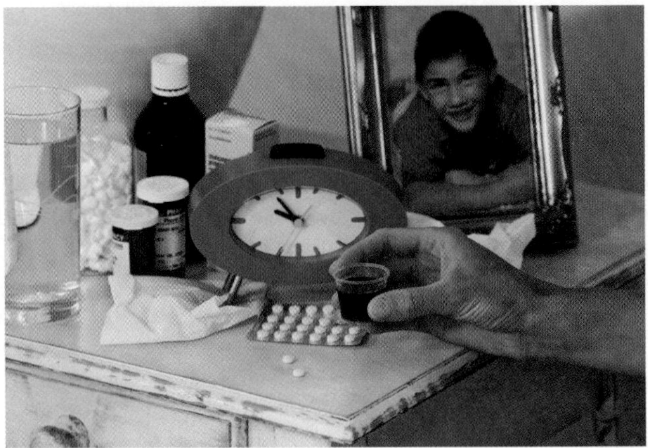

Figure 38-2 Older patients may be taking multiple medications.

Medication Use among the Elderly

[OBJECTIVES 9, 10]

All the medications that a patient is prescribed should be recorded. The elderly often take multiple prescriptions and over-the-counter medications, a condition known as **polypharmacy** (Figure 38-2). These patients frequently cannot recall all the medications they take but instead rely on a written list or organized pill box for proper medication administration.

PARAMEDIC*Pearl*

Writing down an elderly patient's medications, making sure the patient has a list of medications, or bringing all the medication bottles with you to the hospital is important. This usually is the only way to ensure that the ED has an accurate record of the patient's exact medications and dosages.

Polypharmacy is frequently the result of elders being more vulnerable to chronic or acute illnesses (Kelley, 1996). Recognize that in cases of polypharmacy a distinct possibility exists that interactions between the medications may adversely affect the patient. Common herbal or over-the-counter medications such as aspirin, acetaminophen, ibuprofen, and several indigestion agents also are commonly taken but may not be recorded on a list of medications because they have not been prescribed by a physician. These over-the-counter and herbal medications may also adversely interact with other medications the patient is taking, causing harmful side effects.

Although a patient may have a list of prescribed medications, whether the patient is compliant with the dosage

TABLE 38-1 Common Adverse Drug Events and Clinical Outcomes

Drug/Drug Class	Common Adverse Reactions	Common Clinical Outcomes
Antiinflammatory agents	Gastric irritation, ulcers, chronic blood loss, nephrotoxicity	Hemorrhage, anemia, sodium retention, renal failure, may decrease effectiveness of antihypertensive drugs
Aminoglycosides	Renal failure	Increased serum concentration of medications, dialysis
Anticholinergics	Dry mouth, decreased gut motility, bladder hypotonia, decreased cognition, sedation, orthostatic hypotension, blurry vision	Constipation, urinary retention, confusion, instability, and falls
Anticoagulants	Bleeding complications	Hemorrhage
Antidepressants (tricyclic)	Anticholinergic effects, heart block	Falls, confusion, urinary retention
Antipsychotics	Sedation, tardive dyskinesia, dystonia, anticholinergic effects, hypotension	Falls, hip fractures, confusion, social disability
Beta-blockers	Decreased myocardial contractility, decreased cardiac conduction, mild sedation, orthostatic hypotension	Bradycardia, heart failure, possible confusion, falls
Digoxin	Decreased cardiac conduction, GI disturbances	Dysrhythmias, nausea, anorexia
Insulin, sulfonylureas, acarbose (Precose)	Hypoglycemia	Falls, confusion, brain injury
Narcotics	Decreased gut motility, sedation	Confusion, constipation
Sedative-hypnotics	Excessive sedation, cognitive impairment, gait disturbances, impaired psychomotor performance	Falls and fractures, confusion

Reprinted from Kane, R. L., Ouslander, J. G., & Abrass, I. B. (1999). *Essentials of clinical geriatrics* (4th ed.). New York: McGraw-Hill.

schedule must be determined. As the number of prescriptions increases, so does the likelihood of an error in the dosage regimen. By counting the number of pills remaining in a bottle and comparing that to the expected number given the dosage and dispense date, one can usually determine if the patient is adhering to the dosage regimen. Besides simple confusion of the medication schedule, several other predisposing factors may cause the elderly to be less compliant with medications. Poor vision and difficulty reading may lead an elder to misunderstand printed prescription information. Likewise, difficulty hearing may cause an elder to mistake a physician's or pharmacist's instructions. Several elderly also have arthritis or other ailments that inhibit them from easily opening safety caps on medication bottles or administering medicines that come in suppository form.

Falls

[OBJECTIVE 11]

Falls remain a common cause of EMS dispatch in the elderly and are a frequent cause of injury. Approximately 30% of independent individuals older than 65 years are estimated to fall each year, with nearly half suffering multiple falls (Tinetti et al., 1988). The trauma associated with a fall in an elder can be quite serious. Because of the physiologic changes that accompany aging, elders are more likely to sustain more severe soft tissue injury, with extensive bruising, skin tears, and lacerations as well as more serious injuries, including fractures and intracranial bleeding. Although the recovery rate from fractures in a younger population is relatively high, the long-term prognosis of an elderly patient who has sustained a hip fracture is poor, because of the fracture as well as the associated immobilization and hospitalization.

Several intrinsic risk factors predispose the elderly population to falls. When evaluating an elderly patient who has fallen, ascertain whether there is a history of repeated falls; if so, consider if any underlying factors cause these falls. Box 38-2 lists risk factors for falls in the elderly population.

Several strategies have been developed to help reduce the number of falls that the elderly sustain. Many assistive devices, such as canes and walkers, increase the base of support and balance in a patient. These devices should only be used with proper instruction because they can be a hazard when incorrectly used. Several modifications in an elder's house can lessen the risk of falls and create a safer environment. Box 38-3 lists several environmental modifications that reduce the risk of a fall from extrinsic factors.

BOX 38-2 Risk Factors for Falls

- Advanced age
- Alcohol use
- Brain diseases
- CNS problems that may affect balance, such as Parkinson's disease, stroke, tumors, and vertigo.
- Decreased hearing
- Decreased vision
- Dementia
- Depression
- Inaccurate perception of body's position
- Medications that have sedative effects or drug interactions that may cause loss of balance or impaired senses
- Musculoskeletal disorders that lead to an altered gait
- Sensory impairment

CNS, Central nervous system.

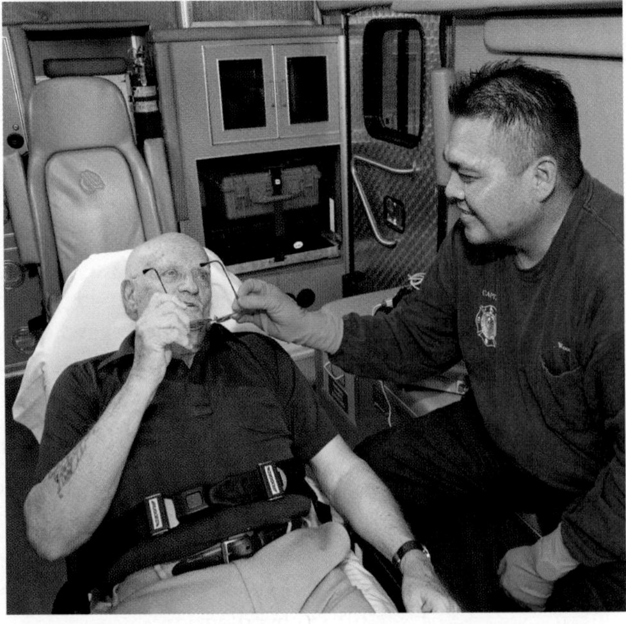

Figure 38-3 Before starting a conversation with an elderly patient, make sure that you are at eye level with the patient and that he or she has hearing aids in and glasses on (if the patient uses these aids).

BOX 38-3 Environmental Modifications to Reduce the Risk of Falls

- Arrange furniture for clear walking paths.
- Install adequate lighting and nightlights.
- Install hand rails where needed, including around tubs, showers, and toilets.
- Remove clutter and any items that may cause someone to trip.
- Remove throw rugs and secure loose carpeting.
- Use nonslip decals in the bathtub and/or provide a shower bench.

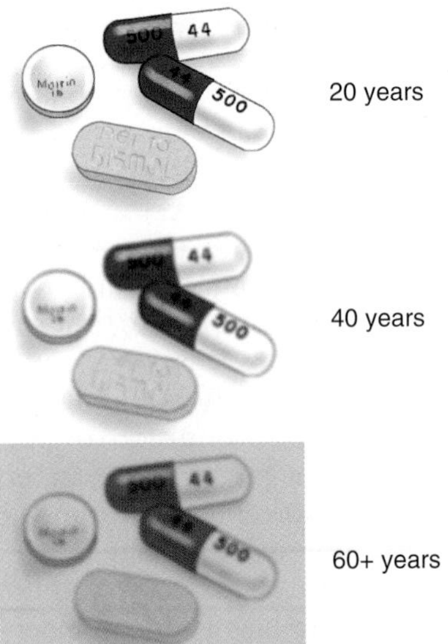

Figure 38-4 Vision comparison: changes in focus, contrast, glare sensitivity, and color discrimination all decrease vision as we age.

Changes with Sensations

[OBJECTIVE 12]

Often the aging process is accompanied by loss of sensory function. These losses affect vision, hearing, speech, and pain perception (Figure 38-3).

Vision

Presbyopia, the inability to see clearly at close proximity, begins at approximately age 40 years and worsens with age. It is the most common vision complaint of adults older than 40 years and often necessitates the use of corrective lenses (Figure 38-4) (Tyson, 1999). Presbyopia is marked by a loss of lens elasticity and impaired accommodation. Similarly, ocular movements and pupillary reaction become more restricted with age, further decreasing visual acuity. As vision slowly worsens, an elder may find reading to be more difficult and require reading or magnifying glasses. They also begin to lose depth perception, have altered color perception, and have increased sensitivity to light and glare. Visual acuity may degrade so that at some point an individual can no longer function as before and may become dependent on others to read and help communicate surroundings. When caring for patients with severe visual loss, always allow them to take your arm as you guide them and describe the immediate environment they are unable to perceive.

Cataracts are an age-related, natural, and painless clouding of the normally transparent lens of the eye. It is the leading cause of preventable blindness in the world, with more than two thirds of the population older than 60 years having some degree of cataracts and 90% of those older than 70 being affected (Tyson, 1999). As the process progresses, the lens slowly hardens and becomes opaque, causing blurred or double vision, spots, or ghost images. Once these visual changes begin affecting lifestyle, surgery often is performed to replace the lens.

Glaucoma is a group of eye diseases that result in vision loss from damage to the optic nerve caused by an increase in ocular pressure. An estimated more than 3 million Americans have glaucoma (Glaucoma Research Foundation, 2006), with the disease causing approximately 120,000 of those to be blind (National Eye Health Program/National Institutes of Health, 2005). The cause of this increased pressure inside the eye is from the drainage canals of the eye becoming blocked. When this slowly occurs over a period of time, the condition is known as *open-angle glaucoma,* a painless process. In angle-closure glaucoma (also known as *acute glaucoma*), the outer edge of the iris covers the drainage canals, causing an acute and drastic increase in intraocular pressure. This is a painful condition that often is worsened or triggered by entering a dark room. Open-angle glaucoma is much more common and, if left untreated, may progress to permanent loss of peripheral vision followed by loss of central vision. Open-angle glaucoma is commonly treated with a combination of eye drops and pills that aim to keep the drainage canals open or decrease the production of fluid in the eye. The treatment for acute-angle closure glaucoma usually involves surgery.

Hearing

A common misconception among the general populace is that all elders have some sort of hearing loss. Although many hearing disorders do affect the elderly more frequently and more adversely, most older patients are able to hear and engage in conversation at a normal volume. Hearing loss is approximately four times more common than vision loss (Snyder & Christmas, 2003). Most of the hearing loss that develops with the aging process affects the higher frequencies. As hearing loss progresses, it impairs the ability of the individual to communicate with others and often may frustrate and even isolate the elder from others. However, with the advent of sophisticated hearing aid devices, many elderly with hearing loss are able to correct this deficit. Unfortunately, persons with specific types of sensorineural hearing loss, in which the nerve pathways that connect the inner ear to the brain are malfunctioning, do not benefit significantly from older hearing aid devices. If a patient depends on hearing aids, ensure that these devices accompany the patient to the hospital.

Speech

As patients age, impairments in verbal communication may occur. This may be a result of difficulty forming words or past medical events such as a cerebrovascular accident. Impairment also may be attributable to difficulty in hearing or with word retrieval, a slowed rate of speech, decreases in fluency, and changes in voice quality. A wide variety of conditions can cause these situations, including dementia, hearing loss, neurologic disorders, organic brain syndromes, laryngeal conditions, or changes in oral structures. When treating patients the paramedic should be compassionate about these conditions because they may be frustrating for the patient. The patient may need extra time to communicate compared with younger individuals; the paramedic must not become impatient in these situations.

Incontinence and Elimination Problems

[OBJECTIVE 13]

Incontinence is an extremely embarrassing problem that plagues some elders and may cause other detrimental conditions. **Incontinence** is the inability to control excretory functions and is most commonly used in reference to bowel or bladder dysfunction. The degree of incontinence varies from very mild to total loss of all control and is never considered normal. If not quickly tended to, the presence of urine or fecal matter against the skin may lead to skin irritation, breakdown, and ultimately infection. Sudden onset of incontinence and back pain (especially in a patient with a history of cancer) necessitates an emergency evaluation for possible spinal cord compression (often from a tumor).

For an individual to remain continent, four factors must be present: (1) a gastrointestinal or genitourinary tract without significant anatomic anomaly, (2) a competent sphincter to stop excretory function adequately when closed, (3) the cognitive capability to control the physical function of withholding excretion, and (4) motivation to remain continent until in an appropriate environment to relieve oneself.

Although advancing age by no means ensures that an individual will become incontinent, several factors of aging predispose some elders to incontinence. As the body ages, bladder capacity naturally decreases and involuntary bladder contractions occur with greater frequency. These physiologic changes, coupled with the fact that many elderly take medications that that may affect bowel or bladder function, contribute to the decreased ability to postpone voiding.

Incontinence is a severely embarrassing condition that can often cripple the self-esteem and social lives of those who are afflicted. Depending on the cause of incontinence, different techniques can manage the issue. For those who have anatomic changes predisposing them to incontinence, surgery often is an option. Over-the-counter absorptive devices are an option used by both active and healthy individuals as well as those who are more debilitated and lack the mobility or cognitive function to use bathroom facilities properly. Several medications treat bladder incontinence. For those who completely lack urinary continence and are at high risk of the adverse consequences of skin irritation and breakdown, indwelling catheters remain an option. However, these catheters often lead to infection, and use should be limited to only the most severe cases.

Although some elders may have incontinence, others have the opposite problem—difficulty eliminating waste material from the gastrointestinal or genitourinary tract. Inability to urinate is most commonly caused by a decrease in the production of urine, medications that cause urinary retention, or an obstruction along the genitourinary tract. The first delineation that must be made in those unable to void is whether the renal system is producing urine that is retained in the bladder. A palpable bladder on abdominal examination suggests that urinary retention is caused by medications or an obstructive process. The most common medications causing urinary retention are anticholinergic agents. The most common obstructive cause of urinary retention in elderly men is prostate enlargement, although kidney stones that become dislodged in the urethra also cause obstruction. Urinary retention can lead to a distended bladder that becomes stretched and quite painful. The treatment for urinary retention is the placement of a catheter into the bladder to drain the urine and relieve the bladder distention.

When the abdominal examination does not reveal a palpable bladder and no suprapubic fullness is felt in an individual who has not urinated in some time, urine may not be produced by the kidneys or the path along the ureters to the bladder is obstructed. Ureteral obstruction is most commonly caused by an obstructing kidney stone and commonly is accompanied by intense unilateral flank pain, costovertebral angle tenderness, and nausea and vomiting. The only reason for urine being completely blocked from entering the bladder is bilateral kidney stones in the ureters, which is extremely rare. If no concern or evidence of genitourinary tract obstruction is present, immediate concern should be that the kidneys are producing urine. This lack of urine production should raise concern for renal failure (a shocklike state causing inadequate blood flow to the kidneys).

Constipation, defined as having less than one bowel movement every 3 days, affects 30% of the population older than 65 years (Bree Johnston et al., 2000). Because most causes of constipation are treatable and improve a patient's well-being, those with this condition should be medically evaluated. Often the addition of exercise, sufficient dietary fiber, adequate hydration, and the use of bulking agents adequately treat constipation. However, more serious causes can lead to decreased fecal elimination, such as colorectal cancer, **volvulus,** or bowel obstruction. A physician will be able to determine if a patient needs a colonoscopy for evaluation for cancer. Volvulus, bowel obstruction, and other disease states that commonly cause difficulty with fecal elimination are usually accompanied by pain.

ASSESSMENT OF THE ELDERLY PATIENT

[OBJECTIVES 14, 15, 16, 17, 18]

Assessment of an older adult is a more complex and time consuming task than evaluation of a younger adult. Patience is vital when attempting to elicit the necessary information. An older adult processes information more slowly than a younger adult does. Most older adults may feel obligated to share information that they believe is important before answering a direct question. In fact, this extra information may be quite helpful in assessing the patient.

Additional facts must be gathered with the geriatric patient compared with their younger counterparts. A social history is important and must include specifics of their living arrangements, family and social support, and baseline level of functioning. For example, an older adult may be able to walk to the ambulance without difficulty. If, however, he or she can recently no longer climb the steps to the bathroom, this represents a significant functional decline that may not have been elicited without precise questioning. Medication history also is a vital component of an older person's history. Prescription medications need to be determined as well as nonprescription drugs and any recent changes in medications. As previously mentioned, polypharmacy is an issue with elderly patients. A complete health assessment of the elderly also includes sleep habits, which often are affected by living situation, illness, and medication as well as a person's ability to care for himself or herself.

Nutritional requirements change as people age, and nutrition directly affects many other areas of health. When people age they undergo a natural decrease in the amount of calories required per day. The elderly are estimated to require one third fewer calories than the average adult. This decline is a result of decreased lean muscle mass and basal metabolic rate (Prentice, 1992). The elderly also exhibit a decreased taste sensation, which contributes to decreased intake. Although caloric requirements decrease, vitamin and mineral requirements are unchanged. This can result in nutritional deficiencies (Chernoff, 1995). These issues often are compounded by chronic illness such as breathing problems, dental issues (missing teeth or improper dentures), medications that affect appetite, and poor mobility, which inhibit an older person's ability to obtain and consume proper nutrition.

The face-to-face assessment of elderly patients is complicated by several factors. Chronic diseases, unusual presentation of disease, and decreased sensory function contribute most to this difficulty. The elderly also tend to keep serious symptoms and chronic disease to themselves and not report them to physicians (Gross et al., 1996; Kriegsmann et al., 1996). When interviewing an older person, speak slowly and clearly. As a matter of respect, always introduce yourself and speak to the *patient,* not a bystander. Gathering information from family and caregivers is important, but this can be done after the patient has already been questioned. Make sure that the patient has his or her eyeglasses and hearing aids in place before questioning, and whenever possible try to explain what and why you are doing something. This will help the patient feel as if he or she is informed and has some level of control in what is happening. Remember that the elderly have been in charge of their lives for many years, and losing that independence in the face of illness is difficult. The patient's surroundings, including whether the home is well kept or cluttered, and risk factors such as multilevel layout and loose rugs, can help health practitioners know whether the patient is safe at home.

Communication with the elderly is challenging but important. As previously mentioned, hearing aids and eyeglasses must be in place. Nonverbal clues used in communication can be just as important as the spoken word. The simple practice of repeating an answer back to the patient can confirm a response or give the patient an opportunity to clarify. This is a good strategy in effective communication with persons of any age. Mostly, whenever possible simply slow down and allow the older person to present the story at his or her own pace. This may slow a response by a few minutes. In most cases, however, that extra information you gain is more critical than the few minutes spent obtaining it. After all, getting the correct history is the responsibility of the EMS provider and can make the difference in early stabilization and treatment or significant delays in care. The physical examination should be thorough and include a brief assessment of mental status, including at a minimum the level of alertness and orientation. More in-depth assessment of mental status can, in most cases, be deferred until the patient reaches the hospital.

Chest pain and shortness of breath are two of the most common reasons for the elderly to use EMS systems. Up to 25% of all transports by EMS of elderly people are because of these two symptoms (Wofford et al., 1995). EMS providers should probe common medical complaints such as history of chronic obstructive pulmonary disease or congestive heart failure when an elderly person reports shortness of breath. This often helps guide initial treatment plans and transport considerations. For example, if a patient has a history of congestive heart failure and is short of breath, keeping the patient sitting up is probably best because a supine position will likely worsen breathing. Chest pain can be caused by many disease processes ranging from simple musculoskeletal pain to more serious illness, such as myocardial infarction, pulmonary embolism, and aortic dissection. Determining the cause in the prehospital setting is usually impossible, so all patients with chest pain should be treated as critical. Local protocols help deliver appropriate and effective care. Other common symptoms include orthopedic injury, weakness, and possible stroke. Before administering any drug, EMS providers must be aware that the effects can be very different in different patients, partly because of the effects of polypharmacy.

MANAGEMENT CONSIDERATIONS FOR THE ELDERLY

[OBJECTIVES 16, 17]

Specific issues related to the prehospital management of older adults must be considered. Elderly airway intervention has unique characteristics. As always, securing a patent airway is the most important intervention in any patient interaction. First determine that no advanced directive or DNR order is in place before performing intubation or other aggressive lifesaving techniques. However, if a clear advanced directive is not immediately present, always treat the patient and then sort out the details of the advanced directive later. If intubation is necessary, identify whether the patient has natural or false teeth. If dentures are present, remove them so they do not obstruct the airway. Advanced life support procedures are the same in the elderly as they are for their younger counterparts. Simply because someone is older does not mean he or she will not survive a cardiac arrest. Age is not an independent predictor of death from prehospital cardiac arrest. Older adults should be resuscitated just as aggressively as younger patients (Bonnin et al., 1993).

The elderly have special needs when considering transport. Many of them have musculoskeletal illnesses that make mobility difficult. Take care to prevent falls getting to and from the stretcher. Extra padding often is necessary to prevent discomfort while on the stretcher. Often older patients and those with osteoporosis have some curvature of the thoracic spine called **kyphosis** (hunchback deformity) and benefit from pillows or extra padding to keep their head elevated while lying on their back. A good rule of thumb is to let the patient guide you and transport in a position of comfort unless necessary immobilization of the spine prevents it. Another management consideration is how to deal with the frequent issue of incontinence in the elderly. Above all, attempt to maintain their dignity and convey to patients that it happens frequently and they should not feel ashamed. Indeed, this problem is often treatable and usually without surgical intervention (Wagg & Malone-Lee, 1998). Specific transport and management considerations are addressed later in this chapter.

Case Scenario—continued

The patient states she does not remember what she was doing when she fell. She says she has history of a heart attack, irregular heartbeat, and appendicitis. She states she takes warfarin, nitroglycerin, and a blood pressure medication. You begin your physical examination with an assessment of her head. You notice that she has a large contusion above her right eye. Her pupils are equal. She has no blood coming from her nose, but she does have bruising behind her right ear. She has clear lung sounds, normal heart sounds, and a soft, nontender abdomen. She has a shortened leg on the right. No bleeding is present from her lower extremities. She has a large laceration on her left arm that is bleeding profusely.

Questions

4. *What is the significance of her medications?*
5. *What do the physical examination findings indicate?*
6. *What is important in the treatment for this patient?*

SYSTEM PATHOPHYSIOLOGY, ASSESSMENT, AND MANAGEMENT

This section discusses the specific pathophysiology, assessment, and management of specific illnesses affecting the major body systems. Remember that most disease states covered in other parts of this book still apply to the elderly, but this section highlights disorders commonly encountered in the elderly population.

Pulmonary Changes in the Elderly

[OBJECTIVES 19 TO 24]

The pulmonary system is greatly affected by the aging process. The kyphosis of the spine that commonly occurs in the elderly makes expanding the lungs more difficult and limits the pulmonary reserve that a patient has when stressed by injury or disease. The aging process also causes decreased strength in the respiratory muscles, causing respiratory fatigue and failure earlier than in younger counterparts. In addition, the elasticity of the lungs and chest wall decreases with age, causing a decrease in tidal volume. As a result, the respiratory rate normally increases in elderly patients to compensate for the decreased tidal volume and maintain an adequate minute volume. This leads to a decrease in the vital capacity making compensation for thoracic trauma or respiratory disorders more difficult. The lung itself ages, and the ability of oxygen to cross the membrane of the lungs into the bloodstream is decreased. For reasons that are not yet understood, the lungs also are at increased risk of bronchoconstriction from asthma and small airway obstruction, such as is seen in long-term smokers. Lifelong exposure to antioxidants, environmental pollutants, and the additive affect of lung infections are possible causes of the decrease in pulmonary function associated with age. Changes also occur in the brain so that elderly people sense hypoxia and increased carbon dioxide differently than do younger patients.

When assessing an elderly person with pulmonary complaint, one of the most useful things is a patient's history of pulmonary disease. A person with a history of chronic obstructive pulmonary disease with shortness of breath and wheezing most likely has disease exacerbation and should be treated accordingly unless something in the story does not fit. Along with that, a good lung examination is useful to determine if wheezing or other findings are present, such as focal sounds, suggesting pneumonia, or crackles, suggesting pulmonary edema. The finding of wheezing or decreased breath sounds helps confirm asthma or chronic obstructive pulmonary disease, but diagnosing pneumonia or pulmonary edema by examination is not reliable, even for physicians (Wipf et al., 1999). When managing pulmonary symptoms, routinely administer oxygen to patients. It is an inexpensive and safe treatment and can potentially improve the situation. Preoxygenation, if the patient requires intubation, provides a much longer period of normal oxygen saturation before hypoxia sets in. If the patient has hypoxia, oxygen is a necessity and should be given to obtain an oxygen saturation of greater than 95%. If a patient continues to have significant hypoxia with maximal oxygen, intubation and positive pressure ventilation may be indicated. Prehospital treatment of chronic obstructive pulmonary disease or asthma is common and appropriate. In most situations, giving a beta-agonist such as albuterol has little risk and can dramatically improve a patient's breathing. In contrast, giving furosemide (Lasix) to someone who may or may not have pulmonary edema can worsen dehydration and may be harmful.

When transporting a patient with shortness of breath, a position of comfort is ideal. Patients are able to determine which position makes breathing easier better than someone else can. A supine position may force the patient to use a more diseased or unhealthy part of the lung and worsen the situation.

Pneumonia

Three to 4 million people contract community-acquired pneumonia each year and approximately 500,000 require hospitalization (Marston et al., 1997). Pneumonia is the leading cause of infection in elderly patients and the fifth leading cause of death (Sims, 1990). Pneumonia is most commonly caused by bacteria such as *Streptococcus pneumoniae* but also can be caused by atypical bacteria and viruses such as influenza. Elderly are at increased risk for pneumonia because of several reasons. First, they often have difficulty swallowing and a weak cough, causing an increased risk for **aspiration** (food particles going into the trachea and lung). The elderly also have a decreased immune response and decreased pulmonary function to fight off early infection of the lungs. This, along with the presence of comorbid disease, makes pneumonia a lethal illness, with a 10% mortality rate for hospitalized elderly patients (Meehan et al., 1997). A large study of hospitalized patients with pneumonia showed an increased risk of death with increasing age (Fine et al., 1997). Institutionalized patients also are at risk for pneumonia because of exposure to many bacteria, the presence of coexisting disease, and often immunocompromised states. Pneumonia vaccination exists and is an important preventive measure for elderly people. Occasionally doctors will prescribe prophylactic antibiotics for patients who are frail and at high risk for acquiring pneumonia.

Diagnosis of pneumonia is difficult in the field. Clues include cough, fever, and shortness of breath. Tachypnea and hypoxia also are often present on physical examination. Treatment in the prehospital setting focuses on adequate oxygen delivery. Oxygen should be delivered to provide adequate oxygen saturation. Tracheal intubation should be used for an inability to oxygenate or to protect the airway in a patient who has severe mental status decline. In a patient who is hypotensive, Intravenous fluid administration helps increase fluid volume so that red blood cells carrying oxygen can be delivered to the tissue. Initiation of early treatment is helpful in patients with severe pneumonia, but many will ultimately require hospital admission for treatment (Meehan et al., 1997).

Chronic Obstructive Pulmonary Disease

Chronic obstructive pulmonary disease (COPD) is a common affliction. According to findings compiled in 2005, approximately 12 million people have been diagnosed with the disease and approximately 12 million more are likely to have COPD but have not be diagnosed. (National Heart, Lung, and Blood Institute, 2007). COPD is predominantly a disease of the elderly, with a prevalence in those older than 65 years fourfold that of those aged 45 to 64 years (Sullivan et al., 2000). Traditional teaching has categorized COPD as either chronic bronchitis or emphysema. The two forms are known today to have much overlap, and the term COPD is generally used for both. Smoking is the major risk factor for COPD. This disease is nearly nonexistent in people who are nonsmokers or without significant exposure to secondhand smoke. In assessing patients, a history of COPD is crucial. In addition, the severity of disease can be gauged by knowing if the patient has ever been intubated for the disease and when he or she was last on oral steroids. Breath sounds can confirm the diagnosis if wheezing is heard, but often only decreased sounds or other focal findings are found, which may be misleading. The history, capnography, and the patient are more reliable at guiding treatment. Determine oxygen saturation, but keep in mind that patients who are working very hard to breathe and in respiratory distress can maintain near-normal oxygen saturation. Albuterol and oxygen are the mainstays of treatment for patients with a history of COPD and worsening shortness of breath. A breathing treatment on the way to the ED often can turn around a patient and dramatically improve breathing. In the ED patients often are given steroids and antibiotics after other diagnoses are excluded. Intubation may be necessary if the patient tires and can no longer sustain the work of breathing.

Pulmonary Embolism

Pulmonary embolism (PE) is a common and often fatal condition that occurs as part of a spectrum of disease along with deep venous thrombosis (DVT). PE has a cumulative probability of 10% in patients aged 80 years and older and an in-hospital mortality rate of 21% in patients aged 65 years and older (Hanson et al., 1997; PIOPED Investigators, 1990). One reason for the high mortality rate of PE is the difficulty with diagnosis. Classic presentations are patients with pleuritic chest pain, shortness of breath, tachypnea, and hemoptysis. Rarely do patients present with this constellation of symptoms. In addition to the fact that patients with a PE rarely exhibit the classic presentation, many pulmonary disorders share common signs and symptoms with a PE, further hampering the diagnosis. Risk factors are important in suspecting the disease and include recent surgery or trauma, immobilization, DVT, and a hypercoagulable state (having a tendency to produce blood clots). Many of these risk factors are present in the elderly. Immobilization is common because of frequent orthopedic injuries, and the presence of hypercoagulable states also increases with age (Price & Ridken, 1997). If PE is suspected, provide supportive care such as intravenous fluid for hypotension or advance life support procedures if indicated. Patients with PE often are anxious because of the degree of shortness of breath and pain. Use a calm voice and reassure the patient to help alleviate fear. Once PE is diagnosed, anticoagulant drugs such as warfarin, heparin, and newer low-molecular-weight heparins such as enoxaparin are effective at preventing increased clot formation. While taking anticoagulants patients have an increased risk of gastrointestinal and intracranial bleeding. This also must be a consideration when treating elderly people with history of PE or DVT.

Cardiology in the Elderly

[OBJECTIVES 25 TO 30]

Multiple changes occur in the cardiovascular system with aging. The large arteries become less elastic and are therefore more rigid. This creates more pressure in the arterial system during systole and causes an increased systolic blood pressure and therefore widened **pulse pressure** (difference between systolic and diastolic blood pressure) (Safar, 1993). The peripheral vasculature also undergoes changes with aging, causing increased peripheral resistance and increased diastolic blood pressure and mean arterial pressure. This increase in hypertension puts the elderly at risk for atherosclerotic disease such as myocardial infarction, stroke, limb ischemia, and mesenteric ischemia. The heart itself also undergoes changes as people age. The left ventricle becomes thickened and stiff as a result of the normal process of aging. In addition, people with hypertension require their heart to pump against higher pressures, which likely is an additional stimulus for left ventricular hypertrophy (Levy et al., 1988).

The heart also has decreased capability to respond to beta-adrenergic stimulus during times of stress and exercise as the body ages (Lakatta, 1980). The heart therefore is unable to compensate and pump blood faster when required. In addition, the blood vessels do not respond as well by contracting and forcing blood to the organs. This, coupled with a lack of venous blood return and multiple medications, make the elderly more prone to postural or orthostatic hypotension (Lipsitz et al., 1990).

The combination of these factors results in a decrease in the patient's myocardial reserve capacity, making compensation for cardiovascular insults more difficult.

When obtaining a history from a patient with a chief complaint related to the cardiovascular system, try to get a sense of his or her cardiovascular fitness. Elderly people who regularly exercise are able to maintain cardiac function much better than their sedentary counterparts (Fleg, 1986). Other important history points are cardiac history, recent changes in exertional tolerance or diet, smoking history, shortness of breath (at rest or at night versus with exertion), palpitations, and medicine use. The examination should focus on the heart, lungs, and peripheral vascular system. Listening to the heart or feeling a central pulse for regularity is important. Feeling peripheral pulses for strength can give a sense of the patient's volume status. Checking pulses in all extremities can detect weakened pulses suggestive of hypotension or isolated absent pulses, which would be seen in limb ischemia or traumatic blood vessel injury. Dehydration can also be gauged by looking at the mouth and appreciating the amount of moisture and saliva present.

Focus management of an elderly patient with a cardiac complaint on maintaining blood pressure and therefore oxygen delivery to the tissues. Deal with airway and ventilation issues first. Common cardiac problems in the elderly include myocardial infarction, heart failure, dysrhythmias, aneurysms, and hypertension. Often these problems require medications to be given. Keep in mind that the elderly have less lean body mass and decreased hepatic and renal function, so medications will not be cleared as quickly as in younger people. Small doses of medications should be used to prevent overmedication. The elderly also have a decreased fluid reserve, so medications that affect the blood pressure, such as nitroglycerin, morphine, or antiarrhythmics, can cause hypotension.

Myocardial Infarction

Coronary artery disease (CAD) is the most common cardiovascular disease in the elderly in the United States, affecting 3.6 million people (Dawson & Adams, 1987). More than half of all people (approximately 60%) hospitalized for acute myocardial infarction (MI) are older than 65 years (Graves, 1991). Coronary artery disease also is much more deadly and debilitating for the elderly. In-hospital mortality rate for MI in the elderly in one study was reported as 19% for those older than 75 years versus 5% in those younger than 75 years (Paul et al., 1996). The most important thing to remember regarding MI in the elderly is that it very well may not present with chest pain, and the likelihood a patient will not have chest pain increases with age (Bayer et al., 1986). In this age group, chest pain is more the exception than the rule for MI. Dyspnea is the most common complaint in elderly patients with MI (Solomon et al., 1989). A series of elderly patients with MI from New York reported that less than 50% of patients older than 75 years with documented MI had chest pain (Muller et al., 1990). Any older person with a complaint from the waist up should prompt consideration for acute MI.

Risk factors in the elderly include increased age, high prevalence of diabetes, and known heart disease. Elderly persons at risk for MI may be taking aspirin or beta-blocking medications, which have both been shown to decrease mortality rate from MI. Given the prevalence and poor outcomes of elderly with CAD, MI should always be considered when treating an older person. Treatment should be as aggressive for the elderly as for their younger counterparts. The benefits and low risk of side effects from aspirin make it a mainstay of treatment for elderly patients with MI. Nitroglycerin also should be used for vasodilation, which may help relieve pain with careful attention to blood pressure and prior use of medications for erectile dysfunction, such as Viagra, which may cause adverse interactions.

Congestive Heart Failure

Congestive heart failure (CHF) **incidence** increases as people age. The Framingham Heart Study found incidences of 8 per 1000 men aged 50 to 59 years and 66 per 1000 men aged 80 to 89 years (Ho et al., 1993). Higher rates of hypertension and CAD in the elderly cause the heart to have either less contractility (left ventricular dysfunction) or stiffness, preventing proper filling of the heart (diastolic dysfunction). In addition to this, pulmonary edema has noncardiac causes as well, such as infection and trauma.

Heart failure often manifests as vague symptoms in the elderly. Weakness is a common complaint that can occur with left heart failure. More classically, shortness of breath, **orthopnea** (sleeping with the head up on pillows or in a chair to prevent lying flat), cough, lower extremity edema, and crackles in the lungs occur. Isolated right heart failure can cause edema and abdominal ascites without the pulmonary symptoms. Nitrates, including nitroglycerin, are the initial drug of choice in normotensive patients with CHF. Nitrates increase venous capacity and relieve the vasoconstriction present in patients with CHF. Caution must be used to avoid hypotension; however, most patients with decompensated CHF are hypertensive. Diuretic use should be minimal in the prehospital arena, especially in the elderly. Although diuretics such as furosemide (Lasix) are the mainstay of treatment, diagnosis of CHF without radiology and laboratory studies can be impossible. Other diseases such as pneumonia and COPD can be significantly worsened by intravenous furosemide, causing worsening dehydration and tissue death when the patient actually needs more fluid (Mosesso et al., 2003).

Dysrhythmias in the Elderly

The prevalence of dysrhythmias increases with age. Atrial fibrillation, the most common dysrhythmia of the elderly, affects approximately 10% of the population older than 80 years (Ryder & Benjamin, 1999). Atrial fibrillation may be caused by structural heart disease that exerts increased stress or pressure on the atria, such as heart failure, hypertensive heart disease, and valvular abnormalities. Other causes of atrial fibrillation include thyroid disorders, recent heart surgery, severe infection, and additional metabolic disturbances. Prolonged atrial fibrillation with tachycardia can cause heart failure as well as syncope and other forms of decreased organ perfusion. Atrial fibrillation without anticoagulation enables clots to form in the atria of the heart and can cause stroke as they are pumped out of the heart.

Other dysrhythmias also are more common in the elderly. Pacemaker cells of the sinoatrial node decrease with age so that only 10% of the cells present at age 20 years are still present at age 80 years. Sick sinus syndrome and sinus arrhythmia are common and can be severe enough to warrant pacemaker placement. Premature ventricular complexes (PVC) are common in the elderly and have many causes. Any condition that causes decreased blood flow to the heart can cause PVCs. Severe electrolyte abnormalities also can cause PVCs and other dysrhythmias.

Any fast or slow dysrhythmia can cause decreased blood flow to the brain and syncope. Cardiac causes of syncope are associated with a 30% 1-year mortality rate and a 50% 5-year mortality rate (Kapoor et al., 1983; Kapoor, 1990). For this reason, syncope in the elderly is a serious symptom and warrants further evaluation to determine a cause. In addition to the poor outcome with cardiac syncope, dysrhythmias are potentially dangerous because they contribute to falls and orthopedic injury and head injury. Falls in the elderly necessitate a search for the cause of the fall.

PARAMEDIC*Pearl*

Evaluation of elderly patients with weakness, falls, palpitations, or syncope should prompt assessment of the patient's blood glucose level and rhythm strip analysis.

Serious dysrhythmias such as ventricular tachycardia or fibrillation, atrial fibrillation with a rapid ventricular response, and supraventricular tachycardia should be treated per advance cardiac life support or system-specific protocols. Tachycardias may occur as a result of fever or dehydration. A small IV fluid challenge in a hypotensive patient with clear lung sounds may be warranted.

PARAMEDIC*Pearl*

All elderly patients with a complaint related to a dysrhythmia should be transported for further evaluation even if they are in a sinus rhythm at the time of evaluation. Dysrhythmias can be transient and recur without warning, causing significant morbidity and death.

Aneurysm

Abdominal aortic aneurysm (AAA) is a condition that increases in incidence with age. Persons younger than 50 years rarely have AAA. One percent of persons aged 54 to 65 years have an aneurysm greater than 4 cm, and the prevalence increases by 2% to 4% every 10 years (Singh et al., 2001; Powell & Greenhalgh, 2003). In addition to age, hypertension, smoking, and atherosclerosis are the major risk factors for AAA. Aneurysms may remain stable for years without rupture, especially aneurysms less than 4 cm, which rarely rupture. Once ruptured, however, mortality rate is high. In a study in Scotland, patients with ruptured AAA had an 80% mortality rate, with the majority of those never making it to the hospital (Adam et al., 1999). In patients who do make it to the ED, abdominal, flank, and back pain are the main symptoms.

All patients with history of AAA and all elderly with abdominal or back pain should have an abdominal examination looking for pulsatile masses and tenderness. Pulses in the lower extremities also should be evaluated to detect absent pulses that can accompany ruptured AAAs. Prehospital care of patients with ruptured AAA should include IV access, IV fluids, and rapid transport. Time is critical in providing a chance of survival in patients with AAA.

Hypertension

More than half of all individuals older than 65 years have hypertension (Wilking et al., 1988). Increased stiffness of the arteries and increased atherosclerosis predispose elderly patients to hypertension, specifically systolic hypertension. Elderly persons with diabetes and obesity are at greater risk for hypertension. Chronic hypertension causes kidney damage and damage to other end organs such as the eyes and heart. Patients can help avoid blood pressure–related issues by taking their medications, avoiding sodium, exercising, and quitting smoking.

Acute hypertensive episodes can cause organ damage and are the main concern in patients with high blood pressure. **Hypertensive emergency** is the current term used to represent acute hypertension with end organ dysfunction. No specific level of blood pressure defines hypertensive emergency. In patients with hypertension, end organ dysfunction may show itself as chest pain, vision changes, mental status changes, vomiting, or urinary complaints. Epistaxis is one symptom that often is accompanied by hypertension. In most instances controlling the bleeding lessens patient anxiety and blood pressure normalizes. Most other hypertensive presentations do not require prehospital medication intervention. However, chest pain associated with hypertension should be treated with nitroglycerin to treat possible cardiac ischemia or infarction.

Neurology in the Elderly

[OBJECTIVES 31 TO 36]

Changes occur in the neurologic system of the elderly. Some of these changes are expected, normal changes with aging and other represent disease processes. The differences must be clarified. As people age some **psychomotor** slowing and slowed reaction time are expected. The elderly also undergo a slight decline in short-term memory that does not interfere with daily activities (Petersen et al., 1992). More severe memory deficit and changes in **cognition** are not normal. A change in cognition represents a disease state such as delirium or dementia that should be addressed so that treatment can be provided.

Assessing the elderly for these cognitive changes can be difficult in a short prehospital interaction. This type of assessment is best conducted over a period of time and if the patient's close family and friends are involved to comment on the changes they have observed. The patient's thinking processes, communication, and memory should be tested in a quiet, calm environment to lessen possible distractions. A mental status examination can be performed in 5 to 10 minutes and is a reliable test of cognition. Determine level of alertness and orientation to person, place, time, and situation. Pay special attention to whether the patient is thinking logically and responding appropriately. Also important is gathering information about recent changes in behavior, ability to perform activities of daily living (bathing, hygiene, food preparation), and the patient's mood. Mood can be assessed simply by asking the patient how he or she feels (e.g., happy, sad, depressed, or angry). While questioning the elderly, keep in mind their decreased reaction time and psychomotor slowing. Be calm, clear, and allow time for them to respond. In addition to the mental changes, neurologic evaluation also should include questions and examination aimed at detecting focal or general weakness, changes in sleeping and eating patterns, and any recent syncopal episodes. This information can provide clues regarding whether a more acute neurologic emergency, such as stroke, is the cause of the complaint.

Management of older adults with neurologic complaints is common for EMS professionals. Specific recommendations are given later in this chapter for cerebrovascular accident, dementia, and delirium. Ensuring that the patient can protect his or her airway is necessary and can be as simple as engaging the patient in conversation. A patient who can speak clearly can protect the airway. If a patient is unable to follow commands and does not have a strong gag reflex, provide airway protection with intubation for the patient to prevent aspiration and hypoxia.

In general, keep the patient calm and provide a quiet environment to prevent further anxiety or agitation.

Cerebrovascular Disease

Cerebrovascular disease is the third leading cause of death in the United States and the leading cause of disability (American Heart Association, 1998; Murray & Lopez, 1997). Two types of ischemic cerebrovascular disease are typically recognized: ischemic stroke and transient ischemic attack. A **cerebrovascular accident** (commonly called a *stroke*) is a sudden change in neurologic function caused by an alteration in cerebral blood flow. An **ischemic stroke** occurs when blood flow in one of the arteries in the brain is blocked. The blockage may be caused by a blood clot, air, amniotic fluid, or a foreign body. A **transient ischemic attack** is the same disease process that resolves, with the patient returning to baseline within 24 hours.

Risk factors include hypertension, smoking, diabetes, and atrial fibrillation, which account for an increased percentage of stroke as people age (Wolf et al., 1991). Prevention is aimed at modifying these risk factors by control of hypertension and diabetes, smoking cessation, diagnosis of atrial fibrillation, and anticoagulation when appropriate.

Acute treatment of stroke is rapidly emerging. The general population is beginning to recognize the time-dependent nature of stroke treatment. For the elderly and all stroke patients, rapid transfer to an ED or stroke center (a hospital that specializes in the management of cerebrovascular diseases) is essential. If the patient is having an ischemic stroke and meets the criteria for its administration, IV tissue plasminogen activator (TPA) is given in the hospital. Currently TPA must be given within 3 hours of symptom onset after obtaining a computed tomographic scan of the head and laboratory work (National Institute of Neurological Disorders and Stroke rt-PA Stroke Study Group, 1995; Marler et al., 2000). This leaves little time for the prehospital phase of treatment. Some stroke centers are able to administer intraarterial TPA or other invasive procedures, which can increase the treatment window to 6 hours.

In patients with possible stroke, prehospital management should be aimed at obtaining a clear history of the time of onset, medical and medication history, and blood glucose determination. In the elderly, obtain a history of the patient's baseline mental status from caregivers or family. This will help the ED staff recognize what are new deficits and what may be old. Because distinguishing ischemic stroke from intracranial hemorrhage is impossible without imaging studies, aspirin is not recommended for possible stroke treatment in the prehospital setting.

Dementia and Delirium

Becoming more forgetful and easily confused often is assumed to be an expected part of aging. Although this is the case regarding forms of dementia, such as Alzheimer's disease, reversible causes of any mental status changes should be considered. In fact, a diagnosis of dementia should not be made until reversible causes have been ruled out.

Understanding the differences between dementia and delirium is critical (Table 38-2). **Dementia** is characterized by a decline in intellectual functioning, sometimes to the extent that the patient cannot perform usual activities of daily living. One of the chief elements of dementia is memory deficit, with the deterioration of intellectual functioning occurring over an extended period of months to years. Several different causes lead to this deterioration, including Alzheimer's disease, Parkinson's disease, vascular dementia, brain tumors, central nervous system trauma, and HIV dementia. These diseases and conditions account for the majority of causes of dementia and currently are irreversible. Although a hallmark of dementia is its irreversibility, some rare reversible causes of dementia, such as vitamin deficiency (e.g., B_{12} and niacin), infection (e.g., neurosyphilis), and normal-pressure hydrocephalus, also occur.

Delirium, on the other hand, is an acute, often reversible, intermittent, global disorder of cognition and/or consciousness that may also be accompanied by emotional or psychomotor disturbances. States of delirium often can be attributed to medication, infection, or metabolic disorder. Common causes of delirium are listed in Box 38-4. The underlying cause of delirium must be identified and immediately treated.

Alzheimer's Disease

[OBJECTIVES 32, 33, 34, 35, 36]

Alzheimer's disease is the most common cause of dementia. An estimated 10% of those older than 65 years and nearly half of those older than 85 years will develop Alzheimer's disease. The disease is marked by gradual memory loss, a decline in the ability to perform daily tasks, disorientation, impairment of judgment, and personality change. As the disease progresses, patients often are unable to care for themselves and require a caregiver. Alzheimer's disease currently has no cure and its cause is unknown. Treatment of Alzheimer's disease is aimed at providing nursing and social care for the patient as well as medications aimed at lessening the symptoms. Psychosocial management helps ease the burdens that the disease places on both the patient and caregivers.

Parkinson's Disease

Parkinson's disease, another common neurologic disorder that often plagues the elderly, is a disorder caused by damage or degeneration of dopamine-producing nerve cells in the basal ganglia portion of the brain. The four cardinal signs of Parkinson's disease are tremors, **bradykinesia,** postural instability, and rigidity. The tremor associated with Parkinson's disease is usually most evident in the hands and is described as "pill rolling." Bradykinesia refers to the fact that those with the disease have difficulty initiating movement or changing the direction of the movement, causing patients to have an overall decrease in voluntary movement. The hallmark sign of bradykinesia in Parkinson's patients is the distinctive

TABLE 38-2 Differences between Delirium and Dementia

	Delirium	Dementia
Onset	Acute or subacute	Insidious
Course	Fluctuating, usually revolves over days to weeks	Progressive
Consciousness level	Often impaired, can fluctuate rapidly	Clear until later stages
Cognitive defects	Poor short-term memory, poor attention span	Poor short-term memory, attention less affected until severe
Hallucinations	Common, especially visual	Often absent
Delusions	Fleeting, nonsystematized	Often absent
Psychomotor activity	Increased, reduced, or unpredictable	Can be normal
Reversibility	Often	Rarely

Reprinted from Northington, W., & Yates, A. (2005). Caring for the aged. *Journal of Emergency Medical Services, 30*(7), 70-85.

BOX 38-4 Common Causes of Delirium

- Acid-base disturbances
- Acute blood loss
- Acute MI
- Acute psychosis
- Abnormally large amounts of nitrogenous waste in the blood (azotemia)
- Congestive heart failure
- Decreased cardiac output
- Dehydration
- Electrolyte abnormalities
- Fecal impaction
- Abnormally large amounts of carbon dioxide in the blood (hypercarbia)
- Hypoglycemia
- Hyperglycemia
- Hypothermia
- Hyperthermia
- Hypoxia
- Infections
- Intoxication
- Medications
- Metabolic disorders
- Small cortical strokes
- Transfer to unfamiliar surroundings
- Urinary retention

MI, Myocardial infarction.

shuffled gait. If left untreated, the disease progresses over several years and leaves the patient with severe weakness and an inability to care for himself or herself. Because Parkinson's disease is associated with decreased levels of dopamine, medications may be prescribed to increase dopamine levels. Administered dopamine does not cross the blood-brain barrier; therefore precursors of dopamine, such as levadopa, are prescribed and subsequently increase dopamine levels. Although medications such as levodopa are aimed at temporarily reversing the symptoms by replenishing dopamine in the brain, Parkinson's disease has no cure. The goal of the treatment is to improve the quality of life by supportive care through counseling, exercise, and special aids in the home.

Endocrinology in the Elderly

[OBJECTIVES 37 TO 42]

Changes in the endocrine system occur with aging. These changes can be part of the natural aging process or part of a disease state. The difference between the two can be difficult to determine. Glucose metabolism and thyroid function are the most important of the endocrine changes for prehospital providers because they are common problems with possible acute presentations. Older people have difficulty using and clearing glucose when compared with younger people for two main reasons. First, tissues are less sensitive to insulin and therefore use glucose to a lesser degree (Roder et al., 2000). Second, some elderly people have a decrease in insulin secretion compared with those who are younger (Chen et al., 1985). These two factors predispose the elderly to glucose intolerance and possible diabetes. Type 2 diabetes in older adults stems from the inability to use the insulin they have rather than an absence of insulin. The thyroid gland secretes less thyroid hormone and the body is slower to convert it to its more active metabolite as the body ages (Oddie et al., 1966; Penzes & Gergely, 1989). This, coupled with an increase of thyroid diseases such as thyroiditis and thyroid nodules, makes hypothyroidism common in the elderly.

When caring for older individuals, note any history of endocrine disorders such as diabetes or thyroid disorders. Checking blood glucose on all diabetics is essential because high and low blood sugar can cause many vague and serious symptoms that should be quickly corrected. Persons taking levothyroxine (Synthroid) are receiving a supplemental thyroid hormone and may become hypothyroid or hyperthyroid. Thyroid complications are difficult to diagnose and recognition of the fact that a patient is at risk by being on thyroid medications can help make this diagnosis.

Diabetes

As the body ages, so does the risk of developing type 2 diabetes. Although the prevalence of type 2 diabetes is 1.4% for those aged 25 to 44 years, at least 10% of those older than 65 years have type 2 diabetes (Kenny et al., 1995). Data from the National Health and Nutrition Examination Survey III suggest up to 20% of people older than 65 years have diabetes. People with diabetes are at risk for injury to the blood vessels and vascular disease that can affect almost any organ. Coronary artery disease, stroke, kidney failure, limb ischemia, and blindness are common complications of diabetes. The risk of death among those with diabetes is twice that of nondiabetics. The risk of heart disease and stroke is two to four times higher in diabetic patients, and it is the leading cause of blindness and kidney failure (Centers for Disease Control and Prevention, 2003). Increasing age, family history, and obesity are the leading risk factors for developing type 2 diabetes. Prevention of this disease is difficult but improvements can be made. People identified as at risk by family history, obesity, or past hyperglycemia can lower their chance of developing diabetes by dietary changes and exercise (Pan et al., 1997; Diabetes Prevention Program Research Group, 2002). Many people with diabetes do not know they have it until a complication develops. Once the disease is diagnosed, lifestyle changes are important, but glucose control should be the aim of treatment. Tight glucose control has been shown to decrease diabetic complications in type 1 and type 2 diabetics. Diabetes Control and Complications Trial

Research Group, 1993; U.K. Prospective Diabetes Study Group, 1998).

Assessing an elderly person with diabetes requires prompt blood glucose determination. Low and high blood glucose can cause many vague and varied symptoms. Assessment also should include what medications they take for their diabetes and any recent changes in medicine or diet. Treatment should be aimed at immediate correction of hypoglycemia with IV dextrose or intramuscular glucagon if IV access cannot be established. In patients with hyperglycemia, start IV fluid administration because it helps lower glucose in patients with hyperglycemia by treating the associated dehydration. Hyperglycemic hyperosmolar nonketotic syndrome is a hyperglycemic state usually found in uncontrolled type 2 diabetes in which dehydration is a major component. This syndrome is similar to diabetic ketoacidosis but differs in how the body uses other fuel when glucose cannot be properly used. Both syndromes are characterized by dehydration, hyperglycemia, and acidosis and should be managed by EMS professionals with IV fluids.

Thyroid Disease

Thyroid disease incidence increases with increasing age. Hypothyroidism affects 5% to 15% of people older than 65 years and hyperthyroidism to the point of thyrotoxicosis occurs more frequently in the elderly (Gussekloo et al., 2004; Ronnov-Jensen & Kirkegaard, 1973). Elderly people with past thyroid disorders who are currently on thyroid replacement therapy are at risk for developing clinical hypothyroidism. Medication noncompliance because of polypharmacy or immobility can create a situation in which elderly patients are not able to take their thyroid medication and develop hypothyroidism. New-onset hypothyroidism can also occur and manifest with vague complaints such as fatigue and cold intolerance, which may be attributed to other illnesses or the aging process itself. Hyperthyroidism presents with vague symptoms such as fatigue and weight loss. Few elderly people have the classic symptoms of tremor, anxiety, and heat intolerance that are common in younger patients (Trivalle et al., 1996).

Identification of the possibility of a thyroid disorder is difficult. It should be suspected in any elderly patient with a vague, unusual complaint, especially if he or she has a history of thyroid problems. Airway and respiratory compromise is rare in thyroid disorders. Aim prehospital treatment at symptom control and transport. The hyperthyroid patient may present with tachycardia, fever, tremor, weight loss, or other vague complaints of weakness. If patients appear dehydrated and are tachycardic, initiate IV fluids. Hypothyroid elderly patients may have fatigue, confusion, cold intolerance, or other vague complaints. Ultimately the treatment for hyperthyroidism is beta-blockers for symptom control and then chemical or surgical correction of the thyroid disorder. Hypothyroidism is treated with thyroid replacement.

Gastroenterology in the Elderly

[OBJECTIVES 43, 44, 45, 46, 47, 48]

The elderly have many changes in the gastrointestinal (GI) system that put them at risk for malnutrition. Malnutrition may affect 30% to 40% of hospitalized patients older than 70 years (Constans et al., 1992). Difficulty with swallowing occurs because of decreased motility of the esophagus and structural problems such as esophageal webs or strictures and cancers (Mendez et al., 1991). Adverse medication effects and a decreased sense of taste also can contribute to decreased appetite and increased malnutrition in the elderly. Gastroesophageal reflux disease (GERD) also is a common and increasing problem for the elderly. It is estimated to affect at least 30% of the elderly population (Spechler, 1992). GERD contributes to poor GI health by causing pain, ulcer disease, aspiration, and even cancer.

Management of elderly patients with GI complaints is difficult. Two factors contribute to the difficulty in managing these patients: the high morbidity and mortality of abdominal disease and the atypical presentations of elderly with abdominal pain. Patients with serious abdominal illness often have vague complaints and can even lack abdominal pain. Surgery is required in 21% to 42% of elderly patients examined in the ED with acute abdominal pain (Marco et al., 1998; Bugliosi et al., 1990). The diagnoses requiring surgery include perforation, obstruction, infection, and malignancy. The elderly present with atypical symptoms because of several reasons. Changes in the nervous system and pain perception alter the elderly patient's ability to localize and characterize pain. Baseline changes in laboratory work, physical examination, the ability to provide an accurate history, and preexisting medical conditions also complicate diagnosis. Accurate diagnosis of abdominal pain in the ED is more difficult in patients older than 65 years than in those younger than 65 years (Kizer & Vassar, 1998).

PARAMEDIC*Pearl*

Abdominal pain in an older adult must be taken seriously.

Prehospital management of an elderly patient with abdominal pain should include a careful, complete examination. Cardiac and pulmonary disorders also can cause abdominal pain, and serious abdominal problems may present with only mental status changes or other vague symptoms. Because of this, any abdominal tenderness with an abnormality in vital signs or mental status change in an elderly patient should be considered a serious condition. Rapid transport and stabilization should be the main focus. In hypotensive patients, consider IV fluids and vasopressors. Pain management in the prehospital setting of abdominal pain is controversial. In the elderly patient, holding narcotics until the patient can be examined by an ED physician is the safest choice. Narcotics have not been shown to change the diagnostic ability of the clinical examination, but in the elderly they could have serious effects on blood pressure or mental status, which can confuse the picture. Long transport times may necessitate narcotic use, but this requires online medical direction or carefully designed protocols.

Gastrointestinal Hemorrhage

Elderly patients are at increased risk for GI hemorrhage. Increased ulcer disease, diverticulitis, and bowel ischemia contribute to this increased incidence (Borum, 1999; Whiteway & Morson, 1985; Rosen, 1999). Symptoms in the elderly can be weakness, shortness of breath, and diarrhea, or they may notice blood in the stool or dark black stool. Treat tachycardia or hypotension as hypovolemia with IV fluid administration. Keep in mind, however, that many older patients are on beta-blocker medication that prevents tachycardia. Elderly patients with GI bleeding are fragile and can quickly decompensate. Two large-bore IVs are required to ensure adequate access for rapid fluid administration. A quick assessment of whether active bleeding from the rectum or continued **melena** is present will help gauge the immediate severity. Active bleeding is life threatening and transportation should not be delayed.

Bowel Obstruction

Obstruction also is a common problem in the elderly. It accounts for 11% to 12% of elderly ED abdominal pain (Kizer & Vassar, 1998; Bugliosi et al., 1990). Prior abdominal surgery puts the elderly at risk for small bowel obstruction. **Incarcerated hernias** also can cause obstruction in all age groups. Signs and symptoms of obstruction usually include vomiting and intermittent abdominal pain, as in younger patients. Bilious emesis (dark green in color) is considered indicative of an obstruction until proven otherwise. Antiemetics can be used successfully by EMS personnel under the order of medical direction. Side effects include drowsiness, akathisia (a feeling of restlessness), and dystonic reactions (uncontrolled head turning or muscular rigidity). Lower dosages of these medications should be used to lessen the chance of an adverse reaction. IV access and IV fluid for the dehydration that often comes with vomiting also may be indicated.

Psychological Disorders in the Elderly

[OBJECTIVE 49]

The elderly are at risk for many of the same psychological illnesses that afflict younger persons. Any elder who exhibits signs of a psychiatric disorder deserves the same evaluation afforded to younger patients. Although several disease states or other factors may affect an elder's psychological state, never assume that psychological abnormalities are simply a manifestation of older age. An evaluation is required to try to diagnose abnormalities and determine any underlying cause.

Depression

[OBJECTIVES 50, 51, 52, 53, 54]

Depression is a common problem among the elderly, estimated to affect approximately 2 million older Americans (Snyder & Christmas, 2003). However, major depression in the elderly is commonly underrecognized and undertreated. Depression in the elderly often may not appear with the usual vegetative symptoms seen in the younger population but may instead be marked by agitation, anxiety, or somatic complaints (Muller-Spahn & Kock, 1994; Box 38-5). The elderly also are more likely to have a chronic illness, financial pressures, loss of physical mobility, bereavement from the death of a close companion, and decreased cognitive function, all risk factors for developing depression (Muller-Spahn & Kock, 1994).

Treatment of depression in the elderly consists of a combination of counseling, medication, and establishment of a social network. Older adults often become isolated and removed from social settings for a variety of reasons. This isolation is a significant factor in the development of depression. Establishing a social network is a commonly used strategy to prevent depression in the elderly.

Suicide

The geriatric population has a higher rate of completed suicides compared with that of the general population. In fact, older adult men have the highest rate of suicide. According to the National Institutes of Health, in 1999 the elderly comprised 12.7% of the population but committed 18.8% of the suicides. Several risk factors for suicide in the elderly population have been identified (Box 38-6).

BOX 38-5 Warning Signs of Possible Depression

- Frequent nonurgent EMS calls
- Frequent ED or physician's office visits
- Physical findings that do not match the severity of the complaint
- Poor hygiene and/or poor housekeeping
- Loss of enjoyment
- No social support network

ED, Emergency department.

BOX 38-6 Risk Factors for Attempted Suicide

- Alcohol abuse and alcohol dependence
- Death of someone close
- Depression
- Isolation
- Loss of purpose
- Sickness

If any concern exists regarding the patient having possible suicidal feelings, you must directly address the issue. No evidence exists that questions concerning suicide increase the risk of suicide. In fact, addressing suicidal thoughts and feelings often allows a patient to open up to you and share some of these deep and painful emotions. After assessing the risk for suicide, you must transport the patient for further medical evaluation. You must take any comments concerning suicide seriously and stay with the suicidal patient at all times, ensuring his safety during transport. Once at the hospital, the prehospital provider must relay the concern that a patient may be suicidal and let the hospital staff know of any explicit statements made indicating that the patient is at risk for committing suicide. Patients exhibiting warning signs of suicide need to be evaluated by a medical professional.

Integumentary Changes with Age

[OBJECTIVES 55 TO 60]

The skin undergoes a general atrophy as people age. It becomes thinner and loses its strength. The epidermis becomes thinner as a result of the layers of cells thinning and a decrease in the number of cells (Newcomer & Young, 1989). Changes in the cells of the epidermis caused by aging and sun exposure put the elderly at increased risk for skin tumors (Elmets & Mukhatat, 1995). The thicker dermis also thins with fewer cells and elastic fibers (Leyden, 1990). The vascularity decreases as well, leading to a decreased response to injury and decreased rate of healing (Montagna & Carlisle, 1979). This increases the elderly person's susceptibility to secondary bacterial infections as well as fungal and viral infections. The layer of subcutaneous fat also decreases in elderly. This decrease, coupled with a loss of elasticity, causes increased risk of skin tears and loss of protection from minor trauma. Appendages within the skin (hair follicles and different types of glands) also change with aging. Hair becomes thinner and glands have decreased function, losing the ability to sweat and compensate for higher temperatures. This is one factor contributing to increased risk of hyperthermia in the elderly.

PARAMEDIC*Pearl*

Because of the normal changes in the skin of the elderly patient and the associated muscle atrophy, the back of the hand is a poor choice in assessing skin turgor. An adequately hydrated patient will likely exhibit "tenting" in this location, leading to a false-positive result. Better locations for assessing skin turgor include the forehead and sternum because these locations maintain their elasticity longer than other parts of the body.

Skin complaints can represent trivial normal changes or signs of underlying emergent conditions. When caring for elderly patients with skin issues, get a sense for how sick the person is systemically. Underlying systemic illness or serious injury is more of an acute risk to the patient than the rash or laceration seen on the skin. Patients with other signs of systemic illness such as abnormal vital signs or change in baseline functioning require immediate transport. Inspect the entire body to look for pressure sores that could cause systemic infection or other lesions unknown to the patient or caregivers. Areas of cellulitis may indicate serious infections. In these cases septic shock is possible and IV access should be obtained and IV fluid administered for anyone with tachycardia or hypotension and no contraindication, such as heart failure or renal failure. Manage lacerations in the elderly just as you would in younger persons. Controlling bleeding is the foremost concern and can be difficult in patients taking blood thinners. This often is accomplished with direct pressure. The use of a gloved finger to apply direct pressure is probably the best method but may not be practical if only a two-person crew is transporting the patient. Pressure dressings can be used but should start with small pieces of gauze located directly over the bleeding site and then built up from there to ensure the pressure is translated to the specific spot of bleeding. Again, if bleeding has been severe, IV fluids are warranted to restore the intravascular volume.

Pressure Ulcers

Pressure ulcers are common in immobile elderly patients. Residents of extended care facilities have a 9% to 13% 1-year incidence of developing a pressure ulcer (Brandeis et al., 1990). The thin, less-vascular skin of the elderly puts them at risk. Constant pressure on a bony area keeps blood from getting to the skin and causes hypoxic tissue to breaks down, creating the sore. Poor nutrition and friction at the weakened site also contribute to make the sores larger and prevent healing. Frequent movement is the best way to prevent pressure ulcers. If a person cannot move on his or her own, frequent turning and careful inspection of the skin are required to prevent and identify skin breakdown. Pressure ulcers are prone to infection and can cause sepsis and death. Treatment of these ulcers includes proper nutrition, local wound care, and sometimes surgical debridement. Presence of pressure ulcers should alert EMS providers to look for other signs of systemic illness and signs of abuse or neglect.

Musculoskeletal Changes with Age

[OBJECTIVES 61 TO 66]

Musculoskeletal problems affect an estimated 35 million people in the United States (United States Bone and Joint Decade, 2006). As the body ages, the skeletal system becomes more brittle and susceptible to injury. The cells that make the bone matrix and cartilage have decreased function. Hormones that regulate bone and soft tissue growth decrease, and a sedentary lifestyle reduces the mechanical stresses required to keep bones and other soft tissues strong (Buckwalter et al., 1993). On average, by the age of 80 years elderly people have lost 30% of their bone mass (Buckwalter et al., 1995). This normal loss of bone is worsened in the elderly with osteoporosis. Other pathologic conditions of aging include osteoarthritis, which limits function in the elderly.

When managing elderly people, keep in mind that their mobility often is decreased from loss of muscle mass, arthritis, and balance problems. Therefore assist the elderly while walking or moving to and from stretchers to prevent falls and injury. The elderly are at increased risk of fracture, and trivial trauma can cause fractures not identified by gross deformity. All injuries should be immobilized for comfort. In addition, the elderly may still be able to function on a broken bone, such as walking on a fractured hip, so maintain a high suspicion for injury. Pain control is important for orthopedic injuries and should be offered to all patients regardless of age with isolated orthopedic injuries.

Osteoarthritis

Osteoarthritis (OA) is one of the most common problems of elderly people. Studies indicate that almost 80% of people will have radiographic evidence of OA by the age of 60 years (Lawrence et al., 1966). Not everyone will develop OA if they live long enough, however. Past the eighth decade of life, the prevalence of OA does not increase. In fact, in persons older than 100 years, only 54% had evidence of OA (Andersen-Ranberg et al., 2001). This suggests that OA is a disease process and not simply a function of normal aging. Common joints involved include the knees, hips, spine, and hands. Overuse of a joint can predispose that joint to OA. Obesity also causes undue stress to joints and increased incidence of OA (Felson et al., 1992). Exercise and increased activity have been shown to decrease symptomatic OA in the elderly (Minor, 1999).

Elderly patients with OA rarely present with acute complications. They may have worsening joint pain that has limited their mobility or pain that they can no longer control with their current medications, prompting them to seek emergency care. Inflamed joints do occur with OA, and emergency personnel must consider other diseases such as gout or septic arthritis as the cause of an acutely inflamed joint. All these conditions occur in the elderly population. Use care when transporting elderly people with joint pain. Transportation in a position of comfort is ideal. If the patient has recent trauma, splinting is appropriate to reduce the pain of movement. If significant pain is present, offer analgesia.

Osteoporosis

Osteoporosis is the most common bone disease in the United States (Wolinsky et al., 1997). It accounts for significant morbidity and mortality in the elderly, contributing to more than 1.3 million fractures per year (Consensus Development Conference, 1993). Osteoporosis is characterized by loss of bone mass and its normal structure. This creates weaker, more brittle bones that are prone to fracture. Age is a large risk factor for decreased bone density. Nearly half of all postmenopausal women have low bone density (Siris et al., 2001). Women are at increased risk of developing osteoporosis because of the rapid decline of estrogen after menopause. White women seem to be at increased risk compared with African American and Asian women (Barrett-Connor et al., 2005). Other risk factors include family history, smoking, and corticosteroid use. Protective factors include high body mass index, estrogen use, exercise, and alcohol use. Medications can be used to prevent further bone loss in patients with osteoporosis. Adequate calcium intake as a child and young adult also helps prevent bone thinning in older age.

Osteoporotic patients can sustain fractures with minimal trauma. Simple falls and minor car accidents can produce life-threatening injuries such as hip and pelvis fracture. Although the fracture may not be deadly, chronic health conditions put these elderly people at risk for other illness (Browner et al., 1996). Elderly people with hip fractures have a 25% 1-year mortality rate, and those who survive have only a 50% chance of returning to their same level of function as before the fracture (Lu-Yao et al., 1994; Magaziner et al., 1990).

Fractures

Fractures in the elderly may be obvious or very difficult to detect. An older person may even be able to walk on a broken hip with minimal discomfort. Any musculoskeletal trauma in a patient with osteoporosis should be treated as if it is a fracture by EMS providers. Also assess neurovascular status beyond the injury. Absent pulses are a sign that arterial injury may have occurred, and prompt treatment is required.

Several actions can be taken to facilitate transfer of the elderly with minor musculoskeletal trauma. Splinting stabilizes the fracture segments to prevent injury to surrounding soft tissue. This also relieves pain by immobilizing the fracture. Pain control with narcotics can create a more comfortable environment for the patient. Removing potential hazards to an elderly person's ambulation can prevent bony injury. Loose rug corners and cluttered homes can cause falls and therefore fractures. If you notice an unsafe environment, report it to the local elderly protection agency so appropriate help can be obtained.

Case Scenario CONCLUSION

You carefully place a cervical collar on this patient. She is logrolled onto a backboard. Her pulses are checked in her right leg at the femoral, dorsalis pedis, and posterior tibial locations. Pulses are present at each site and strong. You start an IV and place the patient on a cardiac monitor. You prepare the patient for transport.

Questions

7. *What can be done as comfort measures for this patient?*
8. *What should be done during transport of this patient?*
9. *What should be included in the written and oral report?*

OTHER CONSIDERATIONS

Toxicology

[OBJECTIVES 67 TO 72]

Patients receive prescription medications to prevent, cure, slow, or eliminate the symptoms of disease. However, although each medication has specific benefits, they also cause drug-related complications. Unfortunately, many elderly individuals experience adverse effects from drug toxicities either inherent in the use of the medication or caused by interactions with other medications or disease states that a patient may have. As previously mentioned, several age-related changes affect pharmacokinetics in the elderly. You should learn and understand how these physiologic changes affect specific medications and may predispose an older person to experience toxicologic effects of the medication.

The first step in the assessment of a patient who is believed to be experiencing toxicologic problems is to identify the offending agent. You must elicit a thorough history, including past medical history and a comprehensive list of all medications (both prescription and over-the-counter) as well as herbal and natural remedies that the patient is taking. The elderly are much more likely to have chronic illnesses that require multiple medications, making the likelihood of drug interactions much more common compared with a younger population. Once a toxicologic event is suspected, first stabilize the patient by using advanced cardiac life support interventions as needed and then identify and address the specific symptoms and treatment needed for the particular toxic incident. All patients experiencing adverse drug effects must be evaluated by a physician so that particular medications or interactions can be identified and corrected.

Beta-Blockers

[OBJECTIVES 73, 74, 75]

Beta-blockers bind to beta-adrenergic receptors throughout the body, blunting the effects of some sympathetic responses. The main therapeutic effects of beta-blockers are to slow the heart rate (negative chronotrope), decrease contractility of the heart muscle (negative inotrope), and reduce blood vessel constriction. These effects efficiently decrease the oxygen demands of the heart and lower systolic blood pressure. Patients most commonly take beta-blockers to treat hypertension or tachycardia or reduce myocardial oxygen demand in patients with coronary artery disease.

Overall, beta-blockers are fairly well tolerated. However, in patients with COPD, beta-blockers may increase breathing difficulty and wheezing. Because beta-blockers decrease heart rate, patients on therapeutic doses can become bradycardic and hypotensive and have feelings of lightheadedness, leading to a syncopal episode. Less commonly, beta-blockers may cause confusion in some elderly patients.

When evaluating a patient taking beta-blockers, remember that the agents slow the heart rate and blunt the tachycardic response normally seen in hypovolemic patients (e.g., hemorrhaging patients) or in those with serious systemic illnesses.

Diuretics

Diuretics, or water pills, work at the level of the kidney to block sodium and fluid resorption, resulting in increased urine output. Diuretics are used to treat excess fluid accumulation and edema throughout the body caused by heart failure, cirrhosis, corticosteroid medication, or kidney disease. Diuretics (particularly hydrochlorothiazide) also may be used to treat hypertension.

Electrolyte abnormalities, such as lowered levels of potassium, sodium, and magnesium, can be seen with any diuretic but are more commonly encountered with the more powerful loop diuretics, such as furosemide (Lasix). These electrolyte abnormalities may lead to life-threatening cardiac dysrhythmias or cause acute mental status changes. Furthermore, they can be even more dangerous in patients who are taking digoxin. Because diuretics have their effect on the kidneys, they must be used with caution in patients with kidney failure and in those who take medications such as lithium, the excretion of which is directly inhibited by loop diuretics.

Digoxin

Digoxin is a heart medication that helps increase the strength of each heart contraction (positive inotropic effect) as well as slow the conduction between the atria and ventricles of the heart (negative chronotropic effect).

It most commonly is prescribed to treat CHF or atrial fibrillation or flutter. Unfortunately, digoxin has a rather narrow therapeutic window. Toxic levels can easily be seen in patients who are taking their normal therapeutic dose. Digoxin is excreted by the kidneys and should be carefully monitored in patients who have declining kidney function.

Patients with low potassium levels (commonly caused by diuretic medications), low magnesium levels, and high calcium levels can present with symptoms of digoxin toxicity even with normal blood levels of the medication. Other common medications, such as quinidine, verapamil, and amiodarone, can increase the blood levels of digoxin and cause toxicity.

The most serious signs of digoxin toxicity include conduction disturbances and cardiac dysrhythmias (such as complete heart block). Other common symptoms seen in digoxin toxicity include abdominal pain, nausea and vomiting, anorexia, and visual changes.

Neuroleptics

Antipsychotic medications (neuroleptics) are occasionally prescribed to elderly individuals who have severe agitation, hallucinations, or other psychiatric disorders resistant to other therapies. Neuroleptic agents block neurotransmitters (e.g., dopamine, norepinephrine, and serotonin) and/or their receptors in the brain. Unfortunately, these medications commonly have anticholinergic effects as well and may lead to dry mouth, sedation, urinary retention, constipation, and hypotension. Patients also often have extrapyramidal symptoms, including involuntary movements, tremors and rigidity, body restlessness, and spastic muscle contractions.

Benzodiazepines

Benzodiazepines are often prescribed for anxiety, insomnia, or agitation. The elderly are much more sensitive to this class of medication, and smaller doses should be used when treating older patients. Common effects seen in the elderly taking benzodiazepines include sedation, ataxia, confusion, and delirium. In general, such long-term treatment and long-acting agents should be avoided in the elderly.

Nonsteroidal Antiinflammatory Drugs

Nonsteroidal antiinflammatory drugs (NSAIDs), such as ibuprofen, naproxen, and aspirin, can have many unwanted, adverse effects in all patients. The most common and one of the more severe adverse effects is gastritis, leading to occult GI bleeding. In fact, elderly individuals taking NSAIDs are nearly five times more likely to die from a GI bleed as elderly people not taking NSAIDs (Griffin et al., 1988). Renal failure also can be attributed to NSAIDs, and their use is discouraged in those with kidney disease.

Many elderly patients who have coronary artery disease take one low-dose aspirin (81 mg) a day for its cardioprotective effects. In an otherwise healthy individual without kidney problems or history of GI bleeding, the cardiac benefits outweigh the risk of this small dose. Although NSAIDs are effective in alleviating inflammatory pain, consider other analgesic medication classes and nonpharmacologic means for pain relief.

Warfarin

Of all anticoagulants, warfarin (Coumadin) is the most commonly used in the outpatient setting. Warfarin is used by patients who currently have a blood clot or are at increased risk of developing clots. Conditions that increase the risk of clot formation and indicate warfarin use include atrial fibrillation, history of heart valve disease or placement of a prosthetic valve, recent surgery or bedridden condition, underlying clotting disorders, or history of a deep vein thrombosis or pulmonary embolus.

Although warfarin decreases the likelihood of pathologic clot formation, it also hinders normal physiologic clotting that stops bleeding. Patients taking warfarin find that their simple cuts and scrapes bleed much longer than when they were not on the medication. This bleeding is of particular concern when it occurs in an area that cannot easily be detected. Patients taking warfarin who fall and strike the head are much more likely to sustain an intracranial bleed. EMS personnel should be vigilant for the signs and symptoms of an intracranial bleed in any patient taking warfarin with even apparently minor injuries. Similarly, patients who have GI bleeding are likely to lose more blood into their GI tract and need immediate medical attention. Thus most patients taking warfarin are told to avoid any NSAID use. If they have a history of ataxia or falls, they will often not be started on warfarin despite other clinical indications.

Narcotics

Narcotics are a highly effective form of analgesia that does not have the same adverse effects that NSAIDs possess. Unfortunately, narcotics have some of the same adverse effects in the elderly as benzodiazepines because such patients often are much more sensitive to side effects, including oversedation, constipation, and confusion.

Nitrates

Nitrate medications such as nitroglycerin act as vasodilators, relaxing smooth muscle in both arteries and veins. This improves coronary collateral circulation and decreases preload and afterload as well as myocardial oxygen demand. Although nitrates are used to reduce the pain related to myocardial ischemia in patients with chest pain, nitrates are not analgesic medications. Current erectile dysfunction medications (e.g., sildenafil, tadalafil, or vardenafil) also work by causing vasodilation. Nitrates should not be given to patients who have ingested these medications in the previous 24 to 48 hours.

Substance Abuse

[OBJECTIVES 76, 77, 78, 79]

An estimated 10% of the elderly population has some sort of chemical dependency, mostly alcohol related, but also abuse of prescription and over-the-counter medications (Adams & Cox, 1995). Substance abuse often goes unrecognized in the older population, and symptoms of alcohol or medication abuse may be attributed to dementia. Substance abuse is likely to affect a person's self-care of a chronic illness. Do your best to detect the signs and symptoms of substance abuse among the elderly and help the patient seek medical help for the addiction.

A wide disparity exists among the common characteristics of elders who abuse alcohol when compared with their younger counterparts. Younger alcoholics are more likely to be disorderly; have a criminal background; and have higher rates of divorce, financial difficulty, and motor vehicle crashes while under the influence (Snyder & Christmas, 2003). Elderly alcoholics, on the other hand, are more likely to live alone, be isolated, and lack social support (Snyder & Christmas, 2003).

Because elders who are substance abusers have different presentations than clinical/their younger equivalents, you must adequately assess the patient. If you have any concern regarding alcoholism, directly address it by asking the patient how much alcohol he or she consumes. Because of the physiologic changes of aging, smaller amounts of alcohol are required to cause intoxication in an elder. The signs of alcohol abuse in the elderly often are quite subtle and can be marked by the vague symptoms of multiple falls, anorexia, insomnia, confusion, mood swings, or hostility. Once recognized, refer an alcoholic elder to the proper resources for help with the addiction (Box 38-7).

Environmental Considerations

[OBJECTIVES 80 TO 85]

As a result of the normal aging processes, the elderly body is less proficient at adapting to environmental surroundings—mainly heat and cold. During temperature fluctuations the hypothalamus acts through physiologic responses to minimize the temperature change of the body. If the hypothalamus detects that the body is cold, it will cause the body to shiver and trigger the release of catecholamines to increase the rate of metabolism so that heat is given off. When the body is hot, the hypothalamus helps lose heat by releasing factors that cause blood vessels near the skin to dilate and cool the blood and increase sweating. The hypothalamus receives information concerning the overall temperature of the body from thermoreceptors in place throughout the body. As the body ages, the density and sensitivity of the thermoreceptors are decreased, blunting and delaying the body's detection and reaction to environmental temperature changes. Unfortunately, because of the financial constraints of a fixed income, many elderly are also unable to afford proper environmental heating and cooling to minimize the work that their bodies have to perform to provide thermoregulation. Treatment of any environmental emergency is aimed at removing the patient from the offending environment and attempting to correct the underlying abnormality.

BOX 38-7 Risk Factors for Substance Abuse

- Depression
- Loss of employment
- Limited monetary resources
- Loneliness
- Poor health

Hypothermia

The elder patient is more likely to be hypothermic because of several physiologic changes associated with aging. The most common reaction that the body uses to combat hypothermia is shivering, the generation of heat as a byproduct of muscle movement. However, as the body ages the amount of muscle mass decreases, causing shivering to be less effective. This, coupled with the fact that older patients also have less insulation (as they develop thinner skin with less subcutaneous fat) and are less efficient at releasing catecholamines to mount a response to decreased environmental temperatures, predisposes the elderly to suffer from hypothermia. Additionally, several medical conditions that are more commonly seen in an older population also place the elderly at a higher risk for hypothermia. Decreased cardiac output, vascular disease, and diabetes have all been implicated in the blunted response that elders have to hypothermia.

Hypothermia is defined as a core body temperature of less than 32° C (89.6° F). The easiest way to measure core body temperature is with a rectal thermometer, a practice not commonly encountered in the prehospital setting. Thus you must be able to assess the typical signs and symptoms of hypothermia. As body temperature decreases, a patient is likely to report being cold and develop shivering; however, as body temperature drops below 33° C (91.4° F), these signs may no longer be present and you will need to suspect hypothermia based on history and the environmental surroundings.

Treatment for hypothermia in the elderly is the same as for younger patients. Remove the elderly patient from the cold environment and address the ABCs. Remove any wet clothing and cover the patient with warm, dry blankets. If available, warmed saline and oxygen also may be used.

Hyperthermia

Hyperthermia is defined as a core body temperature above 38.3° C (101° F). The normal aging process often causes many sweat glands to function poorly or not at all, thus reducing one of the body's important physiologic responses used in cooling. Many medications also play a role in blunting the body's response to hyperthermia. Antihistamines and anticholinergics often reduce sweat output by directly decreasing the function of the hypothalamus as well as blunting the mental ability needed to recognize and avoid the heated environment. Similarly, narcotics and sedatives reduce the mental capacity needed to respond to the heated environment. Diuretics cause fluid loss and may worsen heat emergencies by decreasing total body fluid.

Hyperthermic illnesses are often divided into three categories: heat cramps, heat exhaustion, and heat stroke. Heat cramps are muscular cramps caused by electrolyte imbalances that often are preceded by intense sweating and thirst. Treatment involves moving the patient to a cooler environment and rehydrating through oral intake (including electrolyte drinks) or IV therapy.

Heat exhaustion is more severe than heat cramps and begins to have systemic effects such as nausea, vomiting, increased thirst, and lightheadedness from volume depletion. Although oral fluid replacement may be attempted, most patients require IV fluids and the establishment of an IV should not be delayed while waiting to see if a patient will tolerate oral intake.

Heat stroke, the most serious heat disorder, is characterized by a very high body temperature (usually over 40° C [104° F]). Heat stroke is characterized by the same symptoms seen in heat exhaustion, with the addition of an altered mental status. Typically, those with heat stroke will have an absence of sweating and present with hypotension. Treatment is aimed at managing the ABCs, actively cooling the patient, and administering IV fluids. Because of the serious nature of heat stroke, all patients should have electrocardiographic monitoring.

Trauma in the Elderly

[OBJECTIVES 86, 87, 88, 89, 90]

Trauma is a significant cause of morbidity and mortality in the elderly. Unintentional injury is the leading cause of nonfatal illness in the elderly population (Centers for Disease Control and Prevention, 2002). Unintentional injury is the fifth leading cause of death in all age groups and eighth leading cause of death in those aged 65 years and over (Centers for Disease Control and Prevention, 2005). Blunt trauma in patients aged 65 years and older carries a mortality rate as high as 18% (Knudson et al., 1994). Mortality rates for persons aged 85 years and older are up to nine times higher than for persons aged 25 to 69 years (Traffic Safety Facts, 2003). In addition to the increased mortality rate from injury, disability from the injury also is greater for elderly people. One study found only 17% of geriatric patients sustaining blunt trauma that survived to hospital discharge had return to pre-injury level of function (van Aalst et al., 1991).

Trauma affects the elderly differently than younger patients. Geriatric patients have decreased muscle mass and frequent osteoporosis, creating an increased risk of factures and serious injury with minimal force. Decreased cardiac function inhibits their ability to respond to the cardiovascular stress of serious injury and blood loss (Bass & Seegmiller, 1981). Their impaired kidney function makes adjustment to the blood loss and shift of fluids in the different body compartments difficult. Lung function is often decreased as well, and getting oxygen to the tissues can be impaired. Adult respiratory distress syndrome is a more common complication in geriatric trauma patients than in younger trauma patients (Johnston et al., 2003).

Falls replace motor vehicle crashes as the leading cause of traumatic injury in the elderly population compared with the general population. Assault, abuse, and burns also are significant causes of trauma. Suspect abuse in patients with trauma who are immobile or if other signs of neglect, such as poor hygiene or pressure ulcers, are present. Survey the scene for different types of abuse—physical abuse, neglect, psychological abuse, financial abuse, and self-imposed injury. In the elderly, trauma often is caused by a primarily medical condition such as syncope or MI. Geriatric patients may have a primary event that causes them to fall or lose control of a vehicle and results in traumatic injury. Obtain the specific circumstances around the event from the patient and from observers whenever possible.

Assessment of the geriatric trauma patient differs slightly than that for younger patients. Tachycardia may be blunted by beta-blockers or other medications, so shock may be difficult to identify. Similarly, elderly patients with hypertension may lose significant blood volume, dropping their blood pressure into the "normal" range, incorrectly reassuring medical personnel. Fractures also may be present without significant pain because of decreased pain perception.

As always, airway management should come first in the trauma patient. Identify ill-fitting dentures and remove them if present to eliminate a possible airway obstruction. Supplemental oxygen is recommended for all elderly trauma victims. Administer IV fluid to anyone with significant blood loss or other signs of hypovolemia. Closely watch patients with a history of heart failure or renal failure for signs of pulmonary edema such as hypoxia and crackles on lung examination. Additionally, cardiac monitoring is recommended to identify cardiac rhythm abnormalities, which are common in this population. A formal 12-lead ECG should not routinely be performed because of the delay in transport that may be critical in the trauma patient with severe injuries. If MI is a concern, the severity of injuries must be considered before delaying transport to perform an electrocardiogram. The transport destination should be capable of handling the worst suspected injuries. As stated, elderly trauma patients may have serious injuries without showing classic signs in the early stages. For that reason, always err on the side of safety and transport quickly to a trauma center if the possibility of significant injury exists.

Orthopedic Injuries

Osteoporosis and decreased muscle mass put the elderly at increased risk for fracture. Hip fracture is the most common orthopedic emergency in the elderly and occurs approximately 250,000 times per year in the United States (Barrett-Connor, 1995). Stress fractures also can occur in the hip, pelvis, and other parts of the legs without significant trauma. These fractures are difficult to diagnose because examination and radiographs often are normal (Tountas, 1993). When transporting elderly patients with orthopedic injuries, splinting is necessary and may require bulky padding to fill in unsecured areas. The immobilization will improve comfort and lessen injury to surrounding soft tissue from the jagged bone edges. Patients with severe kyphosis (curved thoracic spine) should have padding under the head or shoulders to relieve stress on the back when they are laid flat. Administer medication for pain per protocol.

Burns

Burns carry a higher mortality rate in older patients than in the general population (O'Keefe et al., 2001). The elderly have more preexisting illnesses, which makes recovery difficult. They also have thinner skin, which is easily damaged by burn. Nutrition also is suboptimal in the elderly. This prevents healing because adequate nutrition is necessary for burn wound repair. Early management of older patients with burn requires close attention to fluid resuscitation. After ensuring airway safety, administer fluids to prevent renal failure from hypovolemia and injury from tissue breakdown products. Assessment of fluid status is best done by monitoring urine output. Keeping urine output at 50 to 100 mL/hr is usually adequate but often is not able to be accomplished in the prehospital setting. Start fluids and administer in a bolus of 1 to 2 L for most short transports. For longer transports, a fixed equation per protocol or consultation with medical direction may be necessary.

Head Injury

Head injury can be a difficult condition to assess in the elderly. Traumatic brain injury is more difficult to recognize and more deadly in the elderly population. Mortality rate for patients older than 70 years is twice that for patients younger than 30 years (Harris et al., 2003). Brain volume decreases with age and allows more room for the brain to move and tear blood vessels. This decreased brain size also allows blood to accumulate before causing symptoms. Significant amounts of blood that would cause severe symptoms in a younger patient may not affect the elderly and give a false sense of security to medical providers soon after the injury. Any head trauma in the elderly must be aggressively treated with transport to a capable facility. Minor trauma also can cause intracranial bleeding because of the blood thinners that many elderly take. In addition to acute trauma, prehospital professionals must be alert to previous trauma because subdural hemorrhages may accumulate over several days to weeks and then cause neurologic symptoms.

Case Scenario SUMMARY

1. *What is your impression of this patient?* This patient has fallen and she is an older adult. Her presentation indicates she may have injured her hip. Her vital signs are stable. She has a contusion above her eye, so head and cervical spine injury should be suspected.
2. *What are important questions in the chief complaint and history?* Ask the patient why she fell. If the patient states she tripped, that provides a good history. If the patient cannot remember, that may indicate a stroke or other cause, such as a dysrhythmia with syncope. The patient's history is important. If the patient has a history of syncope, stroke, or a dysrhythmia, this can provide direction regarding other areas to investigate. Medications also can be important. Anticoagulants can lead to severe bleeding and shock. Blood pressure medications also may lead to syncope if not taken as instructed.
3. *What should be the focus of the physical examination?* The patient should receive a thorough physical examination beginning at the head. Evaluate signs of skull fracture, intracerebral bleeding, and altered mental status. Immobilize the patient's neck and evaluate for pain or boney step-off. Also examine the lungs and heart. Examine the extremities for signs of deformity, bleeding, bruising, capillary refill, pulses, and temperature. Also make sure no deficits would coincide with a spinal cord injury. This patient has head trauma and has fallen from her body height, so a spinal fracture is possible.
4. *What is the significance of her medications?* The patient could experience severe bleeding because she is taking an anticoagulant (warfarin). She has a probable hip fracture and a closed head injury. This information should prompt you to monitor her vital signs continually for shock and altered mental status. She also takes a blood pressure medication, which could have lead to her fall.
5. *What do the physical examination findings indicate?* She has a large contusion over her right eye. She also has bruising behind her right ear. This is called Battle's sign and can be an indication of a basilar skull fracture. The shortened right leg is an indicator of a possible hip

Continued

Case Scenario SUMMARY—continued

fracture. The laceration may bleed profusely because of the anticoagulant she is taking. This injury requires direct pressure to control bleeding and possibly elevation of the extremity.

6. *What is important in the treatment for this patient?* The patient should have her cervical spine immobilized. If she has an intracerebral injury, bleeding may be significant because of the anticoagulant she is taking. Frequently assess the patient's mental status. This can be accomplished by continually talking to the patient. Carefully immobilize the hip. Evaluate the patient's right leg for skin temperature, color, distal pulses, movement, and sensation before and after movement. A pillow splint or long board splint may be appropriate. Give the patient supplemental oxygen and place her on a cardiac monitor. Begin an IV line. Direct pressure with sterile dressings is important to control bleeding from the laceration on the arm.
7. *What can be done as comfort measures for this patient?* Hip fractures can be quite painful. However, because of the patient's possible head injury, administer pain medication with caution in this situation and only after consultation with medical direction. Narcotics may cause a decrease in mental status and impair the patient's neurologic examination at the hospital.
8. *What should be done during transport of this patient?* The patient should receive continual monitoring of mental status, vital signs, and peripheral pulses.
9. *What should be included in the written and oral report?* Clearly document the patient's condition. Include medications, past medical history, events leading up to the event, and the position in which the patient was found. The verbal report should provide information to help the receiving facility prepare for the arrival of the patient. This patient will require radiographs and computed tomography scans of her head. Clearly document any changes in the patient's condition and update the receiving facility.

Chapter Summary

- The elderly population accounts for a significant number (34%) of all EMS responses.
- Most elderly people live independently. When illness makes independent living impossible, some seniors are able afford live-in nursing help or assisted living situations. Nursing home care is usually covered by Medicare and is where many elderly people live in the end stages of life because of severe disability.
- Power of attorney of healthcare and living wills are becoming more prevalent. Unless a clear advanced directive is present, however, prehospital providers should provide aggressive care to all elderly people.
- Changes in drug distribution, decreased drug metabolism, decreased drug excretion, and polypharmacy make adverse drug reactions a common reason for illness in the elderly.
- Make an accurate list of medications the patient is taking or bring the actual bottles of medications with the patient to ensure an accurate medication history. Many elderly people are not able to recall all the medications they are taking.
- Many factors contribute to the increased risk of falling in elderly people. Among these are vision changes, brain diseases, dementia, musculoskeletal disorders, and medication side effects.
- Presbyopia, cataracts, and glaucoma all can cause visual impairment in the elderly and subsequent functional decline.
- Most older patients are able to hear normal conversation. Those with hearing loss often are able to function well with hearing aids. Make sure hearing aids are in place before questioning elderly patients with hearing loss.
- Incontinence is never a result of normal aging. Fecal and urinary incontinence can be caused by severe illness, such as spinal cord compression, and can cause skin breakdown and infection.
- Assessment of an elderly patient must be done carefully because the elderly often process information slower and need a longer time to provide a history.
- Chest pain and shortness of breath are two common presentations for elderly patients and can be caused by numerous illnesses. Every elderly patient with one of these two symptoms should be treated as if he or she has a serious emergency.
- Resuscitation of elderly patients should be done in the same manner as for younger patients and just as aggressively.
- Elderly often are most comfortable while sitting or with extra padding. Transport in the position of comfort for most older patients except when splinting an injury or when spinal precautions are needed.
- The aging process causes decreased strength in respiratory muscles, decreased ability of oxygen to cross into the bloodstream, and increased bronchoconstriction.

- The lung examination is unreliable in determining a cause of shortness of breath. A history of COPD or heart failure should guide initial treatment of shortness of breath in a patient with one of these diagnoses.
- The cardiovascular system of elderly patients is prone to hypertension and coronary artery disease and loses its ability to respond to physiologic stress.
- Coronary artery disease, thoracic and abdominal aneurysms, congestive heart failure, and dysrhythmias are more common in older patients and can be life threatening. Maintain a high level of suspicion for elderly patients regarding cardiovascular emergencies.
- Slight psychomotor slowing is expected in aging, but severe memory deficits and changes in cognition are not normal.
- Acute weakness or change in level of consciousness in an elderly person must be considered an intracranial emergency and necessitates rapid transport because hospital treatment often is time dependent.
- Dementia is a chronic memory problem with long-term declines in intellectual functioning (e.g., Alzheimer's disease); delirium is usually an acute, often reversible, process that produces decreased cognition and level of consciousness.
- Consider hyperglycemia and hypoglycemia in any elderly patient with a history of diabetes or neurologic change. Blood glucose testing should be routine to identify these glucose abnormalities quickly.
- Abdominal and GI emergencies usually manifest atypically in the elderly, with diminished or vague symptoms. Twenty-four percent of elderly patients with acute abdominal pain in the ED require surgery.
- In suspected toxicologic emergencies, obtaining an accurate history and additional information is the most important part of finding a diagnosis.
- Beta-blocker medications are used for hypertension, to control dysrhythmias, or to decrease oxygen demand of the heart tissue. These medications block the ability of the heart to respond to stress by increasing heart rate and contractility.
- Diuretics cause water to be excreted by the kidneys. Adverse reactions include electrolyte abnormalities and dehydration.
- Digoxin is used in CHF to increase contractility of the heart or control the rate of atrial fibrillation. Digoxin can easily reach a toxic level and cause many different cardiac dysrhythmias.
- Warfarin is used in many elderly people to prevent blood clot formation. Some indications for its use are atrial fibrillation, history of blood clots, and artificial heart valves. Patients on warfarin are at increased risk of bleeding.
- Chemical dependency is present in up to 10% of the elderly population. Alcohol accounts for most of this dependency and should be addressed in elderly people in whom it is suspected.
- Decreased muscle mass for shivering and thinner skin for insulation put the elderly at risk for hypothermia.
- Hyperthermia is more prevalent in elderly people because of fewer sweat glands, medication side effects, and a decreased ability to seek a cooler environment.
- Depression is underrecognized in the elderly population; the elderly population also completes suicide more frequently.
- Older patients have thin skin, which is more susceptible to infection, breakdown, and injury from trauma.
- OA affects 80% of patients older than 60 years and causes significant pain and difficulty with mobility.
- Osteoporosis is the most common bone disease in the United States and is characterized by loss of bone density, causing an increased risk of fracture.
- Traumatic injury carries an increased mortality rate in the elderly compared with younger patients. Falls are the most common cause of trauma in the elderly population.
- Older patients have decreased brain volume, which allows blood to accumulate in the skull after head injury without immediate neurologic deficits. Significant intracranial bleeding may not be symptomatic until days after the trauma.

REFERENCES

Adam, D. J., Mohan, I. V., Stuart, W. P., Bain, M., & Bradbury, A. W. (1999). Community and hospital outcome from ruptured abdominal aortic aneurysm within the catchment area of a regional vascular surgical service. *Journal of Vascular Surgery, 30*(5):922-928.

Adams, W. L., & Cox, N. S. (1995). Epidemiology of problem drinking among elderly people. *International Journal of Addiction, 30*(13-14), 1693-1716.

Administration on Aging. (2004). *Aging internet information notes.* Retrieved September 18, 2006, from http://www.aoa.gov.

American Association of Retired Persons. (1999). *A profile of older Americans.* Washington, DC: American Association of Retired Persons.

American Geriatrics Society. (2003). *EMS providers need better training to meet needs of older population.* Retrieved February 26, 2008, from http://www.americangeriatrics.org.

American Heart Association. (1998). *1999 heart and stroke statistical update.* Dallas: American Heart Association.

Andersen-Ranberg, K., Schroll, M., & Jeune, B. (2001). Healthy centenarians do not exist, but autonomous centenarians do: A population-based study of morbidity among Danish centenarians. *Journal of the American Geriatrics Society, 49,* 900-908.

Barrett-Connor, E. (1995). The economic and human costs of osteoporotic fracture. *American Journal of Medicine, 98*(2A), 3S-8S.

Barrett-Connor, E., Siris, E. S., Miller, P. D., Abbott, T. A., Berger, M. L., et al. (2005). Osteoporosis and fracture risk in women of different ethnic groups. *Journal of Bone Mineral Density, 20*(2), 185-194.

Bass, G. R., & Seegmiller, J. E. (1981). Age-related physiologic changes and their clinical significance. *Western Journal of Medicine, 135,* 434.

Bayer, A. J., Chandra, J. S., Farag, R. R., & Pathy, M. S. (1986). Changing presentation of myocardial infarction with increasing old age. *Journal of the American Geriatrics Society, 34,* 263-266.

Bonnin, M. H., Pepe, P. E., & Clark, P. S. (1993). Survival in the elderly after out-of-hospital cardiac arrest. *Critical Care Medicine, 21*(11), 1645-1651.

Borum, M. A. (1999). Peptic-ulcer disease in the elderly. *Clinical Geriatric Medicine, 15,* 457-471.

Brandeis, G. H., Morris, J. N., Nash, D. J., & Lipsitz, L. A. (1990). The epidemiology and natural history of pressure ulcers in elderly nursing home residents. *Journal of the American Medical Association, 264*(22), 2905-2909.

Bree Johnston, C., Goldstein, M. K., & Triadafilopoulos, G. (2000). Constipation, diarrhea, and fecal incontinence. In D. Osterwil, et al. (Eds.). *Comprehensive geriatric assessment,* New York: McGraw-Hill.

Browner, W. S., Pressman, A. R., Nevitt, M. C., & Cummings, S. R. (1996). Mortality following fractures in older women. The study of osteoporotic fractures. *Archives of Internal Medicine, 156*(14), 1521-1525.

Buckwalter, J. A., Glimcher, M. J., Cooper, R. R., & Recker, R. (1995). Bone biology. II: Formation, form, modeling, remodeling, and regulation of cell function. *Journal of Bone and Joint Surgery 77A,* 1276-1289.

Buckwalter, J. A., Woo, S. L.-Y., Boldberg, V. M., Hadley, E. C., Booth, F., Oegema, T. R., et al. (1993). Soft tissue aging and musculoskeletal function. *Journal of Bone and Joint Surgery, 75A,* 1533-1548.

Bugliosi, T. F., Meloy, T. D., & Vukov, L. F. (1990). Acute abdominal pain in the elderly. *Annals of Emergency Medicine, 19,* 1383-1386.

Centers for Disease Control and Prevention. (2004). *National diabetes fact sheet: General information and national estimates on diabetes in the United States, 2003 (rev. ed.).* Atlanta, GA: U.S. Department of Health and Human Services.

Centers for Disease Control and Prevention. (2005). *Web-based injury statistics query and reporting system (WISQARS).* Retrieved February 26, 2008, from http://www.cdc.gov.

Chen, M., Bergman, R. N., Pacini, G., & Porte, D., Jr. (1985). Pathogenesis of age-related glucose intolerance in man: insulin resistance and decreased beta-cell function. *Journal of Clinical Endocrinology and Metabolism, 60*(1), 13-20.

Chernoff, R. (1995). Effects of age on nutrient requirements. *Clinics in Geriatric Medicine, 11*(4), 641-651.

Consensus Development Conference. (1993). Consensus development conference: Diagnosis, prophylaxis, and treatment of osteoporosis. *American Journal of Medicine, 94,* 646.

Constans, T., Bacq, Y., Bréchot, J. F., Guilmot, J. L., Choutet, P., & Lamisse, F. (1992). Protein-energy malnutrition in elderly medical patients. *Journal of the American Geriatric Society, 40,* 263-268.

Dawson, D. A., & Adams, P. F. (1987). *Current estimates from the National Health Interview Survey, United States, 1986,* Hyattsville, MD: National Center for Health Statistics.

Diabetes Control and Complications Trial Research Group. (1993). The effect of intensive treatment of diabetes on the development and progression of long-term complications in insulin-dependent diabetes mellitus. *New England Journal of Medicine, 329,* 977-986.

Diabetes Prevention Program Research Group. (2002). Reduction in the incidence of type 2 diabetes with lifestyle intervention or metformin. *New England Journal of Medicine, 346,* 393-403.

Elmets, C. A., & Mukhatat, H. (1995). Ultraviolet radiation and skin cancer: progress in pathophysiologic mechanisms. *Progress in Dermatology, 30,* 1-16.

Felson, D. T., Zhang, Y., Anthony, J. M., Naimark, A., & Anderson, J. J. (1992). Weight loss reduces the risk for symptomatic knee osteoarthritis in women. *Annals of Internal Medicine, 116,* 535-539.

Fine, M. R., Auble, T. E., Yealy, D. M., Hanusa, B. H., Weissfeld, L. A., Singer, D. E., et al. (1997). A prediction rule to identify low-risk patients with community-acquired pneumonia. *New England Journal of Medicine, 336,* 243-250.

Fleg, J. L. (1986). Alterations in cardiovascular structure and function with advancing age. *American Journal of Cardiology, 57,* 33C-44C.

Glaucoma Research Foundation. (2007). *Glaucoma facts and stats.* Retrieved September 18, 2006, from http://www.glaucoma.org.

Graves, E. J. (1991). *Summary, 1989 national hospital discharge survey: Advance data from vital and health statistics no 199* (p. 112), Hyattsville, MD: National Center for Health Statistics.

Griffin, M. R., Ray, W. A., & Schaffner, W. (1988). Non-steroidal anti-inflammatory drug use and death from peptic ulcer in elderly persons. *Annals of Internal Medicine, 109,* 359-363.

Gross, R., Bentur, N., Einayany, A., Sherf, M., & Epstein, L. (1996). The validity of self-reports on chronic disease: Characteristics of underreporters and implications for the planning of services. *Public Health Review, 24*(2), 167-182.

Gussekloo, J., van Exel, E., de Craen, A. J., Meinders, A. E., Frölich, M., & Westendorp, R. G. (2004). Thyroid status, disability and cognitive function, and survival in old age. *Journal of the American Medical Association, 292*(21), 2591-2599.

Hanson, P. O., Welin, L., Tibblin, G., & Eriksson, H. (1997). Deep vein thrombosis and pulmonary embolism in the general population. "The study of men born in 1913." *Archives of Internal Medicine, 157*(15), 1665-1670.

Harris, C., DiRusso, S., Sullivan, T., & Benzil, D. L. (2003). Mortality risk after head injury increases at 30 years. *Journal of the American College of Surgeons, 197*(5), 711-716.

Ho, K. K., Pinsky, J. L., Kannel, W. B., & Levy, D. (1993). The epidemiology of heart failure: The Framingham Study. *Journal of the American College of Cardiology, 22*(4 suppl A):6A-13A.

Hohl, C. M., Dankoff, J., Colacone, A., & Afilalo, M. (2001). Polypharmacy, adverse drug-related events, and potential adverse drug interactions in elderly patients presenting to an emergency department. *Annals of Emergency Medicine, 38,* 666-671.

Johnston, C. J., Rubenfeld, G. D., & Hudson, L. D. (2003). Effect of age on the development of ARDS in trauma patients. *Chest, 124*(2), 653-659.

Kapoor, W. N. (1990). Evaluation and outcome of patients with syncope. *Medicine, 69*(3), 160-175.

Kapoor, W. N., Karpf, M., Wieand, S., Peterson, J. R., & Levey, G. S. (1983). A prospective evaluation and follow-up of patients with syncope. *New England Journal of Medicine, 309*(4), 197-204.

Kelley, M. (1996). Medications and the visually impaired elderly. *Geriatric Nursing, 18*(4), 6-14.

Kenny, S. J., Aubert, R. E., & Geiss, L. S. (1995). Prevalence and incidence of non-insulin-dependent diabetes (pp. 47-67). In M. I. Harris (Ed.), *Diabetes in America* (2nd ed.). Washington, DC: National Institutes of Health.

Kizer, K. W., & Vassar, M. J. (1998). Emergency department diagnosis of abdominal disorders in the elderly. *American Journal of Emergency Medicine, 16,* 357-362.

Knudson, M. M., Lieberman, J., Morris, J. A., Cushing, B. M., & Stubbs, H. A. (1994). Mortality factors in geriatric blunt trauma patients. *Archives of Surgery, 129,* 448-453.

Kochanek, K. D., Murphy, S. L., Anderson, R. N., & Scott, C. (2004). Deaths: Final data for 2002. *Vital Statistics Report, 53*(5), 21. Retrieved May 10, 2008, from http://www.cdc.gov.

Kreider, R. M., & Simmons, T. (2003). *Marital status: 2000. Census 2000 brief.* Retrieved February 26, 2008, from www.census.gov.

Kriegsman, D. M., Penninx, B. W., van Eijk, J. T., Boeke, A. J., & Deeg, D. J. (1996). Self-reports and general practitioner information of the presence of chronic diseases in community-dwelling elderly. A study on the accuracy of patients' self-reports and on determinants of inaccuracy. *Journal of Clinical Epidemiology, 49*(12), 1407-1417.

Lakatta, E. G. (1980). Age-related alterations in the cardiovascular response to adrenergic mediated stress. *Federal Proceedings, 39,* 3173-3177.

Lawrence, J. S., Bremner, J. M., & Bier, F. (1966). Osteo-arthrosis. Prevalence in the population and relationship between symptoms and x-ray changes. *Annals of the Rheumatic Diseases, 25,* 1-24.

Levy, D., Anderson, K. M., Savage, D. D., Kannel, W. B., Christiansen, J. C., & Castelli, W. P. (1998). Echocardiographically detected left ventricular hypertrophy: Prevalence and risk factors. The Framingham Heart Study. *Annals of Internal Medicine, 108,* 7-13.

Leyden, J. J. (1990). Clinical features of ageing skin. *British Journal of Dermatology, 122,* 1-3.

Lipsitz, L. A., Jonsson, P. V., Marks, B. L., Parker, J. A., Royal, H. D., & Wei, J. Y. (1990). Reduced supine cardiac volumes and diastolic filling rates in elderly patients with chronic medical conditions: implications for postural blood pressure homeostasis. *Journal of the American Geriatric Society, 38,* 103-107.

Lu-Yao, G. L., Baron, J. A., Barrett, J. A., & Fisher, E. S. (1994). Treatment and survival among elderly Americans with hip fractures: A population-based study. *American Journal of Public Health, 84*(8), 1287-1291.

Magaziner, J., Simonsick, E. M., Kashner, T. M., Hebel, J. R., & Kenzora, J. E. (1990). Predictors of functional recovery one year following hospital discharge for hip fracture: A prospective study. *Journal of Gerontology, 45*(3), M101-M107.

Marco, C. A., Schoenfeld, C. N., Keyl, P. M., Menkes, E. D., & Doehring, M. C. (1998). Abdominal pain in geriatric emergency patients: Variables associated with adverse outcomes. *Journal of the Academy of Emergency Medicine, 5,* 1163-1168.

Marler, J. R., Tilley, B. C., Lu, M., Brott, T. G., Lyden, P. C., Grotta, J. C., et al. (2000). Early stroke treatment associated with better outcome: The NINDS rt-PA stroke study. *Neurology, 55*(11), 1649-1655.

Marston, B. J., Plouffe, J. F., File, T. M., Jr, Hackman, B. A., Salstrom, S. J., Lipman, H. B., et al. (1997). Incidence of community-acquired pneumonia requiring hospitalization. Results of a population-based active surveillance study in Ohio. The Community-Based Pneumonia Incidence Study Group. *Archives of Internal Medicine, 157*(15), 1709-1718.

Meehan, T. P., Fine, M. R., Krumholz, H. M., Scinto, J. D., Galusha, D. H., Mockalis, J. T., et al. (1997). Quality of care, process and outcomes in elderly patients with pneumonia. *Journal of the American Medical Association, 278,* 2080-2084.

Mendez, L., Friedman, L. S., & Castell, D. O. (1991). Swallowing disorders in the elderly. *Clinical Geriatric Medicine, 7,* 215-230.

Minor, M. A. (1999). Exercise in the treatment of osteoarthritis. *Rheumatology Clinics of North America, 25,* 397-415.

Montagna, W., & Carlisle, K. (1979). Structural changes in aging human skin. *Journal of Investigative Dermatology, 73,* 47-53.

Mosesso, V. N., Dunford, J., Blackwell, T., & Griswell, J. K. (2003). Prehospital therapy for acute congestive heart failure: State of the art. *Prehospital Emergency Care, 7*(1), 13-23.

Muller, R. T., Gould, L. A., Betzu, R., Vacek, T., & Pradeep, V. (1990). Painless myocardial infarction in the elderly. *American Heart Journal, 19*(1), 202-204.

Muller-Spahn, F., & Kock, C. (1994). Clinical presentation of depression in the elderly. *Gerontology, 40,* 10.

Murray, C. J. L., & Lopez, A. D. (1997). Mortality by cause for eight regions of the world: Global burden of disease study, *The Lancet, 349,* 1269-1276.

National Bureau of Economic Research. (2004). *Social Security and elderly poverty.* Retrieved September 18, 2006, from http://www.ber.org.

National Heart Lung and Blood Institute. (2007). *2007 NHLBI morbidity and mortality chart book.* Retrieved February 26, 2008, from http://www.nhlbi.nih.gov.

National Highway Traffic Safety Information. (2003). *Traffic safety facts 2002: Older population,* Washington, DC: U.S. Department of Transportation.

The National Institute of Neurological Disorders and Stroke rt-PA Stroke Study Group. (1995). Tissue plasminogen activator for acute ischemic stroke. *New England Journal of Medicine, 333*(24), 1581-1587.

Newcomer, B. D., & Young, E. M., Jr. (1989). *Geriatric dermatology: Clinical diagnosis and practical therapy,* New York: Igaku Shoin.

Northington, W., & Yates, A. (2005). Caring for the aged. *Journal of Emergency Medical Services, 30*(7), 70-85.

Oddie, T. H., Meade, J. H., & Fisher, D. A. (1966). An analysis of published data on thyroxine turnover in human subjects. *Journal of Clinical Endocrinology and Metabolism, 26,* 425.

O'Keefe, G. E., Hunt, J. L., & Purdue, G. F. (2001). An evaluation of risk factors for mortality after burn trauma and the identification of gender-dependent differences in outcomes. *Journal of the American College of Surgeons, 192*(2), 153-160.

Pan, X. R., Li, G. W., Hu, Y. H., Wang, J. X., Yang, W. Y., An, Z. X., et al. (1997). Effects of diet and exercise in preventing NIDDM in people with impaired glucose tolerance. The Da Qing IGT and Diabetes Study. *Diabetes Care, 20*(4), 537-544.

Paul, S. D., O'Gara, P. T., Mahjoub, Z. A., DiSalvo, T. G., O'Donnell, C. J., Newell, J. B., et al. (1996). Geriatric patients with acute myocardial infarction: Cardiac risk factor profiles, presentation, thrombolysis, coronary interventions, and prognosis. *American Heart Journal, 131*(4), 710-715.

Penzes, L., & Gergely, I. (1989). Thyroid hormones in the light of general health status of Hungarian centenarians. *Age, 12,* 137.

Petersen, R. C., Smith, G., Kokmen, E., Ivnik, R. J., & Tangalos, E. G. (1992). Memory function in normal aging. *Neurology, 42*(2), 396-401.

PIOPED Investigators. (1990). Value of the ventilation/perfusion scan in acute pulmonary embolism: Results of the prospective investigation of pulmonary embolism diagnosis (PIOPED). *Journal of the American Medical Association, 263,* 2753-2759.

Powell, J. T., & Greenhalgh, R. M. (2003). Clinical practice. Small abdominal aortic aneurysms. *New England Journal of Medicine, 348*(19), 1895-1901.

Prentice, A. M. (1992). Energy Expenditure in the elderly. *European Journal of Clinical Nutrition, 46*(suppl 3), 521-528.

Price, D. T., & Ridken, P. M. (1997). Factor V Leiden mutation and the risks for thromboembolic disease: A clinical perspective. *Annals of Internal Medicine, 127,* 895-903.

Rathore, S. S., Mehta, S. S., Boyko, W. L., Jr., & Schulman, K. A. (1998). Prescription medication use in older Americans: A national report card on prescribing. *Family Medicine, 30,* 733-739.

Røder, M. E., Schwartz, R. S., Prigeon, R. L., & Kahn, S. E. (2000). Reduced pancreatic B cell compensation to the insulin resistance of aging: Impact on proinsulin and insulin levels. *Journal of Clinical Endocrinology and Metabolism, 85*(6), 2275-2280.

Ronnov-Jessen, V., & Kirkegaard, C. (1973). Hyperthyroidism: A disease of old age? *British Medical Journal, 1,* 41-43.

Rosen, A. M. (1999). Gastrointestinal bleeding in the elderly. *Clinical Geriatric Medicine, 15,* 511-525.

Ryder, K. M., & Benjamin, E. J. (1999). Epidemiology and significance of atrial fibrillation. *American Journal of Cardiology, 84,* 131R-138R.

Safar, M. E. (1993). Hemodynamic changes in elderly hypertensive patients. *American Journal of Hypertension, 6*(3 pt 2), 20S-23S.

Sims, R. V. (1990). Bacterial pneumonia in the elderly. *Emergency Medicine Clinics of North America, 8,* 207.

Singh, K., Bønaa, K. H., Jacobsen, B. K., Bjørk, L., & Solberg, S. (2001). Prevalence of and risk factors for abdominal aortic aneurysms in a population-based study: The Tromso Study. *American Journal of Epidemiology, 154*(3), 236-244.

Siris, E. S., Miller, P. D., Barrett-Connor, E., Faulkner, K. G., Wehren, L. E., Abbott, T. A., et al. (2001). Identification and fracture outcomes of undiagnosed low bone mineral density in postmenopausal women: Results from the National Osteoporosis Risk Assessment, *Journal of the American Medical Association, 286*(22), 2815-2822.

Snyder, D. R., & Christmas, C. (Eds.). (2003). *Geriatric education for emergency medical services,* Sudbury, MA: Jones and Barlett.

Solomon, C. G., Lee, T. H., Cook, E. F., Weisberg, M. C., Brand, D. A., Rouan, G. W., et al. (1989). Comparison of clinical presentation of acute myocardial infarction in patients older than 65 years of age to younger patients: The Multicenter Chest Pain Study experience. *American Journal of Cardiology, 63*(12), 772-776.

Spechler, S. J. (1992). Epidemiology and natural history of gastroesophageal reflux disease. *Digestion, 51*(suppl 1), 24-29.

Strange, G. R., & Chen, E. H. (1998). Use of emergency department by elder patients: A five-year follow-up study. *Academic Emergency Medicine, 5,* 1157.

Sullivan, S. D., Ramsey, S. D., & Lee, T. A. (2000). The economic burden of COPD. *Chest, 117*(suppl 2), 5S-9S.

Tinetti, M. E., Speechley, M., & Ginter, S. F. (1988). Risk factors for falls among elderly persons living in the community. *New England Journal of Medicine, 319,* 1701-1707.

Tountas, A. A. (1993). Insufficiency stress fractures of the femoral neck in elderly women. *Clinical Orthopedics and Related Research, 292,* 202-209.

Trivalle, C., Doucet, J., Chassagne, P., Landrin, I., Kadri, N., Menard, J. F., et al. (1996). Differences in the signs and symptoms of hyperthyroidism in older and younger patients. *Journal of the American Geriatric Society, 44,* 50-53.

Tyson, S. R. (1999). *Gerontological nursing care.* Philadelphia: W.B. Saunders.

U.K. Prospective Diabetes Study Group. (1998). Intensive blood-glucose control with sulphonylureas or insulin compared with conventional treatment and risk of complications in patients with type 2 diabetes (UKDPS 33). *The Lancet, 352,* 837-853.

United States Bone and Joint Decade. (2006). *Good moves for life.* Retrieved September 18, 2006, from http://www.usbjd.org.

United States Census Bureau. (2000). *Total population by age and sex for the United States: 2000.* Retrieved September 18, 2006, from http://www.census.gov.

van Aalst, J. A., Morris, J. A., Yates, H. K., Miller, R. S., & Bass, S. M. (1991). Severely injured geriatric patients return to independent living: A study of factors influencing function and independence. *Journal of Trauma, 31,* 1096-1102.

Wagg, A., & Malone-Lee, J. (1998). The management of urinary incontinence in the elderly. *British Journal of Urology, 82*(suppl 1), 11-17.

Whiteway, J., & Morson, B. C. J. (1985). Pathology of ageing: Diverticular disease. *Clinical Gastroenterology, 14,* 829-835.

Wilking, S. V. B., Belanger, A., Kannel, W. B., D'Agostino, R. B., & Steel, K. (1988). Determinants of isolated systolic hypertension. *Journal of the American Medical Association, 260*(23), 3451-3455.

Wipf, J. E., Lipsky, B. A., Boyko, E. J., Takasugi, J., Peugeot, R. L., et al. (1999). Diagnosing pneumonia by physical examination. Relevant or relic? *Archives of Internal Medicine, 159,* 1082-1087.

Wofford, J. L., Moran, W. P., Heuser, M. D., Schwartz, E., Velez, R., & Mittelmark, M. B. (1995). Emergency medical transport of the elderly: A population-based study. *American Journal of Emergency Medicine, 13,* 297-300.

Wolf, P. A., Abbott, R. D., & Kannell, A. B. (1991). Atrial fibrillation as an independent risk factor for stroke: The Framingham Study. *Stroke, 22,* 983-988.

Wolinsky, F. D., Fitzgerald, J. F., & Stump, T. E. (1997). The effect of hip fracture on mortality, hospitalization, and functional status: A prospective study. *American Journal of Public Health, 87*(3), 398-403.

SUGGESTED RESOURCES

Cassel, C. (2003). *Geriatric medicine: An evidence based approach.* New York: Springer.

Kauder, D. R. (2002). Geriatric trauma. In A. B. Peitzman, M. Rhodes, C. W. Schwab, D. M. Yealy, & T. C. Fabian (Eds.), *The trauma manual* (pp. 469-476). Philadelphia: Lippincott Williams & Wilkins.

Sanders, M. J. (Ed.). (2001). *Mosby's paramedic textbook* (2nd ed.). St. Louis: Mosby.

Snyder, D. R., & Christmas, C. (Eds.) (2003). *Geriatric education for emergency medical services.* Sudbury, MA: Jones and Barlett.

Tallis, R. (2003). *Brocklehurst's textbook of geriatric medicine and gerontology.* London: Churchill Livingstone.

Tyson, S. R. (1999). *Gerontological nursing care.* Philadelphia: W.B. Saunders.

The American Geriatrics Society
The Empire State Building
350 Fifth Avenue, Suite 801
New York, NY 10118
Phone: (212) 308-1414
Email: info@americangeriatrics.org
website: http://www.americangeriatrics.org

The Gerontological Society of America
1220 L St. NW, Suite 901
Washington, DC 20005
Phone: (202) 842-1275
Email: geron@geron.org
Website: http://www.geron.org

Chapter Quiz

1. Chest pain and shortness of breath account for what percentage of EMS responses in the elderly?
- **a.** 10%
- **b.** 25%
- **c.** 50%
- **d.** 90%

2. True or False: Elderly people's lungs have an increased ability for oxygen to cross the membrane into the bloodstream.

3. True or False: Elderly people who exercise regularly are able to maintain cardiac function much better than are their sedentary counterparts.

4. Which of the following is true regarding coronary artery disease in the elderly?
- **a.** Approximately one fourth of people hospitalized for MI are older than 65 years.
- **b.** In-hospital mortality rate for patients with MI is the same for younger and elderly patients.
- **c.** Most elderly people (older than 75 years) with MI have chest pain.
- **d.** Risk factors for heart disease in the elderly include diabetes, known coronary disease, and increasing age.

5. What is the leading cause of nonfatal illness in the elderly population?
- **a.** COPD
- **b.** GI hemorrhage
- **c.** MI
- **d.** Unintentional injury

6. As the body ages, the brain ______.
- **a.** becomes larger to accommodate increased oxygen demands
- **b.** loses nerve cells but not overall volume
- **c.** loses volume
- **d.** swells and compress tightly against the skull

7. Beta-blockers are generally not well tolerated in patients with___.
- **a.** COPD
- **b.** dementia
- **c.** hypertension
- **d.** tachycardia

8. The most serious signs of digoxin toxicity are __________.
- **a.** conduction disturbances and cardiac dysrhythmias.
- **b.** depression and other mood disorders.
- **c.** neurologic deficits and lower level of consciousness.
- **d.** weakness and general loss of muscle tone.

9. Which of the following is the most likely cause of delirium?
- **a.** Alzheimer's disease
- **b.** CNS trauma
- **c.** HIV
- **d.** Metabolic disorder

10. Which of the following is typical of dementia?
- **a.** Acute presentation
- **b.** Impaired level of consciousness
- **c.** Poor short-term memory
- **d.** Typically reversible causes

11. Trauma patients older than 85 years_______.
- **a.** account for only a small percentage of traumatic deaths.
- **b.** are less likely to die than trauma patients aged 29 to 65 years.
- **c.** have nine times the mortality rate of patients aged 29 to 65 years.
- **d.** rarely have serious mechanisms of injury.

12. Which of the following contributes to changes in drug distribution with age?
- **a.** Decreased lean muscle mass
- **b.** Decreased liver function
- **c.** Increased drug metabolism
- **d.** Increased total body water

13. An elderly patient with head trauma and no apparent neurologic deficits________.
    a. is able to compensate for longer periods because of increased brain size.
    b. is unlikely to have major intracranial bleeding.
    c. may have less room for bleeding inside the skull than a younger patient.
    d. may still have significant intracranial hemorrhage.

14. Increased vascular resistance leads to________.
    a. hypertension.
    b. increased renal function.
    c. increased ventilatory resistance.
    d. tachycardia.

Terminology

Ageism Stereotypical and often negative bias against older adults.

Aspiration Inhalation of foreign contents into the lungs.

Benzodiazepine Any of a group of minor tranquilizers with a common molecular structure and similar pharmacologic activity, including antianxiety, sedative, hypnotic, amnestic, anticonvulsant, and muscle-relaxing effects.

Bradykinesia Abnormal slowness of muscular movement.

Cataract A partial or complete opacity on or in the lens or lens capsule of the eye, especially one impairing vision or causing blindness.

Cerebrovascular accident Blockage or hemorrhage of a blood vessel in the brain, usually causing focal neurologic deficits; also known as a stroke.

Cognition Operation of the mind by which one becomes aware of objects of thought or perception; includes all aspects of perceiving, thinking, and remembering.

Delirium Short-term and temporary mental confusion and fluctuating level of consciousness, often caused by intoxication from various substances, hypoglycemia, or acute psychiatric episodes.

Dementia Long-term decline in mental faculties such as memory, concentration, and judgment; often seen with degenerative neurologic disorders such as Alzheimer's disease.

Digoxin A medication derived from digitalis that acts by increasing the force of myocardial contraction and the refractory period and decreasing the conduction rate of the atrioventricular node; used to treat heart failure, most supraventricular tachycardias, and cardiogenic shock.

Diuretic An agent that promotes the excretion of urine.

Do-not-resuscitate (DNR) orders Orders limiting cardiopulmonary resuscitation or advanced life support treatment in the case of a cardiac arrest. These orders may be individualized in that they may allow for differing levels of interventions. When individualized, they usually grant or deny permission for chest compressions, intubation or ventilation, and life-saving medications.

Durable power of attorney for healthcare A type of advanced directive that allows an individual to appoint someone to make healthcare decisions for him or her if the person's ability to make these decisions or communicate wishes is lost.

Glaucoma Increased intraocular pressure from a disruption in the normal production and drainage of aqueous humor; causes often are unknown.

Hypertensive emergency Acute hypertension with end organ dysfunction requiring rapid (within 1 hour) lowering of blood pressure to prevent or limit organ damage.

Incarcerated hernia Hernia of the intestine that cannot be returned or reduced by manipulation; it may or may not become strangulated.

Incidence The rate at which a certain event occurs, such as the number of new cases of a specific disease occurring during a certain period in a population at risk.

Incontinence Inability to control excretory functions; usually refers to the involuntary passage of urinary or fecal matter.

Ischemic stroke Lack of perfusion to an area of brain tissue caused by a blood clot, air, amniotic fluid, or a foreign body.

Kyphosis Abnormally increased convexity in the curvature of the thoracic spine as viewed from the side; also called hunchback.

Living will A type of advanced directive with written and signed specific instructions to healthcare providers about the individual's wishes regarding what types of healthcare measures or treatments should be undertaken to prolong life.

Melena The passage of dark and pitchy stools stained with blood pigments or with altered blood.

Orthopnea Dyspnea relieved by assuming an upright position.

Osteoporosis Reduction in the amount of bone mass, which leads to fractures after minimal trauma.

Polypharmacy The concurrent use of several medications.

Terminology—continued

Presbyopia Impairment of vision caused by advancing years or old age; it is caused by diminution of the power of accommodation from loss of elasticity of the crystalline lens.

Psychomotor Pertaining to motor effects of cerebral or psychic activity.

Pulse pressure The difference between the systolic and diastolic blood pressures.

Transient ischemic attack Neurologic dysfunction caused by a temporary blockage in blood flow; by definition, the symptoms resolve within 24 hours.

Volvulus Intestinal obstruction caused by a knotting and twisting of the bowel.

CHAPTER 39

Abuse and Assault

Objectives

After completing this chapter, you will be able to:

1. Discuss the incidence of abuse and assault.
2. Describe the categories of abuse.
3. Discuss examples of intimate partner abuse.
4. Describe characteristics of a person in an abusive relationship.
5. Describe the cycle of violence.
6. Outline techniques for detection of potential violent crime scenes.
7. Describe priorities for crew safety and crime scene awareness.
8. Discuss the assessment and management of the abused patient.
9. Discuss the documentation requirements associated with abuse and assault.
10. Discuss the legal aspects associated with abuse and assault situations.
11. Discuss community resources available to assist victims of abuse or assault.
12. Discuss examples of child abuse and neglect (maltreatment).
13. Identify types of child abuse.
14. Discuss examples of elder abuse.
15. Identify types of elder abuse.
16. Discuss examples of sexual assault.
17. Discuss the assessment and management of a sexual assault patient.
18. Discuss evidence preservation and evidence collection at a crime scene.

Chapter Outline

Case Scenario

You and your partner respond with the fire department to a private residence for an unknown medical problem. On arrival at the address, there is no answer. As you return to your unit, a neighbor runs out of her house and screams, "The baby's in here!" You enter her house and find a limp 6-month-old girl being held by the neighbor. A frightened 15-year-old girl informs you that she was babysitting the infant when the baby suddenly began "gasping for air." The baby is unresponsive and breathing irregularly at a rate of approximately 4 breaths/min. She is pale with blue lips, hands, and feet.

Questions

1. *What is your general impression of this patient?*
2. *What intervention should you initiate at this time?*
3. *What additional questions might be important to ask the babysitter as you continue your assessment?*

You will be exposed to different types of violence in your career. Many violent crimes require EMS personnel who may arrive on the scene before law enforcement personnel. Because of this, each response must carefully be evaluated for crew safety. The violence you encounter may include intimate partner violence, child abuse and/or neglect, sexual assault, and elder abuse.

INTIMATE PARTNER VIOLENCE AND ABUSE

[OBJECTIVE 1]

Intimate partner violence and abuse (IPVA) is a crime. The requirements to report this crime, as well as the criminal charges associated with it, vary from state to state. Be sure to know your local requirements. IPVA is also referred to as *domestic violence, interpersonal violence, battering, marital abuse,* or *family violence.*

IPVA is defined as a learned pattern of assaultive and controlling behavior, including physical, sexual, and psychological attacks as well as economic control, which adults or adolescents use against their intimate partners to gain power and control (Lynch, 2005).

In situations of IPVA, the abuser may display obsessive behaviors and intense affection for the victim. The abuser's control over the victim's life increases as the obsessive behavior progresses. The psychological and/or physical abuse escalates over a period that may vary from weeks to months or even years. Even minor disagreements or behaviors may increase in importance in the abuser's mind and trigger escalation of abusive behavior.

The Domestic Abuse Intervention Program (Duluth, Minn.), uses the wheel model, which exhibits the power and control activities attributed to batterers. The model is in the shape of a wagon wheel, with spokes radiating from the hub. Eight behavioral categories are listed between each spoke; each behavior is used to force the victim to depend on the abuser (Figure 39-1).

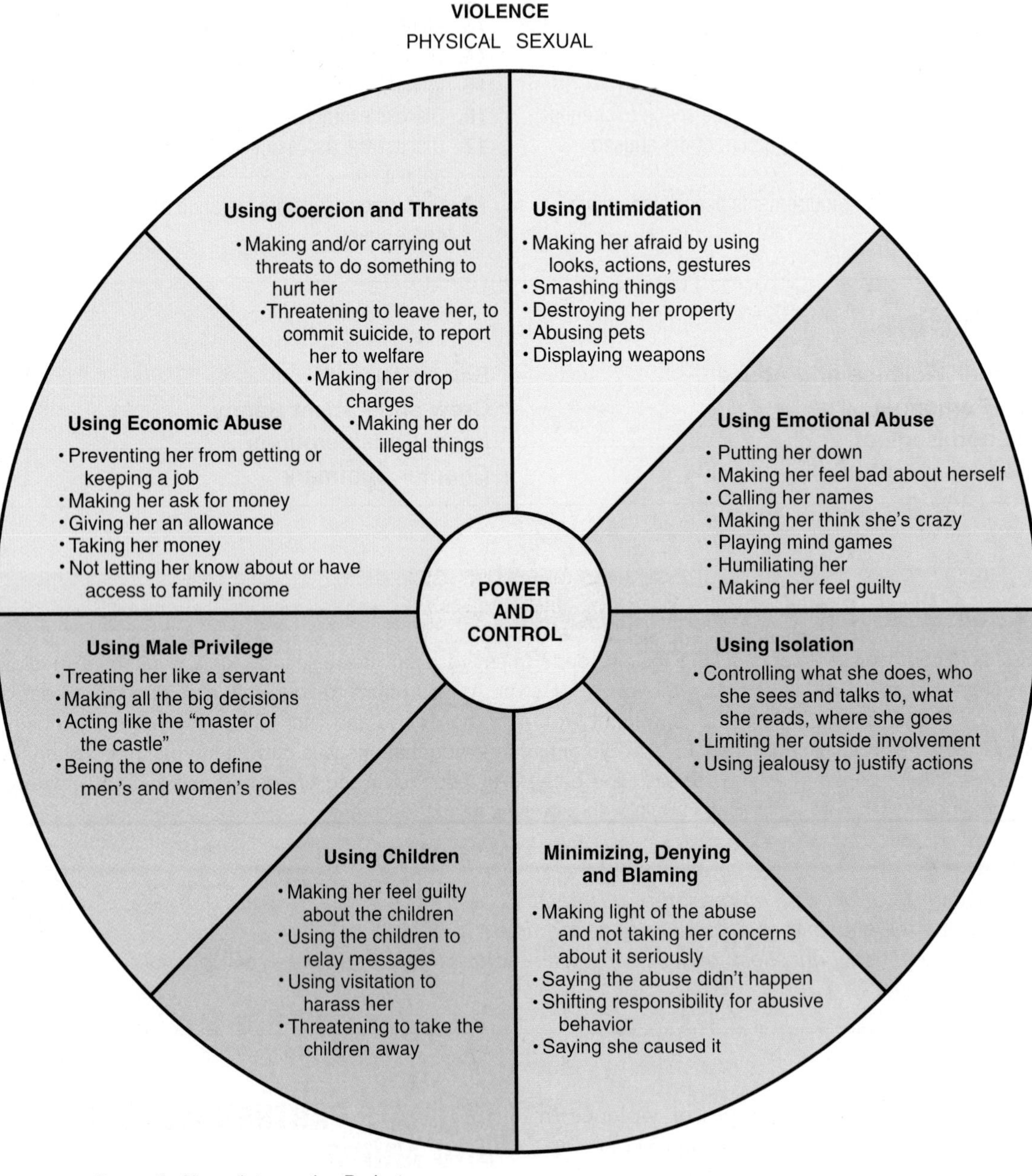
VIOLENCE
PHYSICAL SEXUAL
Using Coercion and Threats
• Making and/or carrying out threats to do something to hurt her
• Threatening to leave her, to commit suicide, to report her to welfare
• Making her drop charges
• Making her do illegal things
Using Intimidation
• Making her afraid by using looks, actions, gestures
• Smashing things
• Destroying her property
• Abusing pets
• Displaying weapons
Using Economic Abuse
• Preventing her from getting or keeping a job
• Making her ask for money
• Giving her an allowance
• Taking her money
• Not letting her know about or have access to family income
Using Emotional Abuse
• Putting her down
• Making her feel bad about herself
• Calling her names
• Making her think she's crazy
• Playing mind games
• Humiliating her
• Making her feel guilty
POWER AND CONTROL
Using Male Privilege
• Treating her like a servant
• Making all the big decisions
• Acting like the "master of the castle"
• Being the one to define men's and women's roles
Using Isolation
• Controlling what she does, who she sees and talks to, what she reads, where she goes
• Limiting her outside involvement
• Using jealousy to justify actions
Using Children
• Making her feel guilty about the children
• Using the children to relay messages
• Using visitation to harass her
• Threatening to take the children away
Minimizing, Denying and Blaming
• Making light of the abuse and not taking her concerns about it seriously
• Saying the abuse didn't happen
• Shifting responsibility for abusive behavior
• Saying she caused it
Domestic Abuse Intervention Project
202 E. Superior Street
Duluth, MN 55802
Phone: 218-722-2781

Figure 39-1 The cycle of violence.

Epidemiology

[OBJECTIVE 2]

It is estimated that there are approximately 1 million cases of IPVA in the United States each year, and perpetrators can be either male or female. However, an estimated 85% to 95% of the victims are female. Abuse can occur between same-sex partners. IPVA does not discriminate among ethnic backgrounds, socioeconomic patterns, or educational levels. People who abuse their intimate partners can include your neighbor, work partner, doctor, supervisor, clergyman, mechanic, co-worker, or best friend. Characteristics of those who abuse their partners are listed in Box 39-1, and risk factors associated with someone becoming an abuser are listed in Box 39-2. IPVA is the leading cause of injuries to women between the ages of 15 and 44 years. One in four women are estimated to be victims of abuse in their lifetimes. More than 5 million women are victims of IPVA in the United States. Incidents may not be reported until after the abuse has occurred several times or is never reported at all. Often incidents are reported as a last resort, and it is estimated that only 10% of cases are reported. Therefore the true number of incidents is not known. The reasons why cases of IPVA are not reported are listed in Box 39-3. Same-sex intimate partner violence occurs for the same reasons that abuse occurs in heterosexual relationships: power and control. The cycle of violence also is the same. One difference that gay and lesbian victims may experience is the lack of an appropriate support network. Normal candidates for support, such as family, friends, co-workers, or clergy may not be aware of the victim's sexual orientation. Fear of confiding in these people or fear of their sexual orientation becoming known to others can be as psychologically devastating as the abuse itself and can even lead to more reluctance to report abuse. Healthcare and judicial systems, which are heterosexually oriented, have traditionally been unsympathetic to gay and lesbian issues. Therefore lesbians and gay men who are abused have much more difficulty finding appropriate support than heterosexual women do. Using these services can be as traumatic as "coming out," which is a major life decision.

BOX 39-1 Characteristics of Those Who Abuse Partners

- Between 18 and 30 years of age
- Low self-esteem
- Witnessed violence in the home as a child
- Believe they are demonstrating discipline
- Do not like being out of control
- Feel there is no alternative
- Inability to back down from conflict
- May feel powerless to change
- Alcohol or drug abuse
- Prone to sudden rage
- Feelings of insecurity or jealousy
- Presence of financial difficulties or difficulty remaining employed
- Abuser may appear charming and loving after the incident

BOX 39-2 Risk Factors for Intimate Partner Violence

- Male is unemployed
- Male uses illegal drugs at least once a year
- Partners have different religious backgrounds
- Family income is below the poverty level
- Partners are unmarried
- Either partner is violent toward children at home
- Male did not graduate from high school
- Male is between 18 and 30 years old
- Male has a blue-collar job, if employed
- Male saw father hit mother

The Cycle of Abuse

[OBJECTIVES 1, 3, 4, 5]

Abuse usually occurs in cycles and may take several forms (Box 39-4). The amount of time between cycles varies from case to case. The cycles may span days, weeks, or even years. The first phase of the abuse cycle begins with intimidation, arguing, verbal and emotional abuse, and isolation tactics. The abuser frightens the victim with looks, actions, or gestures that imply a physical assault may occur. Verbal and emotional abuse may include degrading, name calling, swearing, or embarrassing the victim in public. The abuser may also threaten the victim, the victim's pets, or the victim's children and destroy items that are special to the victim. These tactics are intended to reduce the victim's self-esteem. These behaviors occur in what often is called the **tension-building phase.** During the tension-building phase, the strain in the relationship is high, and heightened anger, blaming, and arguing may occur between the victim and the abuser.

Mind games and humiliation are part of the initial steps in the abuse cycle. Power and control issues continue with increasing isolation. The abuser may begin by

BOX 39-3 Reasons Intimate Partner Violence Is Not Reported

- The patient may fear for herself or her children.
- The patient believes the abuser will change.
- The patient has no other means of financial support.
- The patient has no support structure.
- The patient believes the abuse must be endured to keep the family together.

BOX 39-4 Types of Abuse

Psychological (Emotional) Abuse

The verbal or psychological misuse of another person, including threatening, name calling, ignoring, shaming unfairly, shouting, and cursing; mind games are another form of psychological abuse

Physical Abuse

Harm or injury caused by an intentional physical injury on another person such as punching, kicking, hitting, or biting

Economic (Financial) Abuse

Forcing others from having or keeping a job; forcing control of another person's paycheck; restricting access or forcing conditions on others to receive an allowance; stealing money; not allowing others to know about or have access to economic assets

Neglect

The failure of a caregiver to provide for the needs of an individual in his or her care

Sexual Abuse

Forced and/or coerced sex, violent sexual acts against the victim's will (rape), or withholding sex from the victim; includes fondling, intercourse, incest, rape, sodomy, exhibitionism, sexual exploitation, or exposure to pornography

controlling what the victim reads or watches on television and with whom the victim speaks and visits. The abuser may use other people, including children, to relay messages or act as spies. Religion or citizenship may also be used to control the victim. The abuser may even threaten to self-harm if the victim suggests he or she may leave the relationship.

At some point, the abuse almost always progresses to a form of physical violence. This is considered the second phase in the abuse cycle. It may include sexual assault as well as physical assault. The timeline from verbal to physical abuse can vary greatly depending on the individual case. Physical abuse is never the first form of abuse used by the abuser.

Economic abuse consists of a variety of actions toward the victim, such as intentionally making the victim late for work, not allowing the victim to work, or causing the victim to be fired from a job.

The abuser also may force the victim to work but demand control of the paycheck. This limits the victim's access to money because all purchases go through the abuser. Through paycheck control, the abuser may subtly force the victim to beg for financial resources. The abuser may refuse to allow prescription medications to be filled, refuse to pay bills (thus ruining credit history), refuse to pay child support, or bargain with child support. These threats can be implied or actual. In short, the abuser forbids and prohibits the victim from enjoying any form of financial independence.

The escalating pattern continues until the abuser loses control and pushes, slaps, pinches, hits, or chokes the victim. The victim is blamed for making the abuser behave this way. The abuser does not take responsibility for his or her own actions and subsequently blames the victim for the abuse.

Sexual abuse is common in long-term abusive relationships. This may be in the form of forced and/or coerced sex, violent sexual acts against the victim's will (rape), or the abuser withholding sex from the victim.

After an abusive event, a period of remorse usually follows. The abuser begs for forgiveness, with promises never to abuse again. The abuser's behavior is that of a model partner, often bearing gifts. This period is the third phase in the cycle of abuse. Denial and apologies are the highlights of this phase, which commonly is referred to as the **honeymoon phase.** The abuser's behavior changes for a time. Unfortunately this period does not last, and the cycle of abuse begins again. This repetitive pattern may go on for years (see Figure 39-1).

Why Doesn't the Victim Leave?

Victims do not leave their abusers for many reasons. Perhaps a better question might be, "What are the barriers that prevent victims from leaving?"

- The victim may still be in love with the abuser despite all the abuse.
- The relationship has not always been bad.
- The victim believes he or she can "fix" the abuser.
- The victim hopes that the abuser will change and the abuse will stop.
- The victim may have strong religious convictions that prevent the dissolution of a marriage.

The victim may not be in a financial position to be independent or take care of any children alone. If the victim is not currently employed, the prospect of finding a job may be overwhelming. If the victim needs to leave the home, he or she will need to obtain shelter or be forced to live on the street. Walking away from their homes, possessions, and lives, especially if children are involved, is extremely difficult for victims. Social isolation usually leaves victims without a network of friends to rely on for support.

PARAMEDIC*Pearl*

According to the National Coalition Against Domestic Violence, most battered women have at least one dependent child, are not employed outside the home, lack access to cash or bank accounts, and have no property that is solely theirs.

People in abusive relationships may temporarily leave the situation several times before they leave permanently. Keep in mind that their self-esteem has been shattered such that they no longer believe they are capable of independent living. The most significant reason that victims do not leave an abusive relationship is fear that the abuser will retaliate. The victim fears that the retaliation may be directed at the victim, the victim's family, friends, or pets and may result in more violent or fatal consequences.

PARAMEDIC*Pearl*

An abused victim is estimated to leave the relationship unsuccessfully seven times before leaving permanently.

Characteristics of an Abusive Relationship

[OBJECTIVE 4]

Characteristics of persons in abusive relationships vary but include the following:

- Unrealistic expectations of the relationship
- Difficulty in expressing anger
- Clinical depression
- Repeated attempts to leave the relationship
- Suicidal ideation or attempts
- Use of excessive alcohol or other substances

ROLE OF EMS PERSONNEL

The following is a policy statement of the American College of Emergency Physicians (2000).

The American College of Emergency Physicians (ACEP) believes intimate partner violence is a serious public health problem. Consequently, emergency medical services (EMS) personnel will encounter victims of intimate partner violence. The interactions at the scene, the potential for harm to the healthcare provider, and the need for special documentation and communications differ from other out-of-hospital situations. ACEP believes that training in the evaluation and management of victims of intimate partner violence should be incorporated into the initial and continuing education of EMS personnel. This training should include the recognition of victims and their injuries, and understanding of the patterns of abuse and how this affects care, scene safety, preservation of evidence, and documentation requirements.

Scene Safety

[OBJECTIVES 6, 7]

When you are called to a scene, size-up is essential on arrival. If the situation is potentially violent, notify law enforcement. *Do not enter an environment that is potentially hazardous.* Try to determine whether any weapons or potentially violent people are in the home. Make every attempt to interview the possible abuse victim alone. If no opportunity to speak to the victim alone occurs and you suspect abuse, voice your suspicions to the emergency department staff with any pertinent supportive findings. Have a high index of suspicion if the injuries present do not match the reported mechanism of injury. This requires a detailed examination of the scene and its surrounding environment by EMS and law enforcement professionals. Be alert if you already suspect abuse and the potential abuser is by the victim's side or answers questions for the victim regarding the injuries (Stoy et al., 2005).

Detailed Physical Examination

[OBJECTIVE 8]

You should complete a detailed physical examination of the victim. It may be advisable to have a female assess a female, and have a male assess a male. The most commonly injured areas are sites easily hidden by clothing, such as the chest, abdomen, genitals, and breasts. Other commonly injured areas are the head, neck, face, and pelvis. Keep in mind that accidental injuries are usually distal to the body. Intentional injuries inflicted by others are generally proximal to the body. Additionally patients may attempt to protect the abuser and hide the true cause of their injuries by providing incomplete or inaccurate histories. Often the abuser may appear to be caring and loving after the incident, but may be hesitant to leave the patient alone with the paramedic.

Signs of Injury

Identification of an abused patient can be difficult. Some signs of injury that are distinctive for abuse are listed here (Emergency Nurses Association, 2000). Additional indicators of abuse can be found in Box 39-5.

Patterned Injuries

Patterned injuries leave a distinctive mark, indicating that an object was used in the assault. Cigarette burns, electrical cord whipping, human bites, glove injuries, attempted strangulation, and slaps are common injuries

BOX 39-5 Indicators of Abuse

- Multiple calls to the same address for similar injuries
- Explanations that do not match the injury
- Elusiveness, hesitancy, or nervousness when providing a history of the event
- Delayed care for injuries, particularly if there are indications the patient waited until the partner was not present before calling
- Injuries that occur during pregnancy
- Patients with a history of substance abuse or emotional disorders
- Statements such as "Things have not been going well lately" or "There have been problems at home"

that leave patterns. Be aware of any objects in the environment that might match a pattern of injury (Figure 39-2).

Facial Petechiae

Facial **petechiae,** a tiny pinpoint rash on the upper area of the neck and the face, may indicate near-strangulation or suffocation. Petechiae are caused by venous return that is blocked from the head while arterial pressure remains normal. Petechiae also may be present in mothers after childbirth (Figure 39-3).

Multiple Bruises

Multiple bruised sites in various stages of healing should raise your index of suspicion for abuse (Figure 39-4). Physical abuse is not the only cause for contusions or bruises. Some medications and medical conditions can contribute to bruising, including the following:

- Aspirin
- Nonsteroidal antiinflammatory drugs such as ibuprofen and naproxen
- Warfarin (Coumadin)
- Heparin (ask whether the patient has been recently hospitalized)
- Prednisone
- Valproic acid (Depakene)
- Hemocytopenia

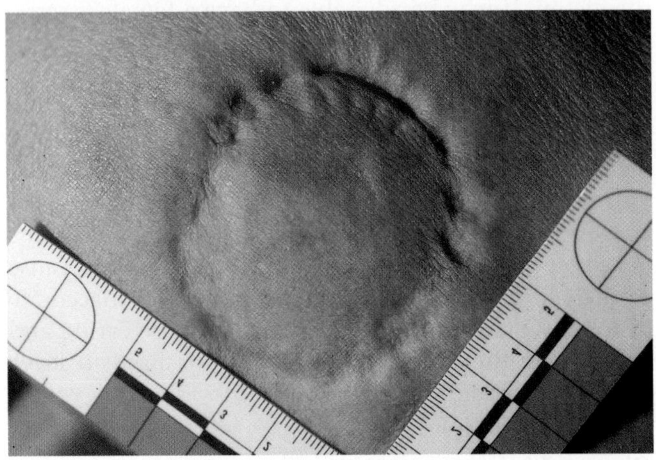

Figure 39-2 Patterned injury.

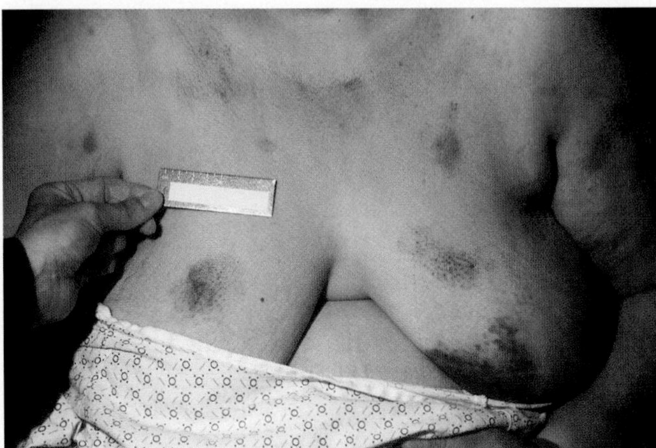

Figure 39-4 Multiple bruises.

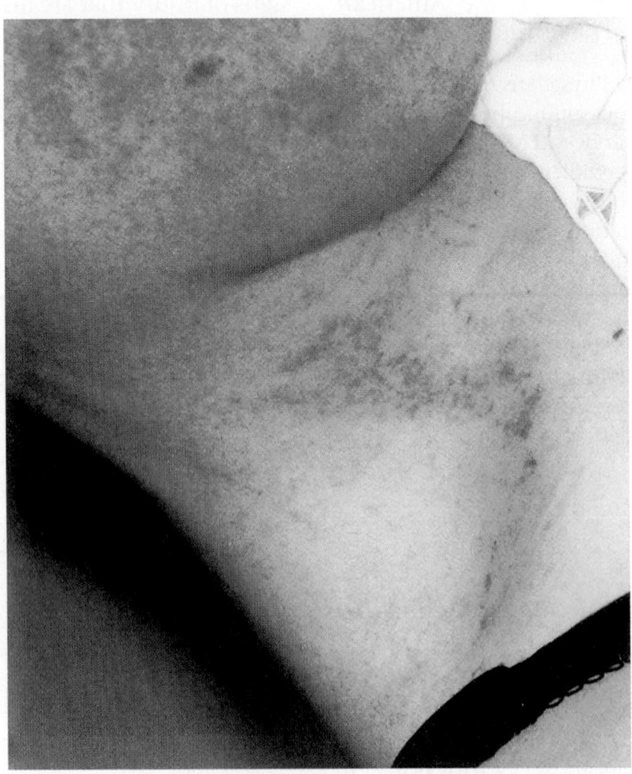

Figure 39-3 Facial petechiae.

Case Scenario—continued

Your partner begins positive-pressure ventilation with a bag-mask device connected to 100% oxygen as you prepare to intubate. You successfully intubate the child's trachea on the third attempt and your partner continues ventilation. The infant's chest rises and falls easily and her color almost immediately improves. When confirming the tube's position you note that lung sounds are moist bilaterally. The babysitter reports that the child was fine, sitting on the floor, when she suddenly "tightened up," arched her back, hit the floor with the back of her head, and became limp and unresponsive. No evidence of trauma is present. When asked, the babysitter states that the floor is carpeted. Vital signs are pulse of 100 beats/min and blood pressure of 70/52 mm Hg. You immediately transfer the infant to the ambulance for transport. The babysitter agrees to accompany the patient to the hospital and rides in the passenger seat next to the driver. You and your partner remain in the patient compartment to provide care.

Questions

4. *Is this patient high priority? Why or why not?*
5. *What are your thoughts about the babysitter's description of the patient "tightening up," arching her back, falling backward, and becoming limp?*
6. *How does the reported mechanism of injury fit into the presentation?*
7. *What treatment will you initiate at this time?*

Multiple, Nontraumatic, and Chronic Complaints

Victims of abuse may have multiple or chronic complaints without signs of injury. Some of the most common complaints include the following:

- Headaches (most common)
- Chest pain
- Vague, nonspecific pain, often of the back, abdomen, and pelvic regions
- Physical symptoms related to stress

These symptoms may appear as depression or anxiety (panic) attacks.

Signs that a person may be a victim of abuse include the following:

- Depression
- Substance abuse
- Chronic tardiness or absences
- Chronic medical complaints
- Inappropriate dress for the climate (i.e., wearing clothes that cover signs of abuse)

Chronic Medical Conditions

The victim of abuse also may have poor control of chronic medical conditions such as diabetes, hypertension, or heart disease because the abuser either does not allow the victim to seek appropriate medical care or may not permit the victim to take medications necessary to control medical conditions. Gastrointestinal symptoms are common in victims of interpersonal violence. Many family physicians now ask patients about the possibility of an unsafe relationship.

Obstetric and Gynecologic Conditions

Sexual abuse may expose women to serious illness. Abused women are particularly at risk for obstetric and gynecologic manifestations such as human immunodeficiency virus (HIV), sexually transmitted diseases, unplanned pregnancy, chronic pelvic pain, or frequent vaginal and urinary tract infections. Abused women may also have miscarriages, multiple abortions, obstetric complications, and delayed prenatal care. Abused women are more likely to give birth to low birth weight infants.

PARAMEDIC*Pearl*

An estimated 67% to 83% of women who are HIV positive are in, or have been in, abusive relationships.

Abuse during pregnancy escalates during the third trimester, usually because the woman begins to focus on her baby and herself instead of the abuser, which is not acceptable to him. Psychiatric presentations are common in victims of IPVA. Victims arrive in emergency departments with complaints such as depression, anxiety, posttraumatic stress disorder, multiple personality disorders, hyperarousal, and suicidal ideations.

Effective Communication

Convey the following messages to victims of IPVA:

- There is no excuse for abuse.
- This is not the victim's fault. Only the abuser is responsible.

- No one deserves to be abused.
- You are there for support, and you believe the victim.

Remember the following points when treating a possible abuse victim:

- Show the victim respect and provide empowerment by allowing the victim to make decisions, regardless of how minor they may seem.
- Listen.
- When possible, have an EMT or paramedic who is the same sex as the victim interview the patient and perform the assessment.
- Provide the referral number or information for an appropriate shelter.
- The victim is more likely to be receptive to intervention before the period of remorse by the abuser.

Educating healthcare professionals and the public to recognize IPVA is the best method to decrease its occurrence (Figure 39-5). Recognizing IPVA when the incident occurs enables the victim to receive help.

Asking the Question

At the time of an incident, you must be knowledgeable enough to "ask the question." You must be direct. The patient must be interviewed alone. The back of an ambulance is an ideal place to interview a potential victim of IPVA.

- Be sure that the victim has *absolute* privacy before asking questions that may endanger someone.
- Do not interview the victim in front of children.
- Anyone accompanying the patient should be considered a potential abuser. Consequently, do not ask questions about abuse until you are alone with the victim.
- If you cannot ask the victim about abuse because of the presence of others, report your suspicions to the staff at the receiving medical facility. Your service should choose a question that each individual

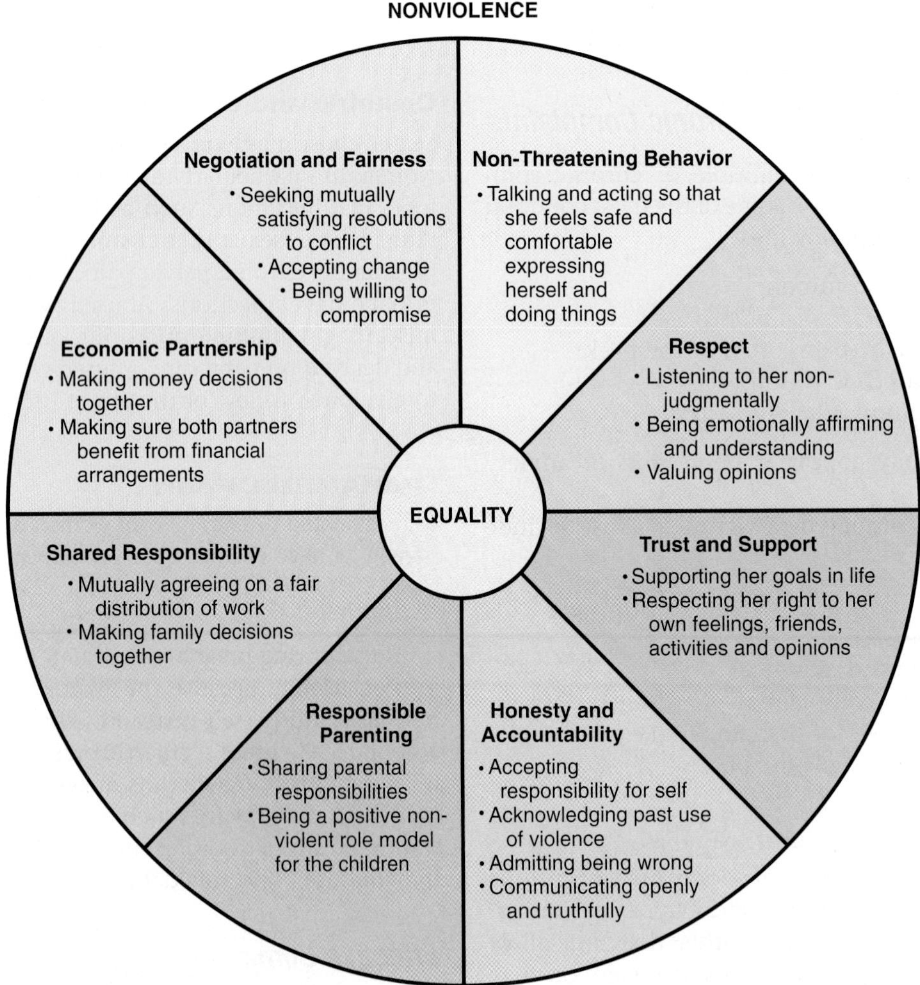

Figure 39-5 Equality wheel from Domestic Abuse Intervention Project.

healthcare professional is comfortable with so that detecting possible abuse is not overlooked. Some examples include the following:

- "Because violence is common in people's lives, we now ask everyone we treat about domestic violence. Have you ever been verbally, physically, economically, or sexually abused?"
- "Because so many people are involved with someone who hits them, threatens them, continually puts them down, or tries to control them, I now ask all of my patients about abuse. Has this ever happened to you?"

The Response

[OBJECTIVES 10, 11]

What should be done when the patient's answer is yes, he or she has been abused? The first thing to do is assess the safety of the situation for the victim. Then notify law enforcement. Be observant of the partner's behavior during your intervention, and *do not leave the victim alone with a suspected abuser.* Do not confront the abuser at the scene. That should be left to law enforcement. Do not put yourself at risk. The victim may listen without acknowledging what is being said and may respond to your question in the negative. Accept his or her response. Many victims of IPVA are ashamed and feel responsible for the abuse. Treat them with respect and let them know where they can get more information if the situation arises. Remain calm, respectful, sensitive, and nonjudgmental with the victim and the abuser.

Responding to your questions about abuse may be difficult for the following groups of people.

Lesbian and Gay Patients. A person's typical support system, such as family, friends, co-workers, or the clergy, may not be aware of the victim's sexual orientation. Fear of confiding in these people or fear of their sexual orientation becoming known to others can be as psychologically devastating as the abuse itself. It can even lead to more reluctance to report abuse.

Non–English-Speaking Patients. Healthcare providers and agencies may lack translators or those knowledgeable about different cultural belief systems. If the victim speaks little or no English, use professionals for translation services. Using family members or acquaintances may expose the victim to danger and provide inaccurate answers to important questions.

Undocumented Immigrants. Immigrants sponsored by their spouses, who are legal residents of the United States, may be reluctant to report abuse because the abuser has threatened to withdraw sponsorship. Additionally, these victims are usually economically dependent on the abuser.

Mental Health or Substance Abuse. Victims with a history of mental health or substance abuse problems may not be reliable historians. Consequently, a victim may feel that claims of abuse might be refuted by an abuser whom authorities may consider more credible.

Victims with Serious Disabilities. Victims with serious disabilities may depend on the abuser for healthcare, shelter, and/or financial support.

Older Adults. Ninety percent of reported abusers of older adults were family members. Two thirds of those were adult children or spouses.

Victims Who May Fear. Perception of an abusive event may be interpreted differently according to the values and traditions of nonmainstream ethnic and religious cultures. Cultural beliefs also may prevent the victim from reporting abuse. Examples include the following:

- Fear that the abuser may be maltreated by law enforcement officials
- Belief that negative life events occur regardless of efforts to prevent them
- Cultural values that focus on the family group as opposed to the individual

Gather information regarding the victim's circumstances to provide to the receiving medical facility. Before transporting the patient, ask the following questions:

- Is the victim's partner present or planning to show up at the receiving facility?
- What does the victim want the ED staff to do if the abuser tries to get the victim to leave the hospital?
- Does the victim want them to call security or the police?
- Does the victim want to leave with the abuser?
- Does the victim want to keep hidden or find a shelter?
- Does someone need to pick up the victim's children?
- Has an order for protection been issued?
- If so, should the abuser be arrested? This may not be up to the victim. It may depend on state regulations.
- Does the victim believe going home with the abuser is a better alternative?
- Does the victim need to be home at a certain time to avoid further abuse?

PARAMEDIC*Pearl*

Studies show that 75% of battered women are beaten after they leave a relationship.

Documentation of Injuries

[OBJECTIVE 9]

Careful and detailed documentation and a report of suspected abuse injuries to the staff at the receiving hospital are important for the victim's safety and follow-up. This should include the presence of injuries and a full description of their appearance, size, and other characteristics. The paramedic must be sure that their documentation is complete and objective, without subjective statements, presumptions, or accusations.

Appropriate documentation is critical because abuse cases may become court cases. In short, do the following:

- Objectively document descriptions of what you see.
- Use the patient's exact words and include them in your report in quotation marks.
- Do not make remarks that cannot be substantiated.
- Write legibly.

Other Considerations

Preserve any physical evidence, such as torn or soiled clothing. Place evidence in a paper bag. Do not use plastic, which may interfere with the preservation of evidence. Do not allow the patient to bathe, shower, or use the bathroom, if at all possible, until arrival at the receiving medical facility. If the victim needs to use the bathroom, ask him or her not to wipe any body parts. Preservation of any evidence discovered at the scene is essential.

You need to know the local resources available for victims of IPVA. Give this information to every potential or suspected victim of abuse. It should include available shelters, crisis centers, advocacy programs, and counseling services.

Unfortunately, the victim may increase substance abuse once the abuse starts. After the victim reports the incident to law enforcement, escalation of the physical abuse is possible, particularly if the two parties continue to reside in the same home.

CHILD ABUSE AND NEGLECT

[OBJECTIVES 12, 13]

In the United States there are nearly 1 million cases of **child maltreatment** reported each year. Like IPVA, child maltreatment spans all social and demographic groups. That being said, there is a greater association in the setting of poverty, alcohol or substance abuse in the household, social isolation, violence in the household, and parental mental illness. Although most people associate child abuse with young children, it can occur from infancy through 18 years of age. The abuse can in fact continue beyond the age of 18; however, at this point it would no longer be considered child abuse. The abuser is often the caregiver of the child such as a parent, foster parent, stepparent, or babysitter; however, other relatives of the child who provide care may be involved.

Characteristics of those who abuse children are listed in Box 39-6. Abusers often have a history of being abused as children as well as a history of rigorous discipline and severe punishment. This establishes a cyclical nature of child abuse, as those children who endure this environment are likely to repeat the pattern as adults. Often the abuser would prefer to use another form of discipline; however, stress and desperation leads them to the same form of discipline they received as a child. Many times the abuser can recognize this pattern and will attempt to seek help before the abuse occurs. This is referred to as the *pre-abuse state.* During this time the adult may make several calls for help within a 24 hour period to support centers or EMS, they may initiate frequent 9-1-1 responses for seemingly inconsequential symptoms, or they may begin to demonstrate behavior indicating they are unable to handle the impending crisis. When faced with these types of situations, the paramedic must be attuned to the possibility that it is a cry for help. In addition to attending to the reported complaint, asking parents if there is anything else bothering them, if they are concerned with the safety of anyone in the household, or if you can be of further assistance may provide the outlet they need to avoid the abusive incident.

BOX 39-6 Characteristics of Those Who Abuse Children

- Is indifferent to the child
- Seldom looks at or touches the child
- Seems unconcerned about the child's injury or prognosis
- Shows no indications of guilt or remorse
- Is openly critical of the child
- Has little perception of how a child feels emotionally or physically
- Blames the child for the injury
- Appears self-centered or preoccupied with himself or herself
- Demonstrates immature behavior

Child maltreatment includes four types of abuse: intentional neglect, and psychological abuse, physical abuse, and sexual abuse (Aehlert, 2005; Emergency Nurses Association, 2004). State laws define what specific acts constitute abuse and neglect. Because laws vary from state to state, you must know the appropriate laws that are in place where you practice.

Neglect is the failure to provide the basic needs to a child. Physical neglect can include lack of food, appropriate clothing for the weather, and inadequate or a lack of medical care. Indicators of neglect include malnutrition, poor growth, poor hygiene, failure to thrive, missed medical appointments, and unsafe living conditions (Figure 39-6). Neglect is the most common cause of all cases of child maltreatment and accounted for 62.8% of all cases of child maltreatment in 2005. There is generally an ongoing pattern of inadequate care that may be recognized by those in close contact with the child. Paramedics are in a unique position to recognize neglect. In addition to the ability to interact with children through their daily activities, paramedics also interact with children at functions such as school presentations or standbys where children are present. Additionally no other members of the health care profession have the opportunity to see the living conditions of their patients, which may provide important clues to the presence of neglect.

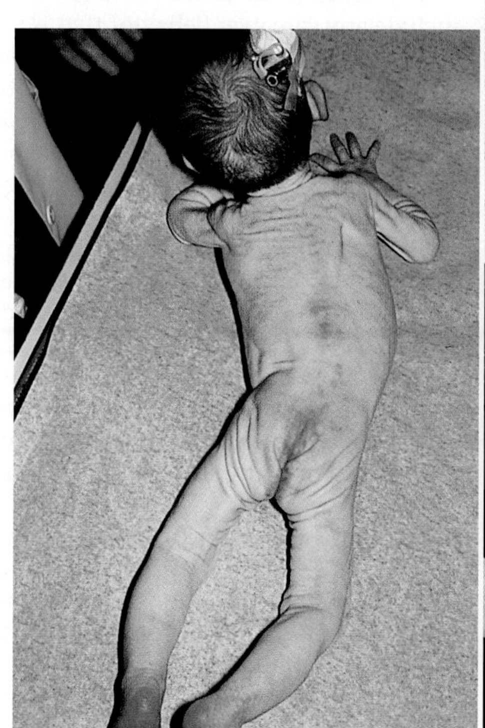
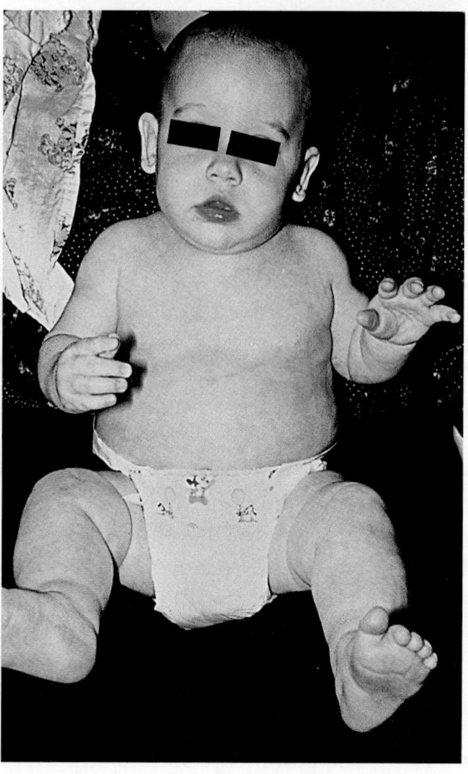

Figure 39-6 Failure to thrive as a result of neglect. **A,** This $4^1/_2$-month-old infant was brought to the emergency department because of congestion. She was found to be below her birth weight and suffering from severe developmental delay. Note the marked loss of subcutaneous tissue manifested by the wrinkled skin folds over her buttocks, shoulders, and upper arms. **B,** Three and one half months after removal from the home, she was well nourished and had caught up developmentally.

If neglect is suspected, it must be reported just as any other type of child maltreatment. Although neglect may seem less serious than other forms of maltreatment, such as physical abuse, it is every bit as dangerous. In fact, in 2005, of the 1460 child fatalities that occurred secondary to maltreatment, neglect was the most common cause and was responsible for 42.2% of these fatalities.

Neglect can be classified as one of four types:

- Physical neglect is responsible for most of the cases of child maltreatment. In these cases the caregiver does not provide the child with the basic necessities of life, including food, clothing, and shelter. Additionally this form of neglect includes abandonment, inadequate supervision, or expulsion from the home without ensuring the child's needs are met (e.g., not making arrangements for the child to live with a responsible relative). These situations endanger the child's development and can result in failure to thrive, physical injury (secondary to being unsupervised, not those inflicted by a caregiver), malnutrition, and illness.
- Medical neglect is the failure to provide appropriate healthcare for a child despite being financially able to do so. In 2005, 2% of all cases of child maltreatment were secondary to medical neglect. There are several situations in which medical neglect occurs. The caregiver may not provide basic healthcare and screenings such as regular childhood physicals and immunizations. The caregiver may not provide recommended treatment for chronic treatable conditions. The caregiver may not provide or seek medical care for the child in an emergency situation. The caregiver may not seek care because of financial considerations; however, this does not include the inability to pay for such services, but rather the desire not to spend the money on the child's healthcare. Another situation that can lead to medical neglect is secondary to religious beliefs. In this situation the caregiver may not provide or seek medical care because of his or her beliefs. Medical neglect can result in poor overall health and compounded medical problems. It is important to note that not all parental decisions based on religious beliefs lead to medical neglect. If the paramedic suspects neglect, the proper authorities must be notified (as in all cases of suspected maltreatment). Child protective service agencies and/or the court system will take steps to provide care for the child in many situations.

- Educational neglect occurs when the child is not allowed to receive adequate education or when the child is allowed to engage in activities that hampers his or her education. This may include not enrolling the child in school, not providing home schooling, or denying recommended special education. Allowing the child to constantly skip school without caregiver intervention to stop the behavior also classifies as educational neglect. This can lead to situations where the child engages in unacceptable behavior and does not acquire essential skills needed for adult life.
- Emotional neglect, also referred to as *psychological abuse,* is discussed later.

Although the nature of emergency medicine dictates that the paramedic will spend less time with child patients than other healthcare providers, teachers, daycare workers, or other individuals in the child's life, it is paramount that indicators of neglect be recognized. Suspicion may be raised with subtle findings or statements. For example if the call is at the child's school and the teacher states that the child is often dressed inappropriately or absent, the paramedic should explore the possibility of neglect. Indicators of neglect may be evident in both the child and the caregivers and are listed in Box 39-7.

Psychological abuse is difficult to detect but may include any caregiver behavior that is meant to make the child feel worthless, unwanted, or unloved or does not provide an environment that allows the healthy emotional development of the child. This type of abuse accounted for 7.1% of reported child abuse cases in 2005. Child and caregiver characteristics in psychological abuse are listed in Box 39-8.

Physical abuse is intentionally inflicting injury to another person; in 2005 physical abuse accounted for 16.6% of reported child abuse cases and 24.1% of deaths secondary to child maltreatment. This is the most obvious form of abuse and often results from severe punishment from an angry or frustrated caregiver. Types of injury may include burns, bites, hitting, shaking, and fractures. Findings consistent with physical abuse are listed in Box 39-9. Head injuries are the most common type of physical abuse and the leading cause of death. Fractures are the second most common injury in physical abuse, but abdominal injury, although rare, is the second leading cause of death. You must be certain to distinguish between injury and certain childhood illnesses. Mongolian spots may be mistaken for bruises, impetigo may look like cigarette burns, and folklore practices such as coining or cupping make linear patterns on the spine or chest. Fractures in children are highly suspicious. Significant force is required for a fracture to occur in a child. Carefully

BOX 39-7 Indicators of Neglect

Indicators of Neglect in the Child

- Untreated injury or illness
- Poor hygiene
- Diaper rash
- Lacks needed medical or dental care
- Lacks sufficient clothing for the weather
- Poor school attendance
- Evidence of prolonged exposure to environmental elements
- The child is chronically tired or hungry
- Malnutrition
- Begging for leftovers or stealing food or money
- Substance abuse
- Constant demands for attention
- Statements of no one to provide care or assuming adult responsibilities
- The child is underdeveloped for the chronological age

Indicators of Neglect in the Caregiver

- Depression or apathy
- Substance abuse
- Irrational behavior
- Indifference to the child

BOX 39-8 Indicators of Psychological Abuse

Child Characteristics

- Developmental delays in the acquisition of speech or motor skills
- Speech disorders
- Weight or height level substantially below norm
- Nervous disorders
- Eating disorders
- Habit disorders (biting, rocking, head-banging)
- Behavioral extremes, such as overly compliant/demanding; withdrawn/aggressive; listless/excitable
- Age-inappropriate behaviors (bedwetting, wetting, soiling)
- Cruel behavior toward children, adults, or animals

Caregiver Characteristics

- Indifference to the child
- Ignoring the child
- Rejection of the child
- Extreme criticism of the child
- Belittlement of the child
- Terrorizing the child, either with severe punishment or playing on fears
- Isolating the child from social contact
- Encouraging illegal or antisocial behavior in the child
- Exposing the child to spousal abuse
- Allowing child substance use or abuse

BOX 39-9 Indicators of Physical Abuse

- Explanations inconsistent with injuries
- Unexplained bruises and welts on the face, throat, upper arms, buttocks, thighs, or lower back
- Unusual patterns or shapes of bruises
- Bruises in various stages of healing
- Bruises on multiple areas of the body that are not explained by normal child behavior
- Defense wounds
- Fading bruises or other injuries after school absences, weekends, or vacations
- Unexplained fractures
- Unexplained burns or patterned burns on the hands, feet, abdomen, or buttocks (e.g., glove or stocking burns secondary to hot water immersion, rope burns, cigarette burns)
- Delayed treatment of burns
- Behavioral extremes or antisocial behavior
- Inappropriate or excessive fear of caretaker
- Reluctance of physical contact
- Reports injury by a caregiver
- Unexplained head injuries
- Unexplained abdominal injuries
- Bite marks that are not from other children

consider the explanation about a fracture if a fracture is obvious or suspected (Figure 39-7). Shaken baby syndrome is the severe shaking of an infant or child without supporting the neck, causing the brain to bounce within the skull cavity, possibly producing a subdural hemorrhage and bleeding within the retina of the eye. Death is almost certain because of the brain trauma.

According to the National Center on Child Abuse and Neglect, child **sexual abuse** is inappropriate adolescent or adult sexual behavior with a child; this accounted for 9.3%, or more than 83,000, of the reported child abuse cases in 2005 and involves both male and female victims. However, it is believed that this number may be higher due to a large number of unreported cases. The age of consent varies from state to state. Sexual assault can be divided into three categories: those that involve touching, those that do not involve touching, and those that involve exploitation. Examples include fondling, incest, rape, sodomy, exposure to pornography, exposure of adult genitals, forcing the child to touch adult genitals, exposure to masturbation, intentional exposure to intercourse, the production of child pornography, and soliciting child prostitution. Report any injury to the perineum, genitals, or internal structures to law enforcement and the receiving hospital (Figure 39-8). Indicators of sexual abuse are listed in Box 39-10. Risk factors for the child

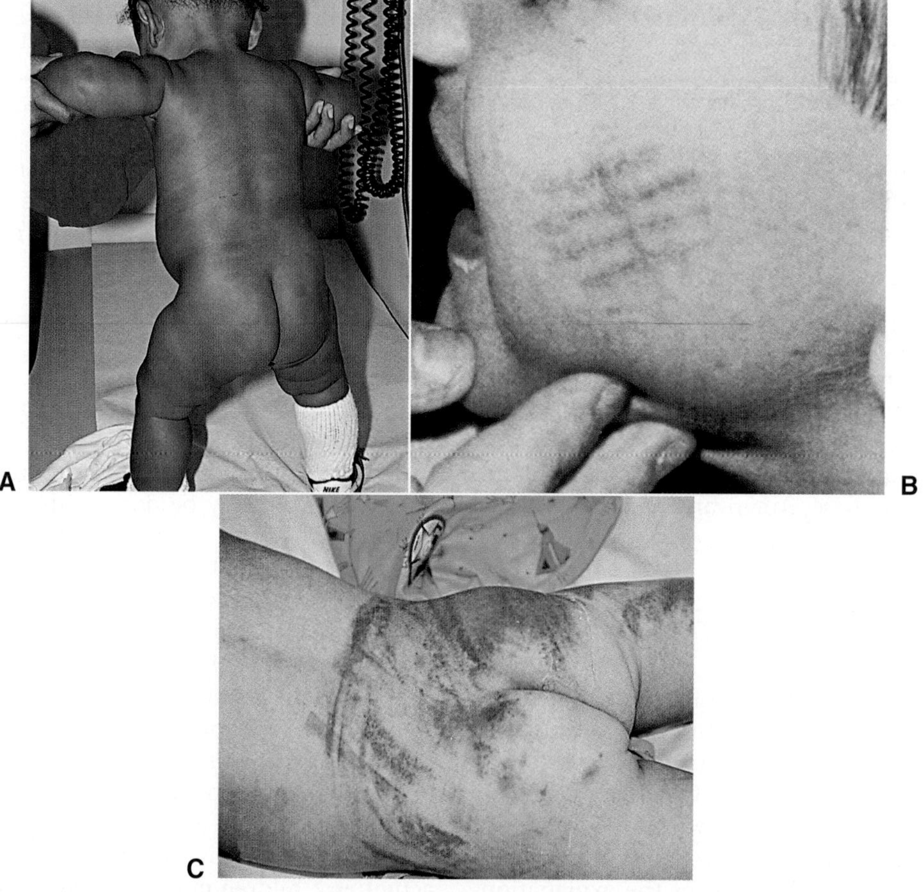

Figure 39-7 **A,** Mongolian spots. **B,** Facial burns of abuse. **C,** Contusions to buttocks.

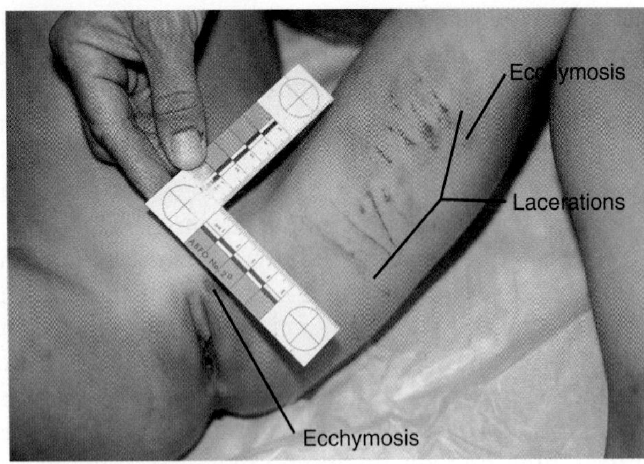

Figure 39-8 Eight-year-old girl after a sexual assault.

BOX 39-10 Indicators of Sexual Abuse

- Complaints of sexual abuse
- Seductive behavior
- Inappropriate or unusual knowledge of sexual concepts for the age
- Torn, stained, or bloody undergarments
- Pain and irritation of the genitals
- Difficulty walking or sitting
- Pregnancy under the age of 14
- Sexually transmitted diseases under the age of 14
- Injury to the genitalia or anal region
- Frequent, unexplained sore throats or yeast or urinary infections
- Regressive behaviors
- Sleep disturbances

BOX 39-11 Child Abuse Risk Factors

Child Risk Factors

- Premature birth or neonatal separation
- Congenital defect
- Developmental disability
- Physical disability
- Chronic illness
- Multiple births

Caregiver Risk Factors

- Often abused as a child
- Young maternal age
- History of mental illness or criminal activity
- Financial stress, unemployment
- Physical illness of parent or child
- Marital or relationship stress
- Low self-esteem, depression
- Substance abuse

BOX 39-12 Indicators of Child Abuse

- Children under 6 years of age are excessively passive
- Children over 6 years of age are aggressive
- Regardless of age, the child does not mind if the caregiver leaves the room
- The child cries hopelessly, or very little, during the examination and treatment
- The child does not look to the caregiver for reassurance
- The child is resistant to physical contact
- The child is extremely apprehensive
- The child appears to be constantly on the alert for danger

and caregiver may increase the potential for child maltreatment. Risk factors are listed in Box 39-11 (U.S. Department of Health and Human Services, Administration on Children, Youth and Families, 2007; Child Welfare Information Gateway, 2006; American Humane Association, 2007).

History and Physical Examination

[OBJECTIVES 8, 9]

While obtaining the history, look for red flags, which are anything that does not fit the situation. If the mechanism of injury does not fit with the injuries seen, you should have a high index of suspicion. Often the child's behavior and relationship with the caregiver will provide important clues regarding the possibility of abuse. If the child readily provides a history that matches the explanation by the caregiver, it is unlikely that abuse was the cause of the injury or illness. Behaviors that may indicate child abuse are listed in Box 39-12.

The physical examination of the potentially maltreated child should ideally be done with your partner present rather than alone. Determining whether an injury is intentional or accidental can be difficult. The paramedic must be familiar with those injuries that are part of normal childhood as opposed to those that are indicative of abuse. The child's developmental stage must be considered in relation to the history of the event, as well as the history of the event and whether medical care was sought at the time of the injury. For example, bruises are common in toddlers and preschool-age children. These bruises often are unilateral and occur on the forehead and bony prominences secondary to normal play activities. Children may even have multiple bruises from multiple falls; again, however, these bruises occur in the areas that are expected for the child's age. Burns that display a pattern consistent with the child spilling a hot liquid are also understandable. A toddler's fracture is a spiral fracture of the tibia that results from the child falling on the affected leg with a twisting motion. Even an adult handprint on a child may have a reasonable explanation. Certain fruit juices, such as citrus juice, will cause a brown discoloration of the skin when exposed to sunlight. If the caregiver had citrus juice on the hands and then placed it on the child, a handprint may appear after exposure to sunlight. Because suspicions of abuse can be emotional for the paramedic and the caregiver (especially if unfounded), the paramedic must take care to consider all possibilities of an injury before attributing it to abuse.

Although the injuries discussed previously have a low index of suspicion of abuse, the paramedic must also be aware of those injuries that have a high suspicion for abuse, such as those listed in Box 39-9. Within this category, head injuries are worthy of particular attention as they are the most common cause of death secondary to physical abuse and generally occur in the setting of shaken baby syndrome. Children may have nonspecific symptoms such as vomiting or seizures and often have no outward signs of head trauma (other than retinal hemorrhages, which are common), nor does the history indicate head trauma. Not only can recognition be difficult for the paramedic, but it has been found that many of these patients are evaluated in the ED setting and the head injury is not discovered. The lack of outward signs of trauma is attributed to the fact that the exterior of the head rarely makes contact with an external object, rather the trauma is caused by the coup-contrecoup mechanism inside the skull, resulting in both intracranial hemorrhages and axonal injuries such as diffuse axonal injury. The classic history given in cases of shaken baby syndrome is one in which the child was sleeping when the caregiver (often a male friend or partner) went to perform some activity in the house. Upon checking on the child the caregiver found that the child had an abnormal outward sign (e.g., apnea, vomiting, seizing). What is omitted from the history is that the child was crying uncontrollably and the caretaker shook the child violently and then put the child to bed where he or she subsequently stopped crying (secondary to the brain injury). More often than not the caregiver will call the mother before seeking medical help (Marx et al., 2006).

Careful documentation of the caregiver's history and the victim's injuries found on examination are essential and should be reported to the receiving hospital and law enforcement. Documentation is critical and should include a description of the scene, general appearance of the child, behavior of those present, and any information available regarding the illness or injury obtained during the physical head-to-toe examination. Mandatory reporting of suspected abuse by paramedics is required in all states.

ELDER ABUSE

[OBJECTIVES 8, 9, 14, 15]

Elder abuse is a significant problem for a highly vulnerable population (Emergency Nurses Association, 2000). Elder abuse was first reported in 1975, and it is estimated that more than 2 million cases of elder abuse occur in the United States each year and that the incidence will continue to grow as the population ages. However, it is also believed that these incidents are underreported and the true annual incidence is unknown (National Center on Elder Abuse, 1997). Factors that are believed to have contributed to the increased incidence of this type of abuse are listed in Box 39-13. The abuser is likely a family member, close friend, or even someone in the healthcare business who is expected to be trustworthy. As with other forms of abuse, elder abuse occurs in all demographic and socioeconomic groups. More often than not the victim lives with the abuser. Geriatric maltreatment often is difficult for the healthcare professional to assess. It can be complicated by preexisting comorbid conditions or those of the normal aging process.

There are three main types of elder abuse, or maltreatment: domestic abuse, institutional abuse, and self-neglect.

Domestic elder abuse is that which occurs in the home of the elderly patient or caregiver. Abusers are most commonly the adult children of the victim, although they may be the spouses, grandchildren, or other relatives and nonrelatives charged with providing care. Neglect is the most common form of domestic elder abuse, and its incidence increased dramatically from 1990 to 1996, during the same time that reported cases of physical abuse declined, as did reported cases of emotional abuse and exploitation (National Center on Elder Abuse, 1997). The typical victim of elder abuse is the female patient who is 78 years of age (National Center on Elder Abuse, 1999), and the gender distribution of the abuser is essentially equally distributed between males and females. More often than not the abuser is dependent on the victim for housing, transportation, or financial support and suffers from cognitive impairment, substance abuse,

BOX 39-13 Factors Contributing to Elder Abuse

- The increased life expectancy of elderly patients with an increase on the dependence of others
- Physical and mental impairments associated with aging
- Decreased productivity
- Limited resources to care for the elderly
- Economic factors such as financial inability to pay for care
- Stress of the middle-age (often children of the patient) caretakers who are responsible for caring for both their parents and their own children

depression, or mental illness (National Center on Elder Abuse, 2002).

There are several theories regarding why domestic elder abuse occurs. One common theory is that the dependency of the victim on the caregiver causes stress in the caregiver, who may lack the knowledge needed to perform the expected functions. As the need for care increases, it is suspected that the stress in the abuser also increases until the abusive incident occurs. However, newer research has challenged this theory, as it has been found that most abusers are in fact dependent on the victim. It also appears that the financial dependency of the abuser on the victim may be a factor in the development of an abusive situation (National Center on Elder Abuse, 2002). Another theory postulates that elderly patients who are in poor health are more likely to be abused than those in good health. There is often a cyclic nature in elder abuse in which tension mounts until the abusive incident occurs; this is followed by a period of calm and reconciliation until the cycle repeats again. A fourth theory is that abusers tend to have more personal problems than nonabusers. This may include financial difficulties, substance abuse problems, or mental impairments. In actuality no single theory can explain the cause of elder abuse; the cause is likely multifactorial and may involve numerous other circumstances that are not part of the current theories regarding elder abuse.

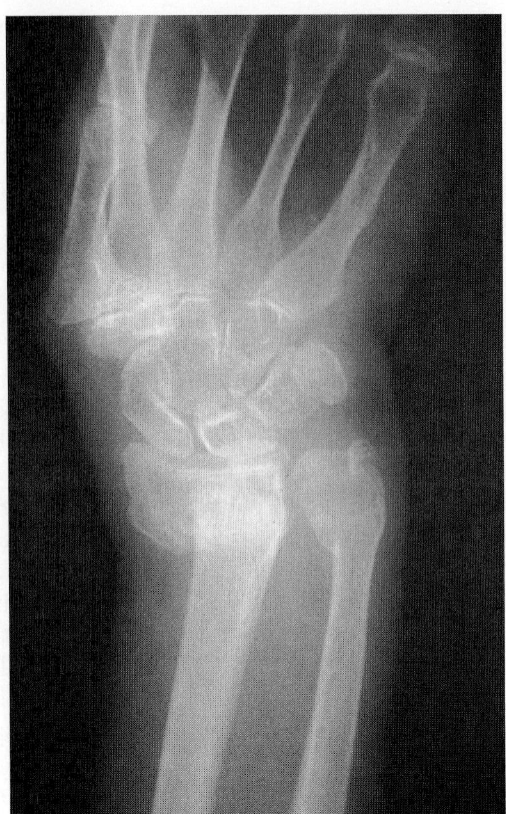

Figure 39-9 Fracture in an older adult.

More than 1.6 million people live in nursing homes, and approximately 1 million live in residential care facilities (Hawes, 2002). Abuse by caregivers in these settings is considered institutional abuse and is usually committed by those who are hired by the facility. These patients often have more significant medical conditions, dementia, and greater needs than their counterparts living at home. They also generally require more assistance in performing normal daily activities. As a result they are more dependent on their caregivers, less able to defend themselves, and at a significant risk for abuse. There are no reliable data regarding the incidence of institutional abuse; however, it is believed to be a significant problem. In interviews with residents of care facilities, many report abuse, rough handling, or witnessing abuse. Additionally many staff of care facilities reported witnessing various forms of abuse (Hawes, 2002). As with any form of abuse, paramedics are obligated to report their suspicions, even when a healthcare facility is involved.

Rather than being abused by another individual, self-neglect occurs when the patient's behavior endangers his or her safety and well-being. This often occurs in the form of refusal to eat, drink, take medications, or perform personal hygiene and other basic necessities of life. However, such activities are not considered self-neglect if the patient is mentally competent and able to understand the consequences of his or her decisions.

Maltreatment is defined as anything that endangers the elderly population, including components similar to those of intimate partner violence. Financial exploitation, deprivation of food or medical care, neglect, intimidation, and physical, sexual, or psychological assault are all possible. Findings associated with the various types of elder abuse are listed in Box 39-14. Physical assault may result in fractures more often than in the younger population because of osteoporosis (Figure 39-9). Psychological abuse may be more difficult to assess; however, witnessing any demeaning or humiliating behavior by the caregiver should concern the EMS crew at the scene. The victim may be reluctant to report because of fear of isolation or loss of control over his or her life. When taking a history and performing an examination, look for signs of malnutrition or dehydration, unexplained fractures, signs of confinement, and head injuries. Careful examination of soft tissue integrity may indicate improper use of restraints if the areas around the wrists or ankles are impaired. Be aware of the verbal and nonverbal interactions between the caregiver and the patient. In addition, take note of the patient's living environment and family dynamics. Attempt to determine if there is unusual tension in the household, if the residence is safe and clean, and if there is adequate food, water, and heat. This information is invaluable in identifying patients at risk for elder abuse and is of great benefit to other healthcare providers. During the history-taking process, acquiring a detailed list of medications is essential. If the patient is slow to respond, consider accidental or intentional overmedication.

The National Committee for the Prevention of Elder Abuse (2005) suggests several ways in which clinicians

BOX 39-14 Indicators of Elder Abuse

Physical Abuse

- Unexplained or inappropriate physical restraint
- A sudden change in behavior
- Unexplained bruises, burns, lacerations, patterned injuries, or other soft tissue injuries
- Unexplained fractures
- Soft tissue injuries in various stages of healing
- Physical signs of punishment
- Complaints of being abused
- Indications of being underdosed or overdosed on medication
- Broken assistive devices such as eye glasses, dentures, or hearing aids

Emotional Abuse

- Complaints or indicators of emotional abuse including:
  - Insults
  - Being treated as a child
  - Threats
  - Humiliation
  - Harassment
- Indicators of forced social isolation
- Sudden withdrawal or decreases in communication
- Increased agitation without a medical explanation
- Behavior generally associated with dementia without medical explanation

Financial Abuse

- Sudden changes in bank accounts or other financial accounts
- Unexpected or abrupt changes in a will or other financial documents
- Sudden and unexplainable transfer of assets to another person
- Disappearance of valuable items or monetary instruments
- Level of care inconsistent with available funds
- Bills not being paid by caregiver despite adequate funds
- Unexplained bank transactions
- Suspicion of forged signatures

Sexual Abuse

- Complaints of sexual abuse
- Unexplained injury to the genitals or anal area
- Bloody, stained, or torn undergarments
- Presence of sexually transmitted disease

Abandonment

- Complaints of being abandoned
- Desertion at a medical facility
- Desertion at a public location

Neglect

- Complaint of substandard care
- Unsanitary living conditions due to the caregiver's neglect
- Lack of care for medical conditions
- Poor personal hygiene due to the caregiver's neglect
- Presence of decubitus ulcers, particularly if untreated
- Evidence of dehydration or malnutrition

Adapted from the National Center on Elder Abuse (2007). *Major types of elder abuse.* Retrieved April 2, 2008, from http://www.ncea.aoa.gov/NCEAroot/Main_Site/FAQ/Basics/Types_Of_Abuse.aspx.

can play a role in early intervention, including the following:

- Identification of somatic signs and symptoms of abuse
- Evaluation of the explanations given for common injuries and conditions (Does the mechanism of injury match what is found on the examination?)
- Assessment of cognitive status and health factors that affect it
- Treatment of injuries that arise from abuse

Documentation is crucial. Legibility and detailed word-for-word comments, in quotes, are extremely helpful in prosecution. Photographic evidence (if possible and appropriate) of the environment and/or injuries also may help law enforcement. As with any crime scene, evidence preservation is necessary.

Mandatory reporting for suspected elder abuse or neglect varies from state to state, so you will need to know the laws where you practice. Education about the signs and symptoms of elder abuse benefits both the crew and community. Active involvement by the EMS staff in addressing findings during a history and physical examination benefits patients and quite possibly will make them feel safe for the first time in a long time.

PARAMEDIC*Pearl*

Although only 42 of the 50 states currently mandate reporting of elder abuse, remember that assault and battery is a crime in all 50 states.

Case Scenario CONCLUSION

En route to the hospital, your partner continues ventilation as you start an intravenous line in the left antecubital fossa. Additional assessment reveals small, sluggishly responsive pupils and bulging fontanels. The cardiac monitor shows sinus tachycardia with no ectopy. SpO_2 on 100% oxygen is 96%. On arrival at the hospital, the infant's condition is unchanged except for an increase in the pulse rate to 130 beats/min. Diagnostic testing in the emergency department revealed a subarachnoid hemorrhage. On further questioning by the hospital staff, the babysitter admitted shaking the baby earlier in the afternoon to get her to stop crying. After stabilization, the patient was flown to a regional tertiary pediatric center. Although she did wake up several days later, the infant had severe permanent neurologic damage. She died of complications almost 1 year later.

Looking back

8. *Do the sluggishly responsive pupils and bulging fontanels relate to your other assessment findings? How?*
9. *If you had known that the baby had been shaken by the babysitter, would you have changed your treatment in any way? Why or why not?*
10. *Given the patient's final disposition, was your treatment appropriate? Why or why not?*

SEXUAL ASSAULT

[OBJECTIVES 6, 7, 11, 16, 17, 18]

Perhaps the most devastating crime that could be perpetrated against another person is that of a **sexual assault** (Lynch, 2005). *Sexual assault* is defined as sexually explicit conduct used as an expression of interpersonal violence against another individual—nonconsenting sexual acts achieved through power and control. Although penetration may be part of a sexual assault, it also includes fondling, kissing, and other forms of touching. *Rape* is defined as an act of violence—nonconsensual sexual aggression involving penetration of a body orifice. The two terms should not be used interchangeably because they have significant legal ramifications depending on the events of the incident.

The incidence of sexual assault continues to increase annually, even in years when the incidence of other violent crimes decreases. Although anyone of any gender and any age can be a victim of sexual assault, women remain the primary victims of this crime. It is unfortunately an extremely common crime, and it is estimated that one in three women and one in seven men will be assaulted during a lifetime. The typical victim is a single female, approximately 20 years of age, who is assaulted by someone she knows, and the younger the victim, the more likely the assailant will be a relative. The "classic view" of an unknown assailant attacking outside is actually one of the less common occurrences in this type of crime. The location of the attack is largely dependent upon the age of the victim. Adults tend to be attacked in their homes, whereas adolescents are assaulted in the attacker's home. Generally weapons are not involved in these assaults; however, in the setting of an attack by a stranger, weapons are typically involved.

When you are first to arrive on the scene of a sexual assault, make every effort to secure and preserve the scene, protect the patient, and afford the victim as much privacy as possible. Depending on local protocols, notify law enforcement on arrival.

After the initial scene size-up and the determination of no life-threatening injuries, assess the patient for minor injuries. Common injuries that may result from a violent sexual assault include abrasions and bruises on the upper limbs, head, and neck (Figure 39-10). Signs of forcible restraint may be evident, such as rope burns or mouth injuries from tape or cloth and petechiae of the face and conjunctiva from choking (Savino & Turveyy,

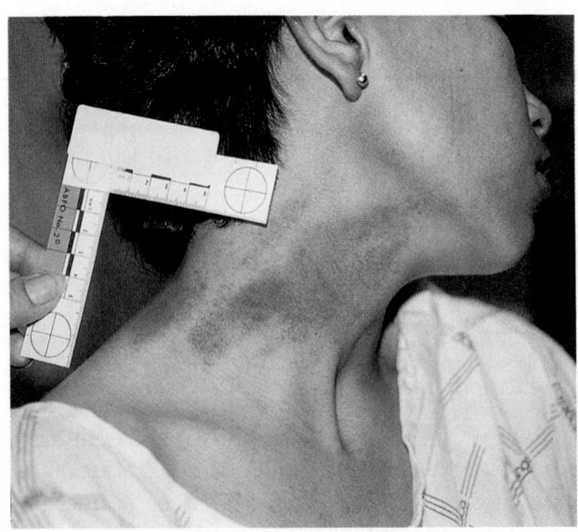

Figure 39-10 Sexual assault: bruising to neck.

2005). The victim may report muscle soreness or stiffness in the shoulders, neck, knee, hip, or back from prolonged positioning that allows sexual penetration. Unless bleeding is profuse, view the genitalia only if absolutely necessary to preserve any evidence that may be present. If possible, a crew member of the same gender should care for the patient. During the history taking and physical examination, remain nonjudgmental, provide support and empathy, calm the patient as much as possible, provide privacy for the patient, and be prepared to answer questions from the victim as directly as possible. The paramedic must understand that anger is a normal part of such an experience and may be directed at the EMS provider. Allow the patient as much control of the situation as possible when appropriate. This may be as simple as asking the patient which partner he or she would prefer to accompany him or her to the hospital and whether he or she would like to lie on the stretcher or sit in the captain's chair (if protocol allows).

Children may also be victims of sexual assault. In these cases the attacker is almost always someone known to them and may be a relative. Although the child may not realize they have been assaulted and may not report the attack, this is a form of sexual abuse. The types of sexual contact, physical findings, and effects are the same as those discussed earlier.

Documentation of what the victim says should be legible, written word for word, and noted by quotes. This information may prove crucial in the courtroom. Do not include personal opinions in the documentation and always follow local protocols for reporting of the assault. Transport the patient to the nearest appropriate facility and ensure safety along the way.

In many communities, sexual assault nurse examiners (SANEs) care for the victims of sexual assault in a specialized manner. The staff of these programs works with other members of a team that address the medical, psychosocial, and legal aspects of the assault. The locations of the examination sites for these victims vary from area to area across the United States. Some of the locations may be within the emergency departments of the hospitals, and others may be in clinic-type centers not associated with one particular hospital. The goal of SANE programs is to work with local law enforcement, EMS, and medical facilities in their respective communities. Protocols vary with each site, but all have specially trained nurses who perform a medical-legal examination. They are responsible for examining the patient, developing a care plan that is specialized based on the findings of the examination, and collecting evidence in accordance with the laws of their locale. They often are called to testify as expert witnesses in court. Knowing your local protocol pertaining to the SANE program, providing that the community in which you work has such a program, can be of great benefit to your patient. Education for both law enforcement and the EMS community regarding the valuable services these programs offer benefits all involved in the care of the sexually assaulted patient (Lynch, 2005).

CREW AND PATIENT SAFETY

[OBJECTIVES 6, 7, 18]

The first priority on any call involving violence or potential violence is personal safety. Law enforcement must be notified as soon as possible if not dispatched on the original call. You must be vigilant in crime scene awareness on arrival and for the duration of the incident. Violence may resume or increase as a crowd develops and additional persons arrive at the scene. This may occur even if law enforcement personnel are on the scene. The responding teams must be aware that the perpetrator may still be on the scene or return to the scene of the crime. EMS crews must take safety precautions because the perpetrator may act violently toward the EMS personnel.

In any violent crime situation, you should not be judgmental. Warning signs of impending violence from those involved can occur. These include becoming verbally abusive to the crew, clenching the fists, or tightening muscles. If the scene becomes dangerous, retreat from the environment until law enforcement can secure the area involved. A safe distance from the area must be a distance that will protect the crew from danger, be out of the line of sight or gunfire, and be far enough away to react to danger if necessary.

As with any incident, collection and preservation of evidence may become part of the call. Once the patient has been assessed and initial treatment has occurred, be observant to the surrounding area. Carry only the necessary equipment, disturb the victim and clothing as little as possible, touch only what is required to care for your patient, and report any findings to the crime scene investigator. If clothing must be removed, preserve it in a paper bag that is sealed, labeled, and turned over to law enforcement personnel. The patient should not be allowed to perform any functions that would destroy evidence, such as urinating, defecating, douching, or bathing; nor should anything be removed from a part of the body that was subject to sexual contact. Ensure you track the history of anything that may become evidence, as this will become an important part of the "chain of evidence" in any subsequent legal proceedings. Provide any evidence to law enforcement and include your name, badge number (if applicable), and unit number, and document the name, badge number, and unit number of the person who received the evidence. In most crime scenes, media personnel present another issue to consider. Be very careful not to make any comments to the press or bystanders about the situation. At a crime scene, EMS personnel are in charge of the patient and law enforcement personnel are in charge of the crime scene (Stoy et al., 2005). In all cases, the EMS team works cohesively with the investigators on the scene.

LEGAL CONSIDERATIONS

[OBJECTIVE 10]

You have legal responsibilities to the patient and the community in which you work. You must follow the guidelines of the scope of practice that is the standard of care in your community. Patient confidentiality is one of the most important matters entrusted to a healthcare professional. Under no circumstances should that trust be broken. When patient transport is required, obtain consent from the patient. If this is not possible, transport under the implied consent rule is still an appropriate response. If the patient is a victim of a violent crime, EMS personnel should do everything possible to preserve evidence and report all findings to the investigator. Paramedics often are required to testify in court in reference to an incident that they were involved in. All personnel must maintain the most current standards of care and be able to present the most professional image while testifying. Continuing education about the legal process will help you become a valuable asset to the criminal process.

Case Scenario SUMMARY

1. *What is your general impression of this patient?* High priority. She is unconscious, unresponsive, and in near respiratory arrest.
2. *What intervention should you initiate at this time?* Secure the airway, assist ventilation, and administer high-flow oxygen. Then perform additional assessment.
3. *What additional questions might be important to ask the babysitter as you continue your assessment?* Helpful answers would include what preceded this episode, especially to determine whether trauma occurred. Any significant past medical history would also be helpful to know.
4. *Is this patient high priority? Why or why not?* Yes. In addition to the obvious alterations in mental and respiratory status, the description of the event suggests the potential for trauma and/or a neurologic disorder.
5. *What are your thoughts about the babysitter's description of the patient "tightening up," arching her back, falling backward, and becoming limp?* The babysitter could be describing a seizure and potential head trauma.
6. *How does the reported mechanism of injury fit into the presentation?* The reported mechanism seems inconsistent with the condition of the child. Although a 6-month-old may be capable of sitting upright on the floor, a fall backward onto carpet wound not likely cause trauma severe enough to produce these symptoms. The disparity between the reported mechanism and the infant's condition increases the index of suspicion for nonaccidental trauma.
7. *What treatment will you initiate at this time?* Immediate transport to a pediatric emergency center is a high priority. En route, continue supportive therapy, including ventilation and establishment of an intravenous line. Given the uncertainly of the mechanism, spinal stabilization might also be considered.
8. *Do the sluggishly responsive pupils and bulging fontanels relate to your other assessment findings? How?* Yes. Bulging fontanels and abnormal pupils suggest increasing intracranial pressure and may be related to other signs of neurologic impairment, such as possible seizure, sudden coma, and unresponsiveness.
9. *If you had known that the baby had been shaken by the babysitter, would you have changed your treatment in any way? Why or why not?* No. Management of the airway, ventilation, and oxygenation are appropriate steps for the management of increasing intracranial pressure.
10. *Given the patient's final disposition, was your treatment appropriate? Why or why not?* Yes. Although local protocols may vary, most would not recommend bypassing an appropriate emergency department to transport this patient directly from the scene to the tertiary pediatric center (which was located in an adjacent city). The patient required stabilization and further diagnostic testing to determine the cause of her sudden neurologic change.

Chapter Summary

- Domestic violence is a tragedy that affects many members of the community every day. It is an epidemic in the United States. A concerted effort from healthcare professionals, social services, the media, and the legal system working together is necessary to end domestic violence in our society. Domestic violence is everyone's problem. The next victim could be someone close to you.
- Interpersonal (intimate) violence may affect the life of every person, either personally or peripherally.
- One in four women will be in an abusive relationship sometime in her life.
- Violence can take many forms: psychological, verbal, physical, or sexual.
- Violence can affect a person of any age, sex, socioeconomic level, ethnicity, or educational level.

- The elderly and children are the most vulnerable populations for unidentified and unresolved abuse.
- Safety is the primary priority at violent crime scenes, and every caution must be used to protect the crew members.
- Reporting requirements vary from state to state regarding the type of abuse or assault. You must be aware of the reporting requirements in your jurisdiction.
- Exact and detailed documentation is essential for all abuse and assault cases.
- Every crime scene needs to be preserved for evidence collection, working collaboratively with law enforcement.

REFERENCES

Aehlert, B. (2005). *Comprehensive pediatric emergency care.* St. Louis: Elsevier.

American College of Emergency Physicians. (2000). *Domestic violence: The role of EMS personnel.* Retrieved October 1, 2006, from www.acep.org.

American Humane Association. (2007). *Child neglect.* Retrieved February 23, 2008, from http://www.americanhumane.org.

Child Welfare Information Gateway. (2006). *Recognizing child abuse and neglect: Signs and symptoms factsheet.* Retrieved March 29, 2008, from http://www.childwelfare.gov.

Emergency Nurses Association. (2000). *Trauma nursing core curriculum* (5th ed.). Lynch, VA: Emergency Nurses Association.

Emergency Nurses Association. (2004). *Emergency nursing pediatric course* (3rd ed.). Lynch, VA: Emergency Nurses Association.

Hawes, C. (2002). *Elder abuse in residential long-term care facilities: What is known about prevalence, causes, and prevention (Testimony before the U.S. Senate Committee on Finance), June 18, 2002.* Retrieved March 29, 2008, from http://finance.senate.gov.

Marx, J., Hockberger, R., & Walls, R. (2006). *Rosen's emergency medicine* (6th ed.). St. Louis: Elsevier.

National Center on Elder Abuse. (1997). *Trends in elder abuse in domestic settings.* Washington, DC: National Center on Elder Abuse.

National Center on Elder Abuse. (1999). *Types of elder abuse in domestic settings,* Washington, DC: National Center on Elder Abuse.

National Center on Elder Abuse (2002). *Domestic abuse in later life.* Washington, DC: National Center on Elder Abuse.

National Committee for the Prevention of Elder Abuse. (2005). *Health and medical professionals.* Retrieved October 1, 2006, from http://www.preventelderabuse.org.

Savino, J. O., & Turveyy, B. E. (2005). *Rape investigation handbook.* St. Louis: Elsevier.

Stoy, W. A., Platt, T. E., & Lejeune, D. A. (2005). *EMT-basic textbook* (2nd ed.). St. Louis: Elsevier.

U.S. Department of Health and Human Services, Administration on Children, Youth, and Families. (2007). *Child maltreatment 2005.* Washington, DC: U.S. Government Printing Office.

SUGGESTED RESOURCES

Burnett, L. B. (2006). *Domestic violence.* Retrieved February 25, 2008, from http://www.emedicine.com.

Child Welfare Information Gateway. http://www.childwelfare.gov.

Gay and Lesbian Medical Association. http://www.glma.org.

Girardin, B. W., Faugno, D. K., Seneski, P. C., Slaughter, L., & Whelan, M. (1997). *Color atlas of sexual assault.* St. Louis: Mosby.

Jensen, L. A. (2000). The cycle of domestic violence and the barriers to treatment. *Nurse Practitioner, 25*(5), 26-29.

National Center on Elder Abuse. http://www.elderabusecenter.org.

National Children's Advocacy Center. http://www.nationalcac.org.

National Committee to Prevent Elder Abuse. http://www.preventelder abuse.org.

National Committee to Prevent Child Abuse. 800-835-2671.

National Organization for Victim Assistance. 800-TRY-NOVA.

National Sexual Violence Resource Center. http://www.nsvrc.org.

National Victim's Constitutional Amendment Network. http://www.nvcan.org.

Parker, B. (2000). Intimate partner violence. *Issues Mental Health Nursing, 1*(2), 145.

Polsky, S. S., & Markowitz, J. (2004). *Color atlas of domestic violence.* St. Louis: Mosby.

U.S. Department of Justice: *Elder justice.* www.usdoj.gov/archive/elderjustice.htm.

U.S. Department of Justice. (2004). *A national protocol for sexual assault medical forensic examinations, adult/adolescents.* Washington, DC: Office of Violence Against Women.

Chapter Quiz

1. The underlying issue with all domestic violent relationships is _____.

a. a desire to nurture another
b. a private family matter
c. loving someone too much
d. power and control

2. Domestic violence is the leading cause of injuries to women between the ages of _____.

a. 15 and 44 years
b. 18 and 45 years
c. 20 and 40 years
d. 30 and 50 years

Chapter Quiz—continued

3. Characteristics or behaviors commonly displayed by the abuser in the prehospital setting are _____.
  a. allowing the victim to answer all questions regarding current illness or injury
  b. appearing charming, concerned, and solicitous of the EMS crew
  c. appearing uncaring and insensitive to the situation
  d. leaving the victim alone with the paramedics

4. The cycle of abuse begins with _____.
  a. control of the victim's finances
  b. forced sexual activities
  c. physical violence
  d. verbal attacks

5. You are dispatched to the home of an injured woman. She is bleeding from her face and has a laceration across her nose and left eyebrow. She states that she had an argument with her husband and it was her fault. He obviously is intoxicated. What is your first consideration?
  a. Administering a breathalyzer to see whether the woman is intoxicated as well
  b. Removing the woman from the home as quickly as possible
  c. Scene safety
  d. Stopping the bleeding

6. You are called to an upscale neighborhood, where the victim is lying on the couch in the living room. You recognize the victim's name as one of the prominent judges in town. The patient is reporting severe gastrointestinal pain. The patient denies any nausea, vomiting, or diarrhea. Past medical history reveals that the patient has been transported to the emergency department for the same complaint on many previous occasions. What should you consider when assessing this patient?
  a. Ask the patient, when alone, if domestic violence is a problem.
  b. Assume that this chronic problem is "all in the patient's head" or that this may be a drug-seeking problem.
  c. Because the patient's complaint is medical, the potential for abuse is low.
  d. Treat this incident as a chronic medical condition and transport the patient.

7. You are dispatched to a call regarding an injury to a child at a private residence in a low-socioeconomic section of the city. On arrival you are greeted by the parent and are informed that the child has suffered burns to the feet. The parent states the child stepped in a bucket of hot cleaning water when the parent was not looking. The child appears to have special needs but is alert and crying. She is easily consoled by the EMS crew. On examination, full-thickness and partial-thickness burns are on the top of the foot only. What might make the crew suspicious that this may be a case of abuse?
  a. Only one caregiver is in the household.
  b. Special needs children are at a lower risk for abuse.
  c. The mechanism of injury does not correlate with the injuries observed.
  d. The victim appears to be poor and the house is dirty.

8. Which ocular finding is associated with shaken baby syndrome?
  a. Conjunctivitis
  b. Glaucoma
  c. Iritis
  d. Retinal hemorrhage

9. Elder abuse may be difficult to assess in the prehospital setting because _____.
  a. it is an infrequent occurrence outside a nursing home
  b. of normal physiologic processes that affect the geriatric population
  c. the caregiver may be the only one capable of answering questions
  d. the elderly fall all the time, so injuries are expected

10. You are dispatched to a scene of a possible sexual assault. On arrival you discover a 27-year-old woman who is curled in the fetal position and is wearing minimal clothing. You notice several footprints surrounding her, and beer bottles are in the vicinity. She is able to answer your questions from across the scene. Your first priority after your initial conversation is to _____.
  a. begin interviewing the patient on arrival about the history of the assault in front of all the bystanders
  b. pick up the patient's clothes and transport them with the patient so that they do not get lost
  c. preserve the crime scene as much as possible while waiting for law enforcement to arrive and secure the scene
  d. treat the patient and transport regardless if law enforcement has arrived

11. While taking the history from a victim of sexual assault, you should _____.
  a. ask for clarification of what the patient is trying to verbalize
  b. delay the head-to-toe exam until arrival at the hospital for the privacy of the patient
  c. document your personal conclusion regarding the incident and whether you believe a sexual assault actually occurred
  d. remain as nonjudgmental as possible

12. When an EMS crew is dispatched to a crime scene, they must ________.

a. assist law enforcement with the evidence collection
b. attempt to capture the perpetrator if still present on the scene and law enforcement has not yet arrived
c. ensure that personal safety is their first priority
d. intervene with any patients despite the evidence of unsafe conditions

13. When considering legal ramifications of any case that the prehospital provider is involved with, the first priority is _____.

a. confidentiality
b. departing the scene as quickly as possible
c. relating the incident, including the patient's name, to others in the station if it was an unusual case
d. speaking to the media about the incident when asked for comments

Terminology

Child maltreatment An all-encompassing term for all types of child abuse and neglect including physical abuse, emotional abuse, sexual abuse, and neglect.

Economic abuse Preventing others from having or keeping a job; forcing control of another's paycheck; restricting access or forcing conditions on others to receive an allowance; stealing money; not allowing others to know about or have access to economic assets.

Honeymoon phase A period of remorse by the abuser, characterized by the abuser's denial and apologies.

Intimate partner violence and abuse (IPVA) Also called *domestic violence,* this is a learned pattern of assaultive and controlling behavior, including physical, sexual, and psychological attacks as well as economic control, which adults or adolescents use against their intimate partners to gain power and control.

Neglect Failure to provide the basic needs to an individual.

Patterned injuries Those that leave a distinctive mark indicating that an object was used in the assault (e.g., cigarette burns, electrical cord whipping, human bites, glove injuries, attempted strangulation, slaps).

Petechiae A tiny pinpoint rash on the upper area of the neck and the face; may indicate near-strangulation or suffocation; caused by an occlusion of venous return from the head while arterial pressure remains normal; may be present in mothers after childbirth.

Physical abuse Inflicting a nonaccidental physical injury on another person such as punching, kicking, hitting, or biting.

Psychological abuse The verbal or psychological misuse of another person, including threatening, name calling, ignoring, shaming unfairly, shouting, and cursing; mind games are another form of psychological abuse.

Sexual abuse Forced and/or coerced sex, violent sexual acts against the victim's will (rape), or withholding sex from the victim; includes fondling, intercourse, incest, rape, sodomy, exhibitionism, sexual exploitation, or exposure to pornography. According to the National Center on Child Abuse and Neglect, to be considered child abuse these acts have to be committed by a person responsible for the care of a child (e.g., babysitter, parent, daycare provider) or related to the child. If a stranger commits these acts, it is considered sexual assault and handled by the police and criminal courts.

Sexual assault Sexually explicit conduct used as an expression of interpersonal violence against another individual; nonconsenting sexual acts achieved through power and control.

Tension-building phase Period when tension in the relationship is high and heightened anger, blaming, and arguing may occur between the victim and the abuser.

CHAPTER 40

Patients with Special Challenges

Objectives

After completing this chapter, you will be able to:

1. Describe the various etiologies and types of hearing impairments.
2. Recognize the patient with a hearing impairment.
3. Anticipate accommodations that may be needed to manage the patient with a hearing impairment.
4. Describe the various etiologies of visual impairments.
5. Recognize the patient with a visual impairment.
6. Anticipate accommodations that may be needed to manage the patient with a visual impairment.
7. Describe the various etiologies and types of speech impairments.
8. Recognize the patient with a speech impairment.
9. Anticipate accommodations that may be needed in order to properly manage the patient with a speech impairment.
10. Describe the various etiologies of obesity.
11. Anticipate accommodations that may be needed to manage the patient with obesity.
12. Describe paraplegia/quadriplegia.
13. Anticipate accommodations that may be needed to manage the patient with paraplegia/quadriplegia.
14. Define *mental illness.*
15. Describe the various etiologies of mental illness.
16. Recognize the presenting signs of the various mental illnesses.
17. Anticipate accommodations that may be needed to manage the patient with a mental illness.
18. Define the term *developmentally disabled.*
19. Recognize the patient with a developmental disability.
20. Anticipate accommodations that may be needed to manage the patient with a developmental disability.
21. Describe Down syndrome.
22. Recognize the patient with Down syndrome.
23. Anticipate accommodations that may be needed to manage the patient with Down syndrome.
24. Describe the various etiologies of emotional impairment.
25. Recognize the patient with emotional impairment.
26. Anticipate accommodations that may be needed to manage the patient with emotional impairment.
27. Define *emotional/mental impairment* (EMI).
28. Recognize the patient with an emotional or mental impairment.
29. Anticipate accommodations that may be needed to manage the patient with an emotional or mental impairment.
30. Describe the following diseases/illnesses:
    - Arthritis
    - Cancer
    - Cerebral palsy
    - Cystic fibrosis
    - Multiple sclerosis
    - Muscular dystrophy
    - Myasthenia gravis
    - Poliomyelitis
    - Spina bifida
    - Patients with a previous head injury
31. Identify the possible presenting sign(s) for the following diseases/illnesses:
    - Arthritis
    - Cancer
    - Cerebral palsy
    - Cystic fibrosis
    - Multiple sclerosis
    - Muscular dystrophy
    - Myasthenia gravis
    - Poliomyelitis
    - Spina bifida
    - Patients with a previous head injury
32. Anticipate accommodations that may be needed in order to properly manage the following patients:
    - Arthritis
    - Cancer
    - Cerebral palsy
    - Cystic fibrosis
    - Multiple sclerosis
    - Muscular dystrophy
    - Myasthenia gravis
    - Poliomyelitis
    - Spina bifida
    - Patients with a previous head injury
33. Define *cultural diversity.*
34. Recognize a patient who is culturally diverse.
35. Anticipate accommodations that may be needed to manage a patient who is culturally diverse.
36. Identify a patient who is terminally ill.
37. Anticipate accommodations that may be needed to manage a patient who is terminally ill.
38. Identify a patient with a communicable disease.
39. Recognize the presenting signs of a patient with a communicable disease.
40. Anticipate accommodations that may be needed to manage a patient with a communicable disease.
41. Recognize sign(s) of financial impairments.
42. Anticipate accommodations that may be needed to manage the patient with a financial impairment.

Chapter Outline

Case Scenario

You have arrived on scene for a 31-year-old man who has cerebral palsy and cannot walk. The patient is deaf and asks you to speak directly at him so that he can read your lips. He is easy to understand when he speaks. He states he has a temperature of 101°F and wants to be seen by a doctor because he doesn't "feel well." His pulse is 118, respirations 20, blood pressure 118/62, and pulse oximetry is 100% on room air. His skin is warm and moist.

Questions

1. *What are some important things to remember when obtaining a history from this patient?*
2. *What is your impression of this patient?*
3. *What should be your next interventions?*
4. *How would your interaction change if this patient were visually impaired versus deaf?*

The purpose of this chapter is to give the paramedic information about how to interact with and treat patients with special challenges. With the increased usage of specialized technology, infants survive life-threatening illnesses and birth anomalies to become productive adult citizens. Children and adults are successfully resuscitated from critical illness or injury only to require rehabilitation or special adaptive devices to function. This population is at a higher risk for emergencies. It is important to be proactive and learn about this unique group before being called to treat them (Figure 40-1).

Many myths and prejudices surround individuals with disabilities. Many people wrongly believe that if something is different about a "part" of a person, the "whole" person is affected. For example, healthcare professionals tend to talk *about* a child with developmental disability instead of talking *to* that child. In this chapter, the paramedic will learn the importance of treating illness or injury first and the disability or special challenge second.

PHYSICAL CHALLENGES

Patients with ongoing physical challenges may require special considerations during the assessment and management process. The following physical challenges are presented in this chapter: hearing impairment, visual impairment, speech impairment, obesity, paraplegia, and quadriplegia.

Hearing Impairment

[OBJECTIVES 1, 2, 3]

Some patients may have preexisting hearing loss. **Deafness** is a complete or partial inability to hear. This impairment ranges from complete hearing loss to a patient who is simply hard of hearing.

For older adults, hearing loss is very common. It is estimated that about one third of Americans older than 60 years and between 40% and 50% of those 75 years and older have some type of hearing loss (National Institute on Deafness and Other Communication Disorders, 2005b).

There are two main types of hearing loss. **Conductive hearing loss** occurs when there is a problem with the transfer of sound from the outer to the inner ear. Sound waves are blocked and cannot reach the cochlea. It may be caused by the accumulation of earwax, infection (e.g., otitis media), or from some type of injury to the eardrum or middle ear (e.g., barotrauma). It is usually temporary and can be reversed by medical treatment of the cause.

Sensorineural hearing loss occurs when the tiny hair cells in the cochlea are damaged or destroyed. In addition, the auditory nerve is damaged such that sounds are not transmitted from the cochlea to the brain. It is usually permanent and may affect the way the patient speaks.

Presbycusis is hearing loss that occurs from changes in the inner ear, auditory nerve, middle ear, or outer ear.

It comes on gradually as the person ages and commonly affects higher-pitched sounds. It can also be caused by loud noise, head injury, heredity, illness, infection, certain prescription drugs (e.g., some antibiotics, aspirin, rapid administration of furosemide), or circulation problems such as high blood pressure. It mainly affects people over the age of 50 and makes it difficult for the person to tolerate loud sounds or to hear what other people say (National Institute on Deafness and Other Communication Disorders, 2005b). See Table 40-1 for a summary of types of hearing loss.

Tinnitus is a ringing, roaring sound, or hissing in the ears that is usually caused by certain medicines, such as aspirin, or exposure to loud noise. It is not a disease but rather a symptom, so it can be present with any type of hearing loss.

Some types of hearing loss occur at birth. There may be an injury during the birthing process or some damage to the fetus as it developed (e.g., a mother who contracted rubella during pregnancy). Other forms show up later in life. **Otosclerosis** is an abnormal growth of bone that prevents structures in the ear from working properly. It is thought to be a hereditary disease.

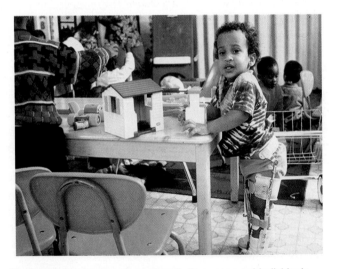

Figure 40-1 Many myths and prejudices surround individuals with disabilities.

Loud noise is one of the most common causes of hearing loss and can permanently damage the inner ear. Every day, more than 30 million Americans are exposed to damaging noises; and about 10 million Americans have already permanently damaged their hearing. Baby boomers are experiencing hearing loss much sooner in their lives than their parents and grandparents did (National Institute on Deafness and Other Communication Disorders, 2005b). This loss is preventable and can be avoided by limiting exposure to noises above 90 decibels in loudness (e.g., loud music, motorcycles, firecrackers, gas lawn mowers, snow blowers).

Communication is usually the greatest challenge. Determine the child's or adult's usual method of communication by talking to the family, school personnel, or long-term care personnel.

- If the patient reads lips, face the person whenever speaking; however, recall that this is not an adequately acquired skill in most persons with congenital deafness, and at best only one third of words are understood.
- Try not to use complicated language or large words.
- Talk at a slow and even pace.
- Do not exaggerate your pronunciation.
- Provide paper and pencil if the patient wants to write a note.
- If the patient uses sign language, ask for help from anyone present. Remember that an injury to the hands or upper extremities may greatly hamper the patient's ability to communicate through sign language.
- Consider using pictures to show basic medical procedures. Laminate pictures of routine treatments, and keep them in the emergency vehicle.

A hearing aid may amplify sound, enabling the person to hear. A whistling noise may be present if the device is not secured into the ear.

A patient with a hearing impairment will notice nonverbal communication much more readily. Remain calm, use a gentle touch when treating the patient, and establish eye contact whenever possible. Actively demonstrate

TABLE 40-1 Hearing Loss Classifications

Type	Conductive	Sensorineural	Combination
Location of problem	Outer/middle ear	Inner ear/auditory nerve	Outer/middle ear and inner ear/ auditory nerve, in combination
Characteristics	Most common Interference with sound volume (loudness)	Sometimes called *perceptive* or *nerve deafness* Sound distortion Trouble identifying one sound from another (discrimination)	Interference with sound transmission, usually in the middle ear and neural pathways

your intent to understand what the patient is trying to communicate.

If the patient has severe deafness, notify the receiving hospital as soon as possible. The hospital can then provide appropriate personnel such as an interpreter to assist the patient. More information regarding communicating with deaf and hard of hearing patients can be found in Chapter 15.

Visual Impairment

[OBJECTIVES 4, 5, 6]

Some patients have preexisting visual impairment that varies from complete loss of sight (blindness) to blurred vision. **Partially sighted** refers to a person who has some type of visual problem and may need assistance. **Low vision** refers to individuals who are unable to read a newspaper at the usual viewing distance even if they use glasses or contact lenses. It is not limited to distance vision and can be a severe visual impairment. **Legally blind** refers to a person who has less than 20/200 vision in at least one eye or has a very limited field of vision (e.g., 20 degrees at its widest point). **Totally blind** refers to anyone who has no vision and uses nonvisual media or reads via Braille (National Dissemination Center for Children with Disabilities, 2004).

Normal vision depends on the uninterrupted passage of light from the front of the eye to the light-sensitive retina at the back of the eye. Anything that obstructs this passage of light can cause vision loss (Box 40-1).

Visual impairments occur in approximately one fifth of people over the age of 70 years. It puts this group of Americans at a greater risk of falls and injuries and is an important cause of disability and limitation of activity in this age group (National Center for Health Statistics, 2005).

A patient who has a central loss of vision is usually aware of the condition. Patients who have a loss of peripheral vision may not realize it until it is well advanced. These are the patients who are more prone to injury. For example, the patient's decreased sight may have caused the injury for which emergency care has been requested, such as injury from a fall that occurred from tripping over an object that was not seen.

These patients may be very frightened during an emergency because they cannot see what is happening. Remember that people with any type of visual impairment may have heightened hearing or smell to compensate for their visual loss.

- Orient the patient to whatever care or treatment is being provided.
- "Lead" ambulatory patients instead of "pushing" them.
- Explain any movements in position, such as moving the stretcher from the home to the back of the ambulance.
- Retrieve visual aids if necessary and take them to the hospital.
- Notify staff at the hospital so that appropriate assistance can be available.

Some individuals with visual impairments use a guide dog for assistance. This animal is not a pet and has been highly trained. The patient may be very concerned about the dog to the point where he or she will not agree to treatment until plans are made for the dog. Make necessary arrangements to transport assistive animals to the hospital. This may be in the ambulance, a supervisor's vehicle, law enforcement, or some other method of immediate transportation. Transportation of the dog should not be deferred "until a family member arrives" or for any other reason. Do not touch a guide dog until the patient releases the dog. If the patient does not wish to have the dog transported to the hospital, enlist the help of a caregiver, friend, or relative to care for the dog. If no one is available and willing to care for the dog, request assistance from the local police to make sure someone assumes responsibility for care of the dog. If the dog was injured, relay that information as well.

BOX 40-1 Causes of Visual Impairments

- Cataracts
- Glaucoma
- Macular problems that result in visual disturbances
- Degeneration of the eyeball, optic nerve, or nerve pathways
- Disease (e.g., diabetes, hypertension)
- Eye or brain injury
- Infection (e.g., cytomegalovirus, herpes simplex virus, bacterial ulcers)
- Vitamin A deficiency in children living in developing countries

Speech Impairment

[OBJECTIVES 7, 8, 9]

Speech impairments include disorders of language, articulation, voice production, or blockage of speech (fluency). All of these can lead to an inability to communicate effectively (Box 40-2).

Language disorders usually result from a stroke, a head injury, or brain tumors that cause damage to the language centers of the brain. These patients often demonstrate **aphasia** or loss of speech with a slowness to understand speech and problems with vocabulary and sentence structure. Expressive and receptive aphasia can appear in both children and adults and may affect their ability to speak and/or to comprehend written or spoken words. Delayed development of language in a child may result from hearing loss, lack of stimulation, or emotional disturbance.

Apraxia is a neurologic disorder that results from dysfunction of the cerebral hemispheres of the brain. This

BOX 40-2 Causes of Speech Impairments

Language Disorders

- Stroke
- Brain tumor
- Head injury
- Hearing loss
- Delayed development
- Lack of stimulation
- Emotional disturbance

Articulation Disorders

- Damage to nerve pathways passing from the brain to muscles in the larynx, mouth, or lips
- Delayed development from hearing problems
- Slow maturation of nervous system

Voice Production Disorders

- Disorders affecting closure of vocal cords
- Hormonal or psychiatric disturbance
- Severe hearing loss

Fluency Disorders

- Stuttering

dysfunction causes an inability to execute skilled voluntary movements despite having the desire to perform the movements and being able to demonstrate normal muscular function associated with the movements. **Verbal apraxia,** or apraxia of speech, is a speech disorder in which the person has difficulty saying what he or she wants to say in a correct and consistent manner. It can be acquired or developmental. Acquired apraxia can happen at any age but usually occurs in adults. Damage to parts of the brain involved in speaking (e.g., due to illness, tumor, head injury, or stroke) cause apraxia, resulting in the loss or impairment of existing speech abilities. Developmental apraxia of speech is present from birth and is diagnosed in children. It can be mild, in which the person only has occasional problems pronouncing words with many syllables, or severe, in which the person may not be able to communicate at all using speech (National Institute on Deafness and Other Communication Disorders, 2005a).

Dysarthria is an articulation disorder in which the patient is not able to produce speech sounds. This disorder results from damage to the nerve pathways passing from the brain to the muscles of the larynx, mouth, or lips. In many instances, the patient's speech will be slurred, indistinct, slow, or nasal. Disorders of articulation may result from brain injury such as cerebral palsy and diseases such as multiple sclerosis. In children, they are commonly the result of delayed development from hearing problems.

Voice production disorders are characterized by hoarseness, harshness, inappropriate pitch, and abnormal nasal resonance. They often result from disorders that affect closure of the vocal cords. Some disorders are caused by hormonal or psychiatric disturbances and by severe hearing loss.

Fluency disorders are not well understood. They are marked by repetitions of single sounds or whole words and by blocking of speech. An example of a fluency disorder is stuttering.

Once a speech impairment has been identified, modify the history taking and assessment process as follows:

- Provide extra time for the patient to respond to questions.
- Avoid displays of impatience.
- Provide a pen and paper if use of these materials will facilitate the communication.

Work with other people at the scene, if available, who know the person's style of communication. Examples of communication styles may include a language notebook with pictures or written words or an electronic communication device such as a portable computer that writes and/or produces words.

BOX 40-3 Body Mass Index

BMI is a measurement tool used to determine excess body weight.

Calculation: (Weight in pounds) divided by (height in inches)^2 × 703 = BMI

For example: Weight = 180 lb, Height = 5′10″ (70″)

Calculation: [180 ÷ (70)^2] × 703 = 25.82

BMI of 25 or more → overweight

BMI of 30 or more → obese

BMI of 40 or more → morbidly obese

From Centers for Disease Control and Prevention, 2008. Retrieved June 5, 2008 from http//www.cdc.gov.

BMI, Body mass index.

Obesity

[OBJECTIVES 10, 11]

Obesity is an excessively high amount of body fat or adipose tissue in relation to lean body mass (Centers for Disease Control and Prevention, 2002). **Overweight** refers to the state of increased body weight in relation to height. **Morbid obesity** is a body mass index (BMI) of 40 or more, which is comparable to being approximately 100 pounds more than ideal weight (Centers for Disease Control and Prevention, 2005).

Body mass index (BMI) is a calculation strongly associated with subcutaneous and total body fat and with skinfold thickness measurements. It is used to screen for childhood obesity and to measure adult obesity (Box 40-3). BMI does not account for muscle mass and can be misleading in weightlifters.

Obesity is a **chronic** disease, has a strong familial component, and is the second leading cause of unneces-

BOX 40-4 Complications of Obesity

Physical Complications

- Arthritis
- Coronary artery disease
- Early disability and death
- Higher risk for impaired mobility
- Hypertension
- Ischemic stroke
- Orthopedic complications caused by bearing excess weight
- Pulmonary dysfunction (including asthma)
- Sleep apnea
- Some forms of cancer
- Type 2 diabetes mellitus

Emotional Complications

- Discrimination at work and school
- Eating disorders
- Feelings of depression and rejection
- Isolated and/or stigmatized socially
- Low self-esteem
- Poor body image

sary death. In the United States, approximately 127 million adults are overweight, 60 million are obese, and 9 million are morbidly obese. Approximately 15.3 percent of children (ages 6 to 11) and 15.5 percent of adolescents (ages 12 to 19) are obese (American Obesity Association, 2005).

Obesity is associated with many other physical complications (Box 40-4). When it becomes severe, it can interfere with normal daily activities and cause bodily pain. Adults may be unable to perform their chosen occupation and become so compromised that they qualify for disability payments.

Treatment for obesity includes weight loss programs, exercise, counseling, medications, and in some cases, surgery. The goal of treatment is permanent weight loss.

Caring for an obese patient may require special considerations.

- The history of present illness and past medical history may be extensive. Allow time to gather the pertinent details.
- Carry equipment that is large enough to accommodate the person's size. A large blood pressure cuff is necessary to get an accurate measurement.
- Be sensitive to the patient who is self-conscious about his or her size.
- Act professional at all times. Do not joke about the patient's weight.
- Request extra personnel as necessary to move the patient to the ambulance as well as from the ambulance into the hospital (Figure 40-2).

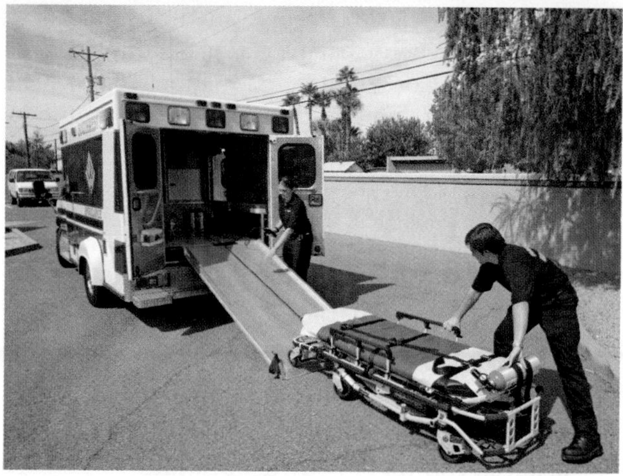

Figure 40-2 Some EMS services have specialized equipment and vehicles to care for bariatric patients.

Paraplegia and Quadriplegia

[OBJECTIVE 12]

Spinal cord injuries damage the spinal cord and result in varying degrees of ability after the injury. Most instances result in some degree of paralysis or weakness. **Paraplegia** is weakness or paralysis of both legs and possibly the trunk. **Quadriplegia** (also called *tetraplegia*) is weakness or paralysis affecting the level below the neck and chest area, involving all four extremities.

Nerve damage to the brain and spinal cord may be caused by a motor vehicle crash, gunshot wound, sports injury, or fall. For example, an injury to the cervical spine and cord from diving into a shallow amount of water can cause quadriplegia. The injury is complete when there is no voluntary movement or sensation below the level of the injury. An incomplete injury may result in some functioning below the primary level of the injury such that the person can move one limb more than the other, feel parts of the body that cannot move, or have more functioning on one side of the body than the other.

Medical illnesses may also cause paralysis or weakness. When a cancerous tumor invades the spinal cord, deterioration of the spinal cord and attached nerves occurs and causes paraplegia or quadriplegia, depending on the level of the tumor.

There are approximately 8000 spinal cord injuries in the United States each year, with the majority of them (82%) involving males between the ages of 16 and 30. Overall, quadriplegia occurs in slightly more than half of all injuries. After age 45, the proportion of people with quadriplegia increases dramatically. After age 60, two thirds of all spinal cord injuries cause quadriplegia. After age 75, 87% of all injuries cause quadriplegia. Approximately 92% of all sports injuries involving the spinal cord result in quadriplegia (The National Spinal Cord Injury Association, 2005).

Approximately 450,000 people in the United States live with some type of paraplegia or quadriplegia (The National Spinal Cord Injury Association, 2005). They usually have other complications in addition to the loss of sensation and/or motor functioning. These include:

- Loss of involuntary functions with very high injuries from C1 to C4 (e.g., the ability to breathe, requiring the use of a mechanical ventilator or diaphragmatic pacemaker)
- Low blood pressure
- Inability to regulate blood pressure effectively
- Dysfunction of bowel and/or bladder
- Sexual dysfunction (decreased fertility in men)
- Reduced control of body temperature
- Inability to sweat below the level of injury, making the person more prone to heat exhaustion and heat stroke
- Chronic pain

PARAMEDIC*Pearl*

Note preexisting paraplegia or quadriplegia in patients who have had a previous spinal cord injury. Also look for areas of weakness.

Special Considerations

[OBJECTIVE 13]

During the assessment, it is important to know whenever possible the type of deficit that existed before the present emergency. Was the patient already paralyzed, or is the numbness and tingling the patient reports a result of the present injury or illness?

The amount of sensation in the body usually varies from person to person. Individuals with no sensation are particularly susceptible to hazards such as burns or other injuries because they cannot feel dangerous things, such as scalding water or hot grease. They also may not feel an ankle being caught in the spokes of a wheelchair. Remember to determine the mechanism of injury and maintain a high level of suspicion for hidden trauma.

The level of bladder and bowel function may also vary. Some people accomplish elimination of waste products through a surgically created opening on the abdomen called a *stoma* or **ostomy.** More common terms *ileostomy* and *colostomy* relate to procedures for fecal elimination. An **ileostomy** is a surgical formation of an opening of the ileum onto the surface of the abdomen, through which fecal matter is emptied. A **colostomy** is a surgical formation of an opening of the colon onto the surface of the abdomen, through which fecal matter is emptied. Feces are collected in special appliances or clear plastic containers that attach directly over the opening. These appliances, or pouches as they are also known, are emptied and changed periodically. Ostomies are covered in more detail in Chapter 42.

If the spinal cord injury was recent, the patient may be at home with a traction device. For a cervical injury, a halo traction device may be in place to stabilize the spine (Figure 40-3). This device may complicate airway management and make patient transport more difficult.

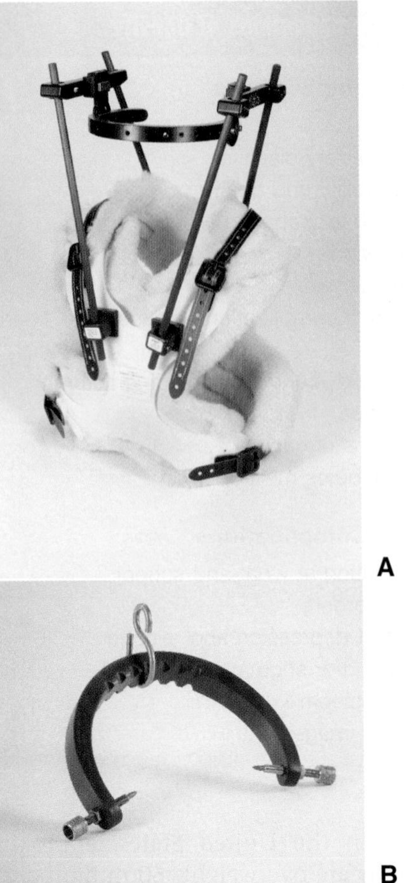

Figure 40-3 Cervical skeletal traction can be applied using a "halo" device. The halo is a metal ring that is secured to the skull with pins and to metal rods attached to a fitted jacket. **A,** Halo device from PMT Corporation (Chanhassen, Minn.). **B,** Traction tong.

Many people with **physical disabilities** use some type of adaptive device, such as a wheelchair, braces, crutches, or a combination of devices. Some people also may use corrective splints at different times during the day or night.

- Ask the patient, family, or caregivers to explain the particular device. Use their knowledge to examine underlying tissue when it is necessary to perform a more thorough physical examination.
- Remember that splints or braces can serve as tools for immobilization if trauma is suspected, as long as there is no damage to the equipment. However, if circulation or breathing is impaired or major bleeding is present, these devices should be removed.
- If a wheelchair is used, make sure someone assumes responsibility for getting it back to the patient's room, home, or personal care facility (Figure 40-4).

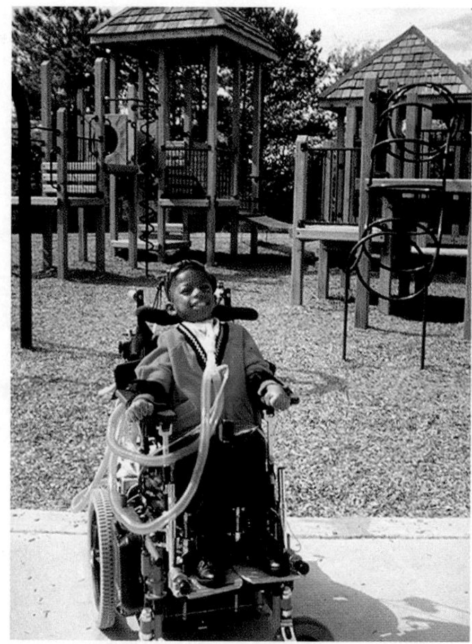

Figure 40-4 Many people with physical disabilities use some type of adaptive device, such as a wheelchair. If a wheelchair is used, make sure someone assumes responsibility for getting it back to the patient's room, home, or personal care facility.

- Additional personnel may be needed to move the patient from the home to the ambulance and from the ambulance to the stretcher in the emergency department.

MENTAL CHALLENGES

Mental Illness

[OBJECTIVES 14, 15]

Mental illness refers to any form of psychiatric disorder (Box 40-5). It is a biologically based brain disorder and can profoundly disrupt a person's thinking, moods, ability to relate to others, feelings, and capacity for coping with the demands of life. Two broad categories are psychoses and neuroses.

Psychoses comprise a group of mental disorders in which the individual loses contact with reality. Psychosis is thought to be related to complex biochemical disease that disorders brain function. Examples include schizophrenia, bipolar disease (also known as *manic-depressive illness*), and organic brain disease.

Neuroses are diseases related to upbringing and personality in which the person remains "in touch" with reality. Neurotic symptoms generally do not limit work or social activity and tend to fluctuate in intensity with stress. Major neurotic disorders include depression, phobias, and obsessive-compulsive behavior.

Mental illnesses commonly strike individuals in the prime of their lives, often during adolescence and young adulthood. The young and the old are especially vulnerable, although all ages are susceptible.

In North America, Europe, and increasingly throughout the world, mental disorders are the leading cause of lost years of productive life. Untreated mental illness costs more than 100 billion dollars each year in the United States (Nation's Voice on Mental Illness, 2005).

BOX 40-5 Types of Mental Illness

- Attention deficit/hyperactivity disorder
- Autism and pervasive developmental disorders
- Bipolar disorder
- Borderline personality disorder
- Major depressive disorder
- Obsessive-compulsive disorder
- Panic and other severe anxiety disorders
- Schizoaffective disorder
- Schizophrenia

Special Considerations

[OBJECTIVES 16, 17]

Recognizing a patient who is mentally challenged may be difficult, especially when caring for patients with mild neuroses whose behavior may be unaffected. Others with disorders that are more serious may present with signs and symptoms consistent with mental illness.

When obtaining the patient history, ask about the following:

- History of mental illness
- Prescribed medications
- Compliance with prescribed medications
- Use of over-the-counter herbal products (e.g., St. John's Wort is used as an antidepressant)
- Concomitant use of alcohol or other drugs

If the patient appears to be paranoid or shows anxious behavior, ask the patient's permission before beginning any assessment or performing any procedure. Once rapport and some form of trust have been established, proceed in the same manner as for a patient who does not have a mental illness (unless the call is related specifically to the mental illness). These patients will experience illness and injury like all other patient groups.

Patients who are dangerous to themselves or others at the scene may need to be chemically or physically restrained. Speak with medical control if needed to receive an order for these procedures. If a patient demonstrates aggressive or combative behavior, summon law enforcement personnel to ensure scene safety.

Developmental Disabilities

[OBJECTIVES 18, 19, 20]

Developmental disabilities involve some degree of impaired adaptation in learning, social adjustment, or maturation. A developmental disability occurs when the brain does not develop properly, resulting in an inability to learn at the usual rate. These impairments generally occur before age 22, and there is a substantial functional limitation in three or more areas of major life activity, such as self-care, receptive and expressive language, learning, mobility, self-direction, capacity for independent living, and economic self-sufficiency. Causes include the following:

- Metabolic disorders
- Infections
- Intracranial hemorrhage
- Anoxia
- Inherited disorders (e.g., Down syndrome)
- Trauma
- Any other entity that damages the brain

Delays may be of varying severity and may affect any or all of the major areas of human achievement. That includes development of the ability:

- To walk upright
- Of fine hand-eye coordination
- Of listening, language, and speech
- Of social interaction

The primary difficulty encountered in emergency medicine is obtaining an accurate and complete history. Maladaptive behaviors may be present in these individuals, further hampering this ability. Accommodations may be necessary when providing patient care. Examples include allowing adequate time for gathering a history, performing assessment and patient management procedures, and preparing the patient for transport. Often nonverbal clues such as facial expressions and body language can be helpful in obtaining a history.

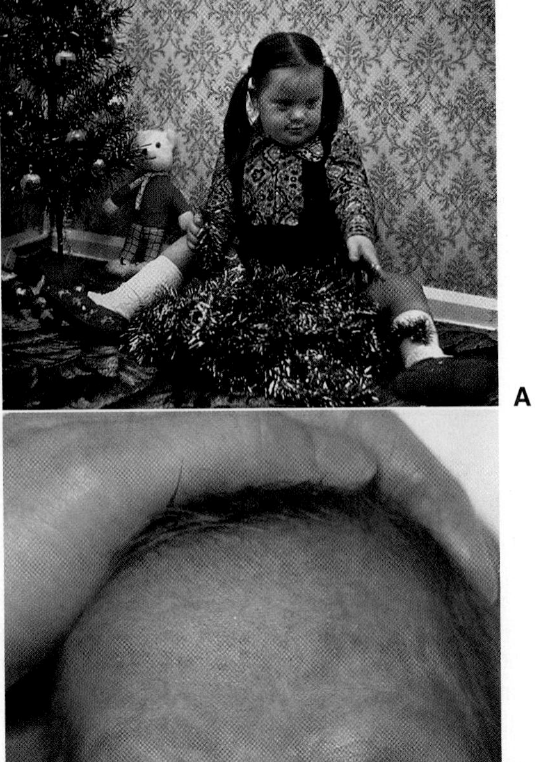

Figure 40-5 **A,** A girl with Down syndrome. **B,** The eyes of an infant with Down syndrome.

Down Syndrome

[OBJECTIVES 21, 22, 23]

Down syndrome is the most common chromosomal abnormality of a generalized syndrome and occurs in one in approximately every 730 live births (Figure 40-5). Because of advancements in clinical treatment and medical technology, up to 80 percent of adults with Down syndrome live to be 55 or older. It is predicted that within the next 10 years, the number of people with Down syndrome will double (National Down Syndrome Society, 2003).

Down syndrome is a developmental disorder that causes **mental retardation.** Children and adults with Down syndrome range from severely retarded to having average intelligence. Most people with Down syndrome, however, have a mild to moderate range of retardation. Trisomy 21 is the most common form because it involves a third chromosome 21. Box 40-6 outlines certain features that are typically seen with Down syndrome.

Up to 50% of people with Down syndrome also have some form of congenital heart defect (National Down Syndrome Society, 2005). Many people have this defect corrected during infancy or childhood yet may still have cardiac problems throughout their lives. Other medical complications include intestinal disorders, hearing defects, and other illnesses.

BOX 40-6 Characteristics of Down Syndrome

- Enlarged anterior fontanel
- Flat nasal bridge
- Flat occiput
- Poor muscle tone
- Mottled skin
- Protruding abdomen
- Small mouth, large or protuding tongue
- Reduced birth weight
- Rounded and small skull
- Short and broad hands with stubby fingers
- Short stature
- Shortened rib cage
- Upward slant to the eyes with short, sparse eyelashes

Several considerations are necessary when treating a patient with Down syndrome.

- Adjust assessment and treatment strategies based on the level of understanding of the person with Down syndrome. Allow extra time to obtain a history and explain procedures whenever possible.
- Because of the large and possibly protruding tongue, airway maneuvers may be more difficult.

- Decreased muscle tone may compromise respiratory expansion. Monitor respirations and respiratory effort closely when an illness or trauma occurs.
- Decreased muscle tone also affects gastric motility, making this patient more prone to vomiting. Have adequate suction equipment readily available.

Emotionally Impaired

[OBJECTIVE 24, 25, 26]

Persons with emotional impairments include those with nervous exhaustion, anxiety neurosis, compulsion neurosis, and hysteria. All of these disorders can result in a wide range of physical or mental symptoms attributed to mental stress in someone who is not psychotic.

It may be difficult to distinguish between symptoms produced by stress and those that indicate serious medical illness. Therefore management should always focus on the chief complaint, and the serious etiology should be assumed.

Signs and symptoms that may result from emotional impairment include somatic complaints such as chest discomfort, tachycardia, dyspnea, choking, and syncope. It is important to gather a complete history from the patient and to perform a thorough examination to rule out serious illness. Prehospital care for these patients, in the absence of serious illness, is primarily supportive and includes calming measures and transport for physician evaluation.

Emotionally/Mentally Impaired

[OBJECTIVES 27, 28]

Emotional/mental impairment (EMI) refers to persons who have impaired intellectual functioning (e.g., mental retardation), which results in an inability to cope with normal responsibilities of life (Table 40-2). In the United States, approximately 3 of every 100 persons has mental retardation (The Arc, 2001). Approximately 613,000 children from ages 6 to 21 have some type of mental retardation and require special education in school (U.S. Department of Education, 2002).

The diagnosis of mental retardation is no longer an automatic sentence for seclusion in a long-term care facility. Children and adults with mental retardation may be involved in the community, hold jobs, vote, and so on, depending on their level of ability.

TABLE 40-2 IQ Classifications

Classification	IQ Score
Borderline intellectual functioning	71-84
Mild mental retardation	55 to approx. 70
Moderate mental retardation	35-40 to 50-55
Severe mental retardation	20-25 to 35-40
Profound mental retardation	Less than 20 or 25

Data from American Psychiatric Association. (1994). *Diagnostic and statistical manual of mental disorders, fourth edition (DSM-IV)*. Arlington, VA: American Psychiatric Association.
IQ, Intelligence quotient.

Special Considerations

[OBJECTIVE 29]

Accommodations that may be necessary during patient care will vary by the patient's level of impairment. Many people with mild impairment show no psychological symptoms other than slowness in carrying out mental tasks. Others with moderate to severe involvement may have limited to absent speech, and neurologic impairments are common. These patients may require extra time and care in patient assessment, management, and transportation.

PATHOLOGIC CHALLENGES

Physical injury and disease may result in pathologic conditions that require special assessment and management skills. Specific pathologic challenges presented here include arthritis, cancer, cerebral palsy, cystic fibrosis, multiple sclerosis, muscular dystrophy, myasthenia gravis, poliomyelitis, spina bifida, and patients with a previous head injury.

Arthritis

[OBJECTIVES 30, 31, 32]

Arthritis is the inflammation of a joint that results in pain, warmth, stiffness, swelling, and redness. The disease has many forms and varies widely in its effects. Two common forms of arthritis are osteoarthritis and rheumatoid arthritis. **Osteoarthritis** results from cartilage loss and wear and tear of the joints. It is common in elderly patients. **Rheumatoid arthritis** is an autoimmune disorder that damages joints and surrounding tissues (Figure 40-6). It is seen in children and adults.

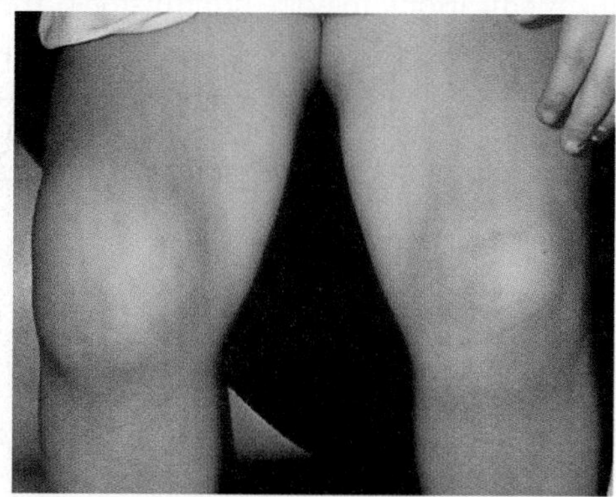

Figure 40-6 This toddler has juvenile rheumatoid arthritis. Note the swelling and slight redness of the child's right knee.

The most common complaint associated with arthritis is pain, which can be acute, chronic, or acute in a patient with a chronic disease. Therefore a complete history should be obtained that includes a prior diagnosis of arthritis if one has been made, as well as compliance with medications, and speed of onset of symptoms. Patients often complain of generalized joint pain as opposed to focal pain that is more commonly associated with tendinitis or bursitis. Patients with arthritis often have decreased range of motion and mobility that may limit the physical examination. However, when possible, the physical examination should include each joint in which the patient complains of pain. Assess for warmth, deformity, range of motion, pain associated with motion, tenderness, and muscle atrophy. Note where these findings are present and, in the setting of pain, the type of movement that causes it—flexion, extension, active, or passive.

Take measures to promote patient comfort whenever possible. Other considerations include:

- Get a complete list of medications, such as analgesics. Consider side effects of current medications before administering pain medications to these patients.
- During movement and transport, take into account the patient's limited mobility. Adjust the equipment to "fit the patient." Do not try to conform the patient to the equipment. When using splints and backboards, extra padding may be necessary to fill all of the voids.

Cancer

[OBJECTIVES 30, 31, 32]

Cancer is a group of diseases that allow for an unrestrained growth of cells in one or more of the body organs or tissues. The malignant tumors most commonly develop in organs and tissues such as the lungs, breasts, intestine, skin, stomach, and pancreas. These cells may also invade the bone marrow, bone, muscle, or the lymphatic system.

Patients with cancer are often very ill, and the signs and symptoms of their disease depend on the cancer's primary site of origin. Try to obtain a thorough history to include a list of all medications. Anticancer drugs and some pain medications may be administered through a surgically implanted port (see information in Chapter 42 about vascular access devices). Transdermal skin patches that contain analgesic agents are also common, and a thorough evaluation should be performed to determine their presence.

Cerebral Palsy

[OBJECTIVES 30, 31, 32]

Cerebral palsy (CP) is a nonprogressive neuromuscular disability in which the person has difficulty controlling the voluntary muscles due to damage to the fetal brain during the later months of pregnancy, during birth, during the newborn period, or in early childhood. It is often diagnosed during the child's first year of life when parents notice unusual muscle tone during holding or feeding difficulties. Disability can range from mild to severe and is fixed, meaning that it does not become progressively worse as the child ages (Figure 40-7). The disorder is common, affecting 1 to 2 people per 1000.

Causes of cerebral palsy include:

- Cerebral dysgenesis or abnormal cerebral development (most common)
- Fetal hypoxia
- Birth trauma
- Maternal infection
- **Kernicterus** or excessive fetal bilirubin; associated with hemolytic disease
- Postpartum encephalitis, meningitis, or head injury

The disorder is often associated with epilepsy and disorders of speech and vision. Intellectual disturbances are common and occur if defects or lesions occur during development of the brain. However, many people with CP have a normal level of intelligence. They are not mentally retarded and may in fact be highly intelligent. Many children with CP develop keen thinking skills because their physical activities are usually limited.

In individuals with severe CP, swallowing may be compromised, which puts them at a higher risk for respiratory difficulties. Airway obstruction can occur from increased secretions or food left in the mouth.

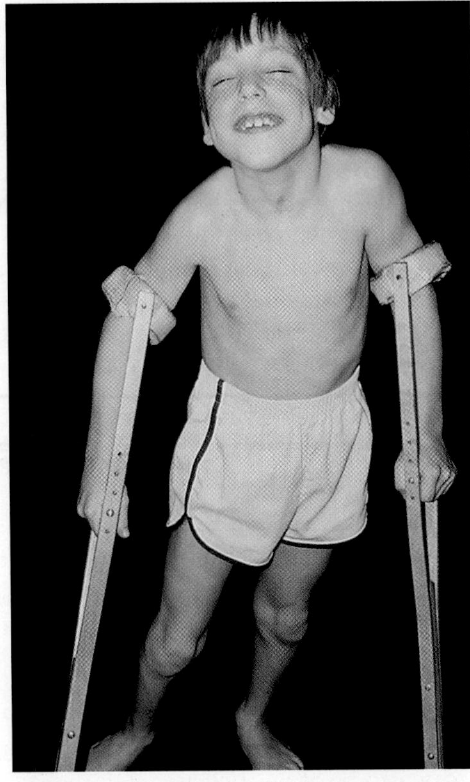

Figure 40-7 Cerebral palsy is a neuromuscular disability consisting of difficulty in controlling the voluntary muscles because of damage to a portion of the brain. This child requires crutches to walk, seizure medication, and a specialized education program.

PARAMEDIC*Pearl*

In patients with cerebral palsy, pay special attention to the respiratory status. Be prepared for airway obstructions caused by increased secretions or food. In addition, be gentle when moving the patient during the physical examination so as not to cause any further harm.

The spastic type of CP accounts for 70% to 80% of cases and presents with the most visual evidence of motor disability. These patients have muscles that are stiff and permanently contracted. Certain muscle groups have an unusually strong tone that can keep portions of the body, particularly the extremities, in characteristic positions. For example, the legs may be crossed with the toes pointed. The patient's fists may be clenched with the upper arm pressed against the wall of the chest. In addition, the head may be extended with the back arched. Deformities of the foot may cause patients to walk on their toes and have associated clonus of the ankle, increased deep tendon reflexes, and a positive Babinski sign. Patients may develop spastic biplegia in which only the lower extremities are affected. This results in atrophy of the lower extremities with disproportionate growth of the upper extremities. In its most severe form, spastic CP can result in spastic quadriplegia in which all the extremities show motor impairment and muscle atrophy. Although approximately 30% of patients with spastic CP will experience a seizure in the first year of life and approximately 25% have cognitive disabilities, those with spastic quadriplegia have an even higher association of seizures and mental retardation.

It is important not to forcefully manipulate the patient with spastic CP when performing the physical examination. Gently attempt to move the extremity to the position desired. If this movement is not possible, document the posturing and continue the assessment. For instance, if the patient's right arm is flexed across the chest, extending the arm to check a blood pressure may not be possible. Use the other arm or document why a blood pressure was not taken if both arms are involved. If possible, wrap a cuff around the patient's thigh and use the popliteal artery behind the knee.

Athetoid CP affects 10% to 20% of patients with CP. It results from damage to the cerebellum or basal ganglia. Because these structures are responsible for smooth coordinated movements, this condition is characterized by slow, involuntary writhing movements of the muscles, particularly those in the face, arms, and torso. These patients may have problems speaking, eating, reaching, and grasping. Swallowing problems may occur secondary to grimacing or protrusion of the tongue. Patients may also be at an increased risk of falls, as they often have difficulty maintaining their posture when sitting or walking.

Ataxic CP affects approximately 5% to 10% of CP patients. It is characterized by low muscle tone, poor coordination of movements, and decreases in depth perception and the sense of balance. As a result these patients often have a wide and unsteady gait with associated tremors. These patients are also at an increased risk of falls and may take longer to perform tasks such as signing paperwork.

Mixed CP affects approximately 10% of CP patients. These patients exhibit signs of both spastic and athetoid CP because of injuries to multiple areas of the brain. Generally these patients show signs of spasticity followed by an increase in involuntary movements. However, other combinations are possible (Marx, 2005).

Cystic Fibrosis

[OBJECTIVES 30, 31, 32]

Cystic fibrosis (CF), or mucoviscidosis, is an inherited metabolic disease of the lungs and digestive system that manifests in childhood. The disease is caused by a defective, recessive gene located on chromosome 7 that is inherited from each parent. The function of this gene is to create a protein called *cystic fibrosis transmembrane regulator,* which regulates chloride channels. In the absence of this protein, chloride is unable to enter cells in amounts necessary for cellular function. The disease occurs in approximately 1 in every 3000 births in Caucasians, and approximately 1 in 25 people in this population are carriers of the gene. It has a much lower incidence in minority populations, occurring in 1 in 17,000 births in African Americans, and 1 in 90,000 births in the Asian population of Hawaii.

The defective gene causes the glands in the lining of the bronchi to produce excessive amounts of thick mucus. Because of defects in the movement of chloride across the epithelium of the airway, there is a reduced ability of the cilia to clear mucus from the airway, a decrease in the antimicrobial abilities of the airway, and an increase in bacterial adhesion in the airway. These factors predispose the patient to chronic lung infections, which, along with progressive lung disease, are the most common causes of morbidity and mortality in patients with CF. In addition the lack of chloride channels in the pancreatic duct does not allow for the normal exchange process that allows the secretion of sodium bicarbonate and water into the pancreatic duct and eventually the duodenum. This leads to the retention of pancreatic enzymes, which causes irreversible destruction of the exocrine portion of the pancreas and can lead to pancreatitis. These enzymes are required for the breakdown of carbohydrates, fats, proteins, and nucleic acids, which ultimately causes them to be absorbed from the small intestine. Because of the lack of these enzymes, patients are not able to absorb these nutrients and can suffer from malabsorption and malnutrition despite a normal diet. These alterations in metabolism cause classic symptoms of CF that include the following:

- Pale, greasy-looking, and foul-smelling stools, often noticeable soon after birth
- Chronic sinusitis and rhinorrhea

- Persistent cough that eventually produces a viscous, purulent, greenish sputum
- Wheezing and shortness of breath
- Lung infections that often develop into pneumonia, bronchiectasis, and bronchitis
- Stunted growth secondary to malabsorption of nutrients
- Abnormally salty sweat
- Failure to thrive (in some cases)
- Late onset of puberty and sterility in 95% of males and 20% of females

Patients often experience pulmonary exacerbations of CF in which there is an increase in their cough, the associated sputum, and weight loss. Over the years these exacerbations become more frequent and lead to further loss of lung function, increase in residual volume, and changes in forced vital capacity and forced expiratory volume, all leading to eventual respiratory failure. Blood may be present in the sputum secondary to infection, and life-threatening hemoptysis is possible. Other signs of chronic hypoxia develop as the patient ages including distal clubbing and cor pulmonale. In addition to the pulmonary aspects of CF, it has several effects on the gastrointestinal tract. This can lead to distal intestinal obstructions causing right lower quadrant pain, a sometimes palpable mass, anorexia, and vomiting. This can mimic appendicitis, which is also common in patients with CF. The exocrine pancreas is destroyed as described previously, but the endocrine pancreas is initially unaffected. However, over time the function of the pancreatic beta cells is impaired, resulting in hyperglycemia and the need for insulin.

During the 1950s the life expectancy of a child with CF was such that they were not expected to survive until elementary school. However, with advances in medicine the life expectancy is now between 30 and 40 years of age. Still, most patients have a permanent colonization of bacteria in the airway leading to chronic pulmonary infection. Diagnosis is generally made by the presence of clinical signs and symptoms and increased levels of chloride in the sweat. This is determined by an analysis of the patient's sweat, or a "sweat test." Older patients and parents of children with CF are usually aware of their disease. Some patients may be oxygen-dependent and require respiratory support as well as suctioning to clear the airway of mucus and secretions.

The goals of respiratory treatment in CF are to increase clearance of mucus from the respiratory system and to reduce respiratory infections. The clearance of mucus is accomplished through the use of percussive therapy to loosen and expel mucus; the inhalation of aerosolized hypertonic saline to promote the movement of water into the respiratory system, thereby thinning mucus; and the administration of inhaled mucolytics. Oral antibiotics are generally administered to reduce respiratory infections; however, in the setting of severe or resistant infections, IV antibiotics are administered. The gastrointestinal effects of CF are often treated with the oral administration of pancreatic enzymes contained in capsules (Braunwald, 2001).

Expect a lengthy history and physical examination because of the nature of the disease and associated medical problems. Some patients will have received heart and lung transplants and may require transfer to specialized medical facilities for treatment.

If parents are unaware of the possibility of CF in the presence of signs and symptoms as previously described, advise the physician at the receiving hospital of any suspicions of the disease.

Multiple Sclerosis

[OBJECTIVES 30, 31, 32]

Multiple sclerosis (MS) is a progressive and incurable autoimmune disease of the central nervous system, whereby scattered patches of myelin in the brain and spinal cord are destroyed. Scarring and destruction of the tissues cause symptoms that range from numbness and tingling to paralysis and incontinence.

The cause of MS is unknown; however, it may have a hereditary, environmental, or viral component. One theory suggests that genetic predisposition interacts with an environmental trigger or an infection to produce T cells oriented to attack the central nervous system, causing areas of scarring called *lesions* or *plaques*, which result from destruction of the myelin sheath, or demyelination. After a long period of inactivity (10 to 20 years), another stressor trigger activates these T cells, which produce a pathologic inflammatory response, resulting in the clinical symptoms of MS. The disease usually begins early in adult life, becomes active for a brief time, and then resumes years later. MS, which affects nearly 350,000 people in the United States, is second only to traumatic injury as a leading cause of neurologic impairment in early adulthood. However, many people with MS lead active, normal lives between exacerbations of their illness.

Signs and symptoms of MS may occur singly or in combination and may last from several weeks to several months (Box 40-7). Attacks vary in intensity and may be precipitated by injury, infection, or physical or emotional stress. Some patients become disabled, bedridden, and incontinent early in middle life. Patients who are disabled also often suffer from painful muscle spasms, constipation, urinary tract infection, skin ulcers, and mood swings.

The neurologic effects of MS can be either positive or negative. Positive effects are the result of the formation of ectopic neurologic impulses, or inappropriate communication between neurons (a "short circuit"). Negative effects result from conduction blocks or conduction delays of the nervous impulses. The presence of blocks and delays can be variable, which explains why the severity of symptoms can vary from day to day and even hour to hour. Symptoms can be variable and in fact may be so subtle that the patient may not seek treatment for years.

BOX 40-7 Signs and Symptoms of Multiple Sclerosis

- Weakness
- Fatigue
- Facial weakness
- Coordination difficulties
- Cerebellar dysfunction
- Loss of dexterity
- Hyperreflexia
- Ataxia
- Increased falls
- Sensory loss
- Paresthesia
- Visual disturbances
- Nystagmus
- Vertigo
- Memory disorders
- Attention difficulties
- Difficulty solving problems
- Impaired judgment
- Urinary urgency
- Urinary hesitancy
- Urinary incontinence
- Constipation
- Impotence
- Extremities that feel heavy and become weak
- Spasticity

Symptoms of MS can be divided into the following major classifications based on the part of the brain affected:

- Changes in mental status and impaired thinking
- Cranial nerve abnormalities
- Difficulties with motor function and sensory function
- Sexual, bowel, and bladder dysfunction

To be diagnosed with this condition, a patient must have at least two clinical episodes of different neurologic symptoms that occurred at different times. Field diagnosis is impossible, and the origin of the call is often for a fall. However, it is a condition to be suspected in young, otherwise healthy patients (especially female) who have recurrent neurologic impairments (with visual changes often being the first described). History-taking will need to be comprehensive to connect the many different symptoms that occur at different times, which at first may not seem to be related. Physical examination should be equally comprehensive because many organ systems are involved. Prehospital treatment involves control of symptoms and supportive care. MS represents a classic case emphasizing the importance of empathetic and sensitive paramedical care even in apparently frustrating cases. Patients with MS can be inappropriately "written off" as psychiatric patients, malingerers, or drug seekers by many providers because of their many vague, migratory, and intermittent neurologic symptoms before the correct diagnosis is made. Long-term management includes medications, physical therapy, and counseling.

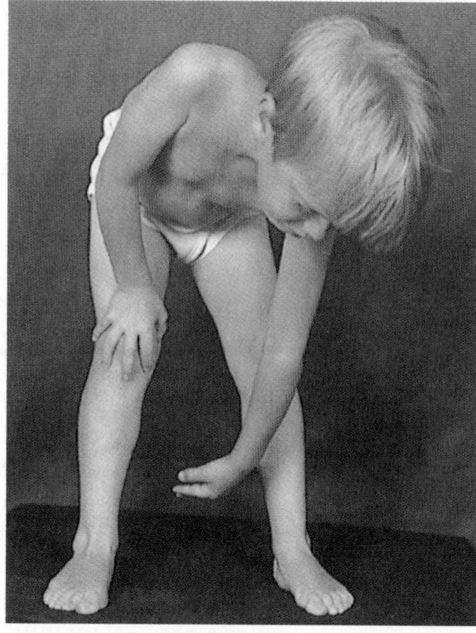

Figure 40-8 Duchenne muscular dystrophy. This 5-year-old boy has difficulty rising from the floor. The support of one hand on the knee is needed to move to an erect position.

Some patients with MS may be difficult to examine and may be unable to provide a complete medical history because of the nature of their illness. Allow extra time for patient assessment and preparation for transport. Do not expect the patient to walk. In severe cases, provide respiratory support as necessary.

Muscular Dystrophy

[OBJECTIVES 30, 31, 32]

Muscular dystrophy is a group of inherited muscle disorders that results in a slow but progressive degeneration of muscle fibers, leading to increasing weakness that spreads over the entire body. The disease is classified according to the age that symptoms first appear, the rate at which the disease progresses and the way in which it is inherited. Muscular dystrophy is incurable.

The most common form is Duchenne muscular dystrophy, caused by a sex-linked, recessive gene that affects mostly males, occurring in approximately 30 of every 100,000 male children (Figure 40-8). The defective gene is responsible for the production of dystrophin, a protein normally found in muscle tissue and the brain. Without dystrophin, muscles develop incorrectly and become weak. It is rarely diagnosed before the age of 3, as it is usually recognized when the child fails to reach normal developmental milestones of muscular activity. Affected children frequently fall and are unable to keep up with their friends when playing.

Signs and symptoms include a child who is slow in learning to sit up, stand, and walk. In order to stand, patients will often roll onto their stomach, push themselves up, and then use their arms to "climb up the legs." This is referred to as *Gower's sign*. Muscles become bulky as they are replaced by fat. Often at approximately 6 years of age the affected child will develop skeletal and spinal abnormalities such as lordosis, or "swayback," and will tend to walk on the toes (toewalking) as a compensation. By age 10, braces are usually needed for walking and joint contractures become evident. By puberty most children will be unable to walk and are confined to wheelchairs. This immobility causes the skeletal muscles and other soft tissues to become contracted, and further atrophy occurs. Because dystrophin is found in the brain, some degree of mental retardation is often seen. Many do not live past their teenage years because of chronic lung infections and heart failure. Others with less common forms of muscular dystrophy, however, may live well into their middle years with varying degrees of muscle weakness.

Accommodations may be required during emergency care depending on the person's age, weight, and severity of the disease. For example, young children will be relatively easy to examine and prepare for transport. Older patients may require additional staff and resources to assist with moving the patient to the ambulance. In severe cases, respiratory support may be indicated.

Myasthenia Gravis

[OBJECTIVES 30, 31, 32]

Myasthenia gravis is an autoimmune disorder in which muscles become weak and tire easily. The disorder is caused by the attack of lymphocytes on the acetylcholine receptors found on the voluntary skeletal muscle side of neuroeffector junctions. Fewer receptors are available to be stimulated, and the antibodies of the immune system often attach to the receptors, blocking them from being stimulated. When the presynaptic neuron releases acetylcholine, instead of stimulating a muscle contraction as normal, the neurotransmitter is blocked. This condition is usually an acquired immunologic disorder, but it can be caused by inherited problems of the neuroeffector junction. The cause of this disorder is believed to be related to the thymus, an endocrine gland important in the body's immunity.

Areas commonly affected include the muscles of the eyes, face, throat, and extremities. It is a rare disease that can begin suddenly or gradually. Myasthenia gravis can occur at any age but usually appears in women between ages 20 and 30 and in men between ages 70 and 80 (Myasthenia Gravis Foundation of America, 2005). It is estimated that there are approximately 36,000 individuals with myasthenia gravis in the United States; however, it is possible this number is higher because many cases are undiagnosed or misdiagnosed.

Classic signs and symptoms include the following:

- Drooping eyelids (ptosis)
- Double vision
- Difficulty speaking
- Facial weakness results in a "snarl" when the patient smiles
- Difficulty in chewing and swallowing
- Difficult extremity movement
- Weakened respiratory muscles

The affected muscles become worse with use but may recover completely with rest. The onset of signs and symptoms can be sudden and may be exacerbated by infection, stress, medications, and menstruation. Often the muscle weakness fluctuates. In many patients it is better in the morning and worsens as the day goes on, particularly in muscles that are extensively used. Myasthenia gravis usually becomes worse over time. The symptoms often go away for periods, only to return. After 15 to 20 years, the condition will become the most severe, and the muscles that are affected most will atrophy and shrink. A myasthenic crisis occurs when the muscles of respiration become involved, causing the respiratory rate and tidal volume to slow until the patient enters into respiratory arrest. This often occurs without any findings other than a history of myasthenia gravis.

Myasthenia gravis can often be controlled with anticholinesterase medications to improve the transmission of nerve impulses in the muscles. Removal of the thymus gland may improve the condition. Immunosuppression is effective in nearly all patients if other methods of treatment are ineffective. In a small number of patients, the disease will progress to paralysis of the throat and respiratory muscles and may lead to death.

Accommodations required for care will vary based on the patient's presentation. In most cases, supportive care and transport will be all that is required. In the presence of respiratory distress, take precautions to ensure an adequate airway, provide ventilatory support, and apply a pulse oximeter, capnography, and cardiac monitor.

Poliomyelitis

[OBJECTIVES 30, 31, 32]

Poliomyelitis is an infectious disease caused by *Poliovirus hominis*. Poliovirus is usually transmitted by direct fecal-oral contact, indirect contact with saliva or feces, respiratory secretions, or contaminated water. The virus enters the body through the mouth, multiplies in the intestine, and then spreads to lymph nodes and the blood. Once multiplied, the virus tends to attack the motor neurons of the spinal cord and brainstem. This can cause signs and symptoms with variable severity, ranging from asymptomatic infection to a febrile illness without neurologic sequelae to aseptic meningitis and finally to paralytic disease including respiratory paralysis and possible death.

The incidence of polio has declined since the Salk and Sabin vaccines were made available in the 1950s. However, the disease may affect adults and indigent children who are not immune, as well as immigrants from other countries. There continue to be sporadic cases each year with the diagnosis of poliomyelitis.

Approximately 95% of infections are asymptomatic. Signs and symptoms of polio that do occur are after an incubation period of 7 to 14 days. In both the nonparalytic and paralytic forms. these symptoms include fever, malaise, headache, and intestinal upset. In the majority of cases, persons with the nonparalytic form of polio recover completely. Paralysis occurs in fewer than 10% of patients, and in this situation extensive paralysis of muscles of the legs and lower trunk can occur.

Post-polio syndrome can affect polio survivors decades after they have recovered from the initial infection, although it does not affect all survivors. The cause is unknown; however, it may be related to the degeneration of nerves in the muscles that survived the initial infection. It is thought that these nerves cannot accommodate the additional stress of compensating for lost nerves and eventually slowly deteriorate. Patients affected by post-polio syndrome experience a new onset of weakness in the same muscles that were affected by the original infection, as well as muscles that did not appear to be affected at the time.

Symptoms include a slow and progressive muscle weakness, generalized fatigue, easily fatigued muscles, and muscle atrophy. Weakness can be asymmetric in some cases. Pain may be present from joint degeneration, and skeletal deformities are common. Patients follow an unpredictable pattern of decline in muscular function. This includes periods of stability in their symptoms followed by the onset of new motor dysfunction. The severity of post-polio syndrome depends on the severity of the initial infection. Patients who had mild symptoms with the original infections will likely have mild symptoms, whereas patients who had severe symptoms with the original infection may develop severe fatigue and muscle atrophy. It is important to note that, when taking a history, many polio survivors were too young to remember the severity of the original infection (National Institute of Neurological Disorders and Strokes, 2007).

Caring for a patient with paralytic polio who has respiratory paralysis may require advanced airway support to ensure adequate ventilation. If the lower body is paralyzed, catheterization of the bladder may be indicated. Additional resources and staff may be needed to prepare the patient for transport. Patients who are experiencing post-polio syndrome may need to be reassured that they are not experiencing polio again and are not contagious to others. As with polio, there is no definitive treatment for post-polio syndrome.

Spina Bifida

[OBJECTIVES 30, 31]

Spina bifida is the number one disabling birth anomaly in the United States. The back portion of the vertebrae fails to close, usually in the area of the baby's lower back. Meninges, the spinal cord, or both may protrude through this opening. Spina bifida is categorized based on the exposure of the meninges and the spinal cord. In spina bifida occulta there is no exposure of these structures, and only a hole exists in the spinal column. Often a small dimple and tuft of hair in the midline lower lumbar region is the only external evidence of this defect. In spina bifida meningocele the spinal cord remains in the spinal column; however, a bulging of the meninges occurs. This creates a pouch, or sac, filled with cerebrospinal fluid and is evident on the exterior lower lumbar spine. A **myelomeningocele** is the most severe form of spina bifida. As with the meningocele, an exterior pouch is present that originates in the hole in the lumbar spine. However. in this case the spinal cord is also protruding from the spine. Hydrocephalus (as described later), epilepsy, cerebral palsy, and developmental delays are commonly associated with this condition.

In most cases, a sac forms on the back of the fetus before birth and is detected when the baby is born. It is usually repaired as soon as the infant is able to undergo surgery, which helps prevent infection and preserve whatever neurologic function remains.

A common occurrence in spina bifida is the presence of **hydrocephalus,** in which cerebrospinal fluid accumulates in the ventricles of the brain. Depending on the type of spina bifida, the child may be at high risk for developing mental retardation and other neurologic complications such as seizures if this fluid buildup is not treated properly.

Hydrocephalus may require lifelong treatment. A shunt or tube is inserted from the brain to another place in the body, such as the peritoneum in the abdomen, to drain the excess fluid. As the child grows, the shunt must be revised or replaced. The shunt can become infected at any time, with the first 2 months after insertion being the time of greatest risk. The patient with an infected shunt will have the usual signs of infection (e.g., fever, irritability) in addition to malfunction of the shunt and abdominal pain (if the shunt ends in the peritoneum). Sepsis, meningitis, bacterial endocarditis, wound infection, and ventriculitis (infection in the ventricles of the brain) are some of the complications that can develop.

Shunts can become blocked, which produces signs of increased intracranial pressure such as a bulging soft spot on the head of an infant, changes in mentation in an older child or adult, headaches, vomiting, lethargy, seizures, or irritability. Immediate evaluation by a physician (i.e., neurologist) is needed. Document the patient's initial neurologic status and any changes that occur during treatment and transport.

Another potential complication is the presence of an **Arnold-Chiari malformation,** which occurs in approximately 90% of patients with spina bifida. The brainstem and cerebellum extend down through the foramen magnum into the cervical portion of the vertebrae. If the patient's head is hyperextended, pressure is put on the brainstem and cerebellum. Apnea may occur as a result of this pressure. Therefore avoid hyperextension of the head and use in-line stabilization when performing airway maneuvers. If the patient needs ongoing airway control, stabilize the cervical spine, just as you would for a trauma patient.

In 1989, latex allergy was found to be a serious problem in children with spina bifida. Because of repeated exposure to products containing latex (e.g., catheters, gloves), children become sensitive to the latex and develop life-threatening allergic reactions. These allergies continue into adulthood.

It is important to know immediately if the patient is sensitive to latex. If a sensitivity or allergy is present, the patient must not be exposed to any latex products or be near equipment with latex (Box 40-8). Assemble a latex-free kit that can be stored in the emergency vehicle for use when needed.

Patients with Previous Head Injuries

[OBJECTIVES 30, 31, 32]

Traumatic brain injury (TBI) can result from many mechanisms of trauma (see Chapter 47). These injuries can affect many cognitive, physical, and psychological skills. Physical deficits can include problems with ambulation, balance, coordination, fine motor skills, strength, and endurace. Cognitive deficits of language and communication, information processing, memory, and perceptual skills are common. Psychological status also is often altered.

Depending on the patient's area of brain injury, obtaining a history and performing assessment and patient care procedures may be very difficult. Interview family members and other caregivers to find out if the patient's actions and responses are typical for him or her, and involve them in managing the patient when appropriate. Expect to spend additional time at the scene to provide care to these patients.

BOX 40-8 Items That May Contain Latex

- Blood pressure cuffs
- Masks
- Stethoscopes
- Airways
- Tops of multi-dose vials
- Tourniquets
- Intravenous tubing
- ECG leads
- Gloves
- Goggles
- Gowns
- Suction tubing
- Syringes

CULTURAL DIVERSITY

[OBJECTIVES 33, 34]

Individuals vary in many ways, and there is enormous diversity in populations of all cultures. **Diversity** refers to differences of any kind such as race, class, religion, gender, sexual preference, personal habitat, and physical ability.

Experiences of health and illness vary widely because of different beliefs, behaviors, and experiences. These differences may conflict with assessment and treatment procedures learned by medical professionals. By demonstrating awareness of cultural issues, the medical provider conveys interest, concern, and respect. Be aware of the eight points outlined in the Cultural Considerations box.

CULTURAL*Considerations*

Treating Patients with Cultural Diversity

Be aware of the following eight points:

1. The individual is the "foreground," and the culture is the "background."
2. Different generations and individuals within the same family may have different sets of beliefs.
3. Not all people identify with their ethnic cultural background.
4. All people share common problems or situations.
5. Respect the integrity of cultural beliefs.
6. Realize that people may not share your explanations of the causes of their ill health but may accept conventional treatments. Do not try to "convert" a patient to another way of thinking to get the desired result.
7. You do not have to agree with every aspect of another's culture, nor does the person have to accept everything about yours, for effective and culturally sensitive healthcare to occur.
8. Recognize your cultural assumptions, prejudices, and belief systems. Do not let them interfere with patient care.

Special Considerations

[OBJECTIVE 35]

Regardless of the patient's cultural background, educational status, occupation, or ability to speak English, most patients will be anxious during an emergent event. Attempt to communicate in English first to determine whether the patient understands or speaks some English words or phrases. Bystanders, co-workers, or family members may be available to provide assistance. In some areas, special translator devices (e.g., the AT&T language line) for patients who do not speak English are available. If the patients does not speak or understand English, attempt to communicate with signs or gestures. Notify the receiving hospital as soon as possible so that arrangements for an interpreter can be made.

If time permits, perform all assessment procedures slowly and with the patient's permission. Be aware that "private space" is culturally defined. It is therefore best to point to the area of the body to be examined before touching the patient. Respect the patient's need for modesty and privacy at the scene and during transport. Chapter 41 contains additional information regarding cultural diversity.

Case Scenario—continued

You begin with the history of the chief complaint. The patient states he has been feeling well until last night. He states that at that time he "started to get right flank pain." He states he is unable to urinate on his own and has to catheterize himself to pass urine. He has a history of urinary tract infections. He has been hospitalized for pneumonia in the past. He does not drink or smoke. Physical examination reveals a patient in mild respiratory distress with moist, warm skin. He has clear lung and heart sounds. He has mild suprapubic abdominal pain.

Questions

5. *What are some appropriate interventions?*
6. *What are the eight pearls in dealing with cultural diversity?*
7. *You discover that this patient may have a mental illness. How does this change your approach?*

PATIENTS WITH TERMINAL ILLNESS

[OBJECTIVE 36]

Patients with **terminal illness** are those with an advanced stage of disease with an unfavorable prognosis or no known cure. Often these encounters will be emotionally charged and require a great deal of empathy and compassion for the patient and his or her loved ones. If emotions at the scene are out of control, make every effort to calm the people involved and take control.

If EMS has been summoned to assess the late stages of a patient's terminal illness or a change in the patient's condition, gather a complete history. Ask the patient or family about advance directives and the appropriateness of resuscitation procedures. Carefully review any documentation presented (e.g., a DNR order) and discuss it with medical direction so that patient care decisions can be made.

Special Considerations

[OBJECTIVE 37]

Care of a patient with a terminal illness often will be primarily supportive and limited to calming and comfort measures. It may involve transport to the hospital for physican evaluation. Many of these patients and their families will be involved in hospice care to help them deal with death and dying.

Pain assessment and the management of pain are important aspects of caring for these patients. Attempt to gather a complete pain medication history. Examine the patient for the presence of transdermal drug patches or other pain-relief devices.

Assess the patient's vital signs, level of consciousness, and medication history before reporting to medical direction. The physician may recommend giving additional analgesics or sedatives to ensure the patient's comfort.

PATIENTS WITH COMMUNICABLE DISEASES

[OBJECTIVE 38]

Exposure to some infectious diseases can pose a significant health risk to EMS providers. It is therefore important to ensure personal protection on *every* emergency response. Required precautions depend on the mode of transmission and the pathogen's ability to create pathologic processes. For example, in some cases gloves provide for necessary protection. In other cases, respiratory barriers will also be indicated. Infectious and communicable diseases are discussed in depth in Chapter 31.

PARAMEDIC*Pearl*

Although medical professionals cannot be provided with a totally risk-free environment, simple measures of protection greatly reduce exposure to pathogenic agents. Using standard precautions is an OSHA requirement for EMS professionals.

Special Considerations

[OBJECTIVES 39, 40]

Some infectious diseases (e.g., AIDS) take a toll on the emotional well-being of affected patients, their families, and their circle of friends. The psychological aspects of providing care to these patients include an emphasis on the following:

- Recognizing each patient as an individual with unique healthcare needs
- Respecting each individual's personal dignity
- Providing considerate, respectful care focused upon the person's individual needs

Case Scenario CONCLUSION

While examining the patient's back, you notice that he has a sacral pressure sore. The patient states he did not know that it was there. He is now complaining of a headache that he rates a 7 of 10.

Looking Back

8. *What should be done for comfort measures?*
9. *What are critical points for the oral and written report?*

FINANCIAL CHALLENGES

[OBJECTIVE 41]

In 2005, 37 million Americans lived in poverty (Table 40-3). In 2005, 46.6 million Americans were without health insurance coverage, up from 45.3 million in 2004. The percentage of people covered by employment-based health insurance decreased between 2004 and 2005, from 59.8 percent to 59.5 percent. The number of people covered by government health insurance programs increased between 2004 and 2005, from 79.4 million to 80.2 million (Table 40-4). The percentage and the number of children (people under 18 years old) without health insurance increased between 2004 and 2005, from 10.8 percent to 11.2 percent and from 7.9 million to 8.3 million, respectively. Children in poverty were more likely to be uninsured than the population of all children in 2005. Statistics show that the likelihood of being covered by health insurance rises with income. In 2005, 75.6 percent of people had health insurance in households with annual incomes of less than $25,000. Health insurance coverage rates increased with higher household income levels to 91.5 percent for those in households with incomes of $75,000 or more (DeNaras-Walt, 2005).

Financial challenges for healthcare can quickly result from the loss of a job and depletion of savings. These challenges, combined with medical conditions that require uninterrupted treatment (e.g., tuberculosis, HIV/AIDS, diabetes, hypertension, and mental disorders) or that occur in the presence of unexpected illness or injury, can deprive the patient of basic healthcare services. In addition, poor health is closely associated with homelessness, in which rates of chronic or acute health problems are extremely high (Box 40-9).

Special Considerations

[OBJECTIVE 42]

Persons with financial challenges often are apprehensive about seeking medical care. Fortunately, the ability to pay for emergency healthcare is not a requirement to access

TABLE 40-3 Number of Americans Living in Poverty

Ages	Number of Americans
All ages	37 million
Under 18 years of age	12.9 million
18 through 64 years of age	20.5 million
65 years of age and older	3.6 million

From DeNaras-Walt, C., Proctor, B. D., & Lee, C. H. (2005). *Income, poverty, and health insurance coverage in the United States*. U.S. Census Bureau, Current Population Reports. Washington, DC: U.S. Government Printing Office, pp 60-231.

TABLE 40-4 Health Insurance in the United States

Insurance Coverages	2004	2005
Number of people WITH health insurance coverage	245.9 million	247.3 million
Number of people WITHOUT health insurance coverage	45.3 million	46.6 million
People covered by government health insurance programs (driven by increases in the number of people covered by Medicaid and Medicare)	79.4 million	80.2 million

From DeNaras-Walt, C., Proctor, B. D., & Lee, C. H. (2006). *Income, poverty, and health insurance coverage in the United States: 2005*. U.S. Census Bureau, Current Population Reports. Washington, DC: U.S. Government Printing Office.

BOX 40-9 Healthcare and Homelessness

- Many homeless people have multiple health problems. In addition to chronic illness, frostbite, leg ulcers, and respiratory infections are common and often are the direct result of homelessness.
- Homeless people are at a greater risk for trauma resulting from muggings, beatings, and rape.
- Homelessness precludes good nutrition, good personal hygiene, and basic first aid.
- Some homeless people with mental disorders may use alcohol or other drugs to self-medicate. Those with addictive disorders are often at risk for HIV and other communicable diseases.

EMS providers. According to *Emergency Medical Services, Agenda for the Future*:

> the focus of public access is the ability to secure prompt and appropriate EMS care regardless of socioeconomic status, age, or special need. For all those who contact EMS with a perceived requirement for care, the subsequent response and level of care provided must be commensurate with the situation (U.S. Department of Transportation National Highway Traffic Safety Administration, 1996).

When caring for a patient with financial challenges who is concerned about the cost of receiving needed healthcare, explain the following:

1. The patient's ability to pay should never be a factor in obtaining emergency healthcare.
2. Federal law mandates that medical screening be provided, regardless of the patient's ability to pay.
3. Payment programs for healthcare services are available in most hospitals.
4. Government services are available to assist patients in paying for healthcare.
5. Free (or near-free) healthcare services are available through local, state, and federally funded organizations.

In cases in which no life-threatening condition exists, the patient with financial challenges should be counseled about alternative facilities for healthcare for his or her present condition and future situations that do not require ambulance transport for emergency department evaluation. For example, provide an approved list of alternative healthcare sites (e.g., a minor-emergency center or health clinic) that can provide medical care at costs that are much less than those charged by emergency departments.

TECHNOLOGIC AIDS

Technology has made a tremendous difference in the lives of many people. This technology includes an array of medical equipment such as apnea monitors, tracheostomies, and gastrostomy tubes and buttons. Patients, families, and caregivers usually receive education about caring for the specific equipment or device while in the hospital before discharge. However, they may experience a great deal of anxiety once the patient returns home.

Once at home, it can be frightening if a malfunction occurs or the device does not operate as it did in the hospital. EMS may be called at the first sign of trouble, especially in the first few weeks during the adjustment phase. The provider may be expected to "save the day" without having actual experience with the equipment in use.

It may be helpful to meet with personnel from the social services departments in the hospitals in your area. Encourage them to notify the ambulance service with whom the patient may be in contact regarding the presence of specialized equipment in the home. These details can precipitate a visit to the residence in which more information is gathered from all parties involved. It may also be helpful to review what procedures should take place if a disaster (e.g., earthquake, tornado, flooding) or other event occurs that can cause a loss of power. Many of the following devices are discussed in detail in Chapter 42.

PARAMEDIC*Pearl*

If special aids are used, make every effort to gather this information before an emergency occurs. Meet with the family and become familiar with the device. Share that information with other members of the service who may respond when help is requested.

Tracheostomy

A tracheostomy may be used as a temporary or permanent device. In some patients it provides protection against secretions that could be aspirated. In other patients, it may be necessary because of direct trauma to the airway, weakened respiratory muscles, or prolonged mechanical ventilation.

Obstruction of the tracheostomy requires immediate action. Difficulty clearing secretions, improper positioning, or incorrect insertion of the tube during replacement may lead to obstruction. Place the patient in a sitting position as long as trauma is not suspected. Removal of the tube and direct suctioning of the stoma may be necessary to relieve the blockage.

Central Venous Access Devices

Some patients who require frequent intravenous medications, repeated blood testing, administration of blood products, or administration of large quantities or concentrations of fluids may have a central venous access device inserted. This device provides extended access to a vein without the need for repeated venipunctures or infusions.

TABLE 40-5 Central Venous Access Devices

Type of Catheter	Benefits	Maintenance Considerations
Peripherally inserted central catheter (PICC)	Used for therapy of short to moderate duration Less costly	Antecubital vein most common site (may limit movement of arm) Risk of infection May become dislodged easily (most are not sutured into place)
Tunneled catheter: Hickman Broviac	Used for long-term therapy Easy to use for self-administered infusions	Daily heparin flushes required Must be clamped or have clamp ready at all times Site must be kept dry Risk of infection Protrudes from body Susceptible to damage May be pulled out May alter patient body image
Implanted ports: Port-A-Cath Infus-A-Port Mediport PowerPort	Used for long-term therapy Reduced risk of infection Only slight bulge on chest; completely under skin Increased safety (under skin and minimal maintenance care) Reduced cost for family Regular physical activity (including swimming) not restricted Heparinized monthly and after each infusion	Must pierce skin to access port Pain associated with needle insertion (may use local anesthetic such as EMLA cream) Special needle (Huber) required to access port Must prepare skin before injection Catheter may dislodge from port, especially if child "plays" with site Generally not allowed to engage in vigorous contact sports Difficult for self-administered infusions

Adapted from Hockenberry, M. (2005). *Wong's essentials of pediatric nursing* (7th ed.). St. Louis: Mosby.
EMLA, Eutectic mixture of local anesthetics.

Several types of devices are available (Table 40-5). Most catheters end at the subclavian vein, superior vena cava, or the right atrium. Some may be used for fluid resuscitation or medication administration in an emergency. Vascular access devices are covered in more detail in Chapter 42.

Vagus Nerve Stimulator

Some patients with seizures that have not responded to medication may have a vagus nerve stimulator in place. These devices are used in patients over 12 years of age and provide a pattern of stimulation to the vagus nerve to stop the progression of seizure activity. The generator is implanted under the skin and can be activated by the patient if necessary. If the patient's heart rate is slow, consider a problem with this stimulator. Relay its presence to the medical direction physician, and monitor the patient's heart rate.

Apnea Monitor

Many infants born prematurely may need an **apnea monitor** at home to warn caregivers of any cessation of breathing. Some monitors also warn of bradycardia and tachycardia. Patches are applied to the baby's chest and connected to the monitor. If the device does not detect a breath within a specific time frame or if the infant's heart rate is too slow or too fast, an alarm sounds.

Many different models are available. Newer apnea monitors are computerized and can store information. A printout can be given to EMS providers or hospital personnel that includes an ECG tracing, heart rate, ventilatory rate, and time. It is best to visit parents before an emergency occurs so that they can show you the features of their child's particular monitor. This visit may also help boost parents' confidence by letting them know that trained members of the healthcare team are available to assist them.

Gastrostomy Tube or Button

People who cannot take food by mouth for an extended period of time may require a **gastrostomy tube** or button for feeding. This device is common in some chronic diseases, central nervous system disorders, disorders of the digestive system, or situations in which the developmental ability of the person hinders feeding.

There are multiple types of gastrostomy tubes and buttons with different methods for inserting and securing them. No unusual measures are necessary from an emergency standpoint. Be aware that if the tube was surgically sutured in place and is now dislodged, additional bleeding will occur inside the stomach. In this situation, further evaluation is necessary by a physician in a hospital setting. Gastrostomy tubes are covered in more detail in Chapter 42.

Special Considerations

When a patient uses a technologic aid, incorporate information about the device into your assessment. Do not be distracted by the equipment because it is still necessary to complete adequate initial and ongoing examinations. For example, if the patient has a tracheostomy, include an inspection of this device as part of the assessment. Is it patent? Are secretions present, and if so, what color are they? Is bleeding present around the tracheostomy site? Request suction equipment to clear away any secretions to maintain patency.

EMERGENCY INFORMATION FORM

If the patient is a child, ask the parent, caregiver, or school nurse if an Emergency Information Form is available (see Chapter 37). During an emergency, this form relays pertinent information that may affect treatment.

ADDITIONAL CONSIDERATIONS

Caring for a patient with special challenges can be intimidating. The equipment may be unfamiliar, or the lack of communication ability on the patient's part may be frustrating. Develop a relationship with the appropriate department at the local hospitals in your service area. Ask them to contact someone at the ambulance service—with the patient's permission, of course—when a person with complex medical needs is being discharged into the community. Whenever possible, make a visit to the person's home, the child's school, or the long-term care facility before an emergency occurs to become somewhat familiar with the situation, the patient, and the associated equipment or devices used to sustain that person outside of the hospital setting.

Keep several considerations in mind when caring for patients with special challenges. A summary of conditions and management issues is provided in Table 40-6.

1. Focus on the patient's abilities, not disabilities. Focusing on what this person is able to do promotes self-esteem and a positive self-image. Be sensitive to the particular situation. Saying to a parent "What is wrong with your child?" or "Your child isn't normal, is he?" may create parental anger and resentment. Asking the parent what is special about his or her child promotes trust and understanding.
2. Avoid using the word *normal*. Normalcy is relative and is not always reflected in growth charts and developmental screening tests. Asking the caregiver, "Is this your mother's usual behavior (or posture or color)?" implies acceptance of the person's health condition and avoids the normal/abnormal merry-go-round.
3. Develop creative means for communication. Never assume that the patient cannot understand what you are saying. Communicate in a manner appropriate to the special challenge. Allow the person to use a communication board or device if he or she is used to doing so. If the patient can read and write, provide pencil and paper so that the patient can write down key words during your examination. Use sign language only if you are skilled in that technique. Speak loudly only if you know that the person is able to hear you at a louder tone. Resist the temptation to shout at someone with a hearing impairment. Shouting usually does not improve the communication and may increase the level of frustration for you and your team members. These techniques open patterns of communication between the patient, family, and emergency care personnel.

   Another crucial level of communication is notification of the receiving facility. Make sure the receiving hospital is aware of the patient's special challenges. In some cases, diversion to a more appropriate facility designed to handle these special circumstances, such as a hospital with a spina bifida program, may be suggested.
4. Treat this patient with the same respect afforded other patients. It is easy to forget the patient's modesty during emergency treatment, especially when an "unusual" physical finding is present or you assume that the patient is not aware of what is happening. Keep exposure to a minimum by using sheets or blankets as appropriate. Also, do not be tempted to "show" the patient's disability to the remainder of the crew or other people at the scene.

   Some patients may not realize that they can refuse repeated examinations and can ask for specific information about their health condition. Serving as the patient's **advocate** assists in the maintenance of dignity. Do not perform needless examinations, and provide as much information as possible.
5. Other factors include the following:
   - When treating the patient with a physical disability, special features of the disability may come into play. For example, a patient with cerebral palsy may routinely have a large amount of secretions that may interfere with airway procedures. Be prepared to suction the airway or provide high-concentration oxygen as necessary. In patients with rigid body parts, do not forcefully manipulate that part to make the

TABLE 40-6 A Sampling of Health Conditions Related to Patients with Special Needs: Implications for Providers of Emergency Care

Special Need	General Characteristics	Treatment Issues
Respiratory conditions	Congenital conditions such as softening of the larynx or trachea, underdeveloped or improperly developed lungs; cystic fibrosis	Perform a complete respiratory assessment; place the patient in a position of comfort Assess the presence and patency of an artificial airway (tracheostomy) Maintain airway patency through suctioning and oxygenation; have replacement trach tubes available (same size and one size smaller) Ask if respiratory status is usual or unusual (i.e., is stridor or the retractions more severe than usual?)
Cardiovascular conditions	Congenital cyanotic heart diseases such as tetralogy of fallot and transposition of the great vessels Congenital acyanotic diseases such as atrial or ventricular septal defects or coarctation of the aorta Other anomalies such as dextrocardia	Ask if the cardiac anomaly has been repaired and if more surgery is needed Ask about the medication schedule and about the use of oxygen at home Ask about the person's usual status (i.e., is the patient more cyanotic or dyspneic than usual?)
Mental retardation	May see physical signs such as unusual formation of teeth or low-set ears; soft neurologic signs such as microcephaly and poor fine or gross motor coordination Cognitive function variable, ranging from educable to needing complete care	Focus on patient's abilities, not disabilities; include patient in conversation whenever possible; ask patient's opinions and concerns
Permanent disabilities	Physical: obvious deformities of limbs, craniofacial malformations, paralysis Sensory: difficulty in hearing, vision, tacticle perceptabilities Cognitive: alterations in thinking abilities	Same as above; ask for help if special equipment is used such as a ventilator, gastrostomy tube, central venous access device, braces, artificial limbs, or a wheelchair
Neurologic conditions	Congenital malformations such as spina bifida and Arnold-Chiari malformation; chromosomal anomalies; Dandy-Walker malformation; hydrocephalus Perinatal causes such as infections, anoxic encephalopathy, birth trauma, cerebral palsy Postnatal causes such as head and spinal cord trauma, neoplasms, demyelinating diseases (multiple sclerosis) Seizure disorders such as infantile spasms, Lennox-Gastaut syndrome, epilepsy	Assess for further findings related to paraplegia or quadriplegia, mental retardation, ileostomy/colostomy, ventriculoperitoneal shunt, spasticity, posturing, seizure activity Conduct a complete neurologic assessment; ask the family what findings are usual or unusual Watch for signs and symptoms of altered neurologic functioning such as increased intracranial pressure or seizures
Neuromuscular conditions	Anterior horn cell diseases such as Werdnig-Hoffmann's disease Neuromuscular function diseases such as myasthenia gravis Muscular dystrophies	Same as neurologic conditions
Immunologic conditions	Acquired such as HIV, hepatitis, leukemia, carcinomas Induced such as immunosuppression for organ transplants (heart, heart-lung, lung, liver, kidneys, visceral), bone marrow transplant, or autoimmune disorders	Isolate patient from other people as much as possible; gather information about the patient's medical schedule Relay informtion about a central venous access device if present Recognize the signs and symptoms of organ rejection and chemotherapy reaction

patient conform to your equipment (e.g., forcing someone with an arched back to lie flat on a long backboard).

- When assessing the patient with special challenges, look for a medical identification bracelet or necklace. Although its absence does not rule out a chronic condition, its presence can be helpful during assessment and treatment.
- Obtain from the parent, caregiver, or other family member a list of the patient's current medications and their schedules. Ask the time of the last dose. Vomiting and diarrhea can alter the medication's absorption. Ask about the presence of side effects.
- Other healthcare professionals may be able to help when caring for the patient with special challenges. Once at the hospital, people such as social services personnel, medical specialists, child life specialists, physical and occupational therapists, and nutritionists can provide the necessary care to help the patient reach his or her potential. Some patients or family members may feel too proud to ask for assistance or may not be able to afford such services. Social service personnel can visit the family in the emergency department and develop a plan for future home care as necessary.

FAMILY INVOLVEMENT

Families of adults and children with special challenges are forced to become experts in the care and treatment of their loved one. Use these resources as much as possible to gather information, assist with treatment, or communicate with the patient. Because they spend a great deal of their time with this person, recognize their knowledge and encourage their participation.

People with special challenges may require frequent prehospital interventions, visits to the emergency department, and hospitalizations. Some patients and families may be familiar with the emergency routine and may seem nonchalant or unconcerned. Others may be overly defensive because of frustration about repeated medical treatments that do not appear to be working. This roller coaster of emotions is typical of families of people with special challenges. Acknowledging the person's frustration and helping to make the situation tolerable strengthens everyone's coping abilities.

If the patient is a child, the siblings of this child may also require attention. Their lives are also disrupted by their sibling's emergency treatments and hospitalizations. They may have anger or resentment that their parents' time is taken up with the child with **special needs.** When they grow older, they may be ashamed of or angry at their "different" brother or sister. Allow the sibling to assist whenever possible, such as retrieving a favorite blanket or stuffed animal, and to ask questions. Praise the brother or sister for helping and being kind. These measures help the sibling to develop a positive self-image, as well as receive some much-needed attention.

PARAMEDIC*Pearl*

Pay special attention to the patient's family, and include them in the care whenever possible. Rely on these resources to assist with communication and explanation of special equipment, for example. Interact with the patient's sibling(s) when present to promote self-esteem.

GUIDELINES FOR DISABILITY AWARENESS

With the passage of the Americans with Disabilities Act in July 1992, people with disabilities have finally received the attention they deserve. These individuals now have legislative support to function in the community alongside their peers without disabilities. However, it will take much longer to educate the public and decrease the discrimination and poor attitudes that still exist. Box 40-10 lists suggestions to help increase awareness and promote equal treatment for everyone.

PARAMEDIC*Pearl*

Think "person first, disability second." Whenever you interact with someone with a disability, think of him or her as a person who just happens to have something unique or different about him or her.

BOX 40-10 Guidelines for Disability Awareness

- Use the word *disability* instead of *handicap.*
- Refer to the person first and the disability second, such as "the child with mental retardation" instead of "the retarded child."
- Use "the child with a disability" instead of "the disabled child."
- Never refer to someone as "wheelchair bound" or "confined to a wheelchair," because a wheelchair actually makes the person more mobile.
- Avoid negative descriptions whenever possible. Do not use "invalid," "afflicted with," or "suffers from." Do not refer to children with Down syndrome as "mongoloids" or to children with epilepsy as "epileptics." Do not call seizures "fits."
- Do not use "normal" to describe people who do not have disabilities. Use "typical" or "people without disabilities."
- Do not refer to a person's disability unless it is relevant.

From Shade, B. R., Rothenberg, M. A., Wertz, E., Jones, S. A., & Collins, T. E. (2002). Special considerations. In *Mosby's EMT-intermediate textbook* (2nd ed.). St. Louis: Mosby.

Case Scenario SUMMARY

1. *What are some important things to remember when obtaining a history from this patient?* Many deaf people use hearing aids to amplify sounds. It is important to ask the patient whether he hears you if you are unsure. Also, ask the patient which form of communication works best. Some basic tips are the following:
   - If the patient reads lips, face the person whenever speaking.
   - Try not to use complicated language or large words.
   - Talk at a slow and even pace and do not exaggerate pronunciation.
   - Provide paper and pencil if the patient wants to write a note.
   - If the patient uses sign language, ask for help from anyone present. Remember that an injury to the hands or upper extremities may greatly hamper the patient's ability to communicate through sign language.
   - Consider using pictures to show basic medical procedures. Laminate pictures of routine treatments, and keep them in the emergency vehicle.
2. *What is your impression of this patient?* This patient requires medical attention. He has a fever with vital signs suggesting infection versus early sepsis. He should receive immediate care and transport.
3. *What should be your next interventions?* Obtain a thorough history, which may reveal the cause of the infection. The patient's chronic illnesses should also be investigated. After obtaining all of this information, a treatment plan should be developed and instituted.
4. *How would your interaction change if this patient were visually impaired versus deaf?* These patients may be very frightened during an emergency because they cannot see what is happening. Remember that people with any type of visual impairment may have heightened hearing or smell to compensate for their visual loss. It is important to explain to the patient who you are and what the overall plan is. As you perform the physical examination, it is important to keep them aware of what you are doing. A few other helpful hints are provided here:
   - Orient the patient to whatever care or treatment is being provided.
   - "Lead" ambulatory patients instead of "pushing" them.
   - Explain any movements in position, such as moving the stretcher from the home to the back of the ambulance.
   - Retrieve visual aids if necessary and take them to the hospital.
   - Notify staff at the receiving facility so that appropriate assistance can be available.
5. *What are some appropriate interventions?* The patient should be packaged for transport. The patient should be given supplemental oxygen and placed on a cardiac monitor. Intravenous access should be established and a fluid bolus should be considered. His blood pressure may normally run low; however, in light of the probable infection, it is important to treat the patient conservatively.
6. What are the eight pearls in dealing with cultural diversity?
   - The individual is the "foreground," and the culture is the "background."
   - Different generations and individuals within the same family may have different sets of beliefs.
   - Not all people identify with their ethnic cultural background.
   - All people share common problems or situations.
   - Respect the integrity of cultural beliefs.
   - Realize that people may not share your explanations of the causes of their ill health but may accept conventional treatments. Do not try to "convert" a patient to another way of thinking to get the desired result.
   - You do not have to agree with every aspect of another's culture, nor does the person have to accept everything about yours, for effective and culturally sensitive healthcare to occur.
   - Recognize your cultural assumptions, prejudices, and belief systems. Do not let them interfere with patient care.
7. *You discover that this patient may have a mental illness. How does this change your approach?* Recognizing a patient who is mentally challenged may be difficult, especially when caring for patients with mild neuroses whose behavior may be unaffected. Some patients may provide a history of anxiety or depression. However, others may not. It is important to be vigilant when working with patients. If you suspect mental illness, ask the patient. If the patient demonstrates any signs of violence, such as defensive posturing, it is important to remove yourself until the scene is safe. Patients with disorders that are more serious may present with signs and symptoms consistent with mental illness.

   When obtaining the patient history, ask about the following:
   - History of mental illness
   - Prescribed medications
   - Compliance with prescribed medications
   - Use of over-the-counter herbal products (e.g., St. John's wort)
   - Concomitant use of alcohol or other drugs

   If the patient appears to be paranoid or shows anxious behavior, ask the patient's permission before beginning any assessment or performing any procedure. Once rapport and some form of trust have been established, proceed in the same manner as for a patient who does not have a mental illness (unless the call is related specifically to the mental illness). These patients will experience illness and injury like all other patient groups.

Patients who are dangerous to themselves or others at the scene may need to be restrained. Follow your local protocols for restraining a patient, which may include speaking with medical direction. If a patient demonstrates aggressive or combative behavior, summon law enforcement personnel to ensure scene safety.

8. *What should be done for comfort measures?* Depending on your local protocols, the patient should receive pain medication if the blood pressure is stable. The patient should also be transported in a position of comfort. A sterile dressing should be applied to the decubitus ulcer.

9. *What are critical points for the oral and written report?* The receiving facility should be given information on this patient including his chief complaint, past history, and current physical examination. This patient may have a urinary tract infection, but it is also important to discuss the decubitus ulcer findings. These are often missed because patients with a disability may be more challenging to move. Any findings on your assessment should be documented. It is also important to document any changes throughout the treatment course. In this case, it would include a discussion on the fever, his vital signs, reassessment, and changes (including development of headache/pain).

Chapter Summary

- Many people now survive life-threatening illness and injury. Therefore individuals with special challenges are present in the community and require additional attention when an emergency occurs.
- Accommodations that may be necessary for a patient with a hearing impairment include retrieving the patient's hearing aid, providing paper and pen to aid in communication, and speaking in clear view of the patient.
- When caring for a patient with a visual impairment, retrieve visual aids and describe all patient care procedures before performing them.
- Allow extra time for the history of a patient with a speech impairment. If appropriate, provide aids such as a pen and paper to assist in communication.
- When caring for a patient who is obese, use appropriately sized diagnostic devices. Secure additional staff members if needed to move the patient for ambulance transport.
- Patients with paraplegia or quadriplegia often will require additional staff to assist with moving special equipment to prepare for ambulance transport.
- Once rapport and trust have been established with a patient who has a mental illness, care for physical ailments should proceed in the standard manner.
- If the patient has a developmental disability, take extra time to explain what is being done even though it seems that the person does not understand you. Use terminology that is appropriate to the patient's level of ability. Allow more time for the assessment, patient care, and preparation for transport.
- The difficulty in assessing patients with emotional impairments is distinguishing between symptoms produced by stress and those caused by serious medical illness.
- Physical injury and disease may result in pathologic conditions that require special assessment and management skills. Solicit information about the patient's current medications and typical level of functioning in the history.
- *Diversity* refers to differences of any kind such as race, class, religion, gender, sexual preference, personal habitat, and physical or mental ability. Good healthcare depends on sensitivity toward these differences.
- If the patient has a physical disability, gather informaton about the circumstances or special equipment involved. Minimize exposure when assessing and treating the patient.
- Often, calls involving the care of a patient with a terminal illness will be emotionally charged encounters that require a great deal of empathy and compassion for the patient and his or her loved ones.
- Some infectious diseases will take a toll on the emotional well-being of affected patients, their families, and loved ones. Be sensitive to the psychological needs of the patient and their families.
- Financial challenges can deprive a patient of basic healthcare services. These patients may be reluctant to seek care for illness or injury.
- If the patient uses specialized equipment, provide reassurance to the patient and family. Make every effort to visit this person before an emergency to get a better understanding of the equipment and why it is being used.
- Pay special attention to family members, and provide support as necessary. Rely on them as a resource, and trust what they tell you. Allow siblings or other family members to assist whenever possible.
- In general, be aware of people with special challenges in the community. Use the appropriate guidelines when interacting with these individuals.

REFERENCES

American Obesity Association. (2005). *Fact sheet: What is obesity?* Washington, DC, 2005. Retrieved October 15, 2006, from http://www.obesity.org.

ARC of the United States. (2004). *Introduction to mental retardation.* Silver Spring, MD: ARC of the United States. Retrieved September 20, 2006, from http://www.thearc.org.

Braunwald, E., Fauci, A., Kasper, D., Hauser, S., Longo, D. L., & Jameson, J. L. (2001). *Harrison's principles of internal medicine* (15th ed.). New York: McGraw-Hill.

Centers for Disease Control and Prevention. (2002). *Defining overweight and obesity.* Atlanta: National Center for Chronic Disease Prevention and Health Promotion.

Centers for Disease Control and Prevention. (2005). *CDC growth charts 2000.* Atlanta: National Center for Chronic Disease Prevention and Health Promotion.

DeNaras-Walt C., Proctor, B. D., & Lee, C. H. (2006). *Income, poverty, and health insurance coverage in the United States; 2005.* U. S. Census Bureau, Current Population Reports, P60-231. Washington, DC: U.S. Government Printing Office.

Hockenberry, M. (2005). *Wong's essentials of pediatric nursing* (7th ed). St. Louis: Mosby.

Marx, J., Hockberger, R., & Walls, R. (2005). *Rosen's emergency medicine: Concepts and clinical practice* (6th ed.) (3 vols.). St. Louis: Mosby.

Myasthenia Gravis Foundation of America. (2005). *Myasthenia gravis: A summary.* St. Paul, MN: Myasthenia Gravis Foundation of America. Retrieved October 15, 2006, from http://www.myasthenia.org.

Nation's Voice on Mental Illness. (2005). *About mental illness.* Arlington, VA: Nation's Voice on Mental Illness. Retrieved October 15, 2006, from http://www.nami.org.

National Center for Health Statistics. (2005). *Trends in vision and hearing among older Americans,* Aging Trends No. 2. Hyattsville, MD: Centers for Disease Control and Prevention, U. S. Department of Health and Human Services. Retrieved October 15, 2006, from http://www.cdc.gov.

National Dissemination Center for Children with Disabilities. (2004). *Visual impairments fact sheet 13.* Washington, DC: U.S. Department of Education, Academy for Educational Development. Retrieved June 6, 2008, from http://www.nichcy.org.

National Down Syndrome Society. (2003). *Down syndrome: myths and truths.* New York: National Down Syndrome Society. Retrieved October 15, 2006, from http://www.ndss.org.

National Down Syndrome Society. (2005). *Questions and answers about Down syndrome.* New York: National Down Syndrome Society. Retrieved October 15, 2006, from http://www.ndss.org.

National Institute on Deafness and Other Communication Disorders. (2005a). *Apraxia of speech.* Washington, DC: National Institutes of Health. Retrieved October 15, 2006, from http://www.nidcd.nih.gov.

National Institute on Deafness and Other Communication Disorders. (2005b). *Hearing, ear infections, and deafness.* Washington, DC: National Institutes of Health. Retrieved October 15, 2006, from http://www.nidcd.nih.gov.

National Institute of Neurological Disorders and Stroke. (2007). *NINDS post-polio syndrome information page.* Washington, DC: National Institutes of Health. Retrieved February 20, 2008, from http://www.ninds.nih.gov.

The National Spinal Cord Injury Association. (2005). *Common questions about spinal cord injury.* Bethesda, MD: The National Spinal Cord Injury Association. Retrieved October 15, 2006, from http://www.spinalcord.org.

U.S. Department of Education. (2002). Twenty-fourth Annual Report to Congress. Washington, DC: The Department. Retrieved October 15, 2006, from http://www.ed.gov.

U.S. Department of Transportation National Highway Traffic Safety Administration, U. S. Department of Health and Human Services. (1996). *Emergency medical services: Agenda for the future.* Washington, DC: U.S. Department of Transportation.

Wertz, E. (2001). *Emergency care of children.* Albany, NY: Delmar Thomson Learning.

SUGGESTED RESOURCES

The Arc of the United States
1010 Wayne Avenue, Suite 650
Silver Spring, MD 20910
301-565-3842
Email: Info@thearc.org
Website: http://www.thearc.org

American Academy of Pediatrics. (1998). Emergency preparedness for children with special health care needs. *Pediatrics 104*(4), e53. Retrieved June 5, 2008, from http://www.aap.org.

American Association on Mental Retardation (AAMR)
444 North Capitol St. NW, Suite 846
Washington, DC 20001-1512
Phone: 800-424-3688
Website: http://www.aamr.org

American Association on Mental Retardation. (2002). *Mental retardation: Definition, classification, and systems of supports* (10th ed). Washington, DC: American Association on Mental Retardation.

American Association on Mental Retardation. (2008). *Fact sheet: Frequently asked questions about mental retardation,* Washington, DC: American Association on Mental Retardation. Retrieved June 5, 2008, from http://www.aamr.org.

American Council of the Blind
1155 15th St. NW, Suite 1004
Washington, DC 20005
Phone: 202-467-5081; 800-424-8666
Email: info@acb.org
Website: http://www.acb.org

American Foundation for the Blind
11 Penn Plaza, Suite 300
New York, NY 10001
Phone (hotline): 800-232-5463
Phone (publications): 800-232-3044
Email: afbinfo@afb.net
Website: http://www.afb.org

American Obesity Association
1250 24th Street NW, Suite 300
Washington, DC 20037
Phone: 202-776-7711
Website: http://www.obesity.org

American Speech-Language-Hearing Association (ASHA)
10801 Rockville Pike
Rockville, MD 20852
Phone: 800-638-8255
TTY: 301-897-0157
Email: actioncenter@asha.org
Website: http://www.asha.org

Developmental Disabilities Assistance and Bill of Rights Act of 2000. PL 106-402. Retrieved June 5, 2008, from http://www.acf.hhs.gov.

Division on Developmental Disabilities
The Council for Exceptional Children
1110 North Glebe Rd., Suite 300
Arlington, VA 22201-5704
Phone: 888-232-7733
TTY: 866-915-5000
Email: cec@cec.sped.org
Website: http://www.dddcec.org

McPherson, M., Arango, P., Fox, H., Lauver, C., McManus, M., Newacheck, P. W., et al. (1998). A new definition of children with special health care needs. *Pediatrics, 102*(1), 137-139.

Myasthenia Gravis Foundation of America
1821 University Ave. West, Suite S256
St. Paul, MN 55104
Phone: 800-541-5454
Website: http://www.myasthenia.org

Nation's Voice for Mental Illness
Colonial Place Three
2107 Wilson Blvd., Suite 300
Arlington, VA 22201-3042
Phone: 703-524-7600
Member Services: 800-950-NAMI
Website: http://www.nami.org

National Center for Health Statistics
3311 Toledo Rd.
Hyattsville, MD 20782
Phone: 301-458-4000
Website: http://www.cdc.gov/nchs/about.htm

National Coalition for the Homeless
2201 P St. NW
Washington, DC 20037
Phone: 202-462-4822
Website: http:/www.nationalhomeless.org

National Coalition for the Homeless. (2003). *People need health care.* Washington, DC: National Coalition for the Homeless. Retrieved June 5, 2008, from http://www.nationalhomeless.org

National Down Syndrome Society
666 Broadway
New York, NY 10012
Phone: 800-221-4602
Email: info@ndss.org
Website: http://www.ndss.org

National Institute on Deafness and Other Communication Disorders
National Institutes of Health
31 Center Dr., MSC 2320
Bethesda, MD 20892-2320
Email: nidcdinfo@nidcd.nih.gov

National Spinal Cord Injury Association
6701 Democracy Blvd., Suite 300-9
Bethesda, MD 20817
Phone: 800-962-9629
Website: http://www.spinalcord.org

Chapter Quiz

1. True or False: When assessing a patient with a speech impairment, it is important to allow adequate time for the patient to respond to questions.

2. List three causes of visual impairment.

____

____

____

3. Conductive deafness is defined as _____.
  a. complete or partial inability to hear based on a behavioral disorder
  b. faulty transportation of sound from the outer to the inner ear
  c. deafness that occurs later in life and may be caused from prolonged exposure to loud noises
  d. sound not being transmitted to the brain because of damage to the structures within the ear

4. What special considerations might an obese patient require?

____

____

____

____

5. True or False: The presence of a medical identification bracelet or necklace may indicate a special challenge.

6. The head is placed in a neutral position when performing airway maneuvers on a patient with spina bifida because:
  a. An Arnold-Chiari malformation may be present.
  b. It makes it easier to use a bag-mask without a partner.
  c. It reduces intracranial pressure.

7. True or False: It is not necessary to explain procedures to a person with a mental illness.

8. Patients with spina bifida are prone to what type of allergy?

9. List three characteristics found in a person with Down syndrome.

____

____

____

10. A ______________ ______________ ______________ may be present in a patient requiring repeated blood testing, frequent intravenous medications, or large quantitites or concentrations of fluids.

11. Patients who cannot eat by mouth for whatever reason may be fed through a/an _____.
  a. colostomy
  b. ileostomy
  c. gastrostomy

12. Prehospital care for patients with emotional impairments _____.
  a. includes specific behavioral interventions
  b. is no different than for other patients
  c. is primarily supportive
  d. is usually transport only

13. Arthritis is the ______________ of a joint.

14. True or False: Cystic fibrosis is an inherited metabolic disease of the heart and lymph system that manifests in early adulthood.

15. Describe signs and symptoms of spinal cord involvement in a patient with multiple sclerosis.

____

____

____

Chapter Quiz—continued

16. The most common form of muscular dystrophy is _____.
    a. Duchenne muscular dystrophy
    b. Fragile X muscular dystrophy
    c. Meniere's muscular dystrophy
    d. Trisomy muscular dystrophy

17. A patient with poliomyelitis may require _____.
    a. advanced airway support to ensure adequate ventilation
    b. aggressive chest physical therapy to loosen secretions
    c. repeated muscular massage to prevent contractures
    d. routine intravenous support to increase blood pressure

18. True or False: A patient with a previous head injury may have cognitive deficits of language, communication, information processing, memory, and perceptual skills.

19. Muscles become weak and tire easily in what disease?
    a. Multiple sclerosis
    b. Muscular dystrophy
    c. Myasthenia gravis
    d. Poliomyelitis

20. True or False: In culturally diverse patients, all people identify specifically with their ethnic cultural background.

21. Personal protection should be used on ___________ emergency response.

Terminology

Advocate A person who assists another person in carrying out desired wishes; a paramedic should function as a patient's advocate in all aspects of prehospital care.

Aphasia Loss of speech.

Apnea monitor A technologic aid used to warn of cessation of breathing in a premature infant; also may warn of bradycardia and tachycardia.

Arnold-Chiari malformation A complication of spina bifida in which the brainstem and cerebellum extend down through the foramen magnum into the cervical portion of the vertebrae.

Arthritis Inflammation of a joint that results in pain, stiffness, swelling, and redness.

Body mass index A calculation strongly associated with subcutaneous and total body fat and with skinfold thickness measurements.

Cancer A group of diseases that allow for an unrestrained growth of cells in one or more of the body organs or tissues.

Cerebral palsy Neuromuscular condition in which the patient has difficulty controlling the voluntary muscles due to damage to a portion of the brain.

Chronic Long, drawn out; applied to a disease that is not acute.

Colostomy Incision in the colon for the purpose of making a temporary or permanent opening between the bowel and the abdominal wall.

Conductive hearing loss Type of deafness that occurs where there is a problem with the transfer of sound from the outer to the inner ear.

Cystic fibrosis (CF) Inherited metabolic disease of the lungs and digestive system that manifests in childhood.

Deafness A complete or partial inability to hear.

Developmental disabilities Disabilities that involve some degree of impaired adaptation in learning, social adjustment, or maturation.

Diversity Differences of any kind such as race, class, religion, gender, sexual preference, personal habitat, and physical ability.

Down syndrome A genetic syndrome characterized by varying degrees of mental retardation and multiple physcial defects.

Dysarthria An articulation disorder in which the patient is not able to produce speech sounds.

Dysphagia Difficulty swallowing.

Emotional/Mental impairment Impaired intellectual functioning such as mental retardation, which results in an inability to cope with normal responsibilities of life.

Gastrostomy tube A tube placed in a person's stomach that allows direct feeding for an extended period of time.

Hydrocephalus "Water on the brain"; can cause increased intracranial pressure if allowed to accumulate.

Ileostomy Surgical creation of a passage through the abdominal wall into the ileum.

Kernicterus Excessive fetal bilirubin; associated with hemolytic disease.

Legally blind Less than 20/200 vision in at least one eye or a very limited field of vision (e.g., 20 degrees at its widest point).

Low vision Level of visual impairment where individuals are unable to read a newspaper at the usual viewing distance even if they use glasses or contact lenses. It is not limited to distance vision and can be a severe visual impairment.

Mental illness Any form of psychiataric disorder.

Mental retardation Developmental disability characterized by a lower than normal IQ.

Morbid obesity Having a Body Mass Index of 40 or more; equates to approximately 100 pounds more than ideal weight.

Multiple sclerosis (MS) Progressive and incurable autoimmune disease of the central nervous system; patches of myelin in the brain and spinal cord are destroyed.

Muscular dystrophy (MD) Inherited muscle disorder that results in a slow but progressive degeneration of muscle fibers.

Myasthenia gravis An autoimmune disorder in which muscles become weak and tire easily.

Myelomeningocele Developmental anomaly of the central nervous system in which a hernial sac containing a portion of the spinal cord, the meninges, and cerebrospinal fluid protrudes through a congenital cleft in the vertebral column; occurs in approximately 2 of every 1000 live births, is readily apparent, and is easily diagnosed at birth.

Neuroses Mental diseases related to upbringing and personality in which the person remains "in touch" with reality.

Obesity An excessively high amount of body fat or adipose tissue in relation to lean body mass.

Osteoarthritis Also known as *degenerative joint disease,* this is a disorder where the cartilaginous covering of the joint surface starts to wear away, resulting in pain and inflammation of a joint.

Ostomy Surgical opening that allows the passage of urine or feces through an incision, or stoma, in the wall of the abdomen.

Otosclerosis Abnormal growth of bone that prevents structures in the ear from working properly; thought to be a hereditary disease.

Overweight State of increased body weight in relation to height.

Paraplegia Paralysis of the lower limbs and possibly the trunk.

Partially sighted Level of vision in persons who have some type of visual problem and may need assistance.

Physical disabilities Disabilities that involve limitation of mobility.

Poliomyelitis An infectious viral disease caused by *Poliovirus hominis,* spread through direct and indirect contact with infected feces and by airborne transmission. It attacks with variable severity ranging from asymptomatic infection to a febrile illness without neurologic sequelae to aseptic meningitis and finally to paralytic disease including respiratory paralysis and possible death.

Presbycusis Hearing loss that occurs from changes in the inner ear, auditory nerve, middle ear, or outer ear; comes on gradually as the person ages.

Psychoses A group of mental disorders in which the individual loses contact with reality; psychosis is thought to be related to complex biochemical disease that disorders brain function. Examples include schizophrenia, bipolar disease (also known as *manic-depressive illness*), and organic brain disease.

Quadriplegia Paralysis affecting all four extremities.

Rheumatoid arthritis A painful, disabling disease in which the body's immune system attacks the joints of the body.

Sensorineural hearing loss A type of deafness that occurs when the tiny hair cells in the cochlea are damaged or destroyed. In addition, there is damage to the auditory nerve so that sounds are not transmitted from the cochlea to the brain.

Special needs Conditions with the potential to interfere with usual growth and development or activities of daily living; may involve physical disabilities, developmental disabilities, chronic illnesses, and forms of technologic support.

Spina bifida The number one disabling birth anomaly in the United States, spina bifida affects the back portion of the vertebrae, which fails to close, usually in the area of the baby's lower back; meninges, the spinal cord, or both may protrude through this opening.

Terminal illness Advanced stage of illness or disease with an unfavorable prognosis and no known cure.

Tinnitus A ringing, roaring sound or hissing in the ears that is usually caused by certain medicines or exposure to loud noise.

Totally blind Description of someone who has no vision and uses nonvisual media or reads via Braille.

Verbal apraxia Speech disorder in which the person has difficulty saying what he or she wants to say in a correct and consistent manner.

CHAPTER 41

Social Issues

Objectives

After completing this chapter, you will be able to:

1. Discuss the impact of cultural differences when rendering patient care.
2. Define codependency and explain its impact on patient care.
3. Discuss the impact poverty has on EMS operations.
4. Discuss the financial burdens placed on patients unable to pay for services as well as society.
5. Understand the impact of homelessness in the United States as it relates to prehospital care.
6. Understand common chronic mental and physiologic illnesses associated with the homeless.

Chapter Outline

Case Scenario

It is 8:20 PM on a summer night and your crew responds to a call by the police department for a "man down" in front of a clothing store. On arrival, the police officer tells you the patient was seen "walking funny" and then sat down in front of the store. The store's owner attempted to chase the man off his property, but the man did not seem to understand or respond. The officer further states that the man seemed incoherent when he arrived on the scene. The officer was preparing to arrest the man for public intoxication when he slumped over and passed out.

The patient is a thin, undernourished man who appears to be in his early 30s. His clothing is dirty, he is unshaven, and he seems to have gone without a shower for several days. No noticeable smell of an alcoholic beverage is on the man's breath.

Questions

1. *What is your initial impression of the patient?*
2. *What additional information do you need to complete your assessment?*
3. *What may be causing the man to appear intoxicated?*

EMS has become an integral part of the chain of patient care. The role of the paramedic also has greatly changed over time. The days of EMS simply being a means of transport to definitive care are gone. Being a great clinician is not enough for the professional paramedic. As the gateway to healthcare for many patients, today's paramedic must possess the skills necessary to provide advanced patient care as well as the skills of understanding, empathy, and compassion when dealing with many social differences seen in today's patients. Regardless of the social issues that you may encounter in practice, remember that everyone deserves the same quality of care, whether they are rich or poor, are able to communicate in English, or are in a difficult social situation. This chapter discusses several key issues today's paramedic must face. Not every paramedic will have to face every issue. Much depends on the part of the country where you live, whether urban or rural environments, and the socioeconomic composition of the residents of your particular area. Nonetheless, you must be able to treat any patient you encounter, and part of that treatment is in understanding and treating social issues without bias.

CULTURAL AWARENESS

[OBJECTIVE 1]

When discussing cultural differences, first understand that the word *culture* refers to behaviors and beliefs of a particular racial, ethnic, social, religious, or age group. EMS professionals learn to care for people in various age groups in EMS education programs but generally only learn about people from various religious and ethnic groups when called to care for them in the community.

According to the Department of Homeland Security *Yearbook of Immigration Statistics* for 2006, more than 1.2 million persons from all over the world obtained legal permanent resident status that year in the United States (Simanski & Rytina, 2006). The other countries on the American continent represented more than 43% of that number; the next largest group emigrated from Asia (32.5%).

Ethnic Values and Traditions

The United States has been called "the great melting pot." Over the years, as waves of immigrants have come to the United States, they have brought with them the values and traditions of their native countries, including healthcare traditions. Western medicine is unfamiliar to many new residents to the United States. Many ethnic cultures value natural (also referred to as *folk*) remedies and find Western medicine vastly different and even uncomfortable. People from cultures that value privacy may find questions that healthcare providers ask intrusive, even offensive, and may be cautious to release personal information about themselves or their family.

Although knowing all the nuances of every ethnic group in the United States is impossible, becoming familiar with the values and traditions of the major ethnic and religious groups in your community is helpful. You may be the first healthcare professional the new resident meets.

Find out whether people in the various ethnic groups make their own healthcare decisions or whether decisions are made by someone else in the family (in many cultures the family elder makes all healthcare decisions), what they consider signs of respect (and disrespect), what folk remedies may be practiced before seeking a Western remedy, rules of modesty, rules of touching, appropriate (and inappropriate) hand gestures, and anything else you can learn that might affect patient care if an emergency arises.

Language barriers are the most common obstacle encountered by healthcare providers. Although asking a relative or friend of the patient to translate seems convenient, this option has a downside. Check your local policies regarding translations. In addition to the potential for violating Health Insurance Portability and Accountability Act rules, asking others to interpret for a patient may result in intentional or unintentional miscommunication by the patient or the translator. For instance, often the children in these households are bilingual, using their native language at home but learning English in school. They can be extremely helpful in an emergency situation. On the other hand, this places the child in a difficult posi-

CULTURAL *Considerations*

Actions and responses to situations depend on a person's cultural and religious background. Many times these may seem inappropriate to those who do not share the same background. In addition, practices of one group may be seen as offensive to another group. Although it would be impossible to list the views of every culture and religion in one chapter, a few examples are:

- Offering the left hand in a greeting, or primarily using the left hand for activities such as taking a pulse, is considered offensive to some Middle Eastern cultures.
- Females of some Middle Eastern cultures will not make eye contact with males, and attempts by males to make eye contact can be considered offensive.
- Individuals who are Jehovah's Witnesses will not accept blood or blood products during medical care.
- Christian Scientists do not believe human intervention should take place during illness.
- In Hispanic cultures the grandmother is often the person who makes medical decisions.
- Many cultures use folk healers such as a *curandrea* in Mexico. This can provide a unique challenge to the paramedic, as Western medicine may conflict with the medical practices of other cultures. As long as your care of the patient is not hindered, you should respect the patient's desire to have these individuals present and allow them to continue their treatment. Showing disrespect or interfering with cultural practices may be interpreted as signs of disrespect. This can lead to confrontations on scene or a request for the paramedic to leave.

In general, the paramedic should be in tune to the patient's verbal and nonverbal responses to the situation. If your patient is continually looking away, you are probably attempting to make too much eye contact. If your patient is constantly backing away from you, he or she likely has a view of personal space that is greater than yours. Finally, the paramedic should be sure not display behaviors of ethnocentrism or cultural imposition. Ethnocentrism is the belief that one's own cultural beliefs are superior to all others, and cultural imposition is the belief that everyone should conform to the individual's beliefs, and as a result those beliefs are imposed on others.

tion, particularly if the patient's health problem is of a nature that an adult would not normally share with his or her children. This may cause the patient to withhold or alter key information and may have a negative effect on how the child perceives his or her role within the family dynamic. In the final analysis, these children can be a tremendous asset in these situations; however, you must realize the potential for inaccurate information and negative effects on the child. If another way to facilitate communication is possible, it may be preferable. Professional services, such as the AT&T Language Line, are invaluable in providing unbiased, accurate translation.

Religious Traditions

Also of importance is being familiar with prominent religious traditions in your community that may affect a person's decision or ability to access healthcare services. Some religions forbid surgeries or infusion of blood or blood products. Other religions prohibit the use of alcohol, including the use of alcohol wipes. Some religions have very strict rules regarding touch by members of the opposite sex. A few religions practice strict dietary laws. Fasting is a practice observed by several religions. Although members of religious sects with health issues are usually exempt from fasting, believers may choose to fast anyway. Those with diabetes or hydration issues may have medical consequences that may warrant a call for EMS. Some religious groups have very strict protocols for dealing with death and dying.

When in doubt about whether any care you are providing is acceptable, ask the patient or family before beginning the care. Many rules are exempt in life-threatening situations.

Case Scenario—continued

Your primary survey reveals a sluggish response to noxious stimuli, an open airway, adequate breathing, and a slow pulse. Your secondary survey reveals no indication of trauma. You and your partner administer oxygen by nonrebreather mask at a rate of 15 L/min. The patient initially fights the application of the mask but finally accepts the device. His responses continue to be sluggish and somewhat uncoordinated. The patient looks at you and attempts to speak, but his words are slurred and incoherent. His skin is pale, cool, and dry. Vital signs are blood pressure, 90/58 mm Hg; pulse, 78 beats/min; and respirations, 14 breaths/min. While assessing the patient and considering the possible causes of his condition and treatment options, a bystander wanders by and states, "This kid is a new one to the streets!" You question the bystander and learn that the patient has just recently been on the street without a home or shelter. The bystander further states that the patient tends to "walk funny, you know, with a shuffle—like he's always drunk and staggering." You press on with your questions, but the bystander has no more information.

Questions

4. *Has your first impression changed?*
5. *What medical conditions might cause the staggering or shuffling gait?*

CODEPENDENCY

[OBJECTIVE 2]

Codependence is a psychological concept defined as putting the needs and wants of others before one's own needs and exhibiting too much and often inappropriate caring behavior. The codependent individual often is involved in a relationship with someone with a drug or alcohol problem, mental illness, or chronic illness. The codependent person feels the need to focus all attention and energy on the individual with the problem, giving up his or her own personal life and even identity to care for the individual. The codependent person may even cover up or deny a problem exists with the individual in his or her care. Codependency creates several challenges for a responding paramedic.

First, this **enabling behavior** may allow a problem to persist, keeping an individual from getting the intervention he or she may need. The codependent individual believes he or she is the only one who truly understands the problem and as such can be the only one to care for the individual. Second, the codependent person may become a victim if the addiction or problem causes an escalation to violence. Because of low self-esteem, the codependent individual may blame himself or herself for an outburst.

For example, you receive a call to an apartment for a victim of battery. Police are on the scene and they requested EMS. On arrival, you find a 36-year-old woman with multiple contusions and lacerations to her face and a 38-year-old man with significant lacerations to his right hand. The man smells of alcohol. You note a shattered glass table in the middle of the living room. The police tell you they were called by a neighbor who heard shouting and then a crash. What are your initial thoughts? Your partner begins assessing and treating the man. While you assess and treat the woman, she tells you it was her fault that he hit her and she does not want to go to the hospital, but please take care of her boyfriend. What do you do now? The challenge EMS faces in these situations is obvious. Of course both patients need to be treated and transported, and both need some form of intervention. The role EMS plays in these situations, beyond treatment for the physical presentations, is to document what was said and share that information with the receiving hospital as it relates to patient care. The hospital then would be in a position to offer help through its social services. However, the single most important aspect when entering a call in which a codependent relationship is discovered or believed to exist is not to be distracted by the relationship. Treat patients based on the assessment findings. A critical patient is a critical patient regardless of the environment from which he or she came. If you encounter resistance through either the patient or the partner, let the police handle it. If the scene escalates to one in which the safety of the EMS crew is in question, get out and immediately call for police backup.

THE POOR AND THOSE IN NEED

[OBJECTIVES 3, 4]

The effects of poverty are felt on multiple levels of society. The upper and middle class support programs for the poor through tax dollars on the federal and state levels. Physically, those hit the hardest are the poor themselves. Poor nutrition, poor living environments, and inadequate access to medical care are primary contributors to ill health among the poor. Research has shown the average life expectancy among the poor is considerably lower than that of other socioeconomic levels.

In urban areas, the poor often rely on emergency departments (EDs) to provide medical care even for minor illnesses or injuries. This practice is one factor that has led to overcrowding in many EDs throughout the country. EMS is directly affected by the practice of visiting an ED for routine care; namely, increases in call volumes over the past few years as well as the potential for not having an ambulance available in the event of a life-threatening medical or trauma situation occurring somewhere else. Increases in call volume lead to the expenditure of more money to keep the ambulances staffed and rolling. Many EMS agencies have difficulty meeting these expenditures, and the revenue generated, if any, is not enough to cover the costs.

The role that economics plays in prehospital care is an unfortunate one. Also unfortunate is the fact that many EMS agencies must charge for their services. However, the greatest misfortune is the mindset that some people "cannot afford the luxury of an ambulance." Consider this situation:

You are called to a home for a woman with difficulty breathing. You are met at the door by an elderly man with a very frightened look on his face. He leads you into the living room where you see an elderly woman sitting on the couch. As you assess your patient, you find her skin is very hot to the touch and flushed. Her lung sounds reveal rhonchi and crackles in all fields. She says she has been sick for a few days. You tell her she needs to go to the hospital for evaluation, that she may have pneumonia. She tells you, "We can't afford an ambulance or for me to go to the hospital. Our insurance won't cover the bill. I'll be okay. I'm going to call my doctor and see if I can get in to see her in a couple of days."

Obviously the woman needs medical attention. You are in a position to provide a portion of the attention she needs, but her mindset is keeping her from getting the much-needed treatment. Your role as a paramedic has taken on a new dimension. Not only are you a caregiver, you also are now a negotiator. The conscientious paramedic must do everything in his or her power and ability to convince the patient to get the attention she needs. This situation, as well as any situation in which economics plays a part in seeking treatment, should be handled with respect but firmness in expressing the importance of getting care.

Case Scenario CONCLUSION

You apply a cardiac monitor, which reveals a sinus rhythm. You assess the man's blood glucose level and find that it is 88 mg/dL; thus the patient is not hypoglycemic. The pulse oximeter shows an oxygen saturation of 98% on oxygen at 15 L/min. The patient's skin does not suggest any febrile condition and he moves his neck without evidence of stiffness or pain. While discussing the patient's condition with your partner, the police officer reaches into the man's pocket and retrieves a small plastic pill bottle containing several pills. The bottle's label indicates the pills are chlorpromazine (Thorazine). Other information on the label reveals the pills were dispensed by the local mental health department early last week.

You and your partner ready the patient for transport. You continue to administer oxygen. You establish IV access with normal saline and, because of the patient's blood pressure, decide to give a 250-mL fluid challenge.

Looking Back

6. *What additional assessment and treatment options for the man should be considered?*
7. *What is your final impression of the patient?*
8. *What treatment options are available for this man?*
9. *What are some things to consider about homelessness in a patient who may be mentally ill?*

HOMELESSNESS

[OBJECTIVES 5, 6]

Homelessness in the United States has reached epic proportions. An estimated 842,000 people are homeless on any given night in February, and 3.5 million experience homelessness during a year (National Coalition for the Homeless, 2007) (Figure 41-1). Of course these figures can only be estimates, and some believe the actual number is much higher. A homeless patient presents the paramedic with unique challenges.

The experience of homelessness causes health problems (frostbite and hypothermia from the cold, communicable diseases from crowded shelter conditions), exacerbates existing illnesses (cuts lead to infection, frostbite results in amputation or even death), and seriously complicates treatment (medications are lost or stolen, health insurance and transportation to health providers are lacking). People who are homeless are sicker and die earlier than those who are housed. A report conducted for the National Health Care for the Homeless Council (2006) found that people experiencing homelessness are three to four times more likely to die prematurely than their housed counterparts.

According to Health Care for the Homeless in Baltimore, Md., approximately 50% of their clients have a treatable addiction, 30% are diagnosed with a major mental illness, and 25% are dually diagnosed with both a mental illness and an addiction. Their clients also have high rates of hypertension, asthma, diabetes, and HIV or AIDS. The most common mental illnesses are schizophrenia, bipolar disorders, and major depression. Most of these mental illnesses and chronic medical illnesses go untreated, contributing to the downward spiral of the homeless patient.

Acute medical conditions add to the harsh environment of the homeless. Assault and rape are common crimes committed on the homeless. Depending on geographic area, the environment itself can be a detriment. Because of these negative factors, the homeless have a mortality rate four times greater than the remainder of the population.

According to Dick and Hillson (2005), "Street people aren't statistics, they're not stupid, and they're not subhuman. They're people. When they get into trouble, they dial 9-1-1 because they have nowhere else to turn." They should know. Dick is a veteran paramedic, author, and major advocate for professional patient care. Hillson, who is Dick's son, was homeless for 2 years and is now an EMT.

Treating a homeless patient can be a challenge for any paramedic, especially when treating a patient with an underlying mental disorder. By following a few simple guidelines when approaching and communicating with a homeless patient, the challenge can be greatly decreased:

- Be empathetic and nonjudgmental to ease the patient's anxiety.
- Remain calm and professional.
- Respect the patient's personal space (Figure 41-2). Stand 3 to 4 feet away in front (far enough away to avoid being kicked) and slightly turn your body in an oblique position to protect yourself.
- Do not speak harshly. A positive tone of voice can go a long way in facilitating treatment.

Be aware that the patient may be armed. Many homeless people carry knives to protect themselves. Also be sensitive and respectful for what few possessions your patient may have. If you work in an area that services a homeless community, carrying large plastic garbage bags in your vehicle may be prudent. This will allow you to bag the patient's possessions and take them to the hospital with him or her. Although what they have may look like a pile of junk in a shopping cart to you, keep in mind that what you see is their home.

In addition to customary standard precautions, Dick and Hillson recommend other steps to take to protect yourself when managing a homeless patient (Box 41-1).

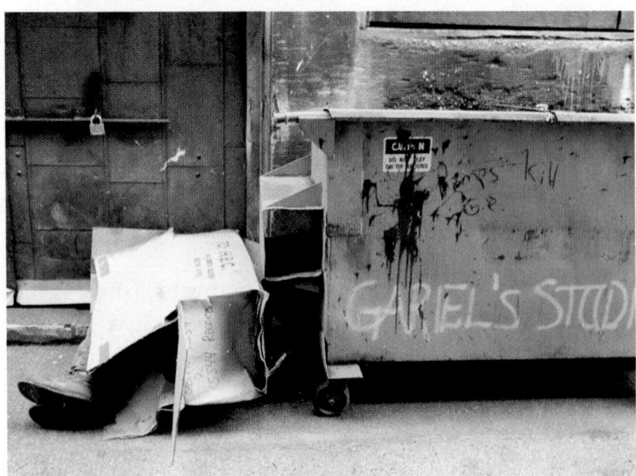

Figure 41-1 Makeshift housing, such as tents, boxes, caves, or boxcars, is used for shelter by the homeless.

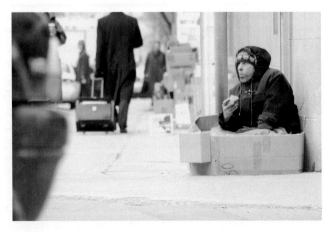

Figure 41-2 Keep in mind that a homeless person's space is his or her home.

Remember, you are in the people business. EMS is the primary care service for the homeless. You have an obligation to treat every patient in his or her time of need to the best of your ability. Do not let homelessness interfere with that patient's right to receive the best care possible.

BOX 41-1 Special Standard Precautions

The uninitiated may wonder how some people can tolerate their own strong body odors. However, if you do not have spare clothing and you do not have access to shower or laundry facilities, you simply wear your garments until they fall apart. The same is true of footwear, blankets, and bedding. That can make a person seem repulsive to even the best field providers, but do your best not to treat street people as though they are untouchables simply because they do not live like you do. On the other hand, consider the possibility of special infection risks that some of them may pose to you as a caregiver. When you are faced with someone who obviously poses a threat (e.g., because of persistent vigorous coughing, obvious major hygiene issues, or purulent skin eruptions), consider the following special practices in addition to your daily standard precautions:

- Provide oxygen by mask any time you suspect that a patient has a respiratory infection. Even in the absence of fever, coughing always warrants this precaution. In fact, consider wearing a mask yourself.
- Think about putting on a gown if you have to carry a patient without a stretcher or stair chair.
- Do you suspect scabies or pediculosis because of extremely poor hygiene, especially if the patient is scratching? Consider applying disposable surgical headgear to the patient's head and wrapping the patient completely in a top sheet on your cot. Also consider wearing a gown.
- Avoid carrying people who can walk unless doing so poses a risk to their medical condition (e.g., if they report non-pleuritic chest pain, shortness of breath, or musculoskeletal pain).
- Clean your door handles, the steering wheel, and the mattress and frame of your ambulance cot with contact cleaner after the call, even if the ambulance needs to be out of service for a few extra minutes.
- Clean your pen thoroughly with alcohol wipes or consider discarding it altogether (if it is disposable) after the call.
- Refrain from using your mouth as an extra hand (this applies to every call).
- Gloves or no gloves, wash your hands thoroughly after the call (this also applies to every call).
- Take precautions on behalf of police and first responders as well as yourself.
- Save some of the plastic bags that most distributors use to deliver newspapers. Cut the closed ends to convert them into sleeves. When you need to obtain a blood pressure on somebody with a hygiene problem, quietly slip a sleeve on the arm first. This can keep the blood pressure cuff clean so you do not have to launder it as often.
- Pressurize the patient compartment with outside air by turning on the air conditioner. Remember, an air conditioner can provide warm as well as cool air, and its intake is filtered.
- Regardless of any precautions you take, be kind.

From Dick, T., & Hillson, D. (2005). Downtown people: Taking care of America's homeless. *Journal of Emergency Medical Services, 30*, 12.

Case Scenario SUMMARY

1. *What is your initial impression of the patient?* Your initial impression is that you have an unconscious male who is in need of medical assistance.
2. *What additional information do you need to complete your assessment?* Additional information needed includes a head-to-toe evaluation and a SAMPLE history, if possible. Vital signs and other diagnostic information might rule out trauma, diabetes, or other conditions that could contribute to the patient's presentation.
3. *What may be causing the man to appear intoxicated?* The appearance of intoxication can be caused by any number of factors, including alcohol, diabetes (insulin shock and ketoacidosis), drug ingestion, stroke, and renal failure.
4. *Has your first impression changed?* An underlying medical condition seems to be contributing to the man's current presentation. The patient's blood pressure is low.
5. *What medical conditions might cause the staggering or shuffling gait?* Gait abnormalities can be congenital or caused by a medical condition such as stroke, meningitis, or Wernicke encephalitis. They also can be caused by drugs or alcohol.
6. *What additional assessment and treatment options for the man should be considered?* Additional information needed includes blood glucose assessment, oxygen saturation, body temperature, and nuchal rigidity. Initial treatment options to be considered include application of a pulse oximeter and cardiac monitor, and intrave-

Continued

Case Scenario SUMMARY—continued

nous access. Count the amount of pills in the bottle and compare the number with the date the prescription was filled and dosage to determine if the patient has been taking his medication correctly. Too little or too much of this type of medicine could account for the patient's current mental state.

7. *What is your final impression of the patient?* A final impression of this patient is a homeless man recently released from psychiatric care. His mental illness and use of chlorpromazine may preclude him from gainful employment or knowledge of resources to help him find food and shelter. The prescription suggests an underlying psychosis such as schizophrenia.
8. *What treatment options are available for this man?* Prehospital care includes oxygen, intravenous access, and monitoring. The patient does not appear violent but should be monitored for behavioral changes while en route to the ED. Because of the patient's confusion, providing reassurance is important to keep him calm. As a paramedic, you also should be aware of the resources available to the homeless and indigent in your area.
9. *What are some things to consider about homelessness in a patient who may be mentally ill?* Homelessness is increasing in the United States. This man is typical of many homeless people. Because of funding shortages, the mentally ill often are released to halfway houses or other facilities that cannot keep them long term. Many persons who are mentally ill cannot afford medication and stop taking their prescribed drugs. When this happens, the mental illness flares and behavioral problems may arise. Because of a lack of facilities and even less money, many mentally ill patients wander the streets.

Chapter Summary

- Paramedics must possess knowledge of key social issues and how those issues could affect treatment.
- Patient populations vary by locale but may include people with ethnic origins and/or religious beliefs unfamiliar to the paramedic. You should become familiar with the values and traditions of the major ethnic and religious groups in your community regarding healthcare.
- The codependent individual often is involved in a relationship with someone with a drug or alcohol problem, mental illness, or chronic illness.
- The codependent person could hinder EMS intervention by covering up for the patient with an acute problem brought on by addiction or illness.
- Economic burdens brought about by poverty affect all levels of society.
- Many poor have chronic medical conditions brought on by poor nutrition and poor living environments.
- Many of the poor have no medical coverage and, as such, must rely on local EDs even for minor illnesses or injuries.
- Paramedics must remember to treat all patients with the same level of respect and care regardless of the presence of social issues.
- An estimated 842,000 people are homeless on any given night in February, and 3.5 million experience homelessness during a year.
- Many homeless individuals also have mental illness and/or an addiction.
- Many homeless have untreated chronic medical conditions.
- Maintain a professional and nonjudgmental demeanor.
- Take additional standard precautions.
- Do not let homelessness interfere with a patient's right to receive the best care possible.

REFERENCES

Dick, T., & Hillson, D. (2005). Downtown people: Taking care of America's homeless. *Journal of Emergency Medical Services, 30,* 12.

Health Care for the Homeless. (n.d.). *Education.* Retrieved May 28, 2007, from http://www.hchmd.org.

National Coalition for the Homeless. (2007). *How many people experienced homelessness? NCH Fact Sheet #2.* Retrieved February 18, 2008, from http://www.nationalhomeless.org.

Simanski, J., & Rytina, N. (2006). *Naturalizations in the United States. Annual flow report, May 2006.* Washington, DC: Office of Immigration Services.

SUGGESTED RESOURCES

Fischer, P., & Breakey, W. (1986). Homelessness and mental health: An overview. *International Journal of Mental Health, 14,* 6-41.

Morse, G. (2000). Community alternatives, St. Louis, Missouri. *Healing Hands,* 4(5).

O'Connell, J. J. (2005). *Premature mortality in homeless populations: A review of the literature.* Nashville, TN: National Health Care for the Homeless Council.

Waxman, L. D., Peterson, K., & McClure, M. (1995). *A status report on hunger and homelessness in America's cities: 1995.* Washington, DC: U.S. Conference of Mayors.

Chapter Quiz

1. According to statistics, how many estimated homeless are there in the United States on any given night?

____

2. True or False: Many homeless individuals also have mental illness and/or an addiction.

3. Define *codependency.*

____

____

4. True or False: A codependent person believes he or she is the only one qualified enough to care for a particular individual.

5. Allowing an individual to continue with a persistent problem, often times interfering with that person getting necessary help, is known as ____________.

6. True or False: Once resettled in the United States, immigrants abandon all aspects of the culture and civilization they left behind.

7. The most common barrier to providing prehospital care with new residents to the United States is ________________________.

8. True or False: The ability to pay for services is the chief criterion for rendering care in EMS.

Terminology

Codependence A psychological concept defined as exhibiting too much and often inappropriate caring behavior.

Enabling behavior Behavior that allows another individual to continue to stay ill.

CHAPTER 42

Care for the Patient with a Chronic Illness

Objectives *After completing this chapter, you will be able to:*

1. Compare the primary objectives of acute care, home care, and hospice care.
2. Summarize the types of home care and the services provided.
3. Compare the primary objectives of the advanced life support (ALS) professional and the home care professional.
4. Differentiate the role of EMS provider from the role of the home care provider.
5. Compare the cost, mortality rate, and quality of care for a given patient in the hospital versus the home care setting.
6. Discuss the aspects of home care that result in enhanced quality of care for a given patient.
7. Identify the importance of home healthcare medicine as related to the ALS level of care.
8. Discuss the aspects of home care that have the potential to become a detriment to the quality of care for a given patient.
9. Given a home care scenario, predict complications requiring ALS intervention and possible hospitalization.
10. Given a series of home care scenarios, determine which patients should receive follow-up home care and which should be transported to an emergency care facility.
11. List pathologic conditions and complications typical to home care patients.
12. Describe airway maintenance devices typically found in the home care environment.
13. List modes of artificial ventilation and prehospital situations where each might be used.
14. Describe devices that provide or enhance alveolar ventilation in the home care setting.
15. Identify failure of ventilatory devices found in the home care setting.
16. List vascular access devices found in the home care setting.
17. Recognize standard central venous access devices used in the home care setting.
18. Describe the basic characteristics of central venous catheters and implantable drug administration ports, complications, and signs of malfunction associated with these devices.
19. List devices found in the home care setting that are used to empty, irrigate, or deliver nutrition or medication to the gastrointestinal or genitourinary tract.
20. Describe the indications, contraindications, and signs of equipment failure for urinary catheters in the prehospital setting.
21. Differentiate home care from acute care as a preferable situation for a given patient scenario.
22. Identify failure of drains.
23. Discuss the significance of palliative care programs related to a patient in a home care setting.
24. Define hospice care, comfort care, and resuscitation attempts as they relate to local practice, law, and policy.
25. List the stages of the grief process and relate them to an individual in hospice care.
26. Given a series of scenarios, demonstrate interaction and support with the family members and support persons for a patient who has died.
27. Discuss the relation between local home care treatment protocols and standard operating procedures and local EMS protocols and standard operating procedures.
28. Discuss differences in an individual's ability to accept and cope with his or her own impending death.
29. Discuss the rights of the terminally ill.

Chapter Outline

Case Scenario

You and your partner respond to a private residence for a "patient with blood in his urine." On arrival, you find a 38-year-old male paraplegic who, according to family members, has had blood in his urine for the past 4 days after replacement of his urinary catheter. The patient has been a paraplegic for the past 10 years after a fracture of the fourth thoracic vertebrae in a motorcycle accident. He has been able to live at home successfully the majority of the time since his accident, with the help of a visiting nurse and significant support from his family. The patient is supine in bed. He is lethargic but responsive to questions and disoriented to time and place. He is pale, warm to the touch, and diaphoretic.

Questions

1. *What is your general impression of this patient?*
2. *What additional assessment will be important to understand better the nature and severity of this patient's condition?*
3. *What intervention should you initiate at this time?*

You may be called to the home of a patient who receives home healthcare or hospice services. This chapter reviews the types of patients you may encounter in the home health setting, common medical equipment used, and specific interventions that may be necessary when caring for these patients. Before performing any of the interventions discussed in this chapter, you must receive the necessary training to perform them. In addition, make sure that you are authorized to perform them per your state and local authorities and medical direction.

OVERVIEW OF HOME HEALTHCARE

Acute Care versus Home Care

[OBJECTIVE 1]

Acute care is short-term medical treatment usually provided in a hospital for patients who have an illness or injury or who are recovering from surgery. The World Health Organization defines **home care** as the provision of health services by formal and informal caregivers in the home to promote, restore, and maintain a person's maximal level of comfort, function, and health, including care toward a dignified death. The first home care agencies were established in the 1880s. During that time, home care focused on preventive care and improving personal hygiene. In 1965, passage of the Social Security Act allowed older adults to receive home healthcare benefits. Some disabled younger Americans were able to receive this benefit beginning in 1973. Hospice benefits were added in 1983. **Hospice** is a care program that provides for the dying and their special needs.

Home Care Providers

[OBJECTIVES 2, 3, 4]

Formal caregivers are professionals who provide healthcare and personal care services in the home and receive compensation for the services they provide. These healthcare professionals provide care to recovering, disabled, chronically ill, or terminally ill persons who need help with activities of daily living. A patient may require only one type of care or a combination of services, depending on condition. Formal caregivers most often include a registered nurse or licensed professional nurse, social worker, and physical therapist. Other healthcare professionals involved in providing care may include respiratory, speech, and occupational therapists.

Informal caregivers who provide care in the home include family, friends, homemakers, and patient companions. The services provided by informal caregivers may include meal preparation, housekeeping duties, escort to physician appointments, help with bathing, or companion services.

Although home care services may be provided by independent providers, most services are provided by home care organizations. According to the U.S. Census Bureau, approximately 20,000 home care organizations existed in 1997. Home care organizations include the following:

- *Home health agencies*. Patients who receive home care require medical, nursing, social, or therapeutic treatment that cannot be easily or effectively provided only by family and friends. Medicare-certified home health agencies must meet federal minimal requirements for patient care and management. Services provided by these agencies are highly supervised and controlled primarily because of Medicare regulatory requirements.
- *Hospices*. Hospice care involves a team of professionals and volunteers who provide care for the terminally ill and support for the patient's family. Hospice care professionals are available 24 hours a day to keep the patient comfortable and make sure that the patient's end-of-life wishes are honored. Most hospices are Medicare certified and state licensed.
- *Homemaker and home care aide (HCA) agencies*. Homemaker and HCA agencies use homemakers and HCAs (also called *caregivers, companions,* and *personal*

attendants) to assist patients with activities of daily living, such as bathing, grooming, and dressing. Depending on the patient's needs, other duties may include housekeeping, laundering, changing bed linens, shopping for food, and preparing meals. Some states require that these agencies be licensed and meet established state standards.
- *Staffing and private-duty agencies*. Staffing and private-duty agencies usually are nursing agencies that offer nursing, homemaker, HCA, and companion services. Depending on the state, these agencies may or may not be licensed or required to meet regulatory requirements.
- *Companies specializing in medical equipment and supplies*. Some companies provide products for use by home care patients. These companies do not provide patient care but deliver their product to the patient's home when needed and teach the patient how to use it properly.

Examples of medical equipment, supplies, and in-home services that may be provided to home care patients are given in Table 42-1.

Home Care Recipients

[OBJECTIVES 5, 6, 7, 8]

The increased use of healthcare services and their associated costs have led to a trend and need to care for patients in the home. The National Association for Home Care estimates that more than 7 million people currently receive home care. Annual expenditures for home care are estimated to be approximately $38 billion. Medicare is the single largest payer of home care services in the United States.

TABLE 42-1 Examples of Medical Equipment, Supplies, and In-Home Services That May Be Provided to Home Care Patients

Equipment, Supplies, or Service	Examples
Medical equipment	Oxygen devices, ventilators, apnea monitors, wheelchairs, beds, walkers
Medical supplies	Mastectomy, ostomy, wound care, and diabetes products; incontinence and urologic supplies
In-home services	Respiratory therapy, infusion therapy, enteral nutrition, nutrition counseling, wound care, chemotherapy, pain management, hospice care; physical, speech, and occupational therapy

Individuals receive home care services for many reasons, including acute illnesses, long-term health conditions, permanent disability, and terminal illness. For example, many older adults elect to remain in their homes as their physical capabilities diminish rather than be placed in a long-term care facility. Patients who are disabled or recuperating from surgery or an acute illness also may receive home healthcare services (Figure 42-1). Chronically ill infants, children, and adults may require sophisticated medical equipment and care that can be provided by healthcare professionals in the home. Terminally ill patients also receive care at home, enabling families to remain together and allowing patients to maintain their dignity at the end of life. Examples of the types of patients who receive home care are listed in Box 42-1. Common medical conditions of home care patients are shown in Table 42-2.

Home care is a cost-effective service (Table 42-3). By allowing the patient to recuperate at home, hospital stays are shortened. However, as hospital stays decrease, increasing numbers of patients need highly skilled services when they return home. As a result, the likelihood that the home care patient will require advanced life support (ALS) EMS care increases.

In addition to cost effectiveness, other advantages of home care include the following:

- Allows the patient to take an active role in his or her own care

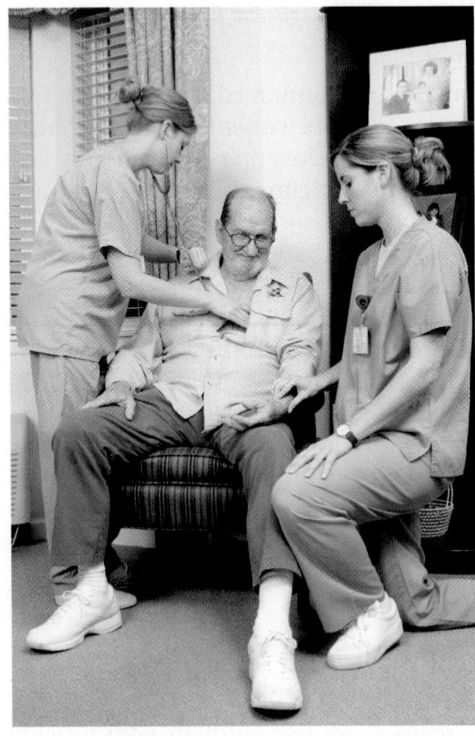

Figure 42-1 Individuals receive home care services for many reasons, including acute illnesses, long-term health conditions, permanent disability, and terminal illness.

BOX 42-1 Types of Patients Who Receive Home Care

- Patients who have mobility problems
- Patients who have a terminal illness
- Patients who have a developmental delay
- Patients who have a congenital condition, such as congenital heart disease
- Patients recuperating from surgery or an acute illness
- Transplant candidates
- Chronically ill infants, children, and adults
- Mothers and newborns
- Patients who require wound care, enteral nutrition, respiratory therapy, physical therapy, chronic pain management, or home chemotherapy
- Psychosocial support of the home care family

TABLE 42-2 Medical Conditions of Home Care Patients

Diagnosis or Condition*	Persons Using Medicare Home Health Agency Services in 2001 (%)
Diseases of the circulatory system	28.6
Diseases of the musculoskeletal system and connective tissue	17.2
Injury and poisoning	15.3
Symptoms, signs, and ill-defined conditions	10.5
Endocrine, nutritional, and metabolic diseases and immunity disorders	9.0
Diseases of the respiratory system	8.8
Disorders of the skin and subcutaneous tissue	6.6
Neoplasms	6.5
Diseases of the digestive system	4.3
Diseases of the nervous system and sense organs	3.9
Diseases of the genitourinary system	3.7
Diseases of the blood and blood-forming organs	2.3
Mental disorders	1.8
Infectious and parasitic diseases	0.8
Congenital anomalies	0.3

Data source: Centers for Medicare & Medicaid Services, Medicare Decision Support Access Facility, *Health Care Financing Review: Medicare and Medicaid Statistical Supplement, 2001.*

*Specific leading diagnostic categories were selected for presentation because of frequency of occurrences or because of special interest.

TABLE 42-3 Comparison of Hospital and Home Health Medicare Charges, 2001-2003

	2001	2002	2003
Hospital charges per day	$3080	$3574	$3838
Home health charges per visit	$105	$108	$109

Modified from National Association for Home Care & Hospice. (2004). *Basic statistics about home care.* Retrieved July 27, 2005, from http://www.nahc.org/NAHC/Research/04HC_Stats.pdf.

- Supplements the care provided by friends and family
- Maintains the patient's dignity and independence

Aspects of home care that have the potential to become a detriment to the quality of care for a patient include the following:

- Unlicensed or improperly trained caregivers
- Unsafe or unprofessional care
- Lack of availability of needed equipment and/or services
- Failure of the home health agency to meet government standards

ALS RESPONSE TO HOME CARE PATIENTS

Typical Responses

[OBJECTIVE 9]

Most patients who receive home care are sick but do not require ongoing care in a hospital or rehabilitation facility. These patients are usually discharged home to continue recuperation with the oversight of a home care agency. Patients who use special medical devices at home, such as a home ventilator, are usually asked to notify their local EMS agency and utility company. These patients may have a medical emergency if the device malfunctions or in case of a power failure. Typical types of home care problems are listed in Box 42-2.

If the patient currently receives home care, a home health professional may be present when you arrive at the patient's home. In fact, this person may be source of the call to 9-1-1. When you arrive, treat the healthcare professional with respect. He or she often can provide valuable information about the patient's illness or condition. For example, the home care professional will know the patient's normal vital signs, assessment findings, and capabilities. This person will be able to tell you if your findings are normal for the patient or different from normal. Use the information the home care professional provides to help assess the seriousness of the patient's current condition.

BOX 42-2 Types of Home Care Problems

Examples of home care problems that usually require intervention by a home health professional or physician include the following:

- Chemotherapy
- Pain management
- Wound care
- Ostomy care
- Hospice or palliative care

Examples of home care problems requiring acute intervention include the following:

- Altered mental status
- Airway complications
- Respiratory failure or acute respiratory events
- Cardiac decompensation or acute cardiac events
- Infection, acute sepsis, or septic complications
- Equipment malfunction
- Gastrointestinal or genitourinary crisis

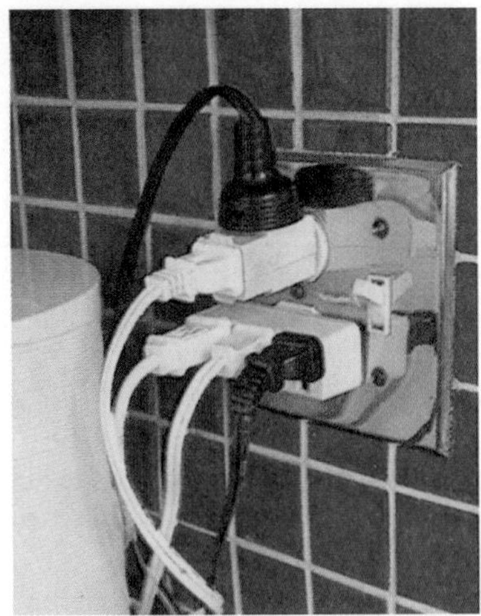

Figure 42-2 Be alert for hazards or obstacles that may be present in a patient's home.

General Principles of Assessment and Management

Scene Size-up

Scene Safety. Scene safety should always be your first priority when arriving to the scene of the home care patient. Treat a call for a home care patient as you would any other in regard to safety. Ensure the scene is safe to enter.

Hazards such as medical supplies, medical equipment, or infectious waste may be present in a patient's home. Be alert for these hazards or other obstacles that may be present (Figure 42-2). For example, a wheelchair, walker, cane, recliner, or bed may block your way as you attempt to gain access to or move a patient. If the patient is receiving home oxygen therapy, long stretches of oxygen tubing often are present on the floor, over or under tables, beds, and/or bedrails. Sharps may be present and may not have been properly disposed. Look for signs that may lead you to believe that infectious waste may be present, such as sharps containers, biohazard bags, gloves, dressings, or ostomy pouches. You may find the patient lying in his or her own feces or urine if immobile. In all situations, take appropriate infection control precautions. If the patient is known to be receiving oxygen therapy or has a respiratory infection, use a mask as you enter the home.

Pets may be present and become agitated and protective of the patient as you enter the home. Ask a family member to remove the pet from the immediate area. The pet may be placed in another room or outside to allow you to examine the patient in a secure environment. Home protection devices, such as firearms and knives, may be present in the patient's home. Be alert and aware of where these objects are located.

Environment. Assess the patient's surroundings. Is the patient able to care for himself or herself? If not, is a family member or other caregiver present to help the patient with daily needs (e.g., food, shelter, elimination, clothing, heat)? Do the patient's physical needs seem to be met adequately? Does the patient appear well nourished? Are the patient's surroundings in overall good condition? If the patient's living conditions are unhealthy or unsafe, notify the receiving facility staff of your findings or contact the appropriate public service agency in your community so that the patient can receive appropriate assistance.

Mechanism of Injury or the Nature of the Illness. Find out why you were called to the patient's home. How does the patient's condition or situation differ today compared with yesterday or last week? Quickly determine if you will need additional equipment or personnel to help you care for the patient.

Initial Assessment

Form a general impression as you approach the patient. Does the patient appear to be awake and alert? What is the patient's muscle tone and body position? What are breathing and effort and skin color? Does the patient appear to be in acute distress? Does the patient appear malnourished? What type of medical equipment is in use? Make mental notes as you begin your assessment.

As you perform the initial assessment, obtain medical information from the patient when possible. If the patient is unable to provide the information, a family member or home health professional often is able to provide it. Ask about the patient's health problems, normal assessment findings, medical devices in use, and current medications.

Home care patients often have medical conditions that make them prone to problems involving their airway, breathing, and circulation. Treat any life-threatening problems as you find them. When assessing the patient's mental status, you need to know what is normal for the patient. An altered mental status and/or reduced responsiveness may be a normal baseline for some home care patients. Compare your assessment findings with the information provided by the patient's caregiver about baseline mental status, behavior, and level of functioning. Does the patient have Alzheimer's disease or dementia? If the patient has had a sudden change in mental status, could it be the result of a recent change in medications, low blood sugar, or a stroke?

Focused History and Physical Examination

Critical problems found during the focused physical examination require rapid assessment and transport. If the patient's condition is not urgent, the focused history and detailed physical examination may be performed on the scene or during transport. Remember to recheck the patient's ABCs (***a***irway, ***b***reathing, ***c***irculation) and mental status frequently throughout the examination.

If the patient is receiving care from a home care agency, find out whether patient care records maintained by the agency or caregiver are available on the scene. These records may be used to compare your assessment and physical examination findings. For example, you may be able to find out the patient's normal vital signs, any recent changes in vital signs or medications, recent hospitalizations, and the patient's medical history. Find out if the patient takes his or her medications as prescribed. Perform ongoing assessments en route to the hospital.

If time permits, perform a detailed physical examination. Inspect, palpate, and auscultate. When assessing the patient's back, legs, and buttocks, look for signs and symptoms of skin breakdown or decubitus wounds. Also note if bruises or injuries on the patient's body indicate abuse or neglect. If these signs are present, be sure to report them to the receiving facility and document them in your prehospital care report.

Other Intervention and Transport Considerations

[OBJECTIVE 10]

Some patients will not require transport but do need home care follow-up or referral to other public service agencies. If transporting the patient to the hospital is necessary, you may need to notify a family member (if not already present) and the patient's physician.

Before leaving the patient's home, be sure to secure it. Lock the doors and windows. Turn off any appliances in use (e.g., stove, oven, coffeemaker). Leave at least one light on in the home if the patient allows it. This will help the patient if he or she returns at night. Bring the patient's purse or wallet to the hospital.

Management and Treatment Plan

Depending on the patient's condition, home health treatment may need to be replaced with ALS care.

Airway and Breathing Considerations

[OBJECTIVE 11]

Dyspnea is common in patients with chronic illnesses because they have difficulty swallowing and handling airway secretions. Excessive airway secretions and salivation may occur because of muscle weakness, brainstem injury, or other diseases and increase the patient's risk of aspiration.

Patients with a tracheostomy or cerebrospinal fluid shunt, patients on home ventilators, and patients with continuous positive airway pressure or bilevel positive airway pressure devices are at risk of airway obstruction.

Some congenital syndromes or diseases are associated with limited cervical motion, making intubation difficult. If a home care patient is on a ventilator, it is connected through a tracheostomy or tracheal tube. If the patient must be transported, you will need to disconnect the ventilator and manually ventilate the patient with a bag-mask device. Some EMS services use automatic transport ventilators. If this is the case in your service area, ensure that the home ventilator settings can be reproduced on the unit per your local protocols.

Circulation Considerations

Patients who depend on a medical device for their survival may have a resting heart rate that varies from what is "normal", which will make assessment for signs of compensated shock difficult to detect. A patient who has congenital heart disease such as tetralogy of Fallot may have chronic peripheral and/or central cyanosis. Check with the patient's caregiver about normal baseline skin color.

A patient who has a vascular access device (i.e., central venous catheter, implanted port, peripherally inserted central catheter) may require assistance because of a dislodged or damaged catheter, catheter obstruction or leakage from the catheter, or complications associated with these devices, such as a pneumothorax. If a home health professional is present, ask for assistance with these devices. The caregiver often is able to flush the lines and cap the ends of the tubing before transport. If the patient is attached to an infusion pump, the device should go with the patient to the hospital. Infusion pumps are used for many reasons, including giving insulin and chemotherapy.

Other Considerations. A home care patient often has a urinary catheter in place. The end of the catheter is usually connected to a drainage bag or leg bag. These devices are portable and must come with the patient to the hospital.

If the patient is using a home healthcare agency, bring any documents that may be present for the physician to use as a comparison to the patient's current condition. If the patient does not have a home healthcare agency, the hospital may need to suggest an agency in your area to assist the patient with home healthcare needs on discharge from the hospital.

If you observed unhealthy or unsafe living conditions at the scene, you may need to refer the patient to a social service agency. If you are not aware of one, be sure to report the conditions to the receiving facility. Document the patient's living conditions in your prehospital care report. The hospital may have a social worker on staff or a contract with a social service agency that can provide help for the patient.

PARAMEDIC*Pearl*

Many home care patients have a sensitivity or allergy to latex because of their repeated exposure to supplies and products made from this material.

Injury Control and Prevention in the Home Care Setting

William Haddon, Jr., a public health physician, is well known for applying principles of public health to injury prevention. He used a scientific approach known as the *epidemiological triangle*. Haddon's theory was that disease might be the direct result of unhealthy interactions among the host, the agent, and the environment. He separated injury-causing events into three subcategories:

1. Pre-event (will the potentially harmful event occur?)
2. Event (did the event cause injury?)
3. Postevent (what was the outcome?)

Haddon's strategy can be applied to the home care setting. For example, the elderly have a known increased risk for falls. Providing education about injury prevention may help reduce the risk of injury or the degree of injury the patient sustains in the event of a fall. When you are called to the home of an older adult, look around and note if potential hazards exist that might increase the patient's risk of falling. Are stairs in the patient's home unsafe? Are handrails broken or missing? Are steps broken or worn? Are the stairs poorly lit? Are throw rugs present that increase the patient's risk of tripping? If so, what resources are available in the community that could be contacted to help make the patient's home safer?

Case Scenario—continued

You administer oxygen at 15 L/min by nonrebreather mask as you continue your assessment. According to the family, the patient is usually alert and oriented but has become increasingly lethargic and confused during the past 1 to 2 days. They also inform you that he often is diaphoretic. Frank blood is visible in the urinary drainage bag. Respiratory distress is not visible, but his pulse is rapid and thready. Breath sound assessment reveals rhonchi in all lobes. Vital signs are pulse, 120 beats/min; blood pressure, 60/52 mm Hg; and respirations, 24 breaths/min. SpO_2 is 92% on room air.

Questions

4. *Is this patient high priority? Why or why not?*
5. *What are some possible causes of the patient's apparent shock? Do these causes relate to the patient's hematuria and altered mental status? Why or why not?*
6. *His family has provided daily care for him for the past 10 years. What emotions do you think they are likely to be experiencing at this time? Why?*
7. *What additional treatment will you provide at this time?*

SPECIFIC ACUTE HOME HEALTH SITUATIONS

Airway and Respiratory Problems

Airway problems in the home care patient may be the result of inadequate bronchial hygiene, inadequate alveolar ventilation, or inadequate alveolar oxygenation.

Inadequate bronchial hygiene may occur because of inadequate suctioning or ineffective airway clearance. This can be caused by a foreign body airway obstruction, cystic fibrosis, or other respiratory disorders.

Inadequate alveolar ventilation usually occurs because of carbon dioxide retention. It can be caused by chronic obstructive pulmonary disease, restrictive pulmonary disease, neuromuscular disorders (e.g., muscular dystrophy, amyotrophic lateral sclerosis, myasthenia gravis), depression of the respiratory control centers, or chest trauma.

Inadequate alveolar oxygenation is a common cause of hypoxia. It can result from pulmonary emboli, atelectasis, pneumonia, emphysema, chronic bronchitis, or acute respiratory distress syndrome.

The patient or caregiver may call for EMS assistance because of the following:

- A change in the patient's normal (baseline) breathing
- Increased respiratory demand (such as a respiratory infection), making current support inadequate
- Increased volume or color of secretions
- Obstructed or malfunctioning airway devices
- Improper application of a medical device to support respirations
- Onset of a fever

Be prepared to protect the patient's airway and provide necessary assistance. Examples of chronic conditions that require home respiratory support are given in Box 42-3.

Oxygen Therapy Found in the Home Setting

[OBJECTIVE 12]

Home Oxygen Therapy. Oxygen is provided in three common ways in the home care setting.

- *Oxygen in cylinders.* Oxygen is usually stored in steel or aluminum cylinders that contain pressurized oxygen. A pressure regulator is used to reduce the pressure in the cylinder to a safe range. A flowmeter is attached to the oxygen cylinder. Adjusting the flowmeter allows control of the liters of oxygen delivered. Oxygen tubing is connected to the cylinder and then attached to the patient to deliver oxygen.
- *Liquid oxygen system.* Liquid oxygen is a cryogenic liquid stored in a specialized vessel and must be filled by a trained professional. The device is more lightweight and therefore more portable than a standard oxygen cylinder (Figure 42-3). It is more expensive than a regular oxygen cylinder. Liquid oxygen supports combustion more readily than oxygen in its gaseous form and poses a greater hazard to the patient.
- *Oxygen concentrator.* An oxygen concentrator is an oxygen delivery machine that extracts oxygen from the air (Figure 42-4). Historically these devices were not portable and required electricity to work. However, there are now small battery-powered oxygen concentrators that are portable, and many are even approved for use on commercial airlines, such as the EverGo (Respironics, Amsterdam, Netherlands). The oxygen supply is endless and is much more cost effective for home care patients. In the setting of non–battery-operated or nonportable devices, the patient must be sure to have a back-up oxygen device in the event of a power failure or need to leave the home.

BOX 42-3 Chronic Conditions That Often Require Home Respiratory Support

- Chronic obstructive pulmonary disease
- Bronchopulmonary dysplasia
- Patients awaiting lung transplant
- Cystic fibrosis
- Sleep apnea

Examples of oxygen delivery devices found in the home care setting include a nasal cannula, oxygen mask, nonrebreather mask, and a tracheostomy collar. A tracheostomy is a small surgical opening (stoma) made from the anterior neck into the trachea between the second through fourth tracheal rings (Figure 42-5). The opening may be temporary or permanent. A tracheostomy may be performed to bypass an upper airway obstruction. It also may be performed in patients who are unable to clear secretions effectively or those who need long-term mechanical ventilation. A tracheostomy collar is a device that delivers high humidity and oxygen to a patient who has a surgical airway. Common complications encountered with tracheostomies are shown in Box 42-4.

Materials used for tracheostomy tubes include Silastic (silicone rubber; Dow Corning, Midland, Mich.), poly-

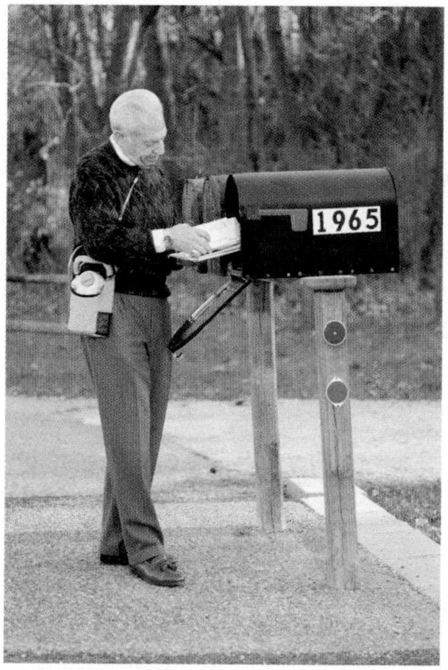

Figure 42-3 Liquid oxygen system.

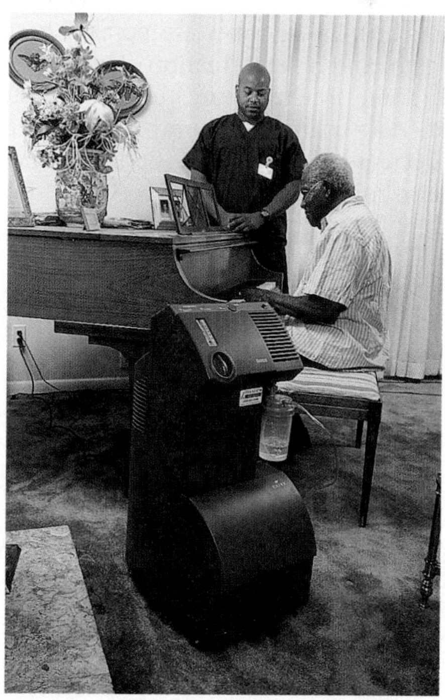

Figure 42-4 Oxygen concentrator.

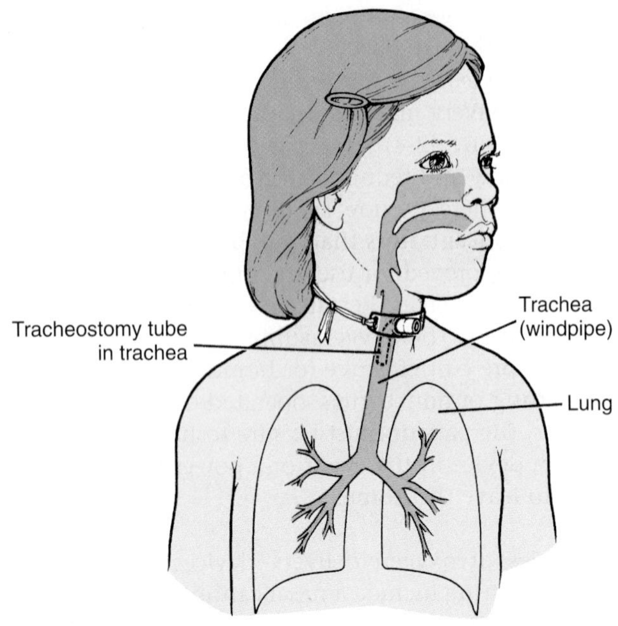

Figure 42-5 Tracheostomy tube in position in the trachea and secured in place.

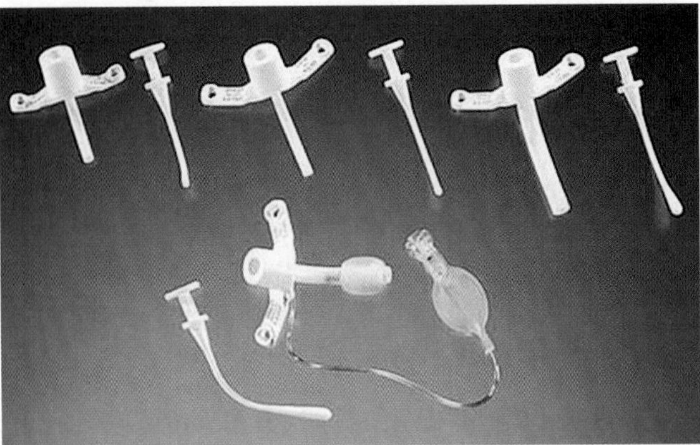

Figure 42-6 Neonatal and pediatric cuffed and uncuffed single-cannula tracheostomy tubes.

BOX 42-4 Common Tracheostomy Tube Complications

- Dislodgement of the tube
- Obstruction of the tube
- Infection

vinylchloride (PVC), stainless steel, and silver metals. Most tubes are made of Silastic or PVC. The tube softens at body temperature, conforming to the shape of the patient's trachea. These tubes are popular because they are lightweight and resist formation of crusted respiratory secretions. Some tracheostomy tubes are custom-made to accommodate unusual anatomy or pathologic conditions. To decrease the possibility of an allergic reaction, some patients require a metal tracheostomy tube. A metal tube contains an inner cannula. All tracheostomy tubes have a standard-size opening or hub outside the patient's neck to enable attachment of a bag-valve device. Metal tracheostomy tubes require an adapter to make this connection.

Tracheostomy tubes have a neck plate (flange) that rests on the patient's neck over the stoma. Holes are present on each side of the neck plate through which soft tracheostomy tube ties are inserted and used to secure the tube in place.

Like tracheal tubes, tracheostomy tubes vary in size. The size of the tube is marked on its sterile packaging and on the flange of the tube. If replacing a tracheostomy tube is necessary, try to use the same length and diameter of tube as the one already in place.

A single-cannula tracheostomy tube has one lumen used for airflow and suctioning of secretions (Figure 42-6). When changing the tube is necessary, a new tube must be inserted quickly because nothing keeps the stoma open once the old tube is removed. When a new tube is inserted, an obturator (stylet) is placed inside the tube to keep the flexible tube from kinking. After the new tube is in position, the obturator is quickly removed to permit ventilation. All neonatal tracheostomy tubes and most pediatric tubes are single-cannula tubes.

A double-cannula tracheostomy tube consists of an outer cannula (main shaft), inner cannula, and an obturator (Figure 42-7). The obturator is used only to guide the outer tube during insertion. When the outer cannula has been inserted, the obturator must be removed to allow ventilation. Once the outer tube is in place, the inner cannula is inserted and locked in place. The inner cannula may be disposable or reusable. A reusable inner cannula must be periodically removed for brief periods for cleaning.

A fenestrated tracheostomy tube helps the patient learn to breathe through the upper airway, expel secretions, and talk. A fenestrated tube has small holes (fenestrations) in the side of the tube (Figure 42-8). When a decannulation cap (plug) is attached to the tracheostomy tube, air flow through the stoma is blocked. Air flow is redirected through the holes in the tube, upward past the vocal cords, and out through the nose and mouth. If the patient cannot breathe through the nose or mouth, the decannulation cap *must* be removed to allow breathing through the stoma.

PARAMEDIC*Pearl*

Assume that any patient who has a tracheostomy and signs of respiratory distress has an obstructed tube.

Home Ventilators

[OBJECTIVE 13]

Long-term mechanical ventilation may be needed for many reasons, including the following:

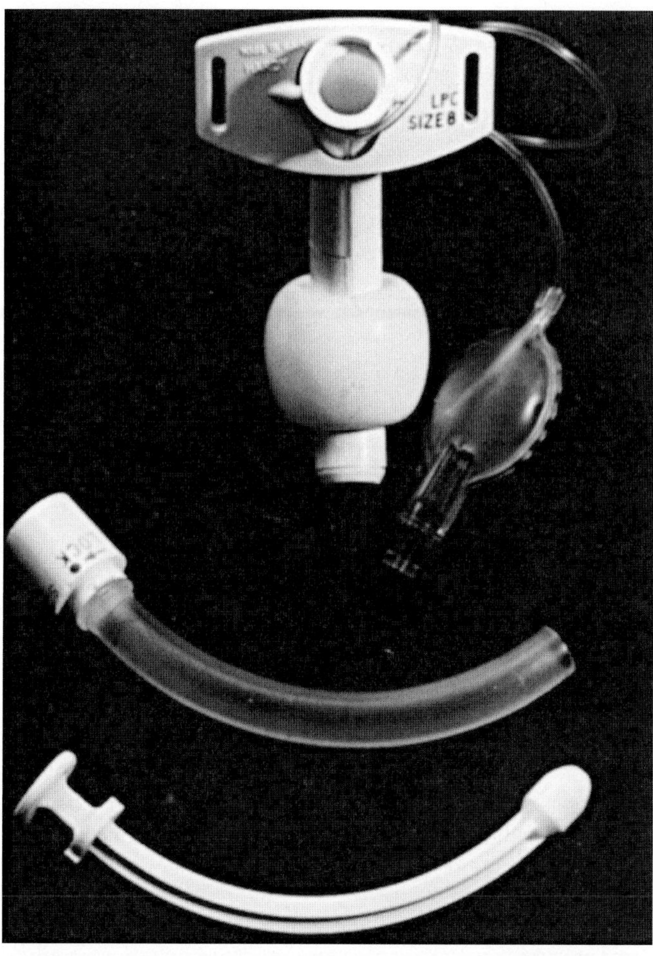

Figure 42-7 Double-cannula tracheostomy tube. Tracheostomy tube *(top)* with inner cannula *(middle)* and obturator *(bottom)*.

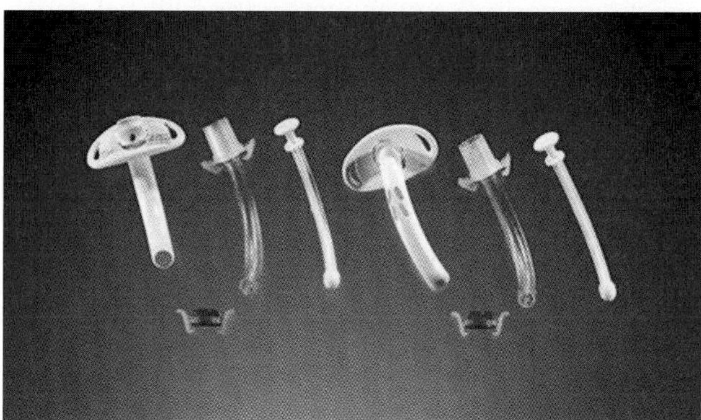

Figure 42-8 Disposable-cannula, cuffless, fenestrated tracheostomy tubes with decannulation caps (shown in *red*).

- Inadequate respiratory drive because of a congenital brain abnormality or brainstem damage
- Weak respiratory muscles from neuromuscular disease
- Cervical spinal cord injury or other conditions that impair the conduction of nerve impulses to respiratory muscles
- Severe chronic pulmonary disease

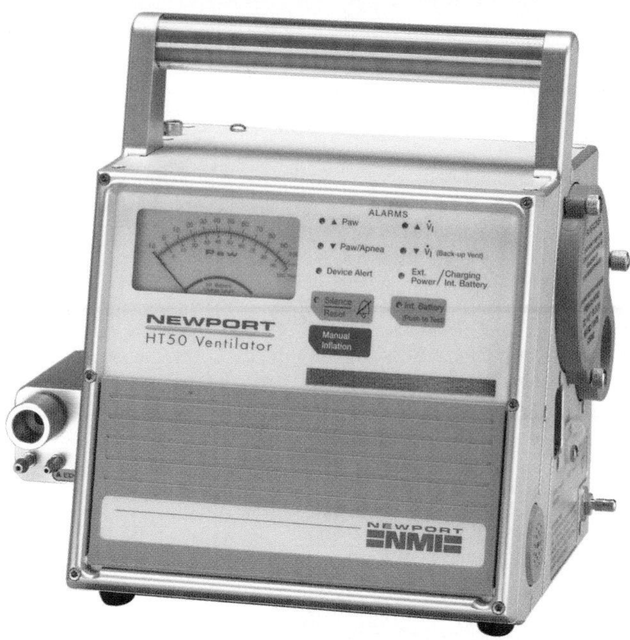

Figure 42-9 Switchable home volume and positive-pressure ventilator.

Some patients require continuous mechanical ventilation; others require intermittent ventilatory support, such as during sleep. Home ventilators are usually one of three types: a volume-regulated ventilator, pressure-regulated ventilator, or negative-pressure ventilator. Volume-regulated and pressure-regulated ventilators are both positive-pressure ventilators.

Positive-Pressure Ventilators. A positive-pressure ventilator forces gas (oxygen) into the lungs. A volume-regulated ventilator ends inspiration after a preset tidal volume has been reached (Figure 42-9). Once the volume has been delivered, the machine allows the patient to exhale before beginning the next cycle. This type of ventilator is one of the most widely used. It delivers a constant tidal volume regardless of changes in airway resistance.

A pressure-regulated ventilator ends inspiration after a preset pressure has been reached (Figure 42-10). Once the pressure is reached, the inspiration stops and the patient exhales. Because the volume of gas delivered by this type of ventilator changes if resistance to air flow changes, the tidal volume delivered may be inconsistent.

Negative-Pressure Ventilators. A negative-pressure ventilator generates intermittent negative pressure, mimicking normal breathing. Patients who have a chest wall deformity, progressive respiratory failure from neuromuscular diseases, or hypoventilation syndromes may use a negative-pressure ventilator. The patient does not require a tracheostomy or tracheal tube to use it.

The Emerson iron lung was a negative-pressure ventilator used during the 1950s for polio patients (Figure 42-11). A common negative-pressure ventilator in use today is the poncho wrap (or jacket) ventilator. It consists

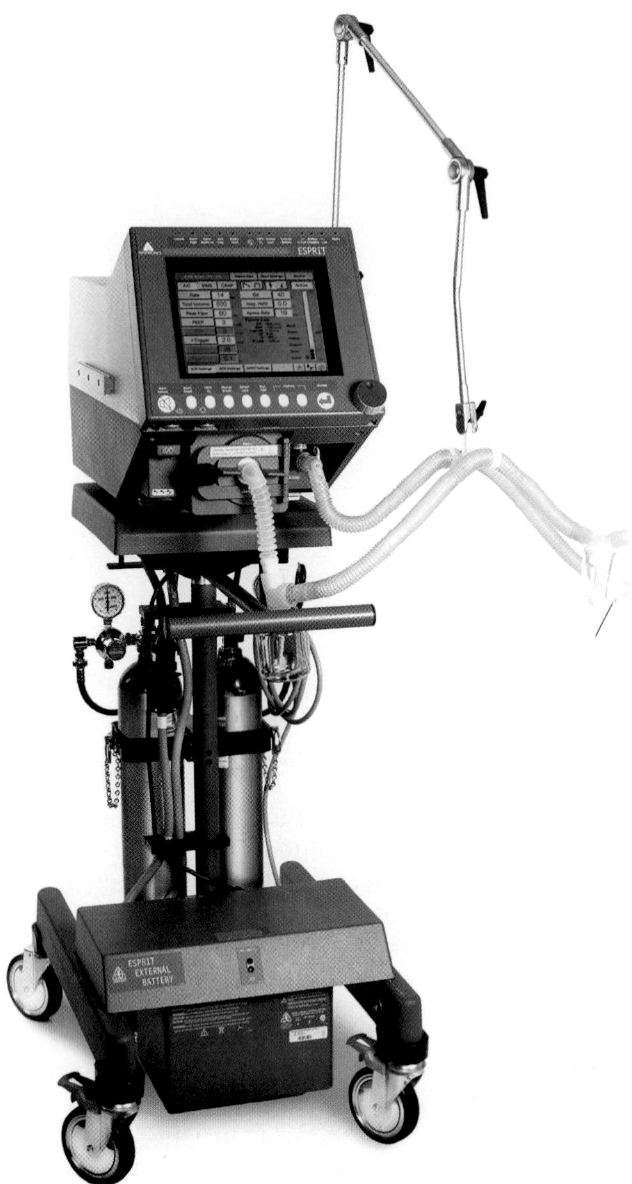

Figure 42-10 Home positive-pressure ventilator.

of a lightweight nylon jacket suspended by a rigid chest piece that fits over the chest and abdomen. The jacket is connected to a negative-pressure generator. Another negative-pressure device is the cuirass (or tortoise shell) ventilator. It consists of a rigid plastic or metal dome that fits over the chest and abdomen. The dome is connected to a negative-pressure generator.

A patient may use more than one type of ventilator. For example, the patient may use a negative-pressure ventilator during the day and a positive-pressure ventilator with a nasal mask at night. A patient may have more than one of the same type of ventilator. For example, a wheelchair-bound patient may use a ventilator mounted on the wheelchair during the day and have another of the same type of ventilator for use while in bed.

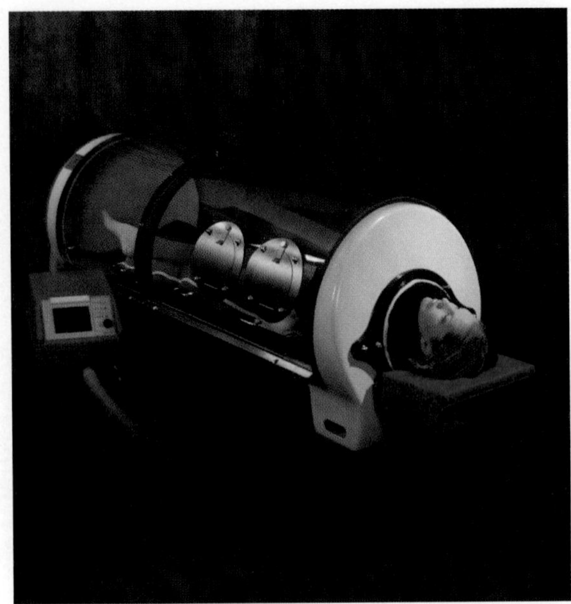

Figure 42-11 Home negative-pressure ventilator.

PARAMEDIC*Pearl*

Patients on ventilators are at risk of developing ventilator-associated pneumonia (VAP). VAP is pneumonia that develops in patients who have been on mechanical ventilation for more than 48 hours. Bacteria are the most common cause of VAP.

Noninvasive Mechanical Ventilation

[OBJECTIVE 14]

Continuous positive airway pressure and bilevel positive airway pressure are noninvasive methods of ventilatory assistance used in spontaneously breathing patients. They do not require a tracheal tube or tracheostomy. A patient who requires noninvasive mechanical ventilation has a higher than average risk for partial or total airway obstruction.

Continuous Positive Airway Pressure. Continuous positive airway pressure (CPAP) is the delivery of slight positive pressure (e.g., blowing through a straw) to prevent airway collapse and improve oxygenation and ventilation. CPAP may be used to assist ventilation in patients with neuromuscular weakness, chronic pulmonary edema, tracheomalacia, or obstructive sleep apnea.

When using mask CPAP, the patient wears a mask that covers the mouth and nose, providing continuous increased airway pressure throughout the respiratory cycle as the patient breathes (Figure 42-12). Nasal CPAP is used for patients who are nose breathers. This device covers only the patient's nose. If the patient opens the mouth while using this device, the pressure may be lost through the mouth and will therefore be ineffective in providing CPAP. Some patients use CPAP continuously, whereas others need it only at night when airway obstruction is most likely.

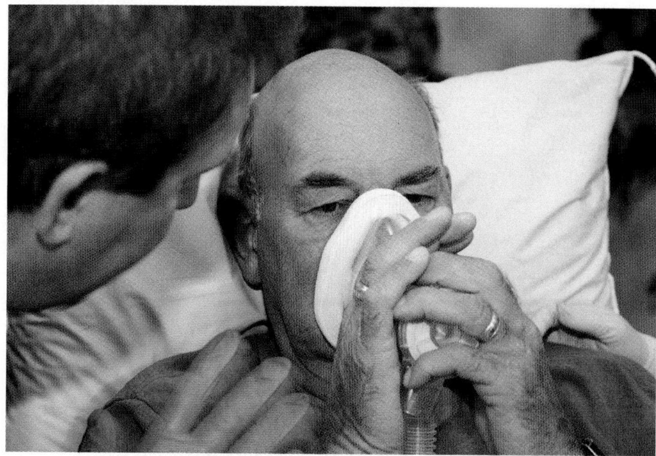

Figure 42-12 Mask continuous positive airway pressure (CPAP).

Bilevel Positive Airway Pressure. Like CPAP, **bilevel positive airway pressure** (BiPAP) is delivered through a tight-fitting mask that fits over either the patient's nose or the mouth and nose. In BiPAP therapy, two (bi) levels of positive pressure are delivered—one during inspiration (to keep the airway open as the patient inhales) and the other (lower) pressure during expiration to reduce the work of exhalation. The BiPAP device can be set to deliver pressure at a set rate or to sense when an inspiratory effort is being made by the patient and deliver a higher pressure during inspiration. BiPAP is used in the treatment of patients with chronic respiratory failure. It may be helpful in the transition from invasive to noninvasive respiratory support.

Assessment Findings

Form a general impression of the patient. Assess the patient's appearance, work of breathing, and circulation to determine the severity of the illness or injury and help you determine the urgency for care. During the initial assessment, assess the patient's work of breathing, tidal volume, peak flow, oxygen saturation, and breath sounds. If the patient has signs of respiratory distress, his or her medical history may help identify the cause of the problem. Consider a lower airway obstruction if the patient has a history of fever and gradual worsening of respiratory status.

If the patient has a tracheostomy, a mucous plug may be the cause if symptoms began suddenly and are accompanied by a change in the consistency of secretions. Consider a displaced or obstructed tracheostomy tube if the patient has signs and symptoms consistent with a possible obstruction (Box 42-5).

BOX 42-5 Signs of Possible Tracheostomy Tube Obstruction

- Altered mental status with restlessness, agitation
- Increased work of breathing
- Raspy noises from tracheostomy tube during breathing
- Change in sounds during respiration
- Diminished breath sounds
- Nasal flaring, retractions
- Difficulty eating or sucking
- Decreased oxygen saturation
- Marked use of accessory muscles
- Poor peripheral perfusion; mottling
- Tachycardia (bradycardia is a late sign)
- Inadequate chest rise during spontaneous or assisted ventilation
- High peak pressure alarm on ventilator
- Difficulty ventilating when providing assisted ventilation
- Cyanosis, bradycardia, and unresponsiveness (late findings)

If the patient is ventilator dependent, a recent change in home ventilator settings or a ventilator malfunction also may cause worsening respiratory symptoms. Ask the patient's caregiver about this possibility.

If the patient is on CPAP or BiPAP, the patient may be removed from the device if it significantly interferes with assessment and interventions. The patient will still be able to breathe but may tire easily. If the patient shows signs of respiratory distress, give supplemental oxygen or assist breathing with a bag-mask device as necessary.

Management and Treatment Plan

Management goals for a patient receiving oxygen therapy and needing emergency care include improving airway patency, ventilation, and oxygenation.

Improving Airway Patency. Improving airway patency may require the following:

- Repositioning airway devices
- Removing secretions from airway devices
- Replacing a home airway device (tracheostomy tube) with an ALS device (tracheal tube)

Clearing an Obstructed Tracheostomy Tube. If you suspect a tracheostomy tube is obstructed, try to ventilate through the tube with a bag-mask device to assess tube patency. If the patient is on a home ventilator, disconnect the tracheostomy tube from the ventilator and attach the tube to the bag-mask device. If compressing the bag is difficult, assess for tube obstruction. Indications for tracheostomy tube suctioning are shown in Box 42-6. Ask the patient's caregiver to provide the suctioning equipment and supplies because the items used in the home are appropriate for the patient's needs.

Begin by placing the patient in a supine position. If the patient is a child, place a small towel roll beneath the shoulders. This helps extend the neck and improve access to the tracheostomy tube.

Examine the tracheostomy tube. Because a tracheostomy bypasses the upper airway, dried secretions can easily accumulate and occlude the tracheostomy despite regular tracheostomy care. Make sure that the tube is properly positioned and the obturator has been removed. If the patient has a fenestrated tube, make sure the decannulation cap has been removed from the tube.

BOX 42-6 Indications for Tracheostomy Tube Suctioning

- Indication by the patient that suctioning is necessary
- Suspected aspiration of gastric or upper airway secretions
- Visible secretions in the airway; secretions bubbling in the tracheostomy tube
- Wheezes, crackles, or gurgling on inspiration or expiration audible to the patient and/or caregiver with or without auscultation
- More frequent or congested-sounding cough
- Inability to clear secretions by coughing
- Altered mental status, restlessness or irritability
- Unexplained increase in work of breathing, respiratory rate, or heart rate
- Decrease in vital capacity and/or oxygen saturation
- Unilateral or bilateral absent or diminished breath sounds
- Cyanosis

Select a suction catheter of appropriate size. It should be no more than half the internal diameter of the tube being suctioned. To determine the correct size of suction catheter for a pediatric patient, use a length-based resuscitation tape or multiply the external diameter of the tracheostomy tube (in millimeters) by two. For example, if the tracheostomy tube is 4 mm in diameter, use an 8F suction catheter. The use of a suction catheter of appropriate size is important to allow the entry of air around the catheter during suctioning. A suction catheter that is too large can obstruct the airway.

Set the suction pressure (portable or wall-mounted) to −100 mm Hg or less. If possible, preoxygenate the patient. Give blow-by oxygen by holding the oxygen tubing close to the opening of the tracheostomy tube. Set the oxygen flow rate to 10 to 15 L/min. If necessary, ventilate the patient's lungs with a bag-mask device by attaching the bag to the tracheostomy tube.

Gently insert the suction catheter into the tracheostomy tube without applying suction (Figure 42-13). Do not use excessive force when inserting the suction catheter because this may damage the soft tissues of the trachea. Insert the catheter no further than 0.5 cm beyond the end of the tracheostomy tube. Once the catheter is in the tracheostomy tube, apply suction while slowly withdrawing the catheter, rolling it between your fingers to suction all sides of the tube. Insertion of the suction catheter and suctioning should take no longer than 10 seconds per attempt. Monitor the patient's heart rate and color throughout the procedure. Stop suctioning immediately if the heart rate begins to slow or if the patient becomes cyanotic.

If suctioning equipment is not immediately available, attempt to clear the obstruction by quickly inserting and removing the obturator. This technique should *not* be used when suctioning equipment is available.

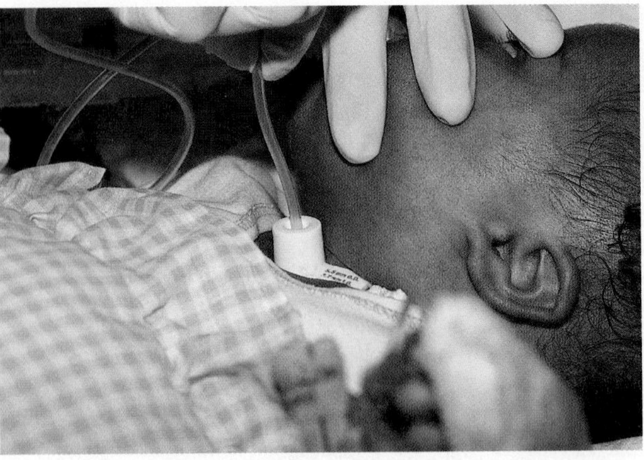

Figure 42-13 Suctioning a tracheostomy tube.

PARAMEDIC*Pearl*

Take care to move a tracheostomy tube as little as possible when cleaning secretions from around it and during suctioning. Movement of the tube irritates the trachea. It also is uncomfortable for the patient.

After suctioning, reassess the patient. Observe the patient's rate and depth of breathing, skin color, heart rate, and mental status. Auscultate breath sounds and assess pulse oximetry, if available. If breathing is adequate, administer oxygen. If breathing is inadequate, suctioning must be repeated. Give oxygen and allow the patient to rest for 30 to 60 seconds (or provide assisted ventilation with high-concentration oxygen) before beginning another attempt. If the patient shows no improvement, prepare to remove and replace the tracheostomy tube.

Removing and Replacing a Tracheostomy Tube. Removal of a tracheostomy tube is called **decannulation.** To remove a tracheostomy tube, begin by assembling and preparing the necessary equipment. Explain the procedure to the patient. Make sure oxygen, suction, and a bag-mask device with mask are immediately available.

Ask the patient's caregiver if a replacement tracheostomy tube is available. If the caregiver is not available, determine the size of the current tracheostomy tube by checking the wings (flanges) of the tube. Try to locate the same size and model of tracheostomy tube. If a similar tube is not available, use a tube of similar size. Select a tube with the same outer diameter as the patient's tube or one-half size smaller. If a tracheostomy tube is unavailable, a tracheal tube with an *outer* diameter equivalent to the patient's tracheostomy tube can be inserted though the stoma in an emergency.

Inspect the new tube for cracks and tears. If the new tube has a cuff, inflate the cuff and check for leaks. Completely deflate the cuff. Avoid touching the part of the tube that will be inserted into the trachea.

Insert the obturator into the new tube. Make sure that it slides in and out easily. The obturator serves as a stylet to guide the tube during insertion. Its blunt tip helps protect the stoma from trauma during insertion. Moisten the new tracheostomy tube with normal saline or a small amount water-soluble lubricant to ease insertion. If time permits, cut tracheostomy ties to the appropriate length. Thread the tracheostomy tie through the flange on one side of the new tube. Some patients use a tracheostomy tube holder that uses hook-and-loop closure material or nylon hooks to secure the tube in place instead of ties (Figure 42-14).

If the existing tube has a deflatable cuff, deflate the cuff by connecting a 5- to 10-mL syringe to the valve on the pilot balloon. With the syringe, aspirate air or water until the pilot balloon collapses. Cutting the pilot balloon will not reliably deflate the cuff.

While holding the tracheostomy tube with one hand, cut or untie the cloth ties that hold the tube in place with the other. Because a cough can dislodge the tracheostomy tube, be sure to hold the tube when the ties are not secure.

If the patient has a single-cannula tracheostomy tube, slowly withdraw the tube (Figure 42-15). If the patient has a double-cannula tracheostomy tube, remove the inner cannula. If the inner cannula is reusable, clean it and reinsert it. The inner cannula of a reusable tube is cleaned with hydrogen peroxide and rinsed with normal saline. If the inner cannula is disposable, remove and discard it and insert a new inner cannula. If replacing the inner cannula fails to clear the airway, remove the outer cannula as well, administer oxygen, and replace both tubes at the same time.

PARAMEDIC*Pearl*

In most patients with a tracheostomy, the upper airway connected to their trachea is patent. This permits bag-mask ventilation and orotracheal intubation if needed. If oxygen is given through the mouth and nose, cover the stoma with sterile gauze.

Administer oxygen until the new tracheostomy tube is inserted. Oxygen can be given directly through the stoma. If airflow can be heard and felt through the upper airway, oxygen can be administered by mask. If significant delay occurs in replacing the tracheostomy tube, the patient may need positive-pressure ventilation. If the upper airway is obstructed, deliver positive-pressure ventilation by ventilating the stoma with a bag-valve device with a neonatal mask (Figure 42-16).

With the obturator in place inside the new tube, gently insert the tube into the stoma with a downward and forward motion that follows the curve of the trachea (Figure 42-17). If necessary, place gentle traction on the skin above or below the stoma to ease insertion. If the tracheostomy tube cannot be easily inserted, withdraw

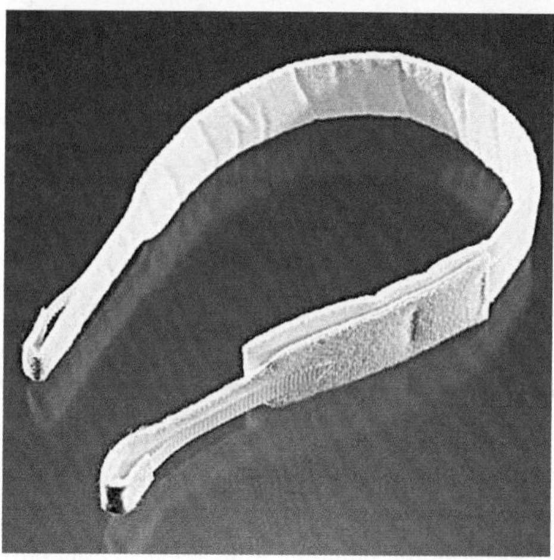

Figure 42-14 Tracheostomy tube holder with hook-and-loop closure material that attaches easily to the flanges on the tracheostomy tube.

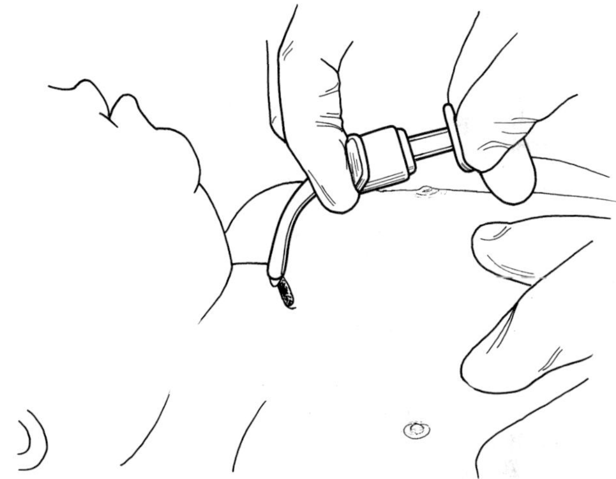

Figure 42-15 Slow withdrawal of the tracheostomy tube.

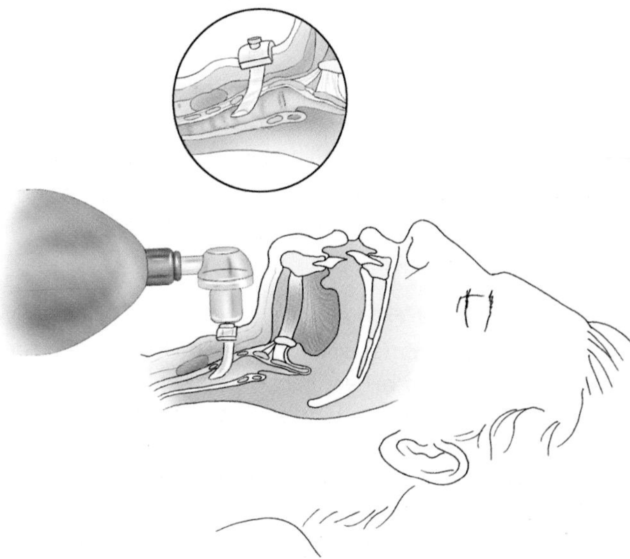

Figure 42-16 Ventilating through a stoma with a bag-valve device.

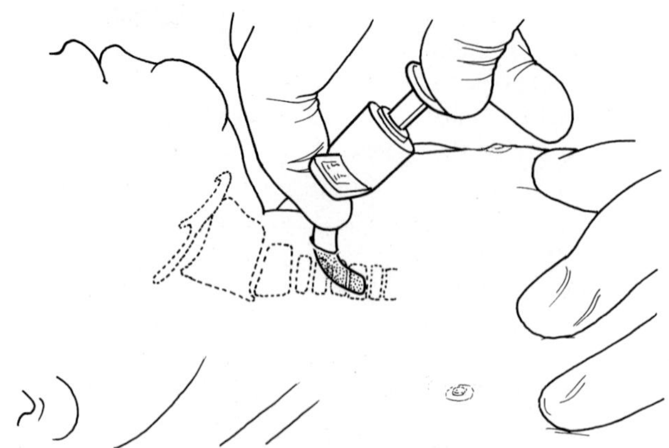

Figure 42-17 With the obturator in place inside the new tracheostomy tube, gently insert the tube into the stoma with a downward motion, following the curve of the trachea.

the tube, administer oxygen, and begin again. If the second attempt is unsuccessful, try a smaller tube. **Never force the tube.** Forcing the tube can create a false tract. After insertion, remove the obturator from the tracheostomy tube.

Connect a bag-mask device to the tracheostomy tube and ventilate the patient's lungs. *Do not let go of the tracheostomy tube* until it has been secured with tracheostomy ties or a tracheostomy tube holder.

Check for proper placement of the tracheostomy tube. Signs of proper placement include equal bilateral chest rise; equal breath sounds (either spontaneous or with assisted ventilation); and improvement in mental status, heart rate, and decreased work of breathing. Signs of improper placement include resistance during insertion of the tube, bleeding from the stoma, lack of chest rise or poor compliance during assisted ventilation, or development of subcutaneous air in the tissues surrounding the stoma.

After confirming proper placement of the tracheostomy tube, secure the tube with tracheostomy ties or a tracheostomy tube holder. The ties or holder should be snug enough that you can place only one finger between the fastening device and the patient's skin.

PARAMEDIC*Pearl*

A suction catheter or feeding tube may be used as a guide to ease insertion of a new tracheostomy tube. Insert the suction catheter through the new tracheostomy tube, then insert the suction catheter into the stoma without applying suction. Slide the tracheostomy tube along the suction catheter and into the stoma until it is in the proper position. *Do not let go of the suction catheter at any time before removing it from the tracheostomy tube.* Withdraw the suction catheter from the tracheostomy tube. Assess the patient.

Placing a Tracheal Tube in a Tracheostomy. If a new tracheostomy tube is not available or if replacement attempts are unsuccessful, try to insert a tracheal tube. Insertion of a tracheal tube is a temporary measure until a tracheostomy tube of the proper size can be replaced. A patient with a tracheostomy may have some airway narrowing, requiring a smaller tracheal tube than usual. Follow these steps to place a tracheal tube through the stoma:

1. Select a tracheal tube that is the same or slightly smaller size than the patient's tracheostomy tube.
2. If the tracheal tube has a cuff, inflate the cuff and check for leaks.
3. Completely deflate the cuff. Avoid touching the part of the tube that will be inserted into the trachea.
4. Moisten the distal end of the tracheal tube with saline or a small amount of water-soluble lubricant.
5. Place the patient in a supine position.
6. If the patient is a child, place a small towel roll beneath the shoulders.
7. If possible, give oxygen just before inserting the tracheal tube.
8. Note the length of the original tracheostomy tube and use it as a guide for depth of insertion of the tracheal tube.
9. Gently slide the tracheal tube through the stoma and into the airway.
10. Direct the tip downward after passing it through the stoma. The insertion depth of the tracheal tube should equal the distance between the flange and the distal tip of the tracheostomy tube.
11. If the tracheal tube is cuffed, inflate the cuff to stabilize the tube and reduce air leakage.
12. Secure the tube in place.

If a tracheostomy tube or tracheal tube cannot be inserted through the stoma, orotracheal intubation can be performed unless an upper airway obstruction is present. If the patient's condition does not improve or if a tracheal tube cannot be inserted, attempt assisted ventilation through the stoma. For best results, attach a neonatal mask to the bag-mask device and place the mask over the stoma. Alternatively, deliver positive-pressure ventilation with a mask placed over the patient's mouth and nose while covering the stoma with a gloved hand to prevent the escape of air.

Improving Oxygenation and Ventilation

[OBJECTIVE 15]

To improve the patient's oxygenation and ventilation, you may need to do the following:

- Remove the patient from a home care device (home oxygen or home ventilator) and use positive-pressure ventilation.

- Replace the oxygen system.
- Change the flow rate of an oxygen delivery device.
- Adjust the settings of a home care device to attempt to improve ventilation.

PARAMEDIC*Pearl*

Do not adjust a patient's home ventilator settings without first consulting medical direction.

If signs of respiratory distress are present in a patient on a ventilator, quickly try to determine the cause and correct the problem. Use the mnemonic DOPE to recall possible reversible causes of acute deterioration in an intubated patient:

- ***D***isplaced tube (right mainstem or esophageal intubation) or ***D***isconnection of the tube or ventilator circuit—reassess tube position and ventilator connections
- ***O***bstructed tube (blood or secretions are obstructing air flow)—suction
- ***P***neumothorax (tension)—needle thoracostomy
- ***E***quipment problem or failure (empty oxygen source, inadvertent change in ventilator settings, low battery)—check equipment and oxygen source

If you suspect ventilator malfunction and you cannot quickly find and correct the problem, take the following steps:

- Disconnect the ventilator tubing from the tracheostomy or tracheal tube.
- Attach a bag-mask device to the tube and provide manual ventilation with supplemental oxygen.
- Watch for equal chest rise and listen for equal breath sounds.
- If the patient's chest rise is shallow, ensure that the bag-mask device is securely connected to the tube. If chest rise does not improve, assess the tube for obstruction.

If the patient is to be transported to the hospital, ensure the patient will have an adequate supply of oxygen throughout the transport. Assistance may be needed when moving the patient because of the oxygen delivery system being used.

Psychological Support and Communication Strategies. Respiratory distress can cause extreme anxiety for the patient and caregiver. When you arrive at the scene, identify yourself and attempt to calm the patient. While working quickly to find the cause of the patient's respiratory distress, let the patient know you are there to help. Be sure to explain the steps of every procedure before you do it.

While providing care for a patient who has a tracheal or tracheostomy tube, keep in mind that the patient may be unable to verbalize concerns, pain, or other issues regarding care to you directly. A patient with a tracheostomy may have a "talking trach." This type of tracheostomy tube has a one-way speaking valve that forces air around the tube, through the vocal cords, and out of the mouth on exhalation, permitting vocalization.

If the patient is alert but unable to speak because of the tube, try alternative methods of communication. For example, ask the patient to blink his or her eyes once for a "yes" answer to your questions and twice for "no." If the patient indicates he or she is in pain, ask the patient to point to where it hurts or blink when you point to or touch the area. Alternately, the patient may be able to relay symptoms by writing on a notepad. Sign language also may be used if you and the patient are both familiar with this type of communication.

Circulatory Problems

Home care patients receive care for many different cardiac conditions, including the following:

- Cardiomyopathy
- Post–myocardial infarction cardiac insufficiency
- Congestive heart failure
- Post–open heart surgery
- Heart transplant
- Heart disease or congenital heart disease
- Stable or unstable angina
- Hypertension

Changes in peripheral circulation may occur because of interrupted arterial and/or venous flow. This can be caused by immobility, swelling, a thrombus, arteriosclerosis, or varicosities.

Vascular Access Devices

[OBJECTIVE 16]

Vascular access devices (VADs) are catheters placed in patients to deliver fluids, medications, blood or blood products, chemotherapy, or nutritional agents and to withdraw blood samples when frequent laboratory tests are required. The catheters are inserted into the central circulation for long-term use, usually for weeks or months. VADs have allowed many patients to be treated as outpatients rather than have prolonged hospital stays. Examples of conditions for which a patient may need a VAD include massive burns, intestinal obstruction, inflammatory bowel disease, AIDS, and cancer chemotherapy.

Although several types of VADs are available, they can be classified into the following four general categories:

- Dialysis shunts
- Central venous catheters
- Implanted ports
- Peripherally inserted central catheters

Dialysis Shunts. Dialysis is a method for removing waste products, such as urea from the blood when the kidneys fail. The two major forms of dialysis are hemodialysis and peritoneal dialysis (see Chapter 27). For patients who have end-stage renal disease (ESRD), adequate vascular access is the most important factor in the delivery of hemodialysis therapy. The most common types of vascular access for hemodialysis, **dialysis shunts,** are the arteriovenous (AV) fistula and AV graft. Because an AV fistula or AV graft join an artery and vein, they also may be called *dialysis shunts.*

An AV fistula is the vascular access route usually used in patients with ESRD. The fistula is surgically created by inserting two cannulae through the skin. One cannula is inserted into a large vein and another into a large artery (Figure 42-18). The blood vessels of the wrist or upper forearm most often are used. When dialysis is not being performed, the cannulae are joined, allowing arterial blood to flow directly into the vein. When dialysis is being performed, the cannulae are separated, allowing the arterial blood to flow to the dialyzer and the dialyzed blood to return from the dialyzer to the circulation through the venous cannula. Approximately 4 to 6 weeks after the procedure, the walls of the vein increase in size and thicken because of the arterial pressure. Thickening of the vessel allows repeated needle sticks, making hemodialysis possible.

Patients who have ESRD often are elderly or have diabetes mellitus. Their veins may be too small, fragile, or arteriosclerotic to create an AV fistula. Instead, a prosthetic graft is used to create an artificial blood vessel that joins an artery and vein. The source of the graft may be a vein from the patient's thigh or artificial material such as polytetrafluoroethylene or Gore-tex (W.L. Gore & Associates, Newark, Del.). An AV graft may be straight or looped. The graft is implanted subcutaneously, usually in the upper arm, lower arm, or thigh (Figure 42-19).

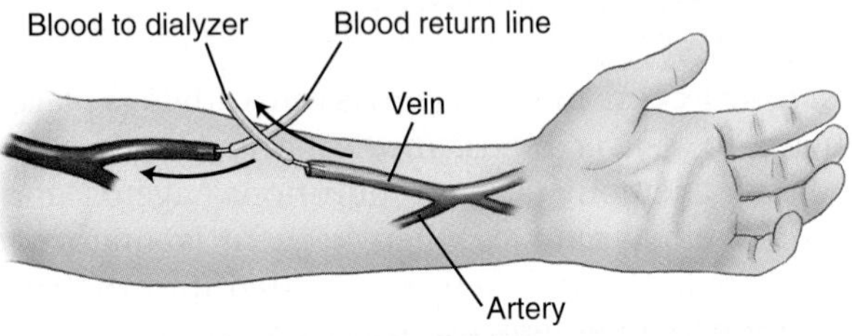

Figure 42-18 Arteriovenous fistula.

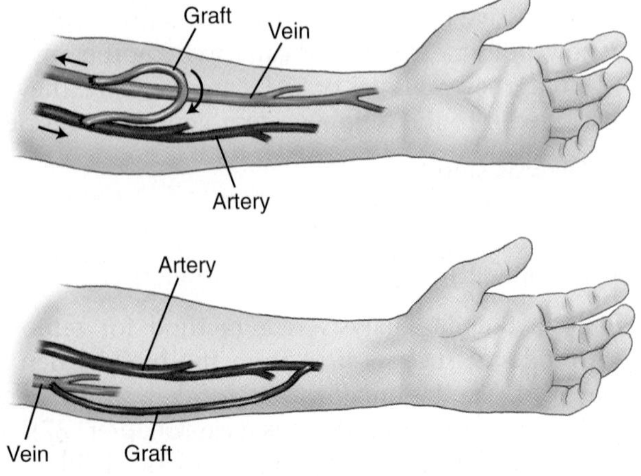

Figure 42-19 Arteriovenous graft.

A patient who receives home (peritoneal) dialysis is usually assisted by a family member or home care professional. Problems may arise such as dialyzer rupture, electrical or mechanical problems, hypotension, shock, or seizures. In addition to the SAMPLE history, be sure to assess the dialysis site, determine how much fluid was removed from the patient during dialysis, and determine how much fluid was replaced before your arrival. This information will be important to the receiving facility staff when caring for the patient.

Central Venous Catheters

[OBJECTIVE 17]

Central venous catheters implanted for long-term use are typically named for the individual who created them (e.g., Broviac, Hickman). These catheters are also called *tunneled catheters.*

A **central venous catheter** is surgically inserted into the external jugular, subclavian, or cephalic veins, with the catheter tip in the superior vena cava, just above the right atrium. The other end of the catheter is tunneled subcutaneously. It exits the skin on the anterior chest wall. A small cuff is located around the catheter approximately 1 inch inside the point where the catheter enters the patient's skin. Fibrous tissue grows around the cuff, anchoring the catheter in place and creating a barrier against infection (Figure 42-20, *A*). The external part of a tunneled catheter may have a single, double, or triple lumen, depending on the patient's treatment needs. A small cap covers each lumen (Figure 42-20, *B*). To ensure that blood clots do not block the catheter's lumen, each lumen is flushed with a diluted heparin solution initially and twice a day when not in use, after each intermittent infusion, after blood drawing, and whenever an infusion is disconnected.

Implanted Ports

[OBJECTIVE 18]

Implanted ports are known by their brand names, such as Portacath, Mediport, or Infusaport. An implanted (or subcutaneous) port is surgically placed completely below the skin, with no parts external to the skin. Like tunneled catheters, a Silastic catheter is inserted into a central vein and advanced so that the tip lies at the junction of the superior vena cava and the right atrium. However, the other end is tunneled subcutaneously and is attached to a port (reservoir). The port can be felt as a raised disk under the skin. To give medications or draw blood, a needle is inserted through the skin overlying the port. The port has titanium or plastic housing and a hard silicone septum that is self-sealing. To extend the life of the septum, a special Huber needle is used to access it (Figure 42-21).

Peripherally Inserted Central Catheters. Peripherally inserted central catheters (PICCs) are not directly inserted into a central vein. Instead, a PICC line is inserted into an antecubital vein and then advanced into the subclavian vein so that the tip lies in the superior vena cava or right atrium. PICC lines also are called *nontunneled catheters* because they enter the skin near the point at which they enter the vein.

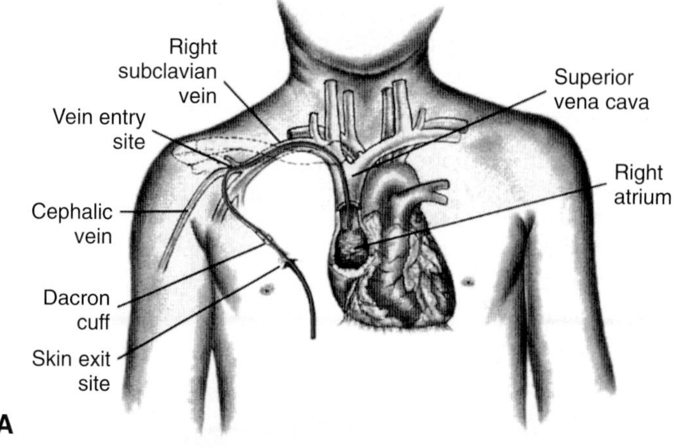

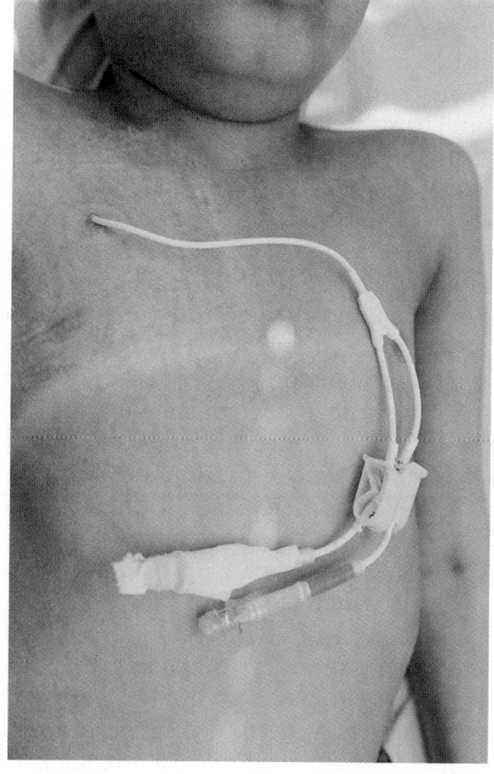

Figure 42-20 **A,** Central venous catheter insertion and exit site. **B,** External venous catheter (note the redness from the dressing site).

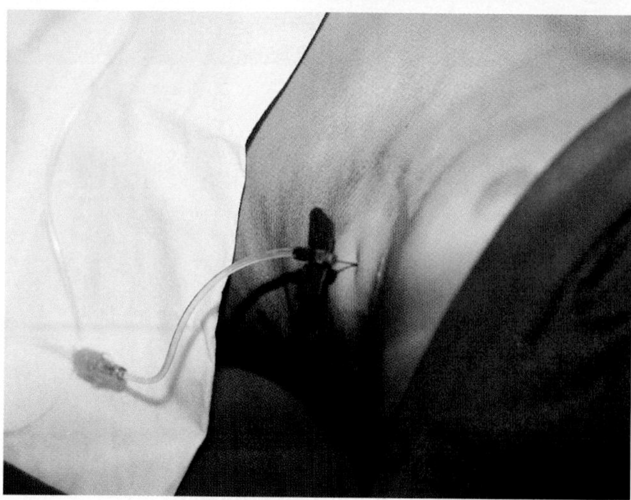

Figure 42-21 To give medications or draw blood through an implanted port, a special Huber needle is used to access the septum of the device.

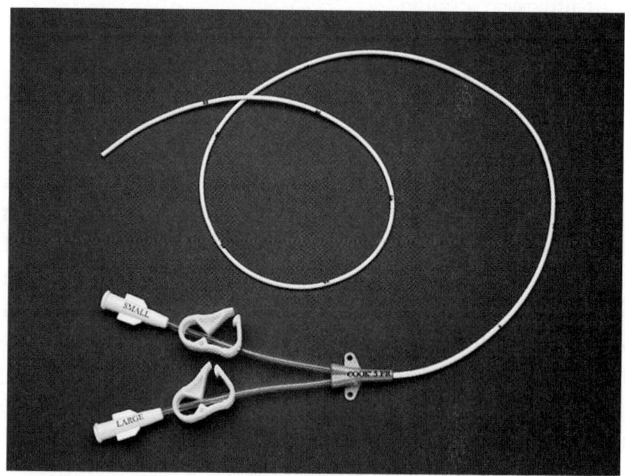

Figure 42-22 Peripherally inserted central catheter (PICC) line.

PICC lines are small (23- to 16-gauge), single- or double-lumen catheters (Figure 42-22). Their small size is helpful for use in infants and small children. A PICC line does not require surgical placement; it can be inserted at the bedside, usually by a specially trained nurse. Complications of PICC lines include infection, catheter dislodgement, bleeding, phlebitis, and catheter clotting. PICC lines have less risk of pneumothorax, hemothorax, or air embolism than centrally placed venous catheters.

Assessment Findings

Potential problems of dialysis shunts include infection, clotting of the shunt, or erosion of the skin around the site. Check the shunt for signs of infection, including redness, swelling, and tenderness or warmth to touch. To reduce the risk of infection, a fistula or graft site must be kept clean and dry. A sterile dressing may be applied to the shunt site. To decrease the risk of clotting, the patient should avoid activities that may decrease blood flow through the shunt. Peripheral intravenous (IV) access and blood pressure cuffs should be avoided in the extremity with the shunt. The patient should not wear constrictive clothing, bracelets, or a watch on the extremity.

If a dialysis shunt is functioning properly, you should be able to feel a good pulse in the shunt. This indicates good blood flow through the entrance portion or artery of the shunt. You should be able to feel a thrill at the end of the shunt. A thrill feels like a cat purring or a buzzing sensation. A thrill indicates good blood flow through the exit portion or vein of the shunt. If you are unable to feel a pulse or thrill, the shunt may be obstructed.

A patient with a long-term indwelling device is at risk for infection. This includes VADs. Signs and symptoms of infection are listed in Box 42-7. If left untreated, an infection may lead to **sepsis.**

BOX 42-7 VADs: Signs of Infection

- Redness at the site
- Drainage from the site (purulent)
- Heat at the site
- Swelling at the site
- Pain at the site
- Fever
- Generalized fatigue or weakness

VAD, Vascular access device.

BOX 42-8 Emergencies Associated with Central Venous Catheters

- Infection or allergic reaction
- Catheter breakage and leakage
- Air embolism
- Infusion errors
- Catheter migration
- Catheter obstruction

A patient who has a VAD is on anticoagulant therapy. Specific types of anticoagulants are used for the VAD that are flushed through the line to prevent clot formation in the tubing or around the tip of the catheter. Some patients also may be prescribed an oral or injectable anticoagulant such as warfarin (Coumadin), enoxaparin (Lovenox), or heparin in addition to the medication used to flush the device. These patients have a higher risk for bleeding complications. Carefully assess the patient for signs of internal and external bleeding.

Management and Treatment Plan

Management of a home care patient who has a circulatory problem should include support of the patient's ABCs. Give oxygen if needed and monitor the patient's vitals signs and ECG.

Emergencies from central venous catheters may result from local or systemic complications associated with their use. Examples of emergencies associated with central venous catheters are listed in Box 42-8.

Injury to a VAD site can cause significant blood loss. If bleeding occurs from an AV fistula, AV graft, or central venous catheter, apply direct pressure as needed to stop the bleeding. If blood loss is severe, treat the patient for shock and immediately transport. In the setting of a broken PICC line that is actively hemorrhaging, the line may be clamped between the broken end and the patient. If using clamps with teeth, such as hemostats, wrap the jaws with gauze to prevent damage to the catheter. The ability to clamp PICC lines in such a manner will vary between localities. As with any procedure or medication, the paramedic must always function within the scope of practice.

BOX 42-9 Air Embolism: Signs and Symptoms

- Altered mental status
- Seizures
- Weakness
- Shortness of breath with clear lung sounds
- Visual disturbances
- Difficulty speaking
- Dizziness
- Headache
- Hemoptysis
- Chest discomfort
- Hypoxia

Hemodynamic compromise may result from circulatory overload. This may result if IV fluids are infused too rapidly or too much fluid is infused. Slow or stop the infusion. Ensure the patient has a patent airway (provide airway support as needed). Unless contraindicated, raise the head of the patient's bed. Give oxygen and apply a cardiac monitor. Give medications as instructed by medical direction.

Hemodynamic compromise also may result from an embolus. An embolus can occur from air, a thrombus, or from dislodgement of a catheter fragment. The patient may be restless or anxious, hypotensive, and/or cyanotic. He or she may have altered mental status. Signs and symptoms of an air embolism are listed in Box 42-9. If you suspect an air embolism, stop the infusion. Place the patient on his or her left side with the head down. This position attempts to keep the embolus in the right side of the heart. Give oxygen, apply a cardiac monitor, and immediately notify medical direction.

Do not give medications or fluids through a VAD unless other methods of vascular access cannot be obtained (e.g., peripheral or central line access), you have received special training to access the device, an emergent condition exists, and medical direction has authorized you to do so.

Gastrointestinal Problems

Some injuries and illnesses may affect the peristaltic movement of the bowel. Conditions associated with increased peristalsis (also called *hyperactive bowel*) include ulcerative colitis, irritable bowel syndrome (IBS), diverticulitis, and Crohn's disease. Increased peristalsis often leads to diarrhea.

Decreased peristalsis (also called *hypoactive bowel*) may be caused by a change of routine or diet, lack of adequate dietary fiber, immobility, pregnancy, inadequate fluid intake, and medications. It also may be associated with many conditions, including diabetes, stroke, multiple sclerosis, Parkinson's disease, and spinal cord injury. Decreased peristalsis often leads to a buildup of stool, resulting in constipation. Gas (flatus) also builds up, resulting in abdominal distention.

Bowel Ostomy

A home care patient may have a bowel ostomy. A bowel **ostomy** is an artificial opening surgically created to get rid of body waste. Examples of bowel ostomies are shown in Figure 42-23. Conditions that may result in a bowel ostomy include congenital bowel abnormalities, cancer, severe Crohn's disease, ulcerative colitis, and abdominal trauma.

An ostomy may be temporary or permanent. During surgery, the intestine is rerouted and a new opening is formed. The opening may be internal or external. An internal tissue pouch may be formed that has a valve nipple opening through which a catheter is passed for emptying. An external opening into the intestine is called a *stoma*. The opening is covered with a pouch that collects waste (Figure 42-24). The patient may have loose stools or diarrhea depending on the location of the intestinal opening. The higher in the intestine (closer to the stomach) the stool is located, the less formed it will be. The pouch must be emptied regularly.

Gastric Tubes and Gastrostomy Tubes

[OBJECTIVE 19]

Gastric tubes and gastrostomy tubes (G-tubes) are used to provide nutrition to patients unable to take food by mouth for an extended period. Conditions for which gastrostomy tubes are used are listed in Box 42-10. A gastric tube is a small tube passed through the nose (nasogastric) or mouth (orogastric) into the stomach (Figure 42-25). The tube is secured to the patient after proper positioning is confirmed. Depending on the patient's needs, a gastric tube may be connected to a feeding pump or suction machine with low suction pressure. Placement of an orogastric or nasogastric tube should be checked after initial insertion, before giving fluids and medications, and again after giving fluids and medications.

BOX 42-10 Conditions for Which Gastrostomy Tubes Are Used

- Difficulty swallowing
- Esophageal atresia
- Severe gastroesophageal reflux
- Esophageal burns or strictures
- Craniofacial abnormalities
- Chronic malabsorption
- Severe failure to thrive
- Severe facial injuries from trauma

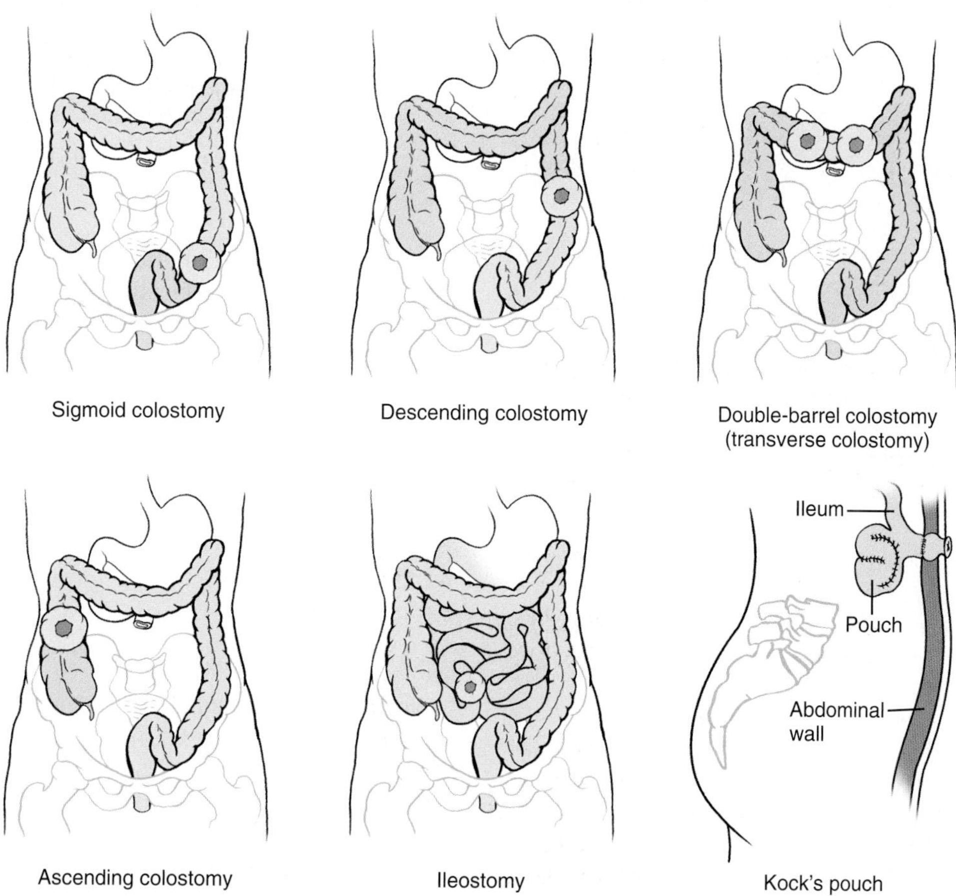

Figure 42-23 Types of bowel ostomies.

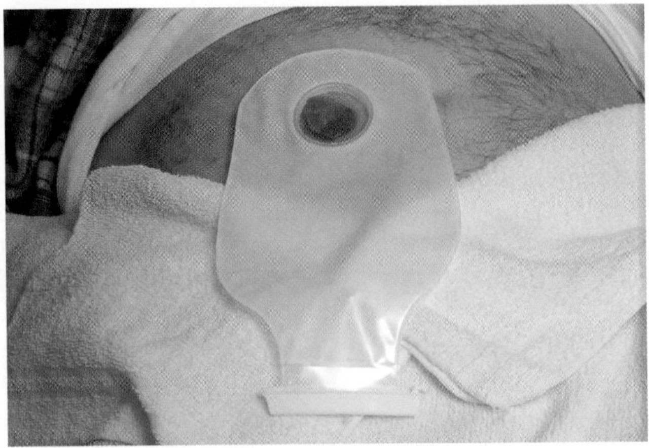

Figure 42-24 A bowel ostomy with an ostomy appliance (collection device) in place.

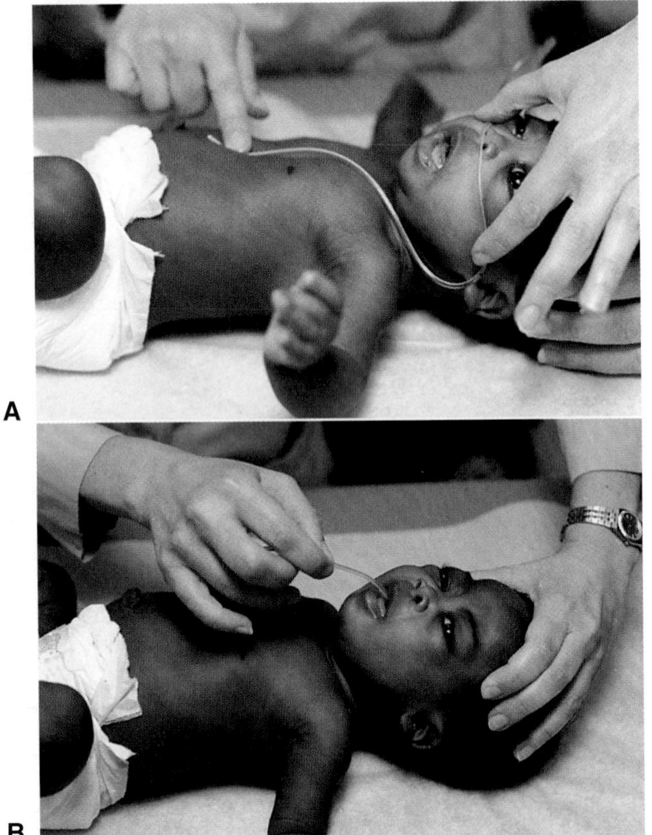

Figure 42-25 **A,** Measuring the tube for an orogastric feeding from the tip of the nose to the earlobe and to the midpoint between the end of the xiphoid process and umbilicus. **B,** Inserting the orogastric tube.

Although the diameter of a gastric tube is small, it is uncomfortable for the patient. It also irritates the nasal and mucous membranes. Many patients with gastric tubes can eat, but they are unable to ingest enough calories. A gastrostomy is performed and a G-tube is inserted when prolonged or permanent enteral nutrition is needed to supplement feedings.

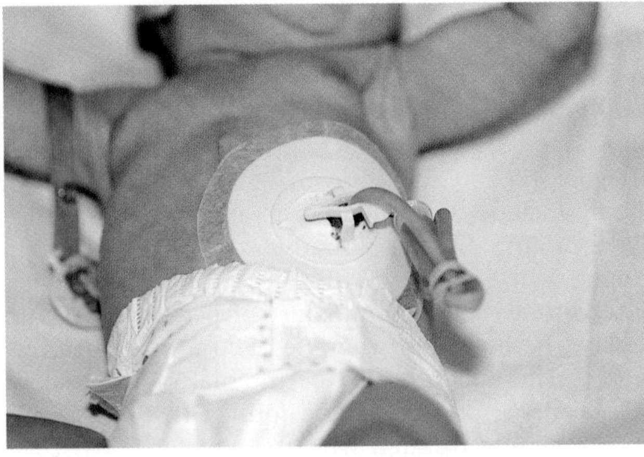

Figure 42-26 Gastrostomy tube.

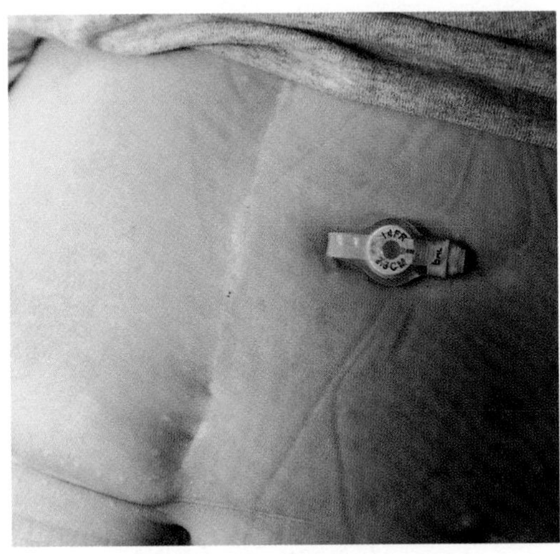

Figure 42-27 Gastrostomy button.

A gastrostomy feeding tube is either a tube or a button (skin-level device) surgically placed into the stomach through the abdominal wall. Initially a full gastrostomy tube is placed (Figure 42-26) and later replaced with a button (Figure 42-27). If the patient has a gastrostomy button, ask the caregiver for the feeding tube adapter if the patient requires evaluation in the emergency department. A jejunostomy tube (J-tube) is another type of feeding tube that passes through the abdomen into the small intestine, bypassing the stomach (Figure 42-28).

PARAMEDIC*Pearl*

Feeding tube adapters are critical, expensive, and specific to the patient's tube. Do not lose them or throw them away!

All feeding tubes have a balloon- or mushroom-shaped tip on the inside of the stomach and a disk, clamp, or crossbar on the outside to keep them in place. If the tip

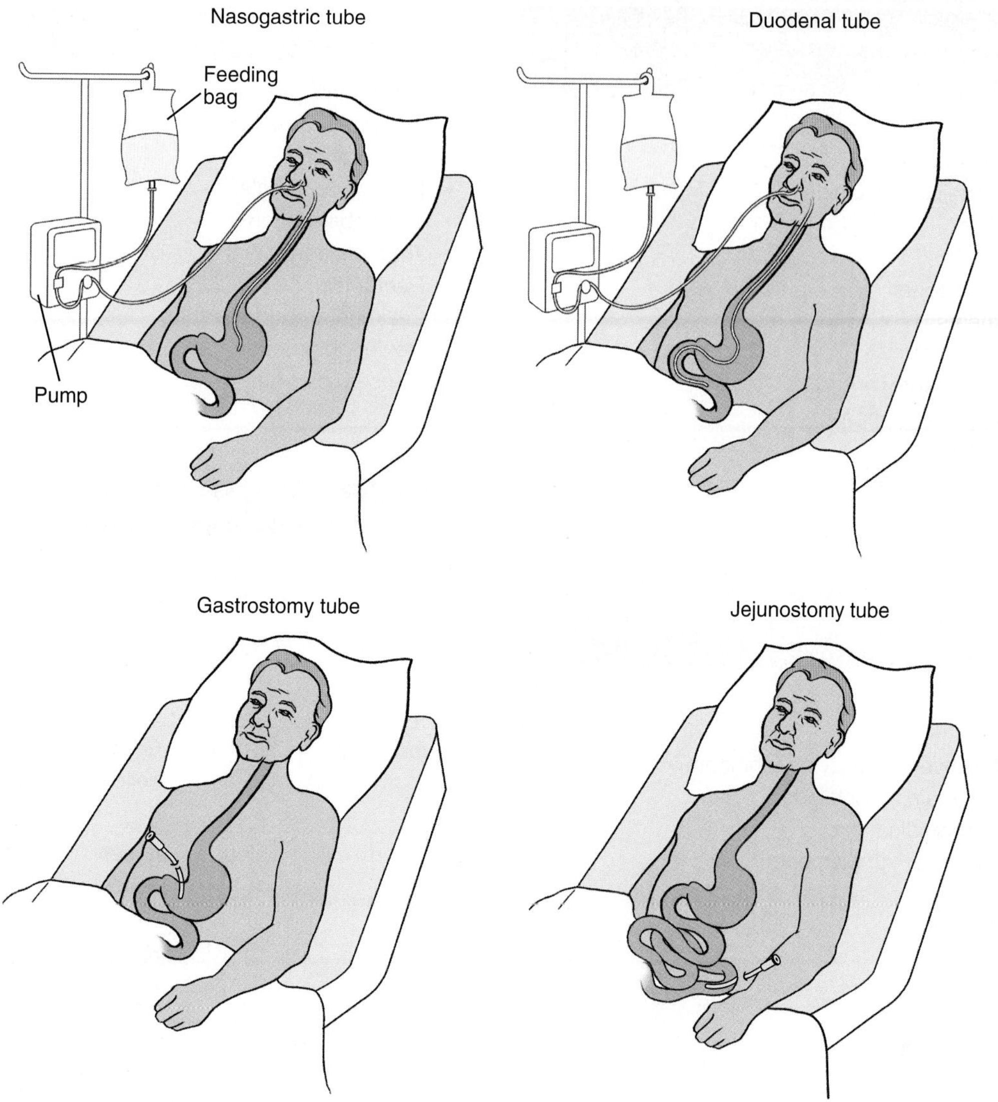

Figure 42-28 Anatomic locations for nasogastric, duodenal, gastrostomy, and jejunostomy tubes.

sinks into the stomach or if the outside disk or clamp is too loose, stomach contents may leak out around the tube. After healing is complete (usually 2 to 3 weeks), a natural tract (fistula) is formed between the stomach and skin that helps hold the tube in place. Percutaneous endoscopic gastrostomy tubes are used more often today instead of surgically placed gastrostomy tubes. These tubes allow the patient more mobility and usually do not require general anesthesia for insertion.

Assessment Findings

Muscle spasm and stretching of the intestinal wall because of gas or excess stool can result in abdominal pain and discomfort. If the patient is reporting abdominal pain, place the patient in a supine position. Assess for signs of abdominal distention. With a stethoscope, listen for bowel sounds in all four quadrants. Gently feel each quadrant for tenderness or masses.

Ask about the patient's bowel habits. When was the patient's last bowel movement? Were the characteristics (color, odor) of the stool normal for the patient? Does the patient have an illness or injury that may contribute to diarrhea or constipation? Does the patient take medications that may cause diarrhea or contribute to constipation? Examples of medications that may contribute to constipation or diarrhea are listed in Boxes 42-11 and 42-12.

The patient with an ostomy may call EMS if he or she experiences abdominal distention or bleeding or needs help changing the ostomy pouch. Distention or bleeding may be signs of a perforated bowel or bowel obstruction. The patient should be transported to the closest appropriate facility for physician evaluation. The ostomy stoma should look pink, like the mucous membranes of the mouth. A stoma that looks pale has a compromised blood supply and needs evaluation by a physician. Check the skin around the stoma for signs of irritation or infection.

BOX 42-11 Medications That May Contribute to Constipation

- Antihistamines
- Calcium channel blockers
- Aluminum-containing antacids
- Antidepressants
- Diuretics
- Lipid-lowering agents
- Iron supplements
- General anesthetics
- Calcium supplements
- Chemotherapy medications
- Narcotic analgesics
- Sedatives

BOX 42-12 Medications That May Contribute to Diarrhea

- Laxatives
- Antibiotics
- Angiotensin-converting enzyme inhibitors
- Magnesium-containing antacids
- Chemotherapy medications
- Vitamin and mineral supplements
- Beta-blockers
- Antidepressants
- Quinidine
- Theophylline
- Diuretics

PARAMEDIC*Pearl*

Because the sight and smell of stool is generally considered unacceptable in adult society, anticipate that the patient will be embarrassed about his or her ostomy. As with all patients, be considerate and professional as you assess and care for the patient.

Management and Treatment Plan

Management of a home care patient who has a gastrointestinal problem should include support of the patient's ABCs. Give oxygen if needed and monitor the patient's vitals signs and ECG.

Common complications of enteral feeding tubes are shown in Box 42-13. Problems that may result from an orogastric or nasogastric tube include a misplaced or displaced tube, plugging of the tube, or equipment failure. If an orogastric or nasogastric tube is in place and the patient is reporting abdominal pain, vomiting, or respiratory distress, check to see if the tube is in proper position.

To check placement of an orogastric or nasogastric tube, inject 10 to 20 mL of air into the tube while listening over the epigastric area with a stethoscope. A swooshing sound should be heard as air enters the stomach. You can also check placement of the tube by aspirating its contents and looking at the color of the aspirate (Table 42-4). Gastric contents are clear to white mucus. Intestinal contents are green and yellow from bile. However, confirming tube placement by visual examination of the color of the aspirate can be unreliable. For example, aspirate from the stomach or lungs may be clear or white. Checking the acidity of the contents is more reliable but impractical in the field setting unless the patient has a pH test kit in the home. Gastric or intestinal drainage that looks like coffee grounds in color and consistency may indicate bleeding.

In the home care setting a gastric tube is usually irrigated by the patient or caregiver after each feeding to prevent clogging of the tube. Despite regular irrigation, the tube may become plugged because of the thick nature of the feeding solution or pill fragments. If you suspect the tube is plugged, irrigating the tube with small amounts (60 mL or less) of normal saline may clear it. Normal saline is used for irrigation because it is isotonic and will

BOX 42-13 Complications of Enteral Feeding Tubes

- Wound infection
- Aspiration of fluids
- Dehydration
- Electrolyte imbalance
- Tube obstruction
- Tube dislodgement
- Peritonitis
- Leakage around the tube
- Bowel obstruction
- Nausea, diarrhea

TABLE 42-4 Normal Aspirates of Intestinal Tubes

Location	pH	Color	Aspirate
Esophagus	6.0-7.0	Clear	Saliva
Stomach	1.0-3.5	Clear White	Hydrochloric acid Water Mucus
Duodenum	7.8-8.3	Green Yellow	Bile Pancreatic enzymes Sodium bicarbonate
Jejunum	≥8.0	Green Yellow	Bile Pancreatic enzymes Sodium bicarbonate
Lung	>6.0	Clear White	Sputum

Reprinted from Shuster, M. H. (1996). Nutrition in the critically ill. In J. M. Clochesy, C. Breu, S. Cardin, A. A. Whittaker, & E. B. Rudy (Eds). *Critical care nursing* (2nd ed.) (p. 1004). Philadelphia: W.B. Saunders.

not upset electrolyte balance. The irrigating solution is drawn into a syringe and slowly injected into the gastric tube. It is then gently aspirated. Check your local protocols to find out if you are permitted to irrigate a gastric tube before doing so.

Equipment failure can occur if a feeding pump (which works similar to an IV infusion pump) or gastric suction device malfunctions. Ensure no obvious blockages or kinks are in the tubing and the device is turned on. If the patient's gastric tube is hooked up to suction but the suction device is not working properly, ensure all connections are tight. Loose connections can allow the entry of air, decreasing the effectiveness of the suction.

Unless contraindicated, a patient who has a gastric tube should be in a semi-Fowler's position. In this position, the tube is less likely to lie against the wall of the stomach. This position also helps prevent reflux of gastric contents, which can lead to aspiration. If the patient shows signs of possible aspiration (e.g., choking, coughing, cyanosis), suction the airway and give oxygen. Monitor the patient's oxygen saturation and cardiac rhythm. Repeat the initial assessment often.

If a gastric tube has become partially dislodged, it can be removed without harming the patient. The tape should be removed from the patient's face and the tube gently pulled out through the nose or mouth. When transferring care of the patient, be sure to tell the receiving healthcare provider of your actions so the tube can be replaced. If positive-pressure ventilations must be given to the patient, the feeding tube can be used to decompress the stomach and relieve pressure on the diaphragm.

If the patient has a gastrostomy tube, look at the insertion site for signs of irritation, infection, or bleeding. Skin irritation is not an emergent problem and can be evaluated by the patient's physician. If signs of infection are present, the patient needs physician evaluation. If bleeding is present, apply direct pressure with a sterile dressing.

Look at the insertion site to see if the tube has become dislodged. Once the tube is out, the fistula will begin to close. It may close completely within 4 to 6 hours. If the tube is dislodged, you may see a small amount of bleeding at the site and stomach contents may leak out of the hole. Cover the hole with a sterile dressing. Avoid using air-tight (occlusive) dressings because moisture builds up under the dressing and can predispose the area to infection. In the emergency department the insertion site will be checked to see if a temporary tube can be inserted.

Genitourinary Problems

Many home care patients are immobile. Immobility increases the patient's likelihood of experiencing problems related to the genitourinary tract.

- *Urinary stasis.* In mobile individuals, gravity helps in the process of emptying the kidneys and bladder. In a patient who is supine for long periods, urine tends to stagnate in the bladder. Stagnant urine promotes the growth of microorganisms that cause infection.
- *Urinary tract infection.* Urinary tract infections (UTIs) are common and occur in patients of all ages. The organism most often associated with UTIs *(Escherichia coli)* is normally found in the colon. *E. coli* may infect the urinary tract by improper perineal care, backward flow of urine (urinary reflux), use of an indwelling urinary catheter, or contamination at the time of bladder catheterization. An untreated UTI may lead to septic complications (urosepsis), which can be treated with antibiotic therapy. Signs and symptoms of UTI are shown in Box 42-14.
- *Urinary retention.* Urinary retention occurs if a patient is unable to empty the bladder completely during urination. For example, a patient confined to bed may be unable to relax enough to empty the bladder completely while lying on a bedpan. Urinary retention may also occur because of a blockage in the urinary tract (e.g., enlarged prostate), medications, infection, spinal cord injury, and after surgery. The patient usually becomes more and more uncomfortable as the bladder becomes distended with urine. The chances of a UTI are increased because of stagnant urine in the urinary tract.

BOX 42-14 UTI: Signs and Symptoms

- Burning sensation or pain during urination (dysuria)
- Back pain
- Cloudy or reddish urine
- Inability to urinate despite the urge to do so
- Fever
- Frequent urination
- General discomfort (malaise)

UTI, Urinary tract infection.

Types of Urinary Catheters

[OBJECTIVE 20]

A home care patient may have a urinary catheter. A physician may order that a urinary catheter be inserted if the patient has urinary retention or incontinence. Urinary catheters are hollow, flexible tubes that come in several sizes and shapes. Most are made of latex or silicone. Some have a Teflon (DuPont, Wilmington, Del.) coating.

External urinary catheters also are called *condom catheters* or *Texas catheters* (Figure 42-29). This type of catheter is used for a man who is incontinent of urine but can urinate on his own. The risk of a bladder infection is less with an external catheter than with an indwelling urinary catheter. An external urinary catheter system consists of a condom catheter and a urine collection bag with drainage tubing or a leg bag. A leg bag is held in place by straps

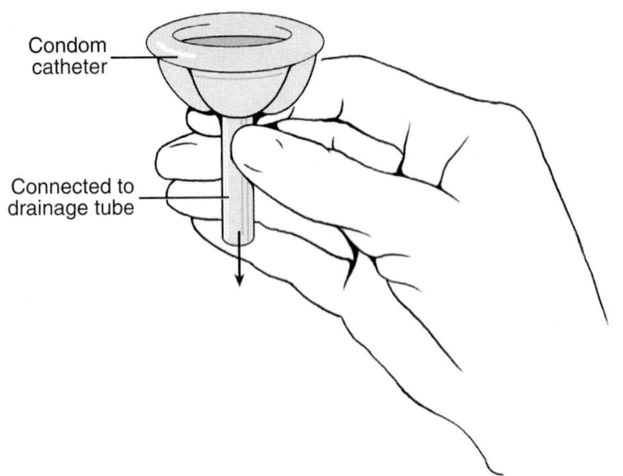

Figure 42-29 An external urinary catheter.

and may be worn under the patient's clothing during the day. The skin surrounding an external urinary catheter may become red and irritated if the catheter is left in place too long.

Indwelling urinary catheters are the most common type of urinary catheter found in the home care setting. An indwelling catheter is inserted into the bladder by sterile technique. It remains in the bladder for extended periods. A Foley catheter is one type of indwelling catheter. It has two lumens. One lumen drains urine, and the other is used to inflate a balloon that holds the catheter in the bladder. Urine continuously drains from the bladder through drainage tubing into a collection bag.

A suprapubic catheter is surgically inserted into the bladder through a cut in the abdominal wall. This type of catheter may be used to drain the bladder in the following situations:

- After gynecologic surgery
- After bladder surgery
- After urethral trauma
- In patients who need long-term catheterization and are sexually active
- In some wheelchair-bound patients

A suprapubic catheter is inserted under a local anesthetic or light general anesthetic. A Foley catheter can be used for suprapubic drainage.

A urostomy is a surgical diversion of the urinary tract to an opening (stoma) on the abdominal wall. A pouch (collection device) is placed over the stoma to collect urine.

Foley Catheter Insertion

Insertion of a Foley catheter may be necessary in the following situations:

- To replace an existing indwelling catheter that is not functioning
- To replace an indwelling catheter that was accidentally removed
- To manage incontinence when other measures have failed
- To relieve urinary retention and provide continuous bladder drainage

Insertion of an indwelling urinary catheter is an invasive procedure and requires a physician order. Before the procedure, assemble all necessary equipment. A Foley catheter insertion set contains the following items:

- Prefilled syringe with sterile water (for inflating the catheter's balloon)
- Sterile gloves
- Antiseptic cleansing solution, cotton balls or gauze squares, and forceps (alternately, the kit may include swab sticks of povidone iodine)
- Water-soluble lubricant
- Sterile drape
- Waterproof absorbent pad
- Sterile drainage tubing and collection bag
- Sterile receptacle or basin (the bottom of the catheterization tray)

The catheter set may or may not include the urinary catheter. An 8F to 10F catheter is generally used for children. A 14F to16F catheter is typically used for women. A 16F to 18F catheter is typically used for men unless a physician orders a larger size.

To reduce the risk of a bladder infection, insertion of an indwelling catheter is a sterile procedure. After the catheter is successfully inserted, be sure that the connections between the urinary catheter and drainage tubing and collection bag are secure.

Assessment Findings

A urinary catheter may become kinked, plugged, or accidentally removed. The patient or caregiver may call EMS if the following occur:

- The urinary catheter falls out.
- Urine is not draining out of the catheter.
- Urine is leaking around the catheter.
- The patient has pain, fever, and abdominal discomfort.
- The area around the catheter is red and sore.
- Bleeding occurs from removal of the catheter.
- Bleeding is present at the site around the catheter.

If urinary retention is present, bladder distention may be visible just above the pubic bone. If the patient has a urinary catheter, note the amount, color, and clarity of urine.

Management and Treatment Plan

[OBJECTIVE 21]

Management of a home care patient who has a genitourinary problem should include support of the patient's ABCs. Give oxygen if needed and monitor the patient's vitals signs and ECG. Transport patients who have persistent discomfort for evaluation by a physician.

If the patient has a urinary catheter in place, make sure the catheter is securely attached to the patient's leg before transport. Be sure to keep the drainage bag below the level of the bladder. If the bag is raised above the level of the patient's bladder, urine can backflow into the bladder, which predisposes the patient to a UTI.

If a suprapubic urinary catheter comes out, it must be replaced within a short time (approximately 20 minutes) or the surgical opening will close. This type of catheter should only be replaced by a healthcare professional specifically trained in this procedure.

Acute Infections

More than 150,000 patients with an infectious disease are cared for in the home care environment each year. The care these patients receive in the hospital is continued at home with the supervision of a home health agency.

Elderly, chronically ill, and homebound patients have an increased rate of infection. Many homebound patients have a decreased ability to perceive pain or perform self-care.

Home care patients with acute infections have an increased mortality rate from sepsis and severe peripheral infections and may have a decreased ability to perceive pain or perform self-care. Conditions for which you may be called that may require emergency care are shown in Box 42-15.

A patient who has decreased peripheral circulation or a chronic illness may have a delayed healing time because of poor tissue perfusion. Patients with poor peripheral circulation sometimes wear elastic stockings to improve circulation to the lower extremities.

A patient who is sedentary or immobile is at high risk for skin breakdown and decubitus ulcers. A decubitus ulcer (bedsore) develops from excessive friction or shearing forces between the skin and another object such as a chair, bed, couch, or sheet. Open decubitus ulcers put the patient at increased risk of infection. Patients who have poor hygiene or poor nutrition also are at risk for skin breakdown and impaired wound healing.

A patient who has an implanted medical device is at risk for infection. The patient should have regular dressing changes to ensure the insertion site is kept clean and dry. The site should be inspected by the patient or a healthcare professional and regularly assessed for signs or symptoms of infection.

Early recognition of signs or symptoms of infection is important and may include the following:

- Fever
- Tachycardia
- Tachypnea
- Fatigue, generalized weakness, malaise
- Decreased appetite
- Nausea, vomiting, diarrhea

Open Wounds

A wound is a break in the skin. Dressings are protective coverings placed over a wound to promote healing, absorb drainage, and protect the wound from infection. Many types of dressings may be found in the home care setting. The type of dressing used varies depending on the location, size, and type of wound; whether infection is present; and the frequency with which dressing changes are needed.

In 1988 a system of classifying wounds according to the colors red, yellow, and black was introduced in the United States. The red, yellow, black system describes a wound in terms of its surface appearance. The type of wound indicates the type of dressing needed.

- A red wound reflects granulation tissue. It consists of connective tissue, new blood vessels, and inflammatory cells. Granulation tissue fills an open wound when it is ready to heal. Wound treatment includes a protective dressing.
- A yellow wound indicates fluid, such as pus, has leaked out of blood vessels into adjoining tissues. Sloughing of the tissue may result in drainage. A yellow wound often becomes infected. It needs frequent cleaning and an absorption dressing changed two to three times per day.
- A black wound reflects hard, dead tissue. The wound must be cleaned of all foreign or unhealthy tissue to heal. Unhealthy tissue may be removed surgically or gradually softened and removed with the use of soaks.

Some wounds are a combination of colors. In these situations, care is given to the most serious wound type first (black), then yellow, and finally the red.

Wounds that contain infected or unhealthy tissue may require irrigation. Irrigation is done using sterile technique to flush material from the wound (Figure 42-30). Wound irrigation requires a physician order. Some wounds require packing with fine mesh gauze. This may

BOX 42-15 Conditions Related To Infection That May Require Emergency Care

- Airway infections in the immunocompromised patient
- Poor peripheral perfusion resulting in decreased healing and increased peripheral infection
- Immobility or sedentary existence, leading to skin breakdown and peripheral infections
- Infection or sepsis from percutaneous and implanted medical devices
- Patient discharged home with open wounds and incisions
- Infection resulting from poor nutrition, hygiene, or ability to care for self
- Abscesses
- Cellulitis

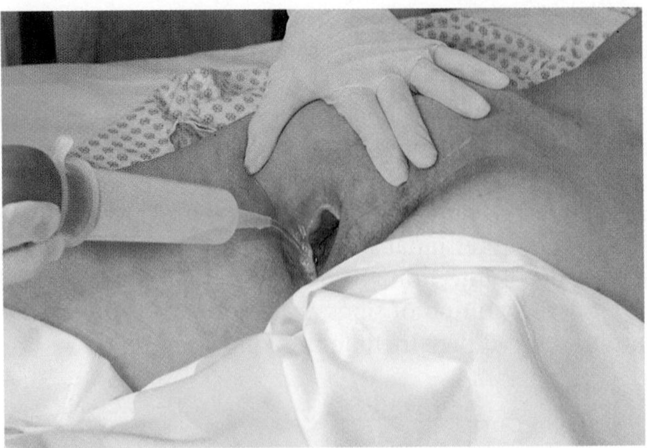

Figure 42-30 Wound irrigation is performed using sterile technique.

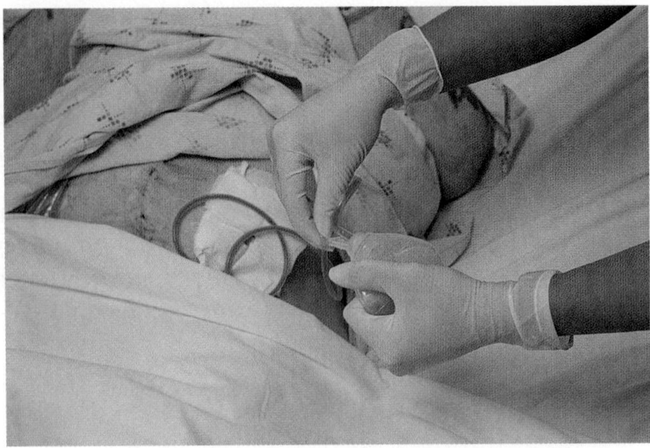

Figure 42-31 Jackson-Pratt drainage system.

be done to clean the wound or stimulate the growth of healthy tissue.

Wounds may be closed with a variety of techniques, including sutures, staples, tape, wire clips, and tissue adhesives. These materials are used to hold the edges of a wound together until the wound heals. The choice of material is based on the patient, the wound, the tissue characteristics, the wound's anatomic location, and the physician's preference.

Decubitus Wounds. Decubitus wounds also are known as *pressure ulcers, pressure sores, decubitus ulcers,* or *bedsores.* A decubitus wound is usually the result of prolonged pressure on a body part. The person's body weight presses on the tissue and skin over a bone, such as the spine, coccyx, hips, heels, or elbows. Blood flow to the area is decreased because the person's body weight traps the skin, soft tissue, and muscle between the bone and another surface, such as a mattress, bedrail, wheelchair, or brace. Without adequate blood flow to the area, the tissue begins to break down and eventually decays. Decubitus wounds can be classified into four stages. This system is used to describe the depth of the wound when the patient is assessed; it is not meant to imply that wounds progress in a step-wise manner from stage 1 to stage 4.

- *Stage 1.* A reddened skin area that does not disappear when you relieve pressure. No break in skin integrity is present. Treatment consists of removing pressure on the area. This is usually accomplished by frequent turning or repositioning and using soft, protective pads and cushions. Adequate nutrition is essential, including vitamin C, protein, and fluids.
- *Stage 2.* A partial thickness break in the skin develops that may resemble a blister, an abrasion, or a shallow crater. Sludge may be present in the wound bed. Treatment involves covering, protecting, and cleaning the affected area.
- *Stage 3.* A full-thickness break in the skin that resembles a deep crater. The subcutaneous tissue is exposed. Because the wound extends through all the skin layers, it is now a potential site of serious infection. Treatment involves maintaining adequate nutrition and hydration; relieving pressure on the affected area; and cleaning, covering, and protecting the wound.
- *Stage 4.* A full-thickness break in the skin that involves underlying muscle, tendons, and bone. If it is not aggressively treated, the wound may become the source of a life-threatening infection. Relieving pressure on the affected area, and cleaning, covering, and protecting the wound are important. However, if the patient does not receive adequate nutrition and hydration, the wound will not heal. Surgery may be needed to remove decayed tissue. Amputation is sometimes necessary.

Drains and Drainage Devices

[OBJECTIVE 22]

Some patients require placement of a drain in a wound during surgery. The drain is used to remove fluid and/or blood from the surgical area. One end of the drain is placed in the wound. The other end of the drain exits the patient through a small slit in the skin made by the surgeon.

A Penrose drain is a soft, tube-shaped piece of rubber or silicone that drains onto a dressing. A Jackson-Pratt drain is shaped like a bulb or lemon (Figure 42-31). When compressed, it applies slight suction and draws fluid from the wound bed. A Hemovac is a disk-shaped drain that works similarly to the Jackson-Pratt drain (Figure 42-32).

Assessment Findings

Assess the patient's skin for signs of inflammation: redness, heat, swelling, and pain. If a wound is present, look for signs of healthy wound healing or signs of infection. Note the size, location, and appearance of the wound. Assess for drainage in or leaking from the wound. If drainage is present, note its type, amount, color, and

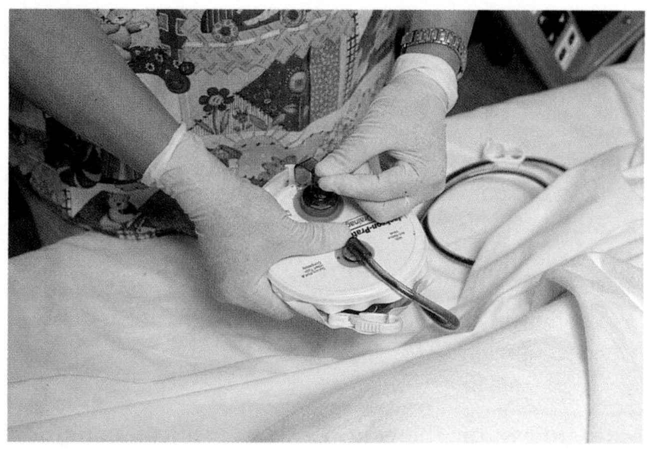

Figure 42-32 Hemovac drainage system.

any odor. If a dressing covers the wound, note if the dressing is dry and intact or if drainage is present.

If a drain is in place, note the amount and color of the drainage. If the patient has a drainage device, check to see if it appears to be working properly.

Management and Treatment Plan

Management of a home care patient who has a wound should include support of the patient's ABCs. Application of a sterile dressing (redressing) may be needed after assessment of the patient's wound. If signs and symptoms of sepsis are present, administer oxygen, start an IV of normal saline, give an IV fluid challenge per medical direction's orders to maintain blood pressure, monitor the patient's vitals signs and ECG, and transport the patient for physician evaluation.

Case Scenario CONCLUSION

En route to the hospital, you start two IVs and administer approximately 2 L normal saline. You also assess the patient's ECG, which reveals sinus tachycardia without ectopy. On arrival at the emergency department, the patient's condition is essentially unchanged, although his pulse has decreased to 104 beats/min and his blood pressure has increased to 84/60 mm Hg. Evaluation in the emergency department reveals a dramatically increased white blood cell count. The patient is admitted to the intensive care unit with a diagnosis of septic shock. Despite aggressive resuscitation, he was unable to be discharged from the hospital and died 2 days after admission of complications related to septic shock.

Looking Back

8. *In addition to infection related to the urinary catheter, what other complications might you expect this patient (who is confined to a bed or wheelchair and is unable to care for himself) to have? How could those complications have contributed to his condition?*
9. *Given the patient's final disposition, was your treatment appropriate? Why or why not?*

MATERNAL AND CHILD CARE

Today many women deliver their babies in the hospital and stay for a period of 24 to 48 hours for an uncomplicated vaginal delivery. Women who deliver their babies by caesarean section usually stay for up to 3 or 4 days. Mothers who deliver their babies by caesarean section have an abdominal incision that needs to be closely monitored for infection.

Problems that may be encountered when mother and newborn return home include the following:

- *Postpartum hemorrhage.* Vaginal bleeding of more than 500 mL after childbirth is considered postpartum hemorrhage. Signs, symptoms, and emergency care for this condition are presented in Chapter 35.
- *Postpartum depression.* Although hormone changes after childbirth appear to play a part, the cause of postpartum depression is not known. The mother may feel unable or unwilling to care for herself and/or her newborn. Symptoms most commonly begin in the first 4 to 6 weeks after delivery. For most women, postpartum depression lasts approximately 1 week, but for some it lasts more than 1 year. Postpartum depression can be successfully treated with psychotherapy, antidepressants, or both.
- *Postpartum infection.* Endometritis is the most common cause of postpartum fever. It is more common after cesarean delivery than after vaginal delivery. Bacteria enter the upper genital tract, peritoneal cavity and, occasionally, the bloodstream because of vaginal examinations during labor and manipulations during surgery. Patients typically have a fever within 36 hours of delivery. Associated findings include malaise, tachycardia, and lower abdominal pain and tenderness. Severe endometritis may result in sepsis. Endometritis is treated with antibiotics.
- *Pulmonary embolus.* Pulmonary embolism is a complication that can occur at any time during or

after pregnancy. It more commonly is seen after cesarean delivery than after vaginal delivery.

- *Infantile apnea.* Apnea is defined as a respiratory pause greater than 20 seconds or a shorter pause associated with cyanosis, pallor, decreased muscle tone (hypotonia), or bradycardia of less than 100 beats/min. Infantile apnea is most common in preterm infants. Causes of apnea in the newborn include infection, prematurity, thermal instability, decreased oxygen delivery, metabolic disorders, central nervous system problems, and maternal or fetal drugs. Most infants who have known periods of apnea are placed on apnea monitors in the home. The caregiver of an infant or child on a home apnea monitor may call EMS to assess the baby after a monitor alarm. Assess the patient to determine life threats and the cause of the alarm. When an apnea monitor is used, sensors are positioned on each side of the patient's chest. The monitor is intended to alarm primarily on the cessation of breathing timed from the last detected breath. Apnea monitors also use indirect methods to detect apnea, such as monitoring of heart rate. False alarms can occur because of a loose lead, low battery, or accidental shut-off. Because many apnea monitors contain a computer chip that can be downloaded to determine if the apnea or high/low heart rate alarms were accurate or caused by artifact, an apnea monitor should be transported with the patient.
- *Septicemia in the newborn.* Newborn sepsis most often is caused by group B streptococcus. The newborn often is infected by the mother. Signs of sepsis in a newborn are unpredictable and vague.

Well-baby checks are essential to the newborn's health. After delivery, the newborn requires frequent examinations, immunizations, and monitoring. Regular examinations also allow the physician to identify any problems in growth and development.

HOSPICE AND COMFORT CARE

[OBJECTIVES 23 TO 29]

When caring for a patient with a terminal illness, recognizing the needs of the patient and family is essential. The *end of life* has been defined as that period when healthcare providers would not be surprised if death occurred within approximately 6 months. End-of-life care issues include the following:

- The patient's choices regarding life support, such as resuscitation and feeding tubes
- The patient's choice to know a terminal diagnosis
- The patient's choice to inform family members of a terminal diagnosis
- The patient's choice to die at home, in the hospital, or in a hospice facility

BOX 42-16 Common End-of-Life Symptoms

- Pain
- Fatigue
- Difficulty breathing
- Loss of appetite
- Muscle wasting (cachexia)
- Nausea
- Depression
- Short-lived episodes of confusion and loss of concentration

Regardless of their underlying medical condition, patients at the end of life experience many of the same symptoms (Box 42-16). These symptoms vary in frequency, intensity, and level of distress. Some patients want treatment for their symptoms, whereas others do not. The primary goal of hospice care is to provide comfort, relieve pain, and promote quality of life rather than extend the length of life.

Pain management in all patients is important. Terminally ill patients may be taking very high doses of medication to control their pain. Overmedication of the patient is possible. The right dose of medication is the dose that provides pain relief without unacceptable side effects. The *patient,* not a caregiver or health care professional, decides whether pain and symptoms have been adequately relieved. If the patient is a part of a hospice program, be sure to make yourself aware of the patient's current medications and therapies.

Palliative care refers to the provision of comfort measures (physical, social, psychological, and spiritual) to terminally ill patients. Palliative care regards death as a natural process and focuses on improving the patient's quality of life as death draws near. Death is neither hastened nor prolonged. **Comfort care** is medical care that is intended to provide relief from pain and discomfort, such as the control of pain with medications.

Hospice care may be provided in familiar surroundings such as the patient's home, in freestanding facilities, or within hospitals. Hospice programs provide many services, including the following:

- Medical care according to the needs of the patient, including physician services and skilled nursing care
- Palliative care and the control of pain and other symptoms with medication
- Spiritual support for the patient and family
- Grief counseling for the family
- Specially trained personnel who have knowledge and experience in the care of the dying and their families

A patient's end-of-life care choices can and should be preplanned. The patient's culture can affect end-of-life choices. In some cultures, confessions of sins or asking forgiveness from those who may have been wronged are important end-of-life concerns. In other cultures, planning or discussing death is considered inappropriate. For example, among the Zuni and Koreans, speaking of a person's impending death is forbidden because it might bring sadness or hasten the patient's death.

In the United States, a patient's consent to cardiopulmonary resuscitation (CPR) is presumed under the theory of implied consent. The presence of an advance directive is a recognized exception to this presumption. An advance directive is a written document recording an individual's decisions concerning medical treatment that is to be applied (or not applied) in the event of the patient's physical or mental inability to communicate these wishes. State law varies on the ability of paramedics and other EMS providers to honor advance directives for healthcare. Most states have adopted specific prehospital **do not resuscitate (DNR)** programs. Most state EMS DNR programs feature EMS specific means of identifying patients with valid DNR orders. These methods often include a DNR bracelet, necklace, form, or card. DNR typically means that the paramedic should withhold cardiac compressions, intubation, artificial ventilation, resuscitative drugs, defibrillation, and other invasive resuscitative measures. This definition varies by state. You should still administer other appropriate care to a DNR patient as indicated. When appropriate, "other care" includes supplemental oxygen, pain control, basic airway management, and other basic steps for a patient's physical comfort.

The patient's culture may affect who should make decisions about the patient's care. For example, Koreans expect the eldest son to decide about a parent's end-of-life care.

When you are called to provide emergency care for a patient with a chronic illness, be sure to determine if a DNR or **do not attempt resuscitation** (DNAR) document exists (see Chapter 4). Challenges may arise when a dying patient with an advance directive (or the patient's family) calls 9-1-1 and the patient has not clearly expressed his or her wishes in the advance directive. Use of vague language such as "no heroic measures" or "no treatment measures that only prolong the process of dying" gives rise to problems with interpretation of the patient's wishes. On the other hand, an advance directive may clearly state that the patient does not wish any resuscitative measures, including CPR, defibrillation, parenteral medications, and so forth. States have begun to address this situation by developing protocols that allow EMS personnel to refrain from resuscitating terminally ill patients who possess a legal document or other approved identifier (e.g., a special bracelet or form) verifying a DNR order.

Cultural Responses to Dying and Death

People from different cultures view death in different ways. Each culture has its own beliefs, standards, and restrictions about dying and death. To help a patient and family with their loss and grief, you must first recognize your own feelings about loss, grief, and death. The stages of grief are presented in Chapter 1.

Providing grief support requires an understanding of how culture influences the grieving process. White Americans usually respond to death with sadness and restrained emotions. Mexican Americans view death as God's will and express their grief openly. Japanese Americans tend to control public expressions of grief. Greek Americans do not view death as the end of life but instead as the last ceremony in the present life. They display their grief openly and often loudly. Black Americans express their grief openly by crying, screaming, praying, and singing. Native Americans may or may not openly express their grief. Muslims may be loud and expressive.

A patient's religion also affects decisions regarding autopsy, organ donation, and after-death rituals. For example, autopsy and organ donation are acceptable to most Hindus. Some Christian Scientists do not seek medical help to prolong life and do not donate body organs. Protestants view organ donation, autopsy, and burial or cremation as individual decisions. Autopsy and organ donation are not acceptable to people of the Jewish faith. Jehovah's Witnesses forbid donation of body organs and an autopsy is acceptable only if legally necessary. Organ donation is acceptable to Muslims, but an autopsy is acceptable only for medical or legal reasons. For Haitian immigrants, organ donation is not viewed as an option.

After the patient has died, people of most cultures find leaving a light on in the room where the body is lying to be comforting. The body should be covered in a clean, white cloth to preserve dignity and modesty; however, the face should not be covered. The deceased's family may wish to wash and dress the body themselves. In many cultures this is a sign of respect for the dead. Jewelry or items associated with the patient's faith or culture should not be removed from the body. For example, Hindus tie a thread around the wrist of the deceased to signify a blessing. Do not remove it. Mormons bury their dead in temple clothes.

If you must touch the body, do so only with gloved hands. Some cultures do not like their dead handled by people from outside their community. For example, non-Hindus should not touch the deceased's body. In some cultures, the body is never left alone. In the Jewish faith, the deceased is never left alone from the time of death until the burial. These are only a few examples of the cultural considerations about dying and death.

PARAMEDIC*Pearl*

The family of a patient who is a part of the hospice program receives bereavement follow-up for 12 to 13 months. The bereaved are contacted by a member of the hospice bereavement program shortly after the death.

Case Scenario SUMMARY

1. *What is your general impression of this patient?* This patient's general impression can be deceiving because differentiating his current episode from his chronic condition is difficult. Hematuria is not considered a life-threatening condition. However, until you have additional information, assume that his diminished mental status, pallor, and diaphoresis are evidence of a serious problem.
2. *What additional assessment will be important to understand better the nature and severity of this patient's condition?* Get reliable information about his baseline mental status and skin color and temperature as well as any recent history of complications. Also helpful would be identifying his current medications and the reasons for any recent changes in medication that might help explain the hematuria or his present condition. Finally, evaluate his circulatory status and vital signs to determine the significance of the pale, diaphoretic skin.
3. *What intervention should you initiate at this time?* You should apply oxygen and prepare to start an IV as you continue your assessment.
4. *Is this patient high priority? Why or why not?* Yes. He has experienced a significant change in his mental status and his vital signs confirm that he is in shock.
5. *What are some possible causes of the patient's apparent shock? Do these causes relate to the patient's hematuria and altered mental status? Why or why not?* Two causes are likely: hypovolemia (potentially caused by blood loss through his urinary tract) or sepsis (related to a possible infection in his urinary tract). Both relate to his hematuria and both could be responsible for his altered mental status.
6. *His family has provided daily care to him for the past 10 years. What emotions do you think they are likely to be experiencing at this time? Why?* Providing care for a chronically ill family member is very demanding and stressful on most families. When complications such as this occur, family members often experience fear (of greater complications, death of their loved ones), anxiety (over the problems a hospitalization may cause, including financial strain), and guilt (believing that they could have prevented the complications if they had done a "better job" caring for him). In some cases, when the symptoms are related to noncompliance on the part of the patient, they also may experience anger.
7. *What additional treatment will you provide at this time?* Increased oxygen administration, cardiac monitoring and infusion of IV fluids to treat shock.
8. *In addition to infection related to the urinary catheter, what other complications might you expect this patient (who is confined to a bed or wheelchair and is unable to care for himself) to have? How could those complications have contributed to his condition?* Prolonged immobility may result in skin breakdown, pneumonia, pulmonary embolus, and reduction in mobility in limbs not affected by paralysis. Skin breakdown and pneumonia may both contribute to infection and sepsis. In addition, patients such as this often have depression and, in some cases, suicidal tendencies.
9. *Given the patient's final disposition, was your treatment appropriate? Why or why not?* Yes, prehospital treatment was appropriate.

Chapter Summary

- Acute care is short-term medical treatment usually provided in a hospital for patients who have an illness or injury or who are recovering from surgery. Home care is the provision of health services by formal and informal caregivers in the home to promote, restore, and maintain a person's maximal level of comfort, function, and health, including care toward a dignified death. Hospice is a care program that provides for the dying and their special needs.
- Examples of home care problems that usually require intervention by a home health professional or physician include chemotherapy, pain management, wound care, ostomy care, and hospice or palliative care. Examples of home care problems requiring acute intervention include altered mental status; airway complications; respiratory failure or acute respiratory events; cardiac decompensation or acute cardiac events; infection, acute sepsis, or septic complications; equipment malfunction; and gastrointestinal or genitourinary crisis. As a paramedic, you should be familiar with types of medical equipment found in the home, their uses, and how to troubleshoot potential problems.

Chapter Quiz

1. List four types of patients who receive home care.

2. What is the difference between CPAP and BiPAP?

3. You are called for a ventilator-dependent patient who has suddenly become restless and agitated. What should you do first?
   a. Perform abdominal thrusts and then start an IV.
   b. Start an IV and then insert an oral airway.
   c. Listen to breath sounds and then ventilate the patient's lungs with a bag-mask device.
   d. Insert an oral airway and then listen to breath sounds.

4. You are caring for a patient who has an air embolus. How should the patient be positioned?
   a. Prone with head turned to the right
   b. Supine with head turned to the left
   c. Left side with head down
   d. Right side with head back

5. List four categories of VADs.

6. The memory aid DOPE can be used to recall possible reversible causes of acute deterioration in an intubated patient. Explain the meaning of each letter and appropriate intervention.

7. True or false: Confirming placement of an orogastric or nasogastric tube is necessary only after initial insertion of the device.

Terminology

Acute care Short-term medical treatment usually provided in a hospital for patients who have an illness or injury or who are recovering from surgery.

Bilevel positive airway pressure (BiPAP) A form of noninvasive, mechanical ventilation in which two (bi) levels of positive pressure are delivered—one during inspiration (to keep the airway open as the patient inhales) and the other (lower) pressure during expiration to reduce the work of exhalation.

Cellulitis Inflammation or infection of the skin tissue usually treated with antibiotic therapy.

Central venous catheter A catheter through a vein to end in the superior vena cava or right atrium of the heart for medication or fluid administration.

Comfort care Medical care intended to provide relief from pain and discomfort, such as the control of pain with medications.

Continuous positive airway pressure (CPAP) Delivery of a steady, gentle flow of air by a medical device through a soft mask worn over the nose (nasal CPAP) or over the mouth and nose (mask CPAP).

Decannulation Removal of a tracheostomy tube.

Dialysis shunt Shunt composed of two plastic tubes (one inserted into an artery, the other into a vein) that stick out of the skin to allow easy access and attachment to a dialysis machine for filtering of waste products from the blood.

Do not resuscitate (DNR)/do not attempt resuscitation (DNAR) Written order signed by a physician stating that, in the event of a cardiac or respiratory arrest, the patient does not wish to be resuscitated.

Home care The provision of health services by formal and informal caregivers in the home to promote, restore, and maintain a person's maximal level of comfort, function, and health, including care toward a dignified death.

Hospice A care program that provides for the dying and their special needs.

Ostomy Surgical opening that allows the passage of urine or feces through an incision, or stoma, in the wall of the abdomen (e.g., gastrostomy, colostomy).

Palliative care Provision of comfort measures (physical, social, psychological, and spiritual) to terminally ill patients.

Peripherally inserted central catheter (PICC line) A thin tube inserted into a peripheral vein (usually

Terminology—continued

the arm) and threaded into the superior vena cava to allow fluid or medication administration.

Sepsis A serious infectious process that may be preceded by an inflammatory response and may lead to a more critical subcategory (septic shock, septicemia); usually treated with antibiotics.

Vascular access device (VAD) Type of IV device used to deliver fluids, medications, blood, or nutritional therapy; usually inserted in patients who require long-term IV therapy.

DIVISION 8

TRAUMA

CHAPTER 43

Trauma Systems and Mechanism of Injury

Objectives

After completing this chapter, you will be able to:

1. Describe the incidence and scope of traumatic injuries and death.
2. Identify the parts of a comprehensive trauma system and describe the roles of each part.
3. Describe the differences in the levels of trauma centers.
4. Describe the considerations for ground versus air transport of a trauma patient.
5. Define the laws of motion and describe their relation to the effects of trauma.
6. Define and describe the roles of kinematics and index of suspicion as additional tools for assessing patients.
7. Describe each type of impact and its effect on the unrestrained victims (e.g., down and under, up and over, compression, deceleration).
8. Describe the role of restraints in injury prevention and injury patterns.
9. Identify and describe the injury patterns associated with motorcycle collisions.
10. Describe the injury patterns associated with vehicle collisions with pedestrians (adult and pediatric pedestrians).
11. Identify and describe the injury patterns associated with sports injuries, blast injuries, and vertical fall injuries.
12. Describe the damage caused by the different types of projectile velocities.

Chapter Outline

Case Scenario

You and your partner are responding with a basic life support (BLS) fire first response unit to a motor vehicle crash in a small town. The BLS unit arrives approximately 5 minutes before your unit and finds a small compact car that was struck on the driver's side in front by a large delivery van. The only patient is the driver of the compact car, who is trapped in a sitting position behind the severely bent steering wheel. He states he was wearing his seatbelt, although it is not in place as you begin your assessment. When the BLS unit arrived the patient was awake; alert and oriented to person, place, time, and event; combative; and screaming "Help me!"

When you arrive, you find a pale, diaphoretic 20-year-old man entrapped behind the steering wheel and door that impinges 2 to 3 feet into the passenger compartment. Because he continues to scream, he is unable to answer questions or follow commands. The fire department informs you that they will have him cut out of the car in 15 minutes.

Questions

1. *What is your general impression of this patient?*
2. *You are 5 minutes from a level III trauma center and 45 minutes from the regional level I trauma center. Describe the factors to consider when deciding the appropriate destination for this patient.*
3. *What additional assessment will be important in the evaluation of this patient? Can you complete any before extrication? Why or why not?*
4. *What intervention should you initiate at this time?*

EPIDEMIOLOGY OF TRAUMA

[OBJECTIVE 1]

Trauma, or unintentional injury, is a significant medical and social issue in every country in the world. In the United States, unintentional injury accounts for millions of healthcare dollars. More importantly, it is a leading cause of death, along with heart disease, cancer, stroke, and chronic lower respiratory diseases (Hoyert et al., 2006) (Box 43-1). The numbers are staggering; trauma or injury-related incidents account for between 100,000 and 160,000 deaths per year (Minino et al., 2006) 27 million emergency department visits per year (National Safety Council [NSC], 2003). Trauma affects all age groups. However, each age group has different causes, or mechanisms of injury, that predominate. For example, trauma (specifically motor vehicle crashes) is the leading cause of death for persons aged 1 to 44 years (Disaster Center, 1998). The "costs of trauma" are far reaching. These include the loss of years of productive life for the trauma patient, financial impact on both families and the healthcare system, the emotional effect on patients and their families, and the financial effects on the community in terms of increased costs of governmental programs or increased insurance costs to pay for trauma care.

BOX 43-1 Cost of Unintentional Injuries

The National Safety Council reports that the economic effect of fatal and nonfatal unintentional injuries amounted to $652.1 billion in 2006. This is equivalent to approximately $2200 per capita, or $5700 per household.

From National Safety Council (2008). *Report on injuries in America: Injury facts.* Retrieved July 11, 2008, from http://www.nsc.org.

Trends in Trauma Deaths

Trauma can be broken into smaller segments of mechanisms of injury that pose the greatest risk of death. The most prevalent mechanisms of injury include motor vehicle crashes (MVCs), falls, poisonings, firearms, and suffocation (Disaster Center, 1998; Minino et al., 2006). In 2003, MVCs accounted for 43,340 deaths, or 26.4% of all injury-related deaths, firearms accounted for 30,136 deaths (18.4% of all injury-related deaths), poisoning for 28,700 deaths (17.5% of all injury-related deaths), and falls for 18,044 deaths (11.0% of all injury-related deaths) (Hoyert et al., 2006) (Figure 43-1). When the injury patterns are examined, an overall annual increase in penetrating trauma compared with blunt trauma is found. Various reasons exist for this phenomenon, including an increase in firearm violence in urban and suburban communities.

PHASES OF TRAUMA CARE

Trauma care is divided into three distinct phases. As a paramedic, you actively participate in the three phases: pre-event, event, and postevent (National Association of Emergency Medical Technicians, 2003). The pre-event phase describes any efforts geared toward reducing injury through prevention. These efforts involve public education activities, such as child safety seat programs, drown-

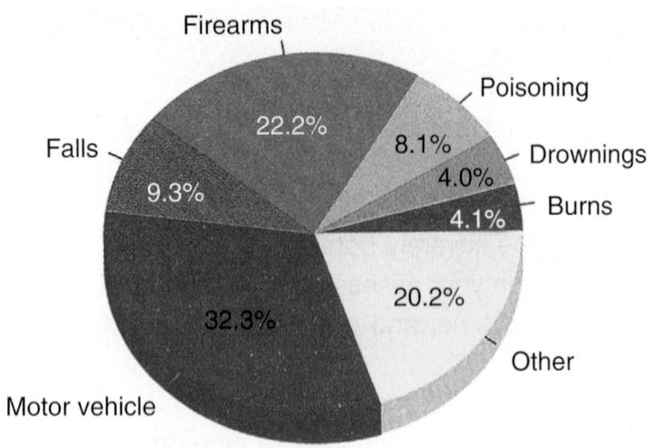

Figure 43-1 Motor vehicle trauma and firearms account for more than half of the deaths that result from trauma and violence.

ing prevention efforts, and fall reduction efforts in the elderly. The pre-event phase embraces the idea that trauma is not usually "an accident"; accidents, by definition, do not carry blame or premeditation. The vast majority of traumatic injuries and deaths are not accidents. They are either acts of omission, or not doing the right thing, or acts of commission, or doing something wrong. Both acts lead to predictable injury.

As a paramedic, you are responsible for being actively involved in ongoing injury prevention programs. Moreover, this is a vital part of your overall responsibility as a professional healthcare provider. Great potential exists to affect people's lives positively through prevention efforts. This has been demonstrated throughout the United States. An additional aspect of prevention activities and programs includes being active with legislative efforts regarding injury prevention at the local, state, and national levels. This may entail working to strengthen helmet laws, drunk driving laws, or working in other areas where the voice of professional paramedics can lend credence and clout to legislative efforts.

The next phase of trauma care is the event phase, during which you interact with people and demonstrate professional attributes. This includes, for example, wearing the appropriate personal protective equipment and wearing safety belts while driving or riding in the patient compartment. Another aspect of this phase includes acting as a mentor and demonstrating good safety practices.

The last phase of trauma care is the postevent phase. In this phase, you perform optimal patient care, make appropriate clinical decisions, carefully treat the patient, and place the patient first in all care decisions. This phase continues until you deliver the patient to the appropriate facility and provide a complete report.

TRAUMA SYSTEMS

[OBJECTIVES 2, 3]

The modern EMS system is comprehensive. It is designed for the prompt and efficient treatment and transport of sick and critically ill patients from the scene of an incident to the appropriate facility. Connected with the EMS system is the supporting trauma system. The trauma system is designed to address the needs of and specifically treat the trauma patient. This trauma system was authorized by the Federal Trauma Care Systems Planning and Development Act of 1990 (Peterson et al., 2003).

According to the "Trauma System Agenda for the Future," a trauma system is an "organized, coordinated effort in a defined geographic area that delivers the full range of care to all injured patients and is integrated with the local public health system."

The parts of a trauma system include the following:

1. Injury prevention
2. Prehospital care
3. Emergency department care
4. Interfacility transport (if needed)
5. Definitive care
6. Trauma critical care
7. Rehabilitation
8. Data collection and trauma registry

As a paramedic, you are an integral link within the trauma system in several areas including injury prevention, prehospital care, interfacility transport, and emergency department care.

Injury prevention efforts are designed to prevent injury or mitigate the effects of trauma. The concept of prevention gives you many opportunities to affect the lives of those in the community in many ways before trauma occurs.

Prehospital care is divided into three aspects: treatment, transportation, and trauma triage guidelines. Treatment is the appropriate care provided on the scene to the patient by you, the paramedic. Transportation involves entering the patient into the trauma system by transporting the patient to the appropriate facility in a safe manner. The final aspect is trauma triage guidelines. These involve medical direction tools that provide guidance for the care of injured persons and their entry into the trauma system in an appropriate manner.

Emergency department care is the patient actually entering the stabilization or definitive care phase of the trauma system.

Interfacility transportation is the transfer of a trauma patient from a facility at a lower level of care to a facility with a higher level of care than the local emergency department.

Definitive care is usually provided at a designated trauma center, where skilled trauma teams staffed by trauma physicians and nurses use their expertise, techniques, and sophisticated equipment to care for the patient.

Trauma critical care is the care provided to the patient during the initial phase of the injury cycle. This is followed by *rehabilitation,* which facilitates the patient's return to as normal function as possible after the injury. The final part of the system is the administrative aspect of *data collection.* During this function, information regarding injury is collected for the analysis of injury patterns, treatment, and overall care.

The key player of the trauma system is the trauma center. This is a specialty hospital designed to address the urgent and critical nature of trauma (Box 43-2).

BOX 43-2 Federal Trauma Care Systems Planning and Development Act

The 1990 Federal Trauma Care Systems Planning and Development Act (PL 101-590) created Title XII of the Public Health Service Act and provided healthcare planning by developing a model trauma care plan. States received funding to develop statewide plans that were consistent with the federal model.

From Peterson, T., Mello, M. J., Broderick, K. B., Lane, P. L., Prince, L. A., Jones, A., et al. (2003). *Trauma care systems 2003.* Retrieved June 25, 2006, from http://www.acep.org.

Trauma centers are designated as level I, II, III, and IV based on the facility's capability of fulfilling staffing requirements. Level I is the most comprehensive. The remaining levels then follow in a decreasing manner to the lowest capable level, designated *level IV* (Table 43-1).

Transfer means transferring the patient from a trauma facility that may not have the capabilities to deal with the extent of the injuries to a higher-level facility that would have the capabilities to treat the injuries.

Transport Considerations

[OBJECTIVE 4]

Paramedics determine the proper level of care and appropriate hospital destination on the basis of the patient's needs and condition. The destination also is based on medical direction advice and protocols and guidelines. First determine the patient's condition and specific need regarding definitive care (level of care). Then determine the most appropriate facility (destination). At this point

TABLE 43-1 Trauma Center Categories

Level	Description	Capabilities	Where
Level I	Regional resource center	Full spectrum of services from prevention programs to patient rehabilitation Serves as the leader in trauma care for a geographic area	Most are found in large, university-based hospitals because of the requirements for patient care, education and teaching programs, and research
Level II	Provides comprehensive trauma care	May not have all resources found in a level I facility Some complex, critical patients may need to be transferred to a level I facility Research is not an essential component	Usually a nonteaching or community hospital
Level III	Designed for communities that do not have immediate availability of a level I or II institution	Provides evaluation, resuscitation, and operative intervention for stabilization When necessary, patients are transferred to a level I or II trauma center for ongoing or more definitive care Should have preexisting relationships and transfer agreements in place with a level I or II trauma center for rapid transfer when necessary	Usually a community hospital
Level IV	Created with rural and remote areas in mind	Provides initial stabilization and transfer of the patient to a level I, II, or III trauma center Should have preexisting relationships and transfer agreements in place with a level I or II trauma center for rapid transfer when necessary	May be a clinic-type facility rather than a hospital

BOX 43-3 Inclusive Systems

According to a draft paper from the Panel on Trauma Care Systems, in 1992 "all hospitals involved in treating injured patients, particularly those in the rural areas, should be in an 'inclusive' system of care facilities. Each facility should provide that level of specialized care within its capability. Regionalization of tertiary trauma care should be accomplished by adherence to trauma care and transfer protocols."

From State of Montana official website, EMS and Trauma System Section. Retrieved March 19, 2008, from http://www.dphhs.mt.gov.

you can make the decision regarding the specific mode of transportation, either ground or air (Box 43-3).

Time

The single most important factor in the survival of trauma patients is the time between the initial injury and definitive care. The term *golden hour* was coined by Dr. R Adams Cowley at the Maryland Shock Trauma Center (later named the R Adams Cowley Shock Trauma Center in his memory). During his work with shock and trauma patients, Cowley found that patients who received surgical care within 1 hour of their injury had a better chance of survival than those who did not. Although there has been debate surrounding the use of exactly 1 hour in determining outcome, there is no debate that rapid access to surgical care is the primary factor in positive outcome. Therefore the current terminology used to define this time is the *golden period.* This means that the patient should be delivered to an appropriate facility as quickly as possible. If it is possible to deliver the patient in 60 minutes, the paramedic should try for 50 minutes; if the system is such that the hospital is 2 hours away, the paramedic should try for 1 hour and 50 minutes.

As important as time is to the trauma patient, patient care should never be sacrificed for speed. The "platinum ten minutes" is used to refer to the 10 minutes the paramedic is allowed on scene with a critical trauma patient. During this time, critical, immediately life-threatening conditions must be treated with the fastest, simplest, yet effective interventions. If, in an attempt to "shave" a few minutes off the scene time, a patient is allowed to become hypoxic by not immediately managing an airway or administering oxygen, the outcome will be worsened. Conversely, time-intensive procedures that do not address immediate life threats, or the provision of advanced procedures when basic procedures are effective, will unnecessarily extend scene time. These procedures are performed during transport.

When making a transport decision, the paramedic must realize that the most appropriate facility may not always be the closest facility. For the comprehensive trauma patient, definitive care is generally surgery and an appropriate facility is one with immediate surgical capabilities. The decision to transport to a closer facility without immediate surgical capabilities may actually delay the patient's access to definitive care. This is due to the fact that time will be spent evaluating the patient, waiting for surgical teams to arrive, and/or arranging transport to an appropriate facility, as well as the time of the second transport itself if needed. These factors of course have to be evaluated in each situation. Although in some systems the paramedic may have several transport choices, other systems may have to transport to "the hospital" as there are no other choices.

Ground Transportation

As a general rule, use ground transportation if the appropriate facility can be reached within a "reasonable" time. Reasonable time is generally derived from the nationally accepted standard of delivering the patient to a trauma center with surgical capabilities within 60 minutes from the time of injury. System-specific issues such as protocols may alter this time frame. The factors involved in deciding to use ground versus air transportation include geographic location, topography, population, weather, availability of resources, traffic conditions, the location of flight services, and time of day. The choice to use ground or air transportation is made by determining which method will deliver the patient to an appropriate facility the fastest.

Aeromedical Transportation

The availability and use of aeromedical services varies widely in the United States. Aeromedical transportation provides rapid response time and a rapid transport to the appropriate care facility. Consider aeromedical transportation in the following situations:

- When time is critical to the patient's condition and aeromedical transportation would deliver the patient to an appropriate facility faster than ground transportation
- When scene times are extended due to extrication or other factors
- When road or traffic conditions would seriously delay the patient's access to definitive care
- When critical care personnel above the level of training of the ground ambulance are needed for the patient's condition

ENERGY

[OBJECTIVE 5]

Physical Laws

The human body is subject to the physical laws of nature that surround it, act on it, and move through it. Trauma is the application of physical energy from an external source onto the human body and the effects of that energy on body systems and parts. The effect of energy applied to the body and the resulting injury depend on the amount and type of energy applied, the speed at which the energy was applied, and the body system or part affected by the applied energy. As a paramedic, you must have a thorough understanding of physical laws to understand the effects of trauma.

1. *Newton's first law of motion:* A body at rest or in motion will stay in that state until acted on by an outside force. An example in terms of trauma would be a vehicle traveling at a rate of 60 mph. The driver also is traveling at 60 mph. When the car makes impact with an object, the car stops but the driver continues to travel at 60 mph. The unrestrained driver is stopped by his or her impact with the steering wheel at a rate of 60 mph.
2. *Conservation of energy:* Energy cannot be created or destroyed; it can only change form. (Energy can only be in the form of chemical, electrical, mechanical, nuclear, or thermal energy.) An example in terms of trauma is how electricity entering the body can take the form of a thermal burn at the site where the electricity entered.
3. *Kinetic energy:* Kinetic energy (KE) equals half the mass of an object multiplied by the velocity (speed) (V) of the object squared (Mass/2 $\times$ V^2) (Box 43-4). Velocity influences kinetic energy more than mass does; in other words, the greater the speed, the greater the energy that is generated. An example in terms of trauma is the velocity of a bullet striking the body, producing a wound disproportionate to the size of the bullet.

BOX 43-4 KE = $\frac{1}{2}M \cdot V^2$

Consider a 150-lb person traveling at 30 mph: KE = 150/2 $\times$ 30^2; KE = 67,500 units. The same 150-lb person traveling at 40 mph: KE = 150/2 $\times$ 40^2; KE = 120,000 units.

4. *Force:* Force = Mass $\times$ Acceleration; Force = Mass $\times$ Deceleration; Mass $\times$ Acceleration = Force = Mass $\times$ Deceleration. Simply put, to accelerate a bullet from the muzzle of a gun, force from the gunpowder explosion is required. Once the bullet is set in motion by this explosion, an equal amount of tissue destruction must occur within the body to stop it as was used to start the bullet moving. An important consideration in the extent of injury is the amount of time the force is delivered, or the speed of deceleration. The faster the delivery of energy (i.e., falling on concrete versus falling in mud), the greater the resulting injury.
5. *Energy law summary:* Motion is created by force (energy exchange). Force (energy exchange) must stop this motion. If such energy exchange occurs within the body, tissue damage is produced (United States Department of Transportation [USDOT], 1998).

ENERGY EXCHANGE

When energy is applied to an object, a corresponding movement of particles occurs within that object. Energy exchange is simply the application of energy onto an object with resulting particle movement. The exact nature of that movement is determined by the density of the material sustaining impact at the surface of the object struck, the speed of the penetrating or impacting object and, to a lesser extent, the shape of the impacted object (Figure 43-2). Energy exchange does not distinguish whether one or both objects are in motion; it works in both cases.

Cavitation

Cavitation is defined as a temporary or permanent opening produced by a force that pushes body tissues laterally away from the tract of a projectile. The effect of cavita-

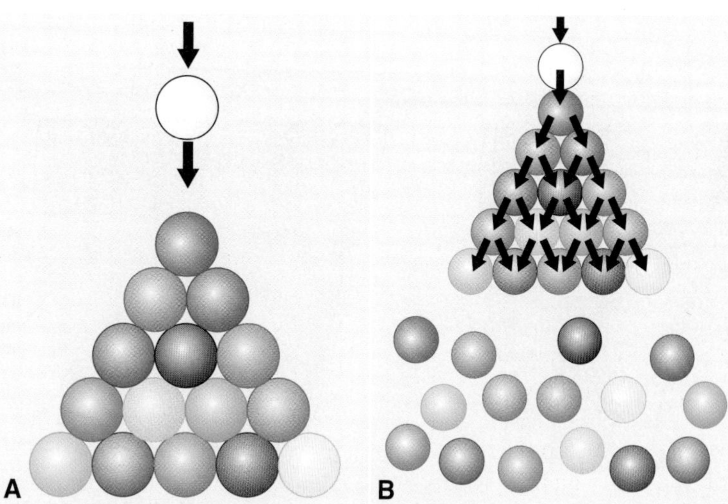

Figure 43-2 A, The energy of a cue ball is transferred to each of the other balls. **B,** The energy exchange pushes the balls apart, or creates a cavity.

tion depends on the density of the object sustaining the impact. According to Anderson, density is "the amount of mass of a substance in a given volume. The greater the mass [is] in a given volume, the greater the density" (2002). To put these definitions in practical terms, cavitation takes into account the speed (velocity) of a penetrating object as it travels through body tissue (density). The body contains three types of density: air (lungs and intestine), water (muscle and most solid organs), and bone. The amount of injury produced therefore is related to the type of organ sustaining impact.

Cavitation can be either temporary or permanent. Temporary cavitation is short lived and produced by stretching of the tissues. The exact limits of stretching depend on the elasticity of the tissue involved. Tissues that are more elastic in nature, such as skeletal muscle, blood vessels, and skin, may be pushed aside after the passage of the projectile. If the projectile strikes inelastic tissue, such as bone or the liver, this tissue or bone may fracture with the passage of the projectile through it. The temporary cavity path produced by projectiles may not be readily apparent.

You can see the permanent cavity of a projectile after the energy exchange between the tissues and the projectile is complete. This type of cavity leads to quick necrosis or death of local cells and tissue at the affected area (United States Department of Defense [DOD], 2004). Permanent cavities are caused by the compression or tearing of the tissue and the destruction of the area around the affected tissue (Figures 43-3 and 43-4).

Dependent Factors

[OBJECTIVE 6]

As previously mentioned, the effects of energy-producing injuries depend on the density and shape of the interacting bodies. This determines how many particles are placed in motion and, in large part, the severity of the injury.

On examination of the density of body organs affected, energy moving through different types of organs and tissues produces different results. For example, energy having an impact on the air-filled organs, such as the lungs or intestinal tract, moves relatively few particles; these are the least dense organs in the body. Next consider the water-dense organs and tissues, such as the liver, spleen, muscle, and vascular system. These objects are relatively denser than air-filled organs. Therefore they will sustain a greater proportional effect because more

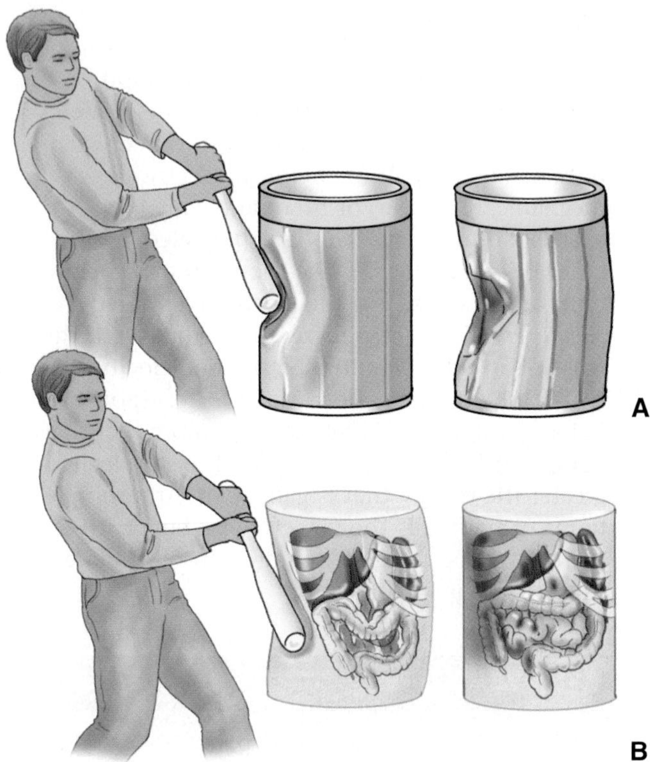

Figure 43-3 A, Swinging a baseball bat into a steel drum leaves a dent, or a cavity, in its side. **B,** Swinging a baseball bat into a piece of foam leaves no visible cavity.

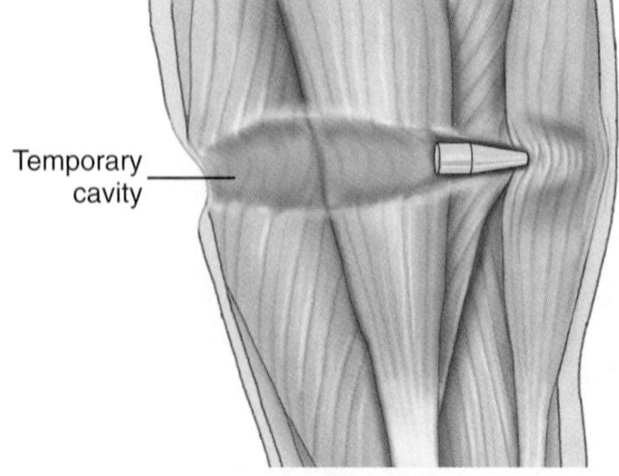

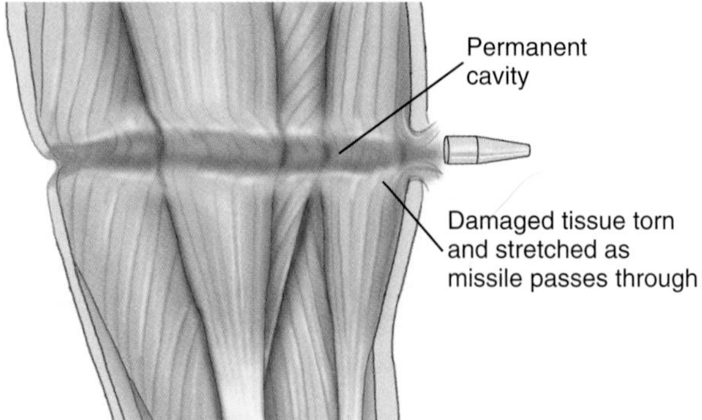

Figure 43-4 Damage to tissue is greater than the permanent cavity that remains from a missile injury. The faster or heavier the missile, the larger the temporary cavity and the greater the zone of tissue damage.

particles are set in motion. Bones, the thickest and densest material in the body, are inflexible organs that, if sustaining impact, will set thick particles in motion.

An additional issue concerns density—the density of the material that makes impact with the body. If the material is not dense, such as foam matting, the resulting injury is relatively less dramatic than if the material had been steel, a very dense material. This means that the paramedic must maintain a high index of suspicion when evaluating trauma patients. Because of the makeup of the human body, a traumatic force may leave nothing more than an area of redness, yet the organs underlying the area, which were in the temporary cavity, may be severely injured.

Another factor must be considered when determining the injury produced by energy applied to the body: the point of impact. As previously mentioned, density and speed are crucial factors. Yet the shape, position, and degree at which the object will fragment or split into many pieces are equally important in determining the effect of the energy on producing injury. Hitting an object flat on will transmit the energy directly through the object. On the other hand, hitting the object with a glancing or oblique impact will lessen the overall injury severity. Hitting a solid object that shatters into many pieces is different from hitting an equally solid item that does not shatter. Shattering or breaking into many pieces adds to the overall injury by causing multiple cavities, each damaging surrounding tissues.

Trauma is generally classified as blunt or penetrating; both can be equally deadly. The significant difference is whether the injury penetrated the skin and, therefore, the tissue. Both types can produce cavitation and tissue destruction. In blunt trauma the tissue is not penetrated, causing the energy to be indirectly communicated through the tissue. Therefore the impacting energy creates a cavitation away from the site and in the direction of impact.

In penetrating trauma the energy is directly communicated through the affected tissue by penetration. In the case of a bullet, the energy creates a cavity 90 degrees outward from the penetration track. The tissue being displaced by the bullet is crushed by the bullet progressing through the tissue, and the energy is applied to the cells within the tissue.

Kinematics

Kinematics is the process of predicting injury patterns based on certain mechanisms. In addition to individual factors, such as age, and protective measures, such as restraint systems, consider the following when evaluating patient care: mechanism of injury, force of energy applied, anatomy, and type of energy (Box 43-5).

BOX 43-5 Kinematics

The *mechanism of injury* involves evaluating the scene, the patient, the paramedic's anticipation that an injury may be present, and actual conditions found at the scene.

The *force of energy* applied relates to the mass of an object and the rate of acceleration or deceleration involved with that object when it sustains impact on the body or if the body is the object in motion.

The *anatomy* relates to what organ or organ system is hit by the force of the energy applied.

The *type of energy* relates to the energy and its physical state, such as electrical, thermal, mechanical, or chemical.

INDEX OF SUSPICION

The **index of suspicion** is the expectation that certain injuries or patterns of injuries have resulted to a body part, organ, or system based on the mechanism of injury and the force of impact to the patient. The index of suspicion, when combined with the physical examination, can lead you to discover critical or other serious injuries.

BLUNT TRAUMA

Blunt trauma injuries are produced by two major forces involved in the impact: shear and compression. Shear, or speed difference, results when one organ or structure moves either faster or slower in relation to other objects in the portion of the body or body system. This can be caused by organs moving faster from deceleration of the body as a whole while the organ or body part continues to move quickly. This can occur, for example, in a car collision in which the body hits the dashboard and the heart still continues to move forward for a fraction of a second. The force applied against the heart and great vessels can tear or shear the heart from the vessels. On the other hand, the shear force can be applied as acceleration, when objects move faster than the organ or body part.

Compression is the force directly applied to an organ or body part. This injury type is accentuated by the length of compression time, force of compression (amount of energy applied), and the area compressed.

Vehicle Collisions

[OBJECTIVE 7]

According to the National Highway Traffic Safety Administration (NHTSA), MVCs are the leading cause of death and injury in the United States for persons aged 1 to 45 years. Moreover, the number of these collisions increased in the years 1999 to 2003 (Disaster Center, 2003). MVCs are significant producers of injury and death because a considerable amount of mass (weight of vehicle) and speed (velocity) is typically involved in a collision. The collision can be divided into three general phases: the vehicle hits the object, the body hits the vehicle, and the organs collide inside the body. With this in mind, MVCs can be organized into five distinct categories: frontal (head on), lateral (side impact), rear end, rotational, and rollover. Each of these types has corresponding general injury patterns.

Frontal (Head-On) Impact

A frontal, or head-on, impact occurs when a vehicle squarely hits another object—such as a tree, wall, or another vehicle—with the front of the vehicle. The speed of the vehicle can be roughly approximated by the extent of damage to the vehicle; the greater the damage, the greater the speed. In such an instance the vehicle comes to an abrupt stop and the occupants continue to move at the speed of the vehicle at the time of impact until they are stopped by the vehicle restraint system, the steering column, or the dashboard. This frontal type of impact generally propels an unrestrained occupant into one of two pathways: down and under, or up and over.

Case Scenario—continued

You begin an evaluation of the patient's head, chest, and arms. You find no visible injuries to the head. Obvious bruising to the anterior chest, normal chest wall excursion and breath sounds, and no apparent trauma to the arms are visible. Although the patient remains awake, he is now oriented only to person and place. The patient continues screaming, "Don't let me die!" Vital signs are pulse, 80 beats/min; respirations, 30 breaths/min. The cardiac monitor shows a sinus rhythm. You are unable to hear or palpate a blood pressure. Jugular venous distention is not present, and the trachea is in a midline position. The patient will not allow placement of a pulse oximeter probe.

Questions

5. *Is this patient high priority? Why or why not?*
6. *Describe the apparent mechanism of injury in this case.*
7. *Given the mechanism of injury, examination findings, and vital signs, what potential injuries can you consider for this patient?*
8. *Has this additional information changed your planned destination? Why or why not?*

Down-and-Under Pathway. In the down-and-under injury pathway, the occupant continues forward toward the steering column or dashboard and moves downward in the seat. For the driver, the leg extended or planted on the floor can twist and produce rotational injury until the knees hit the dashboard. For all occupants, the area surrounding the knee becomes the primary point of impact against the dashboard. If the leg sustains impact slightly below the knee, the tibia is the impact point. In this instance the femur may continue to move forward and simply ride over the tibia. If this occurs, a dislocated knee, torn ligaments, and dislocation of the knee joint likely result (Figure 43-5). Because the popliteal artery lies behind the knee, a blood clot may form, or blood flow distally to the knee may be disrupted. Disruption of blood flow for more than 6 hours could lead to a below-the-knee amputation. Therefore this injury pattern must be reported to the physician so that possible damage to the artery is not overlooked. If the leg hits at or slightly above the knee, the femur is the site of impact. If the femur hits the dashboard, the likely primary injuries include fractured femur, dislocation of the hip (either anterior or posterior), pelvic fracture, and acetabular fracture. These can further lead to secondary injuries, such as blood clots and vascular injury.

Once the knee sustains impact, the body continues forward and hits the steering column, the dashboard, and possibly the windshield. The person may receive similar injuries as in the up-and-over pathway (Figure 43-6).

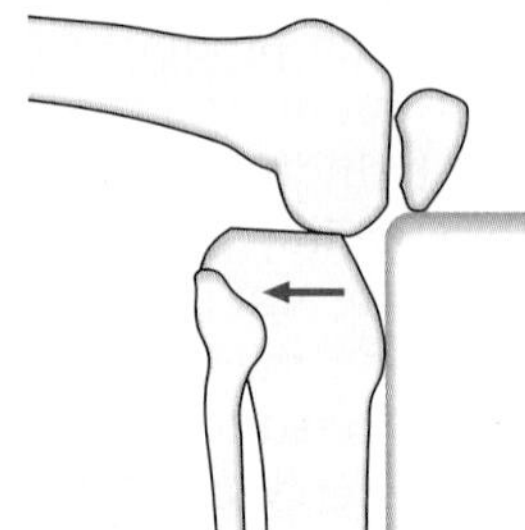

Figure 43-5 The knee has two possible impact points in an MVC: the femur and the tibia.

Although most down-and-under injuries produce considerable evidence of trauma, these injuries initially may be subtle. The only evidence may be the imprint of the knee or leg on the lower dashboard. If you fail to look for this evidence, you will fail to provide this information to the treating physician. As a result, potential serious injuries may not be treated appropriately or in a timely manner.

Up-and-Over Pathway. In the up-and-over pathway the body's forward momentum carries it forward in an upward motion. The head is usually propelled into the windshield, and possibly upward into the roof and rear-

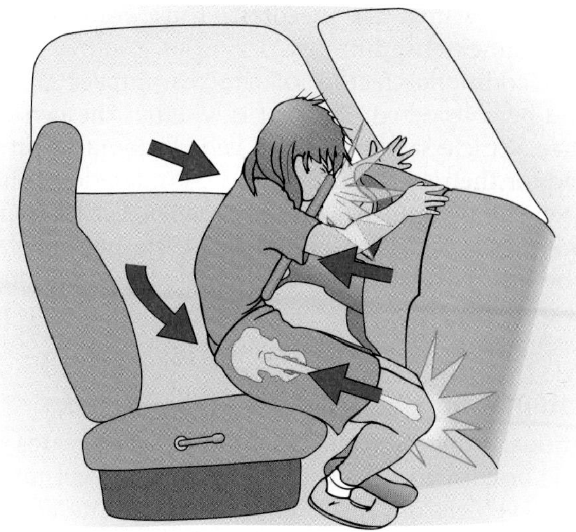

Figure 43-6 The occupant and the vehicle travel forward together. The vehicle stops, and the unrestrained occupant continues forward until something stops that motion.

BOX 43-6 Frontal Impact Body Organ Injury

Head: Skull fractures, cerebral contusion, brainstem stretch or shear, hemorrhage

Neck: Compression fracture of cervical vertebrae, hyperextension injury (posterior element compression and anterior body separation), hyperflexion injury (anterior body compression and posterior element separation)

Thorax:

Chest wall: Compression, fractured ribs to include flail segment, pneumothorax, hemothorax, thoracic spinal fracture

Heart: Myocardial contusion, myocardial rupture, aortic shear at the junction of arch and descending portions, junction of the aortic origin at the aortic valve and at the level of the diaphragm

Abdomen: Diaphragm tear, abdominal wall tear

Liver: Compression and fractured liver, shear injury or tear from ligamentum teres, avulsion of liver from inferior vena cava at the hepatic veins

Spleen: Compression or fracture of spleen and avulsion of pedicle

Gastrointestinal: Rupture of intestines, shear injury, avulsion of mesenteric vessels from aorta or venae cavae, tears along mesenteric vessels, avulsion of vessels from intestine

Gallbladder: Rupture from compression and shear injury caused by avulsion from liver or cystic duct

view mirror. Injury to the head may include open or closed injury, concussion, internal bleeding, compression or flexion and extension cervical spinal injury, lumbar (axial) spinal injury, and facial fractures (Box 43-6).

As the head moves upward, the chest and possibly abdomen are propelled into the steering column. This can produce serious injury to the thoracic wall (ribs and sternum). Primary injuries include fractured ribs, flail chest, pulmonary contusion, myocardial contusion, shearing of great vessels from the heart or lungs, splenic rupture, liver fracture, and diaphragmatic tear, allowing abdominal organs to intrude into the chest. The kidneys may be forced up the vertebral column and torn from their supporting great vessels (Figure 43-7).

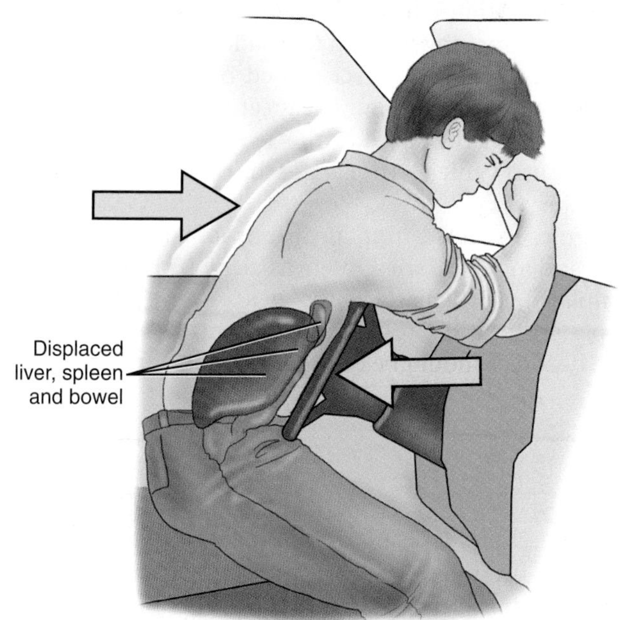

Figure 43-7 Configuration of the seat and position of the occupant can direct the initial force on the upper torso, with the head as the lead point.

Lateral (Side) Impact

Lateral impact occurs when a vehicle collides with another vehicle or strikes an object on the side of the vehicle. In this crash, the injuries depend on whether the vehicle was propelled away from the point of impact or was stopped at the point of impact.

If the damaged vehicle moves away from the impact, the occupants are propelled away from the impact. This causes significant torsion to the head, neck, and torso. If the vehicle stops at the point of impact, the victims absorb the mass of the impact and the impact of the side door as it intrudes into the occupant compartment of the vehicle.

In the side-impact MVC, the occupants may be injured in one of three ways: by the impact of the vehicle itself, by the impact with other passengers in the vehicle, and by the intrusion of the door into the occupant area of the vehicle. Five areas of injury are generally sustained in a lateral impact: neck, head, thorax, abdomen and pelvis, and extremities (Box 43-7; Figure 43-8).

Rear-End Impact

The rear-impact collision occurs when a vehicle is struck from behind by a second vehicle that is moving faster than the first vehicle. The first vehicle that was struck rapidly accelerates forward under the victim with the entire body moving forward in a sudden jerk. This movement or acceleration effect caused by the difference in speeds creates the injuries. The greater the mass at impact (i.e., the faster the speed of the second vehicle colliding with the first vehicle), the greater the potential for damage and injury.

Injuries expected from a rear-impact collision include back and neck injuries, such as flexion and extension (whiplash), particularly if the headrest was not in the proper position to protect the head and neck (Box 43-8). (The headrest should be extended so that the back of the head rests against the headrest, thus preventing the flexion and extension injury.)

Two additional factors of the rear-impact collision should be considered. The first is whether the person in the first vehicle saw the second vehicle about to hit and braced for the impact. The second consideration is if the first vehicle was pushed into another object in front of it. If either aspect is suspected—that the person braced for the impact or that the first vehicle hit something in front of that vehicle—the person may have similar injuries as expected from a front-end collision.

Rotational Impact

Rotational impacts occur when an off-center area of a vehicle or corner of the vehicle strikes an object, such as another vehicle or an immovable object. The end that hits stops moving, and the rest of the vehicle continues to move until the energy of the impact is dissipated. The occupants are usually spun within the vehicle and typically strike the door, the windshield, and other occupants. The resulting injuries are similar to those seen in frontal and lateral impacts. The most severe injuries are usually seen in the victim closest to the point of impact (Box 43-9).

BOX 43-7 Lateral-Impact Body Organ Injury

Head: Skull fracture, cerebral contusion, hemorrhage, brainstem stretch (shear), shear of brain and vessels on the opposite side of the head **(coup contrecoup)**

Neck: Compression (minimal unless head strikes top of passenger compartment or window support), odontoid fracture, rotation injury (see Figure 43-8)

Thorax: Lateral rib fracture and flail chest, pneumothorax, hemothorax, spleen or liver laceration depending on side of vehicle in which occupant was riding, thoracic vertebrae fracture, aortic arch shear at junction of movable arch and descending aorta attached at thoracic spine

Abdomen: Compression of liver or spleen depending on side of impact, kidney injury depending on side of impact, diaphragmatic tear, aortic shear of the renal vessels, shear of splenic vessels

Pelvis: Femoral fracture, femoral head driven through acetabulum, fracture of ilium, sacroiliac fracture

Extremities: Clavicle fracture (compressed between humerus and sternum), lateral compression fracture of humerus

BOX 43-8 Rear-Impact Body Organ Injury

Head: Compression into structures in seat; force of compression depends on force of impact, shear of brain and skull

Neck: Hyperextended with possible ligamentous and tendon stretching

Torso: Usually minimal injury with functional car seat

Extremities: Usually minimal injury because the extremities move with the body

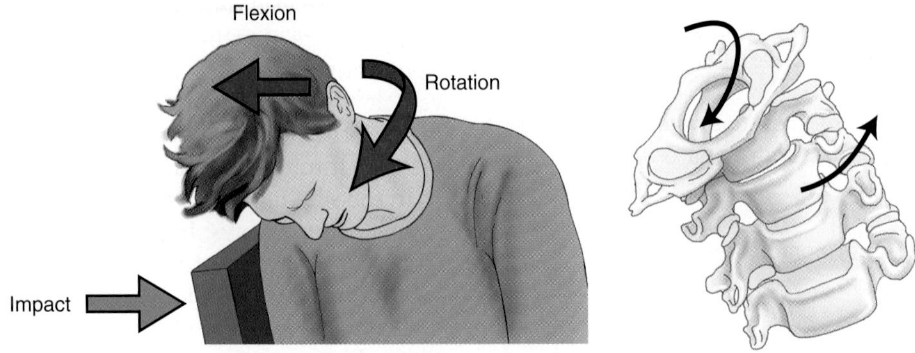

Figure 43-8 The center of gravity of the skull is anterior and superior to its pivot point between the skull and the cervical spine. During a lateral impact, when the torso is rapidly accelerated out from under the head, the head turns toward the point of impact in both lateral and anterior-posterior angles. Such motion separates the vertebral bodies from the side of opposite impact and rotates them apart. Jumped facets, ligaments, tears, and lateral compression fractures result.

BOX 43-9 Rotational Impact Body Organ Injury

Injuries are a combination of those seen in frontal and lateral impact crashes, with an emphasis on the initial impact.

Head: Skull fractures, cerebral contusion, brainstem stretch or shear, hemorrhage (coup contrecoup)

Neck: Compression fracture of cervical vertebrae **(axial compression [loading]),** hyperextension injury (posterior element compression and anterior body separation), hyperflexion injury (anterior body compression and posterior element separation), odontoid fracture, rotation injury

Thorax:

Chest wall: Compression, fractured ribs to include flail segment, pneumothorax, hemothorax, thoracic spinal fracture

Heart: Myocardial contusion, myocardial rupture, aortic shear at the junction of arch and descending portions, junction of the aortic origin at the aortic valve and at the level of the diaphragm

Abdomen: Diaphragm tear, abdominal wall tear

Liver: Compression and fractured liver, shear injury or tear from ligamentum teres, avulsion of liver from inferior vena cava at the hepatic veins

Spleen: Compression or fracture of spleen and avulsion of pedicle (depending on side of vehicle in which occupant was riding), diaphragmatic tear, aortic shear of the renal vessels, shear of splenic vessels

Gastrointestinal: Rupture of intestines, shear injury with avulsion of mesenteric vessels from aorta or venae cavae, tears along mesenteric vessels, avulsion of vessels from intestine

Gallbladder: Rupture from compression and shear injury caused by avulsion from liver or cystic duct

Pelvis: Femoral fracture, femoral head driven through acetabulum, fracture of ilium, sacroiliac fracture

Extremities: Clavicle fracture (compressed between humerus and sternum), lateral compression fracture of humerus

Rollover

In a rollover collision, the occupants tumble around within the vehicle like clothes in a clothes dryer. The victim is injured wherever he or she hits the vehicle as it rolls. Calculating the exact nature of injury based solely on the rollover mechanism is impossible. Generally speaking, the greater the speed of the rollover, the greater the injury. Even if the occupants are restrained, the body's organs are subject to the shear forces of the mass of energy applied in the crash (Box 43-10).

If the occupants are unrestrained, they likely will be ejected from the vehicle as it tumbles. Once ejected, they may be crushed by the vehicle itself or struck by other vehicles.

BOX 43-10 Rollover-Impact Body Organ Injury

Injury patterns are difficult to predict because of the complexity of the crash. The victim may be hit on all sides within the vehicle, causing combinations of injuries consistent with frontal and lateral crashes. Predict injuries by thinking of the first part of the crash rather than the second part. If the victim is ejected, he or she also may be crushed by a vehicle, may have hit trees or other vehicles, and will have injuries consistent with a fall.

Head: Skull fractures, cerebral contusion, brainstem stretch or shear, hemorrhage (coup contrecoup)

Neck: Compression fracture of cervical vertebrae, hyperextension injury (posterior element compression and anterior body separation), hyperflexion injury (anterior body compression and posterior element separation), odontoid fracture, rotation injury

Thorax:

Chest wall: Compression, fractured ribs to include flail segment, pneumothorax, hemothorax, thoracic spinal fracture

Heart: Myocardial contusion, myocardial rupture, aortic shear at the junction of arch and descending portions, junction of the aortic origin at the aortic valve and at the level of the diaphragm

Abdomen: Diaphragm tear, abdominal wall tear

Liver: Compression and fractured liver, shear injury or tear from ligamentum teres, avulsion of liver from inferior vena cava at the hepatic veins

Spleen: Compression or fracture of spleen and avulsion of pedicle (depending on side of vehicle in which occupant was riding), diaphragmatic tear, aortic shear of the renal vessels, shear of splenic vessels

Gastrointestinal: Rupture of intestines, shear injury, avulsion of mesenteric vessels from aorta or venae cavae, tears along mesenteric vessels, avulsion of vessels from intestine

Gallbladder: Rupture from compression and shear injury caused by avulsion from liver or cystic duct

Pelvis: Femoral fracture, femoral head driven through acetabulum, fracture of ilium, sacroiliac fracture

Extremities: Clavicle fracture (compressed between humerus and sternum), lateral compression fracture of humerus

Restraints

[OBJECTIVE 8]

Injury prevention programs, specifically vehicle restraint programs such as the "Buckle Up America" and the "Click it or Ticket" programs, have increased the use of vehicle restraints in the United States. These efforts have steadily shown that they can reduce the number of vehicular deaths. Although the use of seatbelts cannot prevent every death from an MVC, seatbelts have made motor vehicle travel safer. According to NHTSA in a "Buckle Up America" fact sheet, "It is estimated that safety belt use prevented about 15,200 deaths in 2004. Safety belt use prevents untold tragedy to American families and saves billions of dollars in medical expenses and lost productivity costs annually. If all passenger vehicle occupants over age 4 had used safety belts in 2004, NHTSA estimates that nearly 21,000 lives (that is, an additional 5800 lives) could have been saved" (USDOT, 2005a). As of January 31, 2007, 49 states, Puerto Rico, and the District of Columbia have either a primary or secondary seatbelt law. New Hampshire is the only state without an adult seatbelt law (National Conference for State Legislatures, 2008).

A serious threat to unrestrained occupants in MVCs is ejection from the vehicle. Ejection from a vehicle increases rates of mortality and morbidity of the victims. Ejected victims have a sixfold greater chance of death than victims who are not ejected. Moreover, those ejected are more severely injured as well as have poorer long-term outcomes than those who are not ejected (Gongora et al., 2001). Besides having an increased risk of death or serious injury, ejected occupants place other occupants in a vehicle at increased risk of death and serious injury by being propelled through the vehicle and colliding with the other occupants (MacLennan et al., 2004).

Current restraint systems are designed to absorb the energy of an impact before the occupant collides with something hard. They also are designed to limit the distance the body has to travel, thereby decreasing the velocity. Because the mortality rate of persons ejected from a vehicle is high, seatbelts also are designed to keep the occupant in the vehicle and prevent ejection. This decreased velocity, along with keeping the body in the seat, help decrease the potential injuries in an MVC. Restraint systems are effective in all types of MVCs.

Four types of occupant restraint systems are used in the United States: lap belts, shoulder restraints, airbags, and child safety seats.

Lap Belts

The lap belt is the most common restraint system used, with or without concurrent use with shoulder restraints. The benefit of the lap belt is that it holds the lower torso close to the seat and away from the dashboard and steering column. This prevents forward motion of the lower torso in frontal collisions, moves the lower torso with the vehicle in lateral collisions and away from the impact, prevents multiple impacts during rollovers, and prevents ejection.

The lap belt is attached to the floor behind the occupant at a 45-degree angle. It is worn across the iliac crest, adjusted tightly enough to prevent forward motion of the pelvis. When worn properly, the lap belt does not impinge on the soft intraabdominal contents.

The lap belt does have some limitations. It does not support the upper torso during a collision. Moreover, if it is worn improperly, with the belt above the anterior iliac spine (hips), the belt can compress the intraabdominal organs against the belt and the spine. This increases the chances of injury to the liver, spleen, duodenum, and pancreas as well as the spine in the area between T12 and L2. In addition, this force applied to the abdomen during a crash may rupture the diaphragm, causing the abdominal contents to move upward into the chest. A sign of abdominal injury is a lap belt imprint or abrasion on the abdomen (Figure 43-9).

Although the lap belt prevents the lower torso from moving forward in a collision, it does not prevent the upper torso from hitting the steering column, dashboard, or windshield or from twisting and rotating during high-speed collisions. Significant injury can still occur, such as sternal fractures, cardiac tamponade, chest wall injuries, head injuries, and facial trauma.

Shoulder Restraints

Shoulder restraints work along with the lap belt to help prevent the upper torso and head from hitting the steering column, dashboard, or windshield in frontal collisions. By supporting the upper torso, the shoulder restraint prevents hyperflexion or the folding of the body at the waist and the resulting spinal injuries. Additionally, the shoulder restraint moves the upper torso with the vehicle in lateral impacts.

A limitation of the shoulder restraint system includes possible neck injury if it is worn without the lap belt. In addition, the shoulder restraint system is less effective if the occupant is close to the dashboard or steering column.

Moreover, clavicle injury may occur from the position of the strap across the shoulder and chest. During high-speed impact, organ collision inside the body may still occur, resulting in organ injury, cervical fracture, and spinal cord injury. These injuries may occur from the extreme forces involved in the crash.

Airbags

Most vehicles currently on the road have some sort of airbag installed—at the least a frontal driver airbag. Depending on its make and model, the vehicle may have

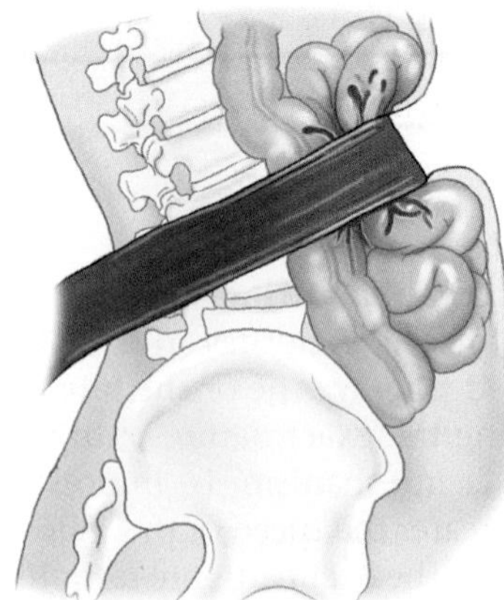

Figure 43-9 A seatbelt incorrectly positioned above the brim of the pelvis allows the abdominal organs to be trapped between the moving posterior wall and the belt. Injuries to the pancreas and other retroperitoneal organs may result, as well as blowout ruptures of the small intestine and colon.

passenger side airbags, side impact airbags, and frontal post (A-post) airbags. Airbags are designed to provide supplemental protection to the lap and shoulder belt combination.

The most common airbag location is in the steering column. This location ideally protects the driver from striking the steering column and dashboard during frontal impacts. These airbags are not designed for lateral impacts, multiple impacts, rear impacts, or rollover collisions. The frontal airbag also may not protect the knee on impact in the collision; therefore the victim may still have leg and pelvis injuries.

Airbags do have limitations. They are minimally effective when used alone. Moreover, they may cause injury if the person is too close (10 inches or closer for the driver, 18 inches for front seat passengers) to the airbag when it deploys. The bag deploys quite rapidly, in fractions of a second. It may cause facial and forearm abrasion injuries as it expands. In addition, the deployed airbag may hide structural damage to the vehicle, such as a fractured steering column, that would aid in assessment of the patient.

Side Airbags. Many newer cars are equipped with side-impact airbags. These airbags work the same as the front airbags, deploying when a sensor is activated by a collision. Three types of side-impact airbags are available: chest or torso, head, and head and chest combination.

Chest or torso side airbags are mounted in the side of the seat or in the door. They are designed to protect an adult in a side-impact collision. Head side airbags are usually installed in the roof rail above the side windows. These airbags may be either curtain or tubular in design. Head and chest combination side airbags, the last type, are usually larger than the head and the chest types and may be installed in the side of the seat or in the door.

PARAMEDIC*Pearl*

Groups at risk for injuries from airbag deployment include infants and children younger than 12 years; short-stature adults less than approximately 5 feet, 2 inches tall; older adults; and special needs persons (i.e., those with modified vehicles).

Most airbag injuries are limited to cuts, abrasions, and bruises. However, these injuries are minor when compared with the potential injury if the airbag did not deploy. Of note, the NHTSA has reported 238 deaths caused by airbags from 1990 through 2002. Most of these deaths occurred because the person was too close to the deploying airbag.

When addressing children and airbags, the National Center for Injury Prevention and Control recommends that children younger than 12 years are safer in the back seat in an appropriate child safety seat and therefore should be placed in the back seat when in a vehicle (2005). Placing a child younger than 12 years in the front seat places the child at risk for injury from airbag deployment. According to the NSC (2004), as of April 2004, 149 children between the ages of 7 days and 11 years have died from airbag-related crashes; 23 of the 149 were infants involved with front airbags.

Be aware of the dangers of airbags when you approach vehicles and during the assessment and extrication of victims. Paramedics and firefighters have been injured by delayed airbag deployment involved in MVCs as well as activation of a second gas canister for a second deployment. According to the National Institute for Occupational Safety and Health (2003), one firefighter has been killed by an airbag.

Child Safety Seats

According to the Centers for Disease Control and Prevention, the leading cause of death for children aged 1 to 9 years is MVCs. For every death, an estimated hundreds more incur permanent disability and injury. In 2004, an estimated 451 lives of children younger than 5 years were saved by child restraint use (USDOT, 2004b).

Four types of child safety seats currently are available: rear-facing infant seats, front-facing safety seats, high-back booster seats, and safety belt or backless safety seats. Some seats may be converted from a rear-facing infant seat to a front-facing toddler seat. The child safety seats work with the seatbelts of the vehicle and other safety devices (anchors) in vehicles manufactured after September 1, 2002, to create a safety system (the Lower Anchors and Tethers for Children [LATCH] system). This system uses a combination of lap belts, shoulder straps, full-body harnesses, and harness-shield devices to protect the child during MVCs.

Predictable injuries from child safety seat use are abdominal trauma, acceleration and deceleration injuries, and neck and spinal injuries. Together these injuries are known as the "seatbelt syndrome" or "lap belt complex." These injuries may be subtle in nature. Moreover, they may be masked compared with the more obvious injuries found in unrestrained children (Davies, 2004).

Of note, although the use of child safety seats has remained high for infants (98%) and toddlers (93%), a negative trend in child safety seat use has occurred over the past few years. In 2002, 83% of children aged 4 to 7 years were restrained. In 2004, that percentage decreased to 73% (USDOT, 2005b).

In addition to the percentage of child safety seat use, other concerns exist regarding children in motor vehicles, including the misguided belief that children in a sport utility vehicle (SUV) are safer than children in passenger cars. In fact, children in SUVs are just as likely to be injured in an MVC as are their passenger car cohorts. However, the manner in which they are injured is different. According to a pediatric hospital study, the potential advantage offered by heavier SUVs is offset by other factors, including the vehicle's increased tendency to roll over (Daly et al., 2006). Another issue of increasing concern is obese children in safety seats. Appropriate seats for these children are quite difficult to find because of age and weight issues. A child may fit a seat based on age but not weight, or the child may fit based on weight but not age. As a result, a child may be placed in a seat that affords less protection and be injured because of improper seat fit (Trifiletti et al., 2006). With these issues in mind, paramedics must continue to work with the community on child safety seat programs to reduce rates of death and injury associated with their use or misuse.

PARAMEDIC*Pearl*

The most common misuses of child restraint systems include age/weight inappropriateness, direction of the safety system, placement of the restraint in relation to airbags, installation and security of the restraint system to the vehicle seat (tight seatbelt), misuse of locking clips for certain vehicle safety belts, fit of vehicle safety belt across child in belt-positioning booster seat, and defective or broken system elements.

From U.S. Department of Transportation (2005). *Traffic safety facts 2005: A compilation of motor vehicle crash data from the fatality analysis reporting system and the general estimates system.* Washington, DC: National Highway Traffic Safety Administration.

The NHTSA recommends that child safety seats be replaced after a moderate or severe vehicle crash. This replacement ensures a continued high level of crash protection for child passengers. The NHTSA recommends that child safety seats do not automatically have to be replaced after a minor crash.

To be regarded as minor, an MVC must meet all the following criteria:

- The vehicle could be driven away from the crash site.
- The vehicle door nearest the safety seat was undamaged.
- No injuries occurred to any of the vehicle occupants.
- The airbags (if present) did not deploy.
- No visible damage has occurred to the safety seat (Box 43-11; Table 43-2).

PEDIATRIC*Pearl*

If during assessment of the child you note that the child is neurologically appropriate, has no obvious thoracic injuries, and the child safety seat appears to be undamaged and intact, you may transport the child in his or her own safety seat.

BOX 43-11 Special Considerations in Transporting Children

- The method or device used to secure children during transport must provide effective restraint without compromising the safety of others on board.
- Younger children and infants who do not require spinal immobilization should be transported in child safety seats appropriate for their size. If you do not have an appropriate safety seat on the ambulance, ask family members if they have one available (preferably one that has not been in an MVC).
- Any time a child is secured to a device, such as a safety seat or spine board, the device must be secured to the stretcher. Ambulance crashes have occurred in which a pediatric patient who was restrained on a spine board that was *not* secured to the stretcher was ejected from the rear cabin, resulting in serious injuries.
- For any patient in whom it is medically appropriate, position the patient on the gurney with the gurney back upright at least at a 45-degree angle. This will optimize transportation safety in the event of an impact or deceleration.
- If the child is secured in a safety seat, secure the seat to the stretcher with at least two belts placed at a 90-degree angle to each other. One strap should be oriented vertically and the other should secure the child seat horizontally to the upright stretcher. Securing the child safety seat to the stretcher with the stretcher back in the upright position has had good results in crash testing conducted to date.
- Restraint systems applied to a flat stretcher are less secure in a crash. If you must use a suboptimal restraint technique such as this, notify the driver to use extra caution during transport. This will help minimize risk.
- Older children who do not require special positioning should be secured on a stretcher that has had the back elevated to an angle of at least 45 degrees.
- Use shoulder harnesses to restrain patients who must be immobilized in the supine position on a back board and therefore cannot have the back of the stretcher elevated for protection.
- *Never* secure the parent and child together on the stretcher. *Never* allow infants or young children to ride in the arms or lap of a parent or rescuer.

Reprinted from the New York University School of Medicine. *Safe transport of children.* http://www.med.nyu.edu/peder/cpem/trippals/38transp.pdf.
MVC, Motor vehicle crash.

Electronic Stability Control Systems

Several automobile manufacturers began to add electronic stability control systems to vehicles in the late 1990s. These electronic systems are designed to prevent potential crash injuries. In other words, they are designed to help the driver of a vehicle avoid crashes and their resulting injuries. They are designed to be used with antilock braking systems and together electronically apply power or decrease power to selected wheels to prevent crashes. They were initially designed to address single-vehicle crash fatality issues, such as losing control and sliding off the highway. However, they have proven effective in decreasing both single- and multiple-vehicle crash fatalities (Kondin et al., 2006).

TABLE 43-2 The Do's and Don'ts of Transporting Children in an Ambulance

Do . . .	Do Not . . .
Drive cautiously at safe speeds and observe traffic laws	Drive at unsafe, high speeds with rapid acceleration, deceleration, and turns
Tightly secure all monitoring devices and other equipment	Leave monitoring devices and other equipment unsecured in moving EMS vehicles
Ensure available restraint systems are used by EMTs and other occupants, including the patient	Allow parents, caregivers, EMTs, or other passengers to be unrestrained during transport
Transport children who are not patients, properly restrained, in an alternate passenger vehicle whenever possible	Allow the child or infant to be held in the parent's, caregiver's, or EMT's lap during transport
Encourage use of the DOT NHTSA Emergency Vehicle Operating Course, National Standard Curriculum	Allow emergency vehicles to be operated by persons who have not completed the DOT Emergency Vehicle Operating Course or equivalent

Reprinted from the U.S. Department of Transportation. (4399). *Do's and don'ts of transporting children in an ambulance*, Washington, DC: National Highway Traffic Safety Administration.
DOT, U.S. Department of Transportation; *NHTSA,* National Highway Traffic Safety Administration.

Organ Collision Injuries

The organs of the body can be injured as a result of deceleration and compression forces (Figures 43-10 to 43-13). You should maintain a high index of suspicion regarding injuries to organs because of the principles of kinematics.

Deceleration Injuries

Recall Newton's first law of motion. Consider how a body organ put into motion after an impact will continue to move. Because the organs were placed in motion from the impact, they will move in opposition to the anatomic structures that attach them to the body. This presents a risk of detaching or separating from their support structures. Injury to the supporting structure, such as vascular pedicle or mesenteric attachment, can lead to rapid blood loss or exsanguinating hemorrhage.

Head Injuries. When the head hits a stationary object, the cranium comes to an abrupt stop. However, the brain inside continues to move until it strikes the skull. This movement can cause the brain tissue to be bruised, lacerated, or crushed, as well as cause blood vessels attached to the brain and skull to be torn, producing intracranial hemorrhage. Other injuries associated with deceleration of the head include central nervous system injury, caused by the stretching of the spinal cord and its attachments, and cervical fracture.

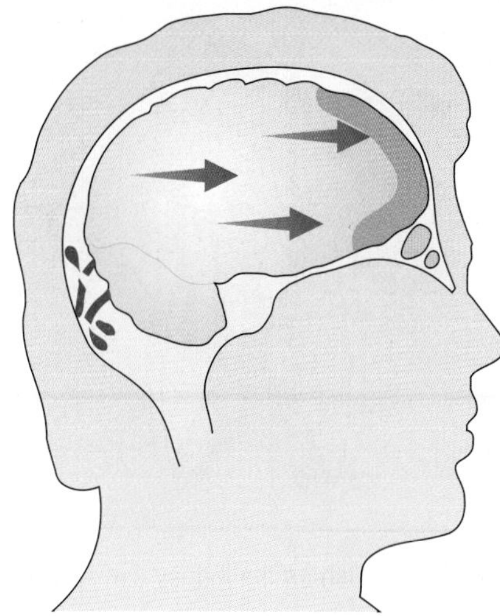

Figure 43-10 As the skull stops its forward motion, the brain continues to move forward. The part of the brain nearest the impact is compressed, bruised, and perhaps even lacerated. The portion farthest from the impact is separated from the skull, with tearing and lacerations of the vessels involved.

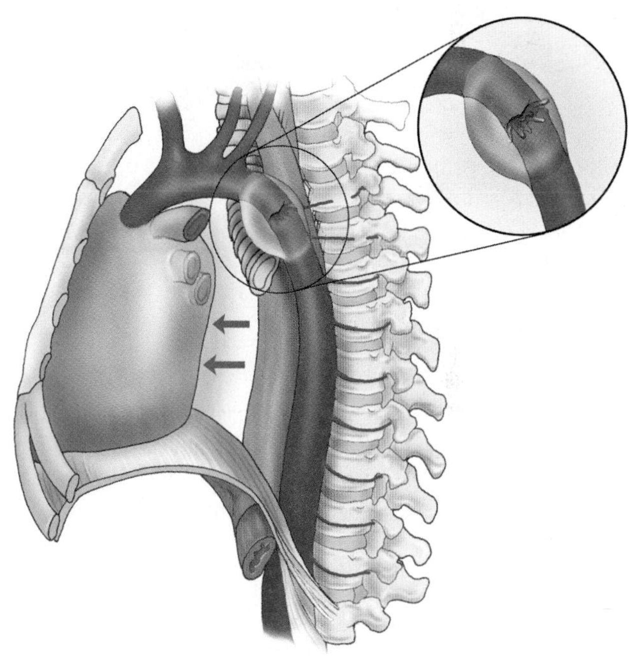

Figure 43-11 The descending aorta is a boxed structure that moves with the thoracic spice. The arch, aorta, and heart are freely moveable. Acceleration of the torso in a lateral impact collision or rapid deceleration of the torso in a frontal impact collision produces a different rate of motion between the arch/heart complex and the descending aorta.

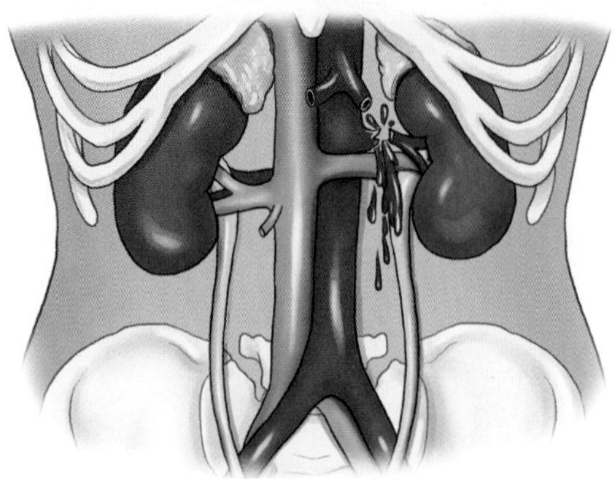

Figure 43-12 Organs such as the kidney can tear away from the abdominal wall.

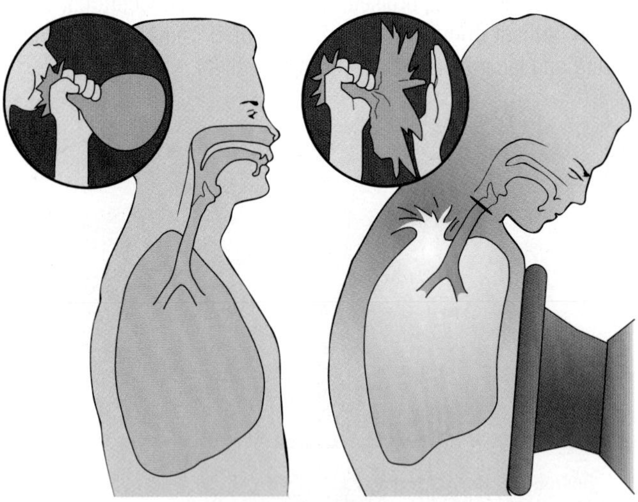

Figure 43-13 Compression of the lung against a closed glottis, by impact on either the anterior or lateral chest wall, produces an effect similar to compressing a paper bag when the opening is closed tightly by the hands. The paper bag ruptures, as does the lung.

Thoracic Injuries. The aorta is often injured by severe deceleration forces because it is affixed at several points. The aorta is fixed proximally by the aortic valve in the descending portion of the aortic arch by the ligamentum arteriosum. The descending aorta also is attached to the thoracic spine. When the thorax hits a stationary object, the heart and aorta continue in motion. This movement is in opposition to the attachment at the lower end of the aortic arch. The aorta is usually sheared at the level of its ligamentum arteriosum attachment. Rupture of the aorta leads to rapid exsanguination. However, transection and dissection through to the internal lining (intima and media of the aorta) can produce tamponade. Patients with this injury often arrive at an emergency department and survive the injury.

Abdominal Injuries. When deceleration forces are applied to the abdomen, intraabdominal organs and retroperitoneal structures (usually the kidneys) are affected. Because of the forward motion of the kidneys, they can shear away from the vascular pedicle attachments. Mesenteric tears can be seen in the small and large intestines from their forward motion. The liver can be separated at its midpoint from its vascular and hepatic duct pedicle as a result of downward and forward motion with deceleration. The spleen is restrained by the diaphragm and abdominal wall attachments. The spleen can tear the splenic capsule with forward motion.

Compression Injuries

Compression forces can injure any portion of the body. This chapter, however, covers only the most susceptible and potentially most serious areas of the body: the head, thorax, and abdomen.

Head Injuries. Compression injuries of the head can result in open- or closed-head fractures, facial fractures, soft tissue injuries, and bone fragment penetration of the brain, as seen in a depressed skull fracture. The associated injuries include brain contusion and brain tissue lacerations. Compression forces to the skull also can produce hemorrhage from fractured bone, from meningeal vessels, or from the brain itself. With any compression force injury to the head, consider cervical fracture and injury to the cervical vertebrae. Compression injury to the head also may produce compression injury to the axial skeleton and hyperextension and hyperflexion injuries.

Thoracic Injuries. Compression injuries to the thorax often involve the lungs and heart. Associated injuries to external structures include fractured ribs and/or sternum, pneumothorax, and hemothorax.

A serious lung injury that can result from compression forces is the rupture of the lungs, commonly called the *paper bag effect*. This occurs when air trapped within the lungs creates an increased intrathoracic pressure that ruptures at a weak point in the lungs. This most commonly occurs when the victim of an MVC sees the crash about to occur and takes an instinctive deep breath, filling the lungs with air closed against the glottis. This formation resembles a paper bag, filled with air; when the victim strikes the steering column, the "paper bag" (lung) bursts. This is thought to account for many instances of pneumothorax after vehicular trauma. In some instances, penetrating ribs may also contribute to pneumothorax after blunt trauma to the chest.

Compression of the heart can occur when the forces pin the heart between the thoracic spine and sternum. Depending on the amount of energy applied, the compression of the contents of the abdomen, and an increase in the pressure in the aorta, the aortic valve can rupture. In addition, compression of the heart between the sternum and spine can cause myocardial contusion, cardiac dysrhythmias, atrial or ventricle rupture, or cardiac tamponade.

Abdominal Injuries. Abdominal cavity compression can result in serious effects, including solid organ rupture, vascular organ hemorrhage, and hollow organ perforation into the peritoneal cavity. Common injuries include rupture of the bladder, especially if full, and lacerations to the liver, spleen, and kidneys.

An effect similar to the paper bag syndrome in the thorax can occur in the abdomen. Increased intraabdominal pressure in the abdominal cavity from compression forces can cause rupture or herniation of the diaphragm and rupture of hollow organs such as the gallbladder, urinary bladder, duodenum, colon, stomach, or small bowel.

Other Motorized Vehicle Collisions

Injuries also can occur from collisions involving other types of motorized vehicles, including motorcycles, all-terrain vehicles (ATVs), snowmobiles, water bikes, jet skis, and farm machinery. This chapter uses motorcycles and ATVs as representative of these other vehicles; these vehicles are popular and cause similar injury patterns. Bicycle injuries are similar to motorcycle injuries; the majority of bicycle-related deaths involve collision with motor vehicles (Kondin et al., 2006). For jet skis or watercraft, the injury possibilities are similar to motorcycle injuries. In addition, consider the additional risk of water-related issues, such as drowning or near-drowning superimposed on the injury.

According to an NHTSA report, 3661 motorcyclists died and 67,000 were injured in highway crashes in 2003 (Society for Public Health Education, 2005). This is part of an increasing trend in motorcycle death and injury rates. An analysis of motorcycle crashes from 1996 to 2000 shows that in 1997, 1 in 20 U.S. road fatalities was a motorcycle rider. In 2001, this figure was 1 in 13. The NHTSA has examined this rise and has provided several possibilities on why this trend is worsening. The average age of the rider is older, rising from 29.3 years in 1990 to 36.3 years in 2001. Another contributing factor is the increased power of motorcycles as a result of increased motor size. In addition, incredibly, five states removed their mandatory helmet laws: Arkansas, Florida, Kentucky, Louisiana, and Texas. The NHTSA showed a significant increase in the number of fatalities in four of these five states, with Florida being the exception (Schneider, 2003) (Table 43-3).

TABLE 43-3 Motorcycle Crash Statistics

Year	Fatal with Helmet	Fatal without Helmet	Severe Injury with Helmet	Severe Injury without Helmet
2000	21	29	37	56
2001	17	36	26	59
2002	17	38	50	77

Smaller motorized vehicles are generally thought to be more dangerous because they do not afford the same level of protection as motorcycles. They offer little protection from the transfer of energy. In fact, these incidents are usually more severe than car crashes. As with other types of MVCs, the predictable injuries depend on the collision.

Motorcycle Collisions

[OBJECTIVE 9]

Motorcycle collisions vary from head-on impact to collision from any angle. These collisions can also include "laying the motorcycle down."

Frontal or Head-On Impact. The motorcycle's center of gravity rests on the front axle and therefore forward of the rider's seat (Figure 43-14). When a motorcycle strikes an object that stops its forward motion, the rest of the motorcycle follows Newton's first law of motion and continues until its motion is stopped by an outside source, such as another vehicle, wall, or road surface. When the motorcycle is involved in a frontal impact, it usually tips forward and propels the rider over the handlebars. Secondary impact with the handlebars or other objects stops the forward motion of the rider. Predictable injuries caused by secondary impact include head and neck trauma and compression to the axial skeleton (axial loading), chest, and abdomen. If the feet remain on the footrests of the motorcycle during impact, the mid-shaft of the femur absorbs the rider's forward momentum, which can cause bilateral femur and lower leg fractures. Serious perineal injuries can occur if the rider's groin strikes the gas tank or the handlebars or if the rider is flipped and hits another surface in a feet-first position (Box 43-12).

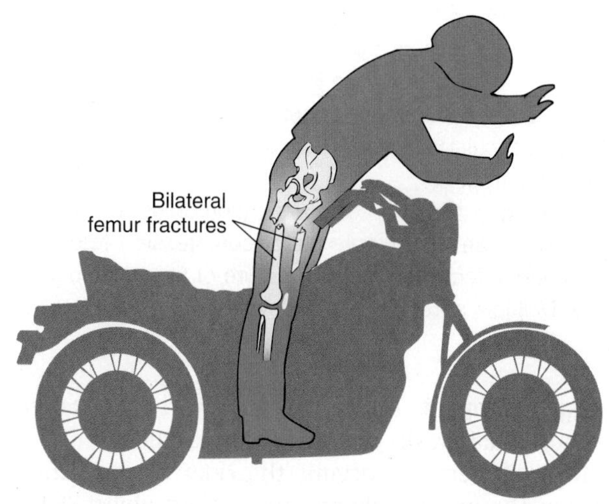

Figure 43-14 The body travels forward and over the motorcycle, with the thighs and femurs hitting the handlebars. The driver can also be "ejected" from the motorcycle.

BOX 43-12 Motorcycle Collision Body Organ Injury

The organs injured and the severity of the injury depend on the speed at the time of impact, the surface struck by the rider, the object struck by the rider, and whether or not the rider was wearing protective gear. In addition to the injuries listed below, the rider may also be at risk for penetrating injury to several of the body or organ areas.

Head: Skull fractures (open or closed), cerebral contusion, brainstem stretch or shear, hemorrhage (coup contrecoup), facial fractures, basilar skull fractures, central nervous system impairment

Neck: Compression fracture of cervical vertebrae, compression of axial vertebrae **(axial load),** hyperextension injury (posterior element compression and anterior body separation), hyperflexion injury (anterior body compression and posterior element separation), odontoid fracture, and rotation injury

Thorax:

Chest wall: Compression, fractured ribs to include flail segment, pneumothorax, hemothorax, thoracic spinal fracture, fractured sternum

Heart: Myocardial contusion, myocardial rupture, aortic shear at the junction of arch and descending portions, junction of the aortic origin at the aortic valve and at the level of the diaphragm

Abdomen: Diaphragm tear, abdominal wall tear, lumbar spine fracture

Liver: Compression and fractured liver, shear injury or tear from ligamentum teres, avulsion of liver from inferior vena cava at the hepatic veins

Spleen: Compression or fracture of spleen and avulsion of pedicle, diaphragmatic tear, aortic shear of the renal vessels, shear of splenic vessels

Gastrointestinal: Rupture of intestines, shear injury with avulsion of mesenteric vessels from aorta or venae cavae, tears along mesenteric vessels, avulsion of vessels from intestine, kidney separation from supporting vessels or structures

Gallbladder: Rupture from compression and shear injury caused by avulsion from liver or cystic duct

Pelvis: Sacroiliac fracture or pelvic fracture

Groin: Testicular avulsion, testicular trauma, penile trauma, vaginal trauma

Extremities: Clavicle fracture (compressed between humerus and sternum), lateral compression fracture of humerus, femoral fracture, fracture of tibia or fibula

Skin: Multiple abrasions and/or avulsions

Angular Impact. Depending on the circumstance of the individual crash, a motorcycle may hit an object at an angle. When this occurs, the rider often is trapped between the motorcycle and the second object. Predictable injuries include crush injuries to the affected side. Examples include open fractures to the femur, tibia, and fibula and dislocation or fracture of the malleolus.

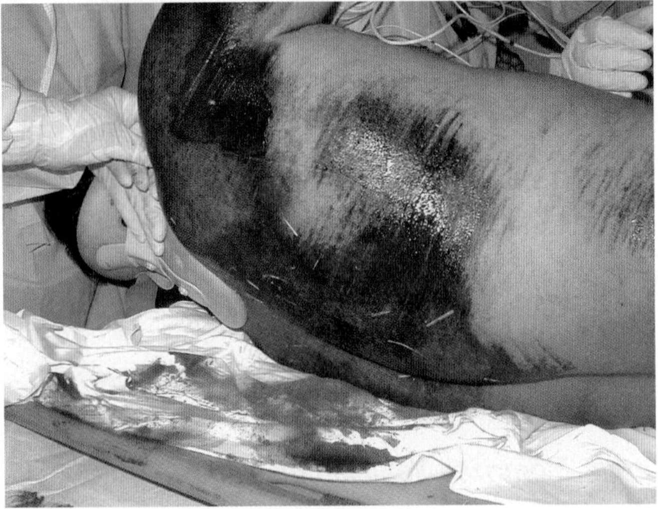

Figure 43-15 Road burns after a motorcycle crash without protective clothing.

"Laying the Motorcycle Down." Motorcycle riders with experience, such as professional riders, often use a tactic called "laying the motorcycle down" to reduce the severity of the injury before they strike an object (Figure 43-15). This protective maneuver separates the rider from the motorcycle, allowing the rider to slide away from the object. Predictable injuries include massive abrasions (road rash) and fractures to the affected side as the rider hits the ground. These fractures can be severe. However, these injuries are generally less serious than those that can occur from hitting an object while still on the motorcycle.

Personal Protection Gear for Riders. Personal protection gear for riders includes helmet, leather boots, eye protection, leather clothing, commercially available nylon padded jackets, and possibly a reflective vest. A rider who does not wear a helmet has a 300% greater chance of severe brain injury (see Table 43-3).

Pedestrian versus Motor Vehicle

[OBJECTIVE 10]

In 2004, 68,000 pedestrians were injured and another 4641 were killed in MVCs in the United States. In addition, according to the USDOT, nearly one fifth of children between the ages of 5 and 9 years killed in MVCs were pedestrians. Because of the nature of the vehicle/pedestrian crash—a large mass striking a relatively small mass—paramedics must have a high index of suspicion for multisystem trauma.

The three main mechanisms of injury (multiple impacts) are involved in auto versus pedestrian collisions. The first impact occurs with the bumper of the vehicle striking the pedestrian's body. The second impact occurs when the pedestrian strikes the hood of the vehicle. The third impact occurs when the pedestrian is bounced off the hood and strikes the ground or another object.

The predictable injuries depend on three important variables: the height of the bumper in relation to the height of the pedestrian, whether the pedestrian is an adult or a child (which affects how the pedestrian typically reacts to the vehicle), and the speed of the vehicle at impact. High speed is not always necessary to produce severe injury. Remember that the mass or size of the objects in relation to each other (big striking little) from the physical laws of motion is important. The larger the mass, the greater the effect. Therefore low-speed impacts should not be discounted during assessment. In a pedestrian versus vehicle collision, also consider whether the pedestrian was hit by another vehicle.

Adult Pedestrian. Most adults faced with the threat of an oncoming vehicle will attempt to protect themselves by turning away from the vehicle. Therefore the majority of injuries are from impact to the lateral or posterior part of the body. During the first impact, the adult usually is struck by the vehicle's bumper at the level of the lower legs, often causing fractures (Figure 43-16).

The second impact occurs as the person falls toward the hood of the vehicle. This results in possible fractures of the pelvis, femur, thorax, and spine. This impact also can produce intraabdominal and intrathoracic injuries (both compression and shear). Also during this second impact the head and neck are flung toward the hood from the force of the impact. This can result in injuries to the head, neck, and cervical spine as well as intracranial hemorrhage.

The third impact occurs when the pedestrian strikes the ground or is propelled against another object. This can result in serious damage to the hip and shoulder of the affected side as the body makes contact with the landing surface. Sudden acceleration or deceleration forces are associated with this impact and can cause fractures; internal hemorrhage; and head, neck, thoracic, and spinal injuries.

Child Pedestrian. The major difference between the adult and child pedestrian involved in a pedestrian/vehicle collision is the protection mechanism triggered (Figure 43-17). The adult turns away from the threat, but the child tends to face the threat; therefore the child's injuries most often are frontal in nature. Because of the child's size in relation to the bumper of the vehicle, the first impact is usually higher up above the knees or around the pelvis. Predictable injuries from the initial impact include fractures of the femur and pelvis as well as internal hemorrhage.

The second impact occurs as the child's thorax hits the hood. This usually flexes the victim's head and neck forward, most likely causing it to strike the hood of the vehicle. Predictable injuries include thoracic trauma, abdominal trauma, facial trauma, head trauma, and neck injury.

The third impact occurs as the child is propelled downward toward the ground or strikes another object. Because of the smaller size of the child in relation to the vehicle, the child may be forced under the vehicle and dragged for some distance. Similar to the adult, the child victim may be struck by other vehicles. Predictable injuries include fractures, possible amputations, internal hemorrhage, and head, neck, thoracic, and spinal injuries. The

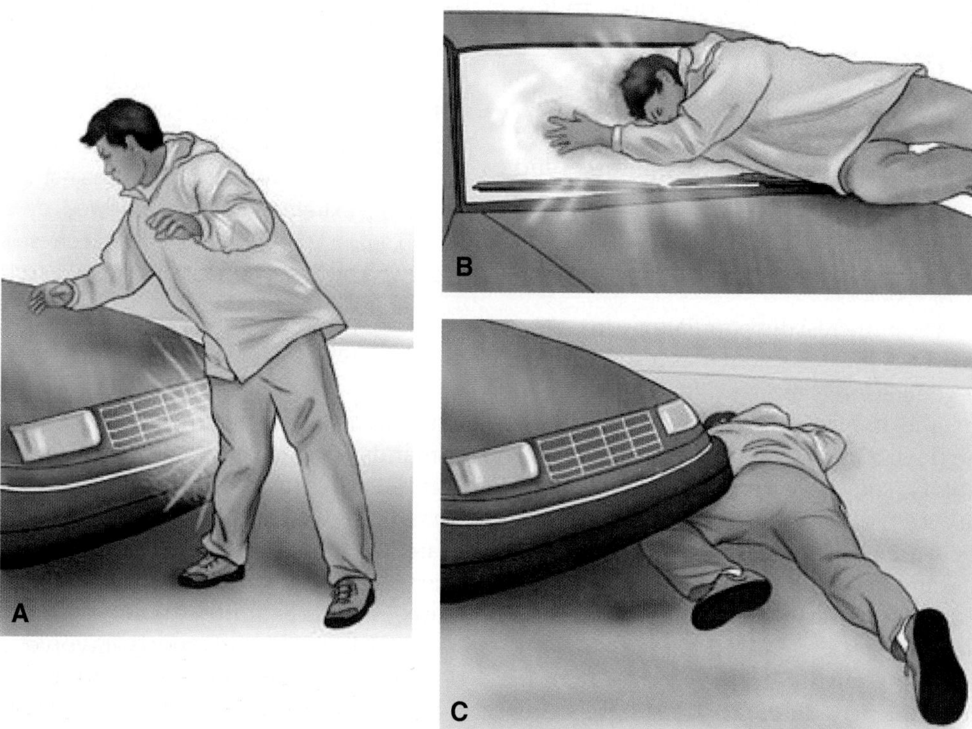

Figure 43-16 Adult struck by a vehicle. **A,** First impact. **B,** Second impact. **C,** Third impact.

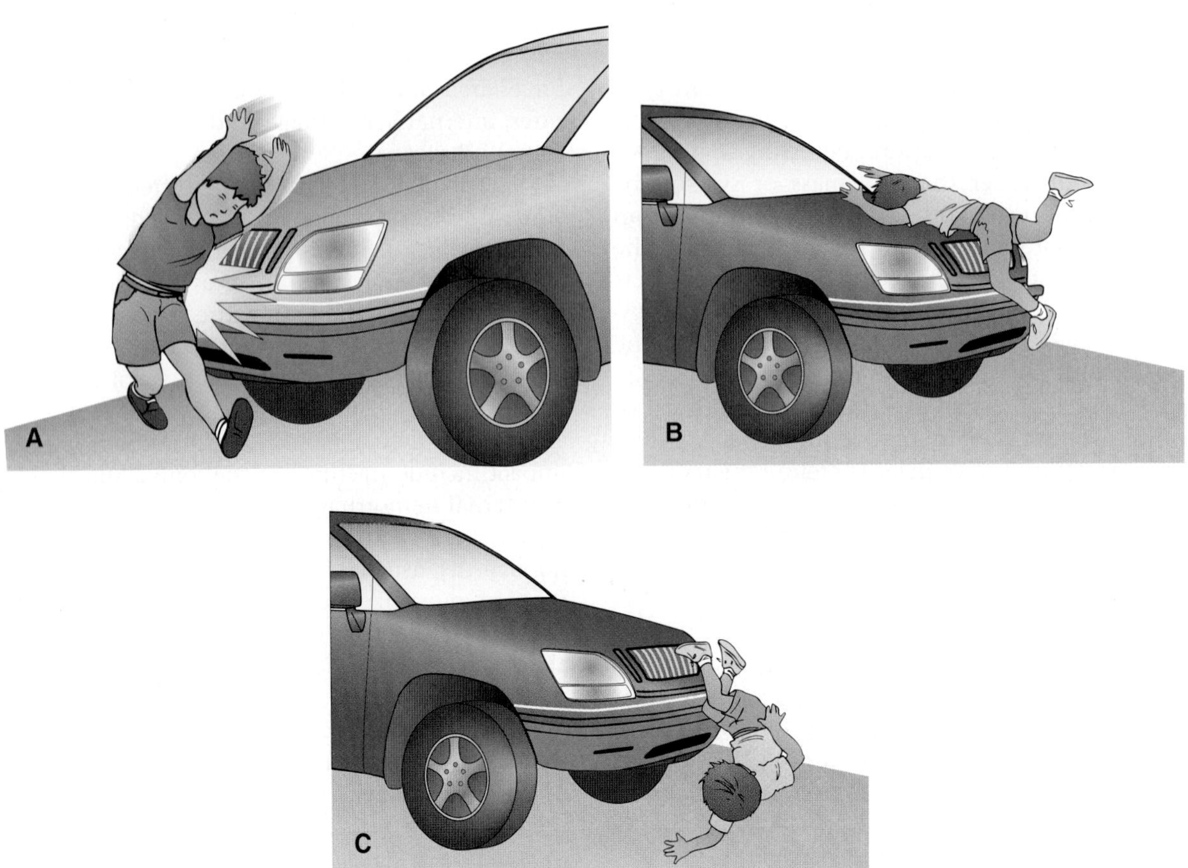

Figure 43-17 Child struck by a vehicle. **A,** First impact. **B,** Second impact. **C,** Third impact.

classic injury pattern associated with auto-pedestrian collisions is called *Waddell's triad,* which is described in Box 43-13.

BOX 43-13 Waddell's Triad

Waddell's Triad is a pattern of injuries commonly found in high-velocity crashes such as those involving motor vehicles, auto-pedestrians, or bicycles. Children typically turn to face a vehicle that is about to strike them. This results in an impact by the vehicle's bumper against the legs that results in lower extremity fracture, followed by an impact of the torso against the vehicle's hood that causes thoracic trauma, followed by the child's falling off the vehicle and striking his or her head on the roadway.

Other Causes of Blunt Trauma

Other causes of blunt trauma include sports injuries and falls.

Sports Injuries

[OBJECTIVE 11]

Sporting activities are an increasing popular pastime. The age of persons involved in sports activities also is rising; the baby-boomer generation is more fitness minded than other generations and is living longer. However, sports often are associated with injuries because of the contact nature of the activity, such as with football, basketball, and hockey. Injury from other sports often is attributable to the high-velocity nature of the sport, such as with downhill skiing, water skiing, bicycling, and rollerblading. Sports offer a range of health benefits but have the potential for serious injury.

Some sports are being taught at younger ages than in the past. As a consequence, different stresses are being placed on the younger athlete's body. These injuries have the potential to be lifelong afflictions and disabilities. One such sport for younger athletes is cheerleading, the demands of which to do more strenuous and more acrobatic stunts lead to higher injury rates. Over the past 17 years, cheerleading accounted for a disproportionate share of sports-related serious injury, accounting for more than 50% of catastrophic injuries to female sports participants (Shields & Smith, 2006).

Injuries related to sports involve acceleration and deceleration, compression, rotation, hyperflexion, and hyperextension. The general principle of kinematics can be used to predict injuries by determining the following:

- What energy forces were applied or transferred to the patient?
- To what body part, organ, or system was the energy applied or transferred?
- What associated injuries should you consider as a result of the energy transferred?
- How sudden was the acceleration or deceleration?
- Was compression, twisting, hyperflexion, or hyperextension involved in the injury?

If the patient used protective equipment, you must examine it for structural integrity, evidence of the amount of force transferred, and whether it operated properly. Examples include inspecting a helmet to see if it cracked during impact, inspecting the frame of a bicycle, and checking skis to see if they are bent or broken.

Vertical Fall Injuries

In 2003 falls accounted for 18,044 deaths and were the fourth leading cause of unintentional injury. In predicting injuries from falls, be sure to consider four aspects of the fall: the height of the fall, the surface of the impact, the objects struck during the fall, and the body part of first impact. More than half in all falls occur in homes; nearly four in five involve a person older than 65 years.

Because of these fours aspects, the number of injuries and deaths attributed to falls and complications of falls is disproportionate to the numbers of elderly in the U.S. population (Fisher et al., 2006; Aschkenasy & Rothenhaus, 2006). Because of this higher rate of significant injury, never dismiss low-velocity falls as insignificant in the elderly (Velmahos et al., 2001). In fact, these falls cause head and spinal injuries that affect the elderly person's quality of life. For these falls, consider transporting the elderly patient to a trauma center because many other injuries may be masked or late in appearing, based on initial trauma presented at the time of injury and a high index of suspicion for complications from the fall (Helling et al., 1999; Bergeron et al., 2006).

Except in the elderly, falls from some levels are rarely associated with fatal injuries, such as falls parallel to the ground. However, falls from distances greater than three times the height of an individual (15 to 20 feet) are more likely to be associated with severe injuries. As a reference, the roof of a one-story house is approximately 15 feet from the ground, and the roof of a two-story house is 30 feet.

Adults who fall more than 15 feet usually fall on their feet. The position of the body on landing is significant. In fact, people who land with straight and locked legs incur a higher degree of injury than those who land with their legs flexed. This concept is taught at all military parachuting schools in the world (Baiju & James, 2003). The flexed legs absorb the shock and the straight legs do not. It is better to land on both legs rather than one leg to absorb the impact because supporting the body is easier with two legs than one (Porter, 2006). If the person locks the legs, the predictable injury from this vertical fall is bilateral calcaneus fractures. As the energy dissipates from the initial impact, the head, torso, and pelvis push downward. The body is forced into flexion. When this occurs, the hip dislocates and compression fractures of the spinal column of the thoracic and lumbar regions occur. Approximately 10% of patients with calcaneus fractures have spinal fractures as well. This injury is referred to as *Don Juan syndrome* (after the literary character) and is described in Box 43-14. If the victim leans forward or tries to break the fall with outstretched hands, bilateral Colles' fractures to the wrist are likely (Figures 43-18 and 43-19). Other injuries associated with this type of fall include fractures of the feet, ankles, femur, acetabulum, and pelvis; compression of the spine (breaking of the "S" and **axial loading**); and shear injuries to the liver, spleen, kidneys, and aorta—the classic deceleration and compression injuries.

BOX 43-14 Don Juan Syndrome

The Don Juan syndrome is a pattern of injuries that occurs commonly in patients who land on their feet after a fall. They suffer bilateral fractures of the calcanei (heel bones) from the initial impact, fractures of the lower legs, knees, femurs, and hips. Compression fractures of the thoracic and lumbar spine can occur as the head and torso continue moving downward.

If the distance fallen is less than 15 feet, most adults land in the position in which they fell. For example, an adult who falls head first will strike the landing surface with the head, arms, or both. Predictable injuries depend on which area strikes first and the route of energy transferred. If the head strikes the surface first, compression injuries such as skull fracture, basilar skull fracture, brain contusion, and laceration occur as well as spinal injuries in the cervical and axial planes. Consider internal injuries, such as aortic shear, kidney fracture or separation from attachment to supporting structures, and spinal injury if the torso is the initial impact area. The severity of the injury also is influenced by the ability of the landing surface to absorb energy. For example, less damage is expected from a fall on a soft, grassy surface than a fall on asphalt or concrete.

Children tend to fall head first, regardless of the distance of the fall, because a child's head is disproportionately larger and heavier. For this reason, suspect significant head injury, such as skull fracture, brain contusion, or intracerebral hemorrhage, in any child who sustains a vertical fall.

BLAST INJURIES

[OBJECTIVES 12, 13]

A blast injury involves damage to a victim exposed to a pressure field or wave. This pressure field or wave is produced by an explosion of volatile substances. Explosive

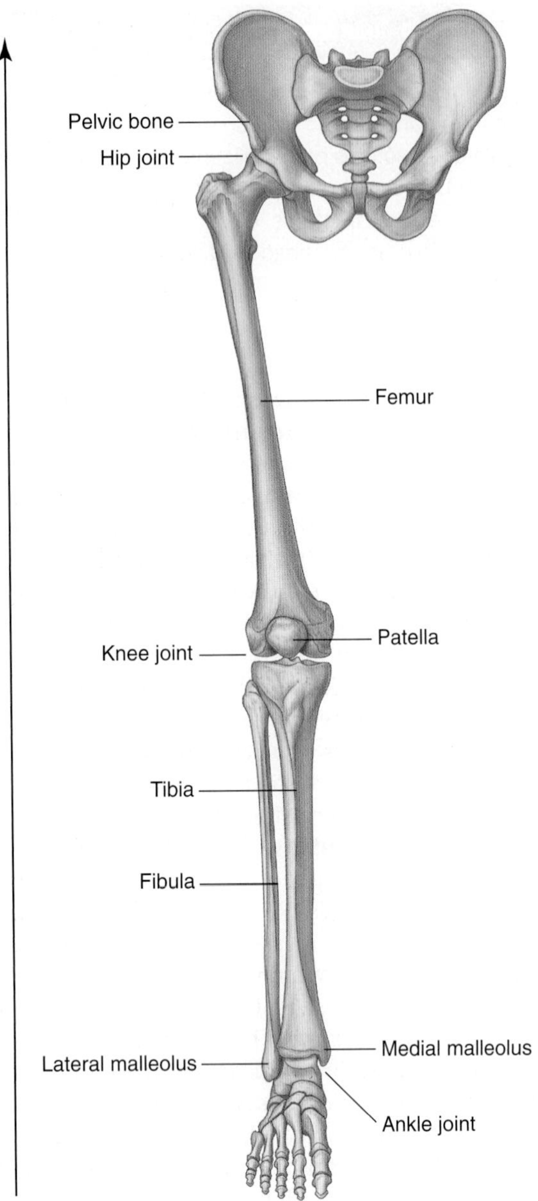

Figure 43-18 Bones and joints of the lower limb.

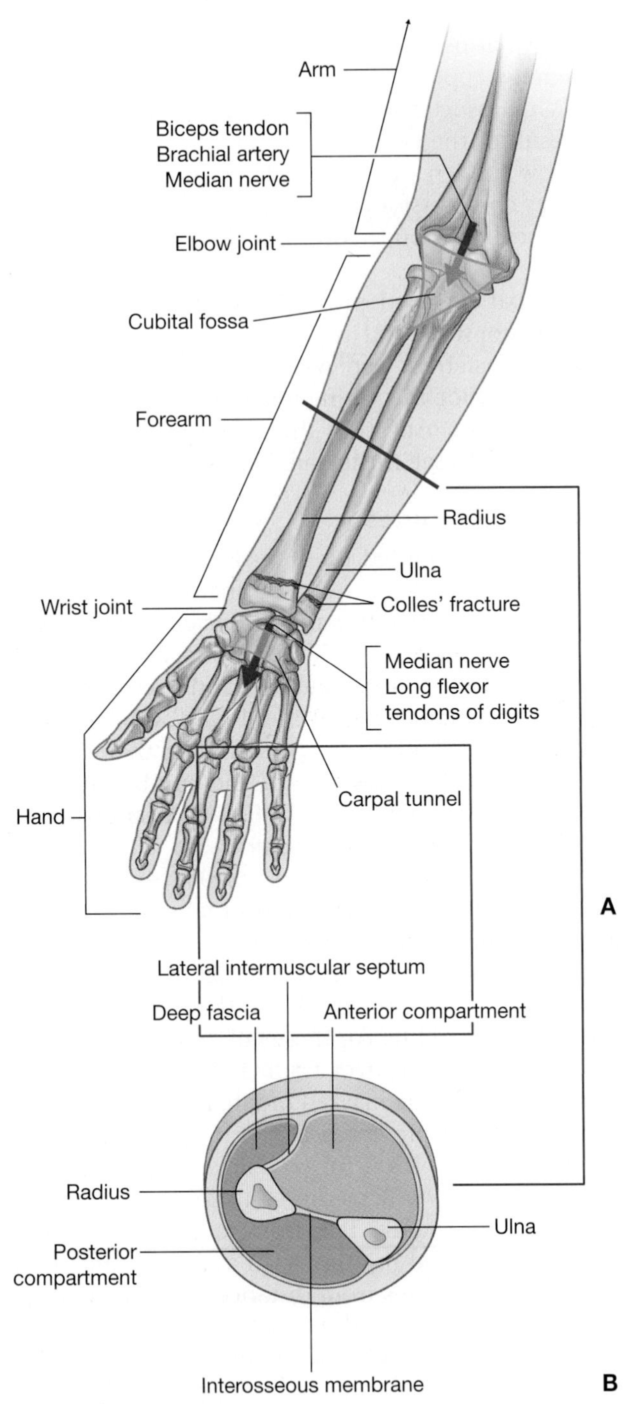

Figure 43-19 Forearm. **A,** Proximal and distal relations of the forearm. **B,** Transverse section though the middle of the forearm.

materials are classified as either low-order explosives (LE) or high-order explosives (HE) (Box 43-15). High-order explosive material is usually reserved for military use. Explosions can occur from a variety of causes, including terrorist attacks, industrial accidents, and motor vehicle crashes. More commonly, explosions are the result of legal industrial activity, such as building demolitions, rock quarrying, and mining. Accidental explosions have occurred at grain elevators, natural gas storage or shipping facilities, natural gas pipelines, and fireworks storage facilities. The intentional detonation of explosives not involving military activities often involves terrorism, either foreign or domestic. These devices typically are designed and deployed to maximize the number of victims involved.

Blast injuries release a large amount of energy almost simultaneously in the forms of pressure and heat. If this energy is confined in a casing (e.g., a bomb), the pressure ruptures the casing and ejects fragments of it and any added material, such as nails or pellets, at a high velocity. The remaining energy is transmitted to the surrounding environment. Depending on the environment, the effects of the blast are magnified and cause secondary problems. This energy can severely injure nearby persons. All conventional explosion–related injuries can be divided into four categories: primary, secondary, tertiary, and quaternary injuries. Each category is defined by the forces

BOX 43-15 High-Order versus Low-Order Explosives

High-order explosives produce a characteristic supersonic overpressurization shock wave. Examples include trinitrotoluene, C-4, Semtex, nitroglycerin, dynamite, and ammonium nitrate fuel oil.

Low-order explosives create a subsonic explosion that does not produce overpressurization. Examples include pipe bombs, gunpowder, and most pure petroleum–based bombs such as Molotov cocktails or aircraft that have been improvised into guided missiles.

High-order and low-order explosives cause different injury patterns.

involved in an explosion. Moreover, each category carries characteristic injuries.

Primary Blast Injuries

Primary blast injuries occur from the pressure wave that rapidly spreads away from the explosion in all directions. The blast wave increases in intensity with the strength of the explosives detonated. It can be greatly intensified when the blast and patient are within a confined space.

Primary blast injuries are only associated with high-energy explosives and result from sudden changes in environmental pressure or overpressure (pressure wave; Figure 43-20). This pressure wave may travel at up to 9000 meters per second and consists of both positive and negative pressure waves. The injuries from blast overpressure depend on the amount of pressure and the length of time of the blast. For instance, if the pressure or duration increases, a corresponding increase in injury will occur (DOD, 2004). The most severe damage occurs when poorly supported tissue is displaced beyond its elastic limit. These injuries usually occur in gas-containing organs such as the lungs **(blast lung syndrome),** gastrointestinal tract, and ears as well as to the central nervous system (Sasser et al., 2006). Predictable injuries to these areas include hearing loss, pulmonary hemorrhage, cerebral air embolism, abdominal hemorrhage, and bowel perforation. Depending on the victim's distance from the blast and the power of the charge, thermal burns also can be sustained.

Secondary Blast Injuries

Secondary blast injuries usually result when victims are struck by flying debris (blast wave). These secondary injuries are the most common category of blast injuries (Arnold et al., 2003). More people sustain these secondary injuries when the blast occurs in an open environment, most likely because the blast is not contained. In military explosives or those used by terrorists, secondary injuries are intentionally maximized by the addition of material to create shrapnel. An example of this is the addition of nails and washers to suitcase bombs and pipe bombs in an effort to increase the potential for injury to persons near the device (Figure 43-21). Obvious injuries are lacerations, fractures, and penetrating injuries from high-velocity flying debris such as nails, pellets, the casing of the device or, in the case of a car bomb, engine or car parts.

Tertiary Blast Injuries

Tertiary blast injuries occur when the victim is propelled through space by the explosion and then strikes a stationary object. These injuries are similar to vertical fall or vehicle ejection injuries. In many cases the deceleration injury from the impact causes more injuries than the acceleration through space because the deceleration is more sudden. Injuries from these forces include abdomi-

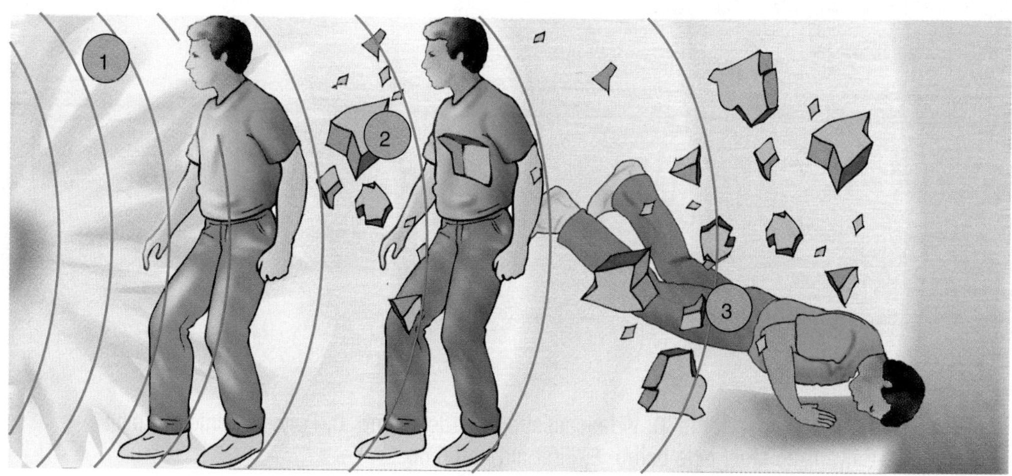

Figure 43-20 Three initial phases of injury that occur during a blast. In the first phase *(1)*, the pressure wave reaches the patient. This is followed by the second phase *(2)*, in which flying debris can become missiles that produce injury. In the third phase *(3)*, the patient becomes a missile and can be thrown into other objects or the ground.

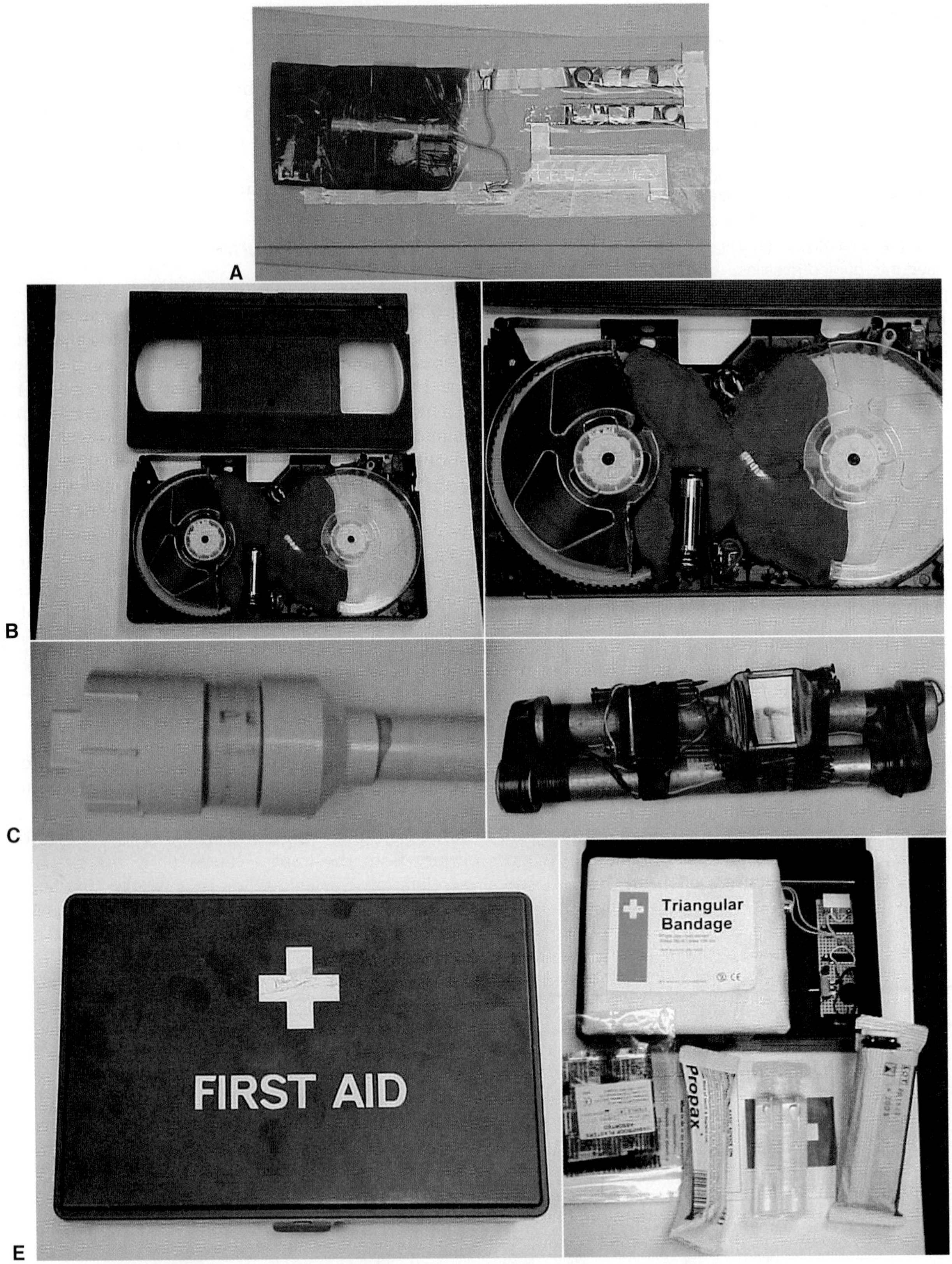

Figure 43-21 **A,** Letter bomb. **B,** Videocassette recorder bomb. **C,** Polyvinyl chloride pipe bomb. **D,** Galvanized steel pipe bomb. **E,** First aid kit bomb.

nal wall injury (abdominal viscera) and central nervous system and musculoskeletal system injuries. Consider immobilization for all victims of explosion.

Quaternary (Miscellaneous) Blast Injuries

Quaternary blast injuries are caused by other environmental effects of the explosion. These can include the blast heat on victims, structural fires, or structural collapse. In the World Trade Center bombing of 1993, 93% of the injuries were inhalation injuries caused by the fires within the building. Other predictable injuries include injury to the eyes, lungs, and soft tissues (Box 43-16).

Quinary Blast Injuries

Quinary blast injuries are the newest categorization of blast injuries. These result from agents added to the explosive such as bacteria, radiation, and chemicals. These types of explosives are often referred to as "dirty bombs." Biologic concerns, such as the human remains that become projectiles in suicide bombings, also fall into this category.

Management of Blast Injuries

The first priority of managing the blast injury patient is to ensure scene safety and comply with order by the law enforcement on scene. This is particularly true in cases of terrorist attack, in which the use of secondary devices, timed to explode during arrival of first responders, is quite common.

After the scene has been made safe, care of the patient is generally driven by the types of injuries caused by the blast. Secondary injuries typically present as multiple punctures, penetrations, or lacerations. Thus care is directed toward control of hemorrhage. Tertiary injuries are similar to those that occur with falls. Therefore the patient should be immobilized and assessed for potential internal injuries and closed soft tissue trauma. Primary effects of the blast present the most difficulty in prehospital assessment and management. These injuries are almost completely internal and therefore are difficult for the paramedic to assess or manage. Rapid transport of blast victims almost always is indicated.

BOX 43-16 Predicted Blast-Related Injuries from Conventional Explosions

Primary

- Confusion
- Dizziness
- Headache
- Increased startle response
- Tinnitus
- Tremors
- Unconsciousness

In Severe Cases (Primary Blast Injuries)

- Abdominal hemorrhage
- Blast lung injury
- Bleeding from ears
- Bowel perforation
- Chest wall injury
  - Rib fracture
  - Sternal fracture
- Hearing loss
- Increased intracranial pressure
- Nose bleeds
- Tympanic membrane rupture

Secondary

- Abrasions
- Extremity fractures
- Eye injuries
- Lacerations
- Penetrating chest and abdominal injuries
  - Hemothorax
  - Perforated bowel
  - Perforated liver
  - Pneumothorax
  - Splenic fractures
- Other penetrating injuries

Tertiary

- Compression fractures of spine
- Flail chest injury
- Hyperextension injuries
- Hyperflexion injuries
- Rib fractures

Quaternary

- Smoke or toxic fume inhalation
- Crush injuries
- Burns from structural fires
- Traumatic amputations may result from any type of blast injury. They are difficult to categorize.

Data from Arnold, J. L., Tsai, M. C., Halpern, P., Smithline, H., Stok, E., & Ersoy, G. (2003). Mass-casualty, terrorist bombings: Epidemiological outcomes, resource utilization, and time course or emergency needs (part I). *Prehospital and Disaster Medicine, 18*(3), 220-234.

Terrorist Bombings

Not every location or every paramedic will experience a terrorist bombing event. However, the likelihood of a bombing occurring has increased over the past few years. Between 1996 and 2002, 44 mass casualty bombing or terrorist incidents occurred worldwide, producing a minimum of 30 casualties, as reported in medical literature. These events involved a variety of explosive material and various quantities (from 2.3 to 5500 kg of explosives) to produce injury and death. Of note, data show that the majority of deaths were immediate. Moreover, relatively few deaths occurred later after the blast (Arnold et al., 2003). This information has implications for understanding the mechanism of such incidents. In fact, it differs from the classic pattern of death reported in general trauma populations.

Case Scenario CONCLUSION

The fire department completes the extrication and transfers the patient to a back board by using manual stabilization. The patient's anxiety and disorientation increase. He is breathing rapidly and deeply and has become even more pale and diaphoretic. Examination reveals a tender abdomen and no abnormalities in the lower extremities. Breath sounds are normal. Vital signs after extrication are pulse, 120 beats/min; blood pressure, 70/56 mm Hg; and respirations, 36 breaths/min. Transport to the nearby level III trauma center takes less than 5 minutes. The patient's condition is unchanged on arrival.

Looking Back

9. *What is the clinical significance of the increasing disorientation? Given the change in vital signs, what is the greatest life threat to this patient?*
10. *What are the advantages to choosing to transport to the level III center? What are the disadvantages?*
11. *What actions could you take during the extrication process to prepare the level III trauma center for the patient and improve the potential for a good outcome?*

PENETRATING TRAUMA

All penetrating objects, regardless of their velocity, cause tissue disruption (penetrating trauma). The tissue damage is a direct result of two types of forces: stretching and crushing. The character of the penetrating object, its speed of penetration, and the type of body tissue it passes through or into (such as lung or muscle) determine which force—crushing or stretching—will predominate.

Cavitation

As previously defined, cavitation is an opening produced by a force that pushes body tissue laterally away from the tract of a projectile. The amount of cavitation produced by a projectile is directly related to the density of the tissue the projectile strikes. Cavitation also is directly related to the ability of the body tissue or organ to return to its original shape and position. As an example, consider a person who receives a high-velocity impact to the abdomen. This person experiences abdominal cavitation at the moment of impact. However, because of the lower density of the abdominal musculature, the cavitation is temporary (cavitation lasts only microseconds). This cavitation is temporary even in the presence of severe intraabdominal injury.

Permanent cavities are produced by penetrating injuries in which the force of the projectile exceeds the tensile strength of the tissue. Tissues with high water density (e.g., liver, spleen, muscle) or solid density (e.g., bone) are more prone to permanent cavitation. Certain injuries, such as stab wounds to the abdomen, can produce cavitations as tissues are displaced in frontal and lateral directions.

Ballistics

The energy created and dissipated by the object into surrounding tissues determines the effect of a projectile on the body. Be sure to consider the principles of kinematics when dealing with penetrating injuries. To review, kinetic energy equals half the mass of an object multiplied by the square of its velocity. Regarding ballistic trauma, doubling the mass doubles the energy; doubling the velocity quadruples the energy. However, this does not always mean that the smaller bullet moving at a higher velocity will increase the amount of tissue damage. Velocity is only one factor in the bullet wound profile. For example, the M16A1 bullet produces the same amount of soft tissue disruption as a .22 long rifle bullet in the first 12 cm of penetration (DOD, 2004).

Damage and Energy Levels of Projectiles

[OBJECTIVE 12]

The injuries caused by penetration trauma result from three energy levels: low, medium, and high. An example of a low-energy projectile is a knife; bullets are medium- and high-energy projectiles.

Low-energy projectiles such as knives, needles, ice picks, tree branches, falling onto rebar at a construction site, and fence posts in an MVC cause tissue damage by their sharp, cutting edges. The amount of tissue crushed in these injuries is usually minimal because the amount of force applied in the wounding process is small. The more blunt the penetrating object, the more force that must be applied to cause penetration. The more force needed to cause penetration, the more tissue is crushed. The damage to tissue and path from low-energy projectiles are usually limited to the pathway of the projectile. However, that pathway can be expanded by movement of the blade or object inside the tissue (e.g., twisting the knife inside the wound).

When evaluating a patient with a stab wound, attempt to identify the weapon used to cause the wound. Do not assume that if the knife or other weapon is impaled in the victim that the position of the knife or weapon is straight down from the point of penetration. The knife or weapon may have been twisted or have moved within the wound, such as in a circular or sawing motion, to produce a worse effect than simple stabbing (Figure 43-22). Twisting of a blade is taught in many military knife fighting courses to produce a greater wound effect because the tissues tend to stick to the metal when it is twisted, shearing associated vasculature and expanding the laceration to solid organs. In addition, consider the possibility of multiple wounds and penetration of multiple body cavities. Maintain a high degree of suspicion of serious injury for stab injuries to the back and flanks. These injuries may be associated with penetrating injuries to hollow organs and injuries to the retroperitoneal organs (kidneys). Penetration injuries of the thorax can involve the abdomen, just as abdominal injuries can involve the thorax.

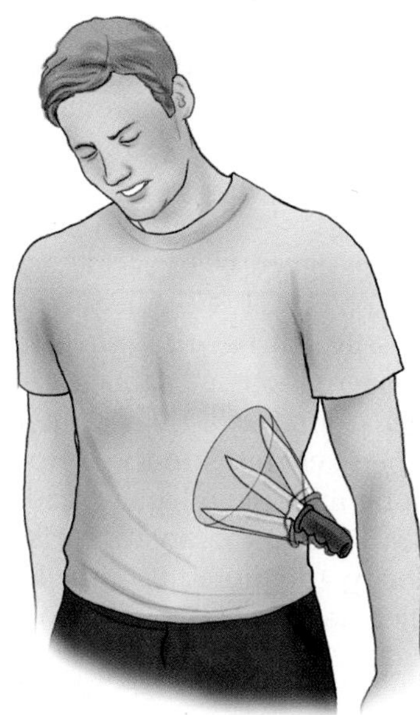

Figure 43-22 Do not assume that an impaled knife or weapon is straight down from the point of penetration. The knife or weapon may have been twisted or moved within the wound to produce a worse effect than simple stabbing.

Firearms can be classified as medium- and high-energy weapons. Medium-energy weapons include handguns and some rifles. High-energy weapons include some civilian hunting rifles and military-style and assault rifles such as the M-16A1/A2, AK-47, or AK-74. Both medium- and high-energy projectiles can produce an injury tract two to three times the diameter of the projectile (Figures 43-23 and 43-24).

Effect of Body Armor on Medium- and High-Energy Projectiles

Some EMS agencies have adopted soft body armor or, for tactical team members, heavier military-style body armor to protect their members from the effects of blunt and/or penetrating trauma. Many services follow the Department of Justice guidelines for the amount of protection warranted in their specific communities (see Chapter 65).

The actual wearing of different body armor types can have implications for determining injuries to the wearer. Experimental data have shown that despite stopping the projectile, the heart, lung, liver, spleen, and spinal cord are still vulnerable to injury. This is simply a result of the rapid, jolting force of the bullet's impact on the body armor and the energy from the projectile not fully dissipating. The energy from the projectile is not fully

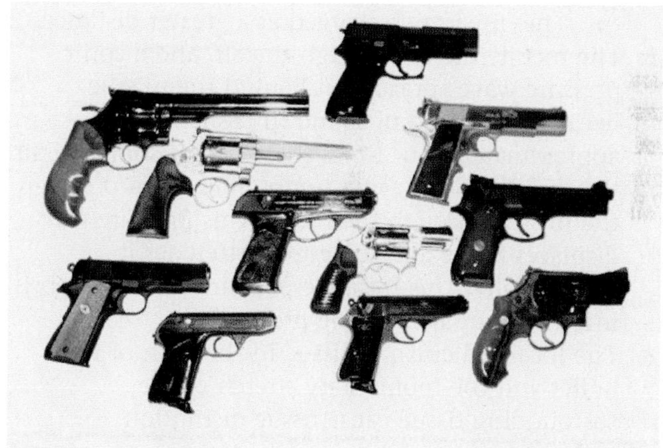

Figure 43-23 Medium-energy weapons are usually guns with short barrels that contain cartridges with less power.

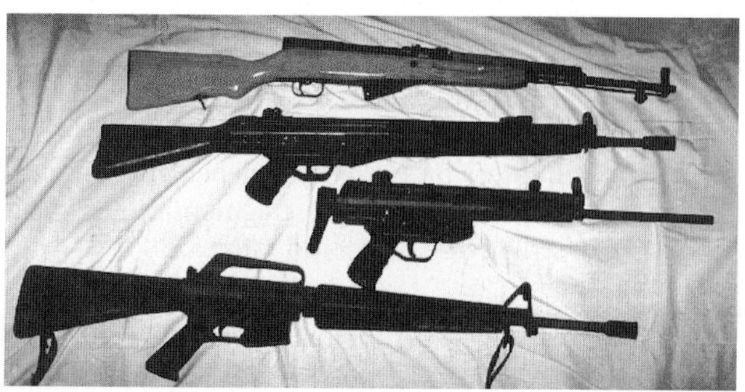

Figure 43-24 High-energy weapons.

transferred by the armor, and the residual energy is transferred into the body. This situation is quite similar to blunt trauma produced by heavier objects; however, it occurs in milliseconds (Roberts et al., 2005). Carefully assess the patient with high-energy projectile injury for subtle signs of internal injury.

Wounding Forces of Medium- and High-Energy Projectiles

A firearm cartridge consists of a metal bullet, gunpowder to propel the bullet, a primer to explode and ignite the gunpowder, and a cartridge case that surrounds these parts. When the trigger is pulled, the hammer inside the weapon strikes the firing pin, which ignites the primer. The gunpowder ignites and forces the bullet to exit the cartridge case. In most cases the bullet travels down a rifled barrel (grooves cut into the barrel to improve accuracy) and exits the weapon.

The mechanism of injury from firearms is related to the energy created and dissipated by the bullet into surrounding tissues. When a firearm is discharged (fired), the following events affect this dissipation of energy and ultimately the wounding forces of the projectile:

1. As the bullet (missile) travels through the air, it experiences wind resistance, or drag. The greater the drag, the greater the slowing effect on the missile. Therefore a firearm discharged at close range usually produces a more severe injury than the same firearm discharged at a greater distance.
2. The missile travels through the air, and a sonic pressure wave spreads out behind the missile. Because the speed of sound in tissue is approximately four times the speed of sound in air, the sonic pressure wave jumps ahead and precedes the missile through the tissue. This pressure wave displaces tissue and sometimes stretches it dramatically. This negative pressure can pull debris into the body behind the projectile.
3. The localized crush of tissue in the path of the bullet and the momentary stretch of the surrounding tissue cause tissue disruption.

When a projectile strikes a body, tissue stretches at the point of impact to allow entry of the penetrating object (temporary cavitation). The energy of the projectile exceeds the tensile strength of the tissue; thus tissue crush occurs, forcing surrounding tissues outward from the path of the projectile (permanent cavitation). The differences in wounds caused by projectiles vary with the amount and location of crushed and stretched tissue. The wounding forces of a projectile depend on the projectile mass, deformation, tumble, fragmentation, type of tissue struck, striking velocity, and range.

Projectile Mass

Tissue crush is limited by the physical size or profile of the projectile. If the bullet strikes point first, the crushed area is no larger than the diameter of the bullet. If the bullet is tilted as it strikes the body, the amount of crushed tissue is no larger than the length and longitudinal cross section of the bullet.

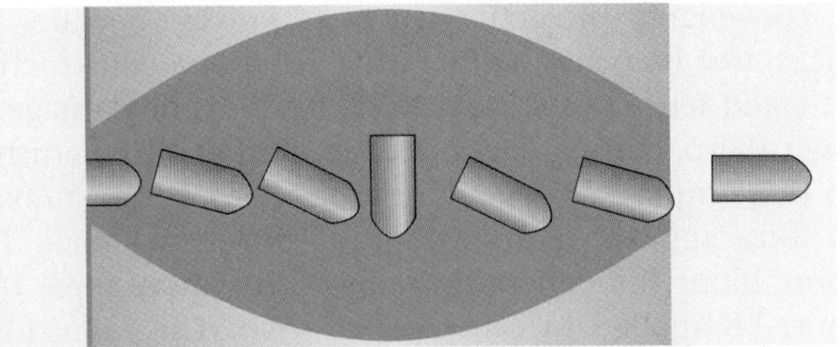

Figure 43-25 The tumble motion of a missile maximizes its damage at 90 degrees.

Deformation

Some firearm bullets deform when striking tissue (e.g., hollow point). The points of these bullets typically flatten on impact. The diameter of the bullet expands, creating a larger area of crushed tissue. The use of these bullets by the military is illegal by international convention. Although expanding bullets are not used by the military, they can be used in automatic weapons (i.e., terrorist or gang activities), allowing for a large amount of very damaging projectiles in a short amount of time.

Tumble

Tumble describes whether a bullet tumbles and assumes a different angle once it enters the body. A wedge-shaped bullet's center of gravity is located nearer the rear of the bullet than its point. When the point strikes an object, it slows rapidly. Momentum continues to carry the bullet forward, with the center of gravity moving to become the leading edge of the bullet. This causes an end-over-end motion, or tumble. As it tumbles, the bullet makes impact with more tissue than when the point was the leading edge. More energy exchange is produced, and greater tissue damage results (Figure 43-25).

Fragmentation

Some bullets are designed to or accidentally break apart when striking an object. This is called *fragmentation*. Each piece of the missile crushes its own path through the tissue, causing extensive tissue damage. These fragments produce a larger frontal area than a single, solid bullet and rapidly disperse energy into the surrounding tissues. Tissues weaken by multiple fragment tracts and the subsequent stretch of the temporary cavity is increased. The higher the velocity, the more likely the bullet is to fragment. If a bullet fragments, no exit wound may occur (Figure 43-26).

Type of Tissue Struck

The disruption of the tissue varies greatly with the tissue type. For example, elastic tissue, such as bowel, lung, and muscle, tolerates stretch better than nonelastic organs such as the liver or spleen.

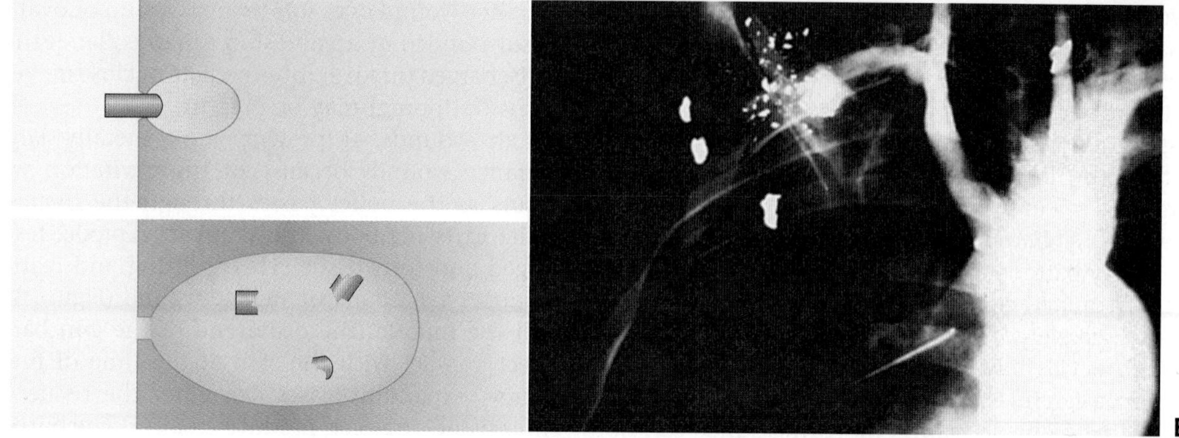

Figure 43-26 **A,** Missile made of soft lead or another component that breaks up will cause damage over a wider area and create maximal absorption of the energy because many more tissue particles sustain impact than with a hard missile. **B,** When the missile breaks up into smaller particles, fragmentation increases its frontal area and increases the energy distribution.

Striking Velocity

The velocity of the bullet is one major determinant of the extent of cavitation and tissue damage. The velocity, to a great degree, and the mass of the projectile determine the crush of tissue. The low-velocity projectile will have little disruptive effect, pushing tissue aside. High-velocity projectiles, however, tend to produce more serious injuries because of the higher energy transfer to tissues.

Range

The difference in distance between the weapon and the target is a key factor in the severity of ballistic trauma. Air resistance (drag) slows the missile significantly, and the force of gravity is exerted on the projectile as it travels toward the target. Therefore increasing the distance between weapon and target decreases the velocity at the time of impact.

If the firearm is discharged (fired) at close range (approximately 3 feet), cavitation can occur from the combustion of powder and the forceful expansion of gases as the bullet leaves the barrel of the gun. The gas and powder can enter the body cavity and cause internal explosion of tissue. This is common with shotgun wounds (versus rifle wounds) because of the configuration of the shotgun. Internal explosion is less common in handguns because of the difference in weaponry. A shotgun does not recoil and discharges all the gases of explosion out of the barrel, whereas many handguns, particularly automatic pistols, expend some energy back through the gas chamber to move the bolt backward and reload the weapon. The expansion of gas only, not powder, can cause extensive tissue damage, especially in an enclosed space such as the skull.

Shotgun Wounds

Shotguns are short-range, low-velocity weapons. They fire multiple lead pellets encased in a larger shell. Each pellet is considered a missile (9 to 400 pellets depending on the size) capable of producing tissue damage. The pattern of the shotgun pellets when fired, or the spread, is controlled by the "choke" of the shotgun. The closer the pattern, the more concentrated the tissue damage. Each shell contains pellets, gunpowder, and a plastic or paper wad that separates the pellets from the gunpowder. This wad, if fired into the skin, increases the potential for infection in shotgun wounds.

The amount of energy transferred to body tissue and the tissue damage that results depend on several factors, including the gauge of the gun (size of the barrel), size of the pellets, powder charge, and the distance from the target. For example, a 12-gauge, full-choke shotgun with number 6 shot (275 pellets) concentrates 95% of the pellets into a 7-inch circle at 10 yards. At close range, a shotgun injury can create extensive tissue damage similar to that of a high-velocity missile weapon.

There are a number of classification systems for shotgun wounds based on distance of the barrel from the patient (measured in meters), number of areas of the body injured, diameter of the wound, and other factors. One classification system divides shotgun wounds into four categories based on distance and penetration. Contact wounds occur when the barrel of the shotgun is in direct contact with the patient resulting in a concentrated entrance wound. In this injury the area around the wound is burned due to the heated gases escaping the barrel. This results in widespread tissue damage with an 85% to 90% morality. Close range wounds create a circular entrance wound that may have gunpowder residue and penetrate beyond the deep fascia. These wounds may also exhibit injury from internal components of the shotgun shell and have a mortality of 15% to 20%. Intermediate range wounds have a wider spread, resulting in a definitive entrance wound surrounded by smaller wounds from individual pellets. This creates both deep and superficial wounds without evidence of gunpowder residue, resulting in a mortality rate of 0% to 5%. Long-range wounds result in a widespread pattern of superficial wounds from individual pellets. These wounds have a mortality of 0%. An alternative representation of this system is to classify shotgun wounds as type I, II, and III wounds. Type III wounds occur when the barrel is less than 3 m from the patient, type II wounds occur when the barrel is 3 to 7 m from the patient, and type I wounds occur when the barrel is greater than 7 m from the patient. Injury patterns and mortality rates are the same as those for contact, close-range, and intermediate-range wounds, respectively.

Although a classification system can provide useful information, a careful examination will be of most benefit in making treatment decisions. Shotgun wounds can be deceiving. A circular wound could be the result of a contact wound with pellets, or an intermediate-range wound could be the result of a single projectile, or slug. The pellets from an intermediate-range wound could penetrate vital organs or vasculature, leading to significant injury. A high index of suspicion for obvious and hidden injuries is required for all shotgun wounds.

Entrance and Exit Wounds

The presence of entrance and exit wounds is affected by several factors, including range, barrel length, caliber, powder, and weapon (Figure 43-27). In general, an entrance wound over soft tissue is round or oval and may be surrounded by an abrasion rim or collar. If the firearm is discharged (fired) at intermediate or close range, powder burns (tattooing) may be present.

Exit wounds, if present, are generally larger than entrance wounds because of the cavitation wave that occurs as the bullet passes through the tissues. As the bullet exits the body, the skin can explode, resulting in ragged and torn tissue. This splitting and tearing often produces a starburst or stellate wound (Figure 43-28).

If the muzzle (the distal end of the gun barrel) is in direct contact with the skin at the time of firearm discharge, expanding gases can enter the tissue. If gasses enter tissue, they can produce crepitus. The burning gases also produce a thermal injury at the entrance site and along the injury tract (Figure 43-29).

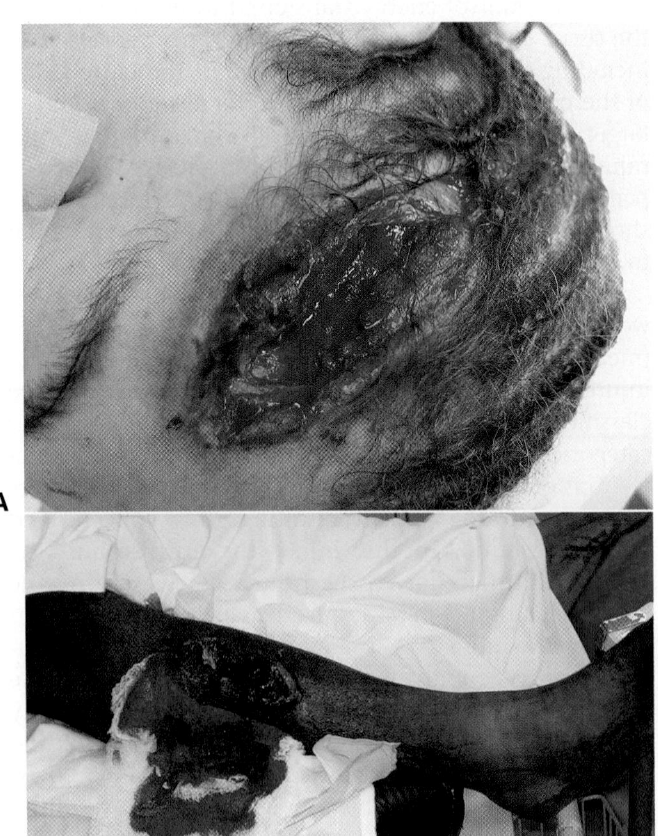

Figure 43-27 **A,** Graze wound from a high-velocity weapon. **B,** High-velocity gunshot wound to the leg demonstrating the large, permanent cavity.

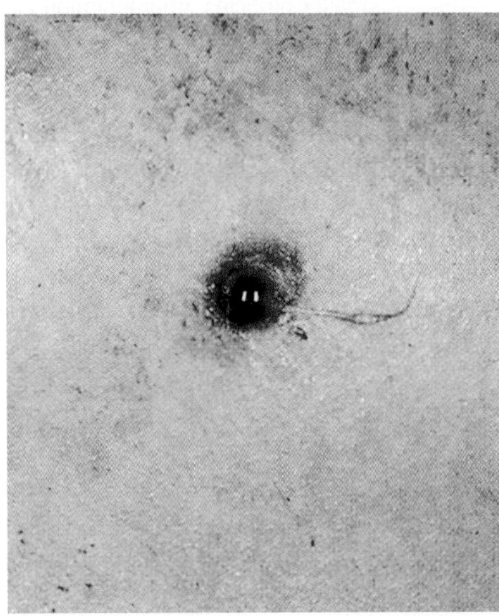

Figure 43-28 The abraded edge of the wound indicates that the bullet traveled from the top right to the bottom left.

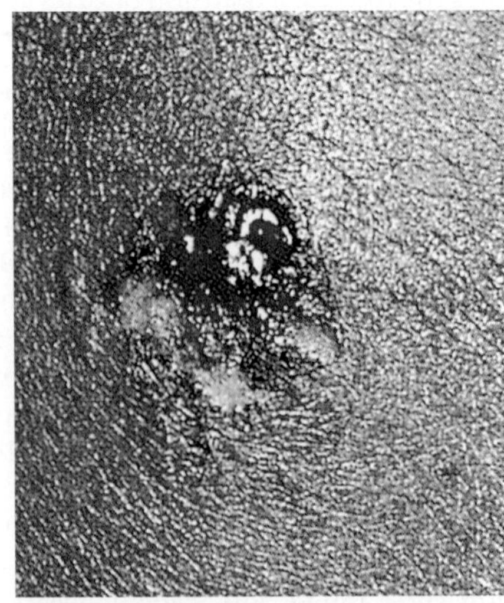

Figure 43-29 Hot gasses coming from the end of a muzzle held in proximity to the skin produce partial-thickness and full-thickness burns on the skin.

PARAMEDIC*Pearl*

Accurate determination of entrance and exit wounds may be difficult in the field. Many EMS physicians, administrators, and educators believe that documenting the total number of penetrating wounds is more important than taking the time to determine whether the wounds are entrance or exit in nature.

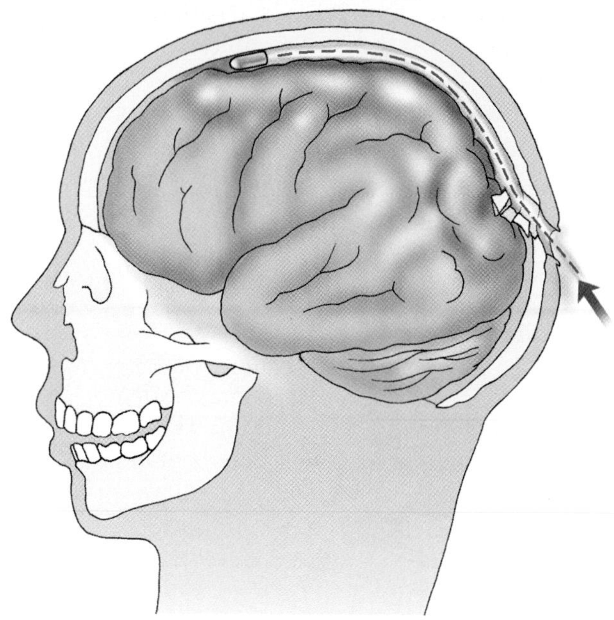

Figure 43-30 The bullet may follow the curvature of the skull.

Special Considerations for Specific Injuries

A thorough physical examination of the patient is required to locate ballistic injuries because the resulting trauma from medium- and high-velocity missiles is unpredictable.

The impact of a projectile is critical in determining the type and severity of injury. Fractions of an inch can make a significant difference in the amount of trauma the patient incurs. These differences often are impossible to distinguish in the field.

Head Injuries

Gunshot wounds to the head are typically devastating because of the direct destruction of brain tissue and subsequent swelling. Patients with head wounds often sustain severe face and neck injuries as well, resulting in major blood loss, difficulty in maintaining airway control, and spinal instability.

As a medium-energy projectile penetrates the skull, the energy is absorbed within the closed space of the cranium. The force of the injury compresses brain tissue against the cranial cavity, often producing plates or sections of bone (think of breaking a plate glass window), which are separated from the brain due to the velocity of the impact. Depending on the specifics of the missile, the bullet may not have enough force to exit the skull after penetration. This is what occurs with .22- and .25-caliber handguns. In these injuries the bullet follows the curvature of the interior of the skull. As it follows the curvature, it produces significant damage (Figure 43-30).

High-velocity wounds to the skull produce massive destruction. Pieces of the skull and brain are typically destroyed. At close range, high-velocity wounds result, in part, from the large quantities of gas produced by combustion of the propellant. If the weapon is held in contact with the head, the gas follows the bullet into the cranial cavity, producing an explosive effect.

Thoracic Injuries

Gunshot wounds to the thorax can result in severe injury to the pulmonary and vascular systems. If the lungs are penetrated by a missile, the pleura and pulmonary parenchyma (the tissue of an organ, as distinguished from supporting and connecting tissue) likely are disrupted, producing pneumothorax. On occasion, the pulmonary defect allows air that cannot be expelled to continue to flow into the thoracic cavity. This subsequent increase in pressure eventually can cause the lung to collapse and a shift in the mediastinum to the unaffected side (tension pneumothorax).

Vascular trauma from penetrating injuries can result in massive internal and external hemorrhage. For example, if the pulmonary artery or vein, venae cavae, or aorta is injured, the patient can bleed to death in minutes. Other vascular injuries from penetrating trauma to the thorax can result in hemothorax and, if the heart is involved, myocardial rupture or pericardial tamponade.

Penetrating injury can cause thoracic trauma in the absence of visible chest wounds. For example, a bullet can enter the abdomen and travel upward through the diaphragm and into the thorax. Evaluate all victims of abdominal gunshot wounds for thoracic injury. Likewise, evaluate all victims of thoracic gunshot wounds for abdominal injury.

Abdominal Injuries

Gunshot wounds to the abdomen usually require surgery to determine the extent of the injury. Penetrating trauma can affect multiple organ systems, causing damage to air-filled and solid organs, vascular injury, trauma to the vertebral column, and spinal cord injury. Assume a serious injury has occurred when managing victims of penetrating abdominal trauma. This should be the rule even if a patient appears to be stable.

Extremity Injuries

Gunshot wounds to the extremities sometimes can be life threatening or result in lifelong disability. Special considerations for these injuries include vascular injury with bleeding into soft tissues and damage to nerves, muscles, and bones. Evaluate any extremity that has sustained penetrating trauma for bone injury, motor and sensory

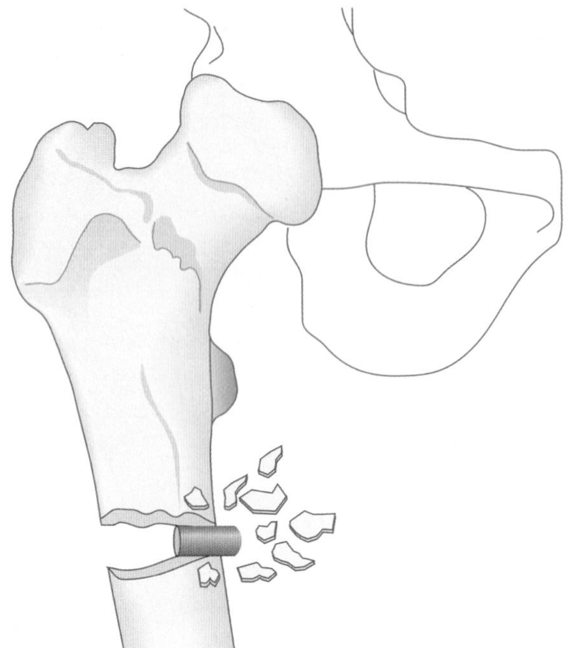

Figure 43-31 Bone fragments become secondary missiles themselves, producing damage by the same mechanism as the original penetrating object.

integrity, and the presence of adequate blood flow (e.g., pulses, capillary refill).

Vessels can be injured when they are struck by the bullet or by the temporary cavitation. Either mechanism can damage the lining of the blood vessel, producing hemorrhage or thrombosis. Penetrating trauma can damage muscle tissue by stretching it as the muscle expands away from the path of the missile. Stretching that exceeds the tensile strength of the muscle produces hemorrhage.

Bone struck by a penetrating object can be deformed and fragmented. If this occurs, the transfer of energy causes pieces of bone to act as secondary missiles, crushing their way through surrounding tissue (Figure 43-31).

Nonlethal or Less-than-Lethal Weapons

Most police departments in the United States and the world have nonlethal or less-than-lethal weapons to control crowds or individuals. These weapons can be broken down into handheld nonelectric devices, such as a baton or an asp (telescoping metal baton); handheld electric devices, such as a taser; rubber or plastic bullets; and shoulder-fire munitions such as beanbags.

The asp or baton is held and swung by one person and is intended to hit another person to subdue him or her. The injury patterns are similar for both weapons, except the asp cannot be used to thrust into a person because it will collapse. The injuries produced are similar to other blunt trauma to the head, neck, hands, arms, shoulders, and legs.

The handheld electronic device, or taser, is used in more than 9800 police departments in the United States alone. This device is designed to disable a person rather than apply lethal force to restrain or stop him or her. The electrical energy is measured in milliamps. The applied energy is believed to go no further than the skin and muscles and therefore has no cardiac side effects. Several deaths have been blamed on handheld electronic devices. However, the deaths have been proven to be primarily related to the substance or factor that made the person agitated and violent. Paramedics should suspect injury patterns related to the underlying or preexisting medical conditions before the delivery of the electricity.

The use of rubber or plastic bullets in crowd dispersal and riot control dates back to their use in Israel and Northern Ireland. In both instances rubber or plastic bullets offered a less-than-lethal option to the police forces with mixed results. The bullets did offer a relatively less-than-lethal option, but their use also resulted in several deaths. Because these bullets are projectiles, they may still penetrate the body. They are generally expected to produce possible lethal effects if the bullets hit at or above the abdomen, depending on variables in body mass, velocity, and angle of impact. Carefully assess the person hit by these projectiles for penetrating injury.

The final type of less-than-lethal weapon is the beanbag projectile. This weapon is a fabric bag filled with shot (metal pellets) fired from a shotgun-type weapon. The desired effect is to disarm or disable the targeted person. These projectiles also are relatively safe, but they can produce penetrating injuries to the thoracic cavity, eye, and abdomen. Also, the force of the bag may produce blunt trauma to the spleen, liver hematoma, cardiac contusions, and even pneumothorax. Be sure to assess fully the person struck with this type of weapon.

GENERAL PRINCIPLES OF TRAUMA MANAGEMENT

Dr. Donald Trunkey has described a trimodal distribution of death among trauma patients, classified as immediate deaths, early deaths, and late deaths. Through his work he determined that 50% of trauma patients die within minutes to 1 hour. Because of the severity of injuries sustained, these patients would likely die despite immediate medical care. Head, chest, and abdominal injuries account for the majority of injuries in this category. The only way to prevent deaths in this category is through injury prevention activities. Patients who fall into the early death group account for 30% of trauma deaths and die within the first 4 hours of the injury. Aggressive prehospital and hospital treatment of these patients, including rapid transport to an appropriate facility, is the key to survival in this group of patients. Late deaths account for 20% of trauma deaths and occur weeks after the initial injury due to related systemic conditions such as multiple organ dysfunction syndrome (MODS), respiratory failure, and infection. The exact causes of systemic failure in these patients remains unknown; however, there is a direct correlation to the development of hypoxia and shock early in the patient's course. In fact, unrecognized hypoxia and shock remains the leading cause of death in trauma patients. It is imperative that the paramedic anticipates these conditions and takes measures to prevent them or immediately treat them when present. Critical actions of the paramedic when treating a trauma patient include scene management, patient prioritization, patient assessment and treatment, and transport to an appropriate facility.

Scene Management

Upon arriving at the scene, a scene size-up must immediately be performed. During this time, assess for potential hazards such as fire, explosion risk, violent situations, exposure to traffic, or other dangers on scene. Take steps to eliminate or mitigate any dangerous conditions before approaching the scene, or wait until appropriate resources are available to ensure the safety of everyone involved in the response.

Once scene safety is established, a global evaluation of the situation is performed. This includes assessing the mechanism involved in the injury. In general, 90% of injuries can be predicted based on the evaluation of mechanism alone. Applying the knowledge and principles described in this chapter will allow the paramedic to quickly and efficiently assess and manage the trauma patient with a minimal scene time. Look for clues to that will provide valuable information regarding the status and criticality of the patient, such as:

- Abnormal body position
- Extensive hemorrhage
- The ability of the patient to make eye contact with you or acknowledge your presence
- Abnormal sounds associated with respirations
- Obvious respiratory compromise
- Spontaneous movement, or absence thereof

PARAMEDIC*Pearl*

If at all possible, do not approach the patient from a direction that would cause him or her to turn the head to look toward you. This could compromise potential injuries to the cervical spine.

Patient Prioritization

As the scene is evaluated, the number of patients must be determined. In the setting of multiple patients, the goal is to do the most good for the most number of patients possible with the available resources. The principles of triage are addressed later in this text; however, in brief, patients should be prioritized in the following order so that patients with life-threatening conditions receive immediate treatment.

- Patients with immediate life threats such as airway compromise or shock
- Patients with threats to the limbs
- Patients with injuries that could result in severe loss of function or disability
- Patients with injuries that will not result in the loss of life, limb, or function
- Patients in traumatic cardiac arrest

Priority is determined by a brief assessment. The paramedic must not get involved with additional assessments or treatments until all patients have been prioritized. Doing so could deny rapid care to the most critically injured patient.

Patient Assessment

Once patient priority, if needed, has been determined, the patient must be assessed. Chapter 17 provides the techniques of physical examination. This section will apply those principles and techniques to the trauma patient. Several terms regarding the phases of patient assessment have been used over the course of EMS education. The terms *primary* and *secondary survey* are used by healthcare professionals and will be used here. Although this nomenclature may be different than terms you may have learned in prior education, the concepts of trauma assessment are essentially the same regardless of terminology.

Primary Survey

The goal of the primary survey is to find and treat immediate life threats. This is accomplished by performing the evaluation in a systematic manner to first determine the greatest threats to life. Although there are exceptions to this order, such as addressing external hemorrhage in a conscious patient who is breathing adequately, the paramedic should follow the sequential steps of assessment the majority of the time. It is important to note that many of these evaluations can be done simultaneously. For example, the respiratory rate, pulse, and skin condition can all be evaluated at the same time. However, altering the order of the evaluation may cause components of the assessment to be overlooked or cause the paramedic to focus on distracting injuries while missing life-threatening ones. With consistent practice the assessment becomes automatic and can be consistently performed quickly regardless of the patient's condition.

Airway. The first consideration of the primary survey is opening and evaluation of the patient's airway with simultaneous stabilization of the cervical spine. Opening the airway is accomplished utilizing the trauma jaw thrust. It is not enough to simply determine if the airway is open, but the airway must be truly evaluated along with potential threats to the airway. Noises indicative of airway compromise, such as snoring, gurgling, or silence, receive immediate treatment. Look in the airway for foreign objects such as gravel, gum, teeth, or any other object that may become an obstruction. Manage the airway as needed with the simplest yet effective measures, saving more advanced and time-intensive interventions for transport. Failure to address and manage the airway by performing other assessments first will lead to hypoxia and hypoxemia.

Breathing. Often performed simultaneously with assessment of the airway, the patient's respiratory condition must be evaluated. The paramedic must avoid the temptation to simply determine whether the patient is breathing. This is wholly inadequate and may result in immediate life threats being overlooked. Instead, determine the effectiveness of the patient's respirations. Evaluate the relative rate, rhythm, and quality. Respirations may be too slow (<10 breaths/min), normal (12 to 20 breaths/min), too fast (20 to 30 breaths/min), or abnormally fast (>30 breaths/min). If the respiratory rate is normal or fast, supplemental oxygen should be immediately administered. If respirations are too slow or abnormally fast, assist ventilations with 100% oxygen and a bag-mask device. In addition to the relative rate, the rhythm and quality of the respirations must be evaluated. Respirations may be of normal rate yet abnormally shallow, leading to ineffective oxygenation. Quickly evaluate the anterior neck for jugular venous distension and the position of the trachea, which may indicate underlying respiratory pathology. Expose, inspect, and palpate the chest wall to determine the presence of injury that may compromise respiration. Be alert for subtle signs that indicate respiratory compromise, such as asymmetric movement, intercostal retractions, or an area of redness that indicates impact to the thoracic wall. Auscultate bilateral breath sounds, noting any discrepancy from side to side or between the upper and lower lobes. At this point in the assessment the auscultation of breath sounds is simply to determine the presence and quality of breath sounds; it should not be a comprehensive assessment. Be sure to consider the depth of respirations when comparing the ventilation status of the upper and lower lobes. Immediately address any causes of respiratory compromise, such as sucking chest wounds or a tension pneumothorax. Injuries that can compromise respiration can occur on the posterior surface of the body. If this is suspected, rolling the patient at this time may be necessary to determine if they are present.

Circulation. To segue into the assessment of circulation, evaluate the color, temperature, and condition of the skin while assessing elements of breathing. As with other elements of the primary survey, the circulatory assessment is composed of more than just evaluating the presence of a pulse. The paramedic should simultaneously evaluate the carotid and radial pulse. Determine the relative rate, rhythm, and quality of the pulse, and note any differences between the quality of the radial and carotid pulses. The pulse may be too slow, normal, too fast, or abnormally fast. Additionally it may be weak, thready, strong, or bounding and may have a regular or irregular pattern. Contrary to popular teachings, the presence of pulses in various locations of the body does not provide quantitative blood pressures; however, these findings do indicate the perfusion status of the body. For example, a radial pulse indicates the body has not shunted blood away from the extremities in compensation for shock, whereas the absence of the radial pulse indicates the opposite. Evaluation of capillary refill, which should be less than 2 seconds, can provide similar information; however, this is less effective, as capillary refill is affected by additional factors such as environmental conditions and preexisting medical conditions. Assess the patient for significant external hemorrhage. The paramedic should be sure to evaluate areas that cannot be seen, such as under the small of the back, the back of the neck, or within heavy clothing and jackets. If significant hemorrhage is located, it needs to be controlled immediately. If the hemorrhage is on the posterior surface, it may be necessary to roll the patient at this time for further evaluation and hemorrhage control. Assess the abdomen, pelvis, and femurs for signs of significant internal hemorrhage.

Disability. Assessment of disability, or assessment of neurologic function, provides valuable information regarding cerebral perfusion. Assessment of neurologic function is more than simply determining if an altered level of consciousness is present. The paramedic must evaluate the patient's response to stimulus. For example, does the patient open the eyes to stimulus? Does the patient respond appropriately or inappropriately to verbal stimulus? Is the response to painful stimuli a push, withdraw, or decorticate or decerebrate posturing? Although the Glasgow coma score may not actually be calculated at this time, the information needed to determine a baseline score is gathered during this step. This information may be critical to healthcare providers who will care for the patient at a later time. Recall that information not gathered is information lost. Assess the pupils to determine if they are equal, round, and reactive to light. Both direct and consensual responses should be evaluated. A gross assessment of pulse, motor, and sensation of all extremities is required during this step to provide information prior to moving the patient. Finally, assess the cervical spine for deformity, step-offs, or crepitus, and apply a cervical collar if indicated. At this point in the assessment (and if in accordance with your medical director and local protocols) the paramedic may determine that spinal immobilization is not indicated. In this case, manual spinal immobilization can be released.

PARAMEDIC*Pearl*

Resist the temptation to immediately place a C-collar on a trauma patient. This not only reduces your ability to evaluate the anterior and posterior neck later in the assessment, but more importantly shifts your focus from what must be evaluated first—the airway, breathing, and circulation.

Exposure. The final step of the primary survey is to expose the remainder of the patient to find any injuries hidden by the clothing. If the pneumatic antishock garment will be used, the entirety of the legs should be evaluated; if not, the assessment can be limited to the femurs at this time. Be cautious of the development of hypothermia and recover the patient as necessary; however, avoiding exposure of the patient can cause injuries to be missed. A prefect example of this is the paramedic crew that was met at the ambulance by a patient who stated he was stabbed. Because he was alert, walking, and talking the crew placed him in the jump-seat for transport. Upon arrival he was brought through triage in the main waiting room of the emergency department. At that time, an evaluation of the patient was performed by the triage nurse, who found nine stab wounds in the patient's flanks. The heavy jacket he was wearing concealed the wounds and contained the subsequent hemorrhage.

Secondary Survey

After finding and addressing all issues with the primary survey, the secondary survey is performed. It is possible that when faced with a multisystem trauma patient, the paramedic may spend his or her entire time with the patient addressing elements of the primary survey. However, the paramedic cannot ignore the secondary survey once the primary survey has been addressed. The timing and location of the secondary survey depends on the type of patient. If the patient is critical, the secondary survey takes place in the back of the ambulance en route to the hospital. If the patient has experienced isolated, noncritical trauma, the secondary survey can take place prior to transport.

The secondary survey, also called a *head-to-toe survey,* is a more detailed assessment of the patient. Its function is to discover injuries that may have been missed during the primary survey and to reevaluate the findings and treatments of the primary survey. Each area of the body is completely evaluated using the techniques described in Chapter 17. During this portion of the assessment quantitative vital signs are obtained as well as a medical history, including medications that may affect how the patient may respond to shock. After both surveys are complete, the paramedic must continually monitor and reassess the patient and any treatments that have been administered.

Packaging and Transport

If the primary survey reveals life-threatening injuries, all further considerations and treatments, such as the secondary survey, quantitative vital signs, and the initiation of IVs, are deferred until transport. The patient should be rapidly packaged on a long spine board, with the posterior surface of the body checked in the process. Assessment of the back is often not performed when extricating seated patients from a motor vehicle. This can result in missed life-threatening injuries and should not occur. After being packaged, the critical patient should be immediately loaded into the ambulance and transported emergently to the nearest appropriate facility. The noncritical patient can be packaged in a careful and methodical manner and transported nonemergently.

Time Management

Although the textual description of the primary survey may make the process seem long, in reality it is not. Although scene time is an important consideration in the setting of multisystem trauma, the assessment and critical interventions cannot be ignored in order to "reduce scene time." It only takes 1 to 2 minutes to perform the primary survey. If interventions are necessary, the time may increase to 3 to 4 minutes. Packaging may take an additional 2 to 3 minutes. This makes a scene time of 6 to 7 minutes or less very achievable. This is not only well within the platinum 10 minutes, but it also does not sacrifice patient care for time.

It has been shown over the last 40 years of prehospital care that simply loading the patient into the ambulance without immediate assessment of life threats leads to poor outcome. It has also been shown that extended scene times lead to poor outcome. Therefore rapid scene times must be tempered with the immediate treatment of life threats for the best possible patient outcome. To put this into perspective, consider the fact that the 6- to 7-minute scene time described previously is considered an acceptable scene time. In an attempt to reduce the scene time to 4 minutes, the paramedic decides to defer all assessment and treatment to the ambulance and only package the patient on scene. Although this may seem reasonable, recall that hypoxic brain injury can occur in as little as 4 to 6 minutes and, as mentioned earlier, hypoxia is one of the leading causes of death in trauma patients. Essentially, in an effort to reduce scene time the paramedic has decreased the patient's chance of survival.

On the other hand, if the patient is not a multisystem trauma patient, the platinum 10 minutes is not applicable and time can be taken to address the patient's injuries along with efforts to reduce discomfort. This may include the splinting of an isolated extremity fracture prior to moving the patient or the administration of analgesia to an elderly patient who has a dislocated hip prior to packaging. In the setting of a motor vehicle accident where the patient has no life-threatening injuries, yet cervical spinal injury is suspected, the goal of treatment is to provide the best possible protection to the spine. In this case, rapid extrication is not indicated and the use of a vest-style immobilization device should be considered.

Case Scenario SUMMARY

1. *What is your general impression of this patient?* High priority based on mechanism of injury and initial presentation. Airway and breathing appear adequate.
2. *You are 5 minutes from a level III trauma center and 45 minutes from the regional level I trauma center. Describe the factors to consider when deciding the appropriate destination for this patient.* Specific destination protocols vary by community. Although mechanism of injury is an important consideration in determining destination facilities, conduct an assessment to establish the extent of injuries before conclusively making this determination. The use of air medical transport and level I trauma centers should be based on clinical data as well as on-scene indicators. Given this mechanism and apparent injuries, this patient should be transported to a level I trauma center if possible. Unfortunately, transport 45 minutes by ground versus 5 minutes to the level III facility is not in the patient's best interests. However, if a helicopter can be summoned early and respond to the scene while the patient is still being extricated (or immediately after), the patient's arrival at the level I trauma center would only be an additional 10 to 15 minutes. The paramedic must rapidly consider these options and **call for the helicopter early** if appropriate. If no helicopter transport is available, this patient should be transported to the Level III center.
3. *What additional assessment will be important in the evaluation of this patient? Can you complete any before extrication? Why or why not?* Effective time management is critical when treating high-priority trauma patients. Examination of the head, neck, chest, and arms can all be completed before extrication, along with vital signs.
4. *What intervention should you initiate at this time?* Manual spinal stabilization, high-flow oxygen, and IV therapy can all be started before extrication if tolerated by the patient. In addition, equipment should be prepared so that the patient can be directly and rapidly immobilized and transferred to a back board and onto the stretcher for rapid transport to the trauma center.
5. *Is this patient high priority? Why or why not?* Yes. His mechanism of injury, increasing disorientation, abnormal vital signs, and obvious chest wall trauma all make this patient a high-priority case.
6. *Describe the apparent mechanism of injury in this case.* The damage to the steering wheel and visible thoracic injuries suggest that this patient experienced an up-and-over mechanism of injury.
7. *Given the mechanism of injury, examination findings, and vital signs, what potential injuries can you consider for this patient?* This patient appears to have primarily experienced thoracic injuries; these could include fractured ribs, aortic injury, flail chest, pulmonary contusion, pneumothorax, tension pneumothorax, pericardial tamponade, or myocardial contusion. His examination and vital signs suggests that his lungs are functioning fairly well, so aortic injury, pericardial tamponade, and myocardial contusion are most likely.
8. *Has this additional information changed your planned destination? Why or why not?* No. If transportation by helicopter to the level I trauma center is not possible, then he should be transported to the local level III center.
9. *What is the clinical significance of the increasing disorientation? Given the change in vital signs, what is the greatest life threat to this patient?* The increasing disorientation and abnormal vital signs signal decreased oxygenation of the brain. Shock is this patient's greatest life threat.
10. *What are the advantages to choosing to transport to the level III center? What are the disadvantages?* Time is the primary advantage. The patient will be in a facility with physicians and advanced diagnostic capability far faster than if ground transport were initiated to the level I center. Initial stabilization, including airway management, placement of chest tubes, vascular access, and blood administration can be rapidly performed. Disadvantages include limited access to trauma specialists, potential delays getting the patient into surgery, and the need (in most cases) to transfer the patient after stabilization to the level I center.
11. *What actions could you take during the extrication process to prepare the level III trauma center for the patient and improve the potential for a good outcome?* Keep them informed so that they can call in the necessary specialists (thoracic surgeon, blood bank personnel, radiology personnel) and notify a helicopter to respond to the hospital to transfer the patient (after stabilization) to the level I center.

Chapter Summary

- Maintain a high index of suspicion for multisystem trauma for pedestrians involved in MVCs. Differences exist between adult and pediatric victims and the body systems involved, even though the essential mechanism is similar.
- Penetrating trauma can affect multiple organ systems, causing damage to air-filled and solid organs, vascular injury, trauma to the vertebral column, and spinal cord injury. Assume a serious injury when managing victims of penetrating trauma.
- Trauma centers are specialty hospitals that have the necessary staff and expertise to deal with serious trauma. They are characterized as level I, II, III, or IV, with level I being the most comprehensive facility.
- Trauma is the leading cause of death in persons aged 1 to 45 years.
- The parts of a comprehensive trauma system include injury prevention, prehospital care, emergency department care, interfacility transport (if needed), definitive care, trauma critical care, rehabilitation, and data collection.
- The physical laws of motion have an effect on trauma:
  - The first law of motion (items in motion will stay in motion until acted on by an outside source) can be seen in unrestrained persons involved in an MVC.
  - Conservation of energy (energy cannot be destroyed but may change state) can be seen in trauma; energy such as electricity has thermal effects on tissue.
  - Kinetic energy (Mass/2 × V^2) relates to trauma; the mass of an object and the velocity are directly related to the amount of damage sustained on the body.
  - Force (Mass × Acceleration = Mass × Deceleration) is the amount of force applied to an object to set it in motion; an equal amount of energy is needed to stop the object. In penetrating injuries, for example, the same amount of force to propel a bullet must be met with the same amount of energy transfer within the body to stop the bullet.
- Base transport decisions regarding ground versus air on the patient's best interests of arriving at the appropriate facility as quickly as possible (approximately 60 minutes). Issues to consider include, but are not limited to, traffic conditions, time of day, weather, delay in transport, and whether the patient needs a higher critical level of care en route.
- Motorcycle collisions can include injury patterns such as those seen in car crashes as well as vertical falls.
- Vehicle collisions can result in multiple injury patterns (e.g., up and over, down and under) that produce highly predictable injuries to organs and organ systems.
- The use of restraint systems in motor vehicles has had a significant impact on decreasing injury and death in MVCs.

REFERENCES

Anderson, K. N. (Ed.). (2002). *Mosby's medical, nursing and allied health dictionary* (6th ed.). St. Louis: Mosby.

Arnold, J. L., Tsai, M. C., Halpern, P., Smithline, H., Stok, E., Ersoy, G. (2003). Mass-casualty, terrorist bombings: Epidemiological outcomes, resource utilization, and time course or emergency needs (part I). *Prehospital and Disaster Medicine, 18*(3), 220-234.

Aschkenasy, M. T., & Rothenhaus, T. C. (2006). Trauma and falls in the elderly. *Emergency Medical Clinics of North America, 24*(2), 413-432.

Baiju, D. S., & James, L. A. (2003). Parachuting: a sport of chance and expense. *Injury, 34*(3), 215-217.

Bergeron, E., Clement, J., Lavoie, A., Ratte, S., Bamvita, J. M., Aumont, F., et al. (2006). A simple fall in the elderly: Not so simple. *Journal of Trauma, 60*(2), 268-273.

Daly, L., Kallan, M., Arbogast, K., & Durbin, D. (2006). Risk of injury to child passengers in sports utility vehicles. *Pediatrics,* 1179-1114.

Davies, K. L. (2004). Buckled-up children: Understanding the mechanism, injuries, management and prevention of seat belt related injuries. *Journal of Trauma Nursing, 11*(1), 16-24.

The Disaster Center. (1998). *Deaths and death rates for the 10 leading causes of death.* Retrieved May 30, 2006, from http://www.disastercenter.com/cdc.

Fisher, A. A., Davis, M. W., Rubenach, S. E., Sivakumaran, S., Smith, P. N., & Budge, M. M. Outcomes for older patients with hip fractures: the impact of orthopedic and geriatric medicine cocare. *Journal of Orthopedic Trauma, 20*(3), 172-178.

Góngora, E., Acosta, J., Wang, D. S., Brandenburg, K., Jablonski, K., & Jordan, M. H. (2001). Analysis of motor vehicle ejection victims admitted to a level I trauma center. *Journal of Trauma, 51,* 5.

Helling, T. S., Watkins, M., Evans, L. L., Nelson, P. W., Shook, J. W., Van Way, C. W., et al. (1999). Low falls: An underappreciated mechanism of injury. *Journal of Trauma, 46*(3), 453-456.

Hoyert, D. L., Heron, M. P., Murphy, S. L., & Hsiang-Ching, K. (2006). *Deaths: Final data for 2003.*

Konkin, D. E., Garraway, N., Hameed, S. M., Brown, D. R., Granger, R., Wheeler, S. et al. (2006). Population-based analysis of severe injuries from non-motorized wheeled vehicles. *American Journal of Surgery, 191*(5), 615-618.

MacLennan, P. A., McGwin, G., Jr., Metzger, J., Moran, S. G., & Rue, L. W. III. (2004). Risk of injury for occupants of motor vehicle crashes from unbelted occupants. *Injury Prevention, 10,* 363-367.

Minino, A. M., Anderson, R. N., Fingerhut, L. A., Boudreault, M. A., & Warner, M. Deaths: Injuries 2002. *National Vital Statistics Report, 54*(10), 1-24.

National Conference of State Legislatures (2008). *State traffic safety legislation, passenger restraints, NHH 802 2008.* Retrieved July 11, 2008, from http://www.ncsl.org.

National Institute for Occupational Safety and Health (2004). *Volunteer fire fighter/fire service products salesman dies after being struck by dislodged rescue airbag—South Dakota.* Retrieved July 11, 2008, from http://www.cdc.gov.

National Safety Council. (2004). *Child passenger safety fact sheet.* Retrieved July 1, 2006, from http://www.nsc.org.

Peterson, T., Mello, M. J., Broderick, K. B., Lane, P. L., Prince, L. A., Jones, A., et al. (2003). *Trauma care systems 2003.* Retrieved June 25, 2006, from http://www.acep.org.

Prehospital Trauma Life Support Committee of the National Association of Emergency Medical Technicians, in Cooperation with the Committee on Trauma of the American College of Surgeons (2007). *PHTLS prehospital trauma life support* (6th ed.). St. Louis: Mosby.

Roberts, J. C., O'Connor, J. V., & Ward, E. E. (2005). Modeling the effect of non-penetrating ballistic impact as a means of detecting behind armor blunt trauma. *Journal of Trauma, 58*(6), 1241-1251.

Sasser, S. M., Sattin, R. W., Hunt, R. C., & Krohmer, J. (2006). Blast lung injury. *Prehospital Emergency Care, 10*(2), 165-172.

Schneider, H. (2003). *An analysis of motorcycle crashes 1996 to 2000*. Baton Rouge, Louisiana State University.

Shields, B. J., & Smith, G. A. (2006). Cheerleading-related injuries to children 5 to 18 years of age: United States 1990-2002. *Pediatrics, 117,* 122-129.

Society for Public Health Education. (2005). *Unintentional injury and violence prevention.* Retrieved June 26, 2006, from http://www.sophe.org.

Trifiletti, L. B., Shields, W., Bishai, D., McDonald, E., Reynaud, F., & Gielen, A. (2006). Tipping the scales: Obese children and child safety seats. *Pediatrics, 117*(4), 1197-1202.

United States Department of Defense. (2004). *Emergency war surgery* (3rd ed.). Washington, DC: U.S. Department of Defense.

United States Department of Transportation. (1998). *Paramedic: National standard curriculum.* Washington, DC: National Highway Traffic Safety Administration.

United States Department of Transportation. (2004a). *Evaluation note.* Washington, DC: National Highway Traffic Safety Administration.

United States Department of Transportation. (2004b). *Traffic safety facts.* Washington, DC: National Highway Traffic Safety Administration.

United States Department of Transportation. (2005a). *Buckle up America and Click It or Ticket—A winning combination.* Washington, DC: National Highway Traffic Safety Administration. Retrieved July 11, 2008, from http://www.nhtsa.dot.gov.

United States Department of Transportation. (2005b). *Research note: Child restraint use in 2004—overall results.* Washington, DC: National Highway Traffic Safety Administration.

Velmahos, G. C., Jindal, A., Chan, L. S., Murray, J. A., Vassiliu, P., Berne, T. V., et al. (2001). "Insignificant" mechanism of injury: Not to be taken lightly. *Journal of the American College of Surgeons, 192*(2), 147-152.

SUGGESTED RESOURCES

Armstrong, E. J. (2005). Distinctive pattered injuries caused by an expandable baton. *American Journal of Forensic Medical Pathology, 26*(2), 168-168.

Bradic, N., Cuculic, D., & Jancic, E. (2003). Terrorism in Croatia. *Prehospital Disaster Medicine, 18*(2), 88-91.

Brassel, K. J., & Nirula, R. (2005). What mechanism justifies abdominal evaluation in motor vehicle crashes? *Journal of Trauma, 59*(5), 1057-1061.

Cannon, L. (2001). Behind armour blunt trauma—An emerging problem. *Journal of the Royal Army Medical Corps, 147*(1), 87-96.

Carrol, A. W., & Soderstrom, C. A. (1978). A new nonpenetrating ballistic injury. *Annals of Surgery, 188*(6), 753-757.

Craig, S. C., & Lee, T. (2000). Attention to detail: Injuries at altitude among U.S. Army Military static line parachutists. *Military Medicine, 165*(4), 268-271.

Cunnigham, P., Rutledge, R., Baker, C. C., & Clancy, T. V. (1997). A comparison of the association of helicopter and ground ambulance transport with the outcome of injury in trauma patients transported from the scene. *Journal of Trauma, 43*(6), 940-946.

De Brito, D., Challoner, K. R., Sehgal, A., & Mallon, W. (2001). The injury pattern of a new law enforcement weapon: The police bean bag. *Annals of Emergency Medicine, 38*(4), 383-390.

Gittelmann, M. A., Pomerantz, W. J., Groner, J. I., Smith, G. A. (2006). Pediatric all-terrain-vehicle-related injuries in Ohio from 1995-2001: Using the injury severity score to determine whether helmets are a solution. *Pediatrics, 117*(6), 2190-2195.

Gondusky, J. S., & Reiter, M. P. (2005). Protecting military convoys in Iraq: An examination of battle injuries sustained by a mechanized battalion during Operation Iraqi Freedom II. *Military Medicine, 170*(6), 546-549.

Farmer, C. M. (2006). Effects of electronic stability control: An update. *Traffic Injury Prevention, 7*(4), 319-324.

Green, P. E, & Woodrooffe, J. (2006). The estimated reduction in the odds of loss-of-control type crashes for sport utility vehicles equipped with electronic stability control. *Journal of Safety Research, 37*(5), 493-499.

Grimal, Q., Naili, S., & Watzky, A. (2005). A high frequency lung injury mechanism in blunt thoracic impact. *Journal of Biomechanics, 38*(6), 1247-1254.

Henderson, J. M., Hunter, S. C., & Bery, W. J. (1993). The biomechanics of the knee during the parachute landing fall. *Military Medicine, 158*(12), 810-816.

Kerr, W. A., Kerns, T. J., Bissell, R. A. (1999). Differences in mortality rates among trauma patients transported by helicopter and ambulance in Maryland. *Prehospital Disaster Medicine, 14*(3), 159-164.

Knapik, J. J., Craig, S. C., Hauret, K. G., & Jones, B. H. (2003). Risk factors for injuries during military parachuting. *Aviation, Space, and Environmental Medicine, 74*(7), 768-774.

Kosashvili, Y., Hiss, J., Davidovic, N., Lin, G., Kalmovic, B., Malamed, E., et al. (2005). Influence of personal armor on distribution of entry wounds: Lessons learned from urban-setting warfare fatalities. *Journal of Trauma, 58*(6), 1236-1240.

Lerner, E. B., & Moscati, R. M. (2001). The golden hour: Scientific fact or medical "urban legend"? *Society for Academic Emergency Medicine, 8*(7), 758-760.

Liden, E., Berlin, R., Janzon, B., Schantz, B., & Seeman, T. (1998). Some observations relating to behind-body armor blunt trauma effects caused by ballistic injuries. *Journal of Trauma, 28*(1 suppl), S145-S148.

Lie, A., Tingvall, C., Krafft, M., & Kullgren, A. (2006). The effectiveness of electronic stability control (ESC) in reducing real life crashes and injuries. *Traffic Injury Prevention, 7*(1), 38-43.

Maguire, K., Hughes, D. M., Fitzpatrick, M. S., Dunn, F., Rocke, L. G., & Baird, C. J. (2007). Injuries caused by the attenuated energy projectile: The latest less lethal option. *Emergency Medicine Journal, 24*(2), 103-105.

National Highway Traffic Safety Administration. (2002). *Costs of injuries resulting from motorcycle crashes: A literature review.* Retrieved June 29, 2006, from http://www.nhtsa.dot.gov.

National Transportation Safety Board. (2005). *Child passenger safety.* Retrieved June 19, 2006, from http://www.ntsb.gov.

Patel, T. H., Wenner, K. A., Price, S. A., Weber, M. A., Leveridge, A., & McAtee, S. J. (2004). A U.S. Army forward surgical team's experience in Operation Iraqi Freedom. *Journal of Trauma, 57*(2), 201-207.

Peleg, K., Rivkind, A., Aharonson-Daniel, L., & Israeli Trauma Group. (2006). Does body armor protect from firearm injuries? *Journal of the American College of Surgeons, 202*(4), 643-648.

Sehgal, A., & Challoner, K. R. (1997). The flexible baton TM-12: A case report involving a new police weapon. *Journal of Emergency Medicine, 15*(6), 789-791.

Steele, J. A., McBride, S. J., Kelly, J., Dearden, C. H., & Rocke, L. G. (1999). Plastic bullet injuries in Northern Ireland: Experiences during a week of civil disturbance. *Journal of Trauma, 46*(4), 711-714.

Tortella, B. J., Sambol, J., Lavery, R. F., Cudihy, K., & Nadzam, G. (1996). A comparison of pediatric and adult trauma patients transported by helicopter and ground EMS: Managed-care consideration. *Air Medicine Journal, 15*(1), 24-28.

Wahl, P., Schreyer, N., & Yersin, B. (2006). Injury pattern of the Flash-Ball, a less-lethal weapon used for law enforcement: Report of two cases and review of the literature. *Journal of Emergency Medicine, 31*(3), 325-330.

Chapter Quiz

1. Which of the following is the leading cause of death for persons aged 1 to 45 years?
   a. Airway obstruction
   b. Poisoning
   c. Trauma
   d. Suicide

2. List the aspects of the trauma system in which the paramedic could play a significant role.
   ____
   ____
   ____

3. Which of the following trauma center level requires research as a component of care?
   a. Level I
   b. Level II
   c. Level III
   d. Level IV

4. Under which of the following situations would the request for air medical transport be appropriate for a critically injured patient?
   a. When the patient requests air medical transport
   b. When paramedics feel uncomfortable treating the patient
   c. When transport by ground would cause a significant delay in receiving care
   d. When transport times are short but additional fluids are needed

5. A vehicle traveling at 60 mph has _________ times the kinetic energy as the same vehicle traveling at 30 mph?
   a. one half
   b. two
   c. four
   d. six

6. Kinematics is the process of _________.
   a. identifying forces
   b. predicting injuries
   c. determining cause
   d. identifying mechanism

7. In which of the following types of impact would you expect to see a patient with bilateral femur fractures?
   a. Lateral
   b. Rotational
   c. Up and over
   d. Down and under

8. Which is the only state that did not have an adult seatbelt law as of January 2007?
   a. Texas
   b. Hawaii
   c. New Mexico
   d. New Hampshire

9. Which of the following types of motorcycle collisions tends to produce the least severe injuries?
   a. Lateral
   b. Head-on
   c. Rear impact
   d. "Laying the bike down"

10. True or False: The major difference between the adult and child pedestrian is the protection mechanism triggered when involved in a pedestrian versus vehicle collision.

Terminology

Axial compression (loading) The application of a force of energy along the axis of the spine, often resulting in compression fractures of the vertebrae.

Blast lung syndrome Injuries to the body from an explosion, characterized by anatomic and physiologic changes from the force generated by the blast wave hitting the body's surface and affecting primarily gas-containing structures (lungs, gastrointestinal tract, and ears).

Coup contrecoup An injury most often associated with a blow to the skull in which the force of the impact is transmitted through the skull bones to the opposite side of the head, where the bruise, fracture, or other sign of injury appears.

Index of suspicion The expectation that certain injuries or patterns of injuries have resulted to a body part, organ, or system based on the mechanism of injury and the force of impact to the patient.

CHAPTER 44

Bleeding

Objectives

After completing this chapter, you will be able to:

1. Describe the etiology, history, and physical findings of external bleeding.
2. Predict hemorrhage on the basis of a patient's mechanism of injury.
3. Distinguish between controlled and uncontrolled hemorrhage.
4. Using the patient history and physical examination findings, develop a treatment plan for a patient with external bleeding.
5. Distinguish between the various techniques for hemorrhage control of open soft tissue injuries, including direct pressure and tourniquet application.
6. Distinguish between the administration rate and amount of intravenous fluid for a patient with controlled hemorrhage and the rate and amount for a patient with uncontrolled hemorrhage.
7. Describe the etiology, history, and physical findings of internal bleeding.
8. Using the patient history and physical examination findings, develop a treatment plan for a patient with internal bleeding.

Chapter Outline

Case Scenario

You and your partner respond to a dormitory on the campus of the local college at the request of the campus police for a patient who is bleeding. Upon arrival the resident director leads you to the third floor, where you see two campus police officers speaking with a male in his early 20s who is bleeding profusely from his right arm with pale skin. Behind the young man is a broken plate glass window, and surrounding him is a large pool of blood. You detect an odor consistent with that of an alcoholic beverage about the patient as he tells you in slurred speech that he has been drinking and he and his girlfriend got into an argument. She left, and in anger he punched the window, putting his arm through it.

Questions

1. *What is your general impression of this patient?*
2. *What additional assessment will be important in the evaluation of this patient?*
3. *What intervention should you initiate at this time?*

As described in prior chapters, **perfusion** is the circulation of blood through an organ structure. Perfusion is critical to the function of the cells, tissues, organs, organ systems, and the body itself as it is through this mechanism that oxygen and nutrients are delivered to the cells and carbon dioxide and other waste products are eliminated. Hemorrhage results from compromised blood vessels causing a loss of blood from the vascular space and an inability for adequate perfusion to occur. In the setting of uncontrolled hemorrhage the patient can quickly enter hypovolemic shock as described in earlier chapters. Therefore in the setting of hemorrhage the goal of the paramedic is to stop the bleeding as quickly and efficiently as possible.

HEMORRHAGE

Bleeding is the escape of blood from a blood vessel. **Hemorrhage** is defined as massive, heavy bleeding. Bleeding or hemorrhage may be external or internal. It may occur suddenly (acutely) or may be associated with a persistent (chronic) condition. Bleeding may occur because of disease or injury involving an artery, vein, or capillary. Causes of major blood loss are listed in Box 44-1.

BOX 44-1 Causes of Major Blood Loss

- Solid organ injury
- Abdominal aortic aneurysm rupture
- Vascular injury
- Penetrating trauma
- Severe gastrointestinal bleeding
- Ruptured liver or spleen
- Hemothorax
- Ruptured ectopic pregnancy
- Arteriovenous malformation
- Bleeding esophageal varices
- Pelvic fracture
- Femur fracture
- Bleeding peptic ulcer
- Placenta previa
- Abruptio placenta
- Scalp lacerations (infants/young children)
- Intracranial hemorrhage (newborn or infant)

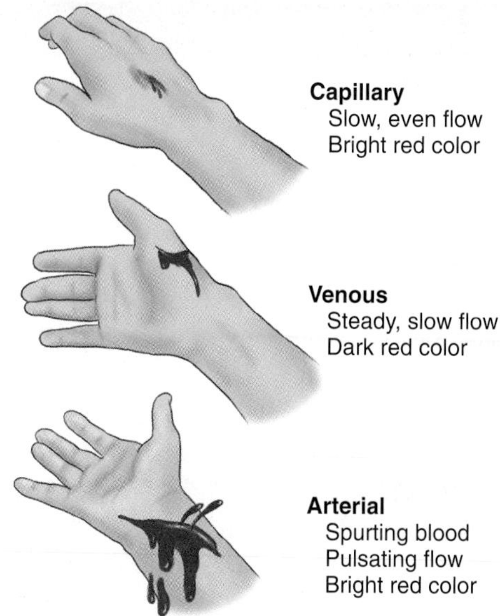

Figure 44-1 Arterial, venous, and capillary bleeding.

External Bleeding

Description and Definition

External bleeding is blood loss that can be seen (observable).

Etiology

[OBJECTIVES 1, 2]

External bleeding may result from many types of injuries, including cuts, scrapes, abrasions, avulsions, amputations stab wounds, gunshot wounds, and open fractures. External bleeding also may result from menstrual bleeding or medical conditions, such as a miscarriage, upper gastrointestinal (GI) bleeding, and lower GI bleeding. Potential causes of bleeding from the nose, ears, or mouth include the following:

- Skull fracture
- Facial trauma
- Digital trauma (nose picking)
- Sinusitis and other upper respiratory tract infections
- Hypertension (high blood pressure)
- Coagulation disorders

When the source of external bleeding involves an artery, blood escaping from the vessel will be bright red because it is rich in oxygen and comes directly from the heart. Because arteries are high-pressure vessels, every contraction of the heart will cause blood to pulse from the wound (Figure 44-1). When a large artery is cut or torn, a person can **exsanguinate** (bleed out) in a matter of minutes.

Venous bleeding is slower and less forceful than arterial bleeding. Blood escaping from a vein flows steadily. It is dark red because the blood in a vein is low in oxygen. A large amount of blood can be lost from a vein. Because of the small size of a capillary, blood will ooze from a damaged capillary. Capillary bleeding is easy to control with direct pressure and usually does not result in uncontrollable hemorrhage.

PARAMEDIC*Pearl*

You must take infection control precautions on every call. However, these precautions are particularly important when you are caring for a patient with signs of external bleeding.

History

Obtain a history from a patient as soon as possible to help identify the mechanism of injury or the nature of the patient's illness. If bleeding is evident or suspected, find out when it started and how long it has been present. The body's blood-clotting ability can be affected by diseases and medications. Ask whether the patient has a history of cancer, hemophilia, or liver disease, which affect the blood's ability to clot. Also ask whether the patient is taking aspirin or blood thinners (anticoagulants), such as warfarin (Coumadin) or enoxaparin (Lovenox), or herbal remedies that may interfere with blood clotting. Examples of drugs that affect blood clotting are shown in Box 44-2. Herbal products such as garlic, ginseng, and gingko also can affect blood clotting.

Physical Findings

The signs of external bleeding depend on the source of the bleeding, the size of the hole in the blood vessel, and the pressure within the vessel. You may see bleeding from a wound or from the ears, nose, mouth, rectum, or other body opening.

The average circulating blood volume is 70 mL/kg. The average circulating blood volumes by age are listed in Table 44-1. In a healthy adult, a loss of 10% to 15% of

BOX 44-2 Drugs That Affect Blood Clotting

- abciximab (ReoPro)
- aspirin
- clopidogrel (Plavix)
- dipyridamole (Persantine)
- enoxaparin (Lovenox)
- eptifibatide (Integrilin)
- ticlopidine (Ticlid)
- tirofiban (Aggrastat)
- warfarin (Coumadin)

TABLE 44-1 Average Circulating Blood Volume by Age

Age	Normal Blood Volume (Average)
Preterm infant	90-105 mL/kg
Term newborn	85 mL/kg
Infant >1 month to 11 months	75 mL/kg
Beyond 1 year	67-75 mL/kg
Adult	55-75 mL/kg

Reprinted from Barkin, R. M., & Rosen, P. (2003). *Emergency pediatrics: A guide to ambulatory care* (6th ed.). *St. Louis: Mosby*.

the blood volume is usually well tolerated. The blood volume in infants and children is proportionately larger than in adults; however, their total blood volume is less than in adults. As a result, a small volume loss can result in signs and symptoms of shock (Boxes 44-3 and 44-4). For example, an 8-kg infant has a proportionately larger blood volume (75 mL/kg), but the total blood vlume is less than that of a 75-kg adult (600 mL versus 5625 mL). The sudden loss of 1 L (1000 mL) of blood in an adult, 0.5 L (500 mL) of blood in a child, and 100 to 200 mL of the blood volume in an infant is considered serious. Assess the severity of blood loss based on the patient's signs and symptoms and your general impression of the amount of blood loss.

Depending on the amount of blood lost and the rate at which it was lost, external bleeding may be accompanied by the following signs and symptoms:

- Dizziness or lightheadedness on sitting or standing
- Pale skin
- Increased heart rate
- Normal to low blood pressure
- Narrow pulse pressure
- Normal mental status, altered mental status, or unresponsiveness

Differential Diagnosis

Differential diagnoses for external bleeding include the following:

- Penetrating trauma
- Hemorrhagic shock
- Hemorrhoids
- Gastric ulcers
- Esophageal varices
- Placenta previa
- Abruptio placentae

Therapeutic Interventions

[OBJECTIVES 3, 4, 5, 6]

When assessing a patient who is bleeding, keep in mind that other injuries or conditions may be present that also will need attention. Systematically search for other injuries or life-threatening conditions. Remove or cut away clothing as needed to find the source of the bleeding while respecting the patient's modesty.

Provide oxygen to maintain an oxygen saturation above 95%. Maintain the airway and provide ventilatory support if needed. If the patient has a simple nosebleed (epistaxis), place him or her in a sitting position leaning forward. Apply direct pressure by pinching the fleshy portion of the nostrils together. If the patient is bleeding from the nose or ears after significant head trauma, refrain from applying pressure to control the bleeding. Apply a loose sterile dressing to collect drainage and limit possible sources of infection.

PARAMEDIC*Pearl*

According to the 2005 American Heart Association resuscitation guidelines, "There is insufficient evidence to recommend for or against the first aid use of pressure points or extremity elevation to control hemorrhage. The efficacy, feasibility, and safety of pressure points to control bleeding have never been subjected to study, and there have been no published studies to determine if elevation of a bleeding extremity helps in bleeding control or causes harm. Using these unproven procedures has the potential to compromise the proven intervention of direct pressure." Check your local protocols about approved methods of bleeding control in your EMS system.

From the American Heart Association (2005). American Heart Association guidelines for cardiopulmonary resuscitation and emergency cardiovascular care, part 14: first aid. *Circulation, 112*(suppl IV), 198.

The most often used and most effective method of controlling external bleeding is applying direct pressure. This should be used as a first-line procedure (Figure 44-2, Skill 44-1). This process involves applying force to the wound to slow the flow of blood from the wound, allowing the body's clotting process to work. At first it can be achieved by using a gloved hand to exert firm pressure directly to the wound until appropriate dressing material can be obtained. Do not delay the application of the pressure to apply dressings. Apply pressure as soon as you detect the presence of hemorrhage. In some cases, par-

BOX 44-3 How Useful Are Orthostatic Vital Signs?

Orthostatic vital signs (also called the *tilt test* or *postural vital signs*) are serial measurements of the patient's pulse and blood pressure with the patient recumbent and then standing. Orthostatic vital signs were first described in 1980 (Knopp et al., 1980). To assess the ability of this technique in detecting acute blood loss, blood was withdrawn from 100 volunteers. In the first group, 450 mL was withdrawn. In the second group, 1000 mL was withdrawn in 500-mL increments. The vital signs were recorded at timed intervals, comparing the values taken when the patient was moved from a supine to a sitting position and a supine to a standing position. Using the criteria of a pulse increase of 30 beats/min or more or severe symptoms (syncope or near syncope), the supine to standing test accurately distinguished a 1000-mL blood loss from no blood loss. These researchers concluded that the major value of this test was in detecting blood loss of 1000 mL or more. They were unable to detect a blood loss of 500 mL consistently when using these criteria. They found that a supine to standing test is more accurate than a supine to sitting evaluation. The supine to sitting test was not reliable for detecting 1000 mL of blood loss.

Orthostatic vital signs have been used for many years to assess for possible volume depletion in patients reporting dizziness, lightheadedness, nausea, vomiting, diarrhea, or GI bleeding. Despite their use, little agreement exists regarding what constitutes a positive or negative test result. If your local protocols or medical direction requires assessment of orthostatic vital signs, the patient should rest quietly in a supine position for 2 to 3 minutes. Do not perform any painful or invasive procedures during the test. Record the patient's blood pressure and pulse. Take two sets of measurements while the patient is supine. Use the second set as the baseline from which to compare later measurements. If the patient is tachycardic while supine, orthostatic vital signs should not be performed. If the patient is not tachycardic, he or she is asked to stand. If the patient feels faint or has extreme dizziness that requires him or her to lie down (regarded as severe symptoms), consider the result positive, stop the test, and help him or her to a supine position. If the patient is not symptomatic, record his or her blood pressure and pulse after he or she has been standing for 1 minute. The "20-10-20" rule was suggested as a guide to determine a positive test result. The rule refers to the expected decrease in systolic blood pressure (up to 20 mm Hg), a rise in diastolic blood pressure of 10 mm Hg, and an increase in heart rate by 20 beats/min. However, the most recent evaluations of data related to orthostatic vital signs concluded that an increase in the pulse rate of more than 30 beats/min or symptoms of decreased blood flow to the brain (dizziness, syncope) in an adult is required to detect hypovolemia from acute blood loss (Gorgas, 2004; McGee et al., 1999). A negative test result indicates only that an acute blood loss of 1000 mL is unlikely. However, a blood loss of 500 mL cannot be excluded (Gorgas, 2004). In children, an orthostatic increase in pulse of more than 25 beats/min constitutes a positive test result. An orthostatic pulse increase of less than 20 beats/min constitutes a negative test result for hypovolemia (Gorgas, 2004; Fuchs & Jaffe, 1987).

Many conditions affect orthostatic vital signs. For example, alcohol ingestion, a meal, increased age, and antihypertensive drugs may cause orthostatic vital sign changes despite a normal blood volume. On the other hand, vital signs may be normal in a patient who is hypovolemic. Based on this information, the usefulness of orthostatic vital signs appears to be limited. Base your treatment decisions on the patient's signs and symptoms. Do not prolong scene times to obtain orthostatic vital signs. Do not attempt to obtain orthostatic vital signs in a patient with a known or suspected spinal injury.

From Fuchs, S. M., & Jaffe, D. M. (1987). Evaluation of the "tilt test" in children. *Annals of Emergency Medicine, 16*(4), 386-390; Gorgas, D. L. (2004). Vital signs measurement. In J. R. Roberts, & J. R. Hedges (Eds.), *Clinical procedures in emergency medicine* (4th ed.) (pp. 14-19). Philadelphia: Elsevier; Knopp, R., Claypool, R., & Leonardi, D. Use of the tilt test in measuring acute blood loss. *Annals of Emergency Medicine, 9*(2), 72-75; and McGee, S., Abernethy, W. B. III, & Simel, D. L. (1999). The rational clinical examination. Is this patient hypovolemic? *Journal of the American Medical Association, 281*(11):1022-1029.

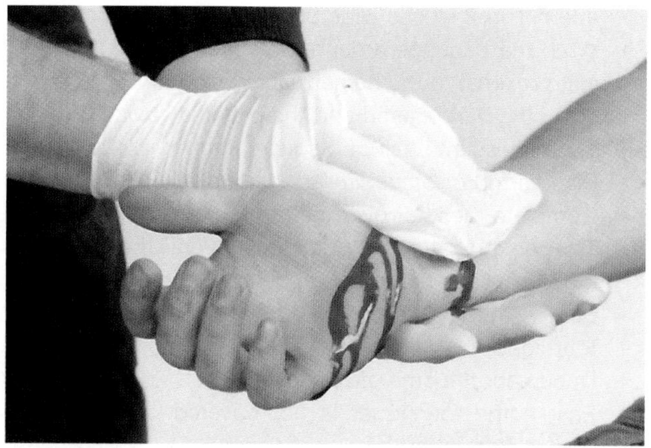

Figure 44-2 Control bleeding by applying direct pressure.

ticularly with injuries to arteries and large veins, you will need to use both hands to apply pressure. As soon as dressing material, typically sterile gauze pad, is available, place it over the wound and reapply pressure. In cases with the potential for air emboli, apply occlusive dressings instead of gauze to the wound.

Maintain the pressure until bleeding is under control. Instead of replacing dressings that become saturated in blood, continue to add additional dressings until the bleeding is controlled. In cases of significant hemorrhage, such as patients with arterial damage, you may consider applying a folded trauma or abdominal dressing to provide enough material to control the bleeding. Do not remove dressings. Removal may result in the rupture of any clot that may have begun to form, reinitiating hemorrhage.

BOX 44-4 Possible Signs and Symptoms of Internal Bleeding

- Anxiety, restlessness, combativeness, or altered mental status
- Weakness, faintness, or dizziness
- Rapid, shallow breathing (with no other respiratory problems present)
- Hypotension
- Rapid, weak pulse
- Pale, cool, clammy skin
- Narrowing pulse pressure
- Excessive thirst
- Pain, tenderness, swelling, or discoloration of suspected site of injury
- Bleeding from the mouth, rectum, vagina, or other body opening
- Vomiting bright-red blood or dark coffee ground–colored blood
- Coughing up blood
- Sudden, severe headache
- Dark, tarry stools (melena) or bloody stools (hematochezia)
- Tender, rigid, and/or distended abdomen

If direct pressure fails to control the hemorrhage or if hands are needed to perform other lifesaving tasks, apply a pressure dressing to the injury. Place a collection of bulky dressings over the wound and firmly wrap the affected region with roller gauze to hold the dressing in place and exert pressure over the wound. The tail of the bandage should be tied tightly enough so that only one finger can slide under the bandage. In cases of extreme hemorrhage, you may need to place a balled-up triangle bandage on top of the dressings before wrapping the injury. This increases the pressure that can be generated. Assess distal pulses to ensure that blood flow has not been cut off by this procedure. The goal is to use the bandage to apply pressure to the wound but not cut off blood supply to the extremity.

If external extremity bleeding cannot be controlled with direct pressure, the next reasonable step in hemorrhage control involves application of a tourniquet. In the event of extreme blood loss that does not respond to any other form of treatment, a tourniquet can be used to prevent exsanguination.

Tourniquets are applied to the affected extremity just proximal to the hemorrhaging wound. To apply the tour-

SKILL 44-1 HEMORRHAGE CONTROL

Step 1 Use appropriate PPE, including, at a minimum, medical examination gloves and protective eyewear.

Step 2 Apply direct pressure to the wound with a gloved hand.

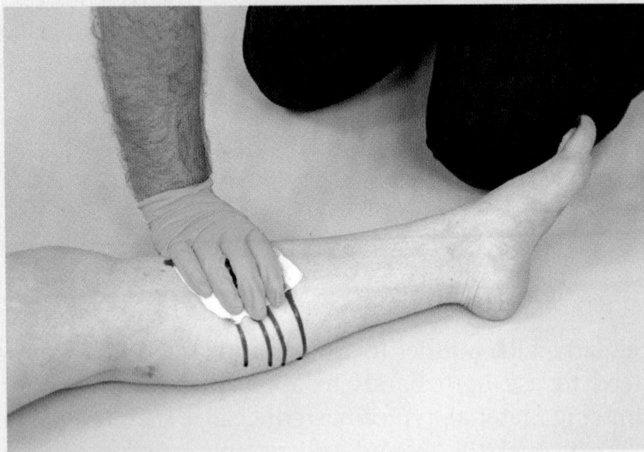

Step 3 Apply sterile dressing material over the wound and reapply direct pressure.

Step 4 Assess for control of the hemorrhage.

Step 5 If the hemorrhage is not controlled, apply pressure dressing to the injury.

- Assess for the presence of a distal pulse.
- Fold triangle bandage to cover the wound completely when placed over it, but no less than 2 inches in width.
- Place the middle of the triangle bandage over the wound and wrap the tails around the extremity.
- Tie the tails into a square knot over the top of the injury; tighten the knot to the point that you can slide only one finger between the triangle bandage and the dressings.
- For extreme hemorrhage, such as that associated with arterial bleeds, consider placing a balled-up triangle bandage on top of the dressing before assessing for a distal pulse to increase the pressure delivered to the injury site.
- Reassess distal pulse to ensure dressing is not acting as a tourniquet; if no pulse is found, loosen the dressing until a pulse is reacquired.

Step 6 Assess for control of the hemorrhage.

Step 7 If the hemorrhage is not controlled, apply a tourniquet.

- Fold a triangle bandage or similar material into a band about 1 to 2 inches wide but no less than 1 inch.
- Wrap the bandage around the extremity and apply it just proximal to the hemorrhaging wound.
- Wrap the bandage around the extremity twice.
- Tie the tails into half of a square knot.
- Place a rod or other similar object on the knot.
- Complete the knot over the rod.
- Turn the rod to tighten the tourniquet until the bleeding stops or distal pulses are absent.
- Secure the rod in place to prevent loosening of the tourniquet.
- Document the time of application.
- Ensure the tourniquet is not covered or otherwise hidden from view.

PPE, Personal protective equipment.

niquet, fold a triangle bandage or other material to form a band that is 1 to 2 inches wide but no less than 1 inch (never use material such as wire or rope). Wrap the band around the extremity twice, and tie the tails together in half of a square knot. Lay on this knot a solid rod or similarly shaped object. Finish tying the knot over this object so that it does not come loose. Rotate the rod to twist the band; continue until the bleeding is controlled or the pulse in the extremity is no longer palpable. The rod should be secure to the extremity to prevent loosening of the tourniquet. If a commercially developed tourniquet is used, follow the manufacturer's recommendation regarding its application. Once placed, carefully document the time of placement and report this to the receiving facility. The tourniquet should never be covered or otherwise obscured to ensure that it is not missed during later assessments.

Once you have placed a tourniquet, do not remove it in the field. Doing so can result in complications similar to crush syndrome and may increase **morbidity** or **mortality.** You often will encounter "tourniquets" applied by well-meaning bystanders. Carefully assess the extremity before modifying such devices. If a pulse is present distally, remove the device and properly manage the wound. If a distal pulse is not present or if you are unable to assess distal circulation, the "tourniquet" should be left in place. When in doubt, discuss the situation with medical direction for resolution.

Depending on the patient's signs and symptoms and the amount of blood lost, intravenous (IV) fluid replacement may be necessary but patient transport should not be delayed to start an IV line. If the patient's breath sounds are clear, an isotonic crystalloid solution (normal saline or Ringer's lactate) is given IV to maintain circulating blood volume. If signs and symptoms of shock are present, two large-bore (14- or 16-gauge), short (1-inch) IV catheters should be used. Although local protocols may vary, the typical goal in the administration of IV fluids is to maintain the systolic blood pressure between 80 and 90 mm Hg unless head trauma is also suspected. In this case the systolic blood pressure must be kept above 90 mm Hg. Check the patient's response by assessing his or her mental status, heart rate, respiratory effort, breath sounds, and blood pressure. If no improvement occurs, give additional fluids until the patient responds appropriately, or as instructed by medical direction. Maintain the patient's normal body temperature. Transport the patient to the closest appropriate medical facility for definitive care.

Patient and Family Education

Instruct anyone who has a wound to make sure his or her immunizations are up to date. A tetanus booster should be given every 10 years. Adults who have never received immunization against tetanus should start with a three-dose series given over a 7- to 12-month period. A tetanus shot is recommended at 5 years if the person has had two or fewer prior immunizations, the wound is heavily contaminated (foreign material), or an extensive crush injury is present.

PARAMEDIC*Pearl*

In infants and children younger than 6 years, dehydration has been strongly correlated with a capillary refill time of more than 3 seconds, which suggests a fluid deficit of more than 100 mL/kg (Saavedra et al., 1991). In adults, capillary refill has no proven diagnostic value when evaluating for hypovolemia (Sinert & Spektor, 2005; McGee et al., 1999).

From McGee, S., Abernethy, W. B. III, & Simel, D. L. (1999). The rational clinical examination. Is this patient hypovolemic? *Journal of the American Medical Association, 281*(11):1022-1029; Saavedra, J. M., Harris, G. D., Li, S., & Finberg, L. (1991). Capillary refilling (skin turgor) in the assessment of dehydration. *American Journal of Diseases in Childhood, 145*(3), 296-298; and Sinert, R., & Spektor, M. (2005). Evidence-based emergency medicine/rational clinical examination abstract. Clinical assessment of hypovolemia. *Annals of Emergency Medicine, 45*(3):327-329.

Case Scenario—continued

The patient is alert, oriented, and cooperative. His airway is clear and his breathing is non-labored. He has a weak and rapid radial pulse, his skin is pale and moist, and he becomes dizzy when he attempts to stand. He tells you he has not eaten in more than 12 hours. He has no significant medical history, and the physical exam reveals a laceration to the underside of his right arm that extends from the wrist to the elbow with exposed muscle tissue. The bleeding is profuse and dark red in color. His vitals reveal a weak radial pulse at 136, a respiratory rate of 18 breaths/min with clear and equal bilateral breath sounds, and a blood pressure of 74/68 mm Hg.

Questions

4. *Is this patient high priority? Why or why not?*
5. *Should you infuse IV fluids? If so, how much?*
6. *If your initial attempts to control the bleeding are unsuccessful, what additional treatment can be considered?*

Internal Bleeding

Description and Definition

Internal bleeding is the escape of blood from blood vessels into tissues and spaces within the body. Because the signs and symptoms of internal bleeding are less obvious than are those of external bleeding, they often are overlooked.

Etiology

[OBJECTIVE 7]

Internal bleeding may be the result of trauma, clotting disorders, rupture of blood vessels, fractures that cause injury to nearby vessels, and many medical conditions. Internal bleeding may be the result of penetrating or blunt trauma. Examples of mechanisms of injury that may result in internal bleeding from blunt trauma include the following:

- Falls
- Motorcycle crashes
- Pedestrian impacts
- Automobile collisions
- Blast injuries

History

The signs and symptoms of internal bleeding may be obvious immediately after an injury occurs to a blood vessel. However, in some cases signs and symptoms may not be present for hours, days, or weeks after the injury. Because internal bleeding has many possible causes, it may not be possible to provide a list of all potential historical details a patient may relay to you. However, a few include the following:

- Suspect internal bleeding in a patient who reports abdominal pain and states he or she feels dizzy or lightheaded upon standing from a supine position.
- Patients with a history of alcohol abuse and those who have liver disease are prone to GI bleeding.
- Consider the possibility of a ruptured ectopic pregnancy in any woman of childbearing age who reports lower abdominal pain.
- Consider the possibility of aortic aneurysm rupture in any patient who reports a "ripping" or "tearing" pain in the back, abdomen, or between the shoulder blades.
- Assume that a patient who says he or she has "the worst headache of my life" has bleeding within his or her head until proven otherwise.

Physical Findings

Suspect internal bleeding on the basis of the patient's mechanism of injury or nature of the illness and the signs and symptoms. Possible signs and symptoms of internal bleeding are given in Box 44-4.

Differential Diagnosis

Differential diagnoses for internal bleeding include the following:

- Solid organ injury
- Vascular injury
- Pelvic fracture
- Closed femur fracture
- Intestinal obstruction
- Aortic aneurysm rupture
- Hemothorax
- Ruptured ectopic pregnancy
- Arteriovenous malformation
- Bleeding esophageal varices
- Peritonitis

Therapeutic Interventions

[OBJECTIVE 8]

Your care for a patient with internal bleeding depends on the source of the bleeding and its severity. Provide airway and ventilatory support. Give supplemental oxygen. Apply a pulse oximeter and use capnography. Maintain oxygen saturation at greater than 95%. Apply the cardiac monitor. Avoid performing additional procedures on the scene that will delay transport to the hospital.

Establish IV access en route to definitive care. If the patient's breath sounds are clear, an IV fluid challenge of isotonic crystalloid solution (normal saline or lactated Ringer's solution) is usually given to maintain circulating blood volume. Although local protocols may vary, the general goal in the administration of IV fluids is to maintain a systolic blood pressure between 80 and 90 mm Hg. Check the patient's response by assessing his or her mental status, heart rate, respiratory effort, breath sounds, and blood pressure. If no improvement occurs, give additional fluids until the patient responds appropriately or as instructed by medical direction. Maintain normal body temperature. A patient who has possible internal bleeding needs rapid transport to the closest facility with immediate surgical capability.

Patient and Family Education

In many cases internal bleeding is the result of a sudden illness or injury and cannot be prevented. Provide emotional support to the patient and his or her family.

PARAMEDIC*Pearl*

Transport a patient who has significant external bleeding or signs of internal bleeding or shock to the closest appropriate medical facility. If the patient refuses care, repeatedly try to persuade him or her to accept the care you want to provide, including transport. Explain to the patient that if his or her condition is not treated, the symptoms may worsen and could result in death. Consider contacting medical direction for advice. If you are unable to convince the patient to receive care, carefully document the patient's refusal.

Case Scenario CONCLUSION

As your partner places the patient on 100% oxygen via a nonrebreather mask, you place direct pressure on the wound with both gloved hands. Your partner then applies a pressure dressing to the entire laceration; however, the wound continues to bleed, soaking through additional layers of gauze pads. You elect to place a tourniquet in a location just above the elbow, which does control the hemorrhage. En route to the emergency department you initiate IV access to the left arm and administer 750 mL of normal saline. Upon arrival at the hospital the patient's color has improved and he has a radial pulse of 110, which is slightly stronger than it was at initial contact; a respiratory rate of 18 breaths per minute; and a blood pressure of 88/68 mm Hg.

Looking Back

7. *Given the change in your patient's condition, was your treatment appropriate? Why or why not?*

Case Scenario SUMMARY

1. *What is your general impression of this patient?* There are many indicators that this patient is high priority. Pale skin is a sign of poor perfusion and indicates that this patient may be in shock. The amount of blood loss indicates that he is hypovolemic and must have the external hemorrhage stopped immediately. A confounding factor is the presence of alcohol in his system. Recall from prior chapters that the clotting cascade is a complex series of reactions that are based on positive feedback. Alcohol interferes with several of these reactions, resulting in an inability of the patient to create clots to control the hemorrhage.

2. *What additional assessment will be important in the evaluation of this patient?* Further evaluation of mental status, skin (for poor skin turgor, cyanosis, and diaphoresis), and vital signs will be important. Although the patient is speaking to you, the airway and adequacy of ventilation must be evaluated. The severity of the laceration and type of hemorrhage (venous or arterial) should also be evaluated.

3. *What intervention should you initiate at this time?* The administration of high-flow oxygen and application of direct pressure to the laceration are the first two treatment actions that should take place.

4. *Is this patient high priority? Why or why not?* The findings of a weak rapid radial pulse, pale, moist skin, and dizziness indicate the presence of hypovolemia. As a result the patient is a high-priority patient.

5. *Should you infuse IV fluids? If so, how much?* Because the patient is hypotensive and experiencing uncontrolled hemorrhage, he is decompensating. Aggressive therapy is important to prevent further deterioration. Although IV fluid infusion remains controversial for individuals in hemorrhagic shock, it is appropriate for this patient and fluid replacement with an isotonic solution is indicated. Although local protocols vary, typical fluid replacement guidelines are to maintain the systolic blood pressure between 80 and 90 mm Hg in this situation.

6. *If your initial attempts to control the bleeding are unsuccessful, what additional treatment can be considered?* The goal in hemorrhage is to control the hemorrhage and stop blood loss as quickly and efficiently as possible. If direct pressure and a pressure dressing are unsuccessful in controlling the hemorrhage, a tourniquet can be considered. Allowing hemorrhage to continue while attempting other methods to control the bleeding can result in unnecessary and potentially detrimental blood loss.

7. *Given the change in your patient's condition, was your treatment appropriate? Why or why not?* Hemorrhage must be controlled as quickly and efficiently as possible. Because direct pressure and a pressure dressing failed to control the hemorrhage, the application of a tourniquet was appropriate. The patient's decreasing pulse and increasing blood pressure indicate an increase in his perfusion status. Although he will require sutures of the laceration and likely will require blood replacement, stopping the hemorrhage will slow the development of hypovolemic shock and allow the patient to maintain as much perfusion as possible to the vital organs.

Chapter Summary

- Internal and external hemorrhage can result from a variety of causes.
- An adequate blood volume is critical to adequate perfusion.
- Uncontrolled blood loss can quickly lead to hypovolemic shock and poor patient outcome.
- The goal of treatment in the hemorrhaging patient is to stop the hemorrhage as quickly and efficiently as possible.
- The patient should not be allowed to continue to bleed while ineffective methods of hemorrhage control are attempted.

REFERENCES

American Heart Association. (2005). American Heart Association guidelines for cardiopulmonary resuscitation and emergency cardiovascular care, part 14: first aid. *Circulation, 112,* IV-198.

Fuchs, S. M., & Jaffe, D. M. (1987). Evaluation of the "tilt test in children." *Annals of Emergency Medicine, 16*(4), 386-390.

Gorgas, D. L. (2004). Vital signs measurement. In J. R. Roberts, & J. R. Hedges (Eds.), *Clinical procedures in emergency medicine* (4th ed.) (pp. 14-19). Philadelphia: Elsevier.

Knopp, R., Claypool, R., & Leonardi, D. Use of the tilt test in measuring acute blood loss. *Annals of Emergency Medicine, 9*(2), 72-75.

McGee, S., Abernethy, W. B. III, & Simel, D. L. (1999). The rational clinical examination. Is this patient hypovolemic? *Journal of the American Medical Association, 281*(11):1022-1029.

Saavedra, J. M., Harris, G. D., Li, S., & Finberg, L. (1991). Capillary refilling (skin turgor) in the assessment of dehydration. *American Journal of Diseases in Childhood, 145*(3), 296-298.

Sinert, R., & Spektor, M. (2005). Evidence-based emergency medicine/rational clinical examination abstract. Clinical assessment of hypovolemia. *Annals of Emergency Medicine, 45*(3):327-329.

SUGGESTED RESOURCES

Guyton, A. C., & Hall, J. E. (2002). *Textbook of medical physiology* (2nd ed.). Philadelphia: Saunders.

Rosen. (2002). *Emergency medicine: Concepts and clinical practice* (6th ed.). St. Louis: Mosby.

Hamilton, G. C. (1991). *Emergency medicine: An approach to clinical problem solving.* Philadelphia: Saunders.

Chapter Quiz

1. Which of the following are signs of internal hemorrhage?
  a. Tachycardia, hypotension, narrowed pulse pressure
  b. Tachycardia, hypertension, narrowed pulse pressure
  c. Tachycardia, hypotension, widened pulse pressure
  d. Tachycardia, hypertension, widened pulse pressure

2. Which of the following types of bleeding presents with bright-red blood that sprays in a pulsating manner?
  a. Arterial bleeding
  b. Venous bleeding
  c. Capillary bleeding
  d. Cellular bleeding

3. What is the first step in controlling external hemorrhage?
  a. Elevation
  b. Tourniquet
  c. Direct pressure
  d. Pressure points

4. Your patient has internal bleeding. Which of the following will benefit your patient the most?
  a. High-flow oxygen
  b. IV isotonic fluid bolus
  c. Pneumatic antishock garment application
  d. Transport to the closest appropriate medical facility

5. Explain the difference between controlled and uncontrolled hemorrhage.

____
____
____

6. List at least 5 signs and symptoms a patient with external bleeding may experience.

____
____
____
____
____

7. What are orthostatic vital signs and what are they used to determine?

____
____

Terminology

Bleeding Escape of blood from a blood vessel.

Exsanguinate Near-complete loss of blood; not conducive with life.

External bleeding Observable blood loss.

Hemorrhage Heavy bleeding.

Internal bleeding Escape of blood from blood vessels into tissues and spaces within the body.

Morbidity State of being diseased; the propensity to cause disease or illness.

Mortality Death.

Orthostatic vital signs Serial measurements of the patient's pulse and blood pressure taken with the patient recumbent, sitting, and standing. Results are used to assess possible volume depletion; also called the *tilt test* or *postural vital signs*.

Perfusion Circulation of blood through an organ or a part of the body.

CHAPTER 45

Soft Tissue Trauma

Objectives

After completing this chapter, you will be able to:

1. Describe the incidence, morbidity, and mortality rates of soft tissue injuries.
2. Describe the layers of the skin, specifically the epidermis and dermis (cutaneous), superficial fascia (subcutaneous), and deep fascia.
3. Identify the major functions of the integumentary system.
4. Describe the anatomy and physiology of joints.
5. Discuss the pathophysiology of wound healing, including hemostasis, inflammation, epithelialization, neovascularization, and collagen synthesis.
6. Describe common interruptions in the wound healing process.
7. Identify wounds that have a high risk for infection or complications.
8. Discuss the pathophysiology of soft tissue injuries.
9. Distinguish between open and closed soft tissue injuries.
10. Distinguish between the types of closed soft tissue injuries.
11. Describe the etiology, history, and physical findings of a closed soft tissue injury.
12. Using the mechanism of injury, patient history, and physical examination findings, develop a treatment plan for a patient with a closed soft tissue injury.
13. Distinguish between the types of open soft tissue injuries.
14. Describe the etiology, history, and physical findings of an open soft tissue injury.
15. Using the mechanism of injury, patient history, and physical examination findings, develop a treatment plan for a patient with an open soft tissue injury.
16. Describe the etiology, history, and physical findings of crush injuries.
17. Using the mechanism of injury, patient history, and physical examination findings, develop a treatment plan for a patient with a crush injury.
18. Discuss the effects of reperfusion and rhabdomyolysis on the body.
19. Define the following conditions: crush injury, crush syndrome, and compartment syndrome.
20. Distinguish between the types of injuries that require the use of an occlusive dressing versus those that require a nonocclusive dressing.
21. Define and discuss the following:
    - Dressings
        - Sterile and nonsterile
        - Occlusive and nonocclusive
        - Adherent and nonadherent
        - Absorbent and nonabsorbent
        - Wet and dry
    - Bandages
        - Absorbent and nonabsorbent
        - Adherent and nonadherent
    - Tourniquets
22. Predict the possible complications of an improperly applied dressing, bandage, or tourniquet.

Chapter Outline

Epidemiology of Soft Tissue Trauma
Standard Precautions Review
Anatomy and Physiology Review
Wound Healing
Pathophysiology and Assessment of Soft Tissue Injuries
Common Soft Tissue Infections
General Management of Soft Tissue Trauma
Documentation of Soft Tissue Injuries
Chapter Summary

Case Scenario

You and your partner respond with the fire department to a construction site for a "man crushed by a concrete block." A supervisor leads you to an area where a crowd has assembled around a young man who appears trapped by a concrete block the size of a refrigerator. His left lower leg and foot are under the block, and he is sitting up yelling to the assembled crowd "get it off me, get it off me!" As you approach him, you see that the fire department is working with several construction workers to attach the block to a crane. The patient has moist skin with normal color and is alert and oriented. He responds to questions and appears to have no respiratory distress. He states that he was guiding the block into position as it was being moved by the crane when it came free and fell approximately 2 to 3 feet onto his leg and foot.

Questions

1. *What is your general impression of this patient?*
2. *What additional assessment is most pertinent at this time?*
3. *What intervention should be initiated before any further assessment is performed?*

The term *soft tissue trauma* can include two different types of injuries: minor superficial wounds caused by everyday living as well as life-threatening conditions such as extensive burns. As a paramedic, you must manage these diverse soft tissue injuries. You will need to identify injuries rapidly that present a threat to life and quickly manage those injuries. One complicating factor is that extremely graphic soft tissue injuries often are not the most serious injuries the patient may have. Therefore you must be able to manage the visible wounds while still assessing for more significant traumatic insults.

EPIDEMIOLOGY OF SOFT TISSUE TRAUMA

Incidence, Mortality, and Morbidity Rates

[OBJECTIVE 1]

When soft tissue injuries are broadly defined, the incidence is quite high because some level of soft tissue involvement is present in nearly every traumatic incident. Even when the term is narrowly defined as cuts or penetrations of the skin, the incidence is still relatively high. In fact, in 2003 these types of injuries were the fifth leading cause of nonfatal injuries in all age groups (Centers for Disease Control and Prevention [CDC], 2003).

Risk Factors

Patients who are most at risk for soft tissue injury are typically small children and the elderly. This is particularly true when children are learning to use bicycles or skates and fall regularly. Despite this generalization, the role of industry must be considered in soft tissue injuries. Calls to industrial sites or assembly plants are common for victims of soft tissue injury. In fact, some careers are predisposed for soft tissue injury, including workers who are required to work from heights, for whom falling is a risk. Additionally, persons with chronic illnesses, especially diabetes, are prone to severe complications after what would seem to be insignificant lower extremity trauma.

PARAMEDIC*Pearl*

Nearly everyone experiences some form of soft tissue trauma during his or her life. However, most individuals do not call for EMS. Therefore when you are called to the scene, approach it as though a life-threatening situation exists until proven otherwise.

Prevention

Injury prevention is morally and financially a better goal than merely providing good care for injuries after they have occurred. Prevention efforts typically focus on programs designed to stop behavior that creates an environment that result in injuries. Examples of these efforts include car seat inspection programs to prevent or reduce injuries to infants in motor vehicle crashes. Additionally, some communities develop elaborate programs to fight drunk driving that combine harsh penalties for offenders with prevention programs such as designated driver services and public education campaigns. Likewise, other community programs have been developed to help end the cycle of domestic abuse among partners and against children through counseling and reeducation. All these programs attempt to prevent injury in the first place. Often many of these programs are in desperate need of resources, both financial and personnel. As a healthcare professional, you should take an active role in injury prevention, perhaps as a volunteer with this type of prevention program.

STANDARD PRECAUTIONS REVIEW

Paramedics are exposed to countless infectious organisms throughout the course of providing patient care. This is particularly true while providing care to the patient with soft tissue injuries. While controlling bleeding and dressing and bandaging wounds, you are at great risk for coming into contact with the patient's blood. Blood may contain infectious organisms that could threaten your health.

While caring for a victim of soft tissue injury, one of your biggest concerns regarding infectious organisms is blood-borne pathogens. Of specific concern are hepatitis B and human immunodeficiency virus (HIV). Both viruses are spread through contact—between infected blood and broken skin or mucous membranes. A second risk of exposure is an accidental needle stick, which can easily occur in the hectic prehospital environment.

Personal Protective Equipment

As with any prevention method, one option to diminish the spread of disease is to interrupt the vector, or the way in which the infectious organism enters the body. With blood-borne illnesses, the vector is direct contact between blood and broken skin or mucous membranes. You can best prevent this occurrence by using appropriate personal protective equipment (PPE) and, most importantly, by practicing good handwashing.

At a minimum, PPE appropriate to managing soft tissue injury includes medical examination gloves. Consider increasing levels of PPE with more extreme forms of soft tissue trauma. If gross contamination is a risk, such as with confined space extrication or when blood is spurting or splashing, you should wear protective eyewear, a mask, and a protective gown. No matter the level of exposure risk or severity of the bleeding encountered, you should *always* thoroughly wash your hands after each patient contact and remove any soiled clothing before returning to service. If soap and water are not available for handwashing, use an alcohol-based hand sanitizer to clean your hands and exposed skin. Once water is available, however, immediately wash your hands and any potentially exposed skin.

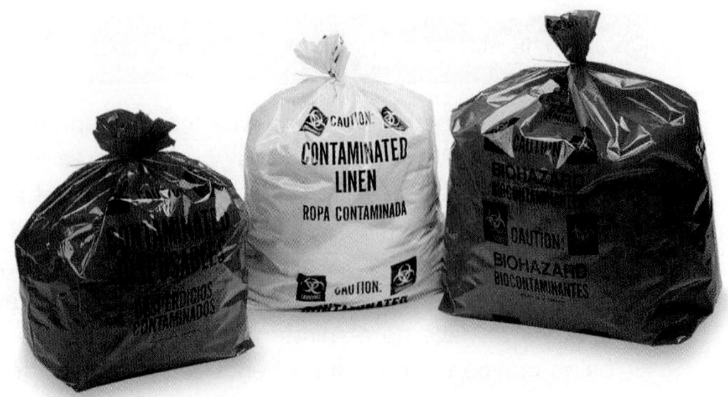

Figure 45-1 Clothing and nondisposable items that are too soiled to clean in the unit should be placed in yellow biohazard bags and taken back to the station. Disposable items used use during patient care should be placed in a red bag for destruction.

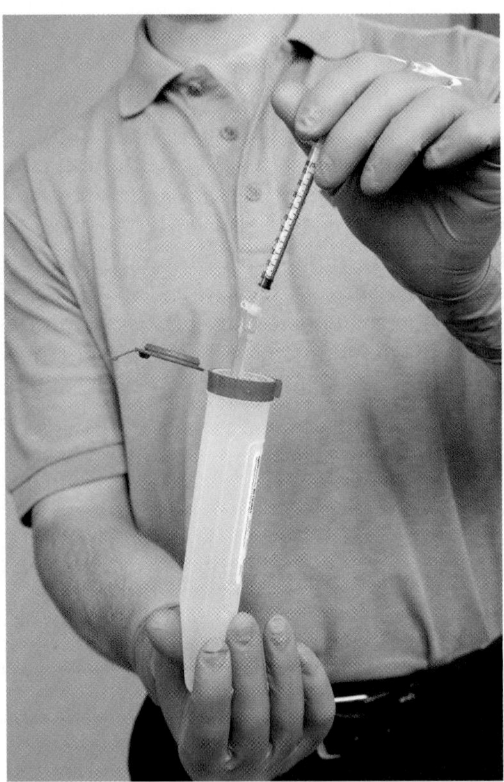

Figure 45-2 All sharps should be placed in an approved sharps container immediately after use. Sharps include needles, scalpels, broken ampules, and any item that could potentially cut or puncture the skin that has been used in the care of a patient.

Disposing of Soiled Material

Place clothing and any nondisposable materials in yellow biohazard bags (Figure 45-1). The contents of these bags are cleaned in accordance with your agency's policy or procedure. Clothing that is so grossly contaminated that it cannot be cleaned and any disposable supplies should all be placed in red biohazard bags. A licensed biohazard waste disposal company will incinerate these bags. Sharps or other similarly dangerous items should be placed in approved sharps containers (Figure 45-2). Once the containers are three-fourths full, they should be sealed and sent for incineration by a licensed biohazard waste disposal company.

ANATOMY AND PHYSIOLOGY REVIEW

[OBJECTIVES 2, 3]

Skin

The skin is a complex organ that serves several important physiologic functions. Its primary role is as a barrier to prevent water loss and the entrance of infectious organisms. In addition, it also regulates the body's temperature. The skin is composed of three layers and an additional protective layer of tissue immediately beneath the skin. These layers all combine to perform the skin's physiologic functions.

The **epidermis** is the external layer of skin. It is composed of constantly developing cells that are formed in the **germinativum** (basal layer) and progress to the **stratum corneum** (outer layer), where they are eventually shed. This outer layer provides the cosmetic appearance of the skin.

Below the epidermis lies the **dermis.** The dermis is a critical area of the skin regarding wound healing. Injuries that occur into the dermis typically result in the formation of a scar. Within the dermis lie sweat glands, **sebaceous glands,** hair follicles, capillary vasculature, and nerve fibers. The dermis is primarily composed of connective tissues, including **collagen** fibers that provide the skin's strength. The size and density of these collagen fibers are the chief means of distinguishing between the **papillary dermis** and the **reticular dermis.** The papillary dermis is composed of loose connective tissue. It primarily houses the vasculature that feeds the germinativum of the epidermis. The reticular dermis is composed of larger and denser collagen fibers and provides much of the skin's elasticity and strength. Additionally, this layer contains most of the skin structures.

Throughout the dermis lie cells crucial to the healing process. Principal among these are the **mast cells.** Mast cells play a significant role in allergic reactions and the inflammatory response to injury. Other cells that play key roles are fibroblasts, macrophages, and **neutrophils.** The role these cells play in inflammation and healing is covered later in this chapter.

The **superficial fascia** is composed of connective tissue that surrounds the subcutaneous fat. This layer serves as a cushioning layer and barrier to infection. Because of its loose makeup, it can easily become infected when it is not properly cleansed before a wound is closed.

Between the outer muscle layer and the superficial fascia lies the **deep fascia.** This thick, dense layer of fibrous connective tissue provides a final layer of defense against infection of internal structures. It also provides support for the underlying anatomy (Huether & McCance, 2004; Marx et al., 2002) (Figure 45-3).

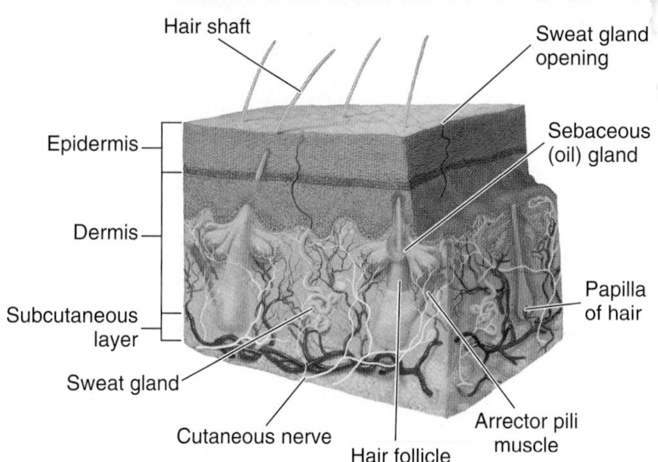

Figure 45-3 Structure of the skin.

Joints

[OBJECTIVE 4]

Throughout the body, bones that provide strength, protection, and mobility are connected in a variety of ways, all of which are collectively referred to as *joints* (Figures 45-4 and 45-5). Joints can be further divided into those that connect two immobile bones together, such as those in the skull; those that allow limited motion, such as the rib joints; and those that allow extensive range of motion, or **synovial joints.** Synovial joints are the joints of greatest concern in the trauma patient. They are composed of the bones' ends held together with tough, fibrous **ligaments.** The ligaments create the joint capsule, which contains the **cartilage** and **synovial fluid.** The cartilage pads the bone ends to prevent them from rubbing against each other during movement. The synovial fluid lubricates the joint. The cartilage is poorly perfused, so injuries that damage cartilage often result in the removal of the damaged tissue. Injuries occur to the joints when they are forced to move beyond their normal range of motion or forced to move too quickly. Injuries can range from mild stretching of the ligaments to tearing of the ligaments and dislocation of the joint.

Tendons connect muscles to muscle and muscles to bone. These tough, fibrous cords of tissue allow muscles to move the bones. Injuries to tendons and muscles can range from mild overstretching of the tissue to tearing of muscle tissue and, in extreme cases, complete disruption of the tendons.

WOUND HEALING

Normal Wound Healing

[OBJECTIVE 5]

Although the healing process is described in the following paragraphs in a step-by-step manner, do not consider it a simple process that always proceeds exactly in that manner. Rather, many of these "steps" occur at the same time and together result in the repair of injured tissue (Figure 45-6).

During the first phase of healing, **hemostasis** occurs immediately after the injury to the tissue. Any damage to tissue will alter the normal anatomy, which causes the release of tissue factors that begin the **coagulation**

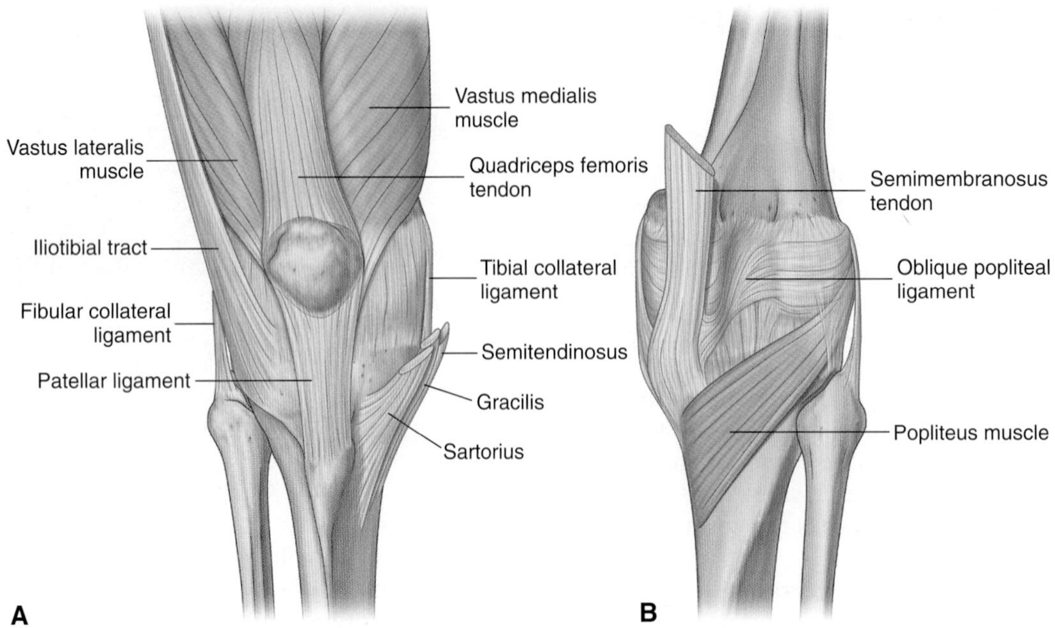

Figure 45-4 Fibrous membrane of the knee joint capsule **A,** Anterior view. **B,** Posterior view.

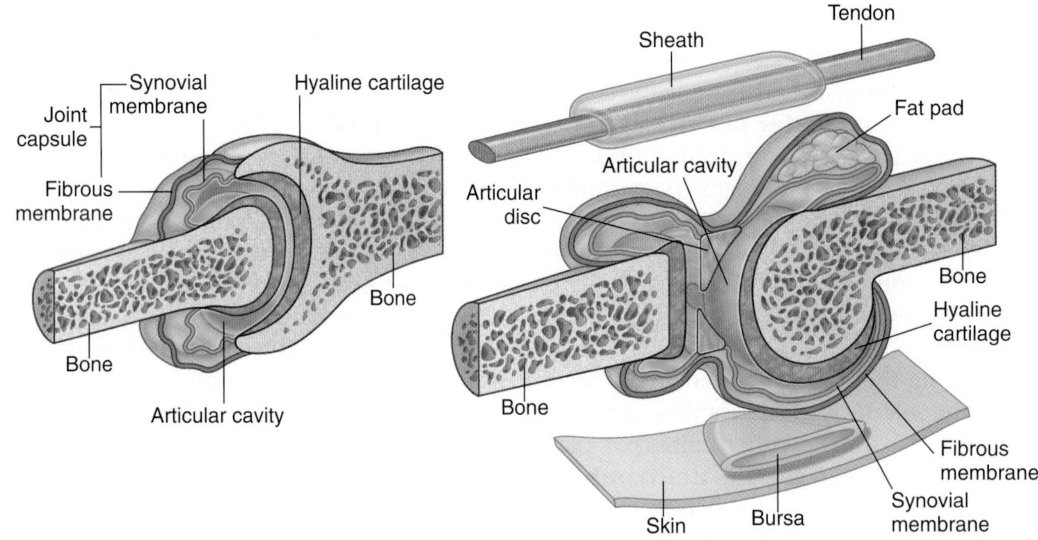

Figure 45-5 Synovial joints.

process. This process generates **fibrin,** which binds with platelets to begin forming a plug in the damaged vessels. Injured capillaries constrict in response to epinephrine and norepinephrine released by the sympathetic division of the autonomic nervous system. Vasoconstriction continues for up to 10 minutes, allowing the clotting process to stop the bleeding.

Tissue injury also stimulates the release of **histamine** from mast cells within the dermis. The release of histamine starts the inflammatory phase of healing by dilating capillaries. This results in increased vascular permeability and increased blood flow to the injured area. Increased permeability allows passage of vascular fluids into the surrounding tissue. Evidence of this process can be seen and felt as the redness, warmth, and onset of swelling that accompanies most injuries.

Increased vascular permeability allows elements of the inflammatory response to move into the damaged tissue and begin attacking invading pathogens. The first among these elements are **granulocytes.** The most common granulocytes are neutrophils. Neutrophils are the first **phagocyte** to attack foreign bodies within the wound. They are short lived and soon replaced by the longer-lived macrophages. Triggered by neutrophils, which release macrophage stimulating factor, **macrophages** are critical to the healing process. They are responsible for the majority of wound cleansing. Additionally, they aid vessel growth by stimulating **endothelial cell** migra-

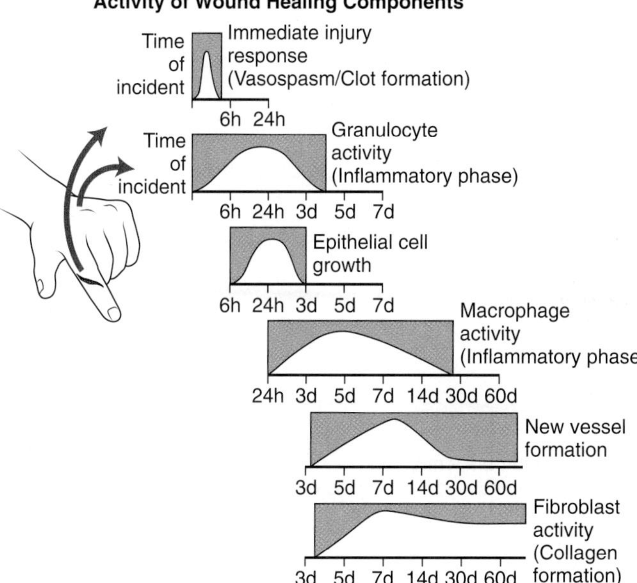

Figure 45-6 The various components of wound healing and their time frames.

tion across the injury. Finally, macrophages help destroy damaged tissue in preparation for the remodeling of the wound.

Within 12 hours of injury, **epithelialization** begins. With this process, cells from the basal layer of the epidermis migrate across the damaged area of tissue. The changes that occurred to cellular structure and connection allow migration across the matrix of fibrin within the wound. The basal layer continues to expand across the injury until the gap is closed. The cells then begin producing the upper layers of epidermis. Despite this apparent regeneration of the epidermis, the new tissue never regains the strength, elasticity, or thickness of uninjured tissue.

The healing wound initially is hypoxic. However, within 3 days new blood vessels have begun to form through the process of **neovascularization.** Stimulated by macrophages, endothelial cells migrate across the injury, forming capillary buds. These buds connect and open, allowing circulation to begin. This process is critical to provide oxygen and nutrients to the newly formed tissue and replace damaged vessels. As the tissue develops, some capillaries join to form larger vessels. This process can last as long as 21 days.

Within 3 to 5 days of injury, **fibroblasts** begin to divide and produce collagen. This protein is essential to the production and strength of connective tissue and skin. The collagen molecules are released by fibroblasts into the tissue, where they align into fibrils and fibers. These structures are initially bound by electrostatic cross links, but stronger covalent bonds are created through the formation of **hydroxylysine,** which can be inhibited by tissue hypoxia and the absence of vitamin C. This process continues for an extended period, with the wound achieving 60% of its ultimate strength within 4 months (Marx et al., 2002; Lawrence et al., 2002) (Figure 45-7).

Interruptions in Wound Healing

[OBJECTIVE 6]

The wound healing process may be interrupted or impaired by a variety of factors. Specifically, consider anatomic conditions near the wound, drugs used by the patient, and preexisting medical conditions. All may significantly affect the healing process.

Anatomic Factors

When evaluating the risk of complications during healing, consider the area of the body in which the wound is located. Areas of poor circulation, such as the feet, may experience delays in healing. Wounds involving the feet have a high risk for infection; wounds in areas of excellent perfusion, such as the face, heal quite well. Wounds in areas of high tension, such as those over joints, may incur repeated high levels of stress. These high levels of stress may cause abnormal scarring or delayed healing.

Skin condition is another factor that may alter the healing process. In particular, darkly pigmented or markedly oily skin is more likely to develop abnormal scars.

Concurrent Drug Use

Many pharmaceuticals can impair the body's ability to heal. Specifically, medications that inhibit the immune or inflammatory response cause delays in the healing process and increase the risk of infection. Some common medications that inhibit healing are provided in Box 45-1. This list of medications should not be seen as

BOX 45-1 Common Medications That Inhibit Healing

Corticosteroids: These medications often are used to treat chronic inflammation. They inhibit all aspects of the healing process through suppression of the immune system and inflammation response.

Nonsteroidal antiinflammatory drugs: Antiinflammatory agents are used to treat conditions that range from inflammatory pain to fever. In over-the-counter form, they often are used to self-treat minor aches and pain. Through their antiinflammatory action, they inhibit the early stages of healing.

Colchicine: This is an antiinflammatory medication primarily used in the treatment of gout. Colchicine inhibits the action of neutrophils.

Anticoagulants: Increased hemorrhage prevents hemostasis. Increased presence of blood components causes increased risk of infection and delays healing.

Antineoplastic agents: Typically used in the treatment of cancerous tumors, these medications inhibit tumor cell growth but also inhibit normal cell growth and the immune response.

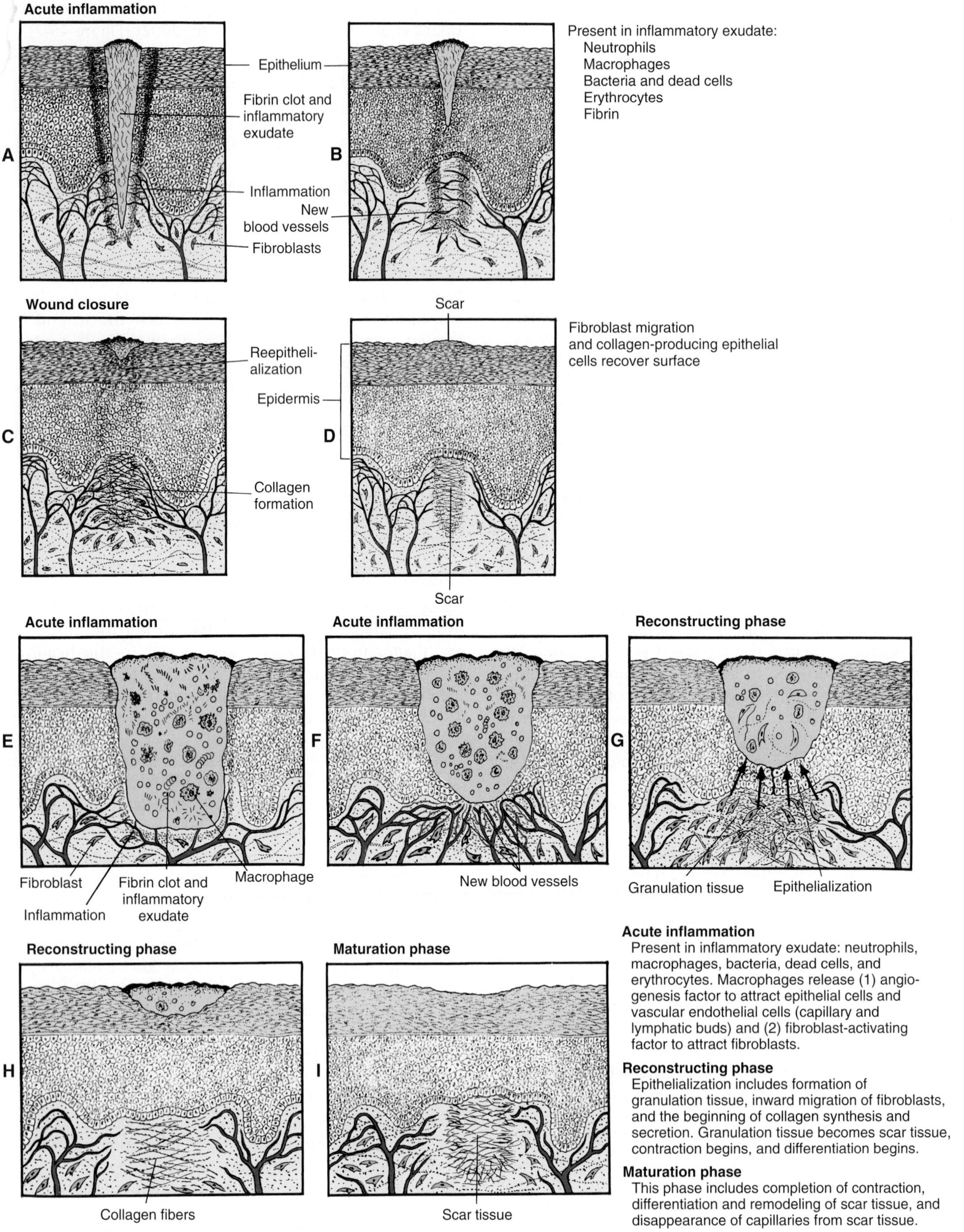

Acute inflammation

A

B

Epithelium

Fibrin clot and inflammatory exudate

Inflammation

New blood vessels

Fibroblasts

Present in inflammatory exudate:
- Neutrophils
- Macrophages
- Bacteria and dead cells
- Erythrocytes
- Fibrin

Wound closure

C

D

Scar

Reepitheli-alization

Epidermis

Collagen formation

Scar

Fibroblast migration and collagen-producing epithelial cells recover surface

Acute inflammation

E

Fibroblast

Inflammation

Fibrin clot and inflammatory exudate

Macrophage

Acute inflammation

F

New blood vessels

Reconstructing phase

G

Granulation tissue

Epithelialization

Reconstructing phase

H

Collagen fibers

Maturation phase

I

Scar tissue

Acute inflammation
Present in inflammatory exudate: neutrophils, macrophages, bacteria, dead cells, and erythrocytes. Macrophages release (1) angiogenesis factor to attract epithelial cells and vascular endothelial cells (capillary and lymphatic buds) and (2) fibroblast-activating factor to attract fibroblasts.

Reconstructing phase
Epithelialization includes formation of granulation tissue, inward migration of fibroblasts, and the beginning of collagen synthesis and secretion. Granulation tissue becomes scar tissue, contraction begins, and differentiation begins.

Maturation phase
This phase includes completion of contraction, differentiation and remodeling of scar tissue, and disappearance of capillaries from scar tissue.

Figure 45-7 Wound repair by primary or secondary intention. **A** to **D,** Healing by primary intention. **E** to **I,** Healing by secondary intention.

comprehensive. Any medication used in the treatment of autoimmune diseases, inflammation, or cancer should be carefully evaluated to determine its possible effect on the healing process.

Medical Conditions and Diseases

Preexisting or concurrent medical conditions can complicate the wound healing process. The ways in which conditions can affect healing vary. However, any condition that causes alteration of the immune system, impairment of circulation, hypoxia, or malnutrition has the possibility to impair healing (Lawrence et al., 2002). Examples of conditions that can affect healing are provided in Box 45-2.

BOX 45-2 Conditions That Can Affect Wound Healing

- Advanced age
- Severe alcoholism
- Acute uremia
- Diabetes
- Severe anemia
- Peripheral vascular disease
- Advanced cancer
- Hepatic failure
- Cardiovascular disease
- Smoking

Case Scenario—continued

As the block is lifted off the patient, he screams in pain. His foot is somewhat deformed, with an 8-inch tissue avulsion on the medial aspect, with bone and tendons visible. Bleeding is minimal. Pedal pulses are absent on the affected foot and normal on the opposite side. The patient states that his only complaint is his left foot. He denies a loss of consciousness with the incident, and states that he was "pinned to the ground" when the block fell but did not get knocked over. He has no pertinent medical history. His pulse is 100 beats/min, blood pressure is 138/80 mm Hg, and respiratory rate is 20 breaths/min. The remainder of the examination is normal.

Questions

4. *Should this patient's spine be immobilized? Why or why not?*
5. *How should the left foot be managed? What additional treatment should be provided?*
6. *The patient is in severe pain. What options exist to help manage his pain, and which do you believe to be most appropriate?*

High-Risk Wounds

[OBJECTIVE 7]

Some wounds present greater risk of infection or complications. These wounds require emergency department (ED) evaluation. Even when they appear insignificant, these wounds may present significant risks. Ensure the safety of the scene before initiating care. This is particularly true in cases of wild animal bites or when the animal has not been located or restrained. Make every attempt to transport patients who have high-risk injuries.

Human Bites

Human saliva is rich in bacteria and can result in extensive infection if the wound is not properly cleansed. In some cases antibiotics are essential in managing the wound. Bite wounds to the hands usually require the administration of antibiotics.

Dog Bites

Dog bites are typically associated with crushing force rather than a puncture. In adults, bites from pet dogs usually do not result in extensive tissue damage or fractures. However, trained attack dogs may cause extreme damage to involved structures. Because of the force of the bite, carefully assess any dog bite in a child for the possibility of serious underlying trauma. Rabies treatment should be considered for bites from dogs showing signs or symptoms of rabies infection or when the animal cannot be evaluated for the disease.

Cat Bites

Cat bites generally involve deep puncture wounds that are difficult to clean. As a result, cat bites are more likely to develop infection than are dog bites. Antibiotics should be considered for cat bites. In addition, the risk of rabies should be evaluated with all cat bites.

Foreign Bodies

Wounds contaminated with foreign bodies are at high risk for infection. In the field, removal of the contamination can be complicated by insufficient lighting and the uncontrolled nature of the prehospital environment. In general, the removal of foreign bodies should not be performed.

Wounds contaminated with organic matter present significant risk for infection. A wound that is contaminated with feces or saliva contains a significant bacterial

BOX 45-3 Potential for Extensive Tissue Damage for Wounds

- Farm or agricultural equipment
- Industrial equipment
- Crushing mechanism of injury
- High-velocity missiles (gunshot wounds, explosions)
- Dragging or sliding at high speeds on pavement

load, **potentiating** infection. This type of wound should be thoroughly cleansed. Additionally, soil can increase the potential of bacteria to cause infection (Marx et al., 2002).

Wounds with Significant Devitalized Tissue

Some causes of injury result in significant tissue damage (Box 45-3). These injuries usually require extensive **debridement** to prevent the development of **necrosis.**

A patient with an extensive soft tissue injury should be transported to the ED for evaluation.

Immunocompromised Patients

In a patient with a compromised immune system, any wound should be considered at high risk for infection and complications. These patients include those on immunosuppressive medications or with advanced cancer, rheumatoid arthritis, or other autoimmune disorder. The risk of infection is further increased in these patients when the wound is located in an area of poor perfusion, such as the foot. Take care to ensure that proper cleansing and dressing of the wound occurs and that a physician evaluates the need for antibiotic therapy.

Poor Peripheral Circulation

Hypoxic tissue results in delayed healing. Moreover, it provides an environment that encourages the proliferation of pathogens. Poor circulation from disease processes, such as diabetes, deep vein thrombosis, or peripheral vascular disease, can dramatically increase the risk for infection. Small wounds on the feet often mark the beginning of the ulceration formation process and require quick attention to prevent complications. Additionally, the use of tobacco, particularly cigarettes, is linked to a slower healing process and increased risk of infection or complications.

Abnormal Scarring

The formation of a scar is the final process of wound healing. It is sometimes referred to as *remodeling*. During this process, wounds contract by healing tissue and collagen fibers begin to reach their ultimate strength. For wounds with little tension or that are not stressed regularly by movement, the scars that form often are difficult to discern from normal tissue or, even when visible, are not significantly raised or pronounced. Unfortunately, some wounds develop abnormal levels of scar formation and produce either a **keloid** or a **hypertrophic scar.**

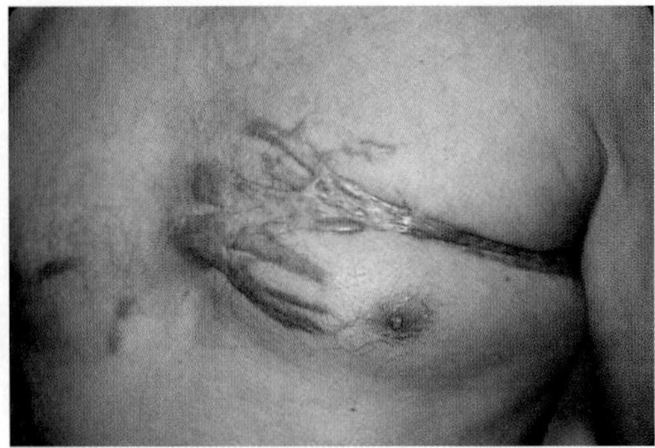

Figure 45-8 Keloid formation.

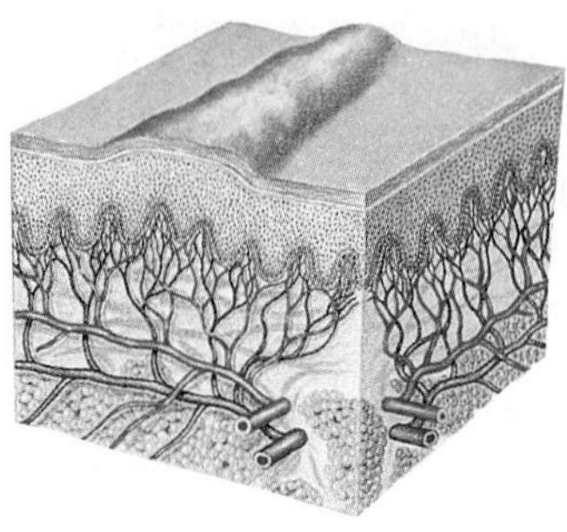

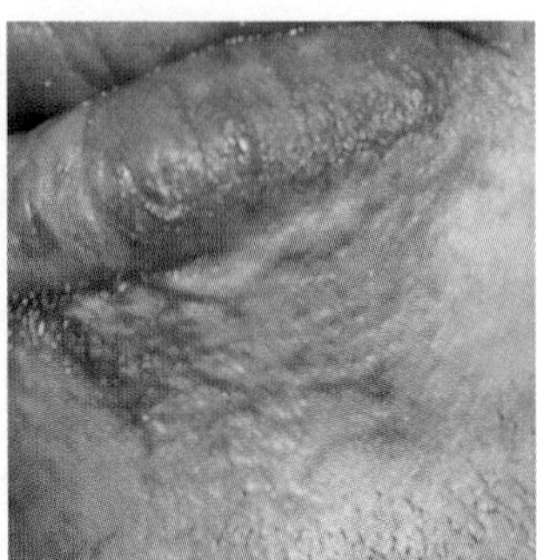

Figure 45-9 Hypertrophic scars form a raised or pronounced scar but stay confined to the original wound margins.

A keloid is an excessive accumulation of scar tissue that extends beyond the original wound borders (Figure 45-8). These are most common on darkly pigmented patients. Most often they form on the ears, upper extremities, lower abdomen, and sternum. Prevention of their formation is difficult; they can appear many months after the injury may seem to have healed. They often are managed through surgical procedures or steroid injections.

Hypertrophic scars occur more commonly (Figure 45-9). They involve excessive amounts of scar tissue that remain within the borders of the original wound. They are slightly raised and may impair function. They commonly form in areas of high tissue stress, such as flexion creases across joints.

Wound Closure

Closure of wounds is usually done with sutures or staples (Box 45-4). The variations in suture types and the techniques used to suture are extensive. Staples are generally reserved for areas not considered cosmetic or where the appearance of the scar is not significant.

BOX 45-4 Wounds Generally Requiring Closure

- Cosmetic regions (e.g., face, lip, eyebrow)
- Gaping wounds
- Wounds over tension areas
- Degloving injuries
- Ring injuries
- Skin tearing

Wounds That Do Not Require Closure

Not all soft tissue injuries require closure. In some cases the injuries may be superficial enough not to warrant transport of the patient. The paramedic should transport the patient to the ED if there is any doubt as to the severity of the injury.

PARAMEDIC*Pearl*

Recognize that even relatively insignificant-appearing trauma may require extensive treatment in the hospital. Several studies have indicated that paramedics may have as high as a 9% error rate in determining whether patients need to be seen in the emergency department (Pointer et al., 2001; Schmidt et al., 2001; Hauswald et al., 2002; Silvestri et al., 2002).

You may encounter patients who have an isolated superficial soft tissue injury. These cases can be managed through a treat-and-release process, but you must comply with local protocol and policy before initiating the release of care. If protocol allows, you are responsible for ensuring that the patient understands the potential risk for infection and scarring for the injury involved. Also inquire about the patient's history of tetanus vaccination. For patients with penetrating trauma who have not received a tetanus vaccine in the last 5 years, strongly encourage them to see their physician for the injection. Finally, instruct the patient on the proper method to cleanse the wound. These instructions should be carefully documented, and the patient should be asked to sign the release as required by your local policy. Although these cases do not present a significant clinical challenge, they represent one of the biggest areas of legal liability paramedics face. Handling the situation and appropriately documenting it are critical. When in doubt, consult medical direction and insist on patient transport. Defending transporting the patient is easier than not transporting a patient.

PATHOPHYSIOLOGY AND ASSESSMENT OF SOFT TISSUE INJURIES

[OBJECTIVES 8, 9]

Soft tissue injury is typically divided into two broad categories, open and closed. These categories are useful when learning the effects of soft tissue trauma and distinguishing between the types of force used to create the trauma. Closed injuries typically result from blows by blunt objects or from falling, whereas sharp instruments often are the cause of penetrating trauma. A type of soft tissue trauma that lies somewhere between the two broad categories is the crush injury. Crush injuries are similar to blunt injuries in their mechanism but, in extreme cases, may involve some rupturing of the skin. Because of their unique nature and the need for specific management procedures, crush injuries are considered later in this chapter.

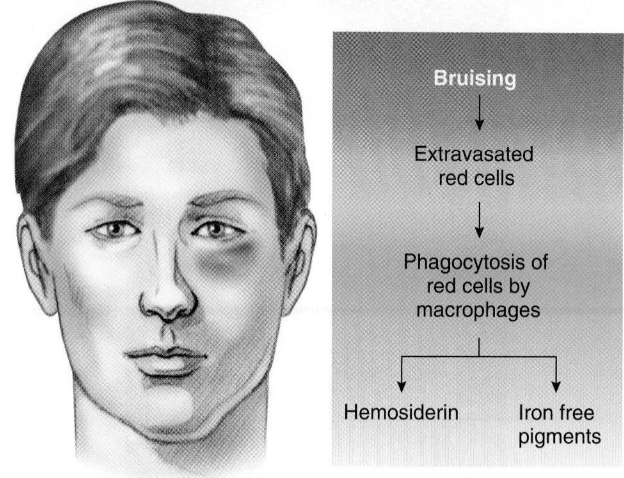

Figure 45-10 Contusion color changes through the healing process.

Closed Soft Tissue Injuries

[OBJECTIVES 10, 11, 12]

Contusion

A contusion is caused by the rupture of small blood vessels and damage to cells within the dermis. Occasionally, however, a contusion can be formed in deeper tissue, such as from a heavy blow. Blood collects within the dermis, creating a blackish-blue mark called **ecchymosis** that fades over time. Contusions may be accompanied by swelling. Although a contusion is not life threatening, it can be an indicator of significant injury to underlying structures or internal **hemorrhage.** Swelling, pain, and discoloration may appear as late as 24 to 48 hours after the injury. Contusions involving deep muscle tissue or organs do not always produce external ecchymosis or swelling. Moreover, they may be detectable only by noting pain on palpation of the injury (Figure 45-10).

PARAMEDIC*Pearl*

When tissue damage occurs deep within the body, the blood may travel along the fascia and appear some distance from the actual injury. This phenomenon is particularly common with ecchymosis associated with joint injuries.

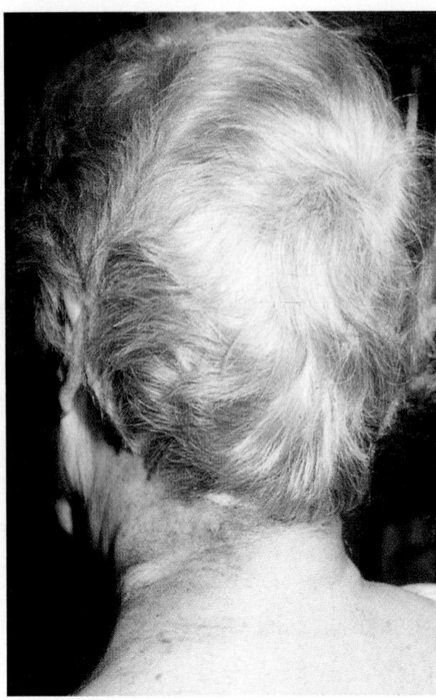

Figure 45-11 Severe hematoma, visible on the occipital area of the scalp, caused by a fall from fainting 3 days before. Blood under the scalp has gravitated down to the neck, causing ecchymosis along its path.

Hematoma

A **hematoma** (literally, "blood tumor") is formed when larger amounts of tissue are damaged or when large veins or arteries are ruptured beneath intact skin. In such cases, a large amount of blood collects beneath the skin, forming a pronounced lump that is pliable on palpation. Bleeding can be significant. In fact, the patient can lose 1 L or more of blood in large hematomas (Figure 45-11).

Management of Closed Soft Tissue Injuries. As a paramedic, your care of closed soft tissue injuries is primarily focused on the possibility of underlying trauma. Except in cases of large hematomas, these injuries are not typically life threatening. However, they are often the only external sign of significant and life-threatening internal trauma.

> **PARAMEDIC*Pearl***
>
> Be sure to assess a victim of closed soft tissue trauma carefully for the possibility of significant internal trauma. Maintain a high index of suspicion.

Sprain

Sprains are common joint injuries. They are caused by forcing a joint beyond its normal range of motion. This results in excessive stretching of the ligaments that form the joint, which can cause irritation to the ligaments and, in severe sprains, result in complete tearing of the ligaments.

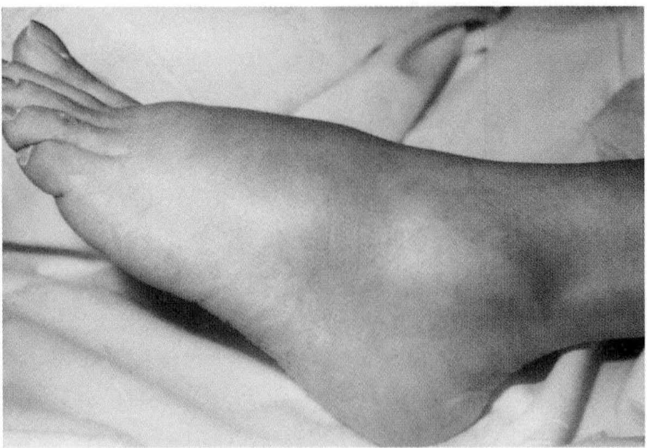

Figure 45-12 Swelling and discoloration of the foot and distal fibula.

Sprains occur more frequently during athletic activity. However, some serious injuries can occur when simply walking. The patient typically has pain at the injured joint, although pain may be minimal when the joint is not being manipulated or bearing weight. Some sprains cause ecchymosis in the area of the joint and can be accompanied by swelling. In the field, ruling out the possibility of fracture or dislocation is difficult. Severe sprains often are accompanied by dislocation of the joint or fracture of the surrounding bones (Figure 45-12).

Strain

Strains involve damage to the muscles or tendons. They are typically the result of sudden, explosive muscular activity. They can be severe, with the muscle or tendon completely torn. Severe strains are typically seen in athletes participating in competitive sports, although they can occur in anyone. Strains also may occur as a result of traumatic injury from motor vehicle crashes, falls, or assaults when sudden movement of an extremity or the head occurs against taut muscles.

Strains typically present with pain to the injured site. In more severe injuries they may present with swelling and bruising and may even feel warm to the touch. In the prehospital setting, determining the severity of a strain is difficult. Patients with significant pain or mechanism of injury should be transported to the ED for evaluation of the injury.

Management of Sprains, Strains, and Joint Injuries. In the prehospital setting, differentiating sprains, strains, and fractures is impossible. Therefore treat all joint injuries as fractures until proven otherwise. Do not allow the patient to place weight on or use the affected extremity. Carefully assess the presence of distal pulse, motor skills, and sensation before and after management. Care of this type of injury is identical to that for fractures. Apply splints to immobilize the bones above and below the affected joint. Moreover, periodically reassess the injury to ensure no nerve or vascular compromise.

Open Soft Tissue Injuries

[OBJECTIVES 13, 14, 15]

Abrasions

Abrasions occur when the skin experiences shearing forces, such as glancing blows, or slides across a hard surface, such as the road. This action results in damage to the outermost skin layers. The wound that results presents with little or no bleeding, though capillary oozing often is present. The wound is quite painful because of the broad area of damage and the involvement of the nerve fibers within the dermis. An additional complication is the contamination often present within the wound. This is particularly true if the injury was caused by sliding on asphalt as a result of a motor vehicle ejection or motorcycle crash. Pieces of gravel or dirt may be embedded within the patient's skin.

Management of Abrasions. Abrasions are rarely life threatening. However, they may distract the patient from more serious injuries. You must not exclusively focus on this injury at the expense of more life-threatening conditions (Figure 45-13). Transport often is indicated even in the absence of significant underlying trauma.

Lacerations

A laceration is a break in the skin that can be superficial or may extend deep into underlying tissue. Lacerations may be **linear,** with regular margins, or **stellate,** with irregular or jagged margins. Lacerations are typically caused by forceful impact with a sharp object. They also may be caused by dull objects that strike with a high level of force. They characteristically have jagged edges and bleed freely. Although they may be isolated, they also can occur along with other soft tissue injuries. Thus be sure to assess the patient carefully for concomitant injuries. Bleeding can be severe and may require aggressive action to control. Closure of the wound may require careful reapproximation of the edges to prevent extensive scar formation (Figure 45-14).

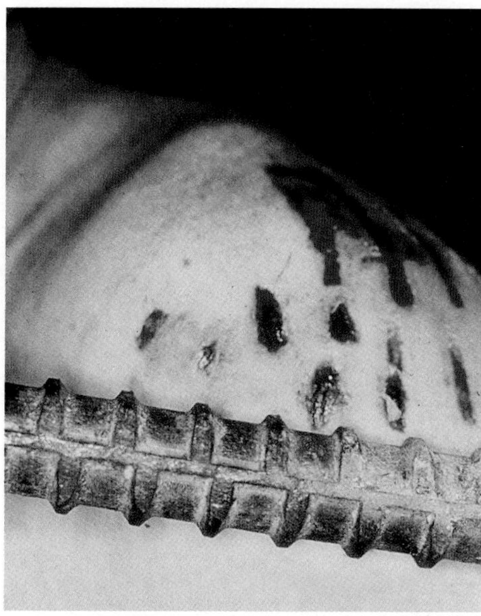

Figure 45-13 Patterned abrasion caused by a piece of rebar. Note the tissue tags at the inferior margins, indicating a downward direction to the blow that caused this injury.

Incisions

Similar to lacerations, incisions may be of varying depth and can bleed extensively. Unlike lacerations, an incision is smooth and even. An incision is usually caused by a sharp object, such as a knife, piece of metal, or scalpel. Incisions tend to heal better and more quickly than lacerations and are normally easier to close (Figure 45-15).

Management of Lacerations and Incisions. Despite their difference in appearance and mechanism of injury, initial care of incisions and lacerations is the same. Your care includes aggressive bleeding control and assessment for other potentially life-threatening injuries. Extensive wound cleansing is not typically performed in the prehospital setting because of a lack of radiograph capability and sufficient lighting to identify foreign material within the wound. In EMS systems with a prehospital wound closure protocol, lacerations present a special challenge because of their irregular borders, which may prohibit prehospital closure attempts. Always follow your local protocol when considering wound closure in the prehospital environment.

Avulsions

Avulsions are flaps of skin or other tissue pulled partially or completely off the patient. The injury is typically dramatic in appearance. It may bleed profusely, particularly if the scalp is involved. This type of injury can range from a minor partial avulsion of skin to an extreme partial or complete avulsion of large areas of skin.

Two particular types of avulsions you will commonly see are degloving injuries and ring injuries. Degloving typically occurs in industrial or agricultural settings. With these injuries, the skin of a finger or the entire hand is forcibly removed, leaving the underlying structures exposed. This can be extremely painful. Degloving also can occur in the lower extremities and feet. Without prompt care, a degloving injury can result in loss of the use of the extremity or even amputation.

Ring injuries are similar to degloving, but they typically occur when a person jumps up to reach a high object or falls from a height and a ring becomes tangled. The finger is then forcibly withdrawn from the ring. This results in the removal of the skin or more tissue from the finger and, in many cases, amputation of the entire finger. Because of the extreme nature of these avulsions, they often are classified as amputations (Figure 45-16).

Amputations

The complete removal of a portion of an entire extremity is called an *amputation.* It may involve any of the extremities or appendages of the body. Moreover, it can result

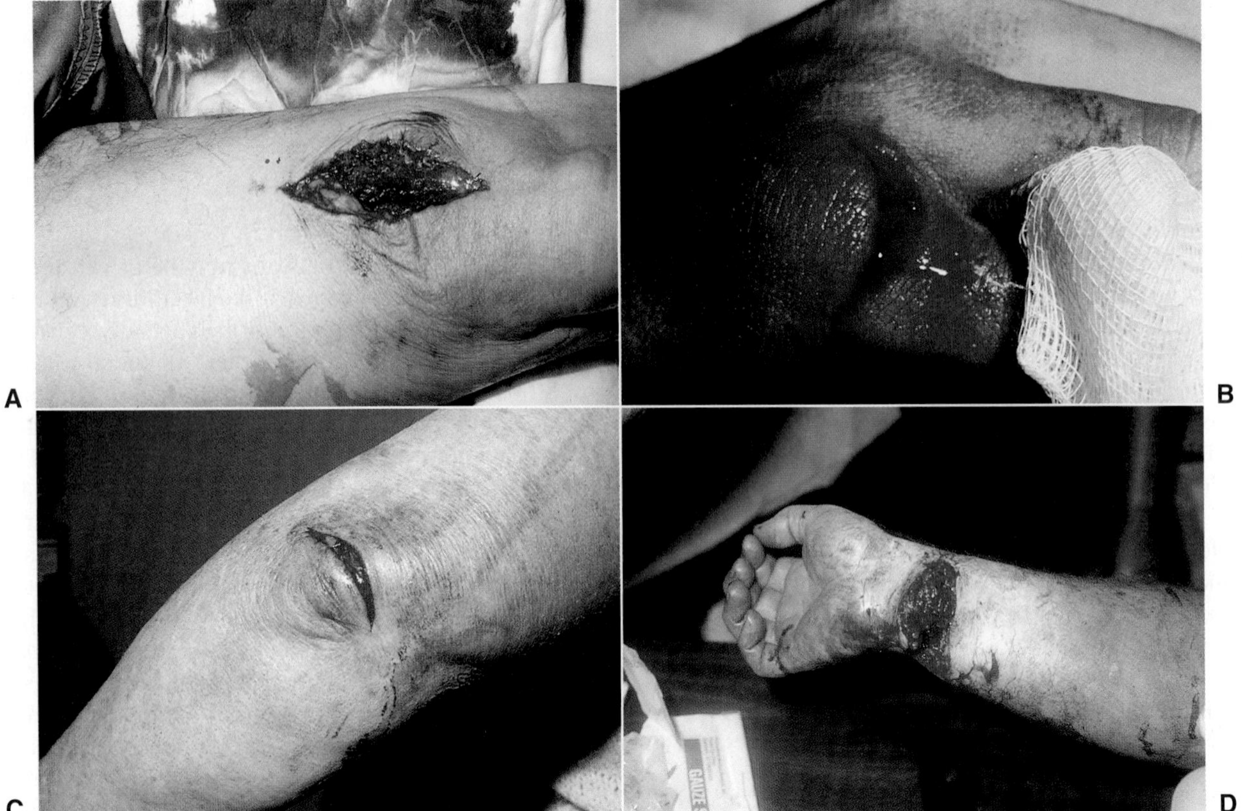

Figure 45-14 **A,** Deep laceration to the thigh caused by a circular saw. **B,** Laceration over the knuckle on the lateral aspect of the hand was caused when the patient struck another person in the teeth. Lacerations in this area suggest contamination from human bite wounds. **C,** Laceration of the elbow caused by a fall on the street. **D,** Laceration to the wrist.

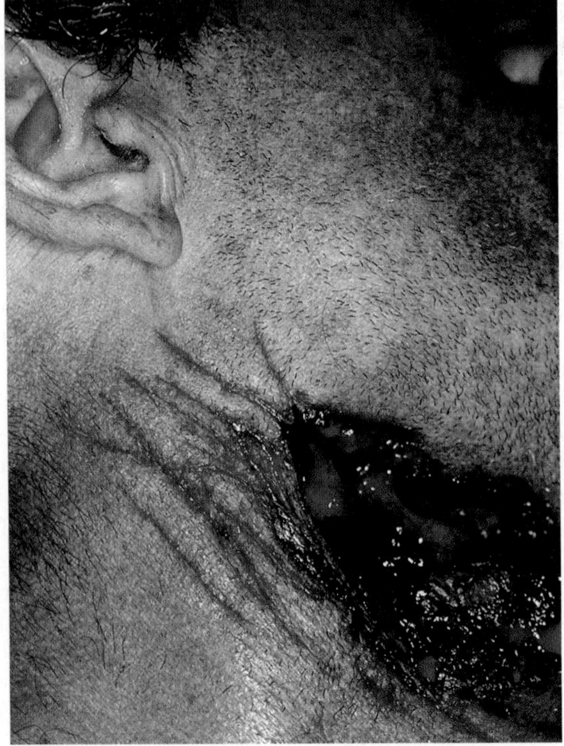

Figure 45-15 Self-inflicted incised wound of the neck with multiple hesitation marks.

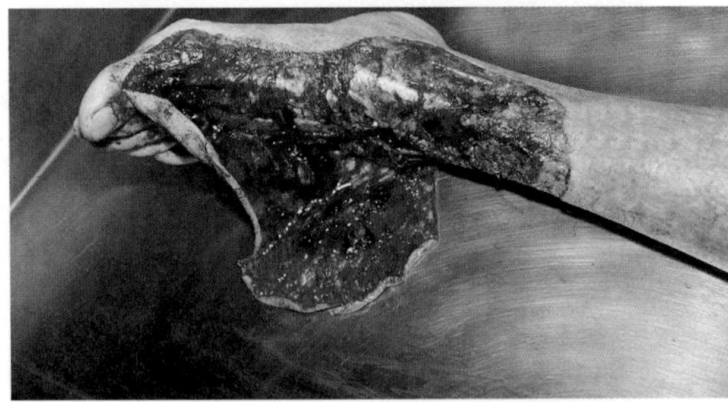

Figure 45-16 Avulsed laceration in motor vehicle crash victim. The victim was the driver, and this injury most likely was caused by the brake pedal.

from a variety of mechanisms. Traumatic amputations usually involve jagged skin, other tissue, and bone at the site of amputation. Bleeding can be severe but also may be minimal depending on the location of the amputation and the damage to adjacent tissue. Not all amputations require tourniquets to control hemorrhage. In fact, tourniquets should not be the first method used to control bleeding. Amputations may be classified as either complete or partial. Degloving injuries sometimes are categorized as a third type of amputation.

Management of Avulsions and Amputations. When caring for traumatic amputations, you must recognize the possibility of replantation of the amputated part and approach these cases as though you had two patients: the victim and the amputated part. Each requires specific care if replantation will be successful. Treatment and transport of the patient should not be delayed to find or care for the amputated part. However, allocating resources to care for and transport the part to the same facility as soon as possible is appropriate (Figure 45-17).

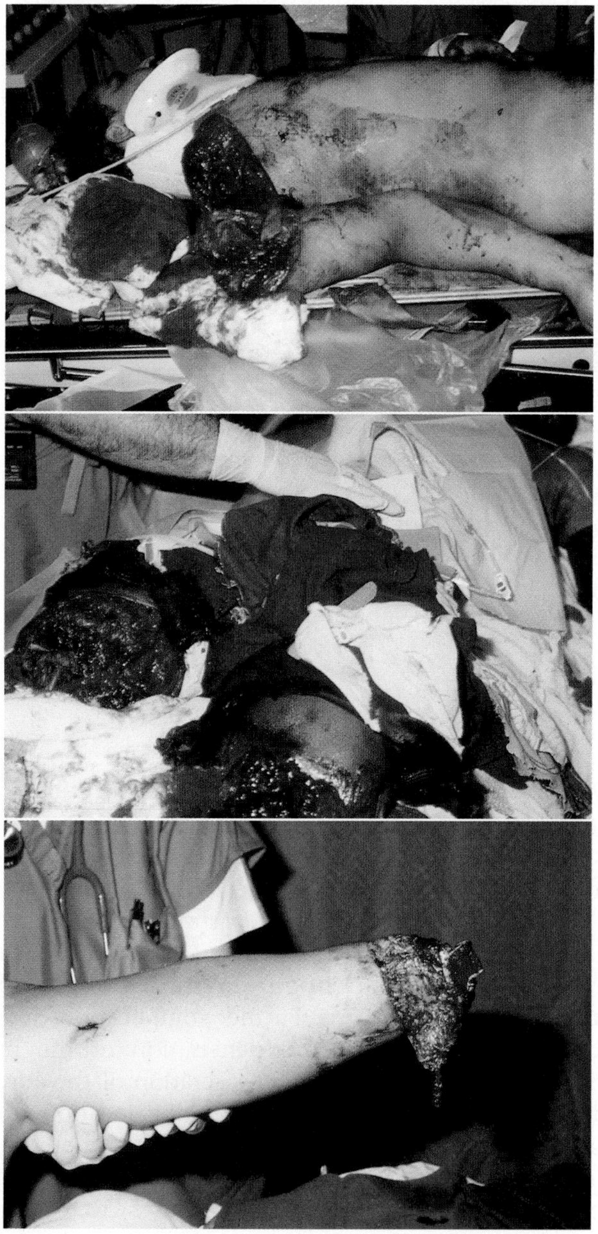

A

B

C

Figure 45-17 A, Amputation of the arm at the shoulder. **B,** Amputation of both legs. **C,** Amputation of the foot.

Amputations and avulsions represent some of the most graphic soft tissue injuries. They threaten the life or limb of a patient and also often result in high anxiety. As previously mentioned, providing the patient with the best opportunity for replantation of the affected part requires two key steps. You must rapidly transport the patient to an appropriate facility and provide proper care of the amputated or avulsed part. Regarding proper transport of the patient, you must be familiar with local medical facilities and their capabilities. Often replantation of the part requires the services of vascular surgeons. Transporting the patient to a facility with that specialty is prudent. When in doubt, consult medical direction and local protocol for assistance with appropriate hospital selection.

PARAMEDIC*Pearl*

Approach a situation involving an amputation as though you have two patients—the actual patient and the amputated or avulsed part.

Care of the amputated or avulsed part depends on the condition of the tissue involved (Skill 45-1). In cases of avulsion in which the tissue is only partially removed, place the tissue in its normal position. Then dress and bandage the injury. Do not remove avulsed tissue. However, some form of irrigation or gross decontamination may be required to remove potentially infectious material (e.g., feces, saliva) from the tissue before bandaging. In cases of complete amputation, locate the part and transport it with the patient to the hospital. If locating the part would extensively delay transport, proceed with taking the patient to the facility. The part should then be transported to the same facility once it is located. Care of the part is designed to prevent further tissue damage and focuses on keeping the part clean and cool during transport. The part should be wrapped with moist sterile dressings and then placed in a sealed plastic bag or similar container. This bag or container should then be placed in a basin of cool water in which ice or ice packs have been added. The part must not be frozen; ensure the water bath is cool but not excessively cold. Additionally, the part should not be directly packed in ice or placed directly in the water. The stump should also be covered with a moist sterile dressing to avoid further contamination. These recommendations may vary, so you must consult your local protocol for the care of amputated parts.

SKILL 45-1 CARE OF AMPUTATED PART

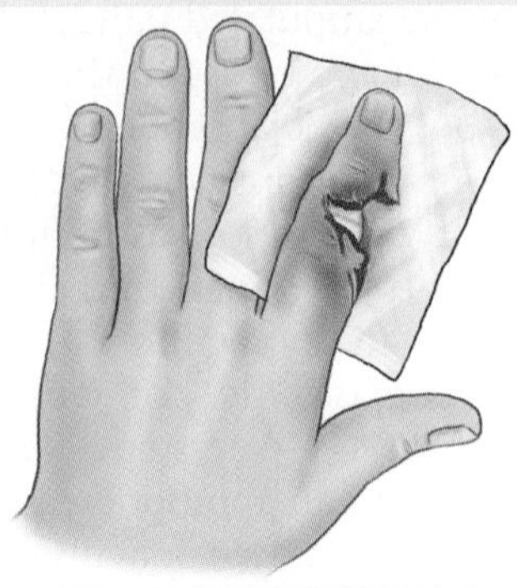

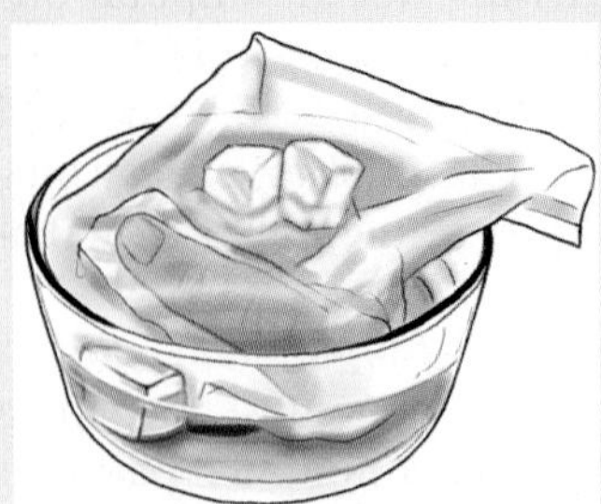

Step 1 Use appropriate PPE, including, at a minimum, medical examination gloves.
Step 2 Control the hemorrhage caused by the amputation.
Step 3 Locate the amputated part.
Step 4 Clean any gross contaminants from the part.
Step 5 Wrap the part in sterile dressings.
Step 6 Place the wrapped part in a sealed plastic bag or similar container.
Step 7 Place the sealed container in a basin of water cooled with ice packs.
Step 8 Do not allow freezing of the part, simply keep the temperature of the water cool.
Step 9 Transport the part with the patient or to the same facility to which the patient is transported.

PPE, Personal protective equipment.

Case Scenario CONCLUSION

You and your partner place the patient on oxygen by nasal cannula at 5 L/min and start an intravenous line (IV). The left ankle is splinted in place with a cardboard splint, and you place moist gauze over the avulsion. You administer 2 mg morphine twice during transport, reducing the patient's pain from a level of 10 out of 10 to 4 out of 10. On arrival at the emergency department, the patient's color is improved, his pulse is 96 beats/min, blood pressure is 112/80 mm Hg, and respiratory rate is 18 breaths/min. The patient is diagnosed with an isolated soft tissue injury to the left foot (no fractures) and is taken to the operating room for definitive repair.

Looking back

7. *Given the patient's final disposition, was your treatment appropriate? Why or why not?*
8. *What are the advantages and disadvantages of aggressive pain management in a patient such as this?*

Punctures and Penetrations

Punctures and penetrations represent potentially life-threatening injuries. Even when these injuries are superficial, they present significant risk for infection or complications. Punctures are caused by a foreign object entering the body. The mechanisms of injury that cause them range from stepping or falling onto a sharp object, such as a nail, to gunshot wounds and stabbings. Bleeding from the wound can be minimal. This may be the case if the wound is located on an extremity or if the wound involves a major compartment that can contain the blood loss, such as the chest. Despite the typically unremarkable external appearance of the wound, internal damage can be extensive, particularly in the chest, abdomen, head, or neck.

Punctures to the chest cavity carry significant risk. These injuries should be considered life threatening until evaluated in the emergency department. Punctures into the chest cavity can cause **simple pneumothorax, hemothorax,** or an **open pneumothorax** with a **sucking chest wound.** Further complications include **tension pneumothorax,** penetration of the heart, **pericardial tamponade,** or laceration of the aorta or subclavian arteries. Depending on the location of the puncture and the course of the injury-causing object, the injuries also can include esophageal, diaphragmatic, or bronchus laceration. Any of these injuries can result from seemingly insignificant puncture wounds. Evaluation of a chest puncture should include determining the size of the object that caused the puncture. For example, determine the caliber of the bullet or length and width of the knife. Particularly in cases of stabbings, consider that extensive movement of the knife's handle was possible while the blade was within the chest. Thus injuries can be extensive even from one stab wound.

As with the thoracic cavity, the abdominal cavity houses many critical structures that are particularly susceptible to penetrating injury. Puncture wounds into the abdomen may cause solid and hollow organ laceration or rupture. In addition, the release of digestive system contents into the abdominal space can result in bacterial infection of the **peritoneum** or chemical irritation, causing **peritonitis.** Some puncture wounds allow portions of the intestines to exit the cavity, creating an evisceration where they protrude from the wound. Assessment of abdominal punctures is complicated by the mobile nature of the skin over the abdomen. This may result in the injury in the skin not lying directly over the injury in the abdominal muscle wall. This can cause you to fail to appreciate the depth of the wound. All puncture wounds to the abdomen should be evaluated in the ED and, as with thoracic wounds, you should attempt to determine the cause of the puncture, the object's size, and the mechanism causing the puncture (Figure 45-18).

Management of Punctures and Penetrations. Your care of punctures and penetrations is typically focused on control of hemorrhage and assessment for potential threats to life. Attempt to identify the size of the object that created the wound to help determine the extent of internal injuries once the patient arrives at the hospital. Notify the police, in accordance with local laws or policy, of all puncture injuries caused by animal bites, assaults, or other possible criminal activity.

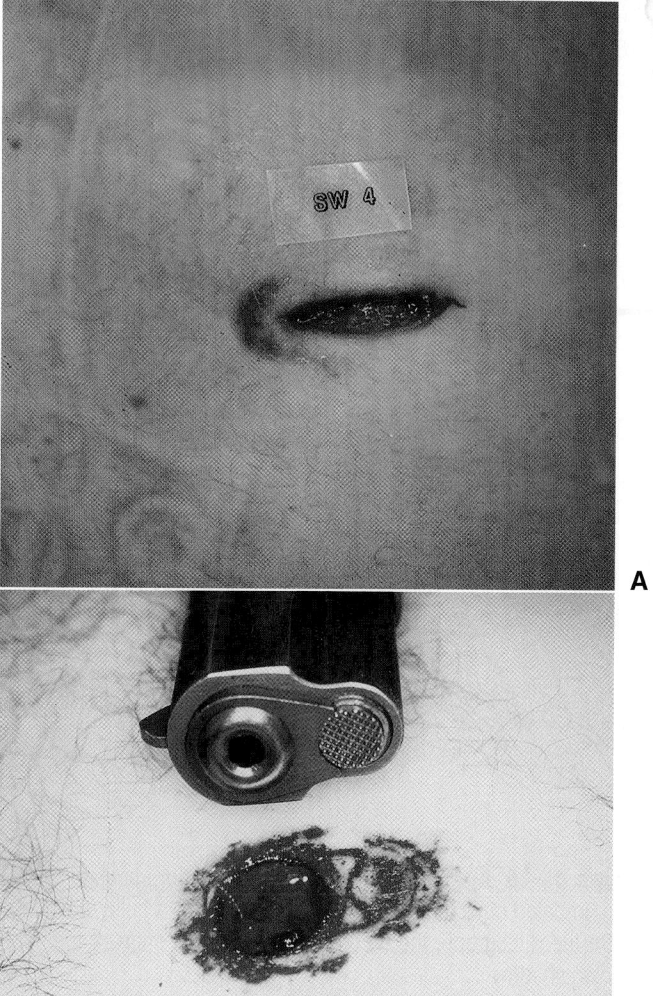

Figure 45-18 By considering mechanism and potential depth, the paramedic can evaluate the potential for serious life threats of puncture wounds. In both instances shown, a significant risk exists of other internal injuries coexisting with the soft tissue injury. **A,** Stab wound with associated hilt mark. Note the sharp margin away from the hilt mark with the blunt margin toward it. A single-edge knife caused this wound. **B,** Contact-range gunshot wound of the chest with a muzzle abrasion.

High-Pressure Injections

A penetration of the body may also occur as a result of high-pressure injection. In the industrial setting, some devices spray liquid material at quite high pressures for the purposes of cleaning, sealing, painting, or lubricating. These agents can be accidentally injected into the hands or arms of a person. This results in an entrance wound that may be draining some of the injected material. Despite their benign appearance, these wounds carry significant risk of complications. Amputation of the extremity often is required. This is particularly true in cases of paint, but less so with water injections.

Management of High-Pressure Injections. Rapidly transport patients with injection injuries to the closest appropriate facility. Consider the area of the body involved when selecting the receiving facility. Ideally, injection injuries to the hand should be managed in a facility that has surgeons who specialize in hand surgery. Additionally, you should provide bleeding control and supportive care.

Impaled Objects

One specific form of puncture wound is when the object that caused the injury remains impaled in the patient. More often than not, the patient (if able) removes the object before EMS arrival. If the object is still in place, do not remove it. The object may actually prevent some hemorrhage by filling the puncture wound. The object should be stabilized to prevent further harm. It should be removed only to protect the patient's airway or by a surgeon in the operating room. Impaled objects present significant prehospital care challenges. They often require trimming of the object to allow transportation (Figure 45-19).

Management of Impaled Objects. Except in extreme cases, patients rarely leave an impaled object in place long enough for EMS to arrive on the scene. When they do leave the object in place, do not remove it because it often acts to tamponade bleeding (Skill 45-2). Additionally, removal of the object can cause further damage to

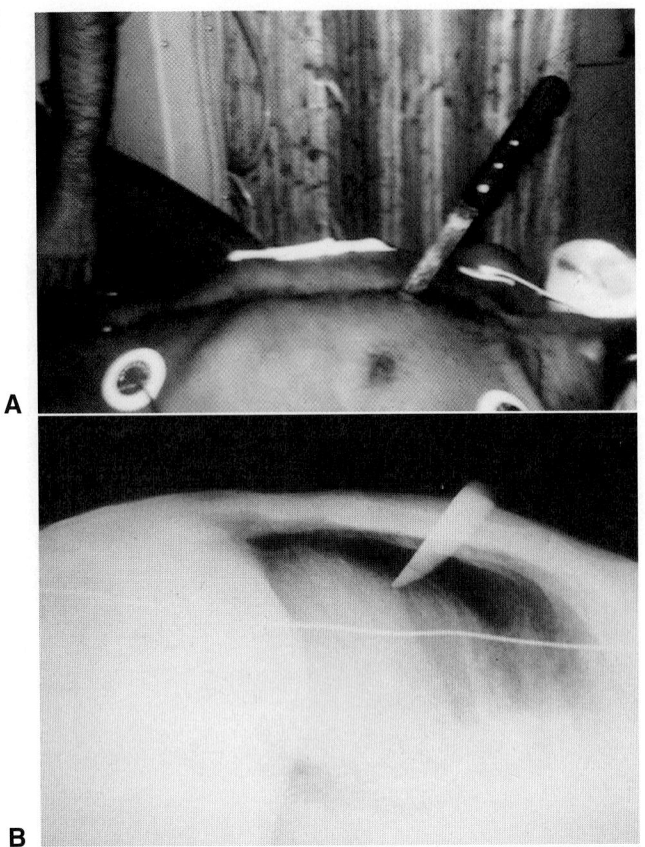

Figure 45-19 **A,** A knife has impaled the anterior chest. In the field, impaled objects are stabilized in place with a bulky dressing. **B,** On the radiograph, the tip of the knife lies just short of the cardiac shadow.

the surrounding structures. Focus prehospital treatment on stabilizing the object in place and transporting the patient with the object to the hospital, preferably a trauma center. This is a simple task when confronted with an impaled knife or similar object. In extreme cases, the surgical team may need to be brought to the patient to remove the object before transport. In every case, consult medical direction before removing the object except when the object obstructs the airway or is so loose that it falls out on its own. Also take care when using devices such as saws and cutting torches to trim the object to a size suitable for transport. In the case of saws, try to minimize the vibration to the patient, although this may be impossible. Also work with the patient to lessen anxiety about having heavy cutting instruments so close to his or her body. In the case of torches, heat transmission and fire are a significant concern. Heat sinks should be used to minimize the transmission of heat to the patient. The fire department should wet the area surrounding the patient before beginning any cutting to prevent fire during the cutting process.

Major Arterial Lacerations

Throughout the body major arteries lie close to the surface of the skin. Many of these locations are used to assess pulse. Wounds in these areas can result in significant bleeding that requires aggressive management. A wound with arterial involvement classically presents with bright-red blood that spurts or flows rapidly from the wound. This type of bleeding can be life threatening and rapidly lead to shock or death if not controlled.

SKILL 45-2 CARE OF IMPALED OBJECT

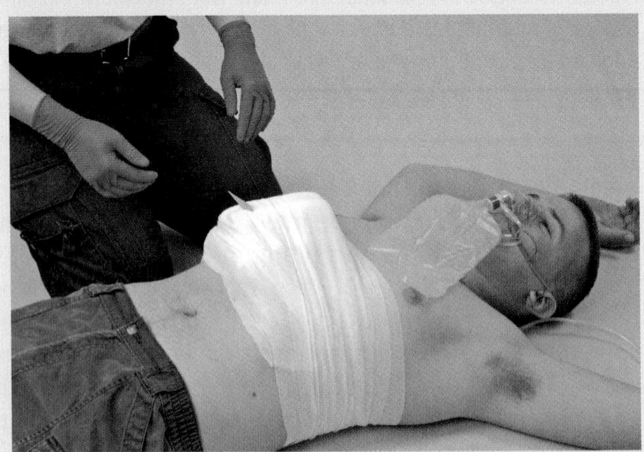

Step 1 Use appropriate PPE, including, at a minimum, medical examination gloves.
Step 2 Assess the injury to ensure the impaled object is not obstructing the airway.
PPE, Personal protective equipment.

Step 3 If the object is obstructing the airway (through the cheek), carefully remove the object.
Step 4 Control the hemorrhage as needed.
Step 5 If the object is not obstructing the airway, stabilize it in place.
Step 6 Place bulky dressings, such as rolls of gauze or folded trauma dressings, around the object to prevent lateral movement.
Step 7 With roller gauze or triangle bandages, secure the bulky dressings to restrict lateral movement of the object.
Step 8 Periodically assess the bandaging to ensure the object is supported and movement is restricted (do not move the object to assess the bandage).
Step 9 If the object is too large to allow transport in the ambulance, work with rescue personnel on scene to trim the object or arrange for alternate transport.

Management of Major Arterial Lacerations. Arterial spasms may slow the pace of bleeding in some injuries. However, aggressive bleeding control measures are usually required to stop blood loss. Additionally, in large arteries such as those in the neck, **air emboli** may form. Occlusive dressings are recommended as part of the management of the wound.

Crush Injuries

[OBJECTIVES 16, 17, 18, 19]

Crush injuries frequently present with little external evidence of the extent of internal trauma. Crushing involves the destruction or damage of large areas of tissue. These injuries often involve complications during the healing process. In addition to an increased risk of infection, crush injuries can result in high pressures within muscle compartments that prevent capillary filling. This can result in widespread tissue hypoxia and cellular damage. Leakage of the contents from damaged muscle cells can result in a condition known as **rhabdomyolysis.** Crush injuries often require aggressive management in the emergency department and can result in loss of the extremity or even death.

Crushing injuries can occur in building collapses after earthquakes, storms, floods, or explosions. They also can be the result of motor vehicle crashes, trench collapse, and industrial accidents. In fact, any prolonged compression of a part of the body may result in a crush injury, including an unconscious person lying on an extremity, prolonged use of a pneumatic antishock garment, an air-splint application, or improperly applied casts.

Crushing can cause extensive damage to muscle tissue and result in major fractures. Additionally, crushing of the chest or abdomen may cause extensive damage to internal organs. In cases involving the chest, a crush injury may result in **traumatic asphyxia** and death. External bleeding may be minimal or even absent, whereas internal hemorrhage can be severe. Finally, crushing force applied to an extremity for a prolonged period may result in the impairment of normal metabolic function of the involved tissue. This impairment is not easily corrected by the restoration of circulation. It often results in a series of events described as **reperfusion phenomenon** that leads to **crush syndrome,** or rhabdomyolysis.

During the crushing phase of injury, blood flow to the extremity is obstructed, resulting in ischemia of the tissue. This, in turn, results in hypoxia at the cellular level, leading to decreased adenosine triphosphate (ATP) production. The lack of ATP results in a decrease in sodium (Na^+) and potassium (K^+), which allows excessive Na^+ and water to flow freely into the cell (Box 45-5 and Figure 45-20).

Restoration of blood flow brings oxygen in contact with the cells, but it also brings an oxygen **free radical** known as *oxygen superoxide*. This free radical attacks the cell membrane through the process of **lipid peroxidation.** This makes the membrane permeable to ions and water, resulting in further stretching of the cell. The damage to the membrane leads to the influx of calcium (Ca^{++}) into the cell and mitochondria. This influx causes mitochondrial swelling and death and ultimately cellular

BOX 45-5 Sodium-Potassium Pump

The sodium-potassium pump involves the active transport of the cation Na^+ to the outside of the cell and the cation K^+ to the inside of the cell. This movement occurs when an ATP molecule is used to stimulate the transport of three Na^+ molecules to the outside of the cell and bring two K^+ molecules into the cell. Movement of sodium to the outside of the cell is essential for the prevention of excessive swelling of the cell, and the corresponding shift of potassium into the cell is essential for enzymatic activity. The combined shift of electrolytes, by placing more ions that are positive outside the cell than inside, creates an electrical potential that allows the excitability of muscle cells (see Figure 45-20).

Reprinted from Thibodeau, G. A., & Patton, K. T. (2003). *Anatomy & physiology (5th ed.)*. St. Louis: Mosby.

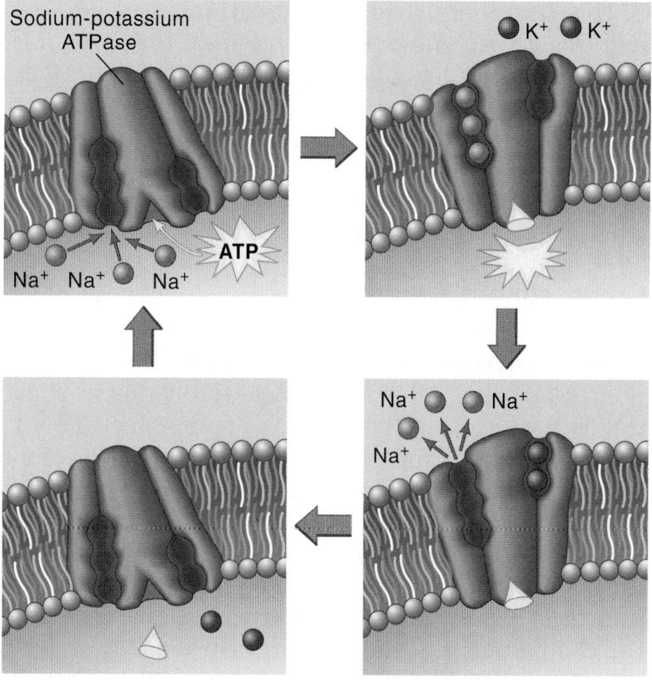

Figure 45-20 Active transport and the sodium-potassium pump. Three Na^+ ions bind to sodium-binding sites on the carrier's inner face. At the same time, an energy-containing adenosine triphosphate (ATP) molecule produced by the cell's mitochondria binds to the carrier. The ATP breaks apart, transferring its stored energy to the carrier. The carrier then changes shape, releases the three Na^+ ions outside the cell, and attracts two K^+ ions to its potassium-binding sites. The carrier then returns to its original shape, releasing the two K^+ ions and the remnant of the ATP molecule to the inside of the cell. The carrier is now ready for another pumping cycle.

death through the breakdown of ATP production within the mitochondria.

The **influx** of water, Na+, and Ca++ into the cells results in extensive cellular swelling. Finally, it results in cellular death accompanied by disruption of the cellular membrane and disintegration of the nuclear membrane. At the same time, an **efflux** of purines occurs from disintegrating cell nuclei as well as K+, **phosphate, lactic acid, thromboplastin, creatine kinase,** and **creatinine** from the cell into extracellular fluid. Additionally, the **myoglobin** within the muscle cells is released into the circulatory system. This combination of factors leads to rhabdomyolysis, or crush syndrome.

Rhabdomyolysis

Efflux causes hyperkalemia, and influx results in hypocalcemia, which when combined with hypovolemia can lead to cardiac toxicity and irritability. This, in turn, complicates the management of the patient. Additionally, the patient will develop hyperuricemia, hyperphosphatemia, metabolic acidosis, and increased serum creatine level, which contribute to the development of renal failure. Another consequence of rhabdomyolysis is disseminated intravascular coagulation (DIC), which results in thrombus formation throughout the vasculature.

The effects of this process on the kidneys are devastating. DIC causes thrombi to form within the glomerular capillaries, resulting in decreased kidney function. Hypovolemia causes the release of catecholamines, further restricting blood flow to the kidneys. Finally, myoglobin, the protein released from the muscle cells, has a nephrotoxic effect. These factors combine to cause acute renal failure.

Compartment Syndrome

Another complication from crush injuries is **compartment syndrome.** Compartment syndrome is the elevation of pressure within the muscle compartment above the level of capillary perfusion, stopping blood flow to the tissue. Compartment syndrome occurs in areas of the body where the fascia compartments that contain muscles are packed closely together, with little room for expansion. The fascia that surrounds muscles is composed of tough, fibrous tissue that does not stretch. When the muscle is crushed, extensive injury to tissue occurs within the compartment. If the compartment remains intact, a risk of pressure occurs as edema develops. If the pressure climbs above capillary hydrostatic pressure (20 mm Hg), ischemia of the muscle develops. Ischemia prolonged for 6 to 8 hours or more leads to tissue hypoxia and ultimately cell death. The extent of soft tissue trauma to the affected extremity can accelerate the process of tissue death. However, it must be appreciated that crush injuries are only one of several causes of compartment syndrome. The two components that lead to the development of compartment syndrome include tissue in a confined space and an increase in pressure in that space. The increase in pressure can result from a decrease in size of the space or an increase in the contents of the space. Decreases in size occur secondary to mechanisms such as limb compression, constrictive dressings, casts, circumferential burns, thermal injuries, and frostbite. Increases in contents occur secondary to mechanisms such as snake bites, hemorrhage, IV infiltration, overuse of muscles, anticoagulation, and orthopedic injury.

Compartment syndrome often manifests with what are considered the "six *P*'s" of ischemia:

- ***P***ain that is out of proportion to the injury
- ***P***aresthesia
- ***P***aralysis
- ***P***uffiness
- ***P***allor
- ***P***ulselessness (late or nonexistent sign)

Patients who sustain crush injuries can present with any level of consciousness, from alert to unresponsive, depending on other injuries. The affected limb initially may appear normal. Assessment of the extremity involved may reveal flaccid paralysis and sensory loss unrelated to peripheral nerve distribution. This paralysis may mimic spinal injury paralysis.

Early in the course of compartment syndrome, the joint distal to the involved muscles may develop rigor. The skin may be taut and have a wooden texture, with loss of voluntary muscle contractions. As the condition progresses, the patient will experience varying combinations of pain, swelling, sensory changes, weakness, and increased pain with passive stretching of the involved muscles. Although the muscle is experiencing significant ischemia, the distal extremity may still be warm and have pulses because it requires much higher compartment pressures to stop arterial blood flow than to stop capillary flow (Box 45-6).

Not all these symptoms are required to diagnose compartment syndrome. The care of closed crush injuries exhibiting signs of compartment syndrome is generally focused on the relief of pressure through fasciotomy. This procedure is done in the ED, so you should transport the patient immediately. In some cases, such as prolonged extrication, bringing surgical personnel to the scene to perform the procedure in an effort to salvage the extremity may be the best option. All crush injuries should be evaluated in the ED because of the delayed onset of many of these conditions. Surgical relief of the pressure is the

BOX 45-6 Six *P*'s of Compartment Syndrome

- *P*ain
- *P*aresthesia
- *P*aralysis
- *P*uffiness
- *P*allor
- *P*ulselessness (late or nonexistent sign)

PARAMEDIC*Pearl*

It is sometimes difficult to understand the differences between crush injury and compartment syndrome. In crush injury, muscle death precedes increased pressures, whereas in compartment syndrome, increased pressure precedes muscle death.

only definitive treatment for compartment syndrome (Haller, 2004; Counselman, 2004).

Management of Crush Syndrome. Crush injuries can lead to complex conditions. These conditions almost always require ED care (Box 45-7).

Throughout the patient encounter, you must ensure the protection of the airway, breathing, and circulation. Death from crush injuries results from several complex biochemical reactions, including crush syndrome, as previously described. This process generally begins after 4 to 6 hours of entrapment secondary to a crushing mechanism. These reactions result from widespread tissue damage combined with reperfusion of the affected area. These combined factors result in the release of acidic compounds and myoglobin from the extremity. When combined, these components work together to damage the kidneys, eventually resulting in renal failure. Hence, your first objective in the management of crush syndrome is to maintain renal function. In the presence of hypovolemia, consult medical direction and consider giving a 1- to 1.5-L fluid bolus. Fluid therapy is important to maintain kidney perfusion. You may need to begin the process of alkalization of the urine. This process alters myoglobin to a form that can be passed through the renal tubules. This is initially accomplished through the addition of sodium bicarbonate to 1 liter of IV fluid. This often is performed in the ED rather than the field. Consult your local protocol to determine if this is begun in the field or reserved for the ED in your area.

In an effort to preserve renal function, care is geared toward a goal of 300 mL/hr of urine production. In some areas, the paramedic will be instructed to mix mannitol with 1 L of IV fluid. Furosemide should not be given because of its tendency to acidify the urine. Depending on protocol, you may be instructed to administer what is considered the "ideal" IV fluid for crush syndrome—dextrose 5% and 0.45% normal saline with sodium bicarbonate and mannitol added. This combination addresses all the goals of initial care by correcting hypovolemia, acidosis, and hyperkalemia and preventing renal failure.

BOX 45-7 Prehospital Goals for Crush Injuries

- Prevent sudden death
- Prevent renal failure
- Salvage limbs
- Initiate care early

Ultimately definitive care will be provided in the emergency department. Thus you should ensure that transport is not unnecessarily delayed.

Management of Crush Injuries. Open crush injuries involve the risks of crush syndrome and a significant risk of infection. Care of these injuries involves normal dressing and bandaging, protection against crush syndrome, and gross decontamination of the wound to prevent the development of life-threatening infection. Every open crush injury should be evaluated in the ED.

In some areas hyperbaric oxygen may be used to treat crush injuries. The goal of this procedure is to expose the patient to the presence of oxygen under higher atmospheric pressure in an effort to get more oxygen to the affected extremity. This treatment has been shown to diminish the extent of tissue necrosis, inhibit lipid peroxidation from oxygen free radicals, and decrease muscle edema. To realize these effects, hyperbaric oxygen must be delivered early. Consult local protocol to determine the availability and use of this treatment in your area for the management of crush injuries.

Blast Injuries

A blast injury involves damage to a victim exposed to a pressure field or wave. Blast injuries are discussed in detail in Chapter 43.

COMMON SOFT TISSUE INFECTIONS

The skin is an important barrier that protects the body from infectious organisms that exist in the environment and even on the surface of the skin itself. Any time that protective barrier is breached, such as from trauma or burns, an opportunity exists for microorganisms to enter the wound and cause infection. Some infections are local and well within the capability of the normal immune system to resolve. However, some are severe enough to develop into life-threatening illness, particularly in patients with compromised immune systems. The failure to recognize and treat these infections can result in loss of function as well as death.

Bacterial Skin Infections

Most common skin infections result from the *Staphylococcus* genus of bacteria, specifically *Staphylococcus aureus,* but may also be caused by beta-hemolytic streptococci. Both types of bacteria are part of the normal bacterial flora of the skin and therefore do not require gross contamination of wounds to cause infection.

The most common infections typically do not result in the activation of EMS, but they may be encountered when conducting examinations of patients reporting other injury or illness. Therefore they are presented here for a more complete range of infectious conditions involving soft tissue. When dealing with any type of open wound or lesion, you must remember to wear gloves and wash your hands. Gloves protect you from exposure and also protect the patient, particularly the immunocompromised patient, from any microorganisms you carry.

Folliculitis

Folliculitis is the infection of hair follicles, most commonly involving the scalp and extremities. It is caused by the collection of bacteria, most commonly *S. aureus*, at the base of the hair, with subsequent invasion of the follicle. Conditions that predispose patients to these infections are prolonged skin moisture, skin trauma, and poor hygiene. Normally presenting as pustules with erythematous borders, these infections rarely cause systemic symptoms. Treatment is typically limited to topical antibiotics, warm soaks and, in severe cases, treatment by a dermatologist.

Furuncles

Furuncles, or boils, often are the result of folliculitis that has spread from the hair follicle to the surrounding dermis. Like folliculitis, the common causative organism is *S. aureus*, and it is unlikely to progress to a systemic infection. Initial presentation is a painful, deep nodule that exhibits redness on the skin and can be 1 to 5 cm in diameter. As the infection progresses, it develops into a tender and **fluctuant nodule.** Incision and drainage may be necessary, and large amounts of pus and necrotic tissue may be expressed during drainage. Any area of the body with hair may develop furuncles, and multiple infections may be present in one area (Figure 45-21).

Carbuncles

Carbuncles result when several furuncles coalesce to form a large area of infection, often connected with channels. They often occur along the back of the neck, upper back, and the interior thighs and are more common in patients with diabetes or suppressed immune systems. They often are treated with warm compresses to cause spontaneous drainage. They can progress to form abscesses, which often require incision and drainage by a physician.

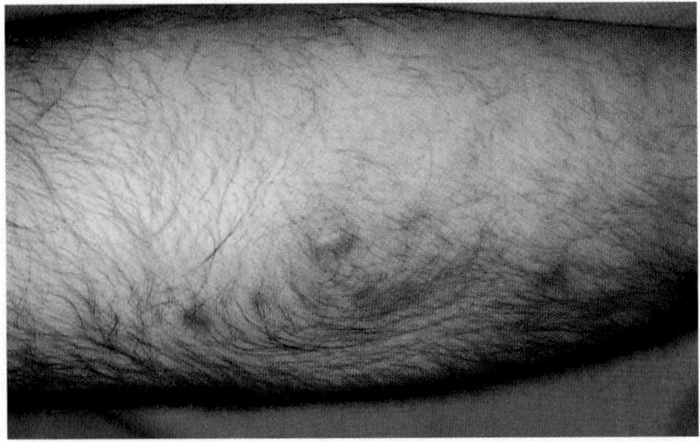

Figure 45-21 Furuncle of the forearm.

Cellulitis

Cellulitis is a local infection of the skin that produces swelling, warmth, and redness to the affected area. This infection is typically caused by staphylococci and streptococci in adults and *Haemophilus influenzae* in children. This infection is commonly associated with patients who have suppressed immune systems or diabetes mellitus. However, it can and does occur in patients of all ages and varying immunity.

Normally the infection does not become systemic. It is treated with antibiotics. Systemic spread is seen more commonly with patients who are immunosuppressed. Evidence of serious infection involves swelling in associated lymph nodes. A particularly serious finding is the presence of high fever and chills. This finding may indicate **bacteremia,** particularly with high-risk patients such as those with suppressed immune systems and diabetes. Prehospital treatment of these patients is focused on supportive care. Do not allow the patient to walk on the affected extremity, which should be elevated during transport.

Necrotizing Cellulitis

The most superficial of the **necrotizing** soft tissue infections is necrotizing cellulitis. This infection involves only the skin and subcutaneous tissue, not the underlying fascia. The common historic findings include recent trauma or surgical treatment to the affected extremity. However, it may spontaneously develop in patients with diabetes. The assessment typically reveals pain and redness to the affected area. The extremity may also exhibit **ecchymosis** or obvious necrosis of the skin and underlying tissue. Vesicles or blebs also may be present. The most common definitive treatment is surgical debridement. Thus prehospital care is typically limited to supporting the patient and dressing and elevating the affected extremity.

Necrotizing Fasciitis

Necrotizing fasciitis is typically a polymicrobial infection widespread throughout the affected area, including the dermis and subcutaneous tissue as well as the underlying fascia. However, it does not spread past the fascia to include the musculature. This infection gained notoriety in the 1990s when the media publicized it as the "flesh-eating bacteria." It is not a new arrival, though, to the world of soft tissue infections. The infection is typically polymicrobial, including a mixture of anaerobic and aerobic bacteria. Occasionally, however, it can be caused by a single organism, typically group A streptococcus.

Patients at greatest risk of contracting necrotizing fasciitis have suppressed immune systems or impaired circulatory function. Predisposing factors include smoking and IV drug abuse. The infection is commonly initiated by soft tissue trauma, surgical incisions, bites, and other breaks in the skin, such as needle punctures, insect bites, or ulcerations. Once the patient is infected, the toxins released from the bacteria cause inflammation of the local blood vessels. This leads to coagulation of blood in the lumen of the vessel. This obstruction results in decreased blood supply, which allows the spread of the infection. Mortality rates are as high as 25% to 50% with this infection.

Patient presentation typically includes severe pain, redness, and possible edema to the affected extremity. Late findings include vesicle formation and crepitus-like sensation. Typically the patient will have a low-grade fever and tachycardia that is disproportionately high in relation to the fever. The infection can progress rapidly, often within hours. Because of the aggressive nature of this infection, prehospital care is focused on support of the patient, immobilization of the affected extremity, and rapid transport to the emergency department. You should not administer any medications that could decrease blood flow to the affected extremity, particularly vasopressors. Aggressive fluid resuscitation is indicated. The treatment course in the hospital likely will involve surgical debridement and possibly hyperbaric oxygen therapy.

Gas Gangrene

Gas gangrene, or clostridial myonecrosis, is a life-threatening infection that typically involves bacteria from the *Clostridium* species. They are large, spore-forming, anaerobic bacteria typically found in the soil, gastrointestinal tract, and female genitourinary tract. These bacteria are common in directly contaminated wounds, particularly soft tissue injuries that create anaerobic environments in tissue, such as crush injuries and those with jagged margins. The immunocompromised patient is at greater risk of contracting this type of infection than is the patient with a normal immune system.

Incubation of the bacteria typically takes 3 days. The initial presentation is heaviness of the affected extremity, brawny (hard) edema, and pain out of proportion to the injury. As the infection progresses, toxins released by the bacteria cause cellular destruction, systemic toxicity, and cardiodepression. The cellular destruction leads to further complications through the release of myoglobin, creatine phosphokinase, and potassium from the cells. The affected extremity will develop a bronze or brown discoloration and have a malodorous **serosanguineous** (blood and serous fluid) **discharge.** Blisters may be present as well. The patient typically presents with a low-grade fever and tachycardia that is higher than would be expected with the fever. The patient also may be disoriented.

As in the case of necrotizing fasciitis, this infection can rapidly progress. Treatment requires surgical debridement and often amputation of the affected extremity. Prehospital care includes aggressive fluid resuscitation and transport to a facility capable of surgical intervention. Hyperbaric oxygen may be used after surgery.

Viral Infections

The majority of common skin infections result from bacterial invasions. However, you will encounter several common viral infections during examination and treatment of patients. These infections typically do not require prehospital treatment and are incidental to the specific chief complaint of the patient.

Herpes Simplex Virus

The two common presentations of infection with the herpes simplex virus are caused by two types of viruses, herpes simplex virus 1 (HSV-1) and herpes simplex virus 2 (HSV-2). HSV-1 typically results in infections of the mouth, such as cold sores or fever blisters. HSV-2, on the other hand, is associated with infections of the genitals. Both viruses infect the nerve ganglion associated with the site of infection. Secondary outbreaks occur with reactivation of the virus, which can occur as a result of stress, exposure to ultraviolet light, skin irritation, fever, or fatigue. The patient's presentation is typically a rash or cluster of inflamed and painful vesicles over the affected area. Before the outbreak, the patient may report **paresthesia,** increased sensitivity, and mild burning. The lesions may last from 2 to 6 weeks as the vesicles rupture and form a crust. HSV-2 infection progresses similarly but typically progresses from vesicles to ulcers within 3 to 4 days. These may be accompanied by pain, weeping, and itching. **Viral shedding** continues throughout the visible outbreak stage (Figure 45-22).

Neither herpes simplex virus currently has a cure. Outbreaks are treated with topical or oral antiviral agents to

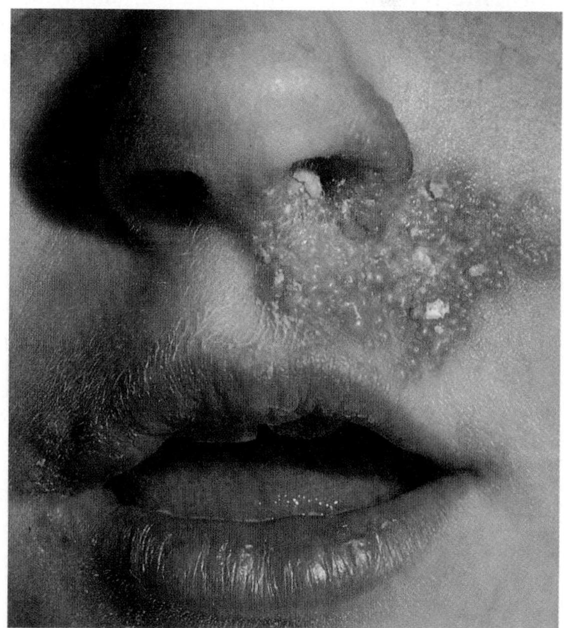

Figure 45-22 Herpes simplex labialis. Typical presentation with tense vesicles appearing on the lips and extending onto the skin.

limit their duration and severity. Some success in controlling outbreaks has been achieved with vaccination. In addition, work continues to develop a prophylactic vaccine.

Herpes Zoster and Varicella

Herpes zoster (shingles) and varicella (chickenpox) are caused by the same virus. The initial infection manifests as chickenpox. After its resolution, the virus lies dormant in trigeminal and dorsal root ganglia. Later in life, the virus reactivates to cause shingles, which initially results in pain and paresthesia localized to a specific dermatome. This is followed by vesicle eruptions along facial, cervical, thoracic, and lumbar dermatomes (Figure 45-23). Herpes zoster infections are more common among the elderly and immunocompromised patients. Treatment is primarily directed to controlling skin irritation through the use of compresses, calamine lotion, and baking soda. Antiviral drugs may be used within 72 hours to prevent postinfection pain, which occurs in approximately 20% of patients.

Hand Infections

Because of the complex structures and critical function of the hand, infections of the hand deserve separate consideration from other soft tissue infections. Whenever possible, most patients with hand injuries or infections that result in EMS activation should be transported to facilities that have access to specialized hand surgeons. Even infections that appear relatively minor may have dire consequences to the continued normal function of the hand. In severe cases, they may result in amputation.

Most hand infections are the result of *Staphylococcus* or *Streptococcus* species infection. However, patients may develop polymicrobial infections with injuries associated with gross contamination of the wound, IV drug abuse, human bites (including self-inflicted bites, such as nail biting), and animal bites. Because of the potential of infection to spread along anatomic compartments of the hand, any infection more severe than paronychia or felons (see below) likely will require surgical intervention.

The general treatment of hand infections and injuries involves proper immobilization. This will help minimize pain and limit worsening of the condition. The proper position of the hand during immobilization can greatly reduce discomfort for the patient and, more importantly, reduce the risk of long-term impairment of hand function. Use splinting material or soft dressings to position the hand in the manner illustrated in Figure 45-24.

Paronychia

Paronychia is an infection of the lateral nail fold or paronychium that occasionally may extend to include the cuticle (Figure 45-25). Typical causes of the infection are minor trauma, such as that associated with nail biting, manicures, and hangnails. *Staphylococcus aureus* is the

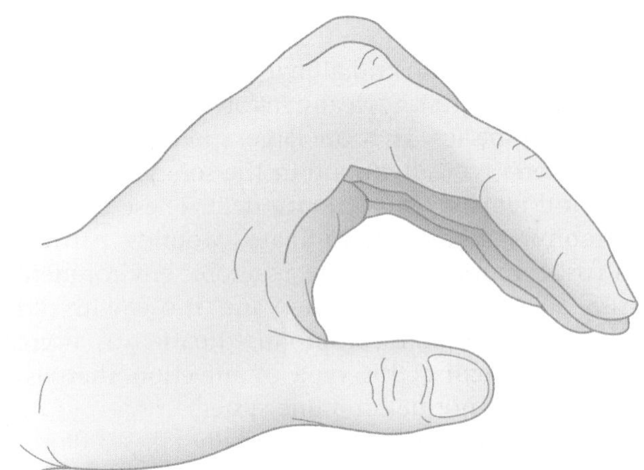

Figure 45-24 The proper position of the hand during immobilization.

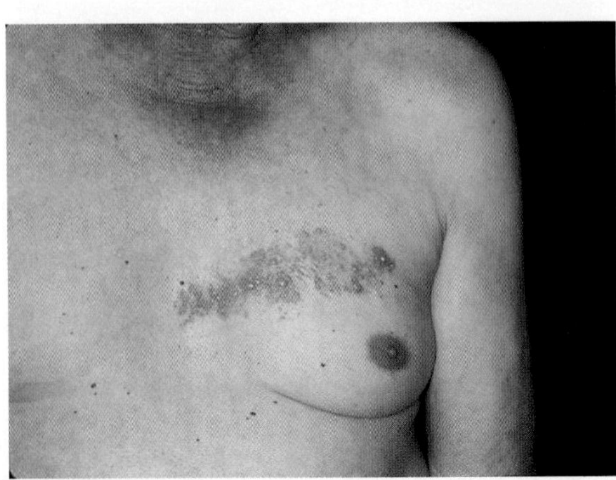

Figure 45-23 Herpes zoster. Diffuse involvement of a dermatome.

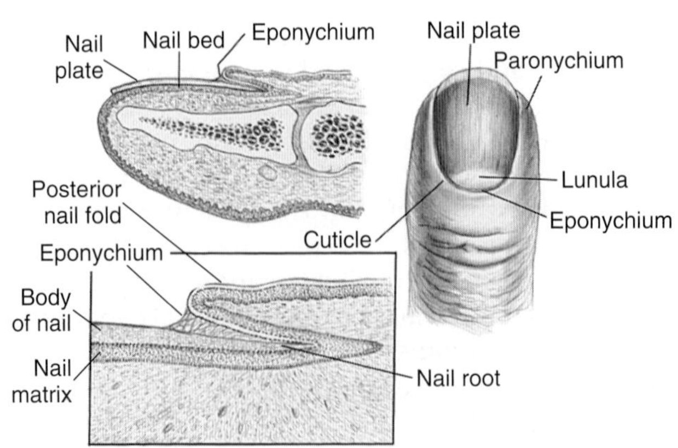

Figure 45-25 Structures of the nail.

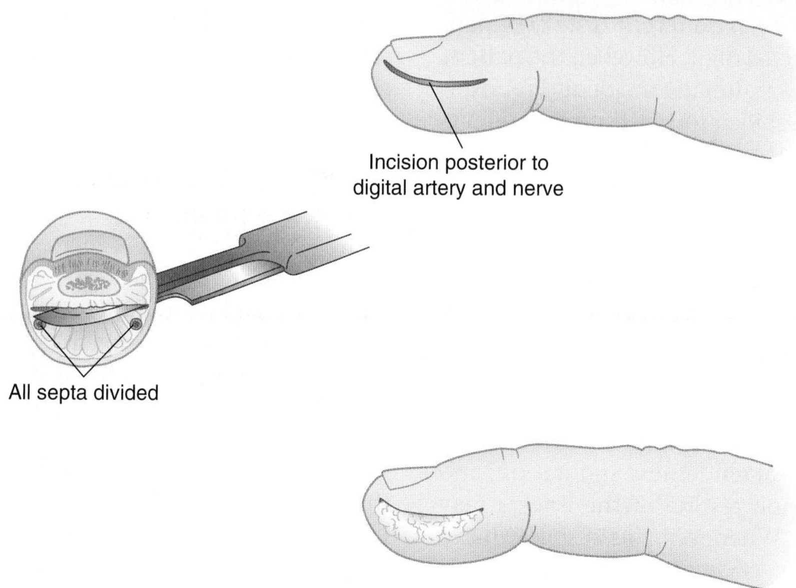

Figure 45-26 Incision and drainage of a felon.

most common infecting agent. Other causative organisms include *Streptococcus* and *Pseudomonas* species. Again, however, the agents may be polymicrobial, particularly in patients with suppressed immune systems or when the wound has been contaminated. Early presentation is a small area of **induration** that is tender and erythematous. At this stage, treatment typically involves warm soaks combined with elevation and topical antibiotics. As the infection progresses, a collection of pus may develop in the fold. This will require drainage in the ED by a physician to resolve the infection. The infection occasionally will involve a portion of the nail and require excision of half or, in severe cases, the entire nail to allow drainage of the infection.

Felon

A felon is a subcutaneous infection of the pulp space of the finger pad. It is characterized by throbbing pain and a red, tense finger pad. This infection typically begins with minor trauma to the dermis. Left untreated, the infection can spread to involve the underlying structures and even develop into **osteomyelitis.** Patients who have swollen, red, and painful finger pads likely will need surgical incision of the abscess and drainage of the pus in the ED (Figure 45-26).

Flexor Tenosynovitis

Flexor tenosynovitis is an infection that involves the flexor tendon sheath (Figure 45-27). These infections can spread rapidly. Failure to identify and manage these infections properly can result in loss of function of the digit or even the hand itself (Box 45-8). This condition should be considered a surgical emergency. Moreover, you should transport the patient to a facility that has specialized hand surgeons available, if possible.

BOX 45-8 Classic Presentation of Flexor Tenosynovitis

- Tenderness over flexor tendon sheath
- Symmetric swelling of the finger
- Pain with passive extension
- Flexed posture of the involved digit at rest

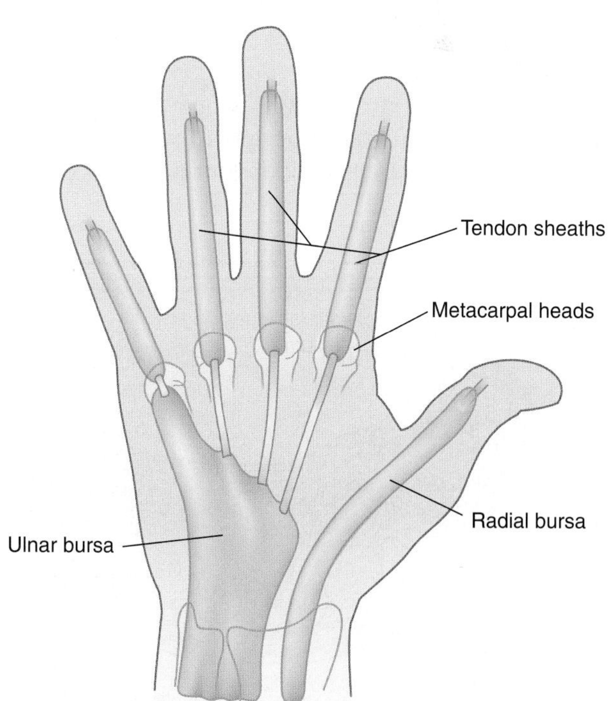

Figure 45-27 Flexor tendon sheath infections can spread rapidly to the radial and ulnar bursae.

The patient typically will have a recent history of penetrating trauma to the affected digit. However, the patient may not actually recall the traumatic incident. Prehospital care is limited to immobilization of the hand, elevation, and transportation to the hospital for likely surgical intervention.

Deep Space Infections

The structure of the hand creates many deep compartments that can become involved in infectious processes (Figure 45-28). Because of the structure of the soft tissues of the palm and dorsal aspects of the hand, dorsal edema is typically present with any infectious process that involves the compartments in the palm. Examination of the infected hand may reveal tenderness, induration, and fluctuance. Range of motion testing of the fingers may produce significant pain. Whenever you suspect that a patient has a deep space infection of the hand, treatment should include immobilization of the hand, elevation, and transportation for surgical consult.

Infection Prevention

Prevention of soft tissue infections is the best long-term strategy. The most effective method for preventing common skin infections and the risk of contaminating patients' wounds is practicing good hygiene, especially regular and thorough handwashing. Most of these infections are caused by bacteria that normally exist in the nares and on the skin. Good handwashing techniques reduce the size of bacteria colonies on your hands and reduce the risk of spreading those colonies to breaches in your own skin or the skin of your patients.

Good Wound Care

Good wound care is essential when managing soft tissue trauma. The use of clean gloves and aseptic techniques greatly reduces the risk of your patients contracting an infection. Removal of debris, when possible, also reduces this risk, as do proper bandaging and dressing techniques.

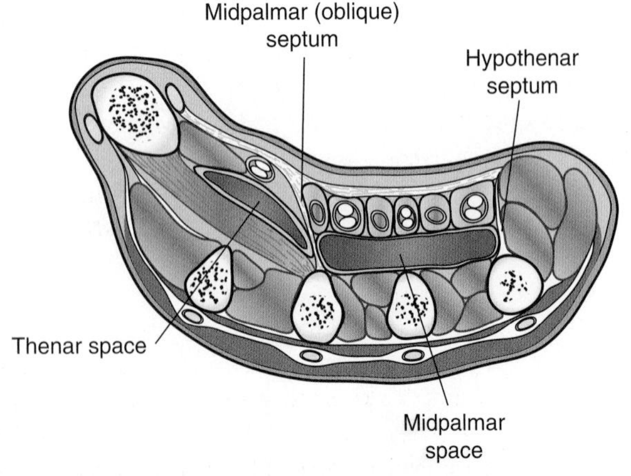

Figure 45-28 Potential mid-palmar compartments.

GENERAL MANAGEMENT OF SOFT TISSUE TRAUMA

[OBJECTIVES 20, 21]

Care of patients with soft tissue trauma begins first with the scene size-up. During this phase, you must evaluate the scene for potential hazards and take steps to eliminate those hazards before entering. The importance of this cannot be overstated. Moreover, the evaluation of safety should begin as soon as the call is assigned to the crew and throughout the time spent on the scene. In particular, situations involving explosions or burns should be considered potentially dangerous if the explosive or fire risk has not been removed. Likewise, cases involving chemical burns present significant risk to the care provider until the patient is properly decontaminated (see Chapter 46). Consider any response for an assault or suicide dangerous until law enforcement has secured the scene.

After assessing for potential dangers, evaluate the scene to determine if additional resources are needed. Consider the number of patients involved and whether any specialized rescue techniques are required. Likewise, attempt to determine the mechanism of injury to anticipate additional injuries or potential complications in the management of the patient. Even though these evaluations are listed as separate steps, they should be performed at the same time as the other components of the scene size-up.

The first priority of managing the patient with soft tissue trauma is to treat underlying life-threatening injuries before treating superficial wounds. Soft tissue trauma is typically not life threatening. However, it may be evidence of more serious internal injuries. The most significant risk to this type of patient is the risk of exsanguinating blood loss and shock. Crucial to managing the patient with soft tissue trauma is assessing for the early signs of shock and aggressively managing shock when it is found. Other life-threatening injuries also may exist, such as those that compromise airway integrity, breathing, or circulation. Although the graphic external soft tissue trauma may capture your attention, you must look for other, potentially more serious injuries.

A key component to managing shock and an important step in managing soft tissue trauma is controlling hemorrhage. Blood loss from soft tissue trauma can range from mild to extreme, depending on the nature of the injury and its locations. Wounds located in the extremities often do not produce life-threatening hemorrhage, but it is possible. For example, a wound to the femoral artery can result in life-threatening hemorrhage. In contrast, wounds to the neck can lead to death in a relatively short period. Methods to control bleeding are discussed in Chapter 44.

PARAMEDIC*Pearl*

When determining the severity of the injury, consider the nature of the bleeding from the wound, the amount of blood already lost, and the proximity of the wound to major vascular structures.

Dressings and Bandages

[OBJECTIVES 20, 21]

After controlling bleeding, apply dressings and bandages to soft tissue injuries. Dressings, which are applied directly to the wound, are used to control bleeding, encourage healing, and prevent infection. Bandages, however, are primarily used to hold the dressing in place and protect against accidental wound contamination. The type of material used to dress a wound depends on the type of wound and the material available for use.

Sterile Dressings. The most common form of dressing on an ambulance is sterile dressings. These have been chemically or radiologically rendered free of bacteria. They are composed primarily of cotton gauze and are packaged in sizes ranging from 2-inch squares to large abdominal or trauma dressings. The most common size is the 4-inch square, commonly known as a 4 × 4. Sterile dressings are typically used when infection is a concern or for direct application to an open wound. This type of dressing often is used, in combination with direct pressure, for primary bleeding control.

Nonsterile Dressings. Another common form of dressing is the nonsterile dressing. These are identical to sterile dressings except that they have not been through the sterilization process. These dressings are clean but are not completely free of bacteria. This type of dressing is primarily used when infection is not a significant concern, particularly to provide bulk when attempting to control bleeding or when cleaning dirt or debris from intact skin. They are normally provided in a package of many 4 × 4 dressings. They are a convenient method to increase the bulk of material rapidly on a heavily bleeding wound or to stabilize impaled objects.

Occlusive Dressings. Most dressing materials used in the prehospital setting are nonocclusive, meaning that air can pass freely through the dressing matrix. This passage of air is not a concern in most injuries. However, wounds that involve the large arteries of the neck or those that open into the chest cavity often require dressings that prevent the free flow of air or are occlusive. The simplest form of occlusive dressing is a plastic sheeting that can be applied over other types of dressings. This is an effective technique when applying moist dressings to exposed organ tissue to prevent drying. The type of dressing most often used to seal wounds into the chest cavity and to cover wounds involving larger arteries is gauze impregnated with petroleum to form an air-proof barrier.

Used properly, these types of dressings can prevent or minimize the entrance of air into the pleural space and the development of pneumothorax with chest trauma. When applied to neck injuries, they can minimize the risk of air emboli. Of note, when applied to chest injuries, the dressing may contribute to the development of a tension pneumothorax. For open chest injuries, tape three sides of the occlusive dressing to create a one-way valve. If signs and symptoms of a tension pneumothorax develop, temporarily remove the dressing to relieve excess pressure. This complication and its management are covered in Chapter 48.

Adherent Dressings. Because dressings used in the prehospital setting are most often used to control hemorrhage, they are typically adherent. This means that they normally become incorporated into the clot and, if left in place, the scab that is formed over the wound. This is initially important to control bleeding but can complicate management of the wound later. Use of this type of material provides additional structure for the body to use for clotting or blocking blood loss. This action is crucial to the control of hemorrhage and is a desirable characteristic of most emergency dressings.

Nonadherent Dressings. Although most of the injuries treated by the paramedic call for the use of adherent dressings, healing in some cases, notably burn patients, can be complicated by adherent dressings. These types of injuries require nonadherent dressing. Such dressing allows wound exudates to pass through them. Nonadherent dressing allows the wound to drain but does not incorporate the dressing into the scab or clot. When managing the burn patient, nonadherent dressings prevent gross contamination of the wounds and do not result in damage to healing tissue when the dressing is removed. Additionally, nonadherent dressings are commonly used after wound closure to allow for drainage away from the wound.

Wet Dressings. For some injuries, wet dressings are the preferable method of management. This is particularly true in cases in which organs are exposed to the air. For safe replantation of organs, the tissue must remain moist and perfused. If the tissue is allowed to dry, salvage is unlikely. When managing a patient with an **abdominal evisceration,** cover the exposed organ tissue with a sterile dressing that has been soaked with sterile saline. Ensure that the dressing remains moist throughout the prehospital phase of treatment. Consider the application of an occlusive dressing over the wet dressing to prevent the evaporation of fluid.

Additionally, wet dressings may be used to enhance the healing process. They enhance healing by creating a wound environment that is supportive of movement of cells across the wound. This is not typically initiated in the prehospital environment, but the use of wet dressings is common in the hospital setting. Except in cases of abdominal evisceration, the majority of dressings applied by paramedics are dry dressings primarily used to control hemorrhage.

Complications

[OBJECTIVE 22]

The complications encountered when bandaging soft tissue injuries often are the result of either too little pressure generated over the wound or too much pressure. In cases in which the bandage is loose or when insufficient direct pressure is applied to the bleeding wound, further hemorrhage can occur. In cases involving major bleeding, this can result in exsanguination. Severe, uncontrolled hemorrhage also may lead to ischemia distal to the injury.

Although too little pressure can result in serious worsening of the patient's condition, excessive pressure also can result in significant harm to the patient. Excessive pressure results from either too much direct pressure, an improperly applied pressure dressing, or swelling that occurs after the bandage has been applied. The increased pressure can result in damage to underlying structures, complicating the patient's recovery.

Wound Cleansing

Most soft tissue injuries in the prehospital setting are treated by applying sterile, absorbent dressing material, typically gauze pads, directly to the wound. Paramedics are not often required to clear debris from a wound before transportation. In the event that a wound is grossly contaminated, particularly with saliva or fecal material, carefully irrigate the wound.

Wound cleansing is best accomplished with at least 500 mL of sterile saline that is directed into the wound under pressure. This effect can be achieved with a 60-mL syringe and an 18-gauge IV catheter (without the needle). The goal is to create a stream of saline that can be used to propel foreign material out of the wound. Commercially prepared devices use IV bags for this procedure. Do not use alcohol, povidone iodine (Betadine), hydrogen peroxide, or similar agents to clean wounds. These chemicals indiscriminately destroy cells, including those needed for healing. Additionally, they all dry the wound, which increases the healing time and the risk for large scar formation.

Bandaging

After cleansing, if indicated, typically use sterile gauze wrappings to secure the dressing over the wound. In the event the patient continues to hemorrhage despite the application of the initial dressing, nonsterile dressings are acceptable to add bulk to the wound area to help clot formation. The bandaging process varies for some areas of the body to prevent injury to adjacent structures or ensure patient comfort.

Head. The shape of the head and the location of the eyes, nose, and mouth present a challenge to the bandaging process. Wounds to the scalp and face often bleed extensively because of the vascular nature of this area. Control of this bleeding is complicated by concerns regarding applying pressure to injuries involving the cranial vault.

You can manage injuries to the top of the head by directly applying sterile dressings to the wound. Gentle but firm pressure may be used if you believe the skull to be intact. If you have any concern or even think a skull fracture is possible beneath the injury, do not apply pressure. The dressing may be held in place with a triangular bandage tied like a pirate's head covering. Roller bandages can be used to secure dressings over wounds to the scalp, but you must take care to ensure the bandage does not cover the victim's eyes, nose, or mouth. It also should not cover the patient's ears, if possible. If the ears must be covered, place a piece of folded gauze behind each ear to prevent the ear from being pushed against the scalp by the bandage.

Face. Injuries to the face present significant challenges to traditional bandaging techniques. Often the best solution is to use tape to hold dressings over relatively small injuries. In cases of bleeding from the nose, or epistaxis, do not have the patient lean his or her head back. This action results in the patient aspirating, or swallowing, blood, which can lead to nausea and, in some cases, vomiting. Instead, have the patient lean forward (when trauma to the cervical spine is not a concern) so that he or she can spit out blood that has run down the back of the throat. Often you can control bleeding from the nose by applying an ice pack to the bridge of the nose or, in some cases, a piece of gauze rolled and placed under the upper lip. Epistaxis can occur from a large vessel or from the posterior chamber, making control of bleeding more difficult. In such cases, the patient must be evaluated in the ED. In some cases, surgery is necessary to control the bleeding.

Bleeding from the ears or mastoid process presents a different problem. In addition to the difficulty in bandaging the wound, bleeding from these areas could be a symptom of more serious head injury. It may actually be a beneficial leaking of fluid from the brain, preventing the development of a dangerously high level of intracranial pressure. For this reason, bleeding from these areas should not be controlled in the prehospital setting. Instead, use gauze to collect the drainage without exerting pressure to the wound.

Neck. Neck injuries represent a potential threat for exsanguination and require aggressive management. This need for aggressive hemorrhage control is complicated by the need to ensure that blood flow to the brain and the structures of the airway is not occluded. Because of this, no bandage should be applied that completely encircles the neck. This is a risk when applied for the purpose of exerting pressure, and any swelling may result in the occlusion of critical structures. In the event that a pressure dressing is necessary, apply an occlusive dressing and support that dressing with bulky nonocclusive dressings. Raise the arm opposite to the injury site and wrap a roller bandage from the injury under the arm and back around the injury several times. Once wrapped in this manner, lower the patient's arm. This exerts pressure on the injury without applying pressure to the noninjured side of the neck. Continuously monitor the patient to ensure the airway is not compromised.

Shoulder. As with neck injuries, wounds to the shoulder represent a challenge when applying bandages. This is attributable to the critical vasculature and nerves located in the axillary region. Additionally, wounds to the shoulder area can, when sufficiently deep enough, compromise the large subclavian arteries or veins, resulting in severe hemorrhage. This compromise typically only occurs with deep penetrating trauma, such as by a knife or a gunshot wound. Bandaging superficial wounds often is best accomplished with tape, but in cases of severe injury use bulky trauma dressing to control bleeding. You can secure the dressing by wrapping roller bandages over the shoulder to the opposite side and back over the shoulder. However, this provides only limited direct pressure. Often manual stabilization of the dressing is all that is effective when continued pressure is necessary to control hemorrhage.

Trunk. Soft tissue trauma to the trunk often is significant because of the underlying internal injuries it may indicate. Carefully assess for the presence of life-threatening internal trauma when treating the patient with soft tissue injuries to the trunk. Often external bleeding is minimal while life-threatening bleeding occurs in the underlying cavity. Always consider penetrating trauma to the trunk as potentially life threatening until proven otherwise. Severe abrasions can occur to the trunk area, particularly in cases of ejection during motor vehicle trauma. These abrasions are rarely treated in the prehospital environment because of the high likelihood of other injuries being present that represent a greater life threat to the patient. The care for these injuries, when other more serious injuries do not demand your attention, should be focused on gross decontamination rather than bandaging.

Groin. As with the trunk, injuries to the groin or pelvic region often occur along with more significant internal injuries. Your provision of care for these injuries should be secondary to the care of serious life-threatening trauma. Still, note that injuries to the groin may result in considerable anxiety and cannot be disregarded. Be prepared to provide significant psychological support to victims of soft tissue injuries to the groin. Bleeding from the vagina could represent serious internal injuries. In the case of pregnancy, it could indicate a serious medical emergency. At no time should the vagina be packed with dressings. Emergency care should include placement of dressings at the vaginal opening to collect the bleeding, but make no efforts at control. Rather, focus on rapid transport to the ED. Examples of types of dressings are shown in Figure 45-29.

DOCUMENTATION OF SOFT TISSUE INJURIES

Documentation is a crucial part of the care of patients with soft tissue trauma. However, most paramedics generally do not consider this a favorite part of the job. Along with providing a mechanism for billing, documentation also serves as a medical record, legal document, and communication device. The medical record is critical for establishing what happened. Moreover, it may be critical as a communication device to ensure that the information discovered during the prehospital assessment is passed along to the emergency department and the rest of the healthcare system. The documents created also serve as a legal record that can be used as evidence in civil and criminal actions regarding the injury. In all three cases, the quality of documentation reflects on the professionalism and competence of you, the paramedic.

A key part of good documentation of patient care is the careful description of the injuries discovered during assessment of the patient. It is understood that you will not discover every injury, as lighting and time are both in limited supply in the prehospital setting. Even so, the injuries that are found should be accurately documented. Diagram complex injuries to provide a reference for when the call is reviewed, sometimes years later.

In addition to specific injuries, be sure to document the patient's response to the treatments provided. For instance, record whether the patient reported any relief of difficulty breathing after pleural decompression or the application of an occlusive dressing. This is relevant information that should be included in the chart. Also document pertinent negatives discovered during the assessment. For example, the fact that a patient with bruising to the chest wall does not report difficult or painful breathing is important. These findings would be considered pertinent negatives. Documenting them proves they were assessed and did not exist.

Finally, carefully document all vital signs recorded during your provision of care to the patient. Remember that a single set of vital signs does not communicate much about the patient's condition. Only a series of signs can detect changes in the patient's status. Be sure to document these changes.

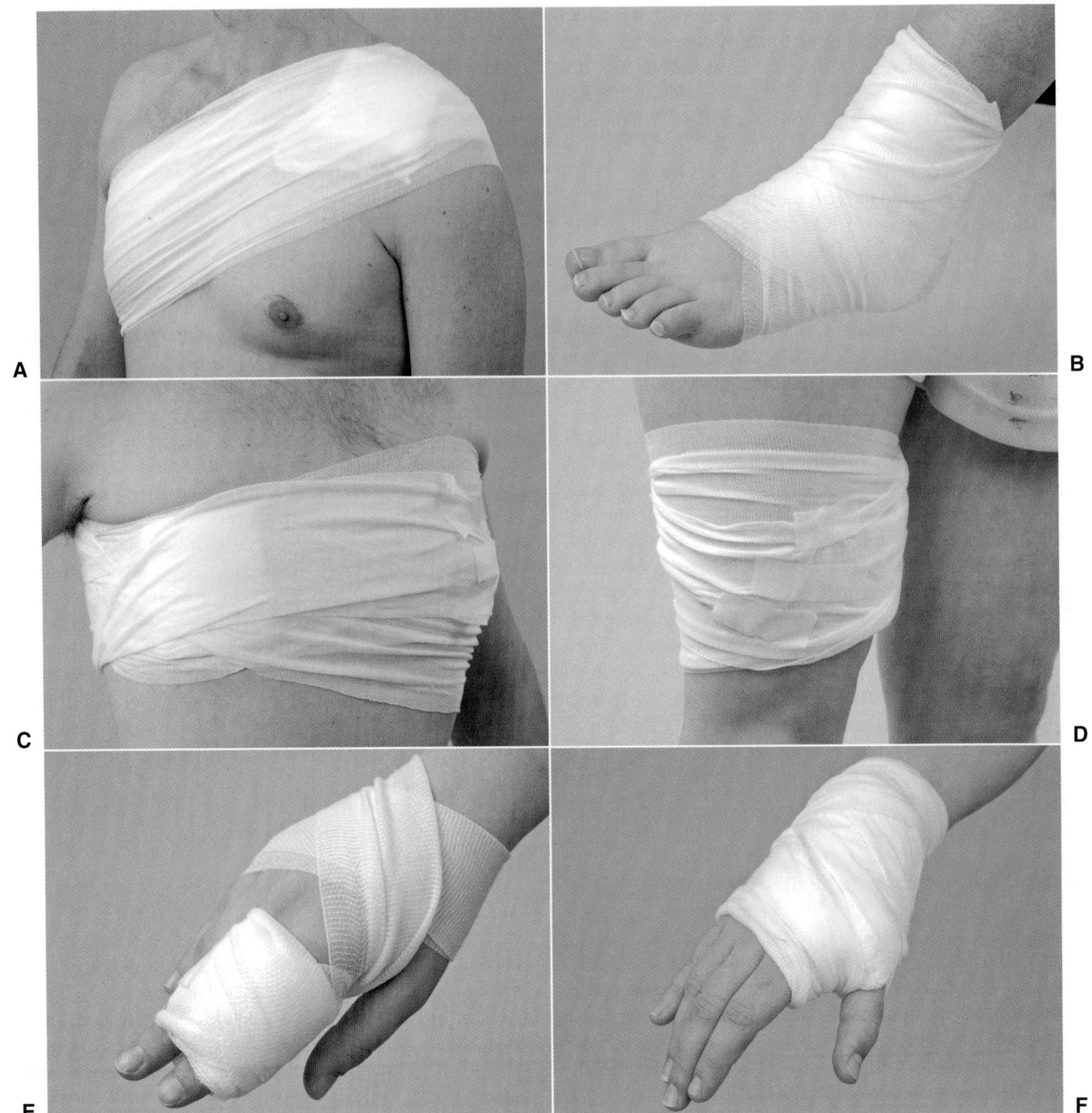

Figure 45-29 Types of dressings. **A,** Shoulder dressing. **B,** Ankle dressing. **C,** Torso dressing. **D,** Thigh dressing. **E,** Finger dressing. **F,** Wrist dressing.

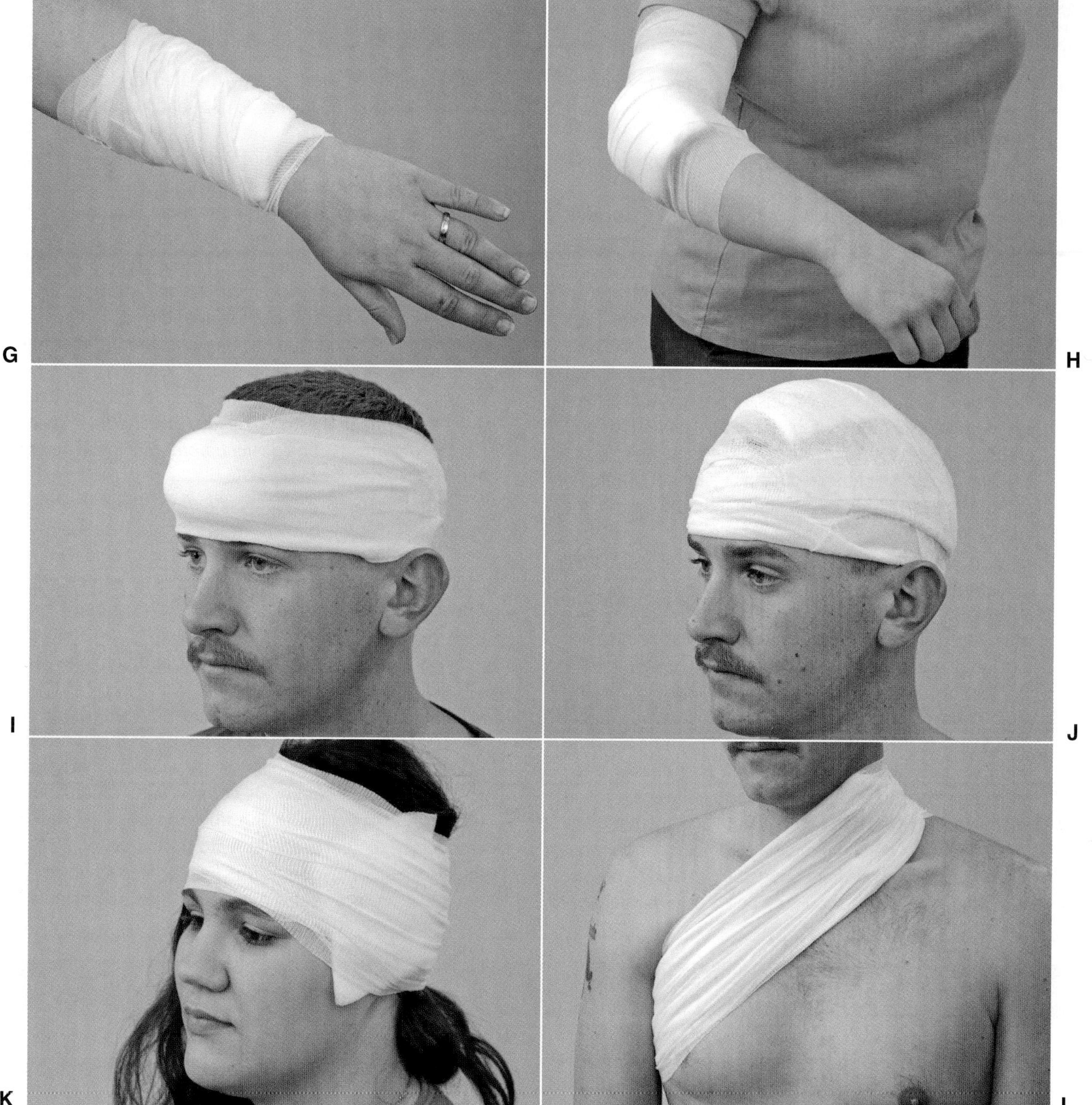

Figure 45-29, cont'd **G,** Forearm dressing. **H,** Elbow dressing. **I,** Forehead dressing. **J,** Scalp dressing. **K,** Ear/mastoid dressing. **L,** Neck dressing.

Case Scenario SUMMARY

1. *What is your general impression of this patient?* Although the patient is obviously in pain, several aspects of the primary survey suggest his condition is not critical. First, his mental status appears normal. He also has normal skin color and appears to be ventilating without difficulty. Beyond his entrapment, severe pain appears to be his greatest problem.

2. *What additional assessment is most pertinent at this time?* This injury appears to be isolated to his left lower leg. Obtaining further information about the mechanism of injury will be important to rule out head and spine involvement and assess the neck, chest, abdomen, and pelvis to be sure they were not injured when he fell.

Continued

Case Scenario SUMMARY—continued

3. *What intervention should be initiated before any further assessment is performed?* High-flow oxygen and manual spinal stabilization should be applied as precautions until you decide whether the patient requires full immobilization.
4. *Should this patient's spine be immobilized? Why or why not?* Local EMS protocols vary widely regarding spinal immobilization of a patient such as this. His physical examination suggests that his injuries are confined to his left lower leg, and he denies any neck or back pain after injury. He is alert and oriented and does not appear to be under the influence of any drugs or alcohol. These factors suggest that spinal stabilization may not be necessary. On the other hand, he was "pinned to the ground" by a huge concrete block, a mechanism that certainly would be capable of causing impact or torsion to the neck or spine. Given the mechanism of injury, spinal stabilization would be a safer choice.
5. *How should the left foot be managed? What additional treatment should be provided?* The deformity and absence of pedal pulses suggests an orthopedic injury with vascular impairment. Principles for management include direct pressure over the avulsion to stop bleeding, immobilization of the injury and adjacent joints, and restoration of perfusion. Initial care will include direct pressure and placement of a dressing over the avulsion and manual stabilization of the foot. High-flow oxygen should be applied and an IV started so that pain medication can be given *before* movement and splinting. The foot should be gently manipulated into a normal anatomic position while monitoring pulses and color. The foot, ankle, and knee should be splinted in normal anatomic position, the foot slightly elevated, and cold packs applied (on top of towels to prevent frostbite) to the injured area.
6. *The patient is in severe pain. What options exist to help manage his pain, and which do you believe to be most appropriate?* Pain relief for orthopedic injuries can be provided by both pharmacologic and nonpharmacologic methods. Nonpharmacologic interventions include positioning (normal anatomic position usually is best), immobilization (to prevent movement of injured tissue), elevation, and cooling (without causing frostbite). Depending on local protocols, morphine, fentanyl, meperidine (Demerol), or nitrous oxide may be used. The best strategy is a combination of methods. Remember to provide IV analgesia *before* manipulating the injured area.
7. *Given the patient's final disposition, was your treatment appropriate? Why or why not?* Overall the treatment was adequate. Given the absence of pulses in the injured extremity, better care could have been provided through the administration of high-flow oxygen (rather than 5 L/min by cannula), positioning of the foot and ankle in a normal anatomic position, and administration of cold packs to reduce swelling.
8. *What are the advantages and disadvantages of aggressive pain management in a patient such as this?* In cases of isolated orthopedic injury, aggressive pain management is important to provide comfort and facilitate positioning and splinting. In the absence of other injuries (especially to the head), a history of drug or alcohol intoxication, or hypotension, pain therapy should be aggressive to provide as much pain relief as possible.

Chapter Summary

- The skin and its structures serve key roles in maintaining body temperature and moisture and protecting the body from disease. Any disruption of the skin caused by trauma can result in significant threats to the patient's life.
- Soft tissue injuries encompass all types of injuries, from superficial to life threatening.
- You must carefully assess a patient's injuries and apply the appropriate knowledge to distinguish superficial from life-threatening soft tissue injuries and provide the proper care.
- Soft tissue injuries can be classified as either open or closed. The critical difference is whether the skin remains intact. Both injuries present the potential for complications when they are not identified and properly managed.
- You will mainly control hemorrhage by applying direct pressure. Check your local protocols regarding approved methods of bleeding control in your EMS system.
- Wound healing can be complicated by age, unrelated medical conditions, wound contamination, location of the injury, and severity of the injury.
- Wound management of open soft tissue injuries is focused on the control of hemorrhage and the protection of the wound from contamination.
- Ultimately you must prioritize the care of injuries to ensure the most life-threatening ones receive the most attention instead of spending excessive amounts of time on insignificant but graphic soft tissue trauma.
- You must take special care when treating amputations, avulsions, chest injuries, abdominal injuries, and crush injuries.

REFERENCES

Centers for Disease Control and Prevention. (2003). *National estimate of the 10 leading causes of nonfatal injury treated in hospital emergency departments: United States 2003*. Washington, DC: Centers for Disease Control and Prevention.

Counselman, F. L. (2004). Rhabdomyolysis. In J. E. Tintinalli, G. D. Klein, J. S. Stapczynski, O. J. Ma, & D. M. Cline (Eds.). *Emergency medicine: A comprehensive study guide* (6th ed.) (pp. 1749-1752). New York: McGraw-Hill.

Folstad, S. G. Soft tissue infections. In J. E. Tintinalli , G. D. Klein, J. S. Stapczynski, O. J. Ma, & D. M. Cline (Eds.). *Emergency medicine: A comprehensive study guide* (6th ed.) (pp. 979-987). New York: McGraw-Hill.

Fourre, M. W. Nontraumatic disorders of the hand. In J. E. Tintinalli, G. D. Klein, J. S. Stapczynski, O. J. Ma, & D. M. Cline (Eds). *Emergency medicine: A comprehensive study guide* (6th ed.) (pp. 1789-1794), New York: McGraw-Hill.

Haller, P. R. Compartment syndrome. In J. E. Tintinalli (Ed.). *Emergency medicine: A comprehensive study guide* (6th ed.) (pp. 1746-1749). New York: McGraw-Hill.

Hauswald, M. D. (2002). Can paramedics safely decide which patients do not need ambulance transport or ED care? *Prehospital Emergency Care, 6*, 383-386.

Huether, S. E., & McCance, K. L. (2004). *Understanding pathophysiology* (3rd ed.) (pp. 1134-1135). St. Louis: Mosby.

Lawrence, W. T. (2002). Acute wound care. In *ACS surgery: Principles and practice* (pp. 1-18). WebMD Inc.

Marx, J. A., Hockberger, R., & Walls, R. (Eds.). *Rosen's emergency medicine: Concepts and clinical practice* (5th ed.) (pp. 737-740). St. Louis: Mosby.

Pointer, J. E., Levitt, M. A., Young, J. C., Promes, S. B., Messana, B. J., & Adèr, M. E. J. (2001). Can paramedics using guidelines accurately triage patients? *Annals of Emergency Medicine, 38*, 268-277.

Schmidt, T. A., Atcheson, R., Federiuk, C., Mann, N. C., Pinney, T., Fuller, D., et al. (2001). Hospital follow-up of patients categorized as not needing an ambulance using set of EMT protocols. *Prehospital Emergency Care, 5*, 366-370.

Silvestri, M. D., Rothrock, S. G., Kennedy, D., Ladde, J., Bryant, M., & Pagane, J. (2002). Can paramedics accurately identify patients who do not require ED care? *Prehospital Emergency Care, 6*, 387-390.

SUGGESTED RESOURCES

Centers for Disease Control and Prevention. (2004). *Injury topics and fact sheets*. Retrieved May 26, 2005, from http://www.cdc.gov.

Marx, J. A. (Ed.). *Rosen's emergency medicine: Concepts and clinical practice* (5th ed.). St. Louis: Mosby.

Tintinalli, J. E., Gabor, M.D., Klein, G. D., Stapczynski, J. S., Ma, O. J., & Cline, D. M. (Eds.). *Emergency medicine: A comprehensive study guide* (6th ed.). New York: McGraw-Hill.

Trott, A. T. (2005). *Wounds and lacerations: Emergency care and closure* (3rd ed.). St. Louis: Mosby.

Chapter Quiz

1. While assessing a patient with soft tissue trauma, the most important action to take is to _______.
- **a.** note every contusion on the patient
- **b.** evaluate all lacerations to determine depth
- **c.** evaluate for underlying life-threatening trauma
- **d.** clean and débride abrasions before transporting

2. You are on the scene of a 33-year-old man who was in a fight at a local bar. The patient is alert and oriented with normal respirations. He is holding a bloody towel to his right arm. On removal of the towel, you see blood spurting from a large laceration. Describe your immediate course of action.

____

____

3. Your patient is a construction worker who was trapped when the sides of a trench he was working in collapsed. He was entrapped for 3 hours and has now been extricated. During your assessment, you note that his right lower leg is firm to the touch and he reports extreme pain when you manipulate his foot. What possibility does your assessment reveal?

____

4. Your patient was injured when a terrorist detonated a suitcase bomb near his seat in the airport. The scene has been secured and you are approaching your patient. As you approach, you recall that you should look for more _______ injuries on this patient than on a patient injured in an accidental explosion.
- **a.** primary
- **b.** secondary
- **c.** tertiary

5. Crush syndrome can occur in any patient who has undergone a prolonged period of crushing to an extremity. The syndrome causes severe physiologic problems, including renal failure and electrolyte derangements within the blood. In addition to a crushing mechanism, what is another mechanism that could result in crush syndrome?
- **a.** Removal of a tourniquet
- **b.** A gunshot wound to the foot
- **c.** A severe laceration to the arm
- **d.** Severe abrasions

6. Bleeding that is dark red and flows heavily is likely to be _____.
- **a.** arterial
- **b.** venous
- **c.** capillary

Chapter Quiz—continued

7. The paramedic most often uses which kind of dressing to manage wounds?
   a. Wet to dry dressings
   b. Nonadherent dressings
   c. Sterile, adherent dressings
   d. Occlusive dressings

8. Your patient has a large laceration to the right lateral neck that is bleeding profusely. You have applied direct pressure with your hand, but you are about to apply dressings to control the hemorrhage. Why should you use an occlusive dressing?

   ____
   ____
   ____

9. Why are patients with cat bites at particularly high risk for infection?

   ____
   ____
   ____

10. Patients with __________ should receive emergency department evaluation for extremity injuries, even when they appear minor, because of potential complications.
    a. athlete's foot
    b. heart disease
    c. diabetes
    d. renal failure

Terminology

Abdominal evisceration An injury in which a severe laceration or incision of the abdomen breaches through all layers of muscle to allow abdominal contents, most often the intestines, to protrude above the surface of the skin.

Air emboli Bubble of air that has entered the vasculature. Emboli can result in damage similar to a clot in the vasculature, typically resulting in brain injury or pulmonary emboli when neck vessels are damaged.

Bacteremia Presence of bacteria in the blood. This condition could progress to septic shock.

Cartilage Connective tissue made up of chondrocytes; exact composition depends on the location and function in the body.

Coagulation Formation of blood clots with the associated increase in blood viscosity.

Collagen A fibrous protein that provides elasticity and strength to skin and the body's connective tissue.

Compartment syndrome A condition in which compartment pressures increase in an injured extremity to the point that capillary circulation is stopped. The condition often is only correctable through surgical opening of the compartment.

Creatine kinase An enzyme in skeletal and cardiac muscles that is released into circulation as a result of tissue damage. Can be used as a laboratory indicator of muscle damage.

Creatinine End product of creatine metabolism. Creatine is released during anaerobic metabolism. Elevated levels of creatinine are common in advanced stages of renal failure.

Crush syndrome Renal failure and shock after crush injuries.

Debridement Removal of foreign material or dead tissue from a wound (pronounced *d' bréd*).

Deep fascia Fibrous, nonelastic connective tissue that forms the boundaries of muscle compartments.

Dermis Located below the epidermis and consisting mainly of connective tissue containing both collagen and elastin fibers; contains specialized nervous tissue that provides sensory information, pain, pressure, touch, and temperature to the central nervous system. Also contains hair follicles, sweat and sebaceous glands, and a large network of blood vessels.

Ecchymosis Collection of blood within the skin that appears blue-black, eventually fading to a greenish-brown and yellow. Commonly called a *bruise*.

Efflux Flowing out of.

Endothelial cells Flat cells that line the blood and lymphatic vessels.

Epidermis Outermost layer of the skin composed of tightly packed epithelial cells.

Epithelialization Migration of basal cells across a wound and the growth of skin over a wound.

Fibrin A threadlike protein formed during the clotting process that crisscrosses the wound opening and forms a matrix that traps blood cells and platelets, thereby creating a clot. Fibrin is formed by the action of thrombin and fibrinogen.

Fibroblast A cell used to form connective tissue.

Fluctuant nodule A movable and compressible mass; typically a pocket of pus or fluid within the dermis.

Free radical A molecule containing an extra electron, which allows it to form potentially harmful bonds with other molecules.

Germinativum Basal layer of the epidermis where the epidermal cells are formed.

Granulocyte A form of leukocyte that attacks foreign material in the wound.

Hematoma Collection of blood beneath the skin or within a body compartment.

Hemorrhage Bleeding.

Hemostasis Stopping a hemorrhage.

Hemothorax Blood within the thoracic cavity, a potentially life-threatening injury

Histamine Substance released by the mast cells that promotes inflammation.

Hydroxylysine An amino acid found in collagen.

Hypertrophic scar Scar that forms with excessive amounts of scar tissue. The scar remains contained by the wound boundaries but may be slightly raised and can impair function.

Induration Hardened mass within the tissue; typically associated with inflammation.

Influx Flowing into.

Keloid An excessive accumulation of scar tissue that extends beyond the original wound margins.

Lactic acid Byproduct of anaerobic metabolism.

Ligaments Fibrous connective tissue that connects bones to bones, forming joint capsules.

Linear laceration Laceration that generally has smooth margins, although not as precise as those of an incision.

Lipid peroxidation Process of cellular membrane destruction from exposure of the membrane to oxygen free radicals.

Lymphocytes A form of leukocyte.

Macrophages Cell of the immune system that can phagocytose foreign material from within the wound.

Mast cells Connective tissue cell that contains histamine; important in initiating the inflammatory response.

Myoglobin A pigment in muscle tissue that serves as an oxygen carrier (also known as *myohemoglobin*).

Necrosis Death of an area of tissue.

Necrotizing Causing the death (necrosis) of tissue.

Neovascularization New blood vessel growth to support healing tissue.

Neutrophil A form of granulocyte that is short lived but often the first to arrive at the site of injury; is capable of phagocytosis.

Open pneumothorax Injury to the thoracic cavity in which the cavity is breached, allowing air into the space between the lung and the chest wall.

Osteomyelitis Infection of the bone.

Papillary dermis Section of the dermis composed of loose connective tissue that contains vasculature that feeds the epidermis.

Paresthesia Tingling of the skin; "pins and needles" feeling.

Pericardial tamponade Life-threatening injury in which blood collects within the pericardium until the increasing pressure prevents the heart from filling with blood, causing death.

Peritoneum Serous membrane that lines the peritoneal cavity.

Peritonitis Inflammation of the peritoneum typically caused by infection or in response to contact with blood or digestive fluids.

Phagocyte A cell that has the ability to ingest and destroy foreign substances.

Phosphate A salt of phosphoric acid that is important in the maintenance of the acid-base balance of the blood.

Potentiating To augment or increase the action of.

Reperfusion phenomenon Series of events that result from the reperfusion of tissue damaged in a crush injury or tissue that is profoundly hypoxic. Can lead to crush syndrome (rhabdomyolysis).

Reticular dermis Section of the dermis composed of larger and denser collagen fibers; provides most of the skin's elasticity and strength. This layer contains most of the skin structures located within the dermis.

Rhabdomyolysis Complex series of events that occur in patients with severe muscle injury, such as that caused by crush injuries. The destruction of the muscle tissues results in a release of cellular material and acidosis that can lead to acute renal failure.

Sebaceous glands Found in the dermis; secrete oil (sebum) in the shaft of the hair follicle and the skin.

Serosanguineous discharge Blood and fluid discharged from the body.

Simple pneumothorax Injury to the thoracic cavity in which a lung is ruptured, allowing air into the space between the chest wall and the lungs.

Stellate laceration A laceration with jagged margins.

Stratum corneum Outer layer of the epidermis where skin cells are shed.

Sucking chest wound Open thoracic injury characterized by air being pulled into and pushed out of the wound during respiration.

Superficial fascia Connective tissue that contains the subcutaneous fat cells.

Synovial fluid Fluid located within the joint capsules of synovial joints; provides lubrication and cushioning during manipulation of the joint.

Synovial joint Freely movable; enclosed by a capsule and synovial membrane.

Tendons Tough, fibrous bands of connective tissues that connect muscle to muscle and muscle to bones.

Tension pneumothorax Life-threatening injury in which air enters the space between the lungs and the chest wall but cannot exit. With each breath, the pressure increases until it prevents ventilation and causes death.

Thromboplastin Blood coagulation factor.

Traumatic asphyxia Life-threatening injury in which the thorax is severely crushed, preventing ventilation; typically results in death.

Viral shedding Release of viruses from an infected host through some vector (e.g., sneezing, coughing, bleeding).

CHAPTER 46

Burn Injury

Objectives

After completing this chapter, you will be able to:

1. Describe the epidemiology, including incidence, mortality and morbidity rates, risk factors, and prevention strategies for the patient with a burn injury.
2. Describe the anatomy and physiology pertinent to burn injuries.
3. Describe the pathophysiologic complications and systemic complications of a burn injury.
4. Identify and describe types of burn injuries, including thermal, inhalational, chemical, and electrical, as well as radiation exposure.
5. Describe the epidemiology of a chemical burn injury and a chemical burn injury to the eye.
6. Describe the specific anatomy and physiology pertinent to a chemical burn injury and a chemical burn injury to the eye.
7. Describe the pathophysiology of a chemical burn injury, including types of chemicals and their burning processes and a chemical burn injury to the eye.
8. Identify and describe the depth classifications of a chemical burn injury.
9. Identify and describe the severity of a chemical burn injury.
10. Describe considerations that affect management and prognosis of the patient with a chemical burn injury and a chemical burn injury to the eye.
11. Discuss mechanisms of burn injury and conditions associated with a chemical burn injury.
12. Describe the management of a chemical burn injury and a chemical burn injury to the eye, including airway and ventilation, circulation, pharmacologic and nonpharmacologic treatment, transport considerations, and psychological support and communication strategies.
13. Describe the epidemiology of an electrical burn injury.
14. Describe the specific anatomy and physiology pertinent to an electrical burn injury.
15. Describe the pathophysiology of an electrical burn injury.
16. Identify and describe the depth classifications of an electrical burn injury.
17. Identify and describe the severity of an electrical burn injury.
18. Describe considerations that affect management and prognosis of the patient with an electrical burn injury.
19. Discuss mechanisms of burn injury and conditions associated with an electrical burn injury.
20. Describe the management of an electrical burn injury, including airway and ventilation, circulation, pharmacologic and nonpharmacologic treatment, transport considerations, and psychological support and communication strategies.
21. Describe special considerations for a pediatric patient with a burn injury.
22. Identify and describe the depth classifications of a radiation exposure.
23. Identify and describe the severity of a radiation exposure.
24. Describe considerations that affect management and prognosis of the patient with a radiation exposure.
25. Discuss mechanisms of burn injury associated with a radiation exposure.
26. Discuss conditions associated with a radiation exposure.
27. Describe the management of a radiation exposure, including airway and ventilation, circulation, pharmacologic and nonpharmacologic treatment, transport considerations, and psychological support and communication strategies.

Chapter Outline

Case Scenario

Dispatch directs you to a house fire. On arrival you notice a 42-year-old man who is burned on his face and arms. You estimate his weight to be 60 kg. He states his house caught on fire and was full of flames. He went from room to room to get his children and wife out of the house. He states he is burned on his face, arms, and chest. He rates his pain a 10 out of 10. He denies any other injury. He is talking in complete sentences and does not appear to have any respiratory distress.

Questions

1. *What is your initial impression of this patient?*
2. *What is your impression of this patient's airway?*
3. *What is critical in the initial investigation of this patient?*

Each year, approximately 1 million people in the United States sustain some type of burn injury. Recent data from the National Burn Repository give specific details about who is burned and by what mechanisms (Miller & Jeng, 2006).

In the United States, men are significantly more likely than women to be burned. Indeed, the epidemiologic evidence indicates that 70% of all burn injuries are sustained by men. The reason for this disparity is related in part to job descriptions (i.e., more men have high-risk jobs such as welding, firefighting, and chemical production than do their female counterparts). In addition, men, especially in the younger population, are more likely to engage in risk-taking behaviors, which can lead to burn injury.

However, worldwide, women are more likely than men to die as a result of burn or fire-related injuries. Women in Southeast Asia have the highest fire-related burn mortality rates in the world (Peden et al., 2002).

The majority (nearly 80%) of all burn injuries are either scald or flame related. The next most common burn injury is contact, followed by chemical and electrical. Table 46-1 lists burn etiologies and their commonalities.

Two groups of patients represent particularly high-risk burns: infants and the elderly. Infants represent 10% of all cases, and the elderly (older than 60 years) represent 14% of all cases. Thus nearly one fourth of all burn cases occur in quite different age groups but with a significant impact on morbidity and mortality. The information provided in this chapter discusses burn etiologies, classifications, and care of the burn patient in the field, including fluid resuscitation, pain control, and wound care. Significant detail is paid to managing inhalation injury and subsequent airway control. The chapter closes with a brief review of the psychosocial and physical and occupational therapy components.

TABLE 46-1 Burn Etiologies in All Age Groups, Aggregated

Burn Etiology	% of Admissions
Flame or fire	46
Scald	32
Contact with a hot object	8
Electrical	4
Chemical	3
Other or unknown	4
Radiation	0.3

Values are rounded and do not include data for nonburn admissions.

BURN ETIOLOGIES

[OBJECTIVE 1]

As previously stated, scald and flame burns account for the majority of all burns. In the case of scalds, patients often are managed in the outpatient setting. This can include the emergency department, urgent care facility, primary care office, or burn clinic. Well known in the burn community is the fact that 90% of all burns may be cared for in the outpatient setting (Brigham, 2000). This is a testament to the feasibility of treating these and other burns.

Flame burns frequently result in admission to burn centers or other inpatient care areas because these burns often are deeper and larger. These burns also frequently require detailed wound care, and many will need a skin graft.

Generally speaking, the mechanisms of injury for burns can be broken down into four distinct but overlapping categories: thermal, chemical, electrical, and radiation. Thermal burns have many causes and are discussed in Box 46-1. Radiation burns are discussed later in this chapter.

BOX 46-1 Causes of Thermal Burns

- **Contact** (with a hot object such as glass, metal)
- **Flame**
- **Flash** (usually caused by the improper use of flammable accelerants, causing the air to become superheated)
- **Scald** (includes all liquids)

Electrical burns and injuries should be considered significant. Although they are not common (accounting for approximately 4% of all burn injuries), they have the potential for devastating, hidden injuries. Electrical injuries are categorized as **high voltage** and **low voltage** injuries to help distinguish the potential for serious injuries. The separation occurs at 1000 V. A burn of more than 1000 V is considered high voltage. At this level of energy, the risk of significant cutaneous injury and internal injury (muscle, spine, and nerve injury) increases.

Chemical injuries are categorized as either **acidic** or basic **(alkaline).** Recall from basic chemistry that the **pH** scale ranges from 0 to 14. A pH of 7 is neutral. A pH less than 7 is acidic and greater than 7 is basic. A change in the pH by a value of 1, either up or down the scale, indicates a 10-fold increase or decrease in the hydrogen ion concentration. An increase in hydrogen concentration means the solution will be more acidic, whereas a decrease in the hydrogen ion concentration means a solution will be more alkaline.

ANATOMY AND PHYSIOLOGY OF THE SKIN

[OBJECTIVE 2]

The skin is among the largest and most complex organs of the human body. Burns injure the skin at various levels. They also have far-reaching effects on the body as a whole, essentially affecting all major organ systems to some extent. This is especially true in large burn injuries.

The skin serves numerous functions. It protects the body from outside invaders (e.g., bacteria, fungi, viruses). It helps regulate body temperature and maintain body fluid homeostasis. These and many other functions make the skin a quite complex organ system.

When skin is viewed beneath a microscope, its distinct layers are visible. These layers, from most superficial to deepest, are the epidermis, dermis, and subcutaneous. Any or all layers may be involved in a burn injury.

The epidermis is the most superficial layer of the skin. It is composed of **keratinized** skin cells. These are cells that were once living but have migrated to the skin's surface, where the cytoplasm of the cell becomes laden with the protein keratin. At the skin's surface, these dead cells function as the first defense against invaders and minor trauma.

The epidermis is secured to the dermis by a complex matrix of proteins and the reticular dermis. Rete pegs hold the two layers together and form a water-tight barrier.

The dermis layer exists beneath the epidermis. The main function of the dermis is that of strength and support. The thickness of the dermis is measured in millimeters. Its thickness varies depending on its location in the body. For example, the dermis of the eyelid is approximately 0.5 mm and is 10 mm on the sole of the foot. In addition, dermal thickness changes with age. In the young and elderly the dermis is thin. It is at its thickest in young adults.

Within the dermis are many structures, including the hair root, shaft, and follicle; nerves; arterioles, venules, and capillaries; lymphatic channels; and sebaceous, scent, and sweat glands and ducts (Figure 46-1). Strength, structure, and flexibility are maintained by collagen and elastic and reticular fibers.

Beneath the dermis is the subcutaneous tissue (superficial fascia), which serves several purposes. It insulates, is a portal for vessels (arterial, venous, and lymphatic) and nerves, and secures the dermis to the underlying muscle **fascia.** As with the dermis, the thickness of the subcutaneous layer depends on its location. Its thickness also is significantly determined by a person's dietary intake, caloric expenditure, and genetic composition. In general, men tend to develop thicker layers of fat around the abdomen, whereas women tend to accumulate fat in the gluteal and thigh regions.

The depth of a burn determines the success of grafting, the amount of scarring, the return to function, and cosmetic outcome. The deeper the burn, the less dermis is available to receive a skin graft. This makes the graft less likely to take and increases scarring. If burns extend to the fat, the removal of the burn down to the underlying fascia will cause cosmetic voids in the natural planes of body contour and remove an important layer of insulation. This, in turn, will make thermal regulation more difficult after the burn injury.

Burn Zones of Injury

A typical burn injury that involves the dermis, subcutaneous, or muscle tissue has three zones of injury (Jackson, 1953). Conceptualizing these zones is important for a complete understanding of burn wound physiology.

In a full-thickness burn wound, the central area of the burn is devoid of blood flow. This tissue is not salvageable and will become visibly necrotic days after the injury. Technically, before necrosis is visible, it already is present. This is known as the **zone of coagulation** (Figure 46-2).

Outside the zone of coagulation is a second zone where blood supply is weak. That is, the capillaries may be damaged, but oxygenated blood can still pass through them to perfuse the surrounding tissues. This is known as the **zone of stasis** or **ischemia.** Be sure to have a clear understanding of this zone. This area is at greatest risk of becoming necrotic if perfusion (i.e., fluid resuscitation) is not restored in a timely manner. If this zone remains ischemic for more than a few hours, it will convert to full-thickness injury, thus extending the zone of coagulation. One of the main goals of fluid resuscitation in burns is preserving the zone of stasis.

Finally, the outermost zone of the burn wound is an area that will most likely remain well perfused. It has a pink or reddened appearance. This is the zone of

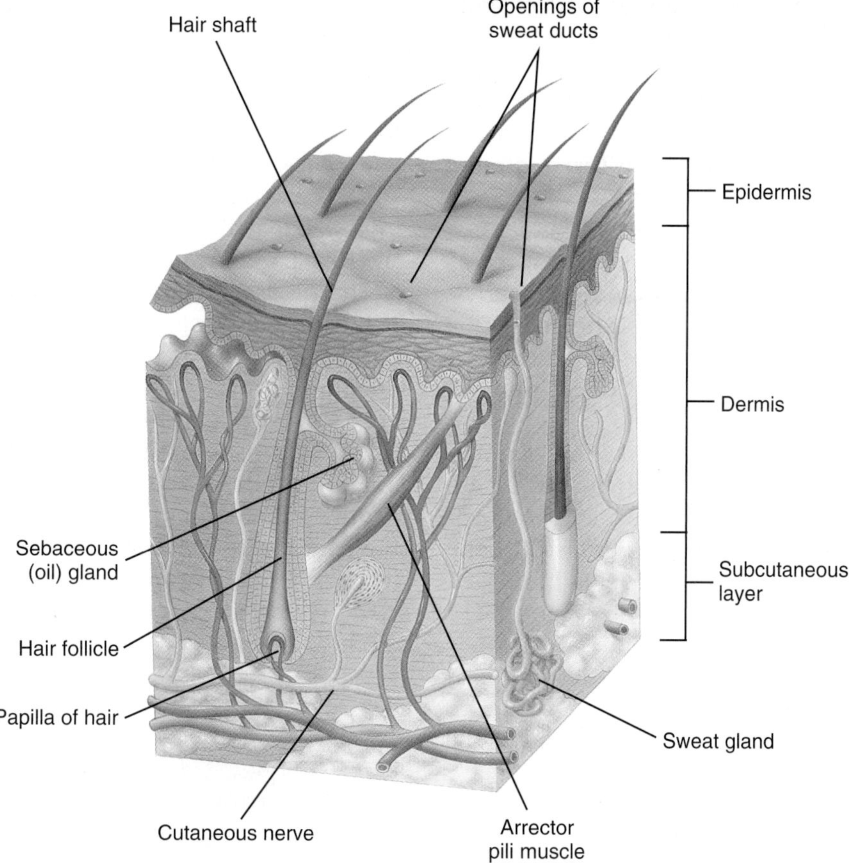

Figure 46-1 Skin structure.

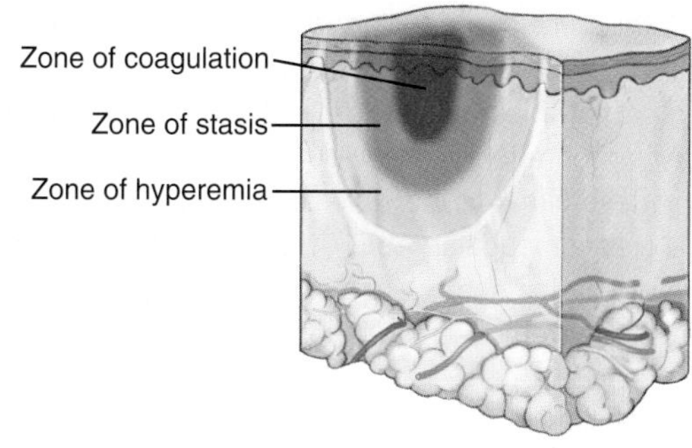

Figure 46-2 Burn zones of injury: zone of coagulation, zone of stasis, zone of hyperemia.

hyperemia. This zone blanches readily when touched. It is also extremely sensitive to touch. Some damage may have occurred to this zone, but by and large it is salvageable.

Burn Depth

When assessing the burn patient, you must take into account the size of the burn, which is measured as **body surface area (BSA),** and the depth of the burn. The burn depth determines whether the burn will heal by itself or require surgical closure.

BOX 46-2 Equivalent Levels of Burn Injury

- First-degree burn = superficial burn
- Second-degree burn = partial-thickness burn
- Third-degree burn = full-thickness burn

As previously described, the skin is composed of the epidermis, dermis, and subcutaneous layers. The epidermis is the thinnest layer. The dermis tends to be approximately 10 times as thick as the epidermis at any given site.

The common nomenclature (naming) of burn depth is well known: first degree, second degree, and third degree. Indeed, healthcare professionals still tend to use these terms when speaking to patients or family members about a burn because these terms are well recognized by the lay public (Box 46-2).

However, the medical nomenclature for burns, as with other illnesses and injuries, is more descriptive. It should be used for the purpose of medical discussion and documentation. For the purpose of this section, the common and medical nomenclature are used together to help you develop an understanding of both.

The best example of a first-degree burn is the common sunburn. Nearly every person, at some point in his or her life, has had excessive exposure to the ultraviolet light rays of the sun, resulting in a burn. These burns are painful both with and without being touched. They have a pink appearance, but blisters do not form. The medical nomenclature for this burn depth is **superficial.** Even in medical circles, the term **first-degree burn** is most often used to describe this level of injury.

Second-degree burns involve any layer of the dermis. Therefore the nomenclature for these burns is **partial thickness.** However, the depth of these burns varies. Furthermore, they depend heavily on location. For this reason, partial-thickness burns are further subcategorized as **superficial partial thickness** or **deep partial thickness.**

Partial-thickness burns are painful. All partial-thickness burns develop a blister (Figure 46-3). Blisters are collections of fluid beneath the epidermis as a result of the disruption of the epidermis from the dermis. Still, the presence of a blister or the loss of the epidermal layer, with subsequent exposure of the dermis, is diagnostic of a partial-thickness burn (Figure 46-4).

Differentiating superficial from deep partial-thickness burns can be difficult, even for the experienced clinician. In fact, the depth of the burn may not immediately be evident. A period of days may pass before depth of penetration of the burn can be determined.

The skin appendages are damaged when a partial-thickness burn occurs. However, they are not damaged to the extent that regeneration cannot occur. Hair shafts and follicles, nerve endings, blood and lymphatic vessels, and sweat and scent glands may have some degree of injury. Still, enough cells remain to allow regeneration of the tissue and organ components.

During assessment, the findings shown in Box 46-3 help distinguish superficial from deep partial-thickness burns.

You will not likely be called on to diagnose superficial versus deep partial-thickness burn injury. However, this information is useful for educational purposes.

Full-thickness (third-degree) burns involve the full depth of the dermis. These burns also may extend into the subcutaneous fat layer. Injuries of this depth cause irreparable damage to hair shafts, nerves, blood vessels, sweat and scent glands, and lymphatic channels of the dermis.

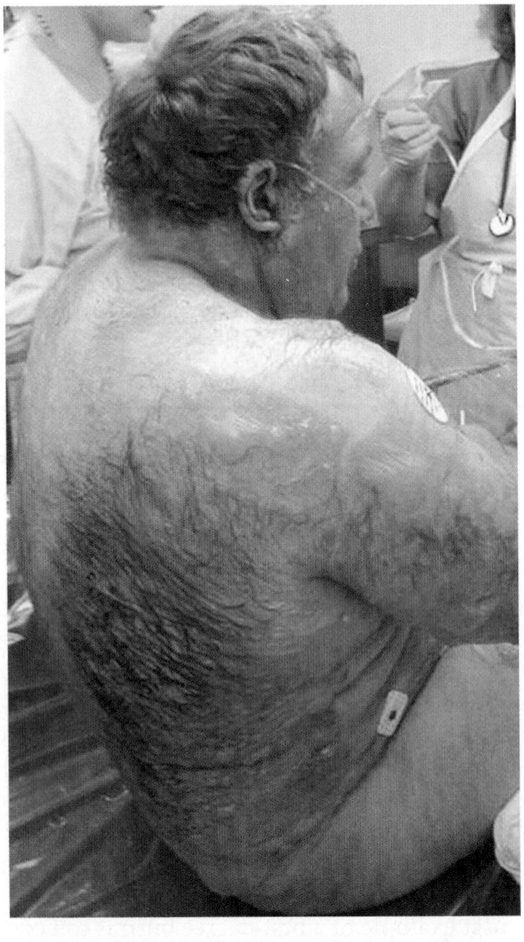

BOX 46-3 Presentation of Superficial versus Deep Partial-Thickness Burns

Superficial partial-thickness burns have a moist, pink appearance. When lightly touched, they are painful and sensate; the patient is able to discern sharp from dull pain. You can test this with a cotton-tipped wooden applicator. In addition, the burn has capillary blanching and brisk refill of the capillaries in the bed of the burn.

Deep partial-thickness burns, in contrast, tend to have a more dry appearance in the wound bed. When tested, the patient is less likely to be able to discern sharp from dull touch. Moreover, capillary refill, if present, is slow to return. Furthermore, if hair shafts are still present, lightly tugging on the shaft easily removes the hair from its follicle.

Figure 46-3 Partial-thickness burn with blisters.

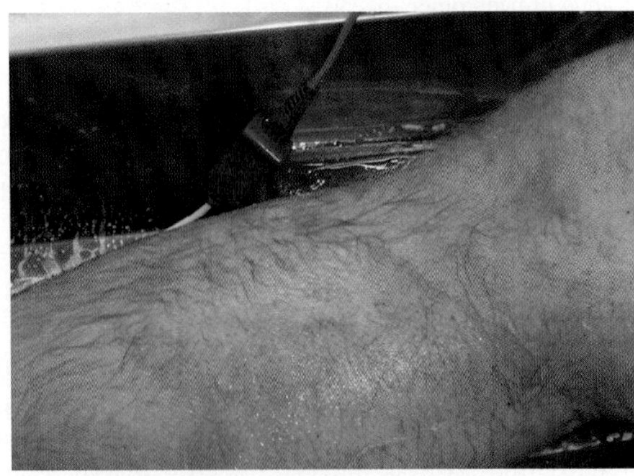

Figure 46-4 Partial-thickness leg burn.

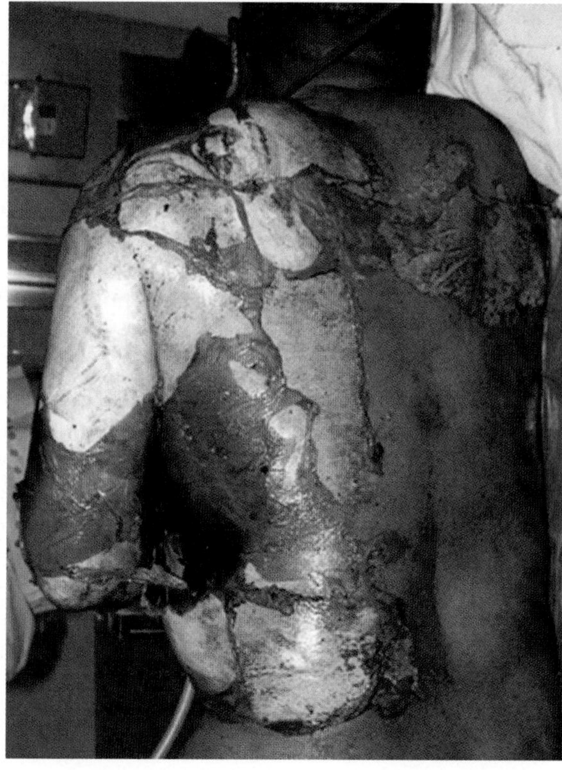

Figure 46-5 Full-thickness burn of the back.

The appearance of the skin in a full-thickness burn is gray and leathery (Figure 46-5). The wounded skin itself is insensate; that is, when sharp pain fibers are stimulated the patient does not feel sharp pain. These burns are not without pain, however. Indeed, most full-thickness burns involve an area around the burn that is partial thickness, markedly edematous, and extremely painful. Finally, the central portion of the burn, which is necrotic, may have a blackened **eschar** (scab).

An extremely deep burn, involving muscle fascia, muscle, and bone, is known as a fourth-degree burn. These burns often occur when the skin is in prolonged contact with a very hot object or extremely high heat in a short period, such as with high-voltage electricity (Figure 46-6). These are devastating injuries that often require amputation.

BURN CLASSIFICATION

Burns may be classified as minor, moderate, or severe (Marx, 2006). Minor burns are those that are:

1. Partial thickness, involving less than 15% of total body surface area (TBSA) in adults, or less than 10% in children or the elderly
2. Full thickness, involving less than 2% TBSA and not involving an area of function such as the face, eyes, hands, feet, or perineum

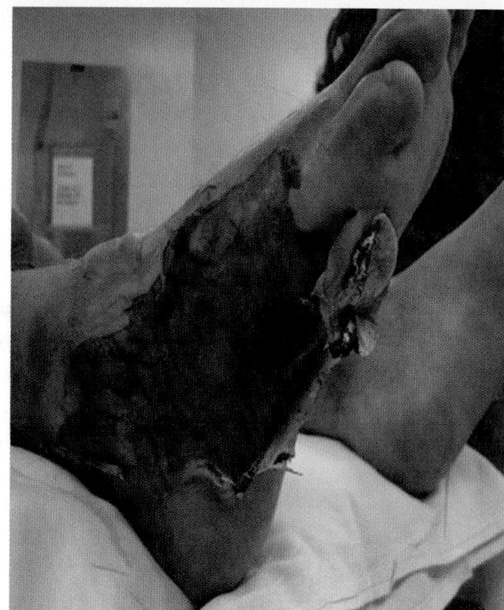

Figure 46-6 Fourth-degree electrical burn.

Moderate burns are those that:

1. Are partial thickness, involving 15% to 25% TBSA in adults, or 10% to 20% in children or the elderly
2. Are full thickness, involving 2% to 10% TBSA, and not involving an area of function such as the face, eyes, hands, feet, or perineum
3. Do not include high voltage electrical injury
4. Are not complicated by inhalation injury
5. Are not complicated by trauma
6. Do not occur in high-risk individuals

Severe (or major) burns are those that:

1. Are partial thickness, involving more than 25% TBSA in adults, or more than 10% TBSA in children younger than 10 and adults older than 50
2. Are full thickness, involving more than 10% TBSA
3. Involve areas of function such as the face, eyes, hands, feet, or perineum
4. Are caustic chemical burns
5. Result from high-voltage electrical injury
6. Are complicated by inhalation injury
7. Are complicated by trauma
8. Occur in high-risk individuals

PATHOPHYSIOLOGY OF BURNED SKIN

[OBJECTIVE 3]

Overview

When assessing burn injuries, the size of the burn is one of the chief factors in evaluating the seriousness of the injury. To assess the burn size accurately, you must use a consistent means to measure the size of the patient's skin. This is known as *body surface area* (BSA) and is calculated by the following equation (Mosteller, 1987):

$$\sqrt{\frac{\text{height (cm)} \times \text{weight (kg)}}{3600}}$$

From the early treatment of burns (resuscitation) through the period of skin grafting, the patient's BSA and the **total body surface area burned (TBSAB)** will repeatedly be referenced for treatment and documentation purposes. This allows a consistent form of documentation familiar to all healthcare providers caring for burn patients.

The percentage of BSA burned plays an important role in a patient's chances of survival. Current data indicate that, as in the past, the size of the burn and the patient's age both predict survival from thermal burn injury (American Burn Association [ABA], 2006). It is less predictive of survival in chemical and electrical burns. The latter two burns have distinct risk factors not related to the TBSAB.

The National Burn Repository Data indicate that the overall survival from burn injury is 95% (Miller & Jeng, 2006). Again, this rate depends on several factors. The presence of inhalation injury, occurrence of multiple organ failure, and preexisting comorbid diseases all play a role in outcome. Indeed, the presence of an inhalation injury alone or in combination with any burn size has a marked, negative impact on survival.

When looking at different age groups, the impact of age and any burn is notable. For example, for ages birth to 59.9 years, inclusive of all burn sizes, the mortality rate ranges from 0.7% to 8%. However, in the next two age groups, 60 to 69.9 years and greater than 70 years, the average mortality rate is 12.8% and 27.6%, respectively. This dramatic increase in these age groups is attributable to comorbid diseases and inherently failing physiology.

Several distinct factors have a significant impact on the patient's survival probability. For example, in the most recent data, 5839 subjects had a documented inhalation injury. Of these, 2087, or 30%, died as a result. The data do not specify whether a concurrent burn injury was present. However, isolated inhalation injuries are relatively uncommon. They account for only 0.3% of all presenting cases in the databank (1995 to 2005). Still, moderate to severe inhalation injury remains an independent predictor of death in all burn patients (ABA, 2006).

Infection and Sepsis

The most common cause of death associated with burn injury is multiple organ failure. Multiple organ failure accounts for more than one fourth of all deaths in burn injury and most commonly is initiated by pneumonia. Pneumonia is, by far, the most common cause of death in the burn patient (ABA, 2006). It is followed by burn shock, pulmonary failure and sepsis, and cardiovascular failure. The implication is that survival is much more likely when only one organ system fails. The mortality rate in intensive care unit patients with four or more organs failing is approximately 80% (Vincent et al., 1998).

Sepsis is a syndrome caused by inflammation and/or infection. It may arise in the lungs (pneumonia), the burn wound (heavy wound colonization occurs in the first 2 to 3 days after the burn injury), or from invasive devices such as intravenous (IV) or urinary catheters. Organisms responsible include the common skin flora *(Staphylococcus, Streptococcus)* and, later, enteric (gastrointestinal) organisms such as *Escherichia coli*, Enterococcus species, and probably the most feared bacterial invader, *Pseudomonas aeruginosa*. This organism is highly virulent and has, over decades, developed significant resistance to numerous potent antibiotics. This organism is well known to cause **invasive wound infections** in burn patients. From there, it spreads through the bloodstream to the lungs, causing pneumonia; the heart, causing valvular infection; and even the brain (abscess) and stomach (ulceration). Another extremely virulent organism is *Acinetobacter* species. This organism may be present in the wound, lungs, and blood and is difficult to treat.

Needless to say, *P. aeruginosa* is among the most feared organisms in the burn unit. Fortunately, science has been able to keep up with the organism's ability to mutate, and several antibiotics, piperacillin-tazobactam, levofloxacin, and tobramycin, are still available and work well to fight the infection. Furthermore, the development of silver-containing wound ointments and, more recently, silver-impregnated dressings has helped keep this organism at bay.

ASSESSMENT AND TREATMENT OF BURNS AND ASSOCIATED INJURIES

[OBJECTIVE 4]

In the field, you must initially assess the burn patient's airway, breathing, and circulation, as you would with any patient. You must then institute therapies to correct any problems. Because inhalation injuries have a significant risk of causing immediate and life-threatening airway edema, the airway must be controlled early.

In brief, the risk of inhalation injury increases in the following settings and circumstances: enclosed space exposure to smoke and/or fire, facial burns, chemical gas exposure, and carbon monoxide exposure. If you note any of the signs or symptoms in Box 46-4, strongly consider early airway control.

BOX 46-4 Signs and Symptoms Suggesting Early Airway Control

- Cough
- Carbonaceous sputum
- Soot on tongue
- Airway stridor
- Dyspnea
- Tachypnea
- Decreased level of consciousness
- Hoarse voice

An important step in the care of the burn patient is gaining venous access. The IV route is the best route for the administration of fluids for resuscitation as well as for analgesics, chemical paralytics, and anxiolytics.

In the setting of a thermal injury, the first and most important step in wound care is to stop the burning process. This seems elementary; however, inexperienced providers often are taken aback by the appearance of the burn and may overlook this critical step.

Burning clothes should be extinguished and cut away. If clothing is adhered to burned skin and has been adequately extinguished, leave the material in place. Then ensure airway control as well as breathing and circulation.

Airway management may present a formidable challenge to even the most skilled paramedic. Airway landmarks are often obscured by edema, abnormal tissue coloration, and soot. The soot can be especially troublesome when trying to identify the normally white vocal cords.

Administer 100% oxygen and establish IV access as soon as possible. IV access will be needed to administer medications and fluids. The ideal site for IV placement is through unburned skin, although this may not be possible. If this is the case, you may place the IV through burned skin.

Ideally, place a large-bore catheter (16 gauge or larger). You can secure the catheter with tape on unburned skin. You can further secure the catheter with gauze roll or self-adherent bandages. If you use elastic bandages of any sort, be careful not to occlude venous return from the extremity.

Wound care should be simple. Dressings must be easily stored with long shelf lives. With a few exceptions, burn wounds should be treated with dry dressings. You do not need to apply water, saline, or other irrigant to the burn wound as long as the burning process has been stopped and no chemical is involved. In fact, prolonged or widespread irrigation or lavage of the burn wound results in many complications. First and foremost, the patient will become hypothermic. This lowering of body temperature results in vasoconstriction, metabolic acidosis, and coagulopathy.

One exception to the rule of no irrigation is the presence of a hot tar burn. Tar is a liquid at several hundred degrees Fahrenheit. For this reason, it traps heat beneath it, causing a prolonged exposure to high heat. Lavage tar until it cools and becomes more solid. Then it will need to be removed. The removal of tar and similar agents is best performed at the hospital, where the proper agents for removal and adequate analgesia are available.

Some novel dressings exist and should be considered, including common kitchen plastic wrap. It has the advantages of not sticking to the wound and helps keep the patient warm, and the wound can be seen through the dressing. Many commercial dressings made of gel material also are available. For smaller burns (less than 5% TBSAB), these dressings provide pain relief and may protect against infection. However, avoid the use of large gel blankets. These may cause hypothermia by conduction of heat from the body as well as vasoconstriction.

Vasoconstriction has several harmful side effects. Most importantly, it decreases blood supply to the zone of ischemia. This could potentially extend the zone of necrosis by disallowing adequate arteriolar and capillary blood flow to the wound bed.

ESTIMATION OF BODY SURFACE AREA

A common language is necessary among burn care providers. One of the most common means to estimate TBSAB is known as the *rule of nines*. These charts, one for adults and one for children, divide the body into segments in multiples of nine. In the case of children, both multiples of nine and numbers divisible by nine are used. The other commonly used documentation chart is the Lund-Browder chart. It, too, has specificities for children and adults. As with the rule of nines, the Lund-Browder chart is widely used in burn care. However, it may be somewhat cumbersome in the prehospital setting because of its variation of BSA based on different age groups.

Whichever chart you use, it should be easily accessible so that you can estimate BSA involved in the burn. Complete the chart and leave a copy with the patient at the hospital.

Another quick reference tool is the patient's palm. The surface area of the patient's palm is estimated to be 1% of the patient's TBSA. Thus for smaller burns the patient's hand can be visualized and "shadowed" over the burn area. Again, this is only a rough estimate and is probably best used for burns encompassing 5% TBSA or less.

Case Scenario—continued

You begin taking a history on this patient. He states he is healthy but does have mild asthma. He denies smoking, alcohol, or drug use. He states he was in the smoke-filled house for about 5 minutes. You begin the physical examination and note that he has a reddened, painful area on the right side of his face. He has singed nasal hairs and some blisters around his nose. He has burns to his neck, chest, and the right arm circumferentially, including the hand and the palm. These burns are blistered and red. He has no burns to his legs, back, left hand, or left arm.

Questions

4. *Which type of burn is on his face?*
5. *What is the significance of the singed nasal hair?*
6. *Which type of burn is on his neck, chest, and arm?*
7. *What is a concern with a circumferential burn?*
8. *What is appropriate initial treatment for this patient?*

CHEMICAL BURNS

[OBJECTIVES 5 TO 12]

Chemical burns present a unique challenge. Literally thousands of chemicals in both industrial and home settings can cause mild, moderate, and severe burn injury. Chemical burns may cause both cutaneous and inhalation and lung injury. Cutaneous injury can result from direct contact with dry, liquid, or gaseous chemicals. Lung injury most commonly occurs when individuals inhale chemicals in the gas form.

For the purposes of definition and for treatment, chemicals are categorized as acids, bases, vesicants, and organics. The categorization of acid or base is based on the pH of the chemical (Box 46-5). The pH is a numeric assignment used to define the **hydrogen ion concentration** of a given chemical.

Vesicants are chemicals that destroy tissue through blistering. The destruction leads to damage to the skin, lungs, and eyes. A well-known vesicant is mustard gas.

Organic chemicals are primarily composed of carbon atoms. They are widely found in everyday life. Examples include paint strippers, paint, wax, and solvents as well as many cleaning, disinfecting, and cosmetic products.

As previously mentioned, chemicals with a pH of less than 7 are acidic. This implies a gradually increasing hydrogen ion concentration. As the numeric values decrease, the hydrogen ion concentration increases. Chemicals with a pH of more than 7 are alkaline; thus they have a relatively lower hydrogen ion concentration. For the sake of reference, normal skin pH is approximately 6.8, or quite near neutral on the acid-base scale.

BOX 46-5 Examples of Acids, Bases, and Organic and Vesicant Chemicals

- **Common acids:** sulfuric acid, hydrochloric acid, hydrofluoric acid, tannic acid
- **Common bases (alkalis):** sodium bicarbonate, calcium carbonate, most soaps, other similar cleaning agents
- **Common organics:** paint stripper, paints, lacquers, cleaning supplies, degreasing and hobby products
- **Common vesicants:** (sulfur) mustard gas, lewisite

Pathophysiology

Whether acid or base, chemicals injure skin and other tissues by physically destroying the components of tissue. Too many potentially dangerous chemicals exist to describe how injury to tissues occurs in each instance. In general, however, chemicals destroy proteins that are integral to cell and tissue support and wreak havoc with intracellular and intercellular communication through ion channels, or they dissolve lipids that are essential to the cellular membrane for the protection of intracellular structures.

Acids are further categorized as either weak or strong. As implied by these descriptors, the relative strength of an acid tends to describe its effect on other matter, such as skin (Box 46-6).

In both acids and bases, tissue injury depends on the pH as well as the attached ionic chemical. Acid exposure creates tissue damage through coagulative necrosis. In this pathologic process the affected cell or tissue maintains its normal size and shape. However, as the cells and tissues die they become more firm and dense than

BOX 46-6 Examples of Strong and Weak Acids

- **Strong acids:** hydrofluoric acid, sulfuric acid, hydrochloric acid (variable pH)
- **Weak acids:** tannic acid, hydrochloric acid (variable pH), acetic acid (vinegar)

surrounding cells and tissues, because their organelles and cellular membranes die.

Weak acids are much less destructive than strong acids. Weak acids have a tendency to "tan" the skin. This is a process used in the leather industry to preserve hides of animals. Interestingly, before current-day standards of care in burns, tannic acid, a weak acid, was used to treat burn injuries. It was thought to provide a protective barrier to the burned skin, thereby decreasing the risk of infection. This is no longer a standard treatment.

Conversely, bases, or alkaline chemicals, are known to be **lipophilic** and cause cellular and tissue death by a process called *liquefactive necrosis*. This means they tend to seek out and bind to fatty substances. Cellular membranes are largely composed of lipids, and deep to the dermis is the subcutaneous fat layer. These cellular membranes are therefore at significant risk for being destroyed from alkaline chemical exposure. This property of alkaline chemicals, lipophilia, causes unseen and ongoing tissue damage as the substance liquefies the cells and moves deeper into the tissues. For this reason alkaline burns tend to be very serious and are more difficult to lavage from the skin and other tissues. This again is because of their ability to bind to fats.

Chemicals in the gaseous form are less likely to cause direct tissue damage. However, the inherent ability of a gas to be absorbed or inhaled systemically cannot be overstated. Gases may be toxic themselves or purely through mass effect. For instance, carbon dioxide is inhaled by all human beings and is relatively inert. Carbon dioxide exists at a very low concentration in the atmosphere. However, in an enclosed space full of only carbon dioxide, hypoxia and subsequent asphyxiation will occur.

When inhaled, other chemical gases, such as chlorine, cause severe damage to the airways and alveoli of the lungs. This subsequently leads to a diffuse inflammatory reaction in the lungs and acute lung injury. The culmination of this injury is, again, hypoxia. In this form, the chemical itself does not cause hypoxia. Rather, the effect of the chemical on the lungs leads to eventual hypoxia.

Vesicants destroy tissue by disrupting proteins that hold membranes together, resulting in widespread blistering of the skin, eyes, and lining of the pulmonary tree. Both sulfur mustard and lewisite were developed for warfare. Both are still available and could potentially be used in a terrorist attack.

Finally, the widespread availability and use of organic solvents and other organically active compounds makes this type of burn injury a possibility in both home and industrial settings. The severity of the injury often depends on the concentration, length of contact, and BSA involved.

Therapeutic Interventions

Because of the vast number of chemicals that exist, developing a treatment plan for each one, or even for a family or group of chemicals, is nearly impossible. Hazardous materials manuals, such as material safety data sheets (MSDSs), provide a great deal of useful information regarding the toxicity of most chemicals. However, specific treatment modalities are significantly lacking in the prehospital setting. Therefore some basic principles of treatment, outlined as follows, apply.

Cutaneous Chemical Exposure

Chemicals that come in contact with the skin may be solid, liquid, or gas. After you ensure the patient's airway, breathing, and circulatory support, initial treatment revolves around removing the chemical from the skin.

Solid chemicals frequently exist in a powder or granular form. In this case, carefully remove the clothing of the exposed person. Note that it is of utmost importance that you protect yourself from becoming exposed to the chemical.

Once the clothing is removed, brush as much of the dry chemical as possible away from the skin. Never do this with your bare hand; use commercially available brushes or even dry towels or similar items. Be careful to remain downwind of the patient to avoid having the chemical blow into your eyes or onto your skin.

Once brushing is complete, begin a thorough lavage. When possible, assess the chemical for its reactivity with water. Some solid chemicals, such as sodium, react violently with water and will cause more injury when combined. Most chemicals, however, can be safely washed away with water. The Centers for Disease Control and Prevention recommend that skin and hair exposed to chemicals be irrigated for 3 to 5 minutes. Gently cleanse chemicals that are oily or oil based with a mild soap and water. If the eye is involved, perform at least 5 minutes of irrigation.

Resist the urge to try to "neutralize" any chemical with another chemical. Neutralization in this manner is not recommended because of the vast numbers of chemicals and their concentrations. This can become an extremely complex process that is neither feasible nor safe to perform, under most circumstances, in the field setting.

A liquid chemical exposure may pose several more problems for managing a patient, including the following:

- Liquids often are colorless, making identification of exposed areas difficult.
- Runoff from lavage will contaminate the surroundings.
- Rapid absorption through the skin and contamination of clothing pose a risk for prolonged exposure to the chemical.

Initiate extensive irrigation or lavage as soon as possible. Hazardous materials units with portable showers and staging areas should be used when possible. This will help prevent you from becoming contaminated, will help contain the chemical once it is washed away, and provides a much more controlled environment. However, the time constraints required for mobilizing a hazardous materials unit may make this approach impractical. Therefore use the resources available for lavage as best you can. Such options may include bottled water, garden hoses, showers, and fire hoses.

In both acid and alkaline exposures, the ultimate goal is to bring the skin pH back as close to normal as possible. This may require large volumes of water and may take a great deal of time. Be aware of the possibility of the patient becoming hypothermic. Take actions to decrease this risk, including irrigating with warm water, removing clothes, reducing exposure to wind currents, and irrigating indoors in inclement weather.

The patient should not remain at the scene of the chemical injury until his or her pH returns to normal. Instead, initiate the treatment and continue it during transport. You must notify the receiving facility of the chemical exposure, the name of the chemical, and the possibility of contaminating the facility. Most hospitals have a contingency plan in place to handle exposures such as this to protect their staff, patients, and the facility from contamination.

Some exceptions to immediate transport exist, however. In situations of mass casualty, in which multiple exposures occur, transporting numerous exposed patients to a single facility may quickly overwhelm resources and put the staff and facility at considerable risk for exposure. This could, in effect, completely debilitate the facility. Therefore in cases of mass casualty a preestablished plan should be used to triage and transport patients to the proper facilities.

Chemical Inhalation

Chemicals in the gaseous form may be inhaled into the lungs. How well these chemicals disperse is based on several factors: wind speed and direction, chemical weight, and containment. For example, carbon dioxide, released into a room, will outnumber oxygen molecules, making the environment toxic. However, in the open atmosphere this is much less likely, and the level of CO_2 will be relatively benign.

Contrast this with chlorine gas. This gas, whether contained in a facility or released in cloud form from a derailed rail car, has the potential to cause widespread illness and injury. Furthermore, many gases change in chemical composition when exposed to changes in the environment, making them more easily absorbed through the skin and inhaled.

With the relatively recent rise in clandestine methamphetamine laboratories, especially in rural areas, injuries from anhydrous ammonia have increased in number. This is a problematic chemical that is extremely caustic. It results in severe cutaneous injury and is readily inhaled in its gas form. Inhalation results in severe lung injury.

Treatment for all chemical injuries revolves around the following basic tenets:

- Remove the exposed patient from the environment.
- Secure the airway.
- Provide supplemental oxygen.
- Assist with ventilation.

In the case of carbon monoxide poisoning, simply moving the patient to an area of low carbon monoxide concentration will have a significant impact. Add to this the administration of supplemental oxygen, and the toxicity of this gas is quite limited.

However, applying the same principles to a chlorine gas exposure, although necessary, will be less effective. This gas, as previously noted, exerts significant toxicity on the lungs. Furthermore, its effects are long lasting and potentially much more life threatening over a longer period.

In summary, the care of chemical burns is relatively simple. The main objectives are to remove the patient from the source of the chemical, then remove the chemical source from the patient. The second part is done with copious water lavage and irrigation.

The priority in any burn patient is airway control, and chemical burns are no exception. Finally, you must ensure your own safety before proceeding with any type of treatment.

Chemical Eye Burns

Given the nature of chemical storage, eye injury from chemical exposure is an unsurprisingly common occurrence. Combined with thermal eye injuries, somewhere between 7% and 18% of all ocular injuries are a result of either chemical or thermal exposure.

As with cutaneous exposure, the two important variables that most affect degree of injury are the concentration (pH) and exposure time of the eyes to the chemical.

Alkalis penetrate more rapidly than acids; as with cutaneous exposure, fat degradation occurs, leading to significant cellular and organ injury. With a pH greater than 11.5, irreversible damage occurs. Treatment of chemical eye burns centers on dilution of the offending agent. Again, a plan for every chemical exposure is not possible, so dilution with water remains the mainstay of therapy. Because of the inherent nature of human beings to close the eyes when any injury occurs, one provider must manually open the injured eyes while another instills the irrigant solution. Commercial products similar to contact lenses are available for irrigation, but getting these attached to the eye without a local anesthetic can be challenging at best. In the field, a bottle of water for irrigation, with one or more holes in the center of the cap, provides a simple solution to prehospital irrigation.

Finally, chemical eye injury has significant psychosocial implications. The patient will undoubtedly be concerned over the potential loss of vision. Calm reassurance is important in these instances. Be mindful of the fact that vision may already be impaired, so the calm and clear spoken word becomes even more important.

Special Considerations

As mentioned, the general treatment of chemical injuries is copious lavage with water and attempts to neutralize chemicals should be avoided. However, for a few specific chemicals, additional treatment to avoid further injury or long-term complications and death is required, or standard treatment is ineffective. Most of these chemicals will be encountered in industrial accidents. One of the best sources of information regarding a chemical, its properties, and treatment will be from those who work with it every day. Most chemical plants have an emergency response team (possibly including advanced life support) that will likely have already initiated treatment upon the arrival of EMS. Be sure to determine what treatment has been provided, what treatment options the emergency response team may have, and what information these specialists can provide about the chemical in question.

Hydroflouric Acid. Hydroflouric acid is an extremely strong acid used in processes such as etching concrete, etching glass, and the production of plastics. In the industrial setting it may be found in concentrations up to 70%. Although primarily used in industry, several preparations may be encountered in the home setting, such as rust removers, and metal cleaners. In these settings the concentration is generally less than 10%; however, exposures to concentrations of 2.5% can cause severe hypocalcemia with resulting cardiac arrhythmias and possibly death, and exposure of any concentration of hydrofluoric acid to 5% of the patient's BSA can cause severe burns.

What is unique about this burn is that the initial burn is a result of the free hydrogen ions (acid), but the burn continues as the fluoride ions penetrate the tissues. As this happens, fluoride binds with calcium in the cell, making it unavailable for cellular function, including the influx of calcium into myocardial cells. This results in significant myocardial dysfunction and eventually death. In high concentrations hydrofluoric acid will leach calcium from the bones, causing demineralization. Associated electrolyte disorders include hypomagnesemia and hyperkalemia; however, it is the hypocalcemia that is of main concern. Knowledge of the effects of this burn as well as the resulting hypocalcemia is crucial, as signs and symptoms may be delayed for several (up to 24) hours. If the paramedic suspects this burn, a thorough history of the use of any cleaning products over the prior 24 hours should be obtained. It is crucial the emergency room physician be notified if hydrofluoric acid exposure is suspected.

PARAMEDIC*Pearl*

Severe hydrofluoric acid burns can be associated with minimal physical signs of injury.

Physical findings associated with exposure to hydrofluoric acid may include pain (described as deep, throbbing, or burning), areas of blanching, erythema, a burn area that is white in color, necrosis, blistering, and signs of hypocalcemia (cardiac dysrhythmias, Trousseau's sign, Chvostek's sign, tetany).

Rapid treatment of hydrofluoric acid exposure is crucial not only to reduce the burn itself, but to slow or avoid associated hypocalcemia and potentially fatal arrhythmias. Initial treatment of burns to the skin consists of flushing the area for 30 minutes. In the setting of ocular exposure the eyes should be irrigated for at least 20 minutes with sterile water or saline. Do not induce vomiting or administer activated charcoal when patients have ingested hydrofluoric acid. The conscious patient can be given 4 to 8 ounces of water as well as 2 to 4 ounces of an antacid containing magnesium and/or calcium. Use caution if the patient vomits, as the emesis will contain hydrofluoric acid. IV administration of calcium gluconate for the treatment of the burn itself is controversial (intraarterial administration is preferred); however, if signs and symptoms of hypocalcemia are present the patient may be treated with IV administration of a 10% calcium gluconate solution. Medical control should always be consulted prior to administering IV calcium to these patients.

Hydrogen Fluoride. Hydrogen fluoride is a colorless, odorless gas that when dissolved in water creates hydrofluoric acid. The main considerations of hydrogen fluoride exposures are identical to those discussed for hydrofluoric acid. However, because it is a gas, hydrogen fluoride exposure is generally an inhalation injury. Although the effects on calcium in the body are the same, hydrogen fluoride exposures do not generally result in burns to the skin. Hydrogen fluoride is rarely encountered outside the industrial setting, where it is mostly used in the production of refrigerants. It is also used in the production of pesticides and fluorescent light bulbs. The pulmonary affects of exposure can include pulmonary edema, bronchoconstriction, and stridor. As with hydrofluoric acid, signs and symptoms of hydrogen fluoride inhalation can be immediate or delayed for several hours (up to 36 hours). Pulmonary injury is also possible from inhaling the vapors of hydrofluoric acid.

Treatment of hydrogen fluoride inhalation includes standard treatment for pulmonary edema and bronchoconstriction. Use caution with bronchodilators, and monitor for and consider the cardiac effects of these medications in relation to the specific patient. In the setting of stridor, standard treatment with 2.25% racemic epinephrine is acceptable.

Alkali Metals. Alkali metals include lithium, sodium, potassium, and rubidium. These metals are highly reactive and are capable of violent exothermic reactions in water. Because of this they are not commonly found in their elemental form in nature but may be encountered in the industrial setting, such as the production of fireworks. Magnesium is an alkaline earth metal that also reacts with water, although not as severely as the alkali metals. Once ignited the alkali metals and magnesium are difficult to extinguish, as they can burn in carbon dioxide and nitrogen environments. Treatments for burns secondary to these metals include removing all contaminated clothing and covering the area with mineral oil or cooking oil. The paramedic must avoid introducing water to the area until it is ensured that all pieces of the metal are removed. Once all the pieces are removed, the burn is treated as any other alkali burn and may be flushed. Because it may be difficult to determine if any pieces of metal are embedded in the patient, it may be safest to assume there are and avoid the use of water until evaluation by the emergency department physician (Kales et al., 1997; Roberts & Hedges, 2004).

Phenol. Phenol is a flammable aromatic acid (based on its chemical structure, not its smell) that has both antiseptic and anesthetic properties. Phenol is used in industrial settings such as the manufacture of synthetic fibers such as nylon or the production of medicines. It is used in procedures such as chemical skin "peels" and several disinfectants, and as a result exposure outside the industrial setting is not uncommon. Because it is present in a number of mouthwashes, throat lozenges, and antiseptic lotions, pediatric patients may be exposed though accidental overdose of these products or through significant skin contact.

As an acid, phenol causes coagulative necrosis; however, it is unique in that weaker concentrations tend to penetrate deeper than strong concentrations. Exposure may be by inhalation, ingestion, or dermal contact. Oral ingestions of 50 to 500 mg/kg can be fatal, as well as exposure of concentrations as low as 5% to 6% to a large enough area of the skin.

Signs and symptoms of phenol exposure will depend on the strength, amount of time of the exposure, and route of entry. Phenol is irritating to the tissues and areas of contact (spill on skin; or via mouth or pharynx) may show burns that are initially red and swollen that later become white and opaque. It is not uncommon for these burns to be painless or numb due to the anesthetic properties of phenol. In the setting of ingestion, abdominal pain is possible as well as nausea, vomiting, and diarrhea. Inhalation injury can result in respiratory distress, tachypnea, pulmonary edema, hypoxia, and cyanosis. Systemic complications are generally secondary to ingestions; however, they can occur after inhalation or significant skin exposure. These can include diaphoresis, dysrhythmias, shock, cardiovascular collapse, tachycardia, hypotension, agitation, seizure, and coma.

There is no specific antidote for phenol; therefore treatment is targeted at reducing absorption, stopping absorption, and treating associated complications. Diluting phenol with water is controversial, as this increases its absorption. Ideally the affected area should be washed with polyethylene glycol 400 (PEG 400) or polyethylene glycol 300 (PEG 300) if available. Although this is not commonly carried in the prehospital setting, it may be available at the location of a call such as an industrial setting that uses large amounts of phenol. Other solutions that can be used are glycerin and isopropyl alcohol. If no other solution is available, copious amounts of water can be used. The patient should be irrigated for at least 15 to 20 minutes, and this should continue until there is no odor of phenol. To avoid additional injury to the esophagus, the patient who has an ingestion exposure should not be encouraged to vomit. Activated charcoal (1 g/kg) can be administered to block further absorption. Support of complications of the airway, breathing, or circulation should be initiated as indicated. There are no deviations from standard treatment of these items. The same holds true for central nervous system disorders such as seizures. Inhalation exposures can cause methemoglobinemia. This can result in hypoxia, cyanosis, and other signs of respiratory collapse that do not respond to oxygen administration. Prompt notification of the emergency room should be made so that the staff can have methylene blue waiting for the arrival of the patient (Agency for Toxic Substances and Disease Registry [ATSDR], 1996; Roberts & Hedges, 2004).

Phosphorus. Primarily used in the manufacture of munitions and fireworks, cleaning products, and pesticides, white phosphorus is a waxy solid that spontaneously ignites and will continue to burn until either all the available oxygen or all the material is consumed. Obviously, without intervention the phosphorus will continue to burn until it has consumed itself. As the material burns, it causes both a thermal burn from the exothermic reaction and an acid burn as the phosphorus is converted into phosphoric acid.

White phosphorus burns often have a garlic odor to them. The burns can be superficial or can be deep if phosphorus is embedded in the skin. Systemic effects generally only occur after ingestion (e.g., suicide attempt); however, white phosphorous can be absorbed through the skin's surface. These conditions may lead to organ failure, specifically of the liver and kidneys, hypocalcemia, and hyperphosphatemia.

Emergency treatment is targeted at stopping the burning process and removing any residual phosphorus if it is practical and safe for the medical provider. As mentioned earlier, in order to stop the burning process the material must be consumed or the oxygen removed. To remove oxygen the affected area should be immersed in water. If this is not possible, it should be covered in dressings soaked with sterile water or saline. The dressings should be kept moist until any residual phosphorus can be removed. The dressings should be carefully monitored to ensure they do not dry. At the emergency department, copper sulfate will be applied to the burned area to make identification and removal of the phosphorus easier (ATSDR, 1997; NAEMT, 2007; Roberts & Hedges, 2004).

Lime. Lime is an alkali that is most commonly found in the form of a powder. When combined with water, a chemical reaction is created that forms heat. As much of the dry lime as possible must be brushed off the patient before irrigating the burn site, while at the same time avoiding further contamination of the patient or responders. When irrigating the area, large amounts of water must be used to flood the area (e.g., using a garden hose). Using small amounts such as an IV bag with tubing will likely not remove the lime and will cause an increase in the severity of the burn.

ELECTRICAL INJURIES

[OBJECTIVES 13 TO 20]

Epidemiology and Demographics

Electrical injuries represent approximately 4% of all burn-related injuries admitted to burn centers. Injuries may be caused by house-type current or high-voltage industrial service. Either type may result in relatively minor or life-threatening injuries.

Etiology

Burns and other trauma (i.e., blunt injuries) commonly occur at the same time. For example, car accidents may cause fires. The patient in these scenarios may incur burn injury as well as orthopedic, chest, and abdominal trauma.

In electrical injuries, unlike many other burn injuries and especially high-voltage injuries, associated musculoskeletal trauma is common. This section reviews the pathophysiology of electrical injuries.

As previously mentioned, electrical injuries are categorized as either low voltage or high voltage. Low-voltage injuries occur when fewer than 1000 V are involved. High-voltage injuries involve more than 1000 V.

Noncommercial (residential) current is an example of low-voltage electricity; it is 60 Hz (60 cycles/sec) of electrical energy.

History

Overhead power lines and lightning are two examples of high-voltage electricity. An important part of your assessment involves knowing the amount of energy that caused the burn. This will help guide you in providing therapy as well as assessing the potential for serious injuries.

Low-voltage electrical injuries commonly occur when someone makes contact with a power source, such as an electrical outlet, in a house. Often these happen when the person is working on an appliance or trying to replace an electrical switch without turning off the power.

Another common occurrence is the **flash electrical burn.** These burns happen when a metal object, such as a screwdriver, makes contact with electrically charged fuses or other similar electrical objects. People often work on fuse or breaker boxes while these items are still charged. Crossing two fuses may cause a brilliant flash. The actual incidence of electrical injury in this setting is low. However, significant burn injury may occur. The temperature of these flashes can reach several thousand degrees Fahrenheit when air particles become superheated. Burns to the face and hands are common, and the eyes also may be involved. Fortunately, these flashes are brief. Furthermore, unless clothing catches fire, severe burns are not frequent occurrences.

Physical Examination

High-Voltage Electrical Injuries

Significant immediate and long-term negative aftereffects are associated with high-voltage electrical injuries. More than 1000 V of energy applied to the skin almost always results in deep burns at the point of contact. The energy then travels through the body, through the path of least resistance, to the grounded point. From there it will exit, again causing thermal injury.

High-voltage contact causes explosive damage to tissues. The energy also may damage skeletal, cardiac, and smooth muscle; bone, nerves, and blood vessels; and skin.

Muscle Damage

Cardiac Injury. The most common immediate cause of death in electrical injury is cardiac arrest as a result of **ventricular fibrillation** (Lee et al., 2000). Energy, both low and high voltage, passing through the cardiac muscle may disrupt the normal conduction impulses of the nodal tissue and bundle branches of the heart. External electrical energy that strikes during a vulnerable period of the cardiac conduction cycle may cause dysrhythmias.

Less commonly, severe cardiac muscle damage occurs as a result of the electrical contact. However, significant structural heart damage has been observed after electrical contact. This, of course, may impair the heart's ability to contract efficiently, resulting in congestive failure.

Skeletal Muscle Injury. As energy travels through the muscle mass, literally thousands of cells are destroyed. This, in turn, causes the intracellular proteins and electrolytes to be released, much of which will reach the circulation.

Myoglobin is a protein within muscle that carries oxygen. When released in large quantities into the bloodstream, these proteins block the small vessels of the kidneys. Clinically, this is recognized by the presence of myoglobin in the urine, a condition known as **myoglobinuria.** Myoglobinuria, if not appropriately treated, ultimately may lead to acute renal failure. This initially will be an acute disease; however, if enough damage occurs, chronic renal failure can result.

In addition to myoglobinuria, the damaged muscle cells release large quantities of potassium. The high serum concentration of this electrolyte can lead to cardiac dysrhythmias as well as central nervous system dysfunction.

The prevention and treatment of myoglobin-induced kidney injury centers on providing the kidneys with adequate fluid volume. In addition, an osmotic diuretic such as mannitol may be given, and the urine may be alkalinized with sodium bicarbonate.

Skeletal Trauma. Long bone and spinal bone trauma is well documented in up to 15% of high-voltage injury patterns. Long bones may fracture under the stress of massive skeletal muscle contraction caused by the energy passing through the body. As with any long bone fracture, blood loss occurs and surrounding tissue damage is almost inevitable.

Similarly, the bones of the vertebral column are at risk for fracture (Layton et al., 1984). Again, massive muscle contraction can pull together these irregularly shaped bones that sit on top of each other in the neck and back. These fractures may result in injury to the spinal cord at any level, causing temporary or permanent paralysis.

In addition to the actual energy of the electrical contact that causes musculoskeletal trauma, many patients involved in these incidents are either thrown or fall long distances. This, in turn, can cause significant injury to the skeleton and any internal organ.

For all patients with electrical contact injuries, perform full spinal immobilization because of the significant risk for vertebral injury. Also splint suspected long bone fractures.

Blood Vessel and Nerve Damage. Damage to blood vessels and nerves can be dangerous and debilitating. This type of damage is most often seen after high-voltage injury. Critical arteries may be damaged, resulting in **intimal** damage, thrombus formation, and vessel occlusion. Without sufficient distal arterial blood flow, tissue loss occurs. Furthermore, the current may be strong enough to **coagulate** blood within vessels. This can occur in all vessel sizes and types. In turn, it will occlude the vessels and subsequently disrupt inflow and outflow.

Electrical contact may damage nerves of all sizes. Depending on the site of contact, the level of energy, and the length of contact time, all portions of the central and peripheral nervous systems are at risk for injury.

High-voltage contact with the head may cause significant intracranial nerve damage. In addition, blood vessels on the surface of the brain may be destroyed, resulting in intracranial hematomas. As in blunt force trauma, these hematomas may become significant **space-occupying lesions.** Furthermore, the lesions may result in severe neurologic dysfunction and death.

Damaged vertebrae may cause spinal cord injury, resulting in partial or complete paralysis. Finally, peripheral nerve damage can significantly impair fine and gross motor and sensory function. These aftereffects often are permanent, leading to a lifetime of disability.

In the long term, high-voltage energy survivors may develop cataracts. In addition, their hearing may be impaired by the nerves that were destroyed by the electrical current. Furthermore, these patients often have a lifetime of pain caused by chronic nerve damage, a condition known as **neuralgia.** It can lead to severe depression and has undoubtedly led to suicide in those affected by this unfortunate disease (Kelly et al., 1999).

Therapeutic Interventions

Before evaluating a patient with an electrical injury, first ensure your own safety. You must assess the scene so that you do not become a victim.

Approach all scenes with extreme caution regardless of the reported mechanism of injury. Downed power lines, electrically charged vehicles, and patients lying on top of electrical sources have all been known to injure and kill would-be rescuers.

Turning off the power source or removing a patient from a live energy source is rarely the job of the paramedic. This would pose significant risk to the rescuer. Textbooks may illustrate the use of a wooden stick or other nonconductive device to remove a power line from a car or from atop the victim. Done properly, the source may be safely removed from the immediate vicinity of the victim. However, this certainly does not remove the energy from the line; therefore all persons involved are still at risk for contact with the power source.

Under ideal circumstances, properly trained professionals from a utility company should be responsible for turning off the power source. The power can be safely turned off with the proper tools and scene access made safe. Fire department personnel also may be trained to turn off electrical service. Always use caution, however, because some circuits are designed to reset themselves after a period of disruption.

Once you safely reach the patient, assess him or her as in any other emergency situation. As always, first ensure the presence of airway patency, breathing, and circulation. Assume spinal trauma for patients who are presumed to have made contact with high-voltage energy or who may have fallen or been thrown. In these cases, perform full spine immobilization. Always follow routine immobilization procedures. In addition, properly immobilize any suspected long bone fractures.

For patients with high-voltage electrical injury, you must initiate IV fluids. As previously described, the product of injured muscle, myoglobin, tends to obstruct the small tubules of the kidneys' nephrons. The patient must be adequately hydrated to maintain adequate flow through the kidneys. This will help lessen the chance of renal damage.

One difficulty in administering fluids to the patient with an electrical burn is that the size of visible burn does not always match the volume of fluid required. In the hospital setting, hourly urine output is measured and, ideally, kept at a volume of 75 to 100 mL/hr. Because having a Foley catheter in place in the prehospital setting is unusual, except for interfacility transfers, IV fluids should be run at a rate of 1000 mL/hr in adults. No consensus currently exists on the rate of fluid administration for adults or children with electrical burns treated in the field. For this reason, local protocol and/or contact with medical control dictates practice. You should treat cutaneous burn injuries sustained from electrical flash or contact the same as thermal burns—with the application of dry dressings.

Lightning Injuries

Each year approximately 100 people in the United States are killed by lightning and more than 250 are injured (Curran & Holle, 1997). Slightly more than half of these injuries occur when the victim is engaged in outdoor, often recreational, activities. The remaining injuries occur in those who work outdoors during storms. A much smaller percentage of lightning injuries happen when lightning travels through walls or telephone lines, injuring someone within the confines of a dwelling. This path may decrease the amount of energy received compared with a direct hit. However, it is dangerous and potentially life threatening nonetheless.

Lightning bolts travel miles through the sky to reach a target. A single bolt of lightning may be as small in diameter as a rope or as wide as 3 feet. The temperature of lightning may reach 50,000° F (Lide, 1996); in comparison, the surface of the sun is approximately 11,000° F).

The injuries sustained from a direct hit by lightning or from lightning splash often are severe. This is a high-voltage injury pattern. As such, treat it in the same manner as any high-voltage injury.

If the injured person is outside when found and lightning strike remains a risk, rapidly stabilize, immobilize, and move the patient to a safer venue, such as the ambulance or a building. The idea that lightning does not strike the same place twice is unfounded because any grounded person or other conductive item will continue to act as a lightning rod.

Scene safety and minimal scene times are paramount in caring for a lightning injury patient due to the fact that lightning has already struck the area. This indicates that lightning is indeed attracted to that area and can easily strike again. All EMS professionals should be familiar with the warning signs of an impending lightning strike, such as a tingling sensation in the hair or skin, the buildup of static electricity, or unusual odors. If you suspect a strike and cannot get out of the environment you should assume the "lightning position." Close your eyes and cover your ears while squatting on the balls of your feet with your head between your knees. This will make you as small a target as possible.

The two mechanisms causing lightning injuries are the electrical current and the secondary blunt trauma as the person is thrown or experiences severe muscle contraction. There are some key differences between lightning injuries and other high-voltage injuries. One of the most striking differences is that burns are rarely obvious in the former. Because of the relatively high resistance of the skin, the lightning may travel across, causing a pattern in the skin known as *ferning* or *Lichtenberg flowers* (Figure 46-7). Other patients may have no sign of electrical injury. If a patient is found unconscious in an area with reported lightning, the possibility of a strike must be included in the paramedic's differential diagnoses, regardless of physical findings. Blunt trauma injuries are treated as any other blunt trauma injury would be. Other injuries include rupture of the tympanic membrane, hearing loss, amnesia, confusion, seizures, and pulmonary contusions, hemorrhages, and edema. The major cause of death from lightning, however, is cardiac arrest, which should be treated as any other cardiac arrest would be. There have been many case reports of multiple people struck by lightning simultaneously. In these settings, because there is a high rate of survival from cardiac arrest secondary to lightning strike, the principle of reverse triage should be employed, and those in cardiac arrest should be treated first.

The specific treatment you provide (splinting, immobilization, and fluid administration) is the same as with other high-voltage injuries.

PEDIATRIC BURN INJURIES

[OBJECTIVE 21]

Description

Children are well recognized as being at high risk for burn injury. In fact, 10% of all burn injuries occur in infants younger than 2 years (ABA, 2006). Inquisitive toddlers are at risk for several burn injury patterns, including scalds (most common; Figure 46-8) and contact burns.

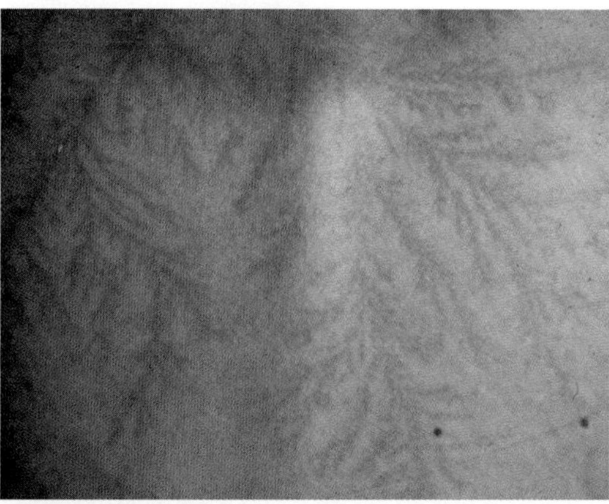

Figure 46-7 Lightning may travel across skin, causing a pattern known as *ferning,* or *Lichtenberg flowers.*

Epidemiology and Demographics

Burn injuries in children most often occur in the home (ABA, 2006) (Box 46-7). As with any trauma in the home, maintain a cautiously suspicious attitude regarding a burned child. Intentional burn injury is an unfortunate but relatively common form of child abuse. Because of this, a physician should evaluate all burn injuries that involve a child. That way, proper burn care can be initiated and an evaluation for the potential for child abuse can be made.

Very young children are at a much greater risk of dying from burn injury than are older children (ABA, 2006), in part because of their limited physiologic reserve. In addition, their immune systems are immature, which puts them at increased risk for complications from infections.

Skin Anatomy

The skin of a child differs in some notable ways from the skin of an adult. First, note the significant differences in the dermal thickness of children. In all areas of the body, the dermis of a child is significantly thinner than the dermis of an adult. Consequently, a partial-thickness burn in an adult is more likely to be full thickness in the child.

BOX 46-7 Most Common Burns in Children Aged 5 Years and Younger

- Scald (approximately 9000/year)
- Contact with hot object (approximately 3000/year)
- Flame or fire (approximately 1500/year)

Physical Examination and Estimating Burn Injury Size in Children

As with adults, the TBSAB in children is based on weight and height. However, children have a disproportionate BSA of the head and extremities compared with adults. Because of this, a separate burn assessment diagram is used in pediatric burns.

When assessing an infant with a burn, note that the surface area of the head is twice that of an adult. In contrast, the extremities occupy a smaller surface area. As previously described, another method for determining TBSAB is the Lund-Browder chart. The chief difference between the rule of nines and the Lund-Browder chart is that the latter is broken down by areas of the body as well as age. That is, adjust for different areas of the body's surface on the basis of how the child changes as he or she grows (Figure 46-9).

Fluid resuscitation and analgesia are examined later in this chapter. However, be sure to understand that, as with adult burns, more fluid is not better for the pediatric burn patient. Children, especially young children, have limited cardiovascular physiologic reserve. Their ventricles are relatively stiff and noncompliant. Excessive volume resuscitation can cause congestive heart failure. Furthermore, children seem to be at an increased risk of developing secondary **abdominal compartment syndrome** (Greenhalgh & Warden, 1994). This phenomenon occurs when fluids administered during the resuscitation of the burn patient accumulate in the peritoneal cavity and the walls of the bowel, causing an increase in the pressure within the abdomen. This, in turn, results in compromise of blood flow to the kidneys as well as diminished return of blood to the right side of the heart. The latter is caused by compression of the abdominal vena cava.

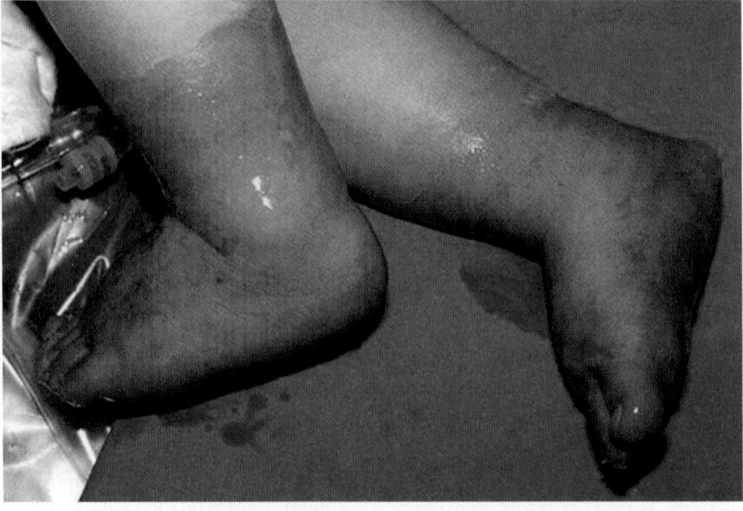

Figure 46-8 Immersion scald burn.

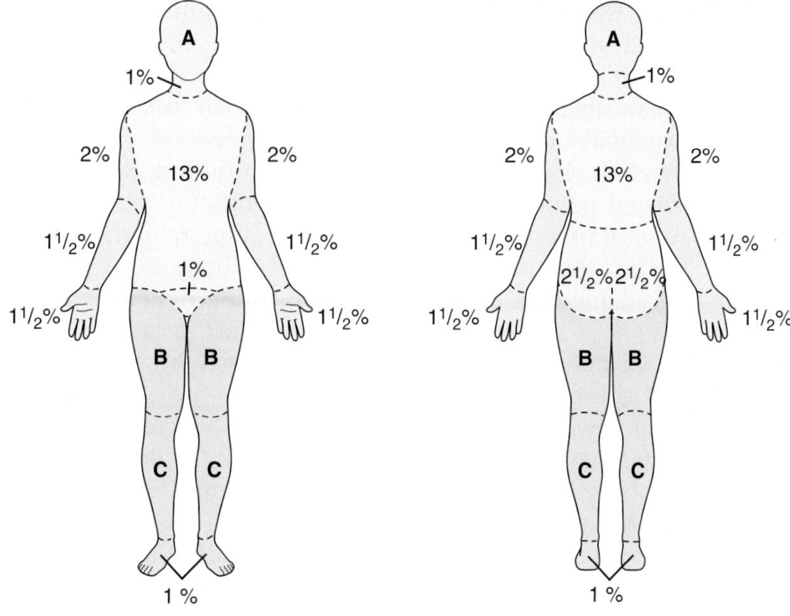

Area	Age 0	1	5	10	15	Adult
A - 1/2 of head	9 1/2%	8 1/2%	6 1/2%	5 1/2%	4 1/2%	3 1/2%
B - 1/2 of one thigh	2 3/4%	3 1/4 %	4%	4 1/4%	4 1/2%	4 1/4%
C - 1/2 of one leg	2 1/2%	2 1/2%	2 3/4%	3%	3 1/4%	3 1/2%

A

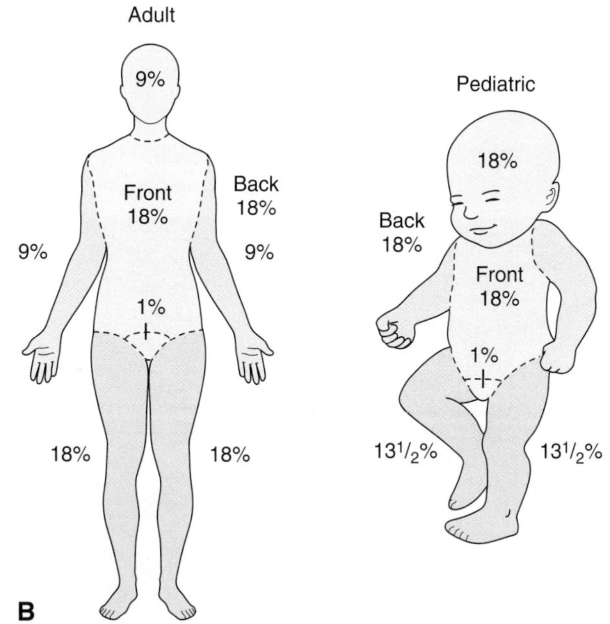

Figure 46-9 **A,** Lund and Browder chart with table showing the relative percentage of body surface area affected by growth. **B,** Adult and pediatric rule of nines.

BURN SHOCK

Burn shock is commonly referred to as *hypovolemic shock*. This term is not entirely accurate; it is a *relative* hypovolemic shock. In reality, burn shock is a **distributive shock.** It is comparable, in many respects, to septic shock.

Burn shock occurs as a result of the loss of plasma from the vascular tree. However, unlike true hypovolemic shock, in which the plasma, water, or blood has been lost from the circulation and often the body, in burns the loss is a result of **capillary leak.** This phenomenon is a result of several factors. First and foremost, capillary integrity is lost because of physical thermal injury to capillaries and larger vessels. Thermal injury causes the destruction of red blood cells, which in large burns (15% to 40% TBSA) contributes to anemia (acute and chronic). As much as 18% of the red cell mass may be lost in the first 24 hours after a burn (Topley et al., 1962). Several factors are involved in the loss of red blood cells. For example, blood loss occurs from surgical procedures, and hormonal factors are involved in the alteration of red blood cell membranes, leading to an increase in their destruction (Hatherill et al., 1986).

However, a more universal loss of fluid occurs as a result of gaps between the cells that comprise the capillary walls. This happens as a result of powerful chemical entities known as **cytokines.** Cytokines are proteins released from the liver, macrophages, and white blood cells in response to injury. Nearly all injuries cause cytokine release, especially severe trauma. However, thermal injuries are known to result in massive cytokine release.

Cytokines affect many organ systems but are particularly effective at causing capillaries to open and leak plasma into the surrounding tissue. This fluid shift causes plasma, which are composed of water and electrolytes, to collect in what is referred to as the **third space.** This is the extravascular and extracellular milieu, also known as the **interstitium.**

This fluid shift causes the easily recognized burn wound edema. In large burns, this can be an impressive sight (Figure 46-10). However, the edema caused by cytokine release is not limited to the burned tissue, as might be expected. Indeed, unburned tissues remote from the burned skin can become quite edematous. The eyes, brain, and bowel all can become engorged with excess fluid. This, in turn, can result in a wide variety of complications.

Laboratory and clinical investigations recently have discovered that cytokines also have an adverse effect on the heart, especially the contractile function of the myocardium (White, 2001). Initially, a rather nebulous factor known as **myocardial depressant factor,** was initially reported to cause a decrease in the contractile force of the heart in an animal burn model. Supporting this finding was the fact that when serum from burned animals was injected into unburned control subjects, the same myocardial depression occurred (Horton, 2001).

More recently, a study has suggested that the factor is probably a well-known cytokine known as **tumor necrosis factor-alpha** (Maass et al., 2005). This cytokine is released in massive quantities in the burn-injured patient. The amount released is related to the size of the burn injury. Clinically, severely burned patients have a markedly diminished **ejection fraction** in the heart, further contributing to burn shock.

To review, burn shock results from two mechanisms. First is a massive capillary leak syndrome, fueled by inflammatory mediators, which results in a distributive shock. Second, inflammatory mediators cause depression of cardiac output. Do not be confused by the fact that in burn shock cardiac function is **hyperdynamic.** In other words, the heart is beating quickly, but the output is insufficient.

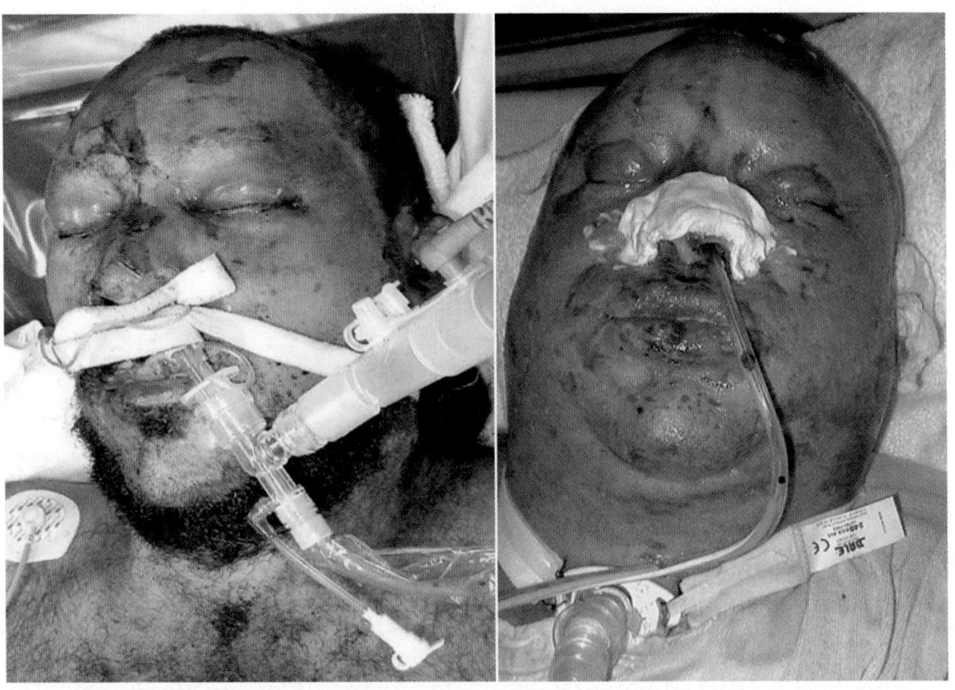

Figure 46-10 Fluid shift in a large burn.

Therapeutic Interventions for Burn Shock: Burn Resuscitation

The inflammatory process leading to burn shock is largely a self-limited process. That is, as time passes, generally within 24 to 48 hours, capillary leak will begin to resolve as a result of an increase in **antiinflammatory mediators** that oppose the effects of the proinflammatory mediators previously described. As a result, capillary leak resolves and the extravascular fluid shifts back into the vascular tree and diuresis occurs.

The resuscitation for burn shock is different from that for other types of shock, such as shock caused by blood loss. In blood loss shock, the objective is to replenish lost intravascular volume and control hemorrhage. Fluid administration is a temporizing measure to sustain perfusion of tissue beds until the loss of blood can be controlled.

In burn shock, however, the course of intravascular volume loss follows a relatively predictable course. As inflammatory mediators increase in concentration, capillary leak increases as well. After this point, the amount of loss begins to decline, interstitial fluid shifts occur, and volume is returned to the vascular tree. This happens over the next 16 to 40 hours. As previously explained, the shift of fluid from extravascular to intravascular causes brisk diuresis in the well-perfused and properly functioning kidney.

A mistake made during the resuscitation of a burn patient outside the burn treatment facility is to give much more fluid than is required and in a very short time frame. Laboratory studies have shown that when crystalloid fluids are administered to a burn patient, they leak out at a rate equal to, or faster than, capillary leak. As this fluid accumulates in the interstitial space, it exerts a **negative pressure** known as *imbibition pressure.* This pressure acts as a vacuum, pulling more fluid from the vascular space at a faster rate than before, further depleting the intravascular volume (Lund & Wiig, 1988).

When excess fluid is administered a vicious cycle results, and the patient never becomes fully resuscitated. Furthermore, the excess fluid accumulates in the extremities and abdominal organs, which may result in a compartment syndrome, damaging a wide range of body parts including skeletal muscle, peripheral nerves, the bowel, and the kidneys. Any or all of these organ systems may then fail. This, in turn, would significantly increase the patient's risk of long-term complications and even death.

The fluid of choice in the resuscitation of the burn patient is lactated Ringer's (LR) solution. However, any balanced salt solution works. A theoretical advantage of LR over normal saline (NS) is that LR has a buffering effect that may improve metabolic acidosis. In fact, the excessive administration of NS may actually worsen metabolic acidosis because the donated chloride ion will cause serum pH to become lower.

One of the most commonly used burn resuscitation formulas is the Parkland burn formula: 4 mL/kg divided by the percentage of TBSAB. In this formula, 4 mL is the volume of fluid administered per kilogram of body weight. The weight of the patient is approximated, as is the TBSAB.

This formula and a similar formula known as the **consensus formula** are calculated and the total volume administered is divided by 2. The resulting number, which is half of the total volume, is administered over the first 8 hours.

The first 8 hours after a burn injury corresponds with the time frame during which the capillary leak rate is the greatest. Therefore picture the volume being administered over this period coinciding with the fluid being lost to the third space. Then, over the next 16-hour period, fluid shifts begin to occur in the opposite direction. During this period of resuscitation the amount of fluid being administered is less, again coinciding with the reverse fluid shifts.

In the formal resuscitation of burned infants (younger than 2 years), a maintenance fluid containing dextrose also is used because very young children have a low reserve of glycogen. Glycogen depletion causes hypoglycemia and subsequent brain damage in this age group. However, in the prehospital setting, where transport times are reasonable, LR or NS will work appropriately.

Following is an example of the consensus formula used for a patient receiving fluid resuscitation for a 40% TBSA burn injury. Assume the patient to weigh 70 kg and be 30 years of age.

$$\text{Consensus formula} = 2 \text{ to } 4\,\text{mL/kg/\% TBSAB}$$

$$4\text{ mL} \times 70 \times 40 = 11{,}200\text{ mL/24 hours}$$

- Half of this (5600 mL) is given over the first 8 hours: 5600/8 = 700 mL/hr.
- Half (5600 mL) is given over the next 16 hours: 5600/16 = 350 mL/hr.
- If the range (of 2 to 4 mL) is used, then the patient would receive 350 mL to 700 mL/hr the first 8 hours and 175 mL to 350 mL/hr over the next 16 hours.

Variation in the formula allows you to adjust the volume you give on the basis of other factors such as age, comorbid conditions, and the burn size. For example, an 80-year-old person will not tolerate large volumes of fluid given quickly, as would be the case at 700 mL/hr. Add to this a "bad heart," and volume overload and congestive heart failure are sure to result (Table 46-2).

Fluid Resuscitation in Pediatric Patients

The resuscitation of the pediatric patient is somewhat more complex than that of the adult because the pediatric patient cannot tolerate large-volume influx as well as an adult. In addition, in the very young child dextrose must be given to prevent glycogen depletion, which will result in hypoglycemia. Also recall that children have relatively stiff and noncompliant left ventricles. Because of this, fluid overload may occur with seemingly safe volumes.

The consensus formula can be used for children, but it frequently underestimates the volume necessary to resuscitate the patient. Follow local protocol regarding this matter. Furthermore, always communicate with a burn center for guidance in caring for burn patients.

TABLE 46-2 Simple Method for Determining Fluid Rate

Age	Rate
<5 Years	150 mL/hr
5-15 Years	250 mL/hr
>15 Years	350 mL/hr

Burn Unit Resuscitation

In practice, burn units tailor the fluid given on the basis of several variables, including hourly urine output, **serum base deficit,** and **serum lactate** level. The latter two variables are a measure of cellular and end-organ perfusion. A more negative base deficit or an increasing lactate level indicates a state of metabolic acidosis and ongoing or worsening cellular hypoxia.

Case Scenario CONCLUSION

You begin by administering supplemental oxygen by nonrebreather mask and establishing two large-bore IVs (avoiding the arm that is burned). You place the patient on the cardiac monitor and prepare him for rapid transport.

Questions

9. *What type of dressings should be placed on the burns?*
10. *What should be done to comfort this patient?*
11. *What is critical to reassess in this patient?*
12. *What are important transport decisions?*

INHALATION INJURY

Description and Definition

Smoke inhalation is a serious and potentially fatal injury pattern seen in patients subjected to enclosed space exposure to the products of combustion or, as previously described, chemicals in the gaseous state. Patients often will have suffered a combination of smoke inhalation and thermal injury to the airways.

As previously noted, the mortality rate from smoke inhalation is approximately 30% (ABA, 2006). This statistic speaks volumes to the seriousness of this injury pattern. As a testament to its significance, consider the fact that most persons who die in house fires die from inhaled toxins, not as a result of the burn injury. Products of combustion, especially carbon monoxide, impair hemoglobin's ability to carry oxygen, causing cellular hypoxia and eventual death.

Airway Anatomy

The airway is divided into upper and lower parts. The **upper airway** is the portion of the respiratory tract above the glottis. The **lower airway** is the portion of the respiratory tract below the glottis.

Upper airway injury affects the oral and nasal cavities, posterior pharynx, and epiglottis. Lower airway injury affects the vocal cords, larynx, trachea, bronchi, bronchioles, and alveoli.

Injury to the upper airway most often results from direct thermal injury; that is, the inhalation of superheated gases. The **mucosa** (lining) of the cavities are thin membranes that are easily damaged by heat. As a result edema and the potential for obstruction exist.

Contrast this to lower airway injury that occurs when the particles and toxins produced during combustion are inhaled. These particles, which vary in size and toxicity, cause damage to the cellular lining of the lower respiratory tract. At this point inhalation injury becomes quite complex. Offending agents damage cells and cause widespread sloughing of the lining of the airways. Combined with mucus, this debris blocks the lower airways, forming concretions that are exceedingly difficult to expectorate. Once the smaller airways are obstructed, lung segment collapse occurs behind the obstruction, preventing oxygen from entering into the segment and carbon dioxide from exiting the lung. As a result, bacteria trapped in the lung will grow uncontrollably, causing severe, often fatal pneumonia.

Finally, carbon monoxide inhalation injury, also a form of **lower airway inhalation injury,** must always be a consideration. Carbon monoxide (CO) is a byproduct of incomplete combustion that is produced in most, if not all, fires. The more incomplete the process of burning, the more CO is produced.

Once inhaled, CO readily crosses the interface between the alveoli and the pulmonary vessels. It binds to hemoglobin with an affinity approximately 200 times that of oxygen. Therefore the patient dies as a result of hypoxia (Box 46-8).

Any and all of these chemicals may be produced in a typical residential structure fire. As such, assume that any person with exposure to smoke has inhaled some degree of these toxins.

History and Physical Examination

When assessing the patient with the potential for inhalation airway injury, keep in mind that time is of the essence. When such an injury is not recognized, airway edema may develop rapidly and cause fatal closure of the trachea or bronchi.

The first step in assessing the patient involves knowing the environment from which the patient came. Any enclosed space exposure to smoke or other toxic byproducts of combustion should lead you to suspect inhalation airway injury.

Visual evaluation of the patient often provides clues to the possibility of inhalation injury (Figure 46-11). A strong indicator of smoke inhalation is the presence of soot around the nose and mouth, in the mouth, or in the posterior pharynx. Add to this the presence of burns to the face and/or singing of the facial hair, and a nearly complete picture of a patient with inhalation injury is formed.

Burns to the face alone are not always predictive of inhalation injury. For example, a person who sustained a flash burn to the face by throwing gasoline on a fire in an outdoor setting is at low risk for inhalation injury because (1) the injury occurred outside (in a nonenclosed space) and (2) the injury happened quickly, thus giving a short exposure time. Many times patients involved in this type of incident have had time to hold their breath and possibly turn slightly away from the flame. This, too, is protective. Still, when in doubt, appropriately treat and observe the patient with any suspected inhalation injury with oxygen and transport for a complete evaluation of the airway.

The next step in assessing for inhalation injury is to listen to the patient. This step involves listening with your ears, not a stethoscope. A patient with involvement of the glottis, vocal cords, and lower airway structures has some distinct findings when listened to for a short period (Box 46-9).

The physical examination you conduct with your stethoscope may disclose rhonchi, rales, and wheezing. Each of these indicates injury to the respiratory tract at a different level. Consider the presence of any of these a red flag.

BOX 46-8 Dangerous Chemicals of Inhalation Injury

- **Carbon monoxide (CO):** A byproduct of incomplete combustion. It is produced in most, if not all, fires. The more incomplete the process of burning, the more CO is produced.
- **Cyanide:** Hydrogen cyanide is produced in fires that involve nitrogen-containing polymers. The toxicity comes from its inhibition of cellular oxygenation. Specifically, it disables the respiratory chain of mitochondria.
- **Hydrogen chloride (HCl):** Produced by the combustion of polyvinyl chloride. It causes severe damage to the respiratory tree and pulmonary edema.
- **Aldehydes:** Chemicals, or chemical byproducts, of wood and kerosene combustion. When inhaled, irritability and edema of the respiratory tract occur.

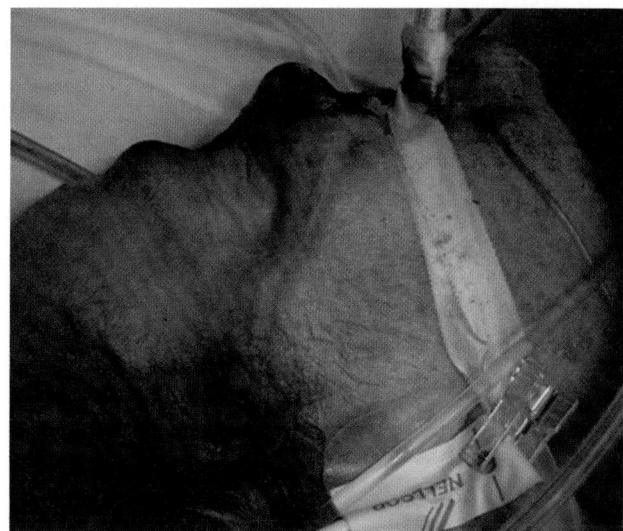

Figure 46-11 This patient sustained an inhalation injury when using home oxygen.

BOX 46-9 Findings Indicating Involvement of Glottis, Vocal Cords, or Lower Airway Structures

- Cough (may be described as "brassy")
- Hoarseness
- Shortness of breath, tachypnea
- Accessory muscle use and stridor

Differential Diagnosis

Comorbid conditions, in the setting of smoke exposure or burn injury, may result in conflicting physical examination findings. For instance, dyspnea, tachypnea, cough, and hypoxia are all hallmarks of asthma, emphysema, and congestive heart failure with pulmonary edema. These and other relatively chronic pulmonary diseases may have acute exacerbations in the setting of a burn or smoke inhalation injury. Relatively small amounts of smoke exposure, which may cause only minimal symptoms in an otherwise healthy person, may precipitate bronchospasm in a patient with asthma. The clinical presentation of this event may have the appearance of severe smoke inhalation instead.

As with any patient presentation, a thorough history will help make clear other potential causes of the patient's distress. Chronic inhaled steroid use and beta-agonist rescue drugs should key the rescuer in to the probability of an underlying pulmonary disease.

Therapeutic Interventions

Without a doubt, a significant inhalation injury will quickly become one of the most challenging and defining moments in any paramedic's career. These patients can progress to acute respiratory failure extremely quickly. Such circumstances can tax the efforts of even the most seasoned provider to secure an airway (Figure 46-12).

The ABCs (***a***irway, ***b***reathing, ***c***irculation) again take precedence over all other injuries when you suspect an inhalation injury. Administer high-flow oxygen immediately and continue it throughout the course of treatment in the field.

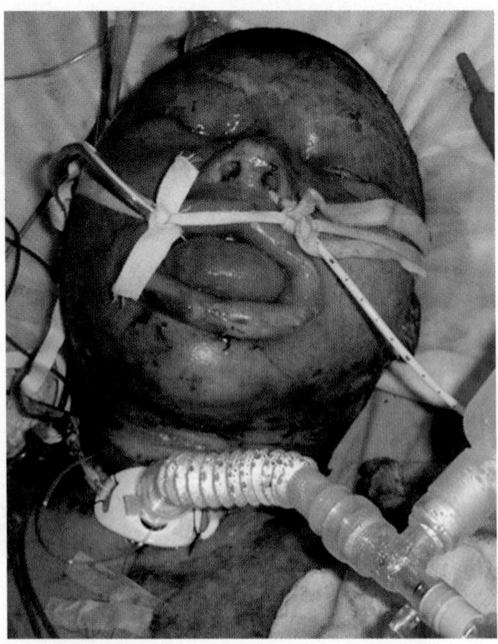

Figure 46-12 Severe inhalation injury.

If endotracheal intubation is necessary, be sure to understand that this may be a "one chance" attempt. Airway edema progresses rapidly, and the anatomic landmarks that were once present may be obscured by soot, edema, and a deep red discoloration of the mucosal tissues. The epiglottis may become markedly edematous, causing complete obliteration of the opening of the glottis. The normally pearl-white vocal cords will be coated with black soot, further disguising what previously has been used as a portal landmark for advancing the tube.

Once you decide to attempt intubation, all necessary equipment must be available, functioning, and at hand for the attempt. This equipment includes a laryngoscope with several different blades, a selection of endotracheal (ET) tubes, high-capacity suction unit, end-tidal carbon dioxide detector, and something to secure the tube. The use of a stylette within the lumen of the tube is a personal choice. You should have an ET tube of the correct size available as well as two additional tubes, one a half size smaller and one a full size smaller than the tube deemed the correct size. If significant edema is present, the correct size of tube may not fit into the trachea.

Once the ET tube is in place, a fast and durable tube-securing device is a must. You may not have another opportunity to intubate the patient. Loss of the tube may prove fatal. Tape does not work well in the presence of facial burns because it will not adhere well. You can use a variety of commercial products; a simple piece of cotton tape (available at most fabric stores) wrapped around the tube and the patient's neck also works well.

If intubation is not required, all patients with a suspected inhalation injury should receive high-flow oxygen by face mask. This is especially important when you suspect CO poisoning.

On room air, the half-life of carboxyhemoglobin (CO bound to hemoglobin) is 250 minutes (more than 4 hours). This is decreased to 40 to 60 minutes when 100% oxygen is administered. If possible, intubate patients who are unable to inspire oxygen effectively, are cyanotic, or are otherwise impaired.

When dealing with the pediatric patient, keep in mind that the airway is much smaller in diameter. Swelling will therefore obstruct the airway much more quickly than in the adult. As such, if intubation is necessary, do it earlier rather than later.

Finally, whether you are considering intubation in the adult or pediatric patient, remember that a secure airway is of utmost importance. Do not be concerned about whether the patient will be successfully extubated once he or she is hospitalized. Most patients intubated in the field who have good pulmonary function before injury can be successfully extubated within hours of arrival in the burn center if necessary.

RADIATION EXPOSURE AND INJURIES

[OBJECTIVES 22 TO 27]

Etiology

Many sources of radiation exposure are present in everyday life. From sun rays (ultraviolet radiation) to nuclear power plants, most prehospital providers can probably count on some source of radiation, outside the hospital, to be present in their communities.

Fortunately accidents at nuclear power plants are relatively rare. Furthermore, with the end of the Cold War came a lessened, albeit not absent, threat of thermonuclear warfare. Current concern surrounds so-called dirty bombs. These are small nuclear weapons designed to be carried into densely populated areas and detonated, releasing ionizing radiation over large areas.

Vehicles marked with the classic "radioactive materials" placard commonly drive city streets and highways. If one of these vehicles becomes involved in a crash, then patients, bystanders, and rescuers could all become injured by radiation exposure.

Epidemiology and Demographics

Serious radiation exposure is a rare cause of burn injury. Nationally, only approximately 0.3% of all burn presentations are from radiation exposure. Certain geographic locations lend themselves to a higher risk of radiation-related accidents. Nevertheless, all responding agencies must have a management plan in place to handle these uncommon but potentially devastating events.

Types of Radioactive Particles

Radioactive particles can be broken down into three types: alpha, beta, and gamma (Health Physics Society, 2006). Alpha particles are large and only travel short distances. They have a very weak ability to penetrate even a sheet of paper. They are, for the most part, not dangerous. However, if exposure were to occur long term, or if the particles were inhaled, ingested, or absorbed, serious damage to internal organs could result.

Beta particles are much smaller, approximately 1/7000 the size of alpha particles. Beta particles have much more energy and the ability to penetrate tissue. When tissue is damaged, such as by trauma, these particles have a much greater propensity to enter the body and cause damage.

For first responders such as paramedics, protection from both alpha and beta particles requires the use of full protective clothing and self-contained breathing apparatus with positive pressure.

Gamma radiation and x-rays are the most dangerous of the three particles. Much good has come from both in many areas of production, industry, and medicine. However, these forces should not be underestimated. As a testament to their power, lead shields must be used to protect a person from the damage that can be caused by these particles.

Gamma particles and x-rays have 10,000 times the power to penetrate compared with alpha particles and 100 times the power of beta particles. Only lead can protect human beings from gamma particles and x-rays. Exposure, even brief, may cause localized burns and severe internal organ injury. Long-term effects include cataracts and a multitude of different cancers.

The amount of radiation emitted is measured in several different ways. For instance, medical x-rays are measured in units known as **roentgens** (named after the physicist who discovered x-rays). Roentgens denote ionizing radiation passing through air, such as when x-rays are used to diagnose illness or injury in patients.

Radiation absorbed dose (rad) is a measurement of ionized radiation absorbed by and active in the body. A roentgen equivalent man, or **rem,** is a number used to assess the effects of radiation on biologic systems (Table 46-3). The sievert (Sv) is a unit for measuring ionizing radiation effective doses. This unit of measurement accounts for the sensitivities of different tissues on a relative scale (Box 46-10).

Therapeutic Intervention: Acute Care for the Radiation-Exposed Patient

By and large, the care you provide is supportive in the setting of radiation exposure. You can treat most symptoms with rest, fluids, and antiemetic medications. More severe exposure involves hospitalization for treatment of immunosuppression, infections, and other negative aftereffects of the exposure.

Decontamination

The decontamination of the rescuer and equipment goes beyond the scope of this text. However, in general, emergencies related to radiation are categorized as either clean or dirty. A *clean event* refers to exposure without contamination; a dirty event is one in which the patient was contaminated by the radiation. Only properly trained hazardous materials personnel should decontaminate the radiation victim.

TABLE 46-3 Symptoms Related to Radiation Exposure

Exposure Level	Symptoms
100 rem	No significant acute symptoms
100-200 rem	Mild symptoms (fatigue, weakness)
>200 rem	Nausea, vomiting, diarrhea
>450 rem	50% mortality within 30 days

Symptoms include hair loss, mucosal ulcerations, skin sloughing, bone marrow suppression, and infections.

BOX 46-10 Personal Protection from Radiation Exposure

- Decrease exposure time; exposure should be minimized for all involved.
- Increase distance from the source; the farther away, the less the dose.
- Use shielding devices; the more dense the material, the better protection it provides. Putting something between you, victims, and bystanders will lessen the exposure risk. This may mean piling mounds of dirt, placing large vehicles in the way, or constructing lead shields. At all times you and other rescuers should wear protective clothing and, when necessary, a self-contained breathing apparatus.
- Limit aggregate quantity. That is, if attire is being removed from the exposed patient(s), do not pile it together. This aggregation will increase the amount of radiation coming from the source. Bag and remove contaminated items from the scene as quickly and safely as possible.

ANALGESIA FOR BURN PATIENTS

Few would argue that burn injuries are among the most painful types of physical trauma anyone can incur. As such, the control of pain caused by the burn injury is of paramount importance. Most advanced providers only require a single interaction with a burn patient to learn quickly that adequate pain control is, perhaps, one of the most difficult battles to win in the arena of analgesia in the field.

Pain Reception and Analgesia

The sensation of pain comes from the injury to tissue with the subsequent activation of nociceptive pain fibers. Nociceptive pain fibers respond to noxious stimuli, such as trauma. Once stimulated, the impulse for pain travels by nerve fibers to the spinal cord, finally reaching the brain. Thus pain is a central nervous system phenomenon initiated by the peripheral nervous system.

The details of pain sensation, transmission, cataloging, chronic pain, and pain control are only recently being better understood. Chronic pain is an especially difficult phenomenon to understand and treat. Acute pain, although more clear, still poses a challenge to the healthcare provider. Pain caused by burn injury comes in both acute and chronic phases. Both can be extraordinarily difficult to treat.

By far, narcotic analgesics are the most commonly used medications to control pain in the setting of the acute burn. Unfortunately, narcotics have, over time, developed a negative reputation because of their highly addictive properties. However, current doctrine holds that, when needed for acute pain control, very little risk exists of a patient becoming addicted to narcotic analgesics.

The most commonly used narcotic for control of acute burn pain is morphine sulfate. This medication has stood the test of time in the arena of burn care analgesia. It is relatively safe and has a predictable mechanism of action. Other narcotic analgesics such as meperidine, fentanyl, and hydromorphone also may be used to control pain in the burn patient. Use caution when administering meperidine. In patients with renal dysfunction, the metabolite of meperidine, normeperidine, can cause seizures.

Fentanyl has the advantage of being a narcotic that does not cause an exaggerated histamine response, as can be seen with morphine, which may cause hypotension and respiratory depression. However, fentanyl has the undesirable side effect of causing chest wall rigidity, usually when given in large doses. This side effect may precipitate a state of respiratory distress and/or failure. Chest wall rigidity is more often reported in the pediatric literature. However, it has been documented in adult patients after a relatively low dose of 55 mcg (Klausner et al., 1988).

Finally, hydromorphone is a potent narcotic analgesic approximately 10 times more potent than morphine. However, it has significant addictive potential and is not routinely carried by prehospital services.

You may find that pain control with any analgesic proves to be a difficult task because of the significant activation of nociceptive pain fibers in the burn-injured area. In addition, the burn patient may have a significant degree of anxiety caused by the injury. Consequently, pain is difficult to control in the burn patient.

Additionally, in larger burns with capillary leak syndrome, the injected drug may not reach the affected tissues. That is, the volume of distribution changes in the burn patient. Therefore more analgesic than would be predicted may be necessary to control pain adequately.

Administration of Analgesics

The preferred route of narcotics administration in the burn patient is the IV route, which provides the best serum levels of drug within a reasonably short period.

IV access may not be readily available in some patients. In these cases, administer the medication by either the intramuscular or subcutaneous routes. Interestingly, in the absence of ill-perfused tissue, the subcutaneous route is nearly as effective as the IV route when giving morphine for pain control. However, in the patient in shock, blood is shunted away from both the muscular and subcutaneous tissue beds, resulting in significantly slowed absorption of the administered medication. When at all possible, the IV route therefore is preferred.

Dosage

In the adult patient of average size and without confounding comorbid conditions, a liberal dosing strategy is suggested. If approved by medical direction, begin dosing with 5 mg of morphine. After establishing that the patient is tolerant (i.e., no nausea, stable vital signs), you can give additional doses of 2 to 4 mg every 5 to 10 minutes (or as per local protocol or medical direction).

With larger burns, expect to give 10 to 20 mg of morphine in the first hour of care. Again, keep in mind that the entire dose of morphine probably will not reach the intended receptors, which may leave the patient with a significant amount of pain.

For children, begin dosing morphine at the recommended weight-based amount. Children should get 0.1 mg/kg morphine if approved by medical direction. As you assess their response to the drug, additional doses can be titrated to effect.

INDICATIONS FOR TRANSPORT OR TRANSFER TO A BURN CENTER

The ABA and the American College of Surgeons have determined that patients with specific types of burns (Box 46-11) should be transported or transferred to a verified burn center. Burn Center Verification indicates that a facility has adhered to stringent standards of care and is capable of managing these complex patients.

Currently fewer than 50% of all burn centers in the United States are verified by the American College of Surgeons and ABA. Therefore patients should be transferred to the burn center that is closest and can accept and provide care for the burn-injured patient.

Some burn centers may not have the capability to care for a major trauma patient. Furthermore, some burn centers may not care for pediatric burns. For these reasons, you must consult the receiving burn center, if at all possible, before transport.

Additionally, burn centers may adopt their own guidelines that may or may not follow those outlined in this text. Be aware of local resources. Moreover, adhere to the local guidelines and protocols related to the care and transportation of burn patients.

BOX 46-11 Criteria for Transport or Transfer to ABA Verified Burn Center

The following types of burns should be referred to a qualified burn center for care:

- Partial thickness burns greater than 10% TBSA
- Burns that involve the face, hands, feet, genitalia, perineum, or major joints
- Third-degree burns in any age group
- Electrical burns, including lightning injury
- Chemical burns
- Inhalation injury
- Burn injury in patients with preexisting medical disorders that could complicate management, prolong recovery, or affect mortality
- Any patients with burns and concomitant trauma (such as fractures) in which the burn injury poses the greatest risk of morbidity or mortality. In such cases, if the trauma poses the greater immediate risk, the patient initially may be stabilized in a trauma center before being transferred to a burn unit. Physician judgment is necessary in such situations and should be in concert with the regional medical control plan and triage protocols.
- Burned children in hospitals without qualified personnel or equipment for the care of children
- Burn injury in patients who will require special social, emotional, or long-term rehabilitative intervention

Reprinted from Committee on Trauma. (2006). *Guidelines for the operations of burn units: Resources for optimal care of the injured patient* (pp 79-86). Chicago: American College of Surgeons.
ABA, American Burn Association; *TBSA*, total body surface area.

CARE IN THE BURN CENTER

Initial Care

Once at the burn center, the patient is reassessed and certain specific indicators of adequate resuscitation are assessed. However, care at the burn center is a continuation of the care begun in the field.

The resuscitation phase of the burn patient is expected to continue for 24 to 48 hours after the acute injury. During this time several other treatments are undertaken, as described in the following section.

Additional Care

Once fluid resuscitation is underway, care of the wound is of primary importance. The burn wound accounts for a continued **hypermetabolic** state. That is, the body, in response to injury, begins to break down protein as a primary energy source after glycogen stores have been exhausted. This is an undesired side effect of burns. Several treatments are available to help diminish this hypermetabolism, although it cannot be stopped.

Within hours of arrival at the burn center, simple debridement of the wound is undertaken. This may entail simple removal of devitalized tissue or, in some centers, burns that are clearly full thickness are surgically excised soon after admission and skin grafting is undertaken (Figure 46-13).

If surgical intervention is not necessary or will be delayed, the wound must be covered with a topical antimicrobial agent to help decrease the burden of bacteria in the burn wound. Burn wounds are not sterile. In fact, most are heavily laden with bacteria within a few days of the burn injury. This accumulation of bacteria on the wound is called the **bioburden.** Without the simple yet crucial step of minimizing wound coloniza-

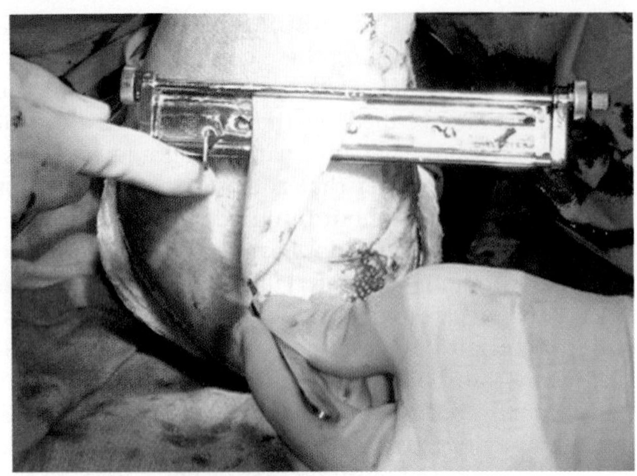

Figure 46-13 Burn excision.

tion, the mortality rate of burn patients increases dramatically.

Nutrition

In burns larger than 15% TBSA, the loss of protein through the wound and through hypermetabolism requires that the patient's nutritional status be supplemented by exogenous proteins, carbohydrates, and fats. The amount of calories needed to replete those lost from the **catabolic** state is far greater than most patients can effectively consume.

Therefore in burns greater than 20% TBSA, a feeding tube is routinely placed into the stomach or small intestine, and nutrition is delivered directly to the gastrointestinal tract. This is done as early as 6 hours after the burn injury occurs. Nearly all studies conducted on burn patients show that early and aggressive nutritional supplementation significantly decreases a multitude of complications. In addition, these supplements are used by the body to help rebuild the structure of the injured skin and aid in the incorporation of grafted skin over the excised burn area, thus closing the open burn wound more quickly.

Surgical Care of the Burn Patient

When burns involve the full thickness of the dermis, surgical intervention is generally required. This is true, with the exception of small burns that will heal without the necessity of a skin graft. Burns that fall into this limited category generally cover far less than 1% TBSA.

Burns that are superficial or deep partial thickness need definitive treatment as well. If an infection occurred, especially an invasive wound infection, the burn could convert to full thickness, thus requiring surgical intervention.

Superficial and deep partial-thickness burns are treated by wound debridement to remove devitalized tissue. The wounds then are covered with any of a variety of commercially available products. Many of these products contain elemental silver, which is an excellent antimicrobial agent. Silver is especially effective against *Pseudomonas* organisms. It is generally nontoxic, with a low side effect profile.

The goal in covering the wound is to keep the bacterial population at a level that can be handled by the body's immune system. This is important in all burns; however, larger burns (i.e., more than 15% TBSA) cause a significant degree of immunosuppression. This, of course, puts the patient at an increased risk for infectious complications.

The environment of the burn center is not sterile. However, hygiene is stressed and is of utmost importance. For this reason, patients with burns are kept relatively isolated from other hospitalized patients. In addition, healthcare providers must maintain good barrier protection during the care of open wounds.

For full-thickness burns, **skin grafting** is often necessary. Purposes of the skin graft include the following:

- Provide coverage and closure of the burn wound
- Decrease incidence of wound infection
- Restore some of the properties of skin
- Remove necrotic tissue **(excision)**
- Decrease protein loss by reversing hypermetabolic state
- Improve the cosmetic appearance (i.e., decrease scarring)

Before 1970 the standard of care was to allow the **eschar** covering a burn wound to separate by bacterial collagenase (enzyme) activity. In effect, the bacteria residing in the wound produce enzymes that destroy the structural protein, collagen. After long periods, the loss of collagen allows the eschar to separate from the wound bed. This resulted in prolonged hospital stays, increased infections, and resulted in poor cosmetic outcome. However, in those days critical care was in its beginning stages, and severely burned patients simply did not often survive.

In the early 1970s the concept known as *early excision and grafting* took hold (Janzekovic, 1970). Patients were recognized to have much better outcomes when the wound was excised and closed with skin grafts as soon as possible. At that time "early" meant within 1 to 2 weeks. Today, the stable burn patient commonly undergoes excision and grafting within 2 to 3 days, if not sooner.

The ideal wound closure is known as **autologous skin grafting.** This technique uses a **dermatome,** a device used to remove healthy skin from somewhere on the body of the burn patient and transfer it to the excised (surgically removed) burn wound bed. Skin grafting in the burn patient is most often done with **split-thickness skin grafts** (Figure 46-14). That is, the thickness of the graft taken is only a fraction of the thickness of the natural dermis. Depending of the location of the

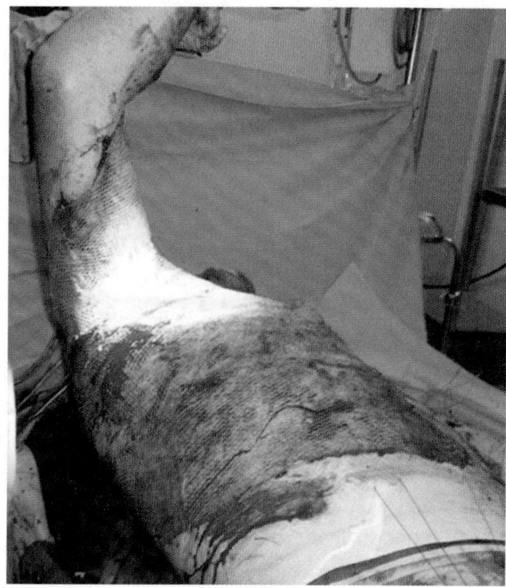

Figure 46-14 Split graft of the chest.

donor skin site and of the site being grafted, the split-thickness graft will be between 4/1000 and 12/10,000 of an inch thick.

To cover larger areas with less skin, such as for a very large burn, the donor skin often is "meshed." This aids in the spreading of the graft and allows the egress of fluid from the wound to the surrounding dressings. Certain areas of the body are covered with nonmeshed skin to improve **cosmesis,** including the face, hands, feet, and neck. However, larger areas can be grafted in this manner if donor skin is available.

PSYCHOSOCIAL ISSUES AND BURN INJURIES

Surviving the burn injury is a small step in the entire process of becoming a burn survivor. Burn injuries are psychologically as well as physically devastating. Burn wounds also leave scars in the mind.

Burn survivors are frequently troubled by nightmares and depression after even relatively minor burn injuries. The constellation of symptoms associated with postburn psychological disorders is known as *posttraumatic stress disorder.* From the beginning of care of the burn survivor, a great deal of focus is centered on the psychological aspects of the injuries, including issues such as chronic pain, body image, depression, and disability.

Survivors need assistance acclimating to home, work, and school. In addition, partner intimacy, environmental climate control, and wound care, to name only a few issues, must be addressed as well.

Long-term problems related to the burn injury include debilitating scar contraction, resulting in possibly numerous corrective plastic surgery procedures, problems acclimating to warm and cold environments (because of the loss of body fat and sweat glands in deep burns), and burn itch. The latter, although seemingly benign, can be the cause of great discomfort and frustration. The itch is caused by an ever-changing wound that undergoes constant reorganization.

Millions of dollars are spent on burn research. The focus of the research covers the gamut of problems associated with burn injuries. Fortunately, because of ever-improving prehospital care, critical care, wound care, and psychological care, burn survivors are seeing a much-improved outcome compared with those who suffered burn injuries decades ago.

BURN PREVENTION

One of the key goals of the ABA is to educate healthcare providers and the public at large about burn prevention. The overwhelming majority of burn injuries are preventable. The goal is to identify groups at greatest risk for burn injury and minimize the risk of being burned through public education. Following are some at-risk groups and the educational process meant to decrease these types of injuries:

- *Scald injury to infants.* Educate parents and other caregivers about proper temperature settings on water heaters and the use of boiling water on stoves and in microwave ovens. Also educate those responsible for bathing infants to prevent bath-related scald injury.
- *Electrical injury in persons not involved in the maintenance of these utilities.* Programs such as "Call Before You Dig" and others help prevent inadvertent contact with underground power and gas lines.
- *Burns related to improper use of petroleum accelerants.* Educational programs have been developed directed at those residing in more rural areas, where trash and debris burning is more common, as well as regarding proper fire-starting techniques for grills and fire pits.
- *Burns related to flammable clothing.* Flammable nightclothes and costume clothing, such as that worn for Halloween, put children especially at risk for burn injuries. The ABA has lobbied tirelessly to change laws regarding the manufacture of these and other similar pieces of attire.

As the saying goes, "an ounce of prevention is worth a pound of cure." This rings true with burn prevention. The number of burn injuries has dramatically declined in the years since the ABA and other prevention-minded organizations have advanced the agenda of burn prevention.

Case Scenario SUMMARY

1. *What is your initial impression of this patient?* The patient has been in a fire for an extended period. The fire was in an enclosed building. Thermal burns are obvious as you approach the patient. In this type of fire, airway complications should be anticipated, so this patient should be treated as a critical patient with rapid assessment, transport, and reassessment.
2. *What is your impression of this patient's airway?* The patient has blisters near his nares and singed nasal hair. This indicates extreme heat near the face. The facial burns also indicate the possibility of airway compromise. The mucosal lining of the airway can be burned by inhaled hot gases. This can cause delayed swelling, which can cause respiratory difficulty, including respiratory failure. This patient's airway may become critical at any moment. Supplemental oxygen with pulse oximetry measurement should be rapidly instituted. Continual assessment of the airway, including breath sounds, is critical. Other signs of possible airway involvement include the following:
   - Cough
   - Carbonaceous sputum
   - Soot on tongue
   - Stridor
   - Dyspnea
   - Tachypnea
   - Decreased level of consciousness
3. *What is critical in the initial investigation of this patient?* The most important thing to remember is that all patients who have been burned should be evaluated for continued burning of the skin. Some patients may not feel the burning continue if nerve damage has occurred. Also, the patient's clothing may continue to burn. A careful assessment of the patient should be done to ensure that the fire is completely out. The patient should have an immediate primary survey with special attention on his airway. Any other life-threatening injuries should also be rapidly treated. Clothing should be cut away from the patient's skin.
4. *What types of burns are on his face?* The patient has a burn to the face that looks like a sunburn. This is a superficial burn. This type of burn is painful with and without tactile stimulation and has a pink appearance but will not exhibit blister formation. Superficial burns typically affect only the epidermis (the outer skin layer).
5. *What is the significance of his singed nasal hair?* Singed nasal hair can indicate superheated gases around the airway, a possible indication of damage to the mucosa of the airway, and should prompt careful monitoring.
6. *What types of burns are on his neck, chest, and arm?* This patient has partial-thickness burns on his neck, chest, and arm. These burns involve any layer of the dermis. Partial-thickness burns are further subcategorized as superficial partial-thickness or deep partial-thickness burns. Partial-thickness burns are painful. All partial-thickness burns develop blisters, which are collections of fluid beneath the epidermis as a result of disruption of the epidermis from the dermis. The presence of a blister or the loss of the epidermal layer, with subsequent exposure of the dermis, is diagnostic of a partial-thickness burn. Differentiating superficial from deep partial-thickness burns can be difficult. In fact, the depth of the burn may not be immediately evident. Days may pass before the burn's depth of penetration is determined.
7. *What is a concern with a circumferential burn?* Circumferential burns can cause a tourniquet effect on the affected part of the body. This injury should be mentioned to medical direction. A circumferential burn typically requires an escharotomy, a method of cutting the skin to allow room for swelling. This is typically done in the emergency department.
8. *What is appropriate initial treatment for this patient?* The patient should receive supplemental oxygen. If the patient's respiratory rate and tidal volume are adequate, a nonrebreather mask should be used. Because the patient has burns to his face, a sterile dressing should be placed under the nonrebreather mask for comfort and to protect the burns.

   All constricting or potentially constricting jewelry should be removed. Unburned areas will swell rapidly and may make rings and other jewelry impossible to get off.

   When calculating a fluid administration rate, use either the Parkland or the consensus formula. According to the Parkland burn formula, 4 mL per kilogram of body weight is multiplied by the TBSAB. The weight of the patient is approximated, as is the TBSAB. With the consensus formula, the patient's weight and TBSAB are calculated and the total volume administered is divided by two. The resulting number, which is half of the total volume, is administered over the first 8 hours. In this scenario, the patient weighs 60 kg. This patient should receive 2 to 4 mL/kg/%TBSAB, or 8160 to 16,320 mL of fluid in 24 hours. Half of this amount should be infused over the first 8 hours. In this scenario, fluids should be infused at a rate of 510 mL/hr to 1020 mL/hr in the field.

   The patient should be placed on a cardiac monitor. Placing the adhesive electrodes should be done with care, and burned skin should be avoided when possible. Care should be taken to avoid hypothermia and any contamination of burned skin. Patients with burns may become hypothermic because of the interruption to the skin. A significant risk for infection also exists because the body's natural barrier to infection has been disrupted. Protecting the skin from contamination is critical.

9. *What type of dressings should be placed on the burns?* Dry sterile dressings are currently the standard of care. The dressings should be placed with a bandage to secure them. Take care to keep the bandages secure but not too tight as to cause pain or constrict circulation.
10. *What should be done to comfort this patient?* Pain from burns can be critical. The patient should receive pain medication per protocol. Morphine sulfate is one of the most commonly used pain medications.
11. *What is critical in reassessment of this patient?* The patient's airway should continually be reassessed. The patient's vital signs also should be closely monitored. Pain control also is important and should frequently be reassessed.
12. *What are important transport decisions?* This patient has potential airway complications. The patient should be rapidly and carefully treated and transported. The receiving facility should have burn capability or at least the ability to stabilize the patient for transfer to a burn center. Treatment should not delay transport unless it is critical.

Chapter Summary

- Approximately 1 million people are burned each year in the United States.
- The majority of burn patients are male.
- Persons at high risk for sustaining burn injuries include infants (10% of all patients), the elderly (14%), and those in high-risk occupations.
- Burns are categorized by their cause, size (BSA involved), and depth.
- The major categories of burns are thermal, chemical, radiation, and electrical.
- BSA, although difficult to estimate in the field, is approximated by using the rule of nines or the Lund-Browder chart. Approximating the size of the burn is critical.
- Burn depth is categorized as superficial thickness (first degree), partial thickness (second degree), or full thickness (third degree).
- The skin is the largest organ in the body and is quite complex. It exists in layers and, as such, these layers correlate with the depth of burn injury. The skin is responsible for, among other functions, controlling body temperature, preventing the invasion of infectious organisms, and maintaining water balance.
- Burns that are partial or full thickness have three zones of injury: (1) zone of coagulation and necrosis (innermost), (2) zone of ischemia (middle, outer zone), and (3) zone of hyperemia (outermost zone). These zones correlate with the potential for spontaneous healing (zone of hyperemia), the potential for spontaneous healing but at risk for complete loss of integrity (zone of ischemia), and loss requiring surgical treatment if larger than 1% or 2% TBSA (zone of coagulation and necrosis).
- Superficial burns are painful, nonblistered, and best represented by the common sunburn.
- Partial-thickness burns are pink, moist appearing, quite painful, and blistered and have an intact blood supply.
- Full-thickness burns have a grayish-white appearance, are insensate, and have lost blood supply.
- Inhalation injury (commonly called *smoke inhalation*) is a serious injury pattern in which the upper and lower airways are compromised by the inhalation of byproducts of combustion. Alone, significant inhalation injury results in a 30% mortality rate.
- The signs of inhalation injury include cough (productive and nonproductive), tachypnea, and hypoxemia.
- The symptoms of inhalation injury include dyspnea, air hunger, and fatigue.
- The treatment of inhalation injury includes high-flow oxygen and intubation if necessary.
- Early intubation is the key to preventing early, devastating loss of airway.
- The treatment of the cutaneous component of burn injury is basic. It involves dry, clean, and sterile dressings; IV fluid resuscitation for burns larger than 15% TBSA; and pain control.
- With the exception of tar and asphalt or chemical burns, lavage or irrigation of burns should not be done. This will result in hypothermia, which substantially increases morbidity in burn patients.
- Cutaneous exposure to chemicals causes varying burn depth, primarily from two factors: pH of the chemical and length of exposure time.
- Chemicals are broadly categorized as either acidic (pH less than 7) or alkaline (pH greater than 7).
- A basic understanding of chemistry is essential for treating chemical burns.
- Chemical and tar burns are the rare exceptions to the "no irrigation" rule in burn care. Chemicals should be diluted to prevent ongoing burn injury. Tar and asphalt burns are cooled with water to prevent ongoing, deep burn injury when trapped heat is contained beneath a blanket of molten material.
- The inhalation of chemicals can cause serious lung injury. Whether trapped within a building containing

Chapter Summary—continued

chemicals in gaseous form or in the outdoors with a widespread chemical cloud, inhalation remains a significant threat to those involved in the initial incident and those responding to the incident.

- Other manners of exposure to chemicals include absorption, ingestion, and injection.
- Electrical injuries may occur in the home, as part of occupational hazards, and in recreation.
- The most common cause of immediate death with electrical injury is ventricular fibrillation.
- Electrical injuries are categorized as either high or low voltage. Energy of less than 1000 V is low voltage, and energy greater than 1000 V is high voltage.
- An example of low voltage is household current; an example of high voltage is lightning.
- Low-voltage injuries cause flash burns and minor muscle or cutaneous injury from direct contact. High-voltage injuries cause devastating muscle, bone, and nerve injury. Long-term effects include kidney damage, paralysis, blindness, and hearing loss.
- High-voltage injuries are treated with spinal and long bone immobilization and aggressive fluid resuscitation.
- Pediatric burn injuries are common. Infants alone account for 10% of all burn injuries (100,000) annually.
- Among the most common burn injuries to children are those caused by scalding hot liquids.
- The dermal portion of the skin of children is much thinner than that of adults. This puts children at increased risk for deep burn injury.
- Fluid resuscitation in children must be undertaken with caution. Children are at significant risk for fluid overload compared with healthy adults because of limited cardiovascular reserve.
- Burn shock is a unique form of shock best characterized as a distributive shock. Its hallmark is capillary leak. Intravascular loss of fluid is in the form of plasma, leaked through capillaries, into the third space.
- Burn shock is treated with fluid resuscitation in a staged manner. That is, fluids are replaced at a rate roughly equal to the rate of loss into the surrounding tissues. Administration is then slowed as fluid moves back into the intravascular space.
- Fluid resuscitation for burn injury is undertaken with a balanced salt solution. The most commonly used fluid is lactated Ringer's solution.
- More fluid in burns is not necessarily better. During resuscitation of the burn patient, fluids should be given in a controlled manner, never as a wide-open therapy.
- The formula used for adult burn resuscitation is known as the *consensus formula*.
- The consensus formula for burn resuscitation calls for 2 to 4 mL/kg/TBSAB of IV fluid given over the first 24 hours after the burn injury.
- Rarely will a significant amount of fluid be given in the prehospital setting.
- Paramedics should understand that an IV rate of more than 250 mL/hour is rarely needed.
- Radiation-associated burn injuries are rare but pose an exceptional danger to both the patient and provider.
- The three types of radioactive particles are alpha, beta, and gamma.
- Of the three types of radioactive particles, gamma radiation is the most dangerous.
- All types of radioactive particles exist in the communities paramedics serve.
- The treatment of radiation exposure focuses on the principles of decreased exposure time, removal from the source, and decontamination. For all types of radiation, aggregate quantity should be limited.
- Pain is a significant problem with all types of burn injury. Controlling pain is an important step in the care of the burn patient.
- The preferred route of administration in the acutely injured burn patient is IV. Subcutaneous and intramuscular routes can be used but are less effective because of the poor perfusion of these tissues.
- The following types of burns should be referred to a qualified burn center for care:
  - Partial-thickness burns of more than 10% TBSA
  - Burns involving the hands, feet, genitalia, face, perineum, or major joints
  - Third-degree burns in any age group
  - Electrical burns, including lightning injury
  - Chemical burns
  - Inhalation injury (with or without burns)
  - Burns with associated trauma of any type
  - Burns in patients with special social, emotional, or long-term rehabilitative needs
  - Burns in children if the current institution lacks qualified personnel or equipment necessary to care for children
- Care at the burn center is a continuation of the care begun in the prehospital setting.
- In addition to ongoing fluid resuscitation, specific wound care (including surgery if needed), nutritional support, occupational and physical therapy, and psychological care are provided by burn centers.
- The goal in the treatment of the burn patient is to restore function, at all levels, to as close to the preburn injury state as possible.
- The surgical care of burn wounds includes simple wound care with debridement; surgical excision of wounds with skin grafting; and reconstructive surgery to restore the normal contour of the body, function of motion, and improve cosmesis.
- One of the key goals of the ABA and the burn centers of the world is prevention. The overwhelming majority of burn injuries are preventable.

REFERENCES

Agency for Toxic Substances and Disease Registry (ATSDR) (2007). *Medical management guidelines for hydrogen fluoride*. Retrieved March 26, 2008, from http://www.atsdr.cdc.gov.

Agency for Toxic Substances and Disease Registry (ATSDR) (2006). *Toxicological profile for phenol*. Retrieved March 26, 2008, from http://www.astdr.cdc.gov.

Agency for Toxic Substances and Disease Registry (ATSDR). (1997). *Toxicological profile for white phosphorus*. Retrieved March 26, 2008, from http://www.astdr.cdc.gov.

Brigham, P. A. (2000). *Burn incidence and treatment in the United States: 2000 fact sheet*. Chicago: American Burn Association.

Curran, E. B., & Holle, R. L. (1997). *Lightning fatalities, injuries and damage reports in the United States from 1959-1994. NOAA Technical Memorandum NWS SR-193*. Washington, DC: National Oceanic and Atmospheric Administration.

Greenhalgh, D. G., & Warden, G. D. (1994). The importance of intra-abdominal pressure measurements in burned children. *Journal of Trauma, 36,* 5.

Hatherill, J. R., Till, G. O., Bruner, L. H., & Ward, P. A. (1986). Thermal injury, intravascular hemolysis, and toxic oxygen products. *Journal of Clinical Investigation, 78,* 629-636.

Health Physics Society, 2006. Terminology. Retrieved March 29, 2008, from http://www.hps.org.

Jackson, D. M. (1953). The diagnosis of the depth of burning. *British Journal of Surgery, 40,* 588.

Janzekovic, Z. (1970). A new concept in the early excision and immediate grafting of burns. *Journal of Trauma, 10*(12), 1103-1108.

Kales, S. N., Polyhronopoulos, G. N., Castro, M. J., Goldman, R. H., & Christiani, D. C. (1997). Injuries caused by hazardous materials accidents. *Annals of Emergency Medicine, 30*(5), 598-603.

Kelly, K. M., Tkachenko, T. A., Pliskin, N. H., Fink, J. W., & Lee, R. C. (1999). Life after electrical injury: Risk factors for psychiatric sequelae. *Annals of the New York Academy of Sciences, 888,* 356-363.

Klausner, J, M., Caspi, J., Lelcuk, S., Khazam, A., Marin, G., Hechtman, H.B., et al. (1988). Delayed muscular rigidity and respiratory depression following fentanyl anesthesia. *Archives of Surgery, 123*(1), 66-67.

Layton, T. R., McMurtry, J. M., & McClain, E. J. (1984). Multiple spine fractures from electric injury. *Journal of Burn Care and Rehabilitation, 5,* 373-375.

Lee, R, C., Zhang, D., & Hannig, J. (2000). Biophysical injury mechanisms in electrical shock trauma. *Annual Review of Biomedical Engineering, 2,* 477-509.

Lide, D. R. (1996). *Handbook of chemistry and physics* (pp 14-33). Boca Raton, FL: CRC Press.

Lund, T., & Wiig, H. (1988). Acute postburn edema: Role of strongly negative interstitial fluid pressure. *American Journal of Physiology, 255*(5 pt 2), H1069-H1074.

Maass, D. L., White, D. J., Sanders B., & Horton, J. W. (2005). Cardiac myocyte calcium accumulation in burn injury: Cause or effect of myocardial contractile dysfunction. *Journal of Burn Care and Rehabilitation, 26*(3), 252-259.

Marx, J., Hockberger, R., & Walls, R. (2006). *Rosen's emergency medicine: Concepts and clinical practice* (6th ed; 3 vols). St. Louis: Mosby.

Miller, S., & Jeng, J. (2006). *National Burn Repository 2005 report*. Chicago: American Burn Association.

Mosteller, R. D. (1987). Simplified calculation of body surface area. *New England Journal of Medicine, 317*(17), 1098.

National Association of Emergency Medical Technicians (NAEMT). (2007). *Prehospital trauma life support (6th ed)* (p 348). St. Louis: Mosby.

Peden, M., McGee, K., & Sharma, G. (2002). *The injury chart book: A graphical overview of the global burden of injuries*. Geneva: World Health Organization.

Roberts, J. R., & Hedges, J. R. (2006). *Clinical procedures in emergency medicine (6th ed)* (pp 766-769). Philadelphia: Saunders.

Topley, E., Jackson, D. M., Cason, J. S., & Davies, J. W. (1962). Assessment of red blood cell loss in the first two days after severe burns. *Annals of Surgery, 155,* 581-590.

Vincent, J. L., de Mendonça, A., Cantraine, F., Moreno, R., Takala, J., Suter, P. M., et al. (1998). Use of the SOFA score to assess the incidence of organ dysfunction/failure in intensive care units: Results of a multicenter, prospective study. *Critical Care Medicine, 26,* 1793-1800.

SUGGESTED RESOURCE

American Burn Association
ABA Central Office—Chicago
625 N. Michigan Ave., Suite 2550
Chicago, IL 60611
Website: http://www.ameriburn.org

Chapter Quiz

1. The outermost layer of the skin is called the ________.
- **a.** dermis
- **b.** epidermis
- **c.** subcutaneous tissue
- **d.** organelle

2. The most common type of burn in the United States is ________.
- **a.** electrical
- **b.** thermal
- **c.** chemical
- **d.** radiation related

3. True or False: The major cause of death from burns is underresuscitation with IV fluids.

4. The innermost area of burn in the zone of injury model is the ________.
- **a.** zone of stasis
- **b.** zone of hyperemia
- **c.** zone of alteration
- **d.** zone of coagulation

5. Full-thickness burns are also known as ________.
- **a.** first degree
- **b.** second degree
- **c.** third degree
- **d.** fourth degree

6. True or False: Partial-thickness burns frequently require skin grafts.

Chapter Quiz—continued

7. An adult has a burn that involves his entire left leg, half of his right arm, and the anterior trunk. According to the rule of nines, his TBSAB is approximately _________.
   a. 30%
   b. 36%
   c. 40%
   d. 48%

8. A child has burns on her entire head and one entire leg. According to the pediatric rule of nines, her TBSAB is _________.
   a. 27%
   b. 32%
   c. 36%
   d. 40%

9. Although fluid volume replacement is somewhat controversial, the paramedic may be directed to perform this treatment. The proper fluid to use in the prehospital setting is _________.
   a. a dextrose solution such as 5% dextrose in water
   b. a colloid
   c. blood (if available)
   d. LR solution

10. True or False: If signs of inhalation burn injury are noted with hoarseness and stridor, ET intubation is contraindicated.

Terminology

Abdominal compartment syndrome Syndrome caused by diffuse intestinal edema, a result of fluid accumulation in the bowel wall. It may be caused by overresuscitation with crystalloids and results in shock and renal failure.

Acidic pH less than 7.0.

Alkaline pH greater than 7.0.

Antiinflammatory mediators Protein entities, often produced in the liver, that act as modulators of the immune response to the proinflammatory response to injury; also called *cytokines*.

Autologous skin grafting The transplantation of skin of one patient from its original location to that of a wound on the same patient, such as a burn. *Autologous* means "derived from the same individual."

Bioburden Accumulation of bacteria in a wound. This does not necessarily imply an infection is present.

Body surface area (BSA) Area of the body covered by skin; measured in square meters.

Capillary leak Loss of intravascular fluid (plasma, water) from a loss of capillary integrity or an opening of gap junctions between the cells of the capillaries. May be caused by thermal injury to capillaries or as a result of the intense inflammatory reaction to burn injury, infection, or physical trauma.

Catabolic Refers to the metabolic breakdown of proteins, lipids, and carbohydrates by the body to produce energy.

Coagulation Formation of blood clots with the associated increase in blood viscosity.

Consensus formula Formula used to calculate the volume of fluid needed to properly resuscitate a burn patient. The formula is 2 to 4 mL/kg/% TBSAB. This is the formula currently regarded by the ABA as the standard of care in adult burn patients. Several other, similar formulas exist that also may be used.

Cosmesis Of or referring to the improvement of physical appearance.

Cytokines Proteins released from the liver, macrophages, and white blood cells in response to injury.

Deep partial-thickness burn A burn in which the mid- or deeper dermis is injured. Results in injury to the deeper hair follicle, glandular, nerve, and blood vessel structures.

Dermatome A device used to remove healthy skin from somewhere on the body of the burn patient for the purpose of transplanting (grafting) at another site, such as an excised burn wound or other open wound.

Distributive shock Inadequate tissue perfusion as a result of fluid shifts between body compartments. Burn shock is a distributive shock in which plasma and water are lost from the vascular tree into the surrounding tissues. This shock also is seen in the setting of sepsis, in which a similar fluid redistribution occurs.

Donor skin site A site on the body from which healthy skin is removed for the purpose of grafting a burn or other open wound.

Ejection fraction Fraction (expressed as a percentage) of blood ejected from the ventricle of the heart with each contraction. Generally at least 60% of the blood entering the ventricle should be forced to the lungs or systemic circulation.

Eschar A thick wound covering that consists of necrotic or otherwise devitalized tissue or cellular components. In a burn wound, this is the burned tissue or skin of the wound.

Excision In reference to burn surgery, this is the sharp, surgical removal of burned tissue that will never regain function. Excision is carried out before skin grafting.

Fascia Anatomically, the tough connective tissue covering of the muscles of the body. Fascia contains the muscles within a compartment.

First-degree burn Superficial burn involving only the epidermis, such as a minor sunburn.

Flash electrical burn A burn resulting from indirect contact with an electrical explosion.

High voltage Greater than 1000 V.

Hydrogen ion concentration Concentration of hydrogen ions in a given solution, such as water or blood; used to calculate the pH of a substance.

Hyperdynamic Excessively forceful or energetic. The term is used to describe shock states in which the heart is pumping aggressively to make up for fluid losses, such as in burn or septic shock.

Hypermetabolic A state or condition of the body characterized by excessive production and utilization of energy molecules such as protein.

Interstitium Extravascular and extracellular milieu; also known as the *third space*.

Intimal In reference to blood vessels, the innermost lining of an artery; composed of a single layer of cells.

Invasive wound infection An infection involving the deeper tissues of a wound that may be destructive to blood vessels and other structures of the skin and soft tissues.

Keratinized Accumulation of the protein keratin within the cytoplasm of skin cells. These cells comprise the epidermis of the skin. These dead cells function as the first defense against invaders and minor trauma.

Lipophilic Substances that tend to seek out and bind to fatty substances.

Lower airway Portion of the respiratory tract below the glottis.

Lower airway inhalation injury Injury to the anatomic portion of the respiratory tree below the level of the glottis. Generally caused by the inhalation of the toxic byproducts of combustion.

Low voltage Less than 1000 V.

Mucosa Layer of cells lining body cavities or organs (e.g., the lining of the mouth and digestive tract). Generally implies a moist surface.

Myocardial depressant factor An inflammatory mediator (cytokine) produced as a result of significant burn injury. This cytokine is known to affect the contractile function of the cardiac ventricles.

Myoglobin A protein within muscle that functions as an oxygen carrier. When released in large quantities into the bloodstream, these proteins block the small vessels of the kidneys.

Myoglobinuria Presence of myoglobin in the urine; almost always a result of a pathologic (disease) state such as widespread muscle injury.

Negative pressure Pressure that acts as a vacuum, pulling more fluid from the vascular space at a faster rate than before, further depleting the intravascular volume; also known as *imbibition pressure*.

Neuralgia Pain caused by chronic nerve damage.

Partial-thickness burn Burns that involve any layer of the dermis. The depth of these burns varies and depends on location, so they are further subcategorized as superficial partial-thickness or deep partial-thickness burns. Also called *second-degree burns*.

pH A numeric assignment used to define the hydrogen ion concentration of a given chemical. The lower the pH, the higher the hydrogen ion concentration and the more acidic the solution.

Potassium The main intracellular ion (electrolyte), with the chemical designation K^+.

rem Roentgen equivalent man.

Roentgens Denote ionizing radiation passing through air.

Serum base deficit Implies that the blood buffer, bicarbonate, is being used to combat a metabolic acidosis. Metabolic acidosis occurs in the setting of numerous shock states, such as burn shock. This number is reported on a standard blood gas assay and is detected in an arterial or venous blood sample.

Serum lactate Measure in the blood; a byproduct of anaerobic metabolism. As such, it is a good measure of end organ and cellular perfusion in shock states. Elevated serum lactate levels, or lactic academia, implies that cells, tissues, or organs are not receiving adequate oxygen to carry out their metabolic activities.

Skin grafting Transplantation of skin, either from the same person or from a cadaver, to the site of a wound, such as a burn.

Space-occupying lesion A mass, such as a tumor or blood collection, within a contained body space, such as the skull.

Split-thickness skin graft A skin graft in which only a fraction of the thickness of the natural dermis is taken.

Superficial burn A burn with a pink appearance that does not exhibit blister formation; painful both with and without tactile stimulation (e.g., sunburn). Also known as a *first-degree burn*.

Superficial partial-thickness burn Burns involving the more superficial dermis. These burns have a moist, pink appearance, and when lightly touched, are painful and sensate. Blood vessels, hair shafts, nerves, and glands may be injured, but not to the extent that regeneration cannot take place.

Terminology—continued

Third space Extravascular and extracellular milieu; also known as the *interstitium.*

Total body surface area burned (TBSAB) Used to describe the amount of the body injured by a burn and expressed as a percentage of the entire BSA.

Tumor necrosis factor-alpha An inflammatory cytokine released in response to a variety of physical trauma, including burns. In burn injuries, massive quantities are produced by the liver; has been implicated as the causative agent in myocardial depression seen in burns.

Upper airway Portion of the respiratory tract above the glottis.

Ventricular fibrillation Disorganized electrical activity of the ventricular conduction system of the heart, resulting in inefficient contractile force. This is the main cause of sudden cardiac death in electrical injuries.

Zone of coagulation In a full-thickness burn wound, the central area of the burn devoid of blood flow. This tissue is not salvageable and becomes visibly necrotic days after the injury.

Zone of stasis or ischemia Outside the zone of coagulation, where blood supply is tenuous. That is, the capillaries may be damaged but oxygenated blood can still pass through them to perfuse the surrounding tissues.

CHAPTER 47

Head and Face Trauma

Objectives

After completing this chapter, you will be able to:

1. Describe the etiology, history, and physical findings of facial injuries.
2. Using the mechanism of injury, patient history, and physical examination findings, develop a treatment plan for a patient with facial injuries.
3. Describe the etiology, history, and physical findings of eye injuries.
4. Using the mechanism of injury, patient history, and physical examination findings, develop a treatment plan for a patient with an eye injury.
5. Describe the etiology, history, and physical findings of ear injuries.
6. Using the mechanism of injury, patient history, and physical examination findings, develop a treatment plan for a patient with an ear injury.
7. Describe the etiology, history, and physical findings of neck injuries.
8. Using the mechanism of injury, patient history, and physical examination findings, develop a treatment plan for a patient with a neck injury.
9. Explain anatomy and relate physiology of the central nervous system to head injuries.
10. Distinguish between head injury and brain injury.
11. Describe the etiology, history, and physical findings of a skull fracture.
12. Using the patient history and physical examination findings, develop a treatment plan for a patient with a skull fracture.
13. Explain the pathophysiology of head and brain injuries.
14. Predict head injuries on the basis of mechanism of injury.
15. Explain the pathophysiology of increasing intracranial pressure and the process involved with each of the levels of increase.
16. Describe the etiology, history, and physical findings of each of the following:
    - Concussion
    - Diffuse axonal injury
    - Cerebral contusion
    - Epidural hematoma
    - Subdural hematoma
    - Intracerebral hemorrhage
    - Subarachnoid hemorrhage
17. Using the patient history and physical examination findings, develop a treatment plan for a patient with any of the following:
    - Concussion
    - Diffuse axonal injury
    - Cerebral contusion
    - Epidural hematoma
    - Subdural hematoma
    - Intracerebral hemorrhage
    - Subarachnoid hemorrhage
18. Develop a management plan for the removal of a helmet for a head-injured patient.

CHAPTER OUTLINE

Case Scenario

You are called to a barn in a rural area for a "patient with head pain." On arrival you find a conscious and alert 66-year-old woman lying on her side in a large pool of blood. She states that she was walking in the barn, thinks she got shot and fell to the ground, then has no memory until her daughter found her. Her only complaint is a headache. Her skin is warm and dry, and she is alert and oriented to person, place, and time. She has a 3- to 4-cm puncture wound on the top of her head that is bleeding profusely. The scalp is swollen in the area surrounding the puncture wound, and some crepitus is evident when palpating the area surrounding the puncture. No exit wound is visible.

Questions

1. *What is your general impression of this patient?*
2. *What physical assessment findings are most pertinent at this time?*
3. *What is the significance of the loss of memory related to the incident?*
4. *What treatment should be initiated immediately?*

In the United States, traumatic brain injuries annually account for 34% of all injury deaths. Including skull and facial fractures, 2 million people sustain a head injury each year. Today 62.3 individuals per 100,000 persons older than 15 years live in society with long-term impairments from a head injury. How you approach this patient population can alter these numbers. Understanding the anatomy and physiology of the head and face as well as the pathophysiology of this group of injuries will better prepare you to make a difference in these patients' outcomes.

MAXILLOFACIAL INJURY

[OBJECTIVES 1, 2]

Anatomy of the Face

Most of the arterial blood supply to the face is from branches of the external carotid artery (Figure 47-1). The facial artery is the major artery that supplies blood to the face. The superficial temporal, mandibular, and maxillary arteries also contribute to the blood supply of the face.

The fifth and seventh cranial nerves are the major nerves of the face. The fifth cranial nerve (CN V) is the trigeminal nerve. It is the major sensory nerve of the head. It also innervates muscles that move the lower jaw. The seventh cranial nerve (CN VII) is the facial nerve. Fibers of the facial nerve innervate the muscles responsible for facial expression. Other cranial nerves that may be associated with facial trauma include the oculomotor and trochlear nerves. The oculomotor nerve (CN III) is responsible for eye movement and pupil constriction. The trochlear nerve (CN IV) is responsible for downward gaze.

Twenty-two bones compose the skull. Of these, eight are cranial bones and 14 are facial bones. The bones of the face are relatively thin but provide protection for the structures behind them.

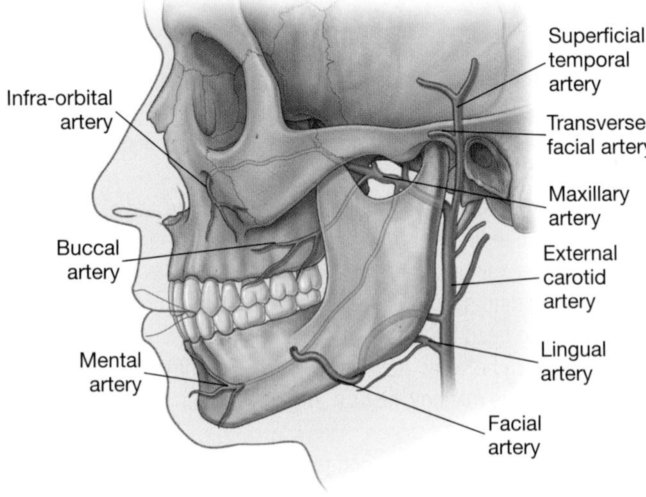

Figure 47-1 Arterial blood supply of the face.

Mechanism of Injury

Facial injuries may be the result of blunt or penetrating trauma. Common mechanisms of injury are shown in Box 47-1. Injuries with which facial trauma is often associated are listed in Box 47-2.

Soft Tissue Injuries

Etiology and Demographics

In the United States motor vehicle crashes (MVCs) are the cause of most facial injuries. However, assaults and personal altercations account for more and more facial injuries. In the elderly, falls account for the greatest number of facial injuries (Brain Injury Association, 2005).

BOX 47-1 Facial Injuries: Mechanisms of Injury

Blunt Trauma

- Motor vehicle crashes
- Motorcycle crashes
- Falls
- Assaults
- Interpersonal violence
- Sports injuries
- Industrial injuries

Penetrating Trauma

- Gunshot wounds
- Stab wounds
- Blasts
- Bites (animal or human)

Toxic Exposure

- Acids
- Alkalis

BOX 47-2 Facial Injuries: Associated Injuries

- Airway compromise
- Cervical spine injury
- Closed head injury
- Vascular injury
- Dental trauma or avulsion

Airbag deployment can cause abrasions to the face, neck, and upper chest. Corneal or sclera injury can occur with airbags as well; however, these are uncommon injuries.

History and Physical Findings

When possible, obtain a history from the patient. Important historical information includes the following:

- Mechanism of injury
- Time the injury occurred
- Signs and symptoms
- Allergies
- Medications
- Last oral intake
- Past medical history
- Events leading up to the injury

To assess facial injuries effectively, take an organized approach to assessment of these patients. As with all injuries, the ABCDs (***a***irway, ***b***reathing, ***c***irculation ***d***isability) are the highest priority. Inspect the facial structures, looking for symmetry and deformity. The face should be symmetric, with only slight variation from side to side. When looking directly at the face, the eyes should appear even and the medial and lateral corners should be level and in line with the top 20% of the **auricles,** or external part of the ears. Some patients may have a dysconjugate gaze that is normal for them. Corners of the mouth should move symmetrically when the patient smiles or talks, and the nose should be relatively straight and midline. Grossly asymmetric facial features are abnormal and should be thoroughly evaluated and documented. Palpate the facial structures with both hands simultaneously, feeling for crepitus or loss of continuity. Palpate the nasal bones and visualize the nasal cavity. Assess jaw movement and alignment by asking the patient to bite down.

Facial lacerations are a common injury. Injury to the facial nerve can result in facial drooping on the affected side. A deep cheek laceration can damage the parotid duct, parotid gland, and branches of the facial nerve. Assessment is vital in determining the extent of nerve damage. If the patient cannot wrinkle his or her forehead on the affected side, suspect damage to the temporal branch of the facial nerve. If the patient is unable to close the eyelid fully, suspect damage to the temporal or zygomatic branch of the facial nerve. If the patient is unable to purse his or her lips, such as to whistle, suspect damage to the buccal branch of the facial nerve. Inability to depress the lower lip indicates possible mandibular branch damage. Excessive facial dressings or a decreased level of consciousness makes assessment of the facial nerve far more difficult.

If the oculomotor nerve is damaged, the patient may be unable to raise an eyelid and have a delayed or absent pupillary response to light. Downward movement of the eye may be absent or limited in the presence of damage to the trochlear nerve.

Lacerations and puncture wounds caused by human and/or animal bites are considered highly contaminated because of bacteria present in the attacker's mouth. These injuries should be inspected for teeth fragments. Abrasions or "road rash" type injuries can be more disfiguring than lacerations to the face because these injuries can cause permanent tattooing or epidermal staining.

Mouth injuries may occur as a result of an MVC, a blow to the mouth or chin, a gunshot wound, a laceration, or a puncture. A lacerated tongue can result in airway compromise because of blood, tissue, or broken or avulsed teeth. Laceration of the mucous membranes of the mouth results in profuse bleeding, compromising the airway. Signs and symptoms of an injury to the mouth include copious bleeding, blood-tinged mucus, and an inability to talk unless leaning forward to allow for drainage.

PARAMEDIC*Pearl*

Because of its abundant blood supply and associated risk of airway compromise, frequent reassessment of the patient with a facial injury is essential.

Therapeutic Interventions

A patient who has facial injuries likely will be agitated or anxious. Calming and reassuring the patient is important. Be sure to explain what you are doing and why as you provide care.

Initial priorities include ensuring an open airway and adequate breathing while taking spinal precautions (Skill 47-1). Spinal precautions are used to minimize

SKILL 47-1 MANUAL STABILIZATION OF THE CERVICAL SPINE

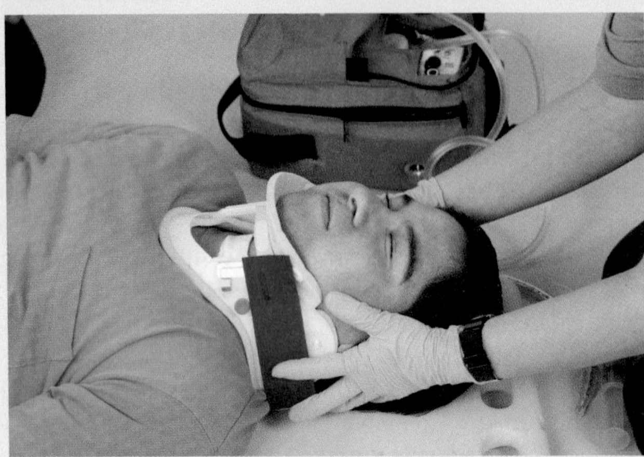

Step 1 Manual stabilization of the head and neck with patient supine.

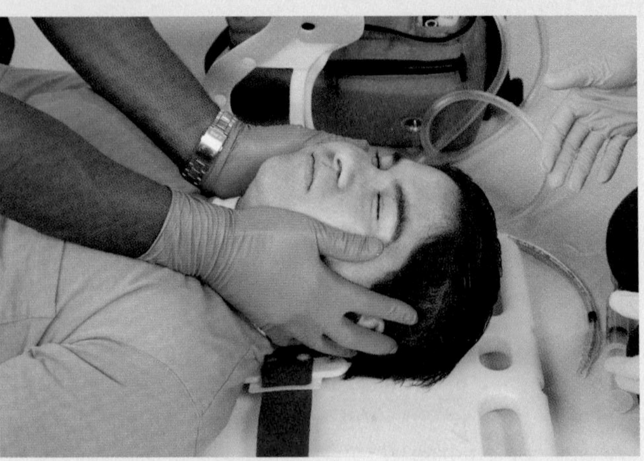

Step 4 Manual stabilization of the head and neck from the front of the patient.

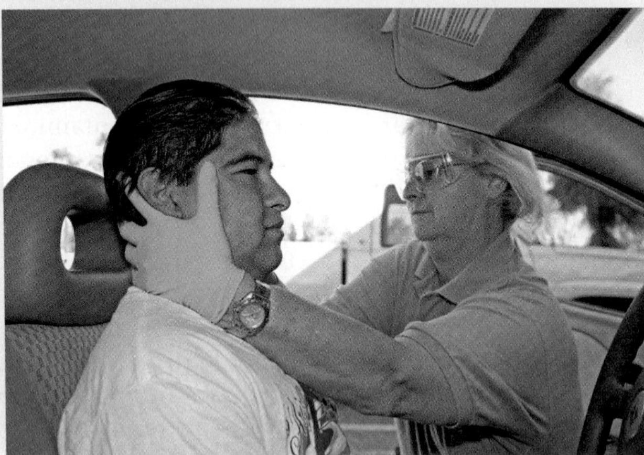

Step 2 Manual stabilization of the head and neck from the patient's side.

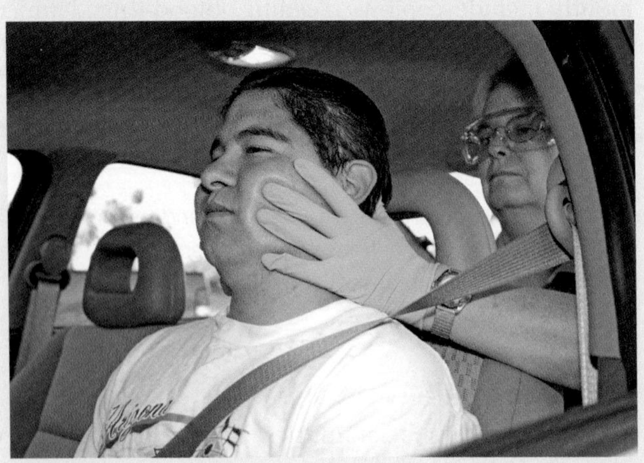

Step 3 Manual stabilization of the head and neck from behind the patient.

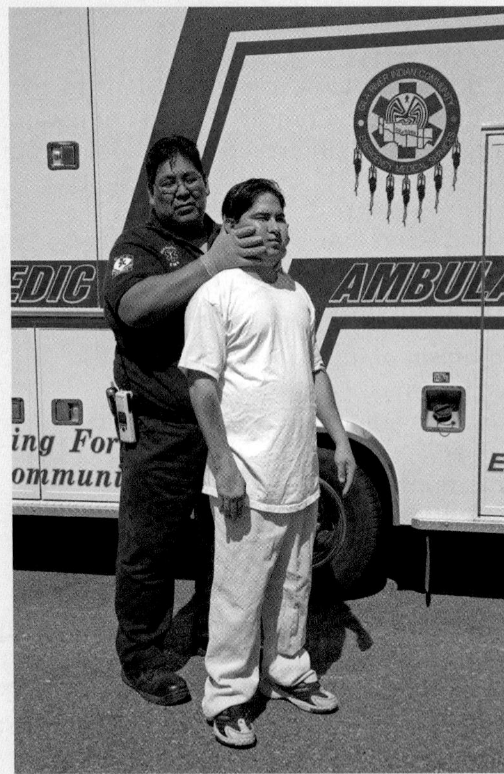

Step 5 Manual stabilization of the head and neck with the patient standing.

movement that could cause injury to the spinal cord. When trauma to the head or neck is suspected or a patient is unresponsive, ask a member of your crew to position the patient's head in a neutral position (eyes facing forward and level) and in line with the body. If the patient complains of pain or resistance is met when moving the head to a neutral position, stop and maintain the head and neck in the position the patient was found. Continue manual stabilization until the patient has been completely secured to a backboard.

The airway must be closely monitored for excessive secretions or bleeding. If present, remove material such as blood and vomitus from the airway with suctioning. If the mandible is displaced for any reason, the anatomic structures that properly align the tongue to maintain the airway are compromised, increasing the likelihood of airway obstruction. Additional factors to consider that can compromise airway patency in patients with facial trauma are alcohol, drugs, and brain injuries. Maintaining a clear airway may require suctioning, intubation, and positioning. In some situations tracheal intubation may not be possible if severe injuries prevent the identification of important landmarks. In an unconscious patient in whom cervical spine injury is not suspected or can be ruled out, the head of the stretcher should be raised approximately 15 to 30 degrees to help avoid aspiration.

Inadequate breathing may require assistance with a bag-mask device. Although bleeding from facial injuries can be profuse, it is usually controlled easily with direct pressure. Contusions of the face usually do not cause problems. However, suspect a fracture at the site until proven otherwise.

PARAMEDIC*Pearl*

Facial Trauma: Patient Management Priorities

- Assume cervical spine injury.
- Relieve airway obstruction.
- Ensure adequate breathing.
- Control bleeding.
- Look for life-threatening injuries.

Nasal and Ear Foreign Bodies

Etiology and Demographics

The nasal cavities are pliable and expandable, so large or multiple objects can be found in the nose. Nasal foreign bodies most commonly occur in children. Common foreign bodies found in the nose and ear are listed in Box 47-3. Nasal foreign bodies from trauma are far less common yet still occur.

Ear foreign bodies most commonly occur in children 9 months of age to 4 years. The foreign body is almost always placed there by the child. Ear wax **(cerumen)** is the most common ear canal obstruction in children and adults. A child is prone to this as a result of the parent or child inserting cotton swabs too far, pushing cerumen or fibers into the canal and impacting them. Older adults are prone to this because of excessive ear wax production and hearing aids blocking the outlet.

BOX 47-3 Common Foreign Bodies Found in the Nose and Ear

- Beads
- Parts of small toys
- Pebbles
- Buttons
- Vegetables
- Crayons
- Bolts
- Screws
- Sticks
- Paper
- Insects

BOX 47-4 Nasal Foreign Body: Possible Signs and Symptoms

- Nosebleed on affected side
- Fever
- Pain
- Swollen nasal mucosa
- Purulent nasal discharge on affected side
- Foul-smelling nasal discharge

BOX 47-5 Ear Foreign Body: Possible Signs and Symptoms

- Bloody or purulent discharge from the affected ear
- Decreased hearing in the affected ear
- Pain or discomfort in the affected ear
- Swelling of the external ear
- Sound of insect buzzing in the ear
- Foul-smelling discharge from the affected ear
- Sensation of fullness or something in the ear

History and Physical Findings

A nasal foreign body may go undiscovered until a foul odor and/or purulent discharge is noticed. Other signs are listed in Box 47-4. Possible signs and symptoms associated with a foreign body in the ear are shown in Box 47-5.

Therapeutic Interventions

In most cases, a foreign body in the ear or nose should be left alone and the patient transported for physician evaluation. Attempt to remove a foreign body from the nose only if the airway is compromised. If the patient shows signs of difficulty breathing, stridor, or altered mental status, consider the possibility of a foreign body airway obstruction and manage the situation immediately.

If the patient is alert, oriented, and cooperative, have him or her block the unobstructed nostril, close the mouth, and forcefully expel air several times. This may cause enough pressure to release a foreign body from the nose.

A patient with an insect trapped in the ear canal often is quite anxious. Provide reassurance as you provide emergency care. A flashlight can be shone into the ear canal in an attempt to draw the insect toward the light.

PARAMEDIC*Pearl*

Never insert anything into the ear canal to remove a foreign body. Without the appropriate equipment, you can damage the patient's eardrum. Do not attempt to remove a vegetable foreign body from the nose or ear by using water or mineral oil. These substances can cause the object to swell, making removal even more difficult.

Orbital Fractures

Anatomy of the Eye

Seven bones help compose the framework of the orbit of the eye (Figure 47-2). The thin and waferlike orbital bones are designed to reduce the weight of the head, but this puts the eyeballs at risk of injury from blunt force trauma to the area. The orbits are cone shaped, with the wide end at the face, narrowing down as it progresses into the skull and ending at a small plate that contains openings for the optic nerve and various blood vessels. The eyes are shaped like a globe and are approximately 1 inch in diameter (Figure 47-3). Because the walls of the orbit are thin, trauma to the face may result in a fracture of one or more orbital bones.

The outside of the eyeball consists of three layers of tissue. The outermost layer consists of a dense, fibrous tissue called the **sclera,** which, as it crosses over the front of the eyeball, becomes the white of the eye and the transparent **cornea.** The **choroid,** or middle layer, is the vascular layer of the eyeball. As this membrane crosses the front of the eye it is seen as the iris, or colored portion of the eye. The innermost membrane layer

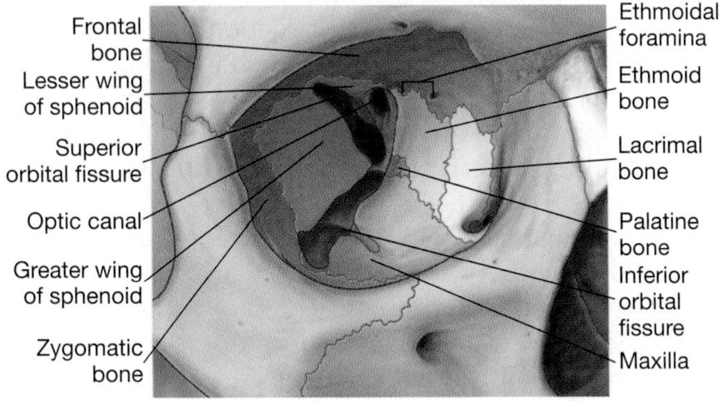

Figure 47-2 Bones of the orbit.

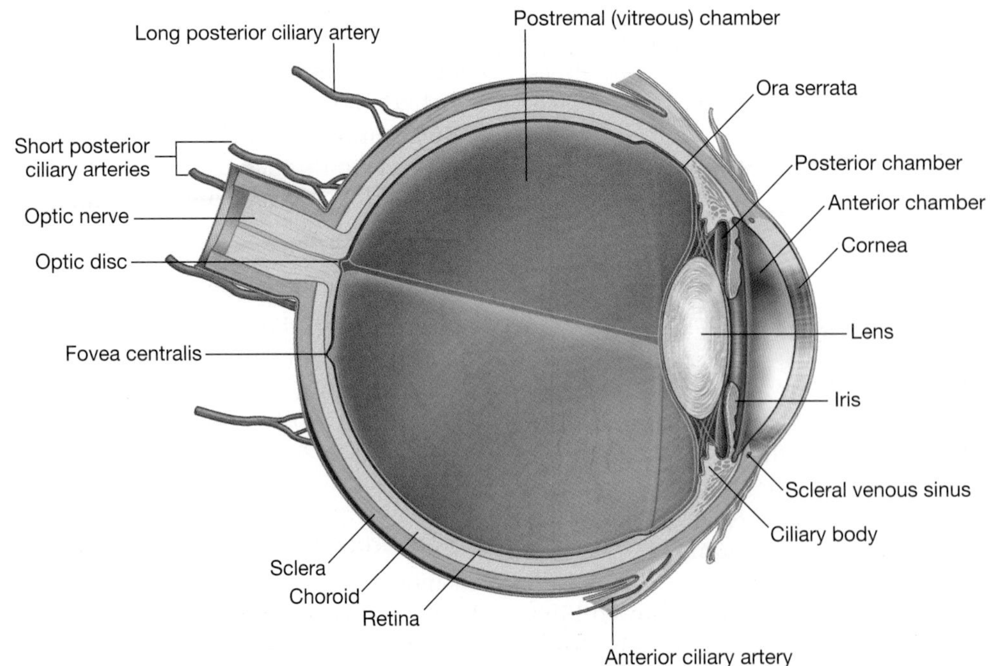

Figure 47-3 The eyeball.

consists of the retina, which covers the posteriormost part of the eyeball.

The inner eye consists of two cavities, anterior and posterior (see Figure 47-3). The anterior cavity contains the anterior and posterior chambers, which are connected by the pupil, or opening in the iris. These chambers are filled with a thin, watery fluid called the **aqueous humor,** which can be regenerated by the body if either chamber becomes injured. The posterior cavity, which is also called the **vitreous chamber,** comprises the remainder of the eyeball, approximately four fifths of the total eye. It is filled with **vitreous humor,** a thick, jellylike substance that cannot be replaced if this part of the eyeball is damaged. The shape of the eyeball is maintained by the hydrostatic pressure exerted on the globe by the aqueous and vitreous humor.

The anterior cavity of the eye protrudes slightly forward. Inside this cavity are the iris and pupil. The iris, the colored portion of the eye, is a continuation of the choroid membrane layer. The pupil is the central opening in the iris. The pupil serves as the connection between the anterior and posterior chambers and also is the structure that allows light and images to enter the vitreous chamber, where they make contact with the retina. The pupil regulates the amount of light that enters the eye by constricting or dilating in response to physiologic or environmental stimuli. Pupillary reactions also can be affected by the autonomic nervous system, medications, and recreational drugs.

Dividing the anterior cavity from the posterior cavity is the lens. The function of the lens is to focus images on the retinal surface. The lens is a transparent group of elastic fibers that contract and relax in response to incoming stimuli, focusing the images on the retina. A cloudiness that results in a loss of transparency in the lens is what causes a cataract. **Myopia,** or nearsightedness, occurs when incoming light focuses in front of the retina and can be caused by poor functioning of the lens and/or an elongation of the eyeball. **Hyperopia,** or farsightedness, occurs when incoming light focuses behind the retina and often is caused by a flattening of the globe and/or poor lens function. As people age the lens becomes less able to accommodate from far to near vision; this condition is called **presbyopia** and often requires older individuals to wear glasses to read. Anyone with symptoms involving the eyes should have his or her visual acuity checked. Box 47-6 reviews how to check visual acuity.

Inside the vitreous chamber are the retinal surfaces, blood vessels, and optic disk. The retina lines the entire surface of the chamber and serves as the focal point for incoming light and images. It contains rods and cones for color vision and nerve fibers that transmit the images to the brain for identification. Assessment of the condition of the retina and blood vessels requires the use of an **ophthalmoscope.** An ophthalmoscope is an instrument with focused light and adjustable magnification. When viewed through an ophthalmoscope, the retina should appear smooth, reddish-purple, and lined with blood vessels. The optic disk, the terminal end of the optic nerve, should appear yellowish in color and have distinct blood vessels at its center on ophthalmic evaluation. The optic disk is often called the *blind spot* because this area contains no retina. To avoid damage to the nerve and because it contains no retina, the optic disk is not located in the direct line of vision; it is typically found in the upper medial quadrant at the back of the eye.

The eyes are surrounded by eyebrows, eyelashes, and eyelids to help protect them from the environment. The eyebrows and eyelashes catch small particles before they can fall into the eye. The eyelids provide the major source of protection for the eye. Any incoming threat causes the eyelids to close to protect the sensitive structures of the eyeball. Examples of conditions that cause the eyelids to close include bright light, foreign matter, or an object that gets too near the eyeball or eyelid. The lining of the eyelids consists of the **conjunctiva,** a continuous layer of tissue that extends from the inside of the upper lid across the eyeball, connecting to the inside of the lower lid. This continuous tissue layer forms the outermost protective layer on the eyeball as well as the sacs that are visible when looking inside the lower lid. The thinness of the conjunctiva allows visualization of the many blood vessels in the area. On darker-skinned individuals this is the best place to observe for pallor. The thinness of the tissue allows rapid absorption of medication or toxic substances from the sac.

The **lacrimal gland** is located on the upper lateral corner of the inside of the eyelid. The lacrimal gland is responsible for making tears and providing the fluid that coats the eyes with each blink. Fluid from the eyes drains

BOX 47-6 Evaluating Visual Acuity

In 1862 Hermann Snellen, a Dutch ophthalmologist, developed the eye chart that is still used today to check visual acuity. Snellen discovered a relation between the size of letters and various distances. The numbers used to describe sight, 20/20, 20/30, and so forth represent the sharpness of sight, not quality of sight. The first letter indicates the distance the individual stands from the chart, and the second number represents the distance the average eye can see the letter. So a person with 20/40 sight is standing at 20 feet and can read letters that the average eye can read at 40 feet.

To test visual acuity, have the patient stand 20 feet from the chart and cover one eye. Ask the patient to read the smallest line of letters possible on the chart. Vision is evaluated for each eye independently and then for both eyes together.

Snellen eye charts are available from most medical equipment supply stores or can be downloaded from the Internet.

through the lacrimal ducts into the nose. Because the tiny porelike opening of the **lacrimal ducts** cannot handle large volumes of fluid, tears and watery eyes drain down the cheek.

Etiology and Demographics

The term *orbital fracture* refers to any fracture that involves the bony cavity containing the eyeball. Orbital fractures may occur as an isolated injury or in conjunction with another injury, such as a zygomatic fracture or fractures of the midface.

An orbital blowout fracture involves the bones of the orbital floor. A typical mechanism of injury involves a fist, tennis ball, or baseball striking the globe of the eye and surrounding soft tissues. (Objects with a larger surface area are unable to compress the globe because of protection by the lower orbital rim surrounding the globe). The impact pushes the globe into the orbit, compressing its contents. The sudden increase in pressure causes a fracture at the weakest point of the orbit, which is usually the orbital floor.

History and Physical Findings

As with any traumatic injury, assess the mechanism of injury for the likelihood of other possible injuries. A patient with an orbital fracture also may have a fracture of the globe and should be assessed for a blowout injury (Box 47-7). A blowout injury can cause muscles, nerves, fat, and connective tissues to become entrapped by the fractured segment. **Entrapment** is assessed by checking the extraocular movements of the eye (Figure 47-4). A patient with a blowout fracture may report double vision and a loss of sensation to the cheek and upper lip. Limited eye motion may be evident (Figure 47-5).

Therapeutic Interventions

Airway, breathing, and circulation are the first priorities. Maintain an open airway by using a jaw thrust without head tilt maneuver, if needed. The use of airway adjuncts, including tracheal intubation, may be necessary. Because of the possibility of intracranial placement of tracheal tubes, severe facial injury is considered a relative contraindication to using the nasotracheal route of intubation. Place the patient on a backboard with a cervical immobilization device if a cervical spine injury is a possibility.

Because the patient's vision will be impaired, be mindful to explain procedures to the patient before performing them. Loose bandages covering both eyes are usually applied to limit movement of either eye. A patient who has an orbital fracture should be instructed to avoid blowing the nose, sneezing, and straining until the eye is repaired. If a blowout fracture is present, surgical intervention is necessary.

Nasal Fractures

Anatomy of the Nose

The primary function of the nose is to support the respiratory system. It also contains **olfactory** nerves that

BOX 47-7 Orbital Blowout Fracture: Signs and Symptoms

- Double vision
- Nosebleed
- Pain
- Soft tissue discoloration of affected eye
- Limited ability to look upward with affected eye
- Crepitus in area of fracture site
- Sunken appearance of affected eye

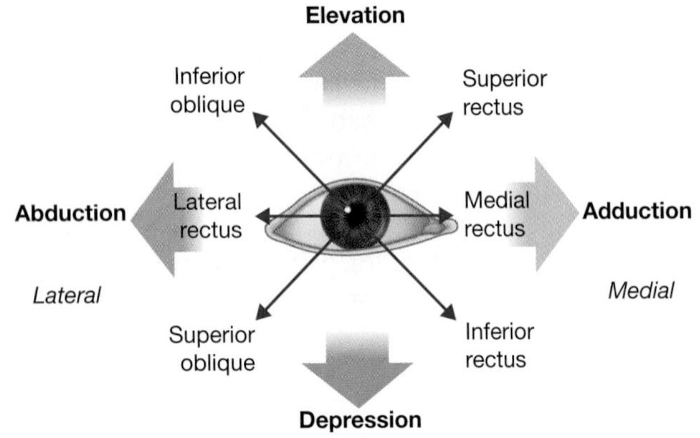

Figure 47-4 Anatomic actions of the eye muscles.

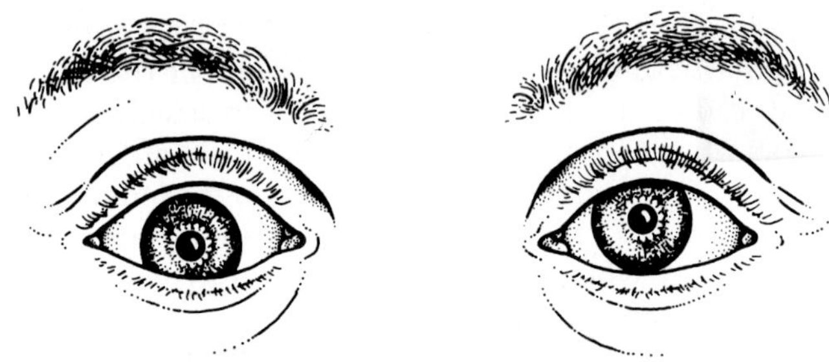

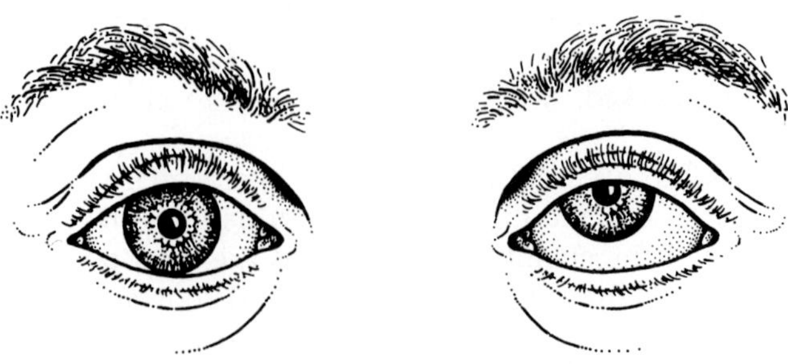

Upward gaze: limitation of motion of right eye

Figure 47-5 Right orbital blowout fracture. Appearance of the eyes and limitation of motion typically present in a blowout fracture are shown.

facilitate smell. The nasal cavity is pyramidal in shape, wider at the base and narrowing toward the top.

Air brought into the body through the nose gets filtered, warmed, and humidified before reaching the lungs, an important function on extremely cold or extremely dry days. The structures of the nose also remove pollen, dirt, and other debris from the air, reducing the amount of it that gets into the lungs. The right and left nasal cavities are the uppermost parts of the respiratory tract. The nasal cavities are separated by a septum that is mainly composed of cartilage and bone and covered by mucous membranes (Figure 47-6). The anterior part of the septum has a rich vascular supply and often is the source of nosebleeds. The hard palate separates the nasal cavities from the oral cavity. Parts of the sphenoid, ethmoid, and frontal bones separate the nasal cavities from the cranial cavity. The lower two thirds of the nose are mostly composed of cartilage. Nasal cartilage gives shape and support to the outer part of the nose. The upper third of the nose is composed of bone. The nasal bone is located between the eyes (Figure 47-7). **Turbinates,** located on the lateral sides of the nasal cavity, are made of bone and soft tissues. Inhaled air passes around, over, and under the turbinates, where it can be humidified and warmed to body temperature by the numerous blood vessels located here.

At the top of the nasal cavity is the olfactory region. This specialty area is lined with **epithelial** cells that contain specialized nerve endings and numerous cilia covered with a thin film of mucus. Various molecules from inhaled air passing by these epithelial cells attach to this surface, stimulating the olfactory receptors. Unlike the eyes and ears, which use nerve impulses to stimulate the brain, the olfactory center consists of chemoreceptors that initiate a direct chemical reaction. The results of the chemical reactions trigger various responses in the brain that allow a smell to be identified.

Next to the nasal cavity are the paranasal sinuses. The maxillary sinuses are located along the lateral wall of the nasal cavity in the maxillary bone. The frontal sinuses are in the frontal bone above the nasal cavity. These cavities are lined with mucous membranes and cilia, which work to facilitate excretion through the nose of fluids or mucus that might build up because of an infection or an allergic response.

Etiology and Demographics

The nose is the most commonly fractured bone of the face. Most nasal fractures are the result of blunt trauma. Nasal fractures can easily become open fractures because of the jagged edges of the nasal structures. Damage can occur to the ethmoid and frontal sinuses, lacrimal ducts, and the orbital margins.

History and Physical Findings

Signs and symptoms of a nasal fracture are listed in Box 47-8. Assessment often reveals edema, deformity, bleeding, crepitus, septal hematomas, and even lacerations. Overlooked nasal fractures can lead to deformities and airway obstructions.

Examine both nares carefully for septal hematomas. A **hematoma** is a localized collection of blood, usually clotted, in a tissue or organ. A septal hematoma presents as a bulging, tense, bluish mass that feels doughy when palpated. A septal hematoma needs to be emergently

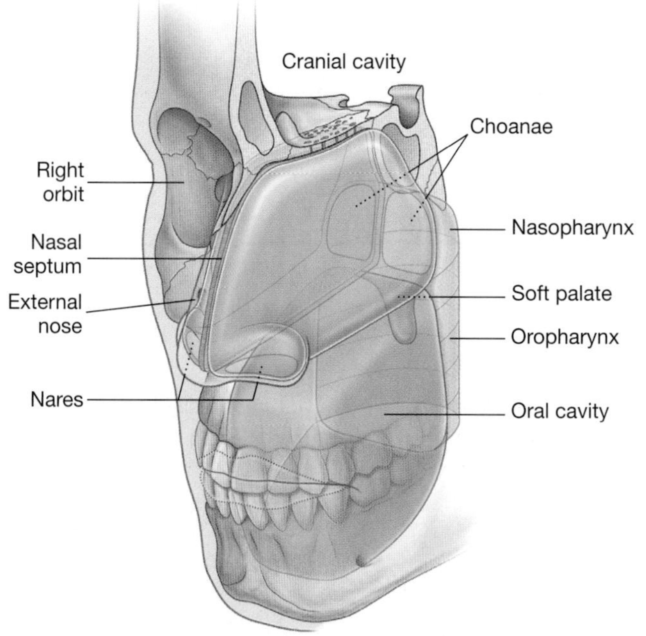

Figure 47-6 Anterolateral view of the nasal cavities and their relation to other cavities.

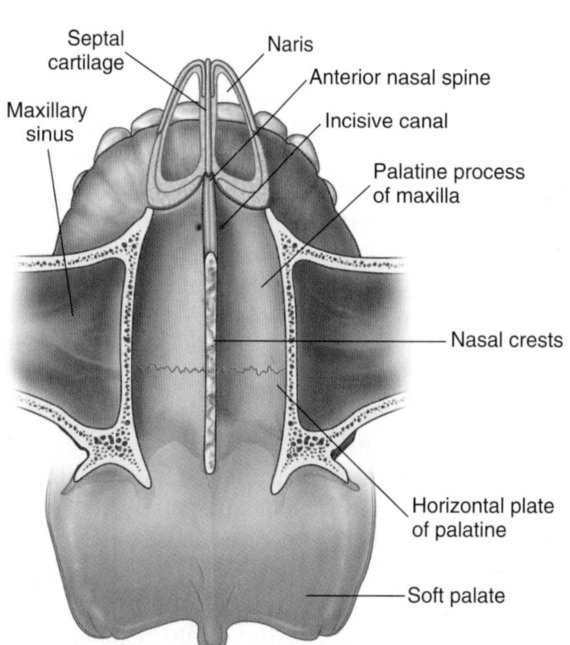

Figure 47-7 Bones of the nasal cavity.

BOX 47-8 Nasal Fractures: Signs and Symptoms

- Swelling
- Nosebleed
- Soft tissue discoloration
- Pain on palpation
- Crepitus on palpation
- Obvious deformity

drained at the hospital to prevent airway obstruction and necrosis of the septal cartilage (Newberry, 2003).

Therapeutic Interventions

Prehospital treatment focuses on airway, breathing, and circulation. Use spinal precautions when providing care. Assess the airway for actual or potential obstruction caused by blood, broken teeth, bone fragments, or other foreign bodies. Suction as needed. Ensure adequate oxygenation and ventilation. A nosebleed (epistaxis) can be severe but usually can be controlled with direct external pressure to the anterior nares. If a skull fracture is suspected and cerebrospinal fluid (CSF) is draining from the nose or ear, do not attempt to slow or stop the flow of fluid. Cover the ear with a loose sterile dressing.

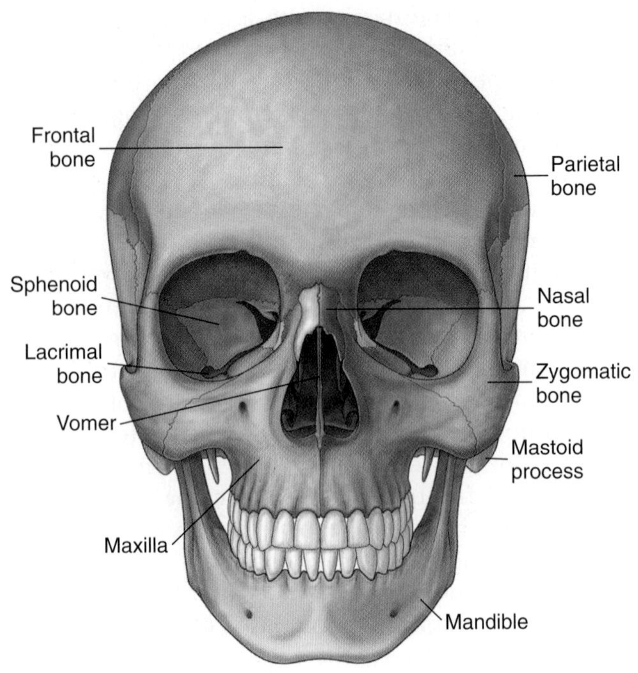

Figure 47-8 Anterior view of the skull.

Zygomatic Fractures

Anatomy of the Cheek

The zygoma (cheekbone) forms the lateral rim of the orbit, so almost all fractures of the zygoma involve the orbit (Figure 47-8). The zygoma meets the lateral skull to form the zygomatic arch.

Etiology and Demographics

Zygomatic fractures are common. This type of fracture is usually the result of an assault or MVC. Interestingly, in altercations the left zygoma is fractured more often than is the right, presumably because of the predominance of right handedness in assailants. Be suspicious of subarachnoid hemorrhage and orbital blowout fractures depending on the mechanism of injury.

Zygoma fractures are categorized as two types: zygomatic arch and tripod fractures. In a zygomatic arch fracture, only the arch itself is fractured. A tripod fracture is a fracture through three suture lines where the zygoma attaches to the facial skeleton.

History and Physical Findings

Signs and symptoms of a zygomatic fracture are listed in Box 47-9. Assessment includes palpating the zygoma for a step-off deformity. Inspection should include looking for asymmetry of the face, swelling and soft tissue discoloration around the eyes, and subconjunctival ecchymosis. If the patient has a fracture of the zygomatic arch, he or she may be unable to open the mouth because of associated pain.

BOX 47-9 Zygomatic Fractures: Signs and Symptoms

- Paresthesia of the anterior cheek
- Facial asymmetry
- Double vision
- Soft tissue swelling and discoloration around the eye
- Pain or tenderness on palpation
- Bleeding from the nose on one side
- Spasm of the muscles used for chewing, resulting in limited movement of the mouth because of pain **(trismus)**
- Step-off deformity
- Sunken globe
- Facial swelling
- Possible CSF draining from the nose
- Unequal pupil height
- Crepitus on palpation
- Obvious deformity

CSF, Cerebrospinal fluid.

PARAMEDIC*Pearl*

A step-off deformity is any fracture or displacement that causes a step if you slide your finger along the normal facial anatomic lines.

Therapeutic Interventions

Maintain an open airway and ensure adequate oxygenation and ventilation. Because significant force is required to produce a zygomatic fracture, use cervical spine precautions when providing care. Loose bandages covering both eyes are usually applied to limit movement of either eye. Continually talking to the patient throughout the assessment and treatment can ease the patient's fears and anxiety.

Maxillary Fractures

Anatomy of the Upper Jaw

The upper jaw bones (maxillae) are paired facial bones located between the orbit and the upper teeth. The left and right maxillae are joined by the intermaxillary suture.

Etiology and Demographics

Maxillary or midface fractures are usually a combination of fractures involving several structures of the face. Significant force is required to fracture this area of the face.

LeFort fractures are fractures involving the maxilla. These fractures usually involve other structures as well. Other terms for each of these fractures are lower third, middle third, and orbital complex fractures. These types of fractures are rarely seen in children because of the flexible, pliable nature of their maxillofacial structures.

A LeFort I fracture results from blunt trauma to the midface, just below the nose. A LeFort II fracture results from blunt trauma aimed at the midface. In a LeFort III fracture, blunt force results in separation of the entire midface from the cranial skeleton.

History and Physical Findings

Patients with LeFort fractures report severe facial pain, anesthesia or paresthesia of the upper lip, and some visual disturbances. Facial swelling, subconjunctival hemorrhage (Figure 47-9), elongation of the face, ecchymosis, periorbital or orbital swelling, facial asymmetry, **epistaxis,** and **malocclusion** will be evident (Box 47-10). Also look for CSF leaking from the nose. You can assess the maxilla by gently, but firmly, grasping the front gum and teeth and trying to move it. If the plate moves at all, suspect a LeFort fracture.

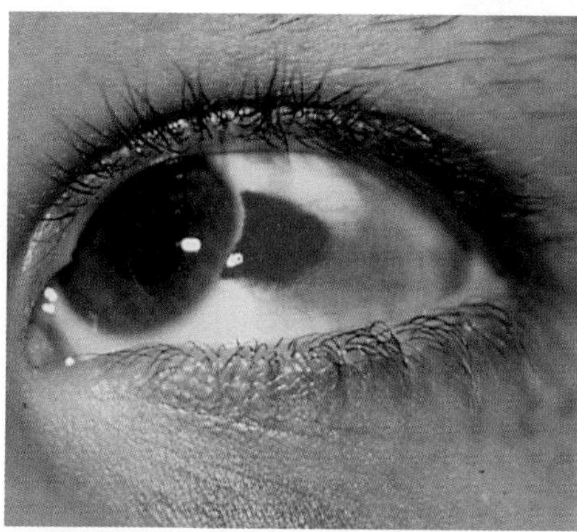

Figure 47-9 Subconjunctival hemorrhage.

LeFort I is a horizontal fracture in which the maxilla is separated from the base of the skull just above the palate but below the zygoma (Figure 47-10). Separation can be unilateral or bilateral. The upper teeth and lower maxilla are a free-floating segment. The fracture, however, may not necessarily be displaced.

LeFort II is a fracture that involves the central maxilla, nasal area, and ethmoid bones. The fracture forms a tripod shape with the apex of the nose. Assessment of the stability of the maxilla in these fractures produces movement of the nose and upper lip but no movement of the orbital complex. The patient with a LeFort II fracture has significant swelling of the nose, lips, and eyes as well subconjunctival hemorrhage and epistaxis. Cervical spine fracture and dislocation also should be suspected. The presence of CSF **rhinorrhea** suggests an open skull fracture. These patients should only be orally suctioned or intubated. Never insert anything nasally on this patient.

LeFort III fractures cause total separation of the head from the face (craniofacial separation). The nose and dental arch can move without frontal bone involvement. The patient will have massive edema, ecchymosis, epistaxis, and malocclusion with a spoon appearance from

BOX 47-10 Maxillary Fractures: Signs and Symptoms

LeFort I

- Malocclusion of the teeth
- Moveable maxilla
- Epistaxis

LeFort II

- Malocclusion of the teeth
- Nose and dental arch move together when manipulated; immobile if impacted
- Midface caved in
- Elongation between eyes and upper lip
- CSF rhinorrhea
- Widening between eyes
- Soft tissue discoloration around the eyes
- Subconjunctival hemorrhage
- Decreased sensation below orbits
- Massive swelling within 2 to 3 hours of injury

LeFort III

- Malocclusion of the teeth
- Movement of maxilla moves entire face separately from cranium ("rocking face")
- CSF rhinorrhea, otorrhea
- Elongated face
- Massive bleeding
- Pain or crepitus over fracture site
- Loss of responsiveness (usually)

CSF, Cerebrospinal fluid.

the profile view of the patient. Assess eye movement to rule out associated injuries. A cribriform plate fracture and associated middle meningeal artery bleeding can compromise airway patency. Suspect cervical spine fracture and dislocation. Other associated injuries may include basilar skull fracture, eye injury, and open or closed head injury.

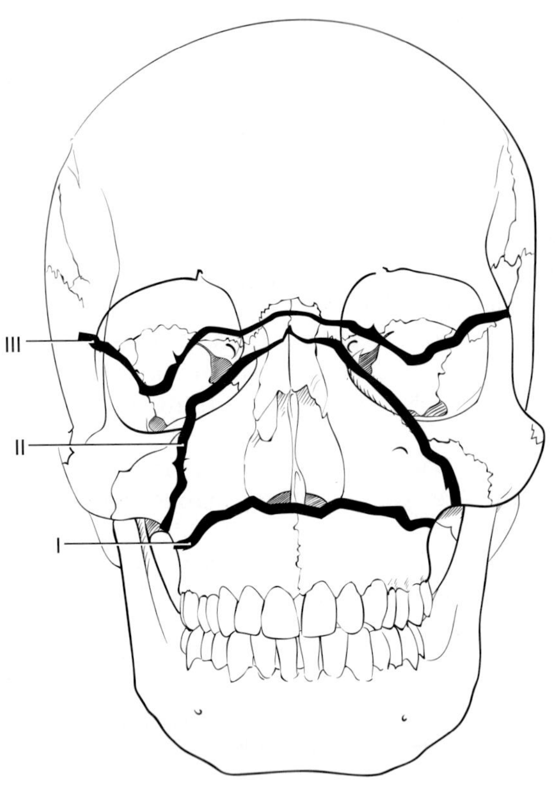

Figure 47-10 Location of LeFort I, II, and III fractures.

Therapeutic Interventions

Because a significant amount of force is required to create a maxillary fracture, cervical spine trauma should be suspected and appropriate precautions taken. Monitor the airway closely in these patients because it quickly may become compromised. Keeping the airway patent is the priority in these patients. Excessive edema and bleeding can make this a challenge. Frequent suctioning is required and orotracheal intubation may be needed. Ice packs may be beneficial to limit the amount of edema to the face and decrease pain (Newberry, 2003).

Mandibular Fractures

Anatomy of the Lower Jaw

The lower jaw (mandible) consists of the body of the mandible anteriorly and the ramus of the mandible posteriorly (Figure 47-11). The body and ramus meet posteriorly to form the angle of the mandible.

Etiology and Demographics

Mandibular fractures are common and are caused by blunt trauma to the face, most often domestic violence altercations and contact sports. A mandibular fracture also can be caused by penetrating trauma such as gunshot wounds, blast injuries, or industrial injuries (e.g., chain saw).

A mandibular fracture is classified by the location of the exact break. From most common to least common, the sites are mandibular angle, condyle, molar, mental, and symphysis. Because the right and left sides of the mandible function as a unit, these patients likely have a reciprocal fracture to the opposite side of the mandible.

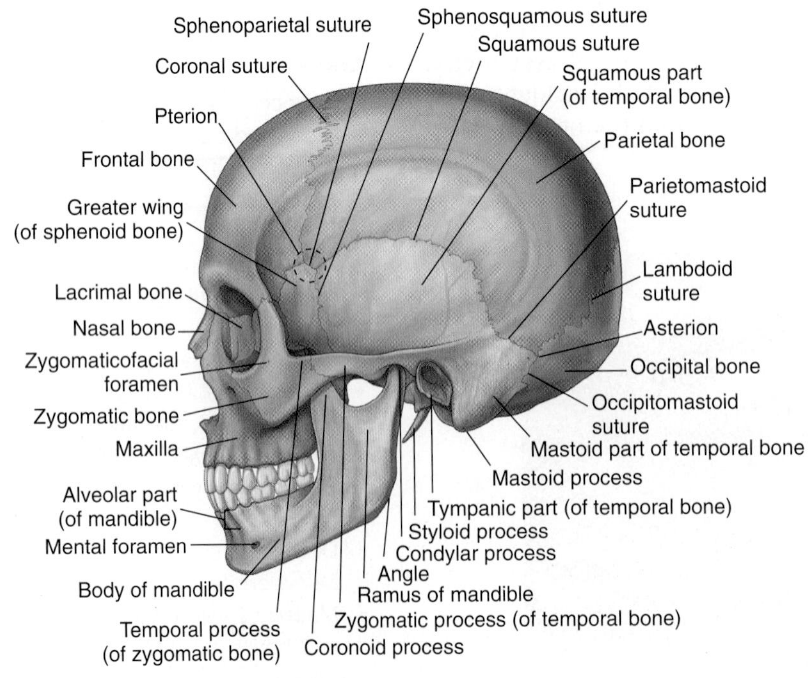

Figure 47-11 Lateral view of the skull.

BOX 47-11 Mandibular Fractures: Signs and Symptoms

- Malocclusion of the teeth
- Trismus
- Facial swelling and/or asymmetry
- Pain or tenderness on palpation
- Loose, missing teeth
- Sublingual swelling
- Soft tissue discoloration over the fracture site
- Crepitus over the fracture site
- Decreased or altered sensation on affected side

History and Physical Findings

Malocclusion of the teeth or misalignment of the jaw curvature is a cardinal sign of a mandibular fracture. Other findings during assessment include point tenderness, crepitus, step-off deformity, trismus, and facial asymmetry (Box 47-11). Remember to inspect the mouth for loose teeth or sublingual swelling and hematomas. Assess the patient for signs of a skull fracture, including inspecting the ear canal and nasal cavity for CSF leakage.

Therapeutic Interventions

Prehospital management remains focused on the ABCs and stabilization of the cervical spine. Patients who have mandibular fractures are at high risk for airway compromise and underlying cervical spine (especially C1 to C4) and brain trauma. Use appropriate spinal precautions when providing care. Suction bone fragments, blood, clots, and vomitus from the airway as needed. Maintain airway, breathing, and circulation. Reassure the patient and provide emotional support.

DENTAL TRAUMA

Anatomy of a Tooth

Children have 20 primary teeth (also called *baby, first, milk,* or *deciduous teeth*) that typically begin to erupt through the gums between the ages of 6 months and 2 years. The primary teeth are gradually replaced by permanent teeth (also called *adult* or *secondary teeth*) between the ages of 6 and 14 years. Wisdom teeth (also called *third molars*) usually erupt between the ages of 17 and 21 years. An adult typically has 32 permanent teeth (16 in the upper jaw and 16 in the lower jaw), 28 if the wisdom teeth have been removed.

The teeth are attached to sockets (alveoli) in arches of bone on the maxillae and mandible. The gums (gingivae) are specialized areas of the oral mucosa that surround the base of the teeth. A tooth has three parts: the crown, the neck, and the root (Figure 47-12). The visible part of the tooth is called the **crown.** The crown is covered with **enamel,** which is the hard, white, outer surface of the tooth. The neck of a tooth connects the crown and root. The root extends into the maxilla or mandible, anchoring the tooth. A tooth may have from one to three roots. The outer surface of the root is covered by a layer of tough tissue called **cementum,** which anchors the root to the periodontal membrane and ligament. The **periodontal membrane and ligament** is a ligamentous attachment between the root of a tooth and the socket of the bone within which it sits. It contains cells that generally begin to die within 60 minutes if a tooth is outside the oral cavity and is not placed in appropriate transport media (Marino et al., 2000).

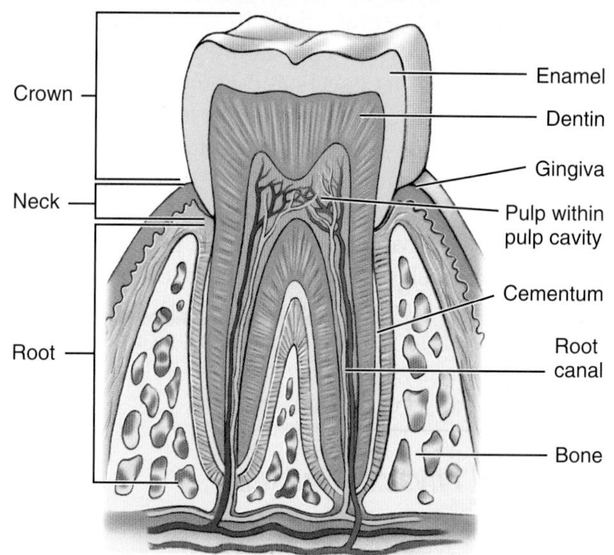

Figure 47-12 Anatomy of a tooth.

The **pulp** is the soft center of the tooth. It contains nerves, blood vessels, and connective tissue. The pulp is highly vascular and has many sensitive nerve endings. When an injury exposes these nerve endings, the patient's tongue, cold water or food, hot water or food, or even air can cause extreme pain. The pulp produces **dentin,** a hard but leaky tissue found under the enamel and cementum of a tooth. Dentin hydrates and cushions the tooth during chewing.

Epidemiology and Demographics

Dental trauma may occur at any age and can range from small enamel chips to loss of entire sections of the jaw. Incidence of dental injuries peaks between 2 and 5 years, a period during which children have just learned to walk and gained independence but still do not have excellent balance. Fractures of the crown of the tooth account for approximately one third of dental injuries to the primary teeth and approximately 75% of injuries to the permanent teeth.

Permanent teeth are usually injured as a result of bicycle, skating, fighting, and playground or sports injuries. Many of the dental injuries in public schools are the result of fighting and pushing, which also are the most common causes of dental injury in young enlisted men; alcohol often is involved. Automobile crashes are a major factor in injuries to teenagers and young adults, whereas individuals with mental retardation or epilepsy often have dental injuries associated with falls. Violent teeth-clenching in drug addicts also can produce dental injuries. Overall, the incidence of dental trauma is twice as great in men compared with women, probably because men are more likely to participate in sports and contact games. With greater involvement in athletic activities, the incidence of dental injuries among women has been on the rise. Finally, family violence—either spousal or child abuse—can cause dental injuries.

History and Physical Findings

Dental trauma is basically divided into two categories: teeth fractures or loosened teeth without other fractures. A chipped tooth is relatively painless. The tooth remains securely in place with a sharp edge where the enamel and insensate area have been broken away. A tooth fracture that involves the dentin of the tooth often is associated with reports of mild discomfort with hot and cold extremes because of some nerve involvement. Tooth fractures that have pulp or nerve exposure are associated with significant pain. A deep fracture of the tooth often involves the root. The patient with this type of fracture has considerable discomfort.

An avulsed tooth has been completely removed from its ligamentous attachments. When confronted with a situation involving an avulsed tooth, consider where the missing tooth might be. Look to see if it may be embedded in the soft tissues of the mouth. If the tooth cannot be found, assume that is was aspirated or swallowed. Be sure to tell the emergency department staff if an avulsed tooth could not be located.

PARAMEDIC*Pearl*

The presence of newly missing or loosened teeth requires reconsideration of the mechanism of injury and the possibility of other injuries.

Therapeutic Interventions

Consider spinal precautions in a patient who has an avulsed tooth, depending on the mechanism of injury and related factors. Maintain airway, breathing, and circulation. Injuries that result in dental trauma often are associated with significant bleeding within the mouth. Closely monitor the airway in these patients because it quickly may become compromised. Frequent suctioning may be needed.

An avulsed tooth may be able to be reimplanted. If you are able to find the avulsed tooth, be careful to handle it only by its crown. The tooth should not be handled by the root. This can damage the periodontal ligament. An avulsed tooth must be placed in an appropriate "tooth saver" solution as quickly as possible. Preferred solutions are milk or the commercially available Save-A-Tooth. A solution such as sterile saline is not ideal; however, it may be used for very short periods (1 hour or less) if a more desirable solution is unavailable. Transport the avulsed tooth and solution in an appropriate container to the hospital with the patient.

EYE TRAUMA

[OBJECTIVES 3, 4]

Corneal Abrasions and Lacerations

Etiology and Demographics

The surface of the cornea is dense but can be easily scratched by something getting into the eye. Typical foreign bodies include dirt, dust, glass, cinders, and contact lenses. Children often get corneal abrasions as a result of playing outside and inadvertently rubbing their eyes too vigorously, but anyone is at risk. Corneal abrasions are the most common eye injuries.

History and Physical Findings

A corneal abrasion usually involves only the eyeball, which will appear reddened and sore. The cause of the abrasion may not be visible, but the patient will report burning in the eye and increased pain when the eye is closed. The patient complains of "something in my eye" or pain on blinking. The reason for the pain is because the scratch exposes several nerves to the elements. A corneal abrasion also causes sensitivity to light (photophobia) and decreased visual acuity.

Small corneal lacerations are treated as corneal abrasions. Large corneal lacerations require surgical intervention to protect the intraocular contents.

Therapeutic Interventions

Prehospital care for a corneal abrasion includes gently rinsing the affected eye with clear fluid. Instead of patching most experts recommend gently covering the eyes to shield them from light and provide comfort. The patient with a corneal laceration should be transported to a definitive care center with an ophthalmologist available.

Burns of the Eye

Etiology and Demographics

The eyes are extremely vulnerable to thermal, chemical, and ultraviolet or flash burns. Because the eyelids react very quickly to incoming danger, most burns are superficial and result in damage only to the cornea. This will result in pain and possibly vision changes if the cornea becomes scarred. Depending on the type of burn, vision changes may be temporary or result in permanent damage. Burns of the eye are an immediate threat to the victim's vision and can cause significant discomfort to

BOX 47-12 Burns of the Eye: Possible Causes

- Chemicals
- Heat
- Radiation
- Lasers
- Infrared rays
- Ultraviolet light

the patient. Causes of burns of the eye are listed in Box 47-12. Treatment depends on the type of burn itself.

Most burns of the eye that are seen in the emergency department are chemical burns. Approximately 15% to 20% of patients with facial burns exhibit ocular injury. Burns of the eye are more common in men than in women. A majority of eye burns are work related. This difference may reflect gender differences in certain occupations, particularly in mining and construction (Cheh et al., 2006).

Thermal burns are the second most common type of eye burn. They result from the presence of any heat source that comes too close to the eye. The resulting damage will be limited to the cornea, but permanent scarring is possible if the source was too intense or left in place for an extended period. As with a corneal abrasion, only the eyeball will appear reddened. But, unlike a corneal abrasion, the surrounding tissue also may show signs of heat exposure, with redness and swelling.

History and Physical Findings

Chemical burns are by far the most damaging to the eye. Individuals at most risk for chemical burns include laboratory technicians and hazardous materials technicians. However, anyone who works with or around chemicals should be considered at risk and receive proper training on how to handle the product and what to do in case of an emergency.

A patient who has a chemical burn to the eye usually has a loss of vision and evidence of facial skin burns. An acid burn generally causes immediate epithelial damage to the cornea. The cornea will appear white and opaque. After the initial damage, no further changes are noted in the cornea because proteins in the tears of the eye act as a barrier to further penetration of the acid. Acidic injuries still cause permanent visual changes.

Alkaline substances are not easily neutralized by the body and penetrate deep into the eye as a result of **emulsification.** Alkaline substances have a devastating effect on the eye. Alkalis can pass into the anterior chamber of eye rapidly (in approximately 5 to 15 minutes), exposing the iris, ciliary body, lens, and other structures to further damage (Cheh et al., 2006). Alkalis are most commonly found in concrete, lye, and drain cleaners. These substances damage each tissue layer of the eye they touch until the substance is removed. The damaged tissues stimulate an inflammatory response, which further damages the tissue by the release of proteolytic enzymes. This is termed *liquefactive necrosis*. Alkaline burns cause permanent scarring of the cornea and sometimes permanent vision loss.

Ultraviolet (UV) burns can occur in individuals exposed to a large amount of UV radiation, such as welders, skiers, ice climbers, and those who sunbathe or use home tanning lights or salon tanning beds. The two most common causes are excessive exposure to UV radiation from the sun (e.g., snow blindness) and unprotected welding. Repeated exposures to the sun without protection, both summer and winter, is another source of UV radiation with long-term results. These patients report pain, a tearing sensation, photophobia, and/or a foreign body sensation up to 6 to 10 hours after the exposure. These are the most painful of all eye burns.

Flash burns are the result of a sudden unshielded exposure to a welding arc or an explosion. The suddenness of the event results in temporary blindness from overstimulation of the retinal surfaces. Flash burns also can result in long-term damage to the corneal surface.

Therapeutic Interventions

Treatment of an acid or alkali burn of the eye involves pain control and continuous flushing of the eyes with normal saline. Patient outcome will improve if the eye can be returned to a normal pH within a few minutes. Flushing of the eyes can be done by using bags of intravenous (IV) fluids and tubing with the flow directed into the affected eye. The eyes should be flushed with a minimum of 2 L or at least 2 hours of continuous flushing. Use of a Morgan Lens (MorTan, Inc., Missoula, Mont.) can make irrigation easier (Skill 47-2). Continue the irrigation until arrival at the hospital, where the pH of eye can be evaluated. Pain control also is important in these patients (Schwartz, 1999). Patients with UV burns of the eye require pain control and possibly eye patching for comfort. UV burns usually heal within 24 to 48 hours after treatment is started. The long-term effect of UV or flash burns may not be known for days or weeks after the injury, depending on the severity of the exposure.

PARAMEDIC*Pearl*

Treatment of all chemical burns must begin immediately to salvage as much of the eye and eyesight as possible.

Eyelid Lacerations

Etiology and Demographics

Eyelid lacerations may be superficial or full thickness. Full-thickness eyelid lacerations can interfere with eyelid function.

History and Physical Findings

An eyelid laceration is usually identified by observation. Do not let an eyelid injury distract you from assessing the rest of the patient's face, head, and neck for injuries.

SKILL 47-2 MORGAN LENS

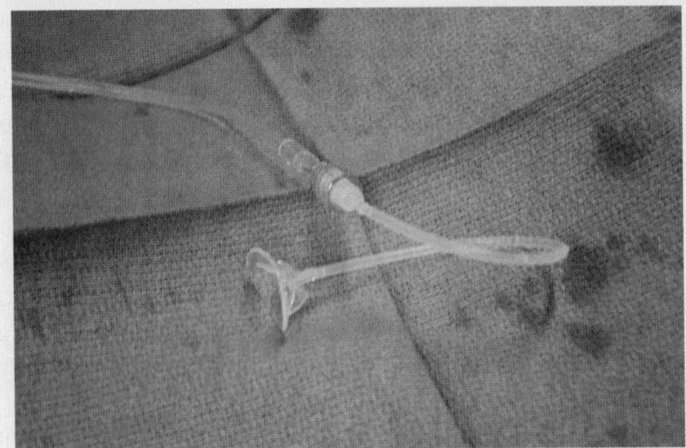

Step 1 A Morgan Lens is used to flush the eye with 0.9% normal saline or Ringer's lactate (check your local protocol).

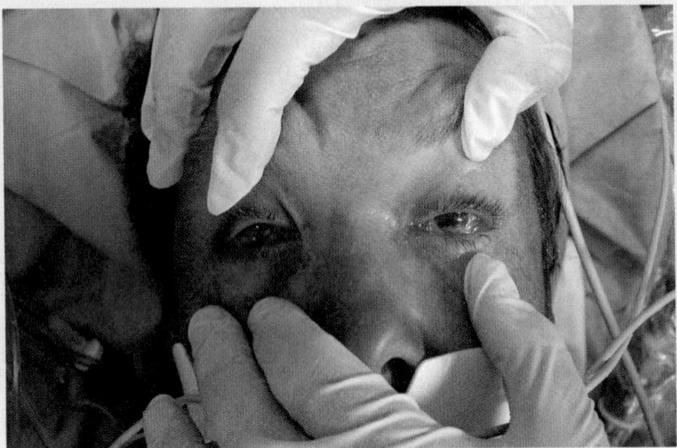

Step 2 Position a container with towels around the patient's head and shoulders to catch the runoff. Attach the Morgan Lens delivery set, IV, or syringe using solution and rate of choice. Start the flow so that the Morgan Lens floats on the fluid (it does not rest on the cornea). Have the patient look down and gently insert the lens under the upper eyelid. Have the patient look up, retract the lower eyelid, and gently insert the lens in place.

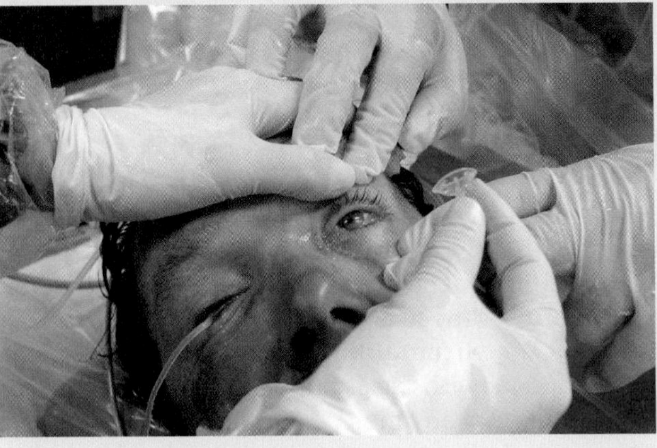

Step 3 Release the lower eyelid over the lens. Once the lens is secure, the fluids are started and the flow adjusted. The patient may feel some discomfort at first. This should ease after the fluids have been running for a few minutes. Most objects and eye injuries require a minimum of 2 hours of flushing or at least 2 L of fluid. Tape the tubing to the patient's forehead to prevent accidental lens removal. *Do not allow the solution to run dry.* Visual acuity should be checked before and after the Morgan Lens procedure is done.

Therapeutic Interventions

A patient with an eyelid laceration must be evaluated by a physician. Prehospital care usually includes controlling bleeding, irrigating the area with saline solution, and applying a sterile dressing. During transport, patching both eyes may be helpful in preventing the patient from further damaging the eyelid.

Corneal Foreign Body

Any object found in the eye on inspection is considered a foreign body. Foreign bodies of the eye are common. Typically the foreign body is a speck of dust or an eyelash. However, wood or steel slivers and fishing hooks are also among the commonly documented foreign bodies found in the eye.

History and Physical Findings

The patient will complain of pain when exposed to light, a burning sensation, and increased pain when the eye is closed. Shining a penlight through the eyelid onto the surface of the eyeball may help detect the presence of a foreign body because the object will appear as a dark shadow on the eye. If the foreign body has penetrated the anterior chamber of the eye, a small amount of vitreous humor will be visible on the eyeball. This can be distinguished from tears because it will be thicker and may be seen as a drop of fluid.

Therapeutic Interventions

A foreign body in the eye is generally removed by flushing the affected eye with clear fluid. Most foreign bodies in the eye are visible on inspection but should never be removed in the prehospital environment. Stabilize the object in place to minimize movement and transport the patient for evaluation by a physician.

Hyphema

Etiology and Demographics

The anterior chamber of the eye contains the iris, which contains numerous small blood vessels. Rupture of one of these small vessels results in bleeding into the anterior chamber (the space between the cornea and the iris) of the eye, called a **hyphema.** They are dramatic in appearance but do not result in permanent damage to the eye.

A hyphema is a result of direct trauma to the globe. The injury is usually a result of blunt trauma but can be a result of a penetrating injury that ruptures blood vessels, which then bleed into the anterior chamber. A hyphema that consists of a dark-colored clot that covers the entire anterior chamber is often called an *eight-ball hyphema.* Because an acute injury usually is associated with bright-red blood in the anterior chamber, the presence of dark blood suggests a nonacute injury.

In the United States the incidence of hyphema is 17 to 20 per 100,000 people per year. Older adults are frequently affected because most intraocular surgery is performed on elderly patients. Younger patients are at risk for hyphema because of other mechanisms such as trauma (Rastogi et al., 2005). African Americans may require closer observation because they may have sickle cell trait or disease and thus have a greater risk of complications.

History and Physical Findings

To visualize the hyphema clearly, shine a penlight from an angle through the anterior chamber. This will highlight the height of the blood in the chamber, differentiating it from blood on the corneal surface. The patient usually will report photophobia, pain, and blurred vision. Patients with hyphema often are drowsy, although the cause of this finding is unclear. Assess the patient for associated injuries, such as a ruptured globe. If a patient with a hyphema has an altered level of consciousness, suspect and treat for a head injury.

Therapeutic Interventions

The force required to cause hyphema should be considered and spinal precautions used. Ask the patient not to cough, strain, or perform any activity that will increase pressure within the eye (intraocular pressure) and subsequently increase bleeding. Be sure to explain to the patient what is happening in the eye, especially before allowing him or her to look in a mirror or lie down. Make sure the patient realizes that when he or she lies down, the blood in the chamber will change position, covering the pupil and making vision blurry. When the patient sits up again, the blood will settle and vision will be restored. The patient should be transported to a hospital for definitive care from an ophthalmologist. Typically no specific treatment is available for a hyphema. The blood is reabsorbed over time.

Penetrating Globe Injuries

Etiology and Demographics

Penetrating and perforating injuries of the ocular structures are a major cause of traumatic vision loss. This type of injury may occur in an industrial setting when a worker fails to wear appropriate protective eyewear. It may also occur as a result of a blast injury (shrapnel), stab wound, or gunshot wound. A penetrating injury of the eye also may occur as a result of an eyelid laceration.

History and Physical Findings

Assessment of a penetrating injury of the eye may reveal a foreign object embedded in the eye or lacerations that resulted from the penetration. Perforation or rupture of the globe may result in a small, shrunken eyeball and an irregularly shaped pupil with a teardrop appearance (teardrop pupil). The pupil may point in the direction of the perforation. A sticky substance (vitreous fluid) may be visible on the eyeball. Hyphema may be present. The patient may report pain, nausea, and a loss of vision.

Therapeutic Interventions

If the injury involves a foreign body impaled in the eye, stabilize the object in place for later removal by a physician. Both eyes should be covered to minimize eye movement. If the injury involves rupture of the globe, carefully place a hard (usually metal or plastic) shield over the affected eye to protect it from additional injury. Cover the other eye to prevent movement.

Never place pressure on the globe. This can cause an outward displacement of the contents of the eye. If instructed to do so by medical direction, give medications for pain relief. Ask the patient not to cough, strain, or perform any activity that will increase pressure within the eye. A patient with a penetrating injury to the eye or globe rupture needs rapid transport to the closest appropriate facility for immediate definitive care.

Retinal Detachment

Etiology and Demographics

Retinal detachment (also called a *retinal tear*) is a separation of the retina from the choroid of the eye. The choroid contains blood vessels that supply the outer layers of the retina with blood. Without a blood supply, the outer retinal tissue layer dies. The vitreous chamber of the eye contains the retinal surface, which wraps around the inside of the eyeball, making a large visual field. These are thin, tissue paper–like structures that can be suddenly dislodged or torn if the eyeball receives significant trauma or can separate more slowly if exposed to many years of stretching. This patient has significant myopia or elongation of the eyeball (Feinberg, 2004). Some long-term health conditions such as diabetes and high blood pressure can result in hemorrhages in the posterior blood vessels, which also can cause separation of the retina from the choroid layer of the eye. Approximately 10,000 people per year are affected by retinal detachments (Feinberg, 2004).

Retinal detachment can be caused by blunt or penetrating trauma or may be spontaneous. It can occur at any age, but it is more common in people older than 40 years. It affects men more often than women and whites more often than African Americans. Retinal detachment may occur months after the original injury.

History and Physical Findings

The patient will report vision changes that may be gradual or sudden. When retinal detachment is sudden, the patient will describe flashes of bright light in the visual field opposite from the damage. Patients with a slower retinal detachment process describe a curtain slowly coming down onto the visual field.

Retinal detachment can result in vision loss to that part of the eye unless the problem is identified and treated early. Unless the retinal detachment is the result of trauma, nothing on external physical examination will alert the provider to a problem. The only way to identify the presence of a retinal detachment is by recognizing the symptoms related by the patient. Vision changes that may accompany retinal detachment are listed in Box 47-13. The patient does not usually report pain.

Therapeutic Interventions

Retinal detachment is a medical emergency that requires rapid treatment to prevent vision loss. Immobilize the head if caused by a traumatic injury and cover both eyes to minimize movement. Transport the patient to a hospital with an ophthalmologist available for definitive care. Patients often are restricted from any activity that results in sudden, rapid, or violent movements of the head. Children will be restricted from most childhood activities until the eye has healed.

BOX 47-13 Retinal Detachment: Possible Vision Changes

- Decreased peripheral vision
- Blurred vision
- Flashes of light (flashers)
- Floating black specks (floaters)
- Curtainlike veil in front of eyes
- Cloudy, gray vision

Traumatic Iritis

Etiology

Traumatic iritis is an inflammation of the iris that results from blunt trauma to the eye.

History and Physical Findings

Assessment of the patient with traumatic iritis usually reveals a reddened eye and a small or distorted pupil. The patient usually reports pain in the eye or brow and is sensitive to light. Excessive tearing sometimes is seen.

Therapeutic Interventions

The patient with traumatic iritis must be evaluated by a physician. Medical direction may order medication for pain relief.

EAR TRAUMA

[OBJECTIVES 5, 6]

Anatomy of the Ear

The ear has three parts (Figure 47-13). The first part, the external or outer ear, is the visible part of the ear. The part of the external ear that sticks out from the side of the head is called the *auricle,* or *pinna.* The auricle is composed cartilage covered with skin and directs sound into the ear canal (Figure 47-14). The lobule of the ear is fleshy and is the only part of the auricle that is not supported by cartilage. The auricle opens into the external auditory canal, which is a passageway for sound waves.

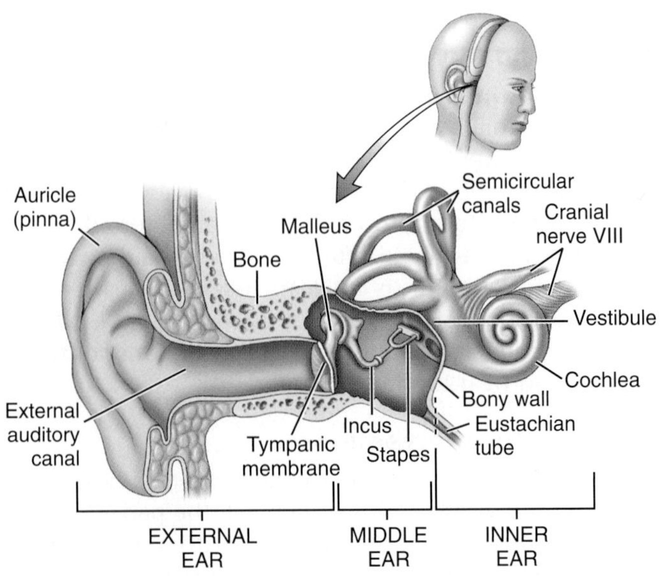

Figure 47-13 Anatomy of the ear.

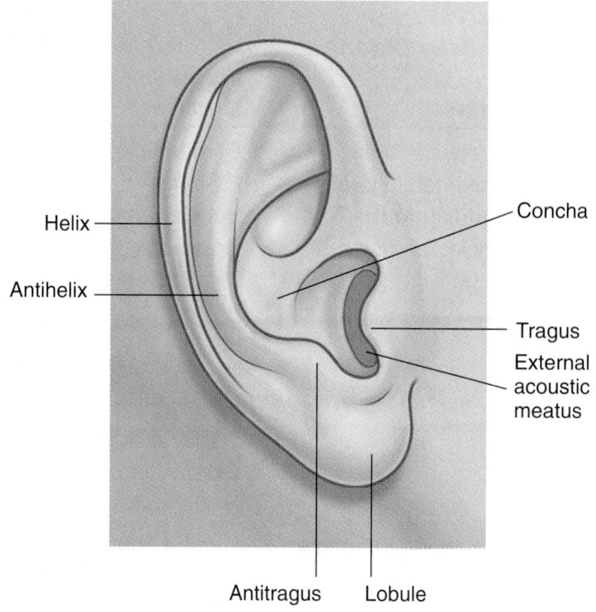

Figure 47-14 Auricle.

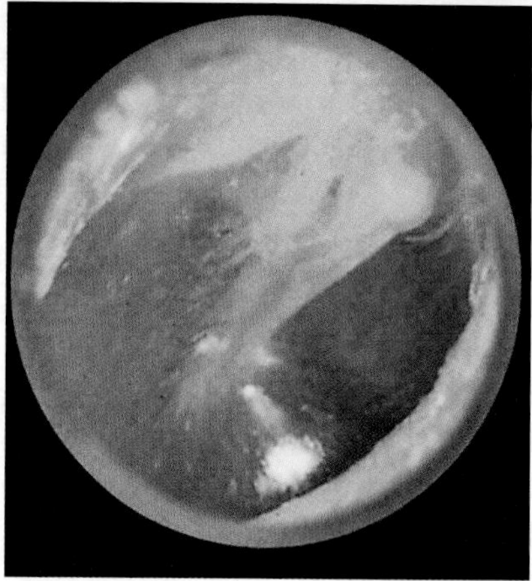

Figure 47-15 Tympanic membrane (eardrum).

Sound waves are amplified as they travel through the external ear canal to the eardrum because the canal narrows as it proceeds inward. The ear canal is considered a mucous membrane. The lateral half of the ear canal contains glands that secrete cerumen (earwax). Cerumen keeps the ear canal moist, inhibits the formation of bacteria, traps dust, and helps protect the delicate structures of the middle ear from cold, wind, and injury.

The second part, the middle ear, is a hollowed-out area of the temporal bone. The function of the middle ear is to transmit vibrations of the tympanic membrane across the middle ear to the inner ear. The middle ear is lined with mucous membranes and filled with air. It is separated from the external canal by the **tympanic membrane,** also known as the *eardrum.* An **otoscope** is used to visualize the deep parts of the external auditory canal. This is a lighted instrument fitted with a cone-shaped piece that directs the light into the canal and onto the tympanic membrane. Seen through an otoscope, the eardrum looks like a thin, translucent, pearly gray oval disk (Figure 47-15). It protects the middle ear and conducts sound vibrations to the three tiniest bones in the body, called the *ossicles.* If the tympanic membrane cannot move freely because of defects or scar tissue on the surface of the membrane or fluid buildup behind the membrane, then the ability to hear with that ear is greatly reduced.

The ossicles are three linked, movable bones: the **malleus** (hammer), **incus** (anvil), and **stapes** (stirrup). The ossicles transmit vibrations from the tympanic membrane to the **oval window,** a membranous structure that separates the middle ear from the inner ear. The **eustachian tube** opens into the middle ear, connecting the middle ear to the pharynx and respiratory system. It is responsible for equalizing pressure between the air outside the ear to that within the middle ear. The eustachian tube is normally closed off by a flap but can be opened by yawning, chewing, or swallowing.

The third part, the inner ear, is composed of a series of fluid-filled tubes within the temporal bone. Within the inner ear is a coiled network of bones called the *bony labyrinth.* The bony labyrinth is composed of the vestibule, semicircular canals, and the cochlea. The **vestibule** and **semicircular canals** contain receptors responsible for balance. The **cochlea** is a tube of bone curled into a snail shape that contains the hearing nerves. Sound vibrations transferred to the inner ear become fluid waves in this cavity, which is lined with **periosteum** and filled with a clear fluid. As the fluid vibrations move through the cochlea and semicircular canals, tiny hairlike structures bend and flex in response to various wavelengths, allowing us to hear various tones. Damage to these tiny, hairlike structures occurs when violent vibrations from excessively loud or prolonged noise enter the cochlea and shears off portions of these structures. Because these hair cells are irreplaceable, permanent hearing loss occurs. Nerve impulses generated in the inner ear travel along the vestibulocochlear nerve (CN VIII) to the brain.

Mechanism of Injury

An ear injury may be a primary injury or secondary to another injury, such as a jaw fracture. Injury to the ear may occur as a result of the following:

- Blunt trauma—MVCs, sports injuries (wrestling, boxing, football, martial arts), interpersonal violence
- Penetrating trauma—gunshot wound, laceration, foreign body, puncture wound
- Blast injuries—explosions
- Pressure injuries—diving

Etiology and Demographics

Lacerations of the outer ear are common. An ear hematoma (also known as *cauliflower ear*), usually occurs as a result of blunt trauma. The most common cause of this injury is sports in young adults and falls in the elderly and children. A ruptured eardrum may occur because of an ear infection, penetrating foreign body, or skull fracture. Because of its position, the external ear is prone to injury from temperature extremes, such as frostbite and burns.

History and Physical Examination Findings

Adequate assessment of the external ear canal and middle ear cannot be done in the field. Bleeding from a laceration of the external ear usually is obvious. Because bleeding from the ear canal usually is less obvious, you must closely examine the ears. Signs and symptoms of a ruptured eardrum may include sharp pain, dizziness, blood or purulent drainage from the ear, and decreased hearing. A patient with an ear infection may experience a relief of pain when built-up fluid is able to drain out through the ruptured eardrum.

Therapeutic Interventions

Maintain airway, breathing, and circulation. If the mechanism of injury warrants it, use spinal precautions when providing care. Reassure the patient and provide emotional support. If an ear laceration is present, control bleeding and gently bandage the ear. A hematoma of the external ear requires definitive care at the hospital. In most cases the hematoma is aspirated with a needle to drain it and promote healing. A draining ear should be loosely covered with a dressing. If CSF is draining from an ear, do not attempt to slow the escape of fluid. Provide additional care as needed for any associated injuries.

NECK TRAUMA

[OBJECTIVES 7, 8]

Anatomy of the Neck

The neck contains many important anatomic structures (Figure 47-16). One method used to identify the structures within the neck and assist in identification of injuries divides the neck into zones. The zones of the neck are shown in Table 47-1 and Figure 47-17. Injuries in zone I can extend into the chest and may be not be easily recognized on physical examination. Injuries in this area are associated with the highest mortality rate. Injuries in zone II are the most common, are usually the most obvious, and have a lower mortality rate than zone I injuries. Injuries in zone III often are difficult for a surgeon to access and repair because many of the structures enter the base of the skull.

TABLE 47-1 Zones of the Neck

Zone	Boundaries	Important Anatomic Structures
I	Area between the cricoid cartilage and extending to the clavicles and sternum	Carotid and vertebral arteries Subclavian veins Brachiocephalic veins Jugular veins Aortic arch Lungs Trachea Esophagus Thoracic duct Cervical spine Spinal cord
II	Area between the angle of the mandible and the cricoid cartilage	Carotid and vertebral arteries Jugular veins Pharynx Larynx Trachea Esophagus Cervical spine Spinal cord
III	Area above the angle of the mandible	Carotid and vertebral arteries Jugular veins Salivary and parotid glands Esophagus Pharynx Trachea Cranial nerves IX to XII Cervical spine Spinal cord

Mechanism of Injury

Trauma to the neck may be the result of a blunt or penetrating injury. Blunt neck trauma is most often caused by MVCs. Compression of the trachea and larynx against the cervical vertebrae can result from improperly worn shoulder seatbelts. Injury to the anterior neck may occur during contact sports such as boxing, wrestling, karate, basketball, football, and hockey. Riding all-terrain vehicles and motorcycles, horseback riding, bicycling, snowmobiling, and snow skiing can result in "clothesline" injuries from striking the neck on an unseen object, such as a wire, rope, or fence (Holleran, 1996). This type of injury can result in separation of the larynx and trachea. Strangulation-type injuries may be caused by clothing, jewelry, or equipment (e.g., a rope or cord) worn around the neck and caught in machinery (Holleran, 1996).

Penetrating neck trauma may be the result of a gunshot wound, stab wound, laceration, or puncture from objects such as a knife, ice pick, screwdriver, or scissors.

Etiology and Demographics

The presence or absence of signs or symptoms of neck trauma can be misleading. For example, only 10% of patients with blunt vascular injury to the neck develop symptoms in the first hour (Levy, 2006).

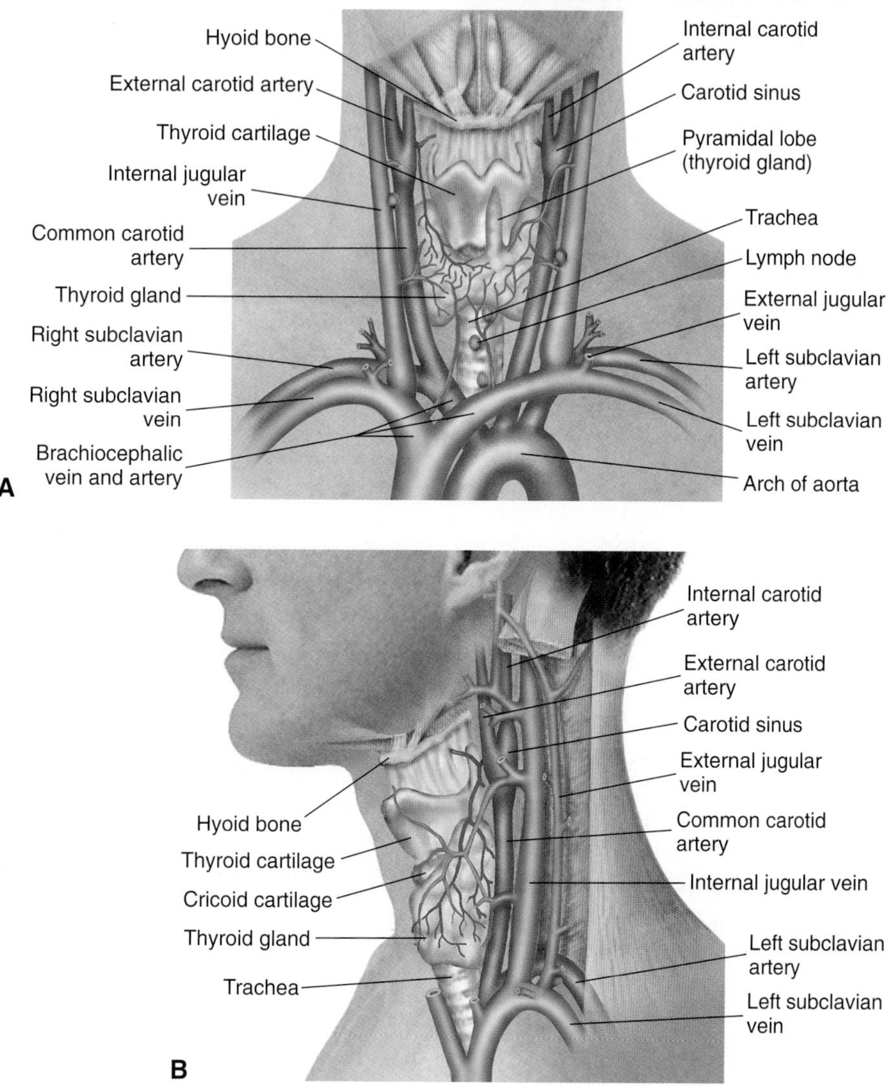

Figure 47-16 Structures of the neck. **A,** Anterior view. **B,** Lateral view.

Compression of the larynx and trachea can result in vocal cord swelling or bruising, disruption of normal airway landmarks, and associated soft tissue swelling. Signs of a tracheal injury include subcutaneous emphysema or hemoptysis. An open wound to the trachea can result in tearing or laceration of nearby blood vessels. If an artery is affected, the blood supply to the brain may be interrupted. This can result in hypoxia and stroke. An open wound with arterial bleeding may cause an air embolism and/or rapid exsanguination. Esophageal trauma may be associated with tracheal fractures, caustic ingestion, or penetrating trauma. Esophageal injuries may be difficult to detect. Injury to the cervical spine can result in vertebral instability and cord interruption, with possible paralysis, paresthesia, or neurogenic shock.

History and Physical Findings

Assessment of the neck should include looking for swelling, lacerations, puncture wounds, soft tissue discoloration, and obvious deformity. Note whether the neck veins appear normal, flat, or distended. Note the use of accessory muscles. Note if signs and symptoms of respiratory distress such as stridor, hoarseness, or dyspnea are present. Listen for a sucking neck wound. Feel for crepitus, subcutaneous emphysema, and tracheal position (Figure 47-18). Signs and symptoms that may be associated with a neck injury are shown in Box 47-14.

When taking a SAMPLE history, be certain to consider the mechanism of injury. For example, attempt to find out when the injury occurred and the circumstances surrounding the event. Attempt to find out if the patient lost consciousness. Note any evidence of drug or alcohol use. Other considerations regarding the mechanism of injury are listed in Box 47-15.

Therapeutic Interventions

Because of the anatomy of the neck, any injury to it can quickly become life threatening. Stabilizing the cervical spine, maintaining an open airway and adequate ventilation, and controlling hemorrhage are the priorities of

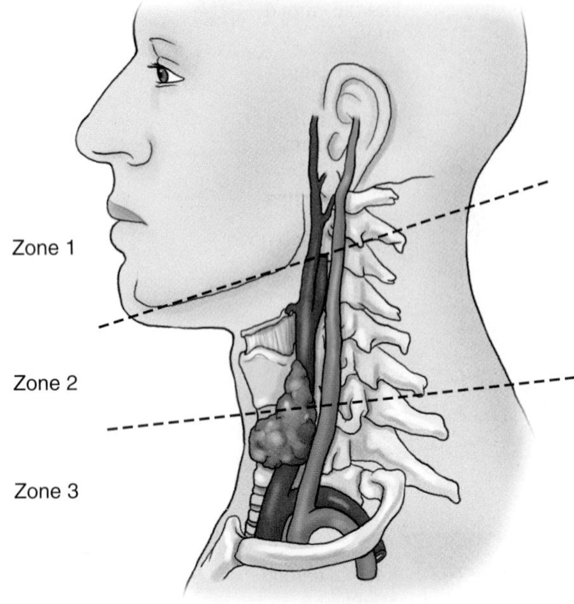

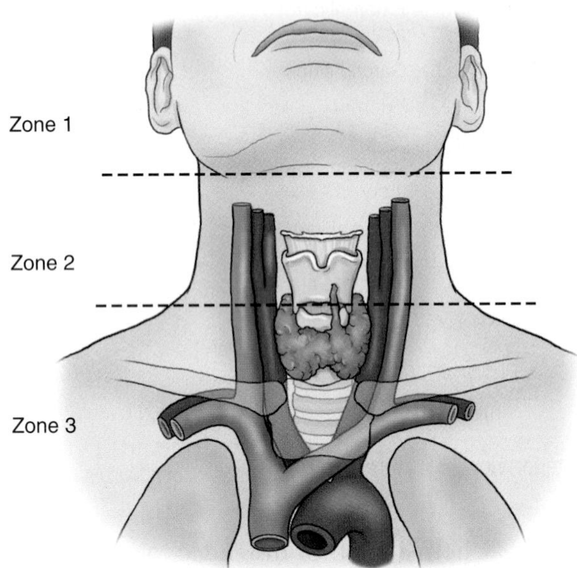

Figure 47-17 Zones of the neck.

care. An injury to the larynx or trachea must be quickly recognized. Suction as needed to remove blood and other matter from the airway. Swelling of the pharynx, larynx, trachea, epiglottis, and vocal cords can result in complete airway obstruction (Holleran, 1996). Tracheal intubation (performed with in-line stabilization of the cervical spine) may be necessary to maintain an open airway. If soft tissue swelling is extreme, "aim for the bubbles" when placing the tracheal tube. If the airway already is obstructed because of massive swelling, surgical cricothyrotomy may be necessary to establish an airway (if permitted by local protocol).

If an open wound to the neck is present, apply an airtight dressing over the neck wound. Do not wrap a dressing completely around the neck. Control hemorrhage by applying direct pressure to the involved

BOX 47-14 Possible Signs and Symptoms Associated with a Neck Injury

Signs

- Pale or cyanotic face
- Bruising of neck
- Redness of neck
- Sucking, hissing, or air frothing through neck wound
- Subcutaneous emphysema
- Hematoma in neck
- Active bleeding (pulsatile bleeding if arterial injury)
- Stridor
- Supraclavicular retractions
- Vocal cord dysfunction (laryngeal nerve injury)
- Weak cough (laryngeal nerve injury)
- Bruit or thrill
- Shock
- Signs of paralysis, paresthesia, or neurogenic shock if spinal cord involved
- Signs of stroke with air emboli or infarct

Symptoms

- Voice changes
- Tickle or feeling of fullness in throat
- Cervical pain
- Weakness
- Numbness
- Hoarseness
- Dyspnea
- Dysphagia

BOX 47-15 Mechanism of Injury Considerations

Motor Vehicle Crash

- Location of patient in the vehicle
- Use of restraints
- Airbag deployment
- Intrusion
- Condition of steering column, windshield

Penetrating Trauma

- Type of weapon involved
- Path of weapon
- Depth of penetration (if able to visualize without invasion of injury)
- Number of wounds
- Underlying anatomy

Strangulation Injury

- Length of time since patient was last seen
- Material involved (scarf, tie, rope, jewelry, cord)
- If hanging injury, drop height

All Injuries

- Alcohol or drug use

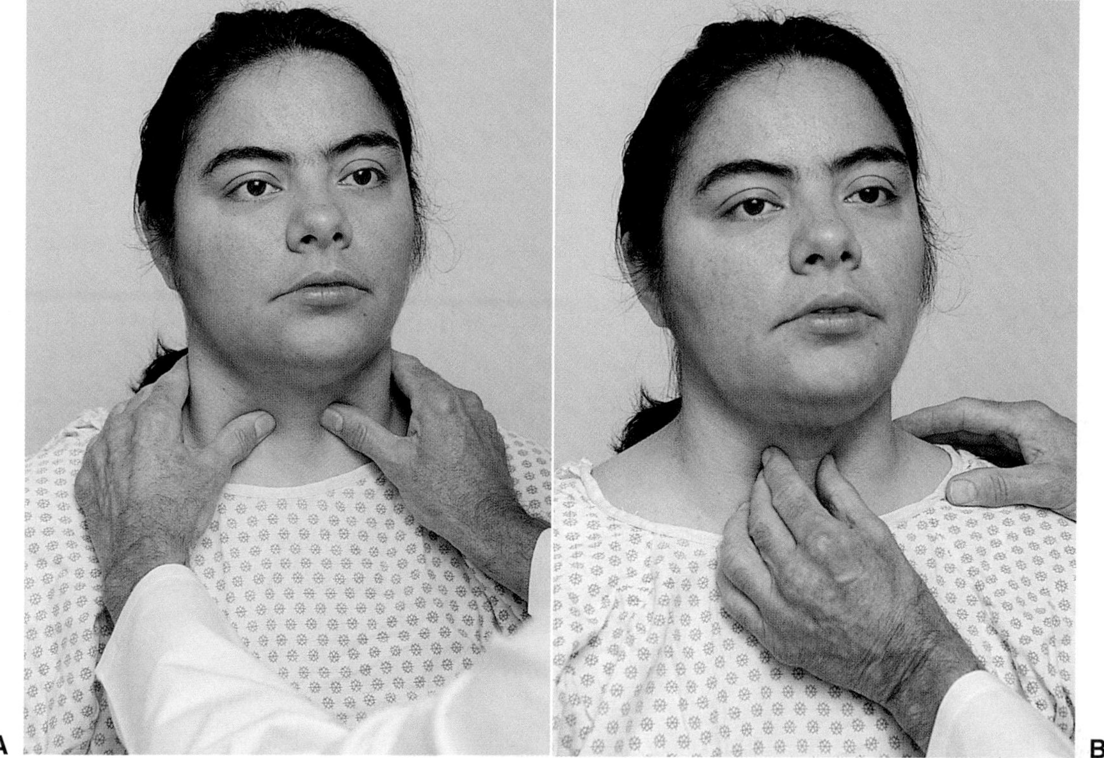

Figure 47-18 A, Position of the thumbs to assess the midline position of the trachea. **B,** Position of the thumb and finger to assess tracheal tugging.

vessel. Establish vascular access en route to definitive care with normal saline or Ringer's lactate. Infuse at a rate per medical direction's instructions to maintain adequate tissue perfusion. If possible, place an IV catheter in the extremity opposite the side of the neck injury in case disruption of the venous circulation on the same side of the body has occurred (Levy, 2006). The patient will need rapid transport to a definitive care facility with appropriate surgical resources, such as a trauma center.

PARAMEDIC*Pearl*

Close monitoring and thorough, frequent reassessment of the patient with a neck injury are necessary.

HEAD TRAUMA

Anatomy of the Scalp and Skull

The role of the scalp is to protect the head from invading organisms, help regulate internal body temperature, and keep extracellular fluid from being lost to evaporation. It also is the typical location for hair. The skin that comprises the scalp is very much like the skin of the face in pigmentation and sensation. It often is difficult to differentiate the hairline in some individuals. Some infants or toddlers may appear bald until approximately age 2 years, whereas others are born with large quantities of hair. Hair growth before birth, as with hair color and eye color, are genetic traits and run in families. Males can begin losing hair as early as their teens, but male-pattern baldness generally begins around age 40 years. As an individual ages, the hair on the head and body begins to thin, primarily because of the changing levels of hormones in the body and nutritional status.

The scalp consists of five layers of tissue that cover the superior, posterior, and lateral areas of the head (Figure 47-19). The outermost layer of the scalp consists of skin covered with hair and containing oil glands. The next layer is dense connective tissue that contains the nerves, arteries, and veins that supply the scalp. Cuts that involve this layer bleed profusely because the dense connective tissue that surrounds the vessels tends to hold the cut vessels open (Drake et al., 2005). The third layer is called the *aponeurotic layer,* which is composed of muscle that attaches just above the eyebrows and at the base of the occiput. The fourth layer is loose connective tissue. The fifth and deepest layer is called the *pericranium,* which is the periosteum of the skull bones.

The skull is divided into two main groups of bones: the facial bones and the bones of the cranium. The cranial bones are composed of a double layer of solid bone separated by a layer of spongy bone. This arrangement gives the skull greater strength. However, the thickness of different cranial bones varies. Therefore their resistance to fracture differs greatly (Frosh et al., 2005).

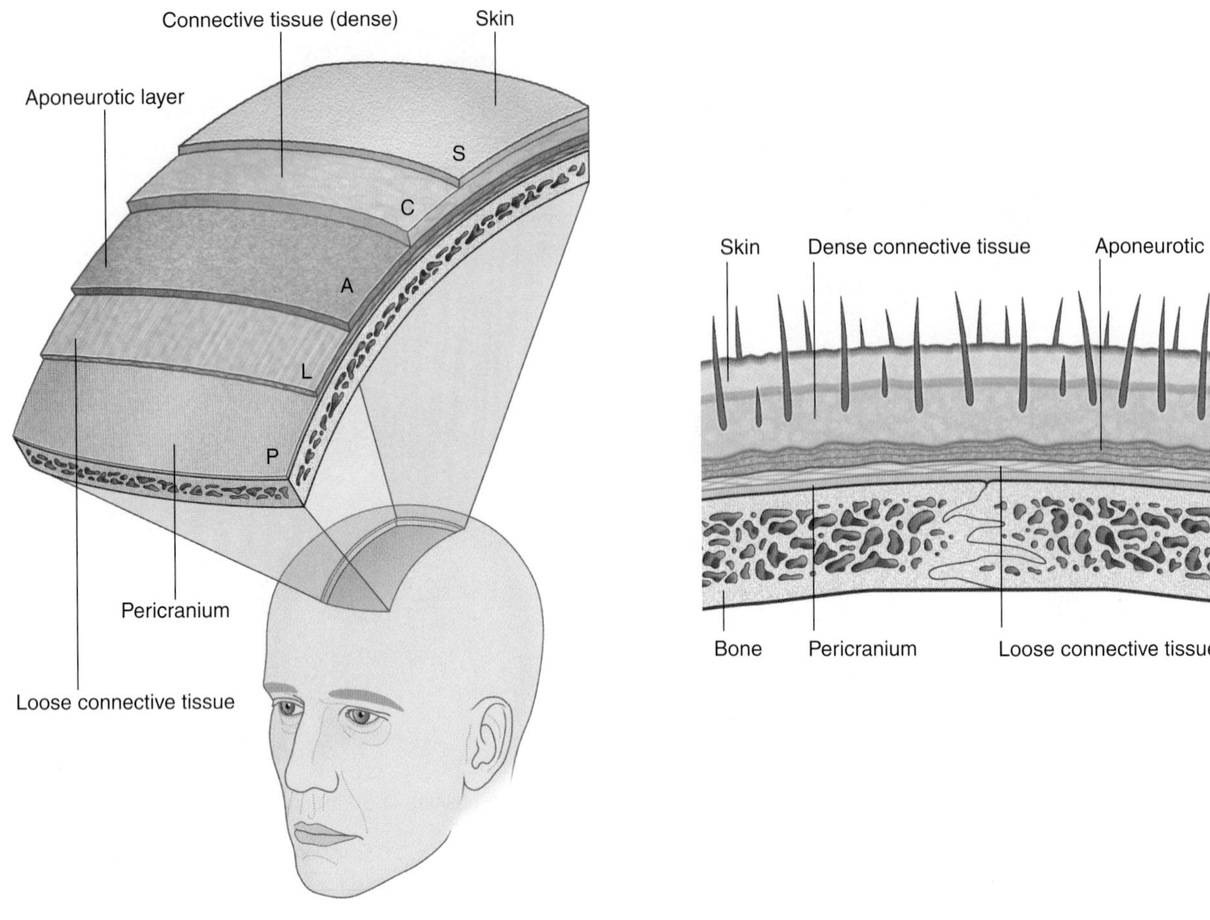

Figure 47-19 The layers of the scalp.

The roof of the skull (the cranial vault) is shaped like a dome and protects the upper portion of the brain. The middle meningeal artery lies under the temporal bone. A fracture of this bone can tear the artery, resulting in an epidural hematoma. The **foramen magnum** is an opening at the base of the skull through which the spinal cord passes (Figure 47-20).

The brain is protected by several layers and structures (Figure 47-21). The **meninges** are three layers of connective tissue coverings that surround and protect the entire central nervous system (CNS). The **dura mater** is the thickest layer of the meninges. The inner, or meningeal, layer of the dura mater is a continuation of the spinal dura mater. The outer, or periosteal, layer is firmly attached to the skull. Beneath the dura mater is the **arachnoid membrane,** a thin, delicate, weblike tissue. The arachnoid membrane runs between the dura mater and the pia mater and forms the subarachnoid space. The subarachnoid space is a fluid-filled area that is smooth on the top but follows all the crevices and cavities of the brain on the bottom. Blood vessels and CSF are in this space. **Cerebrospinal fluid (CSF)** is a clear, watery fluid that circulates beneath the arachnoid membrane and bathes the brain and spinal cord. This fluid cushions and provides some nutrients to the CNS. Large blood vessels supplying the CNS also run through the subarachnoid space. Bleeding into this area can be rapidly fatal. Below the subarachnoid space is the **pia mater,** a delicate membrane that coats the crevices and cavities of the brain and the length of the spinal cord.

Mechanism of Injury

A skull fracture may occur as a result of an MVC, fall, abuse, or an impaled object. Significant force is required to fracture the skull. Fractures of the cranial vault are more common than fractures of the base of the skull.

In fall injuries, the particular skull bone that is fractured is related to the patient's level of responsiveness at the time of the fall. For example, the site of impact when a person falls off a ladder is often the occipital part of the skull. On the other hand, a fall that follows a loss of consciousness, such as in a syncopal episode, commonly results in a frontal impact (Frosh et al., 2005).

Etiology and Demographics

[OBJECTIVES 9 TO 14]

A **head injury** is a traumatic insult to the head that may result in injury to the soft tissue or bony structures of the head and/or brain injury. A head injury may be closed (the result of blunt trauma) or open (the result of penetrating

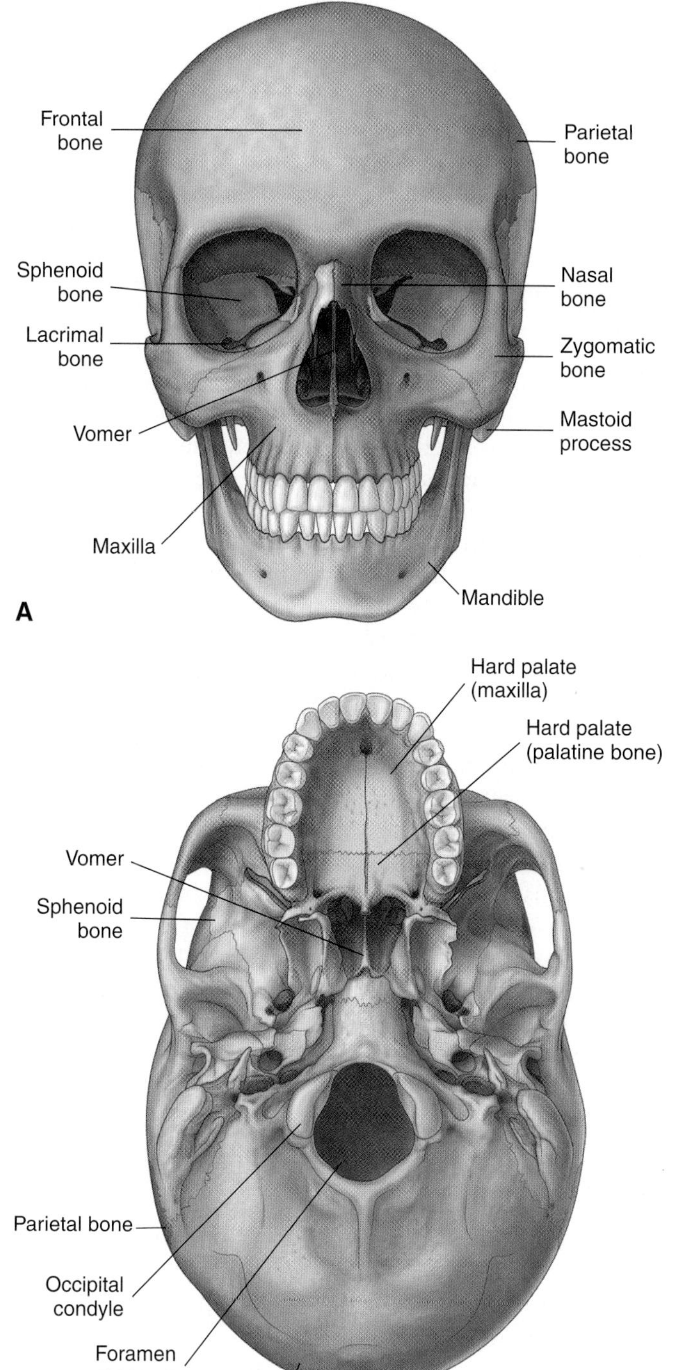

Figure 47-20 Bones of the skull. **A,** Anterior view. **B,** Base of the skull.

trauma). In a closed head injury, the dura remains intact and brain tissue is not exposed to the environment (Figure 47-22). A closed head injury may result in fractures, focal brain injuries, and/or diffuse axonal injuries (discussed later in this chapter). In an open head injury, the dura and cranial contents are penetrated and brain tissue is exposed to the environment (Figure 47-23). Closed head injuries are more common than open head injuries.

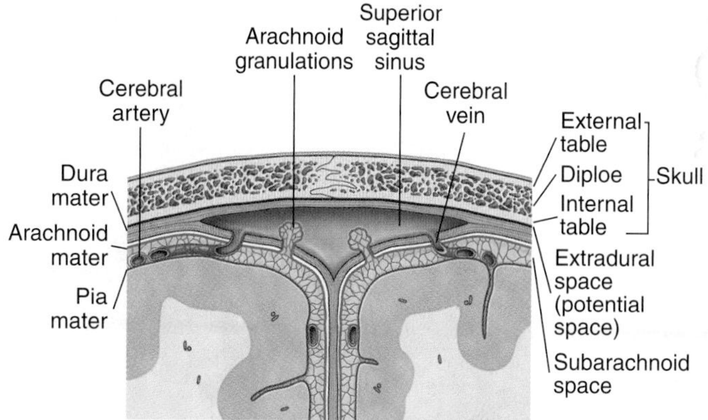

Figure 47-21 The meninges and spaces.

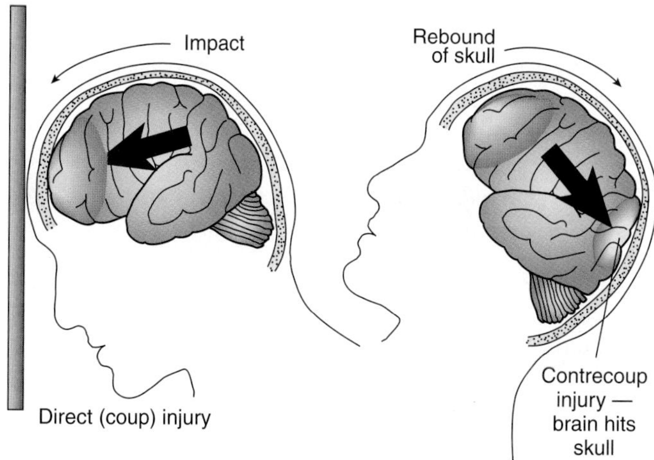

Figure 47-22 A closed head injury occurs when the dura remains intact during the injury and brain tissue is not exposed to the environment but the brain tissue is injured. Blood vessels may rupture because of the force exerted against the skull.

The scalp is designed to provide comfort and some shock absorption to the skull. When struck with enough force the scalp tears, resulting in either a simple laceration or, in more severe cases, a flap laceration, otherwise known as an *avulsion.*

A skull fracture occurs when an object causes enough force to disrupt the integrity of the skull (Box 47-16). In most cases the fracture is less of a concern than the underlying blood clot or bruising of the brain (Marion, 1998). The skull of infants and children is thin and pliable. It is more likely to transfer force to the brain beneath it instead of fracturing and absorbing some of the force along the fracture line.

A **linear skull fracture** (also called a *hairline fracture*) is a line crack in the skull. It is the most common type of skull fracture, especially in children younger than 5 years. It usually results from low-velocity blunt or compression trauma over a wide surface area of the skull. A linear skull fracture does not usually cause significant concern. However, a fracture that runs over the temporal bone may involve injury to the middle meningeal artery.

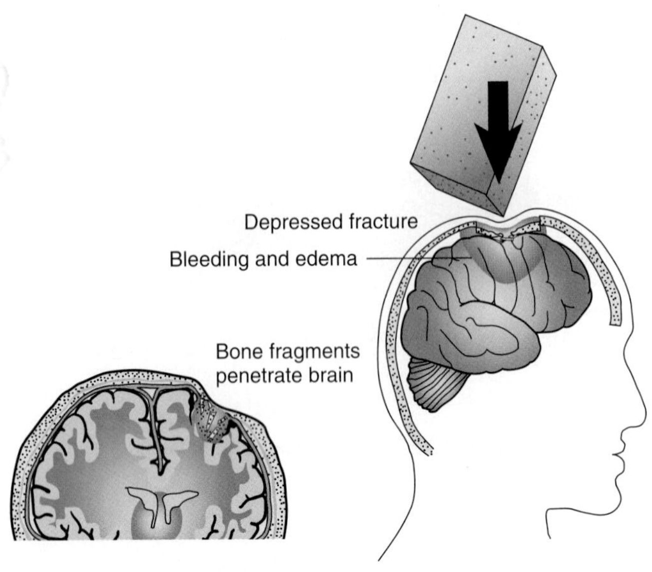

Figure 47-23 In an open head injury, the dura is penetrated, exposing the cranial contents to the environment.

BOX 47-16 Types of Skull Fractures

- Linear
- Depressed
- Basilar
- Comminuted
- Compound (open)

Rupture and hemorrhage of this artery can result in an epidural hematoma.

In a **depressed skull fracture,** pieces of bone are pushed inward and press on brain tissue, sometimes causing tearing of the tissue. This type of fracture usually results from high-velocity blunt or compression trauma to a small surface area of the skull, such as a baseball bat striking the skull. A depressed skull fracture most often is seen in the parietal area. A fracture in this area causes concern because the underlying brain may have been cut or bruised, and the likelihood of intracranial bleeding is higher. Most depressed fractures are also open fractures.

A **compound (open) skull fracture** is a combination of a depressed skull fracture and a scalp laceration. It may occur as a result of blunt or penetrating trauma. In this type of fracture the dura may be torn and brain tissue may be exposed. An open fracture places the patient at high risk for infection.

In a **comminuted skull fracture** the skull bone is broken into multiple fragments. This type of fracture involves moderate-velocity blunt or compression trauma. A **basilar skull fracture** involves the base (floor) of the skull. This type of fracture is usually a result of blunt trauma to the head (especially the mandible). It also can occur when the spinal column is driven into the area where the skull and the first vertebra meet (occipital condyles), such as in a fall on the buttocks (Conley, 1998). Children are particularly prone to basilar skull fractures. A basilar skull fracture may cause a tear in the dura. This can lead to leakage of CSF from the ear or nose. Leakage of CSF indicates that a pathway for infection exists from the environment to the subarachnoid space, increasing the patient's risk of meningitis. A basilar skull fracture typically follows an impact to the back or sides of the head but may occur anywhere along the base of the skull.

History and Physical Findings

Manually stabilize the cervical spine as you begin your assessment. Depressed and open skull fractures are usually found on palpation of the head. Most linear fractures have a bruise or swelling of the soft tissue over the area. However, swelling may not be noticeable if the patient is assessed shortly after the event or if the swelling is underneath the patient's hair. Hematomas in the temporal or parietal regions of the skull may be signs of a fracture.

Inspect and palpate the scalp and skull for DCAP-BLS-TIC (***d***eformities, ***c***ontusions, ***a***brasions, ***p***enetrations/punctures, ***b***urns, ***l***acerations, ***s***welling/edema, ***t***enderness, ***i***nstability, ***c***repitus). Use the pads of your fingers when palpating the head. In a child younger than 14 months, gently palpate the anterior and posterior fontanelles (the "soft spots" of the skull). Feel for any bulging beyond the level of the skull. A bulging fontanel in a quiet infant may indicate increased intracranial pressure. The scalp is highly vascular and often bleeds profusely when cut. Typically this bleeding can be controlled with direct pressure. A scalp laceration can result in significant blood loss in an infant or child. If present, control bleeding as quickly as possible.

Assess for other signs of a head injury. Look in the ears for DCAP-BLS, Battle's sign, and blood or clear fluid. Palpate for tenderness or pain. Inspect the face for DCAP-BLS, singed facial hair, and symmetry of facial expression. Palpate the facial bones, including the orbital rims, zygoma, maxilla, and mandible for DCAP-BLS-TIC. Inspect the eyes for DCAP-BLS, foreign body, hyphema, presence of eyeglasses or contact lenses, raccoon eyes, and swelling around the eyes. Assess pupil size, shape, equality, reactivity to light, and eye movement.

A patient who has a skull fracture may or may not have lost consciousness. Other signs and symptoms will vary depending on associated injuries, such as an epidural hematoma. Signs and symptoms of a basilar skull fracture vary depending on the area fractured. For example, the anterior fossa is above the nasal cavity and the orbits (Figure 47-24). If the fracture involves this area, signs and symptoms typically include the following:

- Epistaxis
- CSF drainage from the nose
- Absence of the sense of smell
- Raccoon eyes (periorbital ecchymosis)
- Visual disturbances
- Subconjunctival hemorrhage

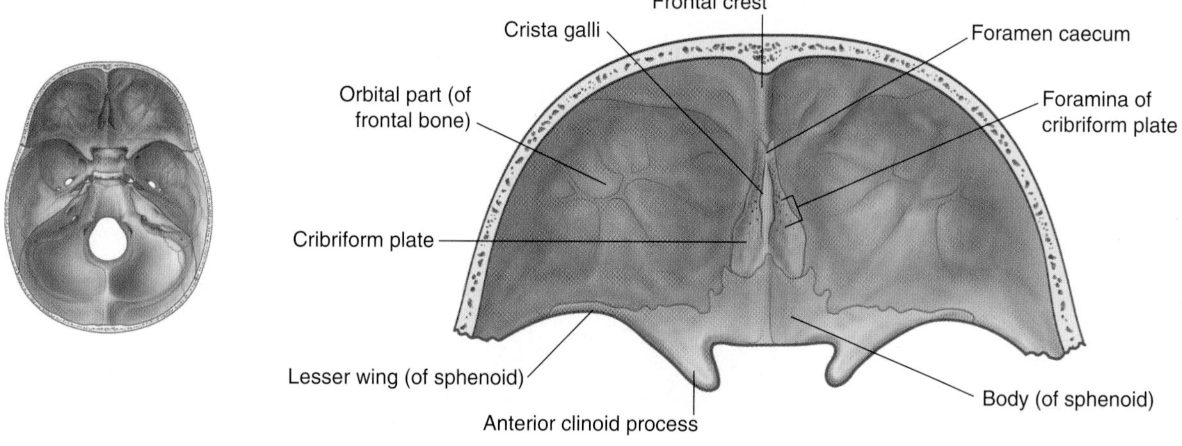

Figure 47-24 Anterior cranial fossa.

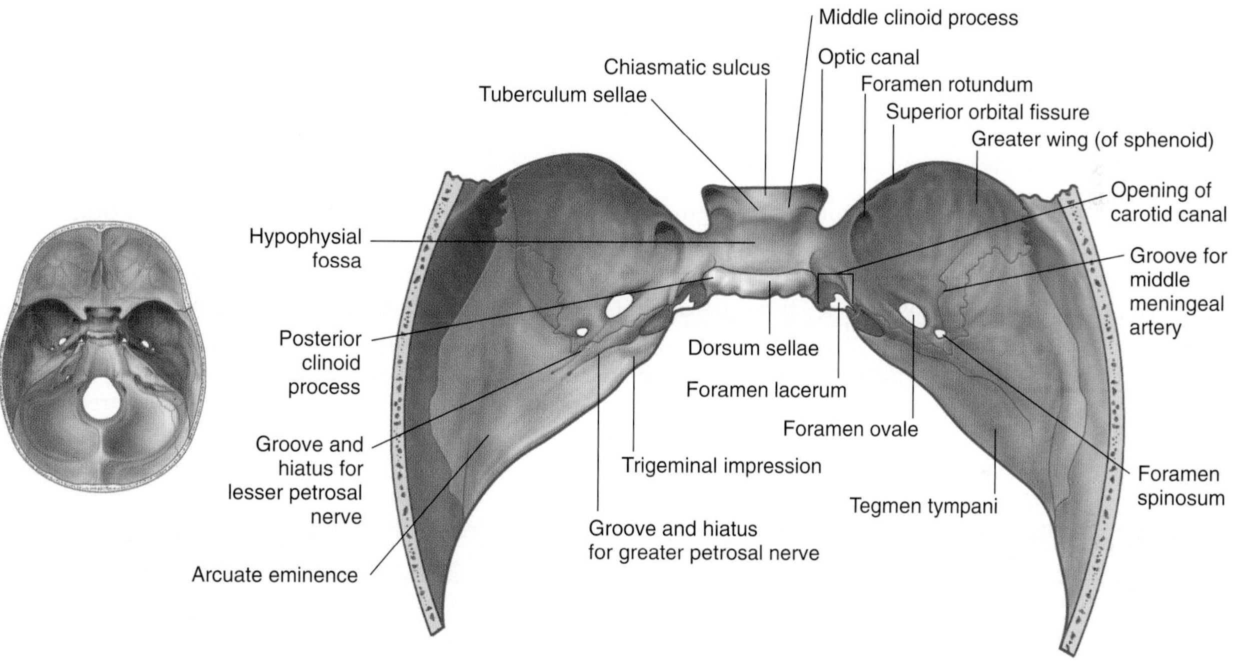

Figure 47-25 Middle cranial fossa.

The middle fossa is composed of parts of the sphenoid and temporal bones (Figure 47-25). The posterior fossa is mostly composed of parts of the temporal and occipital bones and some small areas of the sphenoid and parietal bones (Figure 47-26). If a fracture involves these areas, signs and symptoms often include the following:

- CSF drainage from the ears
- Hearing loss
- Bleeding behind the tympanic membrane (otoscope required to visualize)
- Soft tissue discoloration behind the ear(s) (Battle's sign)
- Injury to facial nerve (facial nerve palsy)

PARAMEDIC*Pearl*

Although frequently cited as a sign of a basilar skull fracture, Battle's sign (soft tissue discoloration over the mastoid bone) is typically not seen for 12 to 36 hours after the injury.

PEDIATRIC*Pearl*

Children are particularly prone to basilar skull fractures.

Therapeutic Interventions

Because a significant amount of force is required to create a skull fracture, cervical spine trauma should be suspected and appropriate precautions taken. Closely monitor

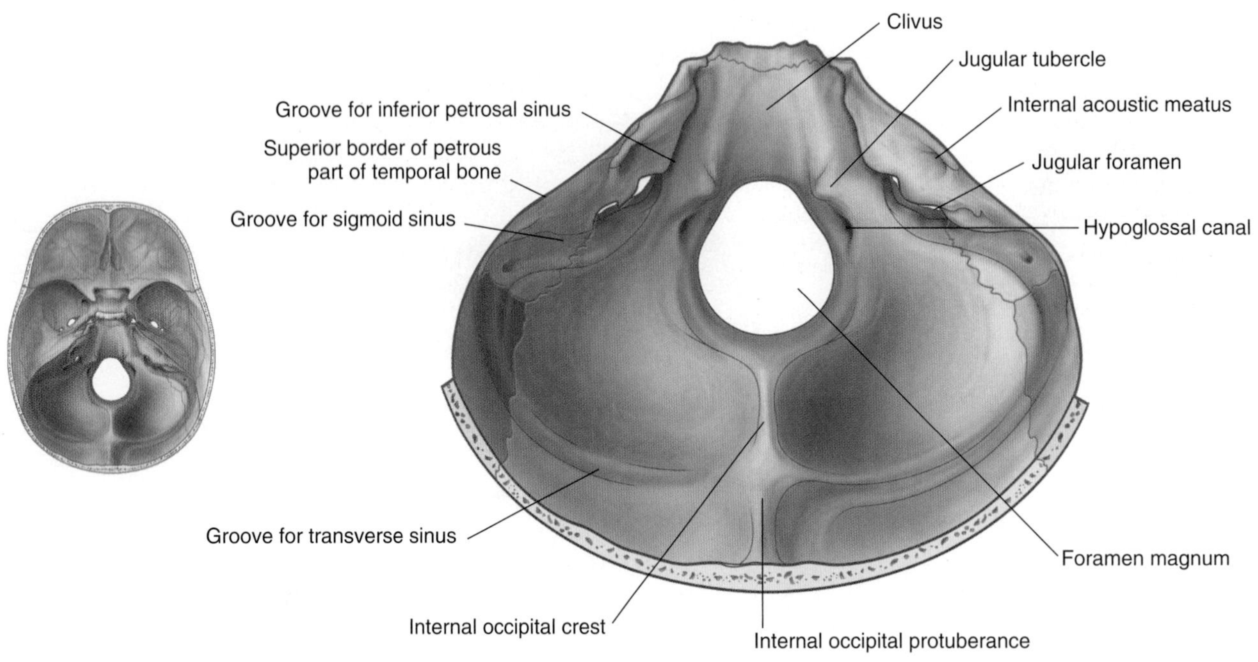

Figure 47-26 Posterior cranial fossa.

the airway in these patients because vomiting is common. If tracheal intubation or insertion of an airway adjunct is necessary to maintain an open airway or ensure adequate breathing, *do not* insert the tube through the nose. If the patient is unresponsive and has no gag reflex, an oral airway may be inserted. If intubation is required, use the oral route with inline spinal stabilization.

A linear skull fracture usually requires only supportive care. If a depressed skull fracture is present, cover the depressed area with a sterile dressing moistened with sterile saline. If CSF drainage is observed from the patient's ears or nose, do not attempt to stop the flow. Cover the ear with a loose sterile dressing. If brain tissue is visible, cover it with a saline-moistened sterile dressing. Transport the patient to the closest appropriate facility for physician evaluation.

Case Scenario—continued

The patient's pupils are equal and round; the right pupil reacts normally to light, whereas the left is nonreactive. The patient does not believe she lost consciousness, although she does not remember the period immediately after falling to the ground. Her right chest wall is slightly tender to palpation; chest movement is symmetric and breath sounds are equal. The patient has type 1 diabetes and also takes furosemide. Her pulse is 120 beats/min, blood pressure is 160/78 mm Hg, and respiratory rate is 20 breaths/min. The remainder of the examination is normal.

Questions

5. *Should this patient be spinally immobilized? Why or why not?*
6. *How should the profuse bleeding from the head be controlled?*
7. *What is the clinical significance of the unresponsive pupil?*
8. *What additional treatment should be provided?*

BRAIN TRAUMA

Anatomy of the Brain

[OBJECTIVE 15]

The brain consists of four main parts: the cerebrum, diencephalon, brainstem, and cerebellum (Figure 47-27). The **cerebrum,** the largest part of the brain, is divided into two hemispheres. Each hemisphere has four main lobes, named after the skull bones that lie immediately above them (Figure 47-28). The cerebral cortex controls voluntary skeletal movement. Injury to this area can result in extremity paresthesia, weakness, and/or paralysis.

The diencephalon includes the thalamus and hypothalamus. The thalamus serves as a relay station or switchboard. It sorts sensory information and then routes it to the brain for processing. The hypothalamus contains centers for vomiting, temperature regulation, and water balance. The brainstem connects the spinal cord with higher brain structures. It is composed of the midbrain, pons, and medulla oblongata. The brainstem contains the nuclei for most of the cranial nerves. It is responsible for vital functions such as coughing, swallowing, respiratory and heart rates, and regulation of blood vessel diameter. The cerebellum controls fine movement, coordinates skeletal muscle movement, and contributes to balance.

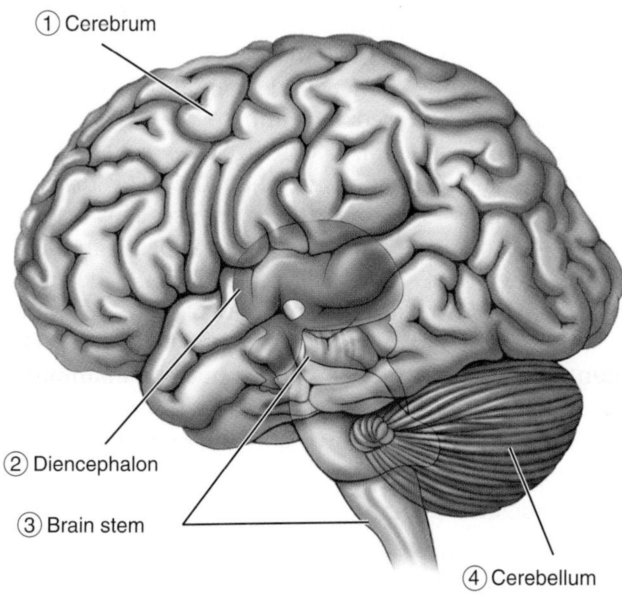

Figure 47-27 The four major areas of the brain.

The **reticular formation** is a collection of nerve cells in the brain responsible for maintaining attention and wakefulness. Deep within the brain are four chambers called *cerebral ventricles*. The ventricles are connected to one another and to the subarachnoid space that surrounds the CNS. CSF is formed by the choroid plexus in the ventricles. The **choroid plexus** is a collection of blood vessels and cells in the ventricles whose function is to produce and maintain appropriate levels of CSF. CSF flows around the brain, through a hole in the center of the spinal cord (the central canal), and the subarachnoid space that surrounds the CNS. It is reabsorbed from the subarachnoid space and then enters the venous bloodstream. Almost half a liter of CSF is produced a day in adults (Drake et al., 2005).

To function properly, the brain must receive a constant supply of oxygen and nutrients, such as glucose. The brain receives approximately 15% to 20% of the cardiac output and consumes approximately 20% of the body's oxygen. The brain receives its blood supply by means of the vertebral and internal carotid arteries. Because the brain is sensitive to decreases in glucose, oxygen, and perfusion, blood flow through the brain (cerebral blood flow) must be maintained at a fairly constant level. If the brain's blood supply is disrupted, the patient may undergo changes in mental status and vital signs, including heart rate, respiratory rate, and blood pressure.

Remember that the cranial cavity houses the brain, its blood vessels, and CSF. Normally the brain occupies approximately 78% of the space within the cranium. Because the skull is a rigid container, an increase in the volume of any of these elements (or the addition of volume) will result in an increase in pressure within the cranial cavity (intracranial pressure) unless something else gives. For example, if blood from a ruptured vessel is added to the contents of the cranial cavity, the amount

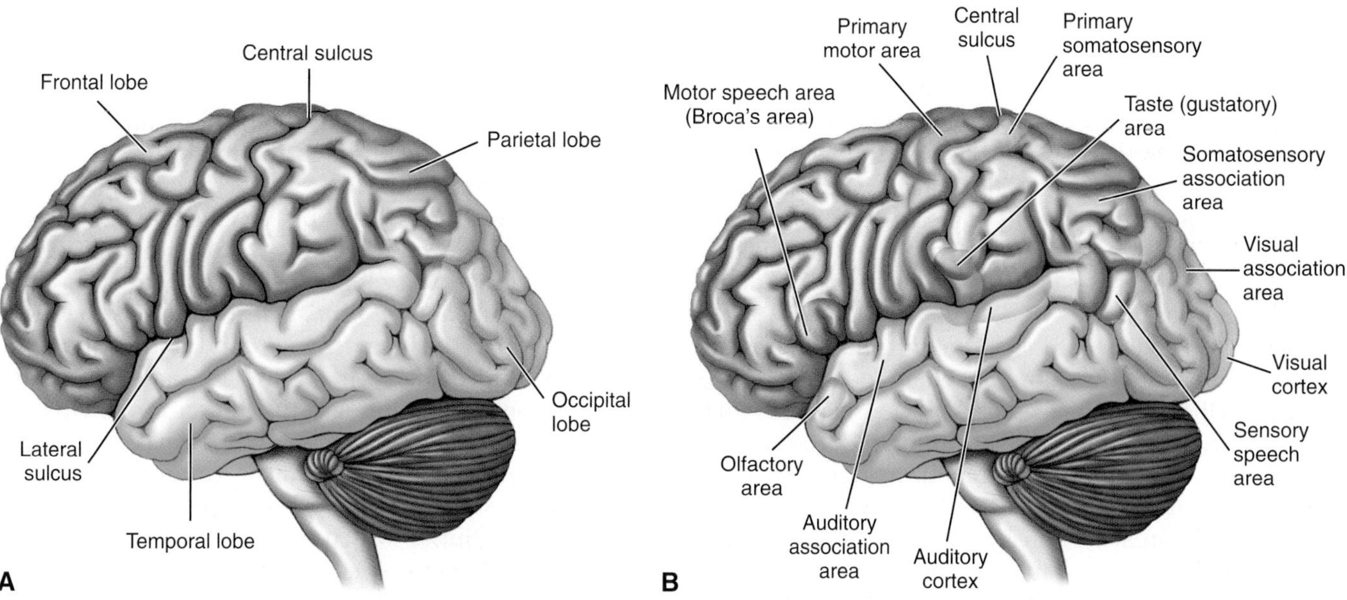

Figure 47-28 **A,** The lobes of the cerebrum. **B,** The functional areas of the cerebrum.

of CSF or the volume of the brain (or both) must decrease to offset it, or intracranial pressure (ICP) will rise.

PARAMEDIC*Pearl*

The brain can compensate for changes in ICP by manipulating one of the three major components of the skull (a decrease in any one of these will lower ICP):

- Brain tissue (occupies 78% of the skull)
- Blood volume (occupies 12%)
- CSF (occupies 10%)

Blood flow through the brain (cerebral blood flow) depends on cerebral perfusion pressure. **Cerebral perfusion pressure (CPP)** is the pressure of the blood filling the arteries of the brain. CPP is determined by the difference between mean arterial blood pressure (MAP) and ICP. MAP is the diastolic blood pressure plus one third of the pulse pressure. The MAP is an indicator of how well the brain is being supplied with nutrients, such as oxygen and glucose. The following formula shows the mathematical relationship between these factors:

$$\text{CPP} = \text{MAP} - \text{ICP}$$

The normal ICP is between 5 and 15 mm Hg, and the normal MAP is between 85 and 95 mm Hg. This results in a normal CPP of 70 to 90 mm Hg. At these pressures the brain receives blood flow, with associated oxygen and glucose, sufficient to meet its metabolic needs. Cerebral blood flow (CBF) and therefore CPP is affected by the diameter of the vessels in the brain.

A mechanism called *autoregulation* refers to the brain's ability to regulate the diameter of the vessels within the brain (and therefore CBF) in response to a wide range of mean arterial pressures (Lucatorto & Taylor, 1993). The brain is able to autoregulate and ensures adequate CBF when the CPP is between 60 and 160 mm Hg. CPP of less than 60 mm Hg results in inadequate perfusion of the brain, whereas pressures greater than 160 mm Hg result in hypertensive encephalopathy. Increased ICP disrupts autoregulation by decreasing CPP based on the mathematical formula above. As CPP decreases, blood vessels within the brain dilate. This increases the volume of blood in the brain. As a result, ICP increases. This further decreases CPP, which leads to further cerebral vasodilation, and so on.

In an effort to combat increasing intracranial pressure the body invokes the Monroe-Kellie Doctrine, or the Monroe-Kellie Principle. As stated previously, the cranial vault is a rigid, nondistensible box that is 100% filled by the brain (78%), CSF, and blood. In response to an expanding intracranial mass the body will attempt to regulate intracranial pressure by expelling CSF and venous blood out of the cranial vault. This creates more space for the mass and keeps ICP within normal limits during the early stages of the expanding mass, which can result in subtle signs and symptoms that are easily missed without a high index of suspicion. As with all compensatory mechanisms, there is a limit to the effectiveness of this process. At the point where no additional CSF or venous blood can be expelled, ICP will increase exponentially.

Once the ICP begins to rise the body will attempt to maintain CPP by increasing the MAP. This will be evidenced by not only an increasing blood pressure (both systolic and diastolic components) but also by a widening pulse pressure. To recognize this pattern it is crucial that the paramedic auscultate a blood pressure, noting both the systolic blood prossure (SBP) and diastolic blood pressure (DBP). Simply palpating a blood pressure will result in the loss of valuable information.

$$\text{MAP} = \text{DBP} + \tfrac{1}{3}\text{PP}$$

Other factors also interfere with CPP. For example, too much carbon dioxide in the blood causes cerebral vasodilation. This results in increased cerebral blood volume, which leads to increased ICP, and so on. Hypotension results in a decreased MAP which causes a decrease in the CPP. As stated previously, when the MAP drops to 60 mm Hg or less, CBF begins to decrease. This leads to cerebral vasodilation, and the cycle repeats itself. In patients older than 12 years, the SBP should be maintained above 90 mm Hg; for patients 5 to 12 years old, the SBP should be maintained above 80 mm Hg; for patients 1 to 5 years old, the SBP should be maintained above 75 mm Hg; and for patients less than 1 year old, the SBP should be maintained above 65 mm Hg.

PARAMEDIC*Pearl*

An SBP of less than 90 mm Hg for any amount of time is one of the most powerful predictors of poor outcome in the setting of a traumatic train injury.

When swelling or bleeding occurs in the brain, the brain sends out signals requesting more oxygen. This triggers a vicious cycle. The more blood that enters the brain, the more oxygen it requires, and the more swelling increases. If the ICP gets too high, the brain tissue has nowhere to go except through the tentorium incinsura, foramen magnum, or both.

Herniation, which is the displacement of brain tissue laterally or downward because of increasing ICP, can result in herniation syndrome. Lateral herniation syndrome, also called *uncal herniation syndrome,* is the most common form. This occurs when a portion of the temporal lobe, called the *uncus,* is displaced laterally before moving downward through the tentorium incinsura. Because the occulomotor nerve (CN III) passes through the tentorium incinsura, it will be compressed by the uncus. This results in the pupil dilation that may be seen in head injuries, which is a strong indicator of herniation. Recall that cranial nerves exert their effect on the same side of the body, whereas spinal nerves exert their effect on the opposite side of the body. As a result the patient will exhibit ipsalateral (same-sided) pupil dilation and contralateral (opposite-sided) motor dysfunction. Early evaluation of the pupils in suspected traumatic brain injury (TBI) is essential, as a unilateral pupil change may only be present from minutes to hours depending on the rate of expansion of the intracranial mass. Herniation that involves brain tissue shifting downward, ultimately compressing the brainstem from above, is called *central herniation syndrome*.

As pressure is exerted on brain tissue, the cerebral cortices and/or the reticular formation are affected. The patient will have an altered level of responsiveness, which may include amnesia of the event, confusion, sluggishness, combativeness, or weakness. When the hypothalamus is affected, vomiting may occur. Bradycardia may result from both pressure on the vagus nerve and the response of the barorceptors to hypertension. The patient may have abnormal respiratory patterns such as Cheyne-Stokes respirations or central neurogenic hyperventilation. As the respiratory center is compressed, the patient may exhibit ataxic respirations. Decorticate (flexion) or decerebrate (extension) posturing may be evident. The patient may have seizures depending on the location of the injury.

By increasing available oxygen, you can help keep ICP within normal (or near normal) levels. Placing the patient on supplemental oxygen tricks the brain into thinking that no damage or less-severe damage has occurred. When you place the patient on oxygen, you are flooding the blood with oxygen molecules, thus displacing the carbon dioxide. As with hypotension, hypoxia is one of the most powerful predictors of poor outcome in patients with a traumatic brain injury. If both hypotension and hypoxia develop, the incidence of poor outcome increases exponentially.

PARAMEDIC*Pearl*

- An oxygen saturation of less than 90% for any amount of time is one of the most powerful predictors of poor outcome in the setting of a TBI.
- Most available resources refer to CO_2 levels in terms of $PaCO_2$. Because $ETCO_2$ levels are more applicable to the paramedic, the CO_2 values presented in this section have been adjusted to represent $ETCO_2$. This adjustment was based on the principle that normal $PaCO_2$ is 35 to 45 mm Hg, whereas normal $ETCO_2$ is 33 to 43 mm Hg because of gas exchange laws.

The levels of carbon dioxide in the blood contribute to this series of events. Capnography is a valuable tool in patients with any type of head injury. Capnography is a noninvasive tool to measure the level of carbon dioxide (CO_2) in the bloodstream. Normal CO_2 levels range from 33 to 43 mm Hg. Whereas increased CO_2 levels will cause cerebral vasodilatation, decreased CO_2 levels will cause cerebral vasoconstriction. In suspected TBI the CO_2 should be maintained at the low end of normal to slightly below normal. Therefore the patient's lungs should be ventilated to maintain the CO_2 between 30 and 35 mm Hg. Recall that increasing the ventilatory rate decreases CO_2 and decreasing the ventilatory rate increases CO_2. In the absence of the ability to monitor CO_2 it is recommended that the adult patient's lungs be ventilated at 10 breaths per minute, the child at 20 breaths per minute, and the infant at 25 breaths per minute to maintain optimal CO_2 levels. If herniation is suspected, evidenced by the dilation of a pupil, a reduction in the Glasgow Coma Scale (GCS) by 2 or more points, or posturing, the patient should be mildly hyperventilated. When performing mild hyperventilation, ensure the patient's CO_2 never falls below 25 mm Hg, as this will result in severe vasoconstriction causing cerebral ischemia. In the absence of the ability to monitor capnography the adult should be ventilated at 20 breaths per minute, the child at 30 breaths per minute, and the infant at 25 breaths per minute.

Signs of increased ICP in an infant include a full fontanelle, altered mental status, periodic episodes of irritability, persistent vomiting, and an inability to fully open the eyes (referred to as the "setting sun" sign). In a child, signs and symptoms include a headache, stiff neck, photophobia, altered mental status, persistent vomiting, symptoms of cranial nerve involvement, Cushing's triad, and decorticate or decerebrate posturing. In decorticate posturing, the legs are extended and the arms are flexed. In decerebrate posturing, all extremities are extended and rotated inward. Progression from decorticate to decerebrate posturing is an ominous sign. Signs and symptoms of increased ICP are shown in Box 47-17.

PARAMEDIC*Pearl*

Changes in the patient's condition will be evident as ICP rises. For example, increases in ICP cause characteristic changes in vital signs, including hypertension (often with a widening pulse pressure), bradycardia, and an irregular breathing pattern. This trio of changes is called *Cushing's triad.* Cushing's triad is a *late* sign of increased ICP; however, its absence does not rule out the presence of increased ICP.

Mechanism of Injury

An injury to the head may or may not result in an injury to the brain. A **brain injury** is defined by the National Head Injury Foundation as "a traumatic insult to the brain capable of producing physical, intellectual, emotional, social, and vocational changes." In essence, a TBI results from a force great enough to cause the brain to be moved inside the skull or the covering to be penetrated—even if the initial blow does not cause visible immediate distress.

BOX 47-17 Levels of Increasing Intracranial Pressure

Cerebral Cortex and Upper Brainstem Involvement

- Blood pressure rises and heart rate begins slowing
- Pupils still reactive
- Cheyne-Stokes respirations
- Initially tries to localize and remove painful stimuli
- Eventually withdraws, then flexion occurs
- All effects reversible at this stage

Middle Brainstem Involvement

- Wide pulse pressure and bradycardia
- Pupils nonreactive or sluggish
- Central neurogenic hyperventilation
- Extension
- Few patients survive with normal cerebral function from this level

Lower Brainstem Involvement

- Pupil dilation (blown pupil) on same side as injury
- Ataxic respirations (erratic, no rhythm) or absent
- Flaccid
- Changing heart rate; irregular, often great, swings in heart rate
- QRS, ST segment, and T-wave changes on cardiac monitor
- Decreased blood pressure, often variable
- Not considered survivable

An injury to the head or brain may be primary, secondary, or tertiary. A primary injury is a direct injury, which means that direct damage was incurred during the actual injury or impact to the head. The injury causes mechanical disruption of cells and changes in vascular permeability. Examples of primary injuries include skull fractures, concussions, contusions, lacerations, axon-shearing injuries, and nerve and vascular damage.

Secondary and tertiary injuries are indirect injuries. A secondary injury is the result of metabolic events caused by the trauma that produce damage to the brain minutes, hours, or days after the initial event. If left untreated, secondary injuries can worsen the primary injury. Examples of secondary injuries include cerebral ischemia and brain edema, which may result from systemic hypotension, hypercapnia, and hypoxemia. Vasospasm, seizures, and meningitis also may produce secondary injury. A tertiary injury is caused by apnea, hypotension, pulmonary resistance, and ECG changes.

Mechanisms of injury that may result in an injury to the brain include MVCs, recreational and sports activities, falls, assaults, firearms, and sharp projectiles (e.g., knives, ice picks, axes, screwdrivers).

BOX 47-18 Concussion: Possible Signs and Symptoms

- Loss of consciousness
- Confusion and disorientation
- Amnesia of the event
- Loss of appetite
- Slurred or jumbled speech
- Difficulty concentrating
- Nausea and vomiting
- Ringing in the ears (tinnitus)
- Headache
- Dazed appearance
- Dizziness
- Irritability
- Pallor
- Unsteadiness
- Visual disturbances

Etiology and Demographics

[OBJECTIVES 16, 17]

General categories of injury include coup, contrecoup, diffuse axonal injury, and focal. A **coup injury** is an injury that occurs directly below the point of impact. A **contrecoup injury** occurs at another site, usually opposite the impact. A **diffuse axonal injury (DAI)** is a shearing, tearing, stretching force of nerve fibers with axonal damage. In a **focal injury,** an injury is limited to a particular area of the brain.

Diffuse Axonal Injury

A **concussion** (or mild DAI) is a brain insult with a transient impairment of consciousness followed by a rapid recovery to baseline neurologic activity. A concussion may occur as a result of a strong, rapid acceleration-deceleration event. It is the most common result after blunt trauma to the head. Concussions are graded on a scale of 1 to 3 as follows:

- Grade 1: Transient confusion, no loss of consciousness, and duration of mental status abnormalities less than 15 minutes.
- Grade 2: Transient confusion, no loss of consciousness, and duration of mental status abnormalities of more than 15 minutes.
- Grade 3: Concussion involving loss of consciousness.

A patient who has experienced a concussion may show signs and symptoms of confusion, disorientation, amnesia of the event, anorexia, vomiting, or pallor soon after the event. The patient may be unable to recall events immediately before (retrograde amnesia) or after (antegrade amnesia) the trauma to the head. Possible signs and symptoms of a concussion are shown in Box 47-18. A concussion rarely leads to significant long-term problems. However, some patients experience **postconcussion syndrome (PCS)** for several weeks to 1 year after the injury with symptoms similar to those of the initial injury.

In a moderate DAI, shearing, stretching, or tearing results in tiny bruises of the brain tissue. The brainstem and reticular formation may be involved, leading to unresponsiveness. A moderate DAI is commonly associated with a basilar skull fracture. A moderate DAI may result in immediate unresponsiveness or persistent confusion, disorientation, and amnesia of the event extending to amnesia of moment-to-moment events. The patient may have a focal deficit. The patient may be unable to concentrate, have frequent periods of anxiety or uncharacteristic mood swings, and have an altered sense of smell long after the event. Most patients survive but neurologic impairment is common.

A severe DAI was formerly called a *brainstem injury.* It involves severe mechanical disruption of many axons in both cerebral hemispheres and extends to the brainstem. A patient with a severe DAI is usually unresponsive for a prolonged period. Posturing is common. Other signs of increased ICP occur depending on the degree of brain damage.

Focal Injuries

Cerebral Contusion. A **cerebral contusion** is a brain injury in which brain tissue is bruised in a local area but does not puncture the pia mater. Bruising may occur at both the area of direct impact (coup) and/or on the side opposite (contrecoup) the impact. A contusion can result from blunt trauma to the head, as in an acceleration-deceleration injury. A contusion also may be found beneath a depressed skull fracture and around penetrating injuries (Conley, 1998).

A patient who has a cerebral contusion may show changes in mental status. Inspection and palpation of the head often reveals swelling of the area. A skull laceration may be present. Confusion or unusual behavior is common. The patient may report a progressive headache and/or photophobia. Assess for signs and symptoms of increased ICP such as an altered level of consciousness, vomiting, pupil changes, and changes in pulse, respiration, and blood pressure. The patient may be unable to form new memories; repetitive phrases are common.

Intracranial Hemorrhage. Bleeding within the brain is classified by the layer of the brain within which it occurs. Types of intracranial hemorrhage include epidural, subdural, intracerebral, and subarachnoid (Box 47-19).

Between the skull and dura mater is a potential space called the *epidural space.* If bleeding occurs and collects in this area, it is called an **epidural hematoma** (Figure 47-29). An epidural hematoma may occur as a result of a fall, MVC, sports injury, or direct blow to the head. In adults, an epidural hematoma almost always is the result of an injury to the middle meningeal artery.

Signs and symptoms associated with an epidural hematoma can be deceptive. At first impact, the force that caused the head injury causes a momentary loss of consciousness (concussion). This is followed by a period in which the patient is awake and alert. This is referred to

BOX 47-19 Types of Intracranial Hemorrhage

- Epidural
- Subdural
- Intracerebral
- Subarachnoid

TYPES OF HEMATOMAS AND THE MENINGES

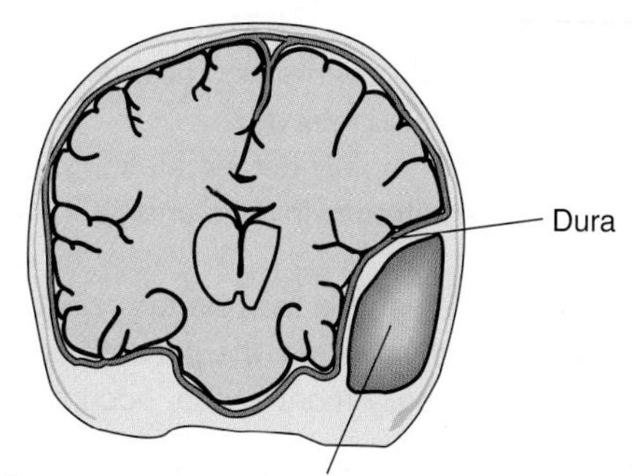

A EXTRADURAL OR EPIDURAL HEMATOMA
Blood fills space between dura and bone

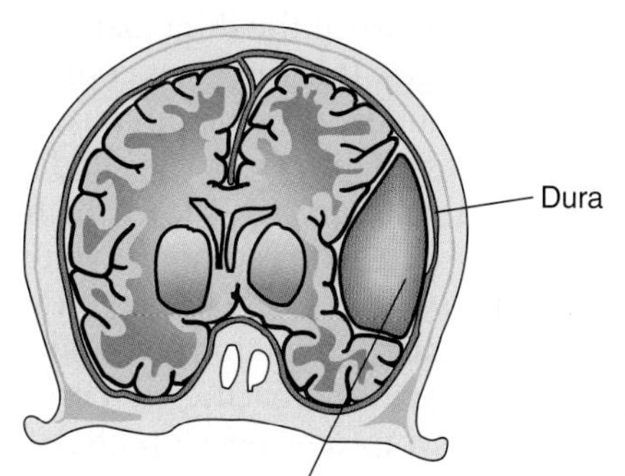

B SUBDURAL HEMATOMA
Blood fills space between dura and arachnoid

Skull bone
Dura
Subdural space
Arachnoid
Brain
Subarachnoid space
Pia

C INTRACEREBRAL HEMATOMA

Figure 47-29 Types of cerebral hematomas and the meninges. **A,** Epidural hematoma. **B,** Subdural hematoma. **C,** Intracerebral hematoma.

as a *lucid interval.* It is often associated with a severe headache. The patient then experiences a rapid decline in mental status, progressing from drowsiness and confusion to coma. This occurs as the hematoma builds up between the skull and the dura and ICP increases. Death will occur if the patient does not quickly receive definitive care at an appropriate facility. Other signs and symptoms include vomiting, early dilation of the pupil on the same side as the impact, and weakness on the side of the body opposite the injury.

PARAMEDIC*Pearl*

Epidural Hematoma

- An estimated 20% to 50% of patients who have an epidural hematoma have a lucid interval.
- The patient's condition often rapidly deteriorates because most epidural hematomas involve arterial bleeding.
- Occasionally an epidural hematoma may be the result of *venous* bleeding. When this occurs, the patient's signs and symptoms are usually more subtle, occurring over a period of days.

A **subdural hematoma** is a collection of blood in the subdural space, which is between the dura mater and arachnoid layer of the meninges. It is the most common type of intracranial bleed. A subdural hematoma usually results from tearing of the veins that cross the subdural space. Possible mechanisms of injury are shown in Box 47-20. Because the source of the bleeding is venous instead of arterial, signs and symptoms are usually slower to develop than in an epidural hematoma. Subdural hematomas are classified as acute, subacute, or chronic depending on how quickly symptoms develop after the injury (Table 47-2).

BOX 47-20 Subdural Hematoma: Possible Mechanisms of Injury

- Motor vehicle crash
- Fall
- Assault
- Sports-related head injury
- Industrial accident
- Shaken baby syndrome

TABLE 47-2 Categories of Subdural Hematoma

Category	Symptom Onset
Acute	≤48 hours of injury
Subacute	2-14 days of injury
Chronic	>14 days of injury

PARAMEDIC*Pearl*

Chronic subdural hematomas are more common in the elderly and alcoholics. Because the patient usually presents with an altered mental status, obtaining a good history and performing a thorough assessment are important. You may find that the patient sustained a head injury days, weeks, or months before the present call for EMS assistance.

Signs and symptoms of a subdural hematoma may include a loss of consciousness immediately after the injury, confusion, headache, drowsiness, a fixed and dilated pupil on the same side as the injury, and weakness on the side of the body opposite the injury. A newborn or infant often presents with seizures, decreased level of consciousness, bulging fontanelle, weak cry, pallor, and vomiting. In children older than 2 to 3 years, signs and symptoms often include pupillary changes, weakness on the side of the body opposite the injury, restlessness, and altered mental status.

GERIATRIC*Considerations*

Signs and symptoms of a subdural hematoma may develop slowly in the elderly because they have larger potential subdural spaces because of cerebral atrophy. Signs and symptoms may rapidly occur in a younger patient with a small subdural space (Holleran, 1996).

From Holleran, R. S. (Ed.). (1996). *Flight nursing: Principles and practice* (2nd ed.). St. Louis: Mosby.

An **intracerebral hematoma** is bleeding within the brain tissue itself. This type of bleeding can occur if blood vessels in the brain are cut from a depressed skull fracture. It may also be caused by rupture or shearing of the blood vessels in blunt trauma or laceration of the vessels in penetrating trauma. Many small, deep intracerebral hemorrhages are associated with other brain injuries (especially DAI). Most intracerebral hematomas from trauma affect the frontal and temporal lobes of the brain. The patient's signs and symptoms depend on the associated injuries and the area involved, the size of the hemorrhage, and whether bleeding continues.

A **subarachnoid hemorrhage** is a collection of blood between the arachnoid layer of the meninges and the pia mater. The patient usually presents with pupil dilation on the side of the injury, severe headache, decreasing level of consciousness, and a stiff neck.

History and Physical Findings

As you begin caring for the patient, keep in mind that determining the specific type of brain injury present may be impossible. Recognizing the presence of a brain injury and beginning immediate care is more important.

PARAMEDIC*Pearl*

The most important assessment you can perform when caring for a brain-injured patient is noting a change in level of consciousness.

An accurate history is vital. Try to find out what the patient was doing. What happened? What is wrong now? What does not seem right? Did the patient lose consciousness? If so, did it happen immediately after the event or later?

A patient with TBI has a cervical spine injury until proven otherwise. Ask a member of your crew to stabilize the cervical spine manually as you begin your assessment. Make sure the patient's airway is open and that he or she is breathing adequately. Check the patient's pulse and control significant bleeding if present. Correct any life-threatening injuries.

A brain-injured patient may have an abnormal rate and pattern of breathing (Figure 47-30). Determine whether an abnormal breathing pattern is present and note whether it changes while the patient is in your care. Determine a GCS score as early as possible and then reassess it often. This will help you detect changes in the patient's condition. The GCS is used to describe a patient's general level of consciousness. The score is a reliable indicator of injury severity and deterioration or improvement in the patient's condition. The GCS is divided into three categories: eye opening, motor response, and verbal response. A patient's response is scored in each category and then added together, with a maximum score of 15 and a minimum score of 3. A GCS score that falls 2 points suggests significant deterioration; urgent patient reassessment is required. The GCS is discussed in more detail in Chapter 23.

PARAMEDIC*Pearl*

Glasgow Coma Score

The initial GCS score often influences treatment, transport, and transfer decisions.

- Score of 3 to 7 = severe injury
- Score of 8 to 12 = moderate injury
- Score of 13 to 15 = mild injury

Assess the patient's vital signs, including the pupils. Watch closely for signs and symptoms of increasing ICP. Reassessment of the patient is required to detect signs of increasing ICP.

PARAMEDIC*Pearl*

It is imperative that the paramedic determine the GCS score during the primary survey so that an accurate baseline can be established and not be missed in the overall patient course. For example, a patient may have a 1-point change in the prehospital setting and a 1-point change in the emergency department, for a total of 2 points. However, if the prehospital change was not noted and the ED course became the baseline, a false impression of the patient's course would occur.

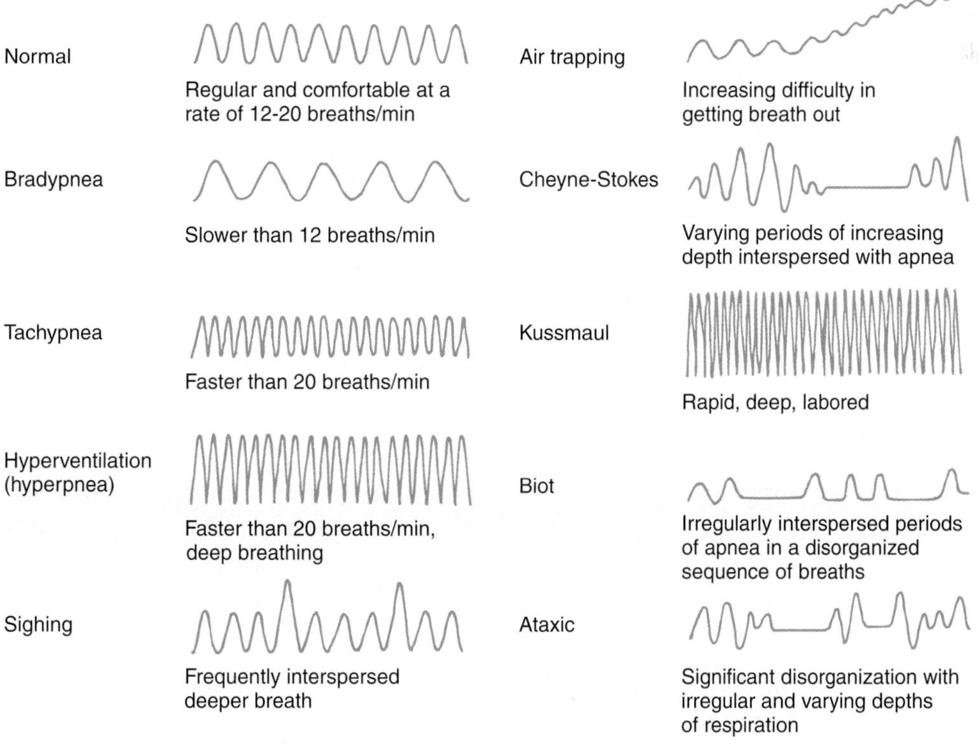
Normal
Regular and comfortable at a rate of 12-20 breaths/min
Bradypnea
Slower than 12 breaths/min
Tachypnea
Faster than 20 breaths/min
Hyperventilation (hyperpnea)
Faster than 20 breaths/min, deep breathing
Sighing
Frequently interspersed deeper breath
Air trapping
Increasing difficulty in getting breath out
Cheyne-Stokes
Varying periods of increasing depth interspersed with apnea
Kussmaul
Rapid, deep, labored
Biot
Irregularly interspersed periods of apnea in a disorganized sequence of breaths
Ataxic
Significant disorganization with irregular and varying depths of respiration

Figure 47-30 Breathing patterns.

Therapeutic Interventions

When caring for a head- or brain-injured patient, the time on the scene should generally not exceed 10 minutes. The patient requires definitive care at a hospital staffed and equipped to handle this type of injury. If your scene time will exceed 10 minutes, contact medical direction with the reason for the delay.

Continue manual stabilization of the cervical spine until the patient has been completely secured to a backboard. Maintain an open airway and ensure the patient's breathing is adequate. Give oxygen and suction as necessary. Attach a pulse oximeter and ECG monitor, and use capnography if it is available. If the patient's breathing is inadequate, assist breathing with a bag-mask device connected to oxygen. Ventilate the lungs of an adult at a rate of 10 breaths/min. Ventilate the lungs of a child at a rate of 20 breaths/min and an infant at 25 breaths/min. These ventilation rates are used when capnography is not available. If capnography is available, it should be used to guide the rate of ventilations. Make sure that you can see gentle chest rise with each ventilation.

PARAMEDIC*Pearl*

For many years hyperventilation was used in the management of severe traumatic brain injuries. Studies have shown that the initial management of a severe brain injury should include ventilation at a normal rate: 1 breath every 5 seconds for an adult and 1 breath every 3 seconds for an infant or child. Hyperventilation should be considered if signs of herniation are present. In most EMS systems, this means ventilation at a rate of 20 breaths/min in adults and 25 breaths/min in children. Hyperventilation is usually considered if a patient has a GCS score of 8 or less accompanied by active seizures and signs of herniation, such as fixed or unequal pupils, decerebrate or decorticate posturing, Cushing's triad, or signs of neurologic deterioration.

Closely monitor the airway and ensure suction is immediately available. Vomiting in the first 30 to 60 minutes after a head injury is common in children. Consider placement of an orogastric tube. Most trauma protocols recommend endotracheal intubation if the patient's GCS score is 8 or less. If intubation is necessary, use the oral route with inline spinal stabilization. If it is a part of your EMS protocol, consider rapid-sequence intubation and the use of lidocaine before the procedure to blunt any increase in ICP.

Establish vascular access. Start an IV of normal saline or Ringer's lactate. Infuse at a rate specified by medical direction or local protocol to prevent hypotension and preserve CPP. The practice of restricting fluids in TBI patients is no longer recommended. The goal in fluid resuscitation is to maintain euvolemia and, as mentioned previously, to avoid hypotension. Assess the patient's serum glucose level to rule out a diabetic emergency. Avoid giving glucose or glucagon unless hypoglycemia (less than 60 mg/dL) is confirmed. If hypotension (systolic blood pressure of less than 90 mm Hg) is present, look for internal bleeding, as an isolated TBI will almost never present with hypotension. Elevate the head of the stretcher or backboard approximately 15 to 30 degrees. Treat seizures if present. Rapidly transport the patient to the closest appropriate facility for definitive care. Patients who are combative, agitated, or fighting against immobilization will cause an increase in their ICP and potentially worsen existing injuries. Sedation or chemical restraint, discussed later in this chapter, may be considered in these situations. Always weigh the risks and benefits of these procedures and consult with medical direction as needed before performing them.

Helmet Removal Considerations

[OBJECTIVE 18]

The purpose of a helmet is to protect the head and brain; however, the cervical spine remains vulnerable to injury. Whether to remove a helmet is a controversial subject. Several factors must be considered (Table 47-3).

Many sports helmets have a removable face mask to allow access for airway control. Also, athletic trainers have multiple apparatuses to immobilize the athlete's spine with the helmet in place. Automobile racing drivers may also have an onboard immobilization device to secure their head and neck in line, such as the HANS (head and neck support racing driver safety device). Such devices also need to be removed with minimal movement of the cervical spine.

TABLE 47-3 Helmet Removal Considerations

Consideration	Do Not Remove Helmet	Remove Helmet
Fit	Good fit with little or no movement	Poor fit, allows movement
Airway and breathing	No problems, easy access	Restriction of airway or access
Spinal immobilization	Able to immobilize in a neutral position (without hyperflexion or hyperextension) effectively with helmet in place	Unable to immobilize in a neutral position (without hyperflexion or hyperextension) with helmet in place

Case Scenario CONCLUSION

Bleeding from the puncture wound was adequately controlled with direct pressure to the margins of the wound. The patient is spinally immobilized and placed on oxygen by nonrebreather mask at 15 L. On arrival at the emergency department, the patient's mental status is unchanged and her pulse is 94 beats/min, blood pressure is 150/90 mm Hg, and respiratory rate is 18 breaths/min. Diagnostic testing reveals that the patient has a 6- to 8-cm depressed skull fracture with no accompanying brain injury. The patient is taken to the operating room for debridement of the wound and repair of the fractures. It is ultimately determined that she was struck in the head with a hammer.

Looking Back

9. *Given the patient's final disposition, was your treatment appropriate? Why or why not?*

Restraints

In specific situations, medical direction may give orders for mechanical or chemical restraint. **Restraints** are typically used for patients who display behaviors harmful to themselves or others. However, medical direction may instruct you to use them in clinically justified situations. For example, restraints may be used in incapacitated persons who require emergency medical care, such as a head-injured patient or a patient in shock.

When a patient is restrained, he or she must be monitored *at all times* during treatment and transport. This includes assessment and monitoring of the patient's airway, breathing, and vital signs, including pulse oximetry. If mechanical restraints are used, circulation to the extremities should be assessed at least every 10 minutes.

EMS agencies typically have policies and procedures pertaining to the use of restraints. These policies generally specify the type of mechanical and chemical restraints acceptable for use as well as acceptable positions in which the patient may be placed. A patient must be positioned in a manner that does not compromise the airway or breathing. Furthermore, restraints should not be positioned in such a way as to prevent proper assessment of the patient's medical condition.

If restraints are used, be sure to carefully document the following:

- The reason the patient was restrained
- The name of the physician who provided online medical direction
- The type of restraint used
- The position of the patient during treatment and transport
- Information indicating regular monitoring of the patient's airway, breathing, circulation, and vital signs (including pulse oximetry)
- Assessment findings pertaining to the patient's distal pulses while restrained
- The total time the patient was restrained while in your care
- The patient's condition at the time of transfer of care

Mechanical Patient Restraint. It is advisable to have online medical direction to restrain a patient. To restrain the patient mechanically, have plenty of trained and competent help. Try to have at least four people to assist in restraining the patient (one for each extremity). Act quickly and directly toward limiting the patient's abilities. Have one person communicate with the patient throughout the process, explaining what is being done and why. Avoid placing the patient face down if possible. This limits access to the patient medically. Prevention of aspiration can be accomplished by having the head of the bed raised at least 30 degrees. The patient can be prevented from spitting by simply placing a mask over his or her mouth. Continually communicate with and reassess the patient to monitor for any changes in behavior or medical condition. Frequently check and adjust the restraints to facilitate a secure patient and optimal circulation to all extremities.

Chemical Patient Restraint. Chemical patient restraint can compromise a patient's airway control more severely than other forms of restraint. Again, it is advisable to receive online medical direction for chemical restraint application. Often chemical restraints can be more effective and occasionally safer to the patient and caregivers than physical restraints. Intramuscular or IV is the most common form of administration of chemical restraints. However, newer oral instant application chemical sedatives are available, such as dissolving tablets and a rapid-absorbing liquid version of several antipsychotics. Frequent reassessment and evaluation are required to check for any changes in behavior or medical status of the patient. A patient should never be transported face down with application of restraints because of risk of aspiration. The head of the stretcher should be raised at least 30 degrees.

Case Scenario SUMMARY

1. *What is your general impression of this patient?* Despite the dramatic nature of this woman's head injury, she is remarkably stable with warm, dry skin and good mental status. Her most apparent high-risk problem is bleeding from the head wound as well as the potential for development of increased ICP.
2. *What physical assessment findings are most pertinent at this time?* Signs related to head injury and shock are most important at this time: mental status, skin color, and vital signs.
3. *What is the significance of the loss of memory related to the incident?* The presence of amnesia for the event defines a loss of consciousness at the time of the event and suggests that she at least has suffered a cerebral concussion.
4. *What treatment should be initiated immediately?* High-flow oxygen and manual spinal immobilization pending additional assessment.
5. *Should this patient be spinally immobilized? Why or why not?* Yes. The uncertainty regarding the mechanism of injury, her apparent loss of consciousness, and her age all lead to an increased potential for vertebral injury.
6. *How should the profuse bleeding from the head be controlled?* Because of the crepitus and apparent skull fracture, a dressing should be applied to the puncture wound and pressure applied circumferentially rather than directly over the wound.
7. *What is the clinical significance of the unresponsive pupil?* Changes in papillary function may signal increasing ICP. However, because the patient is alert and oriented, in this case it is likely a preexisting condition or evidence of an isolated eye injury. Pupillary changes related to increasing ICP occur *after* the patient becomes combative or unconscious.
8. *What additional treatment should be provided?* High-flow oxygen should be continued and her respiratory status monitored (because of her tender right chest). An IV should be established. Her mental status, skin color, temperature, and blood pressure all suggest she is not in severe shock, so IV fluid administration should be minimal unless her condition changes. She should be rapidly transported to a trauma facility that has neurosurgical capabilities.
9. *Given the patient's final disposition, was your treatment appropriate? Why or why not?* With the exception of initiating an IV, the treatment provided was adequate. The reduction in pulse rate and blood pressure confirms that her on-scene tachycardia was not caused by shock.

Chapter Summary

- Facial injuries may be the result of blunt or penetrating trauma. Airbag deployment can cause abrasions to the face, neck, and upper chest.
- An orbital fracture is any fracture that involves the bony cavity containing the eyeball. Orbital fractures may occur as an isolated injury or in conjunction with another injury, such as a zygomatic fracture or fractures of the midface.
- The nose is the most commonly fractured bone of the face. Most nasal fractures are the result of blunt trauma.
- Zygomatic fractures are common and are usually the result of an assault or MVC. Maxillary or midface fractures are usually a combination of fractures involving several structures of the face. Significant force is required to fracture this area of the face.
- Mandibular fractures are common. They are caused by blunt trauma to the face, most commonly domestic violence and contact sports. A mandibular fracture also can be caused by penetrating trauma, such as gunshot wounds, blast injuries, or industrial injuries (e.g., chain saw).
- Two million brain injuries occur every year. Most brain injuries are mild, with a ratio of 8:1:1 (mild/moderate/severe). Assessment is the key to proper care and evaluation of the injury. Correctly identifying and prioritizing injuries can greatly improve patient outcome. Appropriately treat injuries, always assessing airway, breathing, circulation, and deficits. Never occlude the nose or ear, especially if CSF fluid leaks are present.
- In loss of consciousness with facial or head injuries, protect the spinal cord.
- If in doubt, treat the patient for a traumatic brain injury.

REFERENCES

Brain Injury Association of America. (2005). *Types of brain injury.* Retrieved December 20, 2007, from http://www.biausa.org.

Cheh, A. I., Reenstra-Buras, W. R., Rosen, C., & Swisher, L. (2006). *Ocular burns.* Retrieved September 17, 2006, from http://www.emedicine.com.

Conley, R. L. (1998). Head injury. In E. W. Bayley & S. A. Turcke (Eds.). *A comprehensive curriculum for trauma nursing* (2nd ed.). Park Ridge, IL: Roadrunner Press.

Drake, R., Vogl, W., & Mitchell, A. W. M. (2005). *Gray's anatomy for students*. Philadelphia: Elsevier.

Frosh, M. P., Anthony, D. C., & De Girolami, U. (2005). The central nervous system. In V. Kumar, A. K. Abbas, & Fausto, N. (Eds.). *Robbins and Cotran pathologic basis of disease* (7th ed.). Philadelphia: Elsevier.

Holleran, R. S. (Ed.). (1996). *Flight nursing: Principles and practice (2nd ed.).* St. Louis: Mosby.

Levy, D. (2006). *Neck trauma*. Retrieved September 17, 2006, from http://www.emedicine.com.

Lucatorto, M., & Taylor, J. E. Sensory/perceptual: Responsiveness and vision. In Neff, J. A., & Kidd, P. S. (Eds.). *Trauma nursing: The art and science* (pp. 263-324). St. Louis: Mosby.

Marino, T. G., West, L. A., Liewehr, F. R., Mailhot, J. M., Buxton, T. B., Runner, R. R., et al. (2000). Determination of periodontal ligament cell viability in long shelf-life milk. *Journal of Endodontics 26*(12), 699-702.

Marion, D. W. (1998). Head injury. In A. B. Peitzman, M. Rhodes, C. W. Schwab, & D. Yealy (Eds.). *The trauma manual* (pp. 134-141). Philadelphia: Lippincott-Raven.

Newberry, L. (2003). *Sheehy's emergency nursing* (5th ed.). St. Louis: Mosby.

Rastogi, S., Garcia-Valenzuela, E., & Allen, M. (2005). *Postoperative hyphema*. Retrieved December 12, 2007, from http://www.emedicine.com.

Schwartz, G. R. (1999). *Principles and practice of emergency medicine* (4th ed.). Santa Fe, NM: Williams & Wilkins.

SUGGESTED RESOURCES

Brain Injury Association of America
8201 Greensboro Dr., Suite 611
McLean, VA 22102
Phone: 703-761-0750
Website: http://www.biausa.org

Evans, R. W., & Wilberger, J. E. (2003). Traumatic disorders. In C. M. Goetz (Ed.). *Textbook of clinical neurology* (2nd ed.) (pp. 1129-1151). St. Louis: Elsevier.

Headway: The Brain Injury Association
4 King Edward Court
King Edward St.
Nottingham NG1 1EW
United Kingdom
Phone: 0115 924 0800
Website: http://www.headway.org.uk

McQuillan K. A., VonRueden, K. T., Hartsock, R. L., Flynn, M. B., Whalen, E. (2002). *Trauma nursing: From resuscitation through rehabilitation* (3rd ed.). St. Louis: Harcourt Health.

Moore, E. E., Feliciano, D. V., & Mattox, K. L. (2004). *Trauma* (5th ed.). New York: McGraw-Hill.

National Eye Institute. (2006). *Retinal detachment*. Retrieved September 17, 2006, from http://www.nei.nih.gov.

National Eye Institute
2020 Vision Place
Bethesda, MD 20892-3655
Phone: 301-496-5248
Website: http://www.nei.nih.gov

Qureshi, N. H., & Harsh, I. V. G. (2005). *Skull fracture*. Retrieved December 20, 2007, from http://www.emedicine.com.

The Saskatchewan Brain Injury Association (SBIA)
2310 Louise Ave.
Saskatoon, SK S7J 2C7
Canada
Phone: 306-373-1555
Fax: 306-373-5655
Website: http://www.sbia.ca

Shepard, S. (2004). *Head trauma*. Retrieved December 20, 2007, from http://www.emedicine.com.

Skalletta, T. (2005). *Subdural hematoma*. Retrieved December 20, 2007, from http://www.emedicine.com.

Tintinalli, J. E., Kelen, G. D., & Stapczynski, J. S. (2004). *Emergency medicine: A comprehensive study guide* (6th ed.). New York: McGraw-Hill.

Trauma.org: Website: http://www.trauma.org

Ullman, J. S., & Sin, A. (2005). *Epidural hemorrhage*. Retrieved December 20, 2007, from http://www.emedicine.com/med/topic2898.htm.

University of Michigan Health System. (2005). *Ruptured eardrum (perforated tympanic membrane)*. Retrieved September 17, 2006, from http://www.med.umich.edu.

Wasserman, J. R., & Koenigsberg, R. A. (2004). *Diffuse axonal injury*. Retrieved December 20, 2007, from http://www.emedicine.com.

Chapter Quiz

1. List the areas assessed when using the GCS.

____

____

____

2. True or False: All head injuries need to be treated as if the patient had a cervical spine injury.

3. A 40-year-old man was involved in a fight and sustained a blow to the left side of the head. He is now showing signs of increased ICP. Which of the following signs is consistent with compression of the oculomotor nerve?

- **a.** Constriction of the pupil on the right side
- **b.** Dilation of the pupil on the left side
- **c.** Constriction of the pupil on the left side
- **d.** Dilation of the pupil on the right side

4. Cushing's triad is associated with ______________________.

- **a.** increased ICP
- **b.** mandibular fracture
- **c.** nasal foreign body
- **d.** concussion

5. True or False: A burn to the eye involving an alkali is typically more serious than a burn involving an acid.

6. CSF drainage from the nose or ears is a possible sign of _____.

- **a.** zygoma fracture
- **b.** orbital blowout injury
- **c.** meningeal artery injury
- **d.** basilar skull fracture

Chapter Quiz—continued

7. Signs of increased ICP include ______________________.
   a. altered mental status, unequal pupils, decreased heart rate, and increased blood pressure
   b. agitation, tachycardia, and hypotension
   c. altered mental status, irregular pulse, Battle's sign, and hypotension
   d. unresponsiveness, raccoon eyes, and Battle's sign

8. True or False: All head injuries are potentially life-threatening.

9. True or False: All patients with any type of helmet need to have the helmet removed immediately.

10. Which of the following injuries is usually associated with arterial bleeding?
    a. Moderate diffuse axonal injury
    b. Basilar skull fracture
    c. Subdural hematoma
    d. Epidural hematoma

Terminology

Aqueous humor Fluid that fills the anterior chamber of the eye; maintains intraocular pressure.

Arachnoid membrane Weblike middle layer of the meninges.

Auricle Also called the *pinna;* outer ear.

Basilar skull fracture Loss of integrity to the bony structures of the base of the skull.

Brain injury A traumatic insult to the brain capable of producing physical, intellectual, emotional, social, and vocational changes.

Cementum A layer of tough tissue that anchors the root of a tooth to the periodontal membrane/ligament.

Cerebral contusion A brain injury in which brain tissue is bruised in a local area but does not puncture the pia mater.

Cerebral perfusion pressure (CPP) Pressure inside the cerebral arteries and an indicator of brain perfusion; CPP = MAP – ICP.

Cerebrospinal fluid (CSF) Fluid that bathes, protects, and nourishes the CNS.

Cerebrum Largest part of the brain; divided into right and left hemispheres.

Cerumen Earwax.

Choroid Vascular layer of the eyeball.

Choroid plexus Group of specialized cells in the ventricles of the brain; filters blood through cerebral capillaries to create the CSF.

Cochlea Bony structure in the inner ear resembling a tiny snail shell.

Comminuted skull fracture Breakage of a bone or bones of the skull into multiple fragments.

Compound skull fracture Open skull fracture.

Concussion A brain injury with a transient impairment of consciousness followed by a rapid recovery to baseline neurologic activity.

Conjunctiva Thin, transparent mucous membrane that covers the inner surface of the eyelids and the outer surface of the sclera.

Contrecoup injury An injury at another site, usually opposite the point of impact.

Cornea Avascular, transparent structure that permits light through to the interior of the eye.

Coup injury An injury directly below the point of impact.

Crown The visible part of a tooth.

Dentin A hard but porous tissue found under the enamel and cementum of a tooth.

Depressed skull fracture A fracture of the skull with inward displacement of bone fragments.

Diffuse axonal injury (DAI) A type of brain injury caused by shearing forces that occur between different parts of the brain as a result of rotational acceleration.

Dura mater Toughest layer of the meninges; top layer.

Emulsification The breakdown of fats on the skin surface by alkaloids, creating a soapy substance; penetrates deeply.

Enamel Hard, white outer surface of a tooth.

Entrapment A state of being pinned or entrapped.

Epidural hematoma A collection of blood between the skull and dura mater.

Epistaxis Bloody nose.

Epithelial tissue Covers most of the internal and external surfaces of the body.

Eustachian tube A small tube connecting the middle ear to the posterior nasopharynx; allows the ear to adjust to atmospheric pressure.

Focal injury An injury limited to a particular area of the brain.

Foramen magnum The opening at the base of the skull through which the spinal cord passes.

Head injury A traumatic insult to the head that may result in injury to the soft tissue or bony structures of the head and/or brain injury.

Hematoma Collection of blood beneath the skin or within a body compartment.

Herniation The shifting of brain tissue laterally or downward because of increasing ICP.

Hyperopia Farsightedness; difficulty seeing objects close to the person.

Hyphema Blood in the anterior chamber of the eye.

Incus The anvil-shaped bone located between the malleus and stapes in the middle ear.

Intracerebral hematoma Bleeding within the brain tissue itself.

Lacrimal ducts Small openings at the medial edge of the eye; drain holes for water from the surface of the eye.

Lacrimal gland One of a pair of glands situated superior and lateral to the eyeball; secretes lacrimal fluid.

Linear skull fracture A line crack in the skull.

Malleus Hammer-shaped bone located at the front of the middle ear; receives vibrations from the tympanic membrane.

Malocclusion The condition in which the teeth of the upper and lower jaws do not line up.

Meninges Covering of the brain and spinal cord; layers include the dura mater, arachnoid, and pia mater.

Myopia Nearsightedness; difficulty seeing objects at a distance.

Olfactory Sense of smell.

Ophthalmoscope An instrument used to examine the inner parts of the eye; consists of an adjustable light and multiple magnification lenses.

Otoscope An instrument used to examine the inner ear; consists of a light source and magnifying lens; the tip is covered with a disposable cone.

Oval window A membranous structure that separates the middle ear from the inner ear.

Periodontal membrane/ligament Ligamentous attachment between the root of a tooth and the socket of the bone within which it sits.

Periosteum The fibrous connective tissue rich in nerve endings that envelopes bone.

Pia mater Last meningeal layer; adheres to the CNS.

Postconcussion syndrome Symptoms of a concussion that persist for weeks to 1 year after an initial injury to the head.

Presbyopia Loss of function of the lens to adjust to close reading; usual onset in middle age.

Pulp Center of a tooth that contains nerves, blood vessels, and connective tissue.

Restraint Any mechanism that physically restricts an individual's freedom of movement, physical activity, or normal access to his or her body.

Reticular formation A cloud of neurons in the brainstem and midbrain responsible for maintaining consciousness.

Retinal detachment A condition in which the retina is lifted or pulled from its normal position, resulting in a loss of vision.

Rhinorrhea Persistent discharge of fluid (such as blood or CSF) from the nose.

Sclera Firm, opaque, white outer layer of the eye; helps maintain the shape of the eye.

Semicircular canals Three bony, fluid-filled loops in the internal ear; involved in balance of the body.

Stapes The stirrup-shaped bone that links the middle ear to the inner ear; connects to the malleus and incus.

Subarachnoid hemorrhage A collection of blood between the arachnoid layer of the meninges and the pia mater.

Subdural hematoma A collection of blood in the subdural space, which is between the dura mater and arachnoid layer of the meninges.

Traumatic iritis An inflammation of the iris caused by blunt trauma to the eye.

Trismus Spasm of the muscles used for chewing, resulting in limited movement of the mouth because of pain.

Turbinates Large folds found in the nasal cavity; highly vascular area in the nose that warms and humidifies inhaled air.

Tympanic membrane A thin, translucent, pearly gray oval disk that protects the middle ear and conducts sound vibrations; eardrum.

Vestibule Space or a cavity that serves as the entrance to the inner ear.

Vitreous chamber The most posterior chamber of the eyeball.

Vitreous humor Thick, jellylike substance that fills the vitreous chamber of the eyeball.

CHAPTER 48

Spinal Trauma

Objectives

After completing this chapter, you will be able to:

1. Describe the incidence, morbidity, and mortality rates of spinal injuries in the trauma patient.
2. Describe the anatomy and physiology of the following structures related to spinal injuries:
   - Cervical
   - Thoracic
   - Lumbar
   - Sacrum
   - Coccyx
   - Spinal cord
   - Nerve tract
   - Dermatome
3. Predict spinal injuries on the basis of mechanism of injury.
4. Describe the pathophysiology of spinal injuries.
5. Explain traumatic and nontraumatic spinal injuries.
6. Describe the assessment findings associated with spinal injuries.
7. Integrate pathophysiologic principles to the assessment of a patient with a spinal injury.
8. Differentiate spinal injuries on the basis of assessment and history.
9. Formulate a field impression on the basis of assessment findings.
10. Develop a patient management plan on the basis of field impression.
11. Describe the assessment findings associated with traumatic spinal injuries.
12. Describe the management of spinal injuries.
13. Integrate pathophysiologic principles to the assessment of a patient with a traumatic spinal injury.
14. Describe the pathophysiology of traumatic spinal injury related to the following:
    - Spinal shock
    - Neurogenic shock
    - Tetraplegia and paraplegia
    - Incomplete cord injury and cord syndromes
      - Central cord syndrome
      - Anterior cord syndrome
      - Brown-Séquard syndrome
      - Cauda equina syndrome
      - Conus medullaris syndrome
      - Spinal cord injury without radiologic abnormality
15. Differentiate traumatic and nontraumatic spinal injuries on the basis of assessment and history.
16. Describe the pathophysiology of nontraumatic spinal injury, including the following:
    - Low back pain
    - Herniated intervertebral disk
    - Spinal cord tumors
    - Degenerative disk disease
    - Spondylosis
17. Describe the assessment findings associated with nontraumatic spinal injuries.
18. Describe the management of nontraumatic spinal injuries.
19. Integrate pathophysiologic principles to the assessment of a patient with nontraumatic spinal injury.
20. Formulate a field impression for nontraumatic spinal injury on the basis of assessment findings.
21. Develop a patient management plan for nontraumatic spinal injury on the basis of field impression.

Chapter Outline

Incidence, Morbidity, and Mortality Rates of Spine Trauma
Spinal Anatomy and Physiology
Mechanism of Injury
Spinal Injury Assessment
Pathophysiology of Spinal Injury
Types of Spine Injury
General Management of Spinal Injuries
Assessment and Management of Nontraumatic Spinal Conditions
Medications Used in Spinal Cord Injury Management
Documenting Your Assessment and Care of the Spine-Injured Patient
Chapter Summary

Case Scenario

A 19-year-old male patient has slipped off of a ladder while painting a house. He fell approximately 20 feet. He states that he landed on his back, he has pain in his back, and he cannot move his legs. He denies any loss of consciousness. You notice that he is lying flat on his back in the supine position.

Questions

1. *What are your initial thoughts regarding this patient?*
2. *What is your impression of the mechanism of injury?*
3. *What should be done for initial treatment?*

INCIDENCE, MORBIDITY, AND MORTALITY RATES OF SPINE TRAUMA

[OBJECTIVE 1]

Spinal cord injury (SCI) is a suddenly occurring, debilitating injury that often devastates a patient's lifestyle. Each year 11,000 new cases of SCI are reported, excluding cases resulting in a death at the scene. Approximately 250,000 people in the United States live with disabilities after an SCI. The typical SCI patient is a 28-year-old unmarried white man; however, the evidence and data about spine injury have been collected only since 1973.

Most SCIs occur in the area of the cervical spine, with the next most common in the lumbar region. This is logical considering the anatomy of the human body. The cervical vertebrae support the bowling ball–like head, are the smallest vertebrae, and have no additional protection. The lumbar region, although it includes the largest vertebrae, has no additional support or protection. The thoracic region, which has the fewest injuries, has additional support from the ribs.

Motor vehicle crashes (MVCs) account for 48% of all reported cases of SCI, with falls being the next most common mechanism (23%). Acts of violence—primarily gunshot wounds (14%) and sporting injuries (9%)—round out the top four SCI mechanisms. Approximately 18% of these injuries result in complete **tetraplegia** (formerly called *quadriplegia*), paralysis of all four extremities, requiring complete care of the patient for the remainder of his or her life (Figure 48-1) (National SCI Statistical Center, 2006).

Spinal cord injuries often are permanent debilitating injuries, resulting in poor prospects for return to an independent life. Generally, the treatments are preinjury education and prevention. Seatbelt use campaigns involving local media, law enforcement, and EMS to encourage and develop habitual use of passive restraint devices by all passengers in an automobile reduce the likelihood of injury during an MVC, especially a rollover incident. Awareness and education about the safe and appropriate use of firearms, anger management education and intervention, and positive conflict resolution programs have the potential to affect rates of SCI as a result of violence.

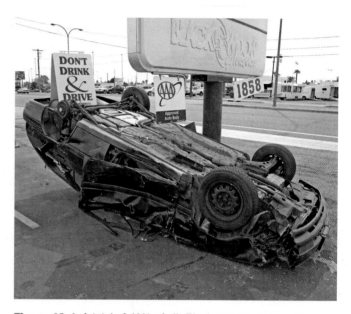

Figure 48-1 A total of 48% of all spinal cord injuries are the result of a motor vehicle crash.

Safety education programs and campaigns for coaches and parents involved in sporting activities as well as the use of adequate protective equipment attempt to prevent spine injury on the playing field. The paramedic should play a role in these activities.

SPINAL ANATOMY AND PHYSIOLOGY

Spinal Column

[OBJECTIVE 2]

The spinal column is composed of 33 bones called **vertebrae.** The vertebrae are grouped and divided into five sections. The sections include seven **cervical** vertebrae, 12 **thoracic** vertebrae, five **lumbar** vertebrae, five **sacral** vertebrae (which are fused together in adults to form the **sacrum**), and four **coccygeal** vertebrae (also fused together in adults to form the **coccyx**). Each vertebra is identified by its region (e.g., cervical, thoracic) and then given a number. Thus the first vertebra is cervical 1, or C1. Starting at C1 and following the spinal column inferiorly, each vertebra progressively gets larger than the previous. This is because each vertebra must support more weight than the bone above it. The fifth lumbar vertebra is the largest, after which the sacral and coccygeal vertebrae get progressively smaller until the most distal coccygeal vertebrae, the tailbone (Figure 48-2).

Each vertebra consists of an anterior solid body, called the *vertebral body,* which is the weight-bearing component of the spine. The posterior, or rear-facing, side of the vertebrae does support some weight but is much smaller. It is called the *vertebral arch.* Many bony prominences—the transverse process, superior articular process, inferior articular process, and spinous process—and the lamina combine to form the posterior vertebrae (Figure 48-3).

When you palpate the midline of the spine, you are feeling the spinous process—remember this later during

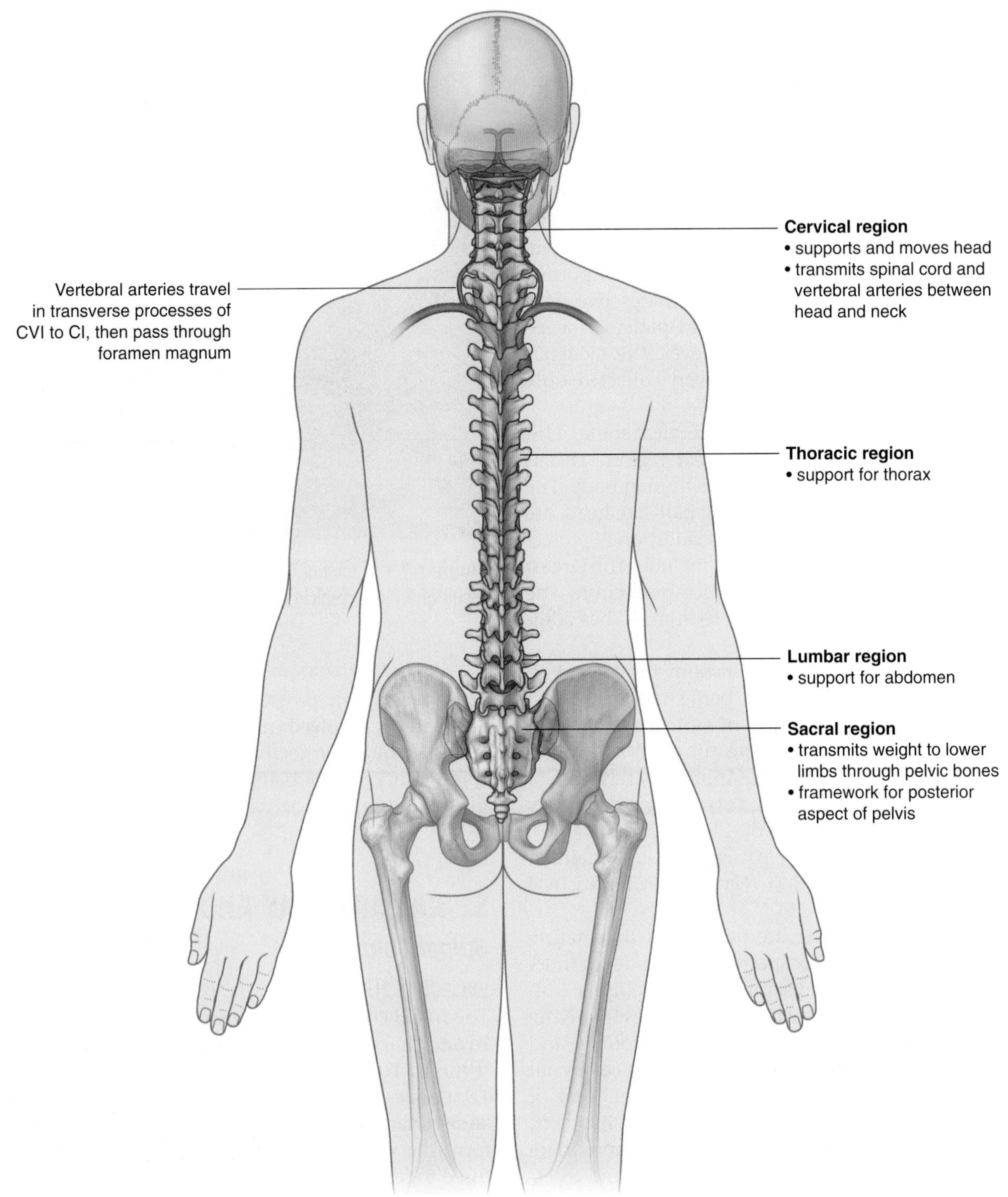
Vertebral arteries travel in transverse processes of CVI to CI, then pass through foramen magnum
Cervical region
• supports and moves head
• transmits spinal cord and vertebral arteries between head and neck
Thoracic region
• support for thorax
Lumbar region
• support for abdomen
Sacral region
• transmits weight to lower limbs through pelvic bones
• framework for posterior aspect of pelvis

Figure 48-2 The spinal column.

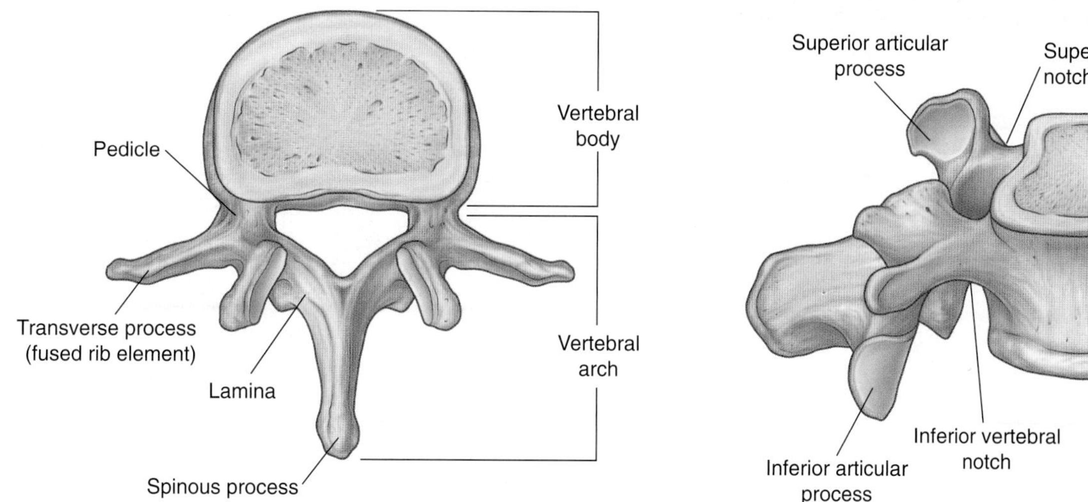

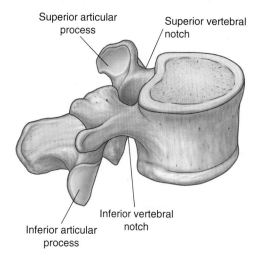

Figure 48-3 A vertebra.

the discussion on spine examination. The vertebral arch serves as a connection point for muscles and ligaments, allows movement by acting as a lever for muscles, and is the site of interlocking articulation between multiple vertebrae. Thoracic vertebrae also articulate with ribs at the vertebral arch. Finally, a supportive cartilaginous intervertebral disk rests between each vertebra to provide padding and space for flexibility (Drake et al., 2005).

PARAMEDIC*Pearl*

When you palpate the midline of the spine along the back, you are feeling the spinous process of each vertebra.

The first and second cervical vertebrae—named the **atlas** and **axis,** respectively—are highly specialized, providing support for the head and permitting it to articulate with the spinal column. The atlas permits the head to nod and rotate left to right; however, its most distinguishing feature is the lack of a vertebral body (Figure 48-4). C2, the axis, has a unique part called the *odontoid process,* which protrudes superiorly. The atlas rotates around the odontoid process, which allows its free movement while also keeping the atlas stable on the spinal column (Drake et al., 2005).

Ligaments connecting the vertebrae provide support during flexion and extension, whereas ligaments between the laminae provide support during lateral flexion. A space, or foramen, is between the vertebral body and vertebral arch on each vertebra and is called the **vertebral foramen.** When all vertebrae are aligned, this space forms a large canal running the length of the spinal column. This space is maximized when the spine is straight (aligned). As the body turns, twists, and bends, the size of the canal becomes slightly smaller, but not dangerously small during normal movement. The spinal cord is housed within this canal, protected by the vertebrae. A transverse foramen also runs along the side of each vertebra, through which the spinal nerves pass and innervate the body (Sanders & McKenna, 2005).

Spinal Cord

The spinal cord and brain comprise the central nervous system (CNS). Well protected by the spinal column, the spinal cord leaves the skull through the foramen magnum and extends through the spinal column. The average adult's spinal cord ends at the level of the disk between the second and third lumbar vertebrae. This "end" of the spinal cord is known as the **conus medullaris.** A group of spinal nerves continue to travel through the remainder of the spinal column. This group of nerves is called the **cauda equina** and is not part of the spinal cord. At birth, the spinal cord extends lower, to the third lumbar vertebrae (Kahn, 2005).

Physically, the spinal cord has a texture similar to a carrot, with many long, stringlike strands running through it. A cross-sectional view reveals that the spinal cord is fairly organized (Figure 48-5). The cord has a central canal surrounded by white and gray matter. The central gray matter is identified by its characteristic H shape. There are three projections, or horns, of gray matter on each side of the column, called the *anterior, lateral,* and *posterior horns,* respectively. The gray matter is rich in nerve bodies and is primarily responsible for motor function. Surrounding the gray matter is the nerve cell–rich white matter. White matter has multiple functions and is divided by the gray matter into three columns on each side, known as the *anterior, lateral,* and *posterior (dorsal) funiculi.* Lateral and posterior white matter both return sensory signals from the body to the brain, whereas the anterior white matter, like the gray matter, carries motor signals to the body. The funiculi contain both ascending and descending tracts, which are named for their origination and termination (Figure 48-6). Each tract of the spinal cord carries specific signals, and their functions are described as follows.

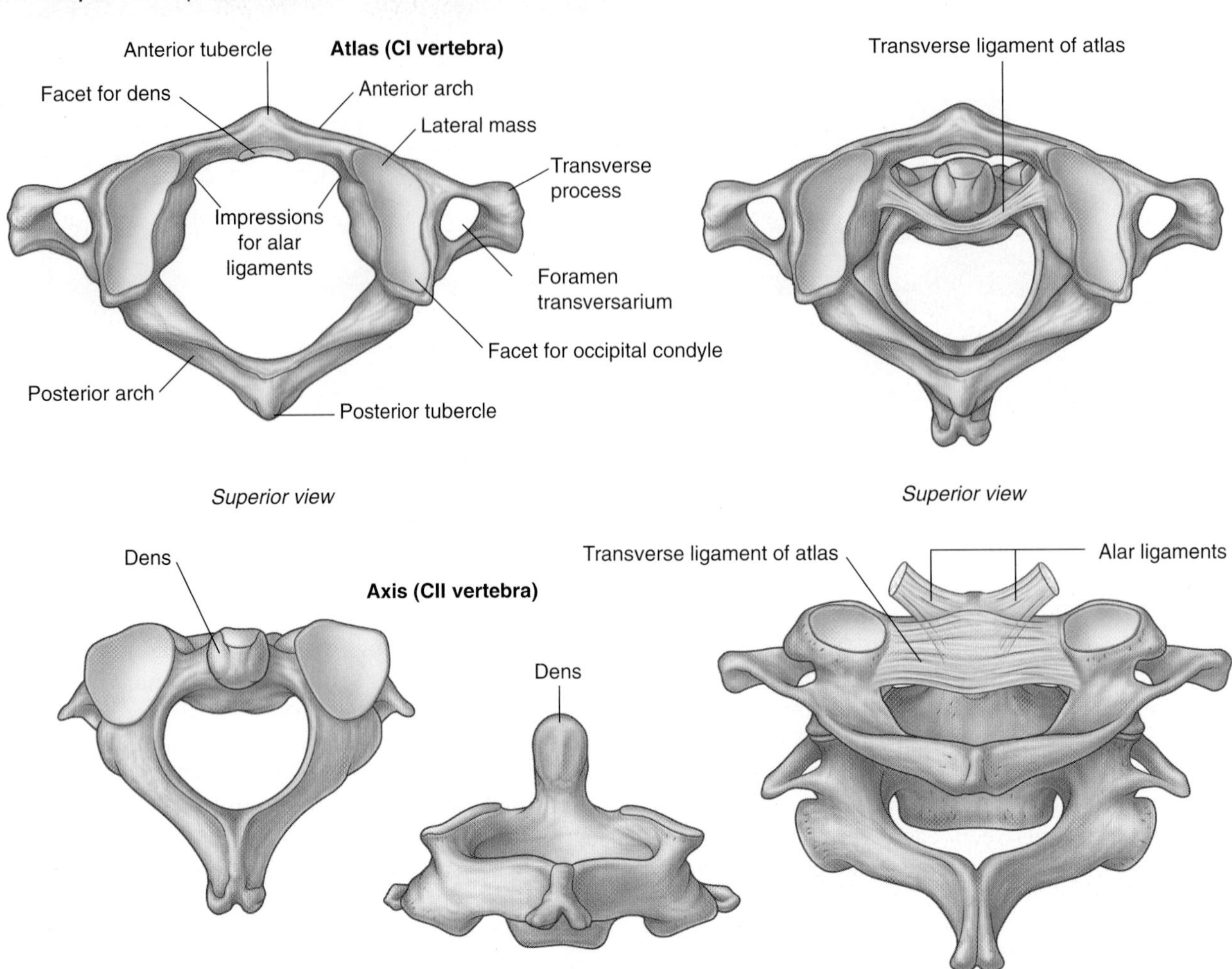

Figure 48-4 The atlas and the axis.

Ascending tracts transmit impulses and sensations from the body to the brain.

- *Fasciculus gracilis and fasciculus cuneatus:* The posterior funiculi, which may also be referred to as the *dorsal column–medial lemniscus system,* contains the fasciculus gracilis and fasciculus cuneatus tracts. These tracts conduct sensations of discrimination such as light touch and pressure, two-point discrimination, vibration, and proprioception. **Proprioception** is the ability to sense the location of body parts relative to the rest of the body (Gondim, 2006). These tracts travel the same side of the spinal cord as the impulses they receive and do not cross to the opposite side of the body until they reach the medulla. Although this does result in the right brain sensing impulses from the left body and the left brain sensing impulses from the right body, in the setting of injury to these tracts the physical deficits will be ipsilateral, or on the same side as the injury
- *Spinothalamic tracts:* The anterior spinothalamic tract and lateral spinothalamic tract lie within the anterior and lateral funiculi, respectively. Although these two tracts represent a cruder system than the dorsal column–medial lemniscus tract, there are certain sensations only they transmit. The anterior spinothalamic tract transmits crude touch and pressure while the lateral spinothalamic tract transmits tickle, itch, pain, and temperature sensations. These tracts travel on the opposite side of the body compared with the impulses they receive. This not only results in the right brain sensing impulses from the left body and vice versa, but in the setting of injury, physical deficits will be contralateral, or on the opposite side of the injury.
- *Spinocerebellar tracts:* The spinocerebellar tracts are found near the lateral funiculi and have both posterior and anterior tracts. The fibers of the posterior spinocerebellar tract are uncrossed and are more numerous than the anterior spinocerebellar tract fibers. The posterior spinocerebellar tract transmits sensations associated with motor function, equilibrium, proprioception, muscle tone, and movement of the limbs. The fibers of the anterior spinocerebellar tract are mostly crossed (although some fibers do remain uncrossed) and receive less information than the posterior tract.

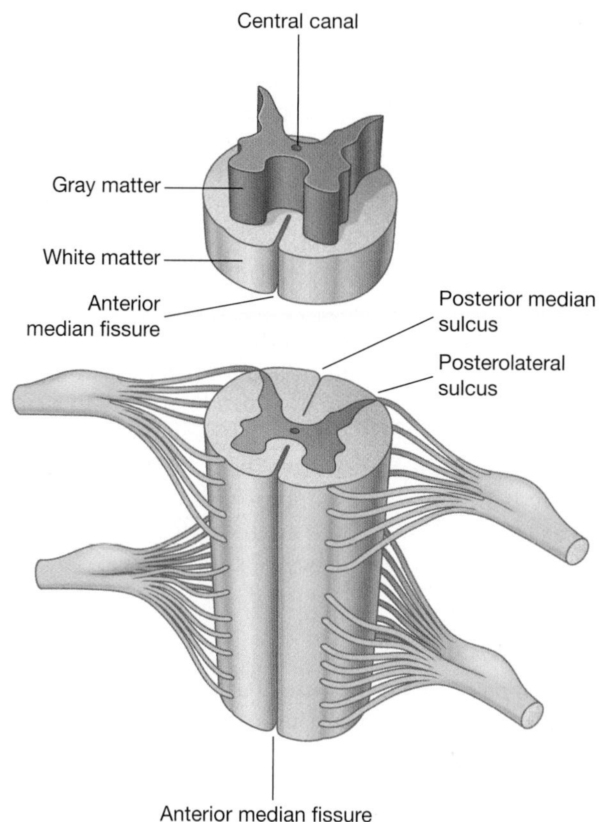

Figure 48-5 A cross-sectional view of the spinal cord. Note the H-shaped pattern to the central cord canal.

The anterior tract is stimulated by motor signals arriving from the brain through the corticospinal tracts and from internal motor pattern generators in the cord itself. The main function of the anterior tract is to provide feedback to the brain that motor signals have arrived to the anterior horns of the gray matter.

Descending tracts transmit motor impulses from the brain to the body.

- *Corticospinal tracts:* The corticospinal tracts, also called the *pyramidal tracts,* originate in the cortex and descend through the anterior and lateral funiculi. Most of the fibers of the corticospinal tract cross to the side of the body to which they transmit impulses at the level of the medulla, becoming the lateral corticospinal tract. Those fibers that do not cross at the level of the medulla continue down the same side of the cord as the side of the brain they originated in, becoming the anterior corticospinal tract. However, the fibers of the anterior corticospinal tract also cross to the side of the body opposite (contralateral) to their origination in the brain. This generally occurs in the neck or upper thoracic region. Both tracts transmit motor impulses from the cortex to the spinal nerves, where they are then distributed to the voluntary muscles. The majority of the fibers of the corticospinal tract terminate at interneurons near the gray matter of

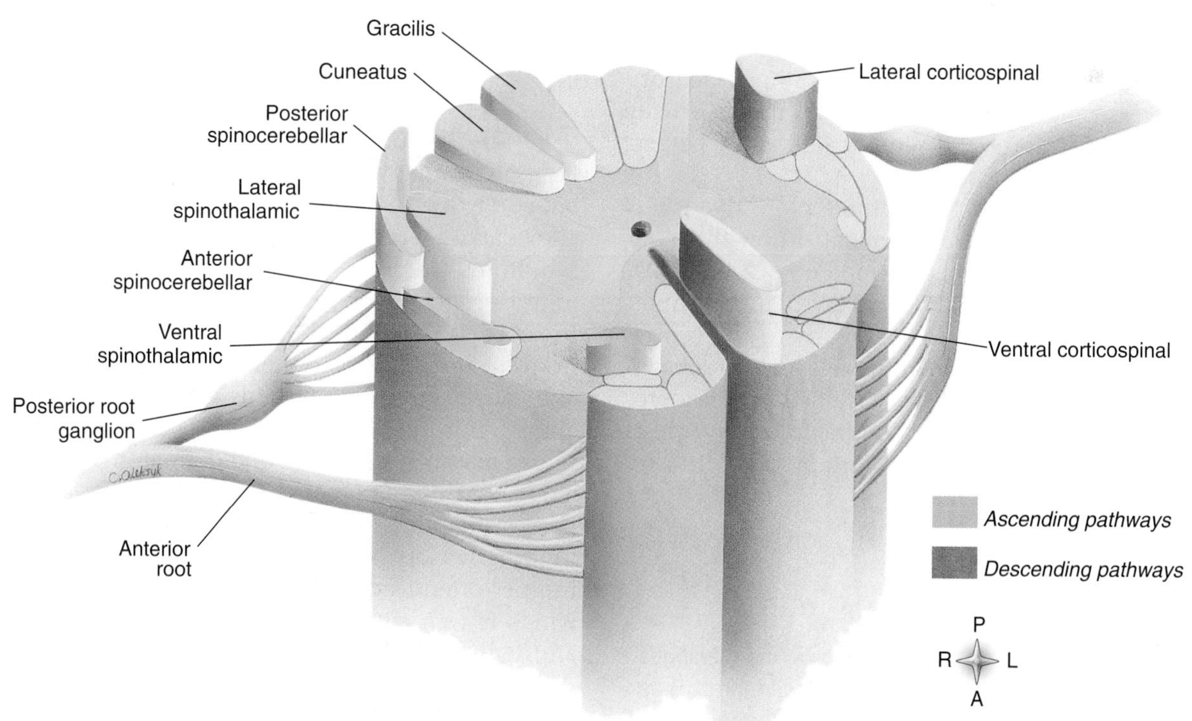

Figure 48-6 Major ascending (sensory) tracts, shown here only on the left, are highlighted in blue. Major descending (motor) tracts, shown here only on the right, are highlighted in red.

the spinal cord. However, those fibers that are responsible for the fine motor function of the fingers and hands terminate directly on the anterior horn(s) of the gray matter, allowing fine motor control. When these tracts are injured, physical findings such as loss of motor control will occur on the same (ipsilateral) side as the injury.

- *Extrapyramidal tracts:* Although the corticospinal tracts are primarily responsible for voluntary movement, additional tracts play a role in motor activity. Often called the *extrapyramidal system,* the extrapyramidal tracts are not well defined and lie outside the pyramidal system. They are responsible for some degree of movement and posture that are not under the control of the pyramidal system, as well as control of the sweat glands.
- *Reticulospinal tracts:* The lateral reticulospinal tract is located in the lateral funiculi. The majority of these fibers cross at the level of the medulla, but a few do not. The medial reticulospinal tract is contained in the anterior funiculi, and these fibers do not cross to the opposite side of the body once they leave the brain. These tracts transmit impulses to the body that control muscular tone and the activity of the sweat glands.
- *Rubrospinal tracts:* Upon leaving the brain, these tracts immediately cross to the opposite side of the body and travel down the lateral funiculi. Their primary function is to transmit impulses from the brain that control muscle coordination and posture.

It is important to understand the physical arrangement of the spinal cord because cord injury to only one region may only have certain effects. For example, a partial posterior cord injury may only impair sensory skills, whereas motor skills would remain intact. This is why both specific motor and sensory tests must be performed during a spinal assessment.

The entire CNS is protected by three protective layers called *meninges.* An easy way to remember how the meningeal layers sit is to remember the mnemonic **CNS-PAD.** The meninges pad the central nervous system. The innermost layer, the ***p***ia mater, adheres tightly to the central nervous system. The middle meningeal layer is the ***a***rachnoid layer. The subarachnoid space is filled with cerebrospinal fluid (CSF)—the cushion. The arachnoid layer rests on the innermost part of the outermost and thickest meningeal layer, the ***d***ura mater.

PARAMEDIC*Pearl*

Although the spinal cord ends at the L1 disk, the meninges and CSF continue to the second sacral vertebra. Thus spinal taps can safely draw off CSF when performed in the lower lumbar region without danger of damaging the spinal cord.

Spinal Nerves

The peripheral nervous system is a series of one-way signal pathways to and from the spinal cord to other body tissues. Sensory nerves take signals from throughout the body and transmit the signal to the CNS. After processing a signal, the CNS may transmit response to all or a part of the body through the motor nerves. Motor nerves transmit signals from the CNS to the body. Both sensory and motor nerves transmit their signals in one direction.

Nerve roots leave the spinal cord at the base of each vertebra and distribute autonomic information and motor signals along a distinct and organized pathway to a single region of the body. This same pathway collects sensory signals, which are transmitted back to the CNS. Each pathway is innervated by one of the 31 pairs of **spinal nerves** (Figure 48-7). There are 8 cervical, 12 thoracic, 5 lumbar, 5 sacral, and 1 coccygeal spinal nerve.

PARAMEDIC*Pearl*

The term *pair of spinal nerves* is used because each nerve affects a body region on only half of the body. The other half of the pair affects the same region on the other half of the body.

These regions can be closely followed and identified, another important step in assessing spinal cord injuries. A **myotome** is a region of skeletal muscle innervated by a single spinal nerve. A **dermatome** is a specific region of skin that a spinal nerve innervates. Myotomes are more difficult to assess. As a result, they are more commonly evaluated by physicians. However, the paramedic must be familiar with dermatomes and their regions.

Dermatomes

Become familiar with the 29 dermatomes throughout the body (Figure 48-8). Familiarity with the dermatomes allows an understanding of the presentation of a patient's symptoms when the spinal cord is injured. Spinal cord injuries generally do not result in a block of impairment to a specific part of the body (e.g., numbness and tingling from the knee down); rather, some impairment of motor and sensory skills is found as well as numbness or tingling following the path of a specific dermatome. An injury may be isolated to one dermatome or may begin along that dermatome and continue inferiorly. Injured nerves manifest with motor impairment (myotome injury), sensory impairment, or both. Musculoskeletal injuries often lead to neurovascular bundle impairment, which is seen with a loss of circulation as well as motor and sensory skills distal to the injury site.

PARAMEDIC*Pearl*

The paramedic must understand the difference between cranial nerves and spinal nerves.

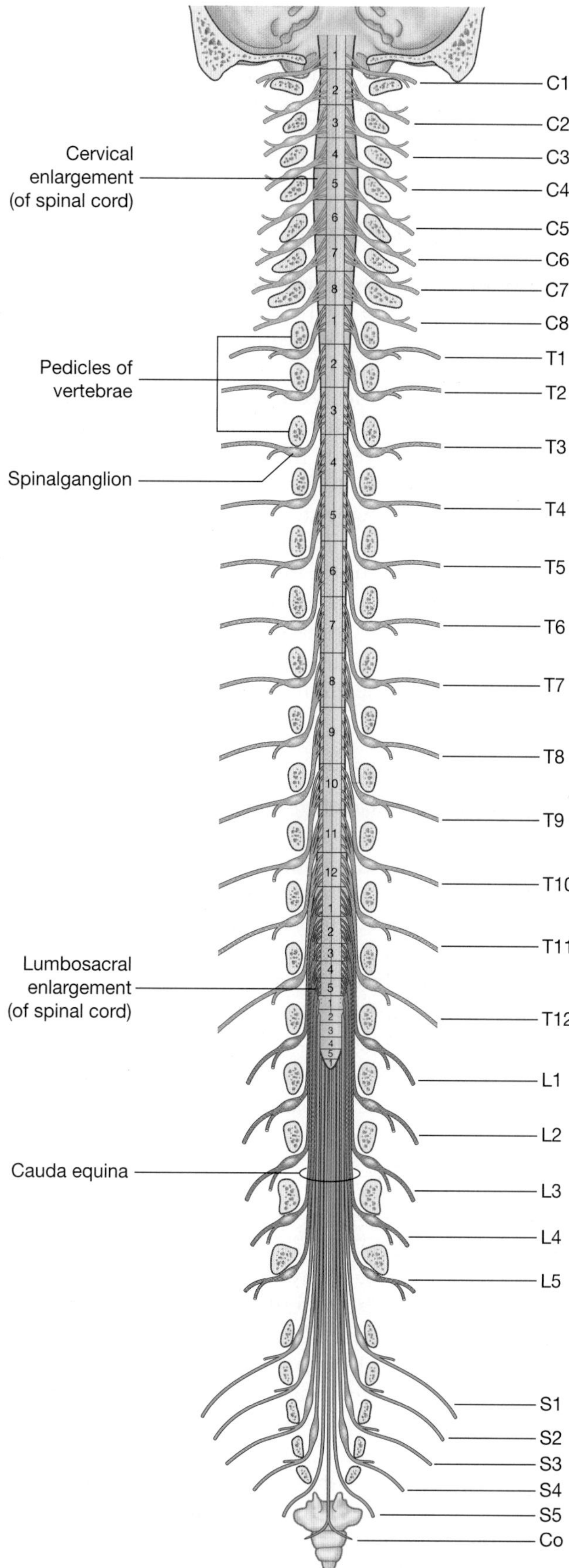

Figure 48-7 The spinal nerves.

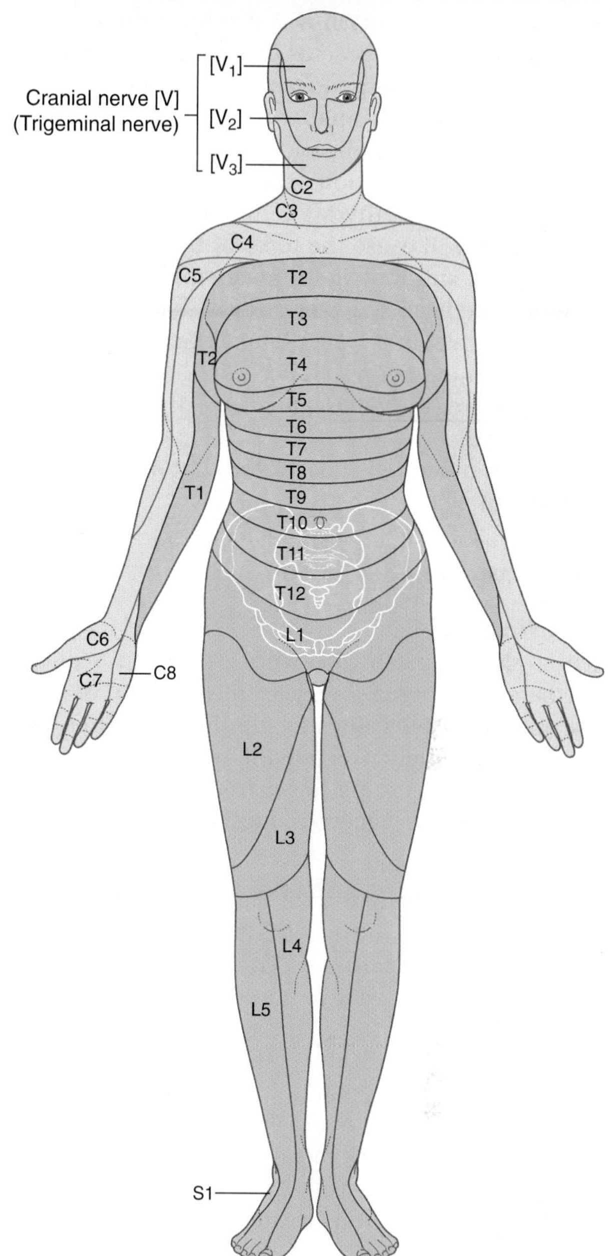

Figure 48-8 Dermatomes of the human body.

MECHANISM OF INJURY

[OBJECTIVES 3, 4]

Any sudden force or change in direction or speed can cause the head and body to move in opposite directions or force the torso to twist, flex, or extend in a way that may cause spinal fracture or SCI. Blunt or penetrating trauma directly to the spinal column can cause vertebral fracture, SCI, or both. When assessing the mechanism of injury, the paramedic must decide if sufficient force occurred to cause injury to the spinal column or cord. Following are some basic principles that can guide the paramedic while assessing the mechanism of injury:

- Any object in motion will stay in motion in a straight line unless acted on by an outside force with enough energy to cause a shift in motion or direction. For example, the head is perched on top of the spinal column and will, in general, move in the opposite direction of force applied to the spinal column. Any MVC involving a rear-end collision will cause the torso of the occupant in the front automobile to move rapidly forward while the head snaps or "whips" backward.
- Speed, mass, and weight are all factors in the diffusion of energy.
- The greater the force, the greater the injury potential.
- Lack of neurologic deficit does not automatically rule out SCI.

Obvious Mechanism of Injury

[OBJECTIVE 5]

Often a skilled paramedic who arrives on scene can immediately recognize a clear mechanism of injury. These incidents typically include direct trauma to the head or spine, sudden acceleration or deceleration, or high-velocity penetrating forces (e.g., gunshot wounds). Examples of these types of mechanisms include the following:

- An MVC with significant damage to either or any of the vehicles, intrusion into the driver or passenger compartment, engine displacement, bending of the vehicle frame, or vehicle rollover with ejection
- An MVC in which the patient's head strikes the windshield
- Ejection from a moving vehicle
- A pedestrian struck by an automobile
- Any motorcycle crash
- In adults, a fall from greater than three times the patient's height
- Contact sports injuries, such as in football, wrestling, or boxing
- Shallow water diving injury

PARAMEDIC*Pearl*

When assessing a patient who has fallen down stairs, calculate the linear distance of the angled stair steps and not the vertical distance from top to bottom. Also assess whether the steps are padded (e.g., carpet) to dampen the forces.

Traditionally, patients with a clear mechanism of injury for a spine injury received full spine immobilization. Recognition of these mechanisms of injury remains critical and, when required, these patients should receive full spine immobilization. The more current treatment for these patients (when authorized by medical direction) is a thorough spine assessment and spinal stabilization only when the spine cannot be cleared. However, selective spinal immobilization is region dependent and, as always, paramedics must follow state and regional standards of care.

Uncertain Mechanism of Injury

Determining whether a mechanism of injury is significant enough to injure the patient's spine can be difficult. These less-obvious mechanisms require further assessment and questioning of the patient, bystanders, and other emergency medical responders. Isolated or focused injuries, in the absence of an obvious mechanism of injury, may not require full immobilization. In the process of obtaining a full history, no mechanism for a spine injury may become evident. For example, a broken ankle that occurred from the patient stepping into a hole while running is generally not a mechanism that would result in a spine injury. When no mechanism of injury exists for a spine injury, full spine stabilization is not required. Perform a thorough spine assessment if you cannot safely determine that no mechanism of spine injury exists.

PARAMEDIC*Pearl*

The terms *spine stabilization* and *immobilization* often are easily interchanged even though they have different meanings. Spinal immobilization means the *complete* elimination of any spine movement; this technical skill is nearly impossible. Spine stabilization refers to the control over the spine and its heavy weight centers and the elimination of as much unnecessary and preventable spine movement as possible. This can be accomplished through manual or hands-on stabilization of the head, shoulders, and hips or with mechanical stabilization—a cervical collar and long board.

Comorbid Factors

When determining whether the patient's mechanism of injury is significant enough to cause a spinal injury, consider medical history. Many medical conditions can significantly increase the potential for spinal column and cord injury. The patient's age also should be a consideration. Newborns and neonates have not developed the muscle tone to control head movement during an incident, have an underdeveloped spinal column, and are unable to communicate pain level. Older adults may have osteoporosis or osteoarthritis, making them more vulnerable to vertebral fractures during a fall.

Box 48-1 summarizes medical conditions that can cause low bone density. Patients with low bone density are more prone to fracture than those with normal bone density given the same mechanism of injury. Other conditions that increase the risk of SCI include the following (Gondim, 2006):

BOX 48-1 Risk Factors for Low Bone Density

- Alcohol abuse
- Asian or Caucasian race
- Cigarette smoking
- Diabetes, liver disease, kidney disease
- Family history of osteoporosis
- History of fractures
- Inactive lifestyle
- Use of steroids, barbiturates, anticonvulsants, or thyroid replacement hormones

- Spinal stenosis
- Multiple current medical conditions
- Rheumatoid arthritis
- Down syndrome
- Neck dystonia or torticollis
- Congenital neck abnormalities

SPINAL INJURY ASSESSMENT

General Assessment of the Spine-Injured Patient

[OBJECTIVES 6, 7]

The assessment of the potentially spine-injured patient begins during the scene size-up as you evaluate potential hazards and the mechanism of injury. You must be able to recognize an obvious mechanism of injury for a spine injury and prepare to control the cervical spine immediately with manual stabilization. In addition to assuming control over head movement, be mindful of shoulder and hip motions as well. Movement of any of these weight centers will result in movement of the spine.

PARAMEDIC*Pearl*

Spine stabilization requires control over the entire spinal column and the three weight centers that affect the spine's motion: the head, shoulders, and hips. Simply controlling the head does not protect the entire spinal column.

If you determine that airway management is needed for the patient who has a mechanism of injury for a spinal injury, open the airway with a jaw thrust without head tilt maneuver. If the airway cannot be opened with this maneuver, use a head tilt/chin lift. While protecting the spine, perform initial and focused assessments as you would for any other patient. Apply a cervical collar as soon as possible to help reduce cervical spine movement.

Specific Assessments to Determine Spine Injury

[OBJECTIVE 8]

A good assessment of the mechanism of injury is obtained through a complete patient assessment. Whenever you determine that the mechanism of injury is significant enough to have caused a spine injury, a detailed spine assessment must be performed. The detailed spine assessment can safely and accurately determine when no spine injury exists and also reveal when a spinal column and/or cord injury has occurred. When you determine that a patient has sustained a spine injury, you must determine the extent of spine injury while initiating transport to an appropriate trauma facility and continuing your assessment en route. A detailed spine assessment and its components are not performed as part of a routine patient assessment. Rather, think of these assessments as a treatment for a positive mechanism of injury for a spine injury.

PARAMEDIC*Pearl*

The spine assessment and its components are not performed during a routine physical examination. They are performed separately after managing other injuries that may distract from the patient's ability to provide accurate feedback during the assessment. The spine assessment is a stand-alone examination.

Detailed Spine Assessment

[OBJECTIVES 9, 10, 11, 12, 13]

The detailed spine assessment consists of the following three important parts used to rule out spinal injury (Box 48-2):

1. A reliable patient
2. A clear history
3. A clear physical examination

All three components must be present to rule out a spine injury (Box 48-3). Take the time to complete each component. Failure to do so could result in clearing a spine that you should not clear.

To perform a spine assessment accurately, you must have a reliable patient. Reliable patients are conscious; awake; alert and oriented to person, place, time, and event (A&O×4). A reliable patient also is cooperative, sober, not anxious, and does not have a distracting injury. Determining the presence or absence of a **distracting injury** is somewhat subjective. Generally, if the patient is focused on the pain or discomfort of a specific injury (e.g., a dislocated ankle), then it is distracting. Other examples of distracting injuries include impaled objects, open fractures, severe abdominal pain, and respiratory distress. When a patient has a distracting injury, manage it. Proper care and management of the injury may reduce the discomfort to a tolerable level so that the injury is no longer distracting. This is particularly true for long bone

BOX 48-2 Spine Assessment

This specific spine assessment is one of many well-documented assessments used throughout the United States. Peter Goth, MD, and Jeffery Isaac, PA-C, developed this particular spine assessment during the 1980s while founding Wilderness Medical Associates (www.wildmed.com). Their research was designed to prevent patients from needless placement on back boards for extended periods when being evacuated from remote and rural environments. Since Isaac and Goth designed this spine assessment, it has been published in *The Outward Bound Wilderness First-Aid Handbook* and *Wilderness and Rescue Medicine.* Furthermore, the company's Wilderness First Responder, Wilderness-EMT, and Wilderness-ALS students have been taught and successfully used this assessment throughout the world. In recent years, Maine EMS and Michigan EMS both have adopted this spine assessment for use by their EMS professionals.

The NEXUS study on cervical spine injuries, released in 2000, reinforced the safety and efficiency of the techniques of this spine assessment. It reviewed more than 34,000 patients with a mechanism of injury that could cause a spine injury and studied a five-step approach to evaluating for spine injury without radiographs. The five-step approach was nearly identical to the steps included in the Wilderness Medical Associates spine assessment detailed in this chapter.

Consider the following: more than hundreds of thousands of U.S. patients are immobilized by EMS professionals annually, and 97% of them do not have any spinal column or cord injury. Many studies have demonstrated that less than 4% of patients sustaining blunt trauma have a spine injury. Determine if protocols exist in your area that permit clearing the spine in stable patients in the field.

BOX 48-3 Components of the Spine Assessment

Reliable patient: A&O×4, cooperative, sober, no anxiety, no distracting injury

Clear history: No spine pain, numbness, tingling, or sensations of electrical shooting

Clear physical: No spine tenderness; intact motor and sensory skills

A&O×4, Alert and oriented to person, place, time, and event.

injuries. Before splinting, long bone injuries often are quite painful. However, when placed in their anatomic position, padded, and splinted, the pain often substantially decreases. Performing a spine assessment on an unreliable patient may give false results. Distracting injuries may prevent the patient from sensing spine pain or tenderness. Once you determine that the patient is reliable, continue with the spinal assessment by evaluating the patient's spine history.

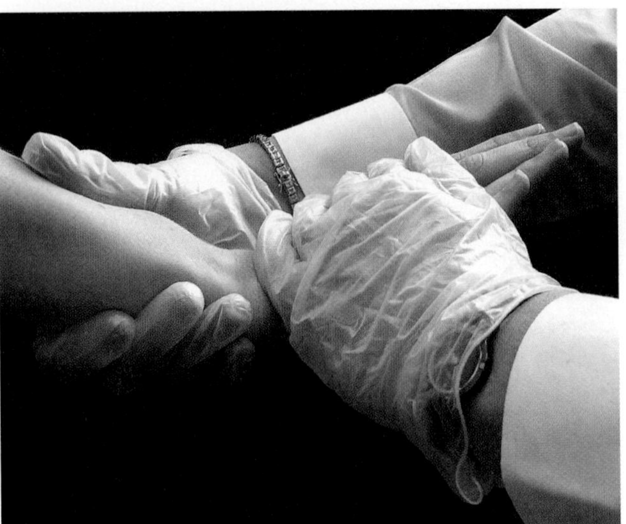

Figure 48-9 Evaluate wrist extension against pressure during the spine assessment.

Obtaining a clear history requires the patient's focus and attention. Ask the reliable patient two simple questions: "Do you have any numbness, tingling, or sensations of electrical activity anywhere in your body?" and "Do you have any pain in your spine?" Differentiate back and spine pain. Many patients chronically have sore or painful back muscles. However, they do not have bone pain. To do this accurately, ask the patient to close his or her eyes and focus on each vertebra. Have the patient mentally walk down each vertebra and sense whether any single vertebra hurts. A painful vertebra indicates a spinal *column* injury, whereas the presence of any numbness, tingling, or sensations of electricity shooting down an extremity indicate an SCI. If either is present complete the assessment, but full spinal stabilization is indicated because the spine cannot be cleared.

The third portion of the spine assessment is the physical examination. During the spine examination, palpate each vertebra from C1 to L5 for tenderness (pain on palpation). Press firmly on the posterior spinous process. Doing so will illicit pain if any part of the vertebra is fractured. The presence of tenderness indicates a spinal column injury. Finally, perform a distal motor and sensory examination.

During both the motor and sensory examination, compare the patient's extremities for bilateral symmetry. Full spinal stabilization is required whenever asymmetry is found during the examination and when the patient cannot complete the examination. Begin the motor examination by comparing the upper extremities for either wrist extension or finger abduction (both) against moderate resistance. Both of these motor skills test the function of the distal nerve roots that innervate the upper extremities. To test wrist extension, stabilize the wrist firmly in one hand and apply pressure to the posterior of the patient's hand. Ask the patient to extend the hand upward against your pressure (Figure 48-9). Test one arm, then compare it to the other. Test finger abduction when then patient cannot extend one or both of the wrists, such as with a splinted wrist injury. Ask the patient to spread the fingers apart and resist your attempt to squeeze his or her index and ring fingers together (Figure 48-10). The patient should be able to apply equal resistance on both extremities.

Lower extremity motor function is tested with the flexion *and* extension of either the great toe or the ankle. Note that this is different from the upper extremity examination, which only tests extension. Apply moderate pressure to the top of both feet at the same time and have the patient pull the feet upward (Figure 48-11). Immediately place your hands on the bottom of the feet and have the patient push the feet downward, as if pushing on the gas pedal of a car. Both sides should have equal strength. Use the same process with only the great toe for patients with ankle injuries as well as the mechanism for a spine injury (Figure 48-12).

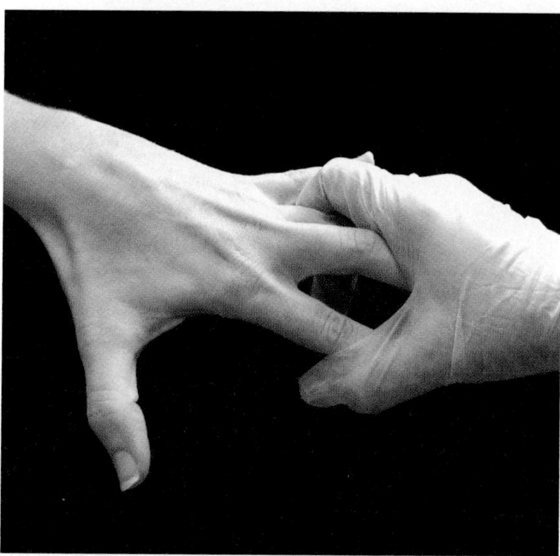

Figure 48-10 Evaluate finger abduction against pressure during the spine assessment.

A sensory examination is the final portion of the spine assessment. The patient must be able to differentiate sharp (pain) and soft/light touch sensations at the distal end of each extremity. This tests the **free nerve endings,** the pain-sensing nerve ending in the skin, and the **Meissner corpuscle,** which senses light touch. Before beginning the assessment, obtain objects capable of triggering these senses in the skin. You will need a cotton ball or piece of gauze to test light touch and a safety needle or sharp tweezers to test pain. Remember, you are not testing pressure-sensing nerve endings. You are trying to trigger only the pain and light touch nerves. Be sure that your patient can differentiate the sharp and light touch sensations by testing them on the patient's forehead (Figure 48-13). Press one of the objects against the top and lateral sides of the hands and ask the patient if he or she senses pain or light touch (Figure 48-14). Repeat the test randomly, alternating between your two objects at least four to five times before moving on to the next extremity. Perform the sensory examination along the anterolateral surface of the foot or ankle (Figure 48-15). Your patient must be able to differentiate pain and light touch consistently in each extremity. Suspect an SCI if the patient

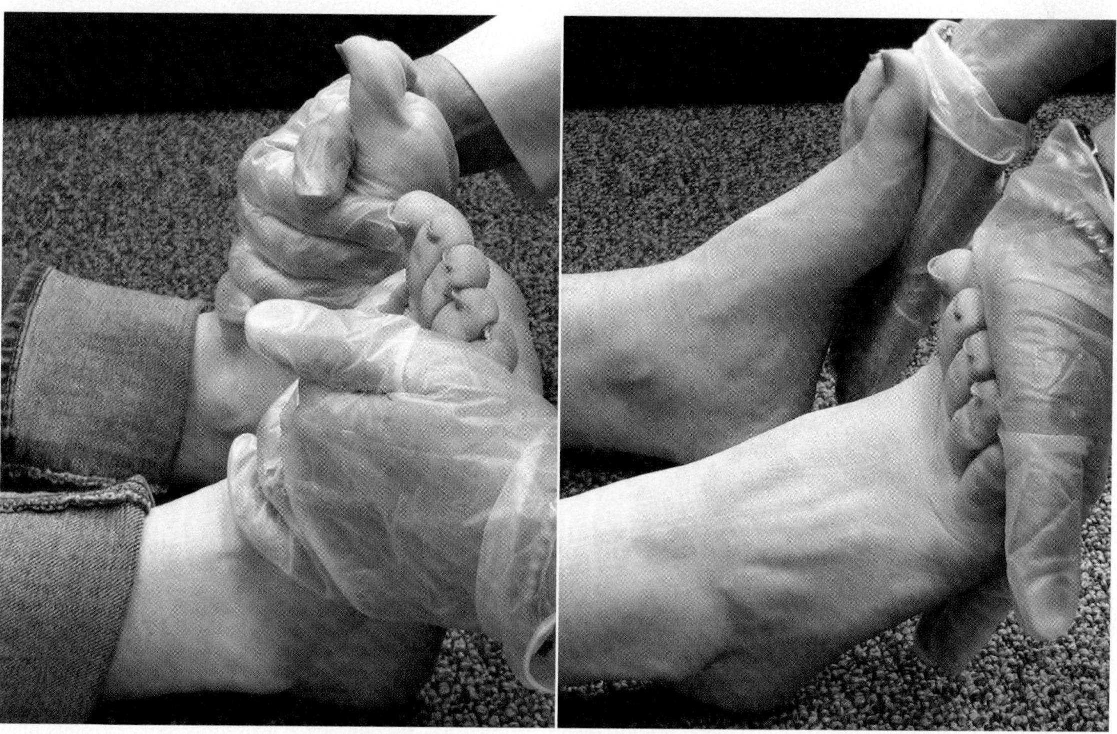

Figure 48-11 Evaluate ankle flexion and extension during the spine assessment.

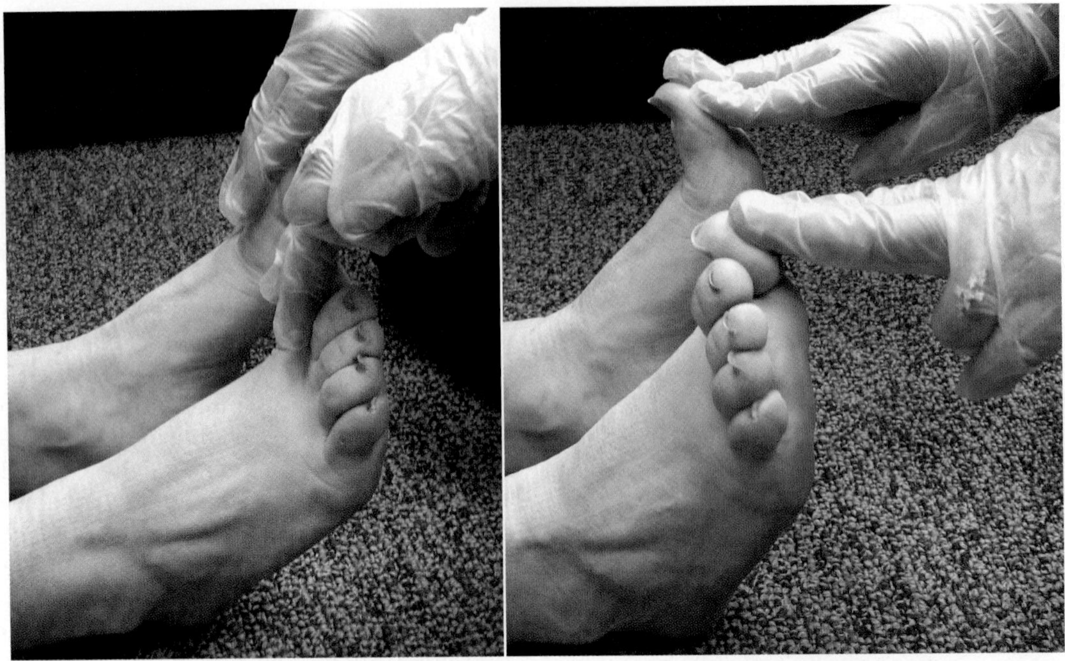

Figure 48-12 Evaluate great toe flexion and extension during the spine assessment.

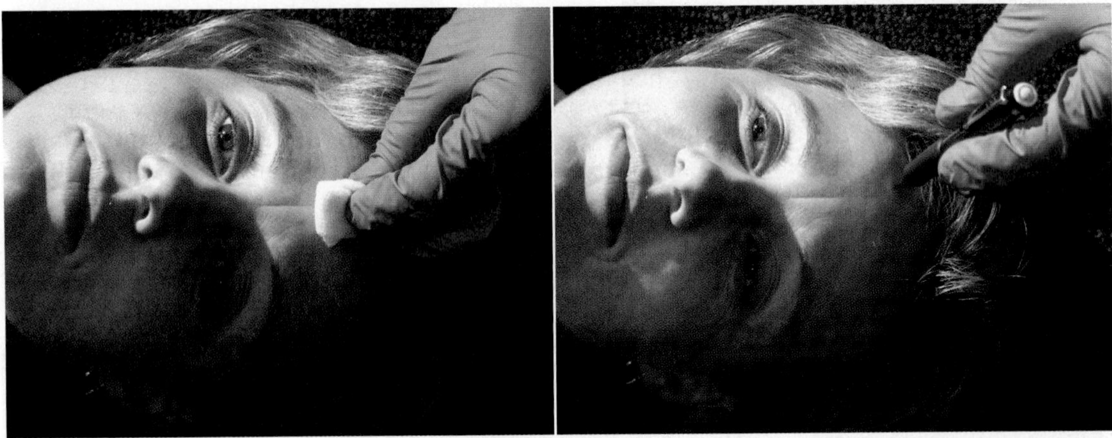

Figure 48-13 Ensure the patient can differentiate the objects you selected by testing them on the patient's forehead.

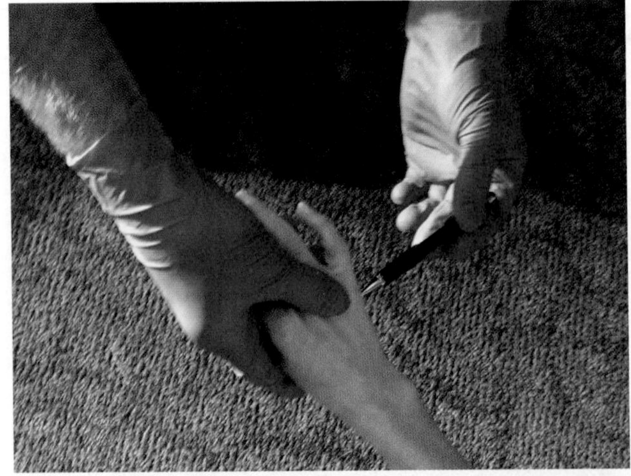

Figure 48-14 Test upper extremity sensory skills along the lateral aspect of the hand.

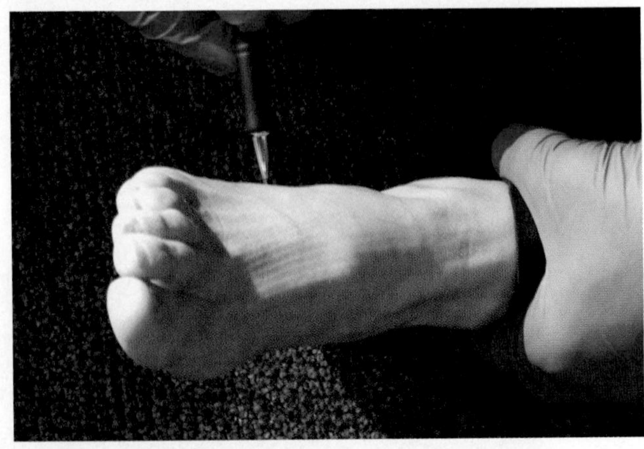

Figure 48-15 Test lower extremity sensory skills along the lateral aspect of the foot and/or ankle.

cannot differentiate pain and light touch in one or more extremities. Full spine stabilization is indicated in these situations.

PARAMEDIC*Pearl*

Assessing pain and light touch sensation along the anterior and lateral sides of the distal extremities is important because you are testing the most distal dermatome along each extremity.

Patients who are reliable, have a clear history, and have a clear physical examination do not need full spine stabilization. Unnecessarily immobilizing patients may cause the following:

- Increased patient discomfort
- Impaired ventilatory ability
- Increased risk of soft tissue injury
- Increased safety risk to healthcare professionals
- Difficulties for the hospital staff when examining the patient

However, any spine pain or spine tenderness indicates a spinal column injury, necessitating spine stabilization. Impaired motor or sensory skills or the presence of any numbness, tingling, or electrical sensation suggests SCI. Document your assessment findings, why spinal stabilization was or was not needed, and the findings that indicated that stabilization was or was not needed. Differentiate a suspected spinal column injury from SCI or if you suspect both. When assessment findings indicate an SCI, find out the extent of injury.

PARAMEDIC*Pearl*

Do not confuse loss of motor function and sensation from a musculoskeletal injury with loss of motor function associated with an SCI. Musculoskeletal injuries generally have a loss of pulses, movement, and sensation beginning at the injury site and moving distally. Spinal cord injuries cause impaired motor and sensory skills along one or more nerve roots and do not cause a loss of circulation. Thus you may see numbness and loss of sensation beginning at the shoulder and along the lateral side of the arms.

Further Spinal Cord Injury Assessments

[OBJECTIVES 11, 12, 13]

Assess the spine-injured patient in the same way as each trauma patient. During the detailed physical examination, visually inspect the neck and back to look for deformities, bruises, lacerations, and abrasions. After completing the spine assessment, identify an SCI and consider performing a few additional assessments.

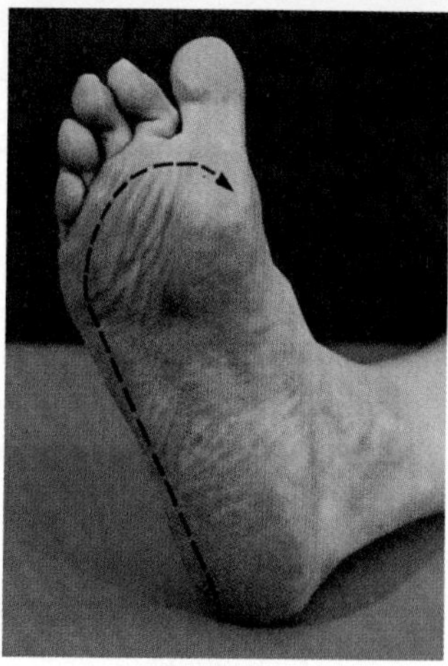

Figure 48-16 Check to determine the presence or absence of Babinski's sign.

Dermatome Assessment. Dermatomes are the areas of skin innervated by spinal nerves. Assessment of dermatomes reliably indicates the level of SCI. Begin at the feet, track up the legs and then the arms, toward the spine until you reach a level where the patient has intact sensation and motor function. Track this level to the spinal column and identify the vertebra to which you have tracked. This is the level of the SCI. It is not necessarily the level of spinal column injury.

Babinski's Sign. Check for **Babinski's sign** by scraping your pen or trauma shears along the plantar side of the foot, moving from the heel toward the toes (Figure 48-16). If the great toe flexes toward the head, and the rest of the toes fan apart, this is a present Babinski's sign. Babinski's sign is an abnormal finding except in infants younger than 14 months of age (it is normal in these infants). Its presence indicates an upper spinal column injury (Russell & Triola, 2006). Babinski's sign is reported as either present or absent.

Strength Scale. When a motor deficit is noted, evaluate strength present compared with the opposite limb by using a chart endorsed by the American Spinal Injury Association (Table 48-1). The lower the score, the more serious the suspected SCI.

Assessing the Pediatric Patient with a Potential Spine Injury

Much less force is needed to injure the spinal column and cord of a child. Their vertebrae are still growing; the younger the child, the higher the percentage of spinal column made of cartilage, not bone. As children age, more spinal bone forms. The softer cartilage offers the spinal cord less protection than do fully developed vertebrae. Because of this, children can injure the spinal cord

TABLE 48-1 Motor Strength in Spinal Cord Injury

Strength Score	Motor Activity
0	No movements or contractions
1	Minimal movement
2	Limited movement, but no movement against gravity or resistance
3	Active movement against gravity, not resistance
4	Active movement against some resistance
5	Active movement against full resistance

Data from Schreiber, D. (2006). *Spinal cord injuries*. Retrieved November 15, 2006, from http://www.emedicine.com.

without fracturing a vertebra. This is known as *spinal cord injury without radiologic abnormalities*.

When you evaluate the mechanism of injury, remember that forces that may not injure an adult's spine may easily injure a child's spine because the child's spinal column (particularly the cervical spine) is not as developed or as strong as the adults. Thus a child's cervical spine is more susceptible to whipping forces, such as those that occur during sudden speed changes. Children younger than 8 years are more likely to sustain an upper cervical SCI than any other spinal region. As patients age, injuries tend to occur lower in the cervical region.

PARAMEDIC*Pearl*

Increased vulnerability does not suggest that column and cord injuries are more common in children. Given a similar mechanism of injury (e.g., a fall down a flight of stairs), the adult is injured more often than the child.

In general, assessing a potentially spine-injured child should begin at the feet and slowly progress toward the head. This approach helps keep the child calm, gains trust, and reduces the risk of aggravating an unseen injury. The presence of a trusted adult will help keep the child calm during the assessment. You can perform a complete spine assessment on any pediatric patient you can clearly communicate with, who will follow commands, and whom you determine to be reliable. If you cannot reliably communicate with the child, he or she cannot listen to your commands, or if he or she is not cooperative, spinal stabilization will be required. Remember to follow your state and regional standards of care regarding pediatric spinal stabilization.

PEDIATRIC*Pearl*

Pediatric patients often require extra padding beneath their shoulders to maintain their cervical spine in a neutral position.

Assessing the Older Adult with a Potential Spine Injury

As people age, bones become more brittle and easily broken. A seemingly minor fall by an older adult may result in a spinal column injury with spinal cord trauma. Osteoporosis, arthritic joints, and slowing reflexes can combine to cause an older patient to fall, unrestrained, onto a hard surface and possibly sustain a severe injury. Patients who use a cane, walker, or wheelchair often fall more easily than do younger patients. Use caution during your evaluation. Many patients may not sense pain as well as younger adults because of prior disease-induced nerve damage or the general aging process. Carefully review the patient's history to identify any potential mechanism of injury that could cause a spine injury. Many medical conditions, such as a stroke, transient ischemia attack, hypoglycemia, and Parkinson's disease, can mimic an SCI. Remember: when in doubt, immobilize.

Assessing the Pregnant Patient with a Potential Spine Injury

The pregnant patient with a mechanism of injury that could injure the spine will be anxious about her injury as well as her unborn child. Instill confidence by keeping calm and providing reassurance to the patient. Avoid placing her in a supine position, especially during the third trimester of pregnancy. The fetus can compress on the major vessels of the abdomen, causing significant hypotension as well as numbness, tingling, and loss of sensation in the lower extremities. Assess and, if necessary, immobilize the pregnant patient on her left side. Take extra time to differentiate back pain associated with the pregnancy from spine pain caused by trauma.

PARAMEDIC*Pearl*

Rather than immobilizing the pregnant patient supine and then tilting the board, consider positioning the patient on her side while on the board and providing extra padding under her head, sides, and between the legs.

The following information pertaining to the patient's obstetric history also must be obtained:

- What was the date of your last menstrual cycle?

- Is this your first pregnancy?
- Do you have other children?
- Are you receiving prenatal care? Where?
- Does your physician expect any problems with this pregnancy?
- What is your due date or expected date of confinement?

Assessing the Obese Patient with a Potential Spine Injury

Many special considerations are necessary when assessing and immobilizing an obese patient. Obese patients who fall have more force acting on the spine caused by excess weight, although that is not as much of a factor as speed. Next, consider if you can effectively evaluate the spine. If you cannot touch each vertebra, then you cannot complete a spine assessment. Make every attempt to perform a thorough assessment. If the patient does have a spine injury, estimate his or her mass and ability to breathe adequately in a supine position. Obese patients may (1) exceed the weight limitations of the equipment used to immobilize them and (2) may be too large to be safely secured onto a device. Immobilization of the obese spine-injured patient may be impossible. It may also be a serious risk to you, the rescuer. If this situation arises, focus on controlling the spine by eliminating as much movement as possible.

The patient's weight and size must be considered when immobilizing him or her into neutral spinal alignment. Weight and size also determine the number of other rescuers needed to safely move the patient. You must be aware of any weight limitations or size restrictions on the equipment used in your jurisdiction.

PARAMEDIC*Pearl*

If appropriate, consider transport to facilities that have bariatric medicine programs. These programs are becoming more common in larger cities and represent a better level of care for the bariatric patient.

Assessing the Special Needs Patient with a Potential Spine Injury

Patients with preexisting paralysis or spinal cord damage may fall, be involved in an MVC that may reinjure an old lesion, or may injure previously uninjured areas of the spinal cord. New onset of paralysis may be overlooked or erroneously mistaken for existing paralysis because of the old injury. If any of these patients is involved in an accident that could injure the spine, perform a spine assessment and immobilize the patient. Assume the presence of a new injury or reinjury.

Handicapped individuals driving specially equipped vehicles may be a challenge to disentangle and immobilize because an entanglement may involve lifting equipment, locked wheelchairs with vehicle controls in place, and unique operating equipment near the steering column. Work with the patient for proper and safe extrication. These patients will know their equipment the best.

Do not assume you cannot communicate with or understand a patient with a cognitive learning disability such as mental retardation or Down syndrome. Often they can understand you and work with you to assess any potential spine injury. If a long-term care worker is on scene, he or she may be able to understand the patient's answers to your questions. If the patient cannot understand your questions, carefully consider immobilization. If you cannot explain to the patient what you intend to do and immobilization scares the patient, the process may cause him or her to become combative and lead to further injury. If you can safely limit spine movement by having the patient rest calmly and comfortably on your stretcher, then that may be the safest thing for the patient.

Ongoing Assessment

As you proceed with the treatment plan, you must continue to reevaluate the patient. Stable patients must have their vital signs reassessed every 15 minutes. Unstable and potentially unstable patients should have vital signs reassessed at least every 5 minutes. Remember to track vital signs over time. Patients with an SCI may have very abnormal vital signs because of impaired sympathetic nervous system function.

If you splint and manage any musculoskeletal injuries before assessing the spine, be sure to recheck pulses, movement, and sensation (PMS) after splinting. Reassess motor and sensory skills after immobilization of a spine-injured patient. Traditionally PMS is reassessed. However, PMS is not an accurate assessment of spinal cord function. Instead, reassess the specific motor skills and quickly check for sensory skills. Not all sensory skills need to be reassessed because you have already determined that a spine injury probably exists. Document your findings.

PARAMEDIC*Pearl*

When you determine that a patient is unstable—such as with suspected internal bleeding, a traumatic brain injury, or multiple proximal long bone injuries—do not spend time on scene performing a spine assessment. Instead, provide immediate stabilization and perform a spine assessment en route to the hospital during a rapid transport.

Case Scenario—continued

You begin by having your partner secure the cervical spine. The primary survey is initiated. The patient is awake and alert. His airway is patent and he has no obvious signs of head trauma. His breathing is regular and his skin is warm and dry. Vital signs are blood pressure, 94/68 mm Hg; pulse, 70 beats/min; respiratory rate, 22 breaths/min and nonlabored; and pulse oximetry, 98%.

He states he was on his ladder painting when he slipped and fell. During the secondary survey you notice that he has normal heart tones, clear lung sounds, a soft abdomen, and a stable pelvis but a deformity of the left femur. He has no sensation below his waist.

Questions

4. *Is this a primary or secondary cord injury?*
5. *Discuss the significance of the left femur deformity.*
6. *Where is his injury most likely located?*
7. *Describe the differences among cord contusion, concussion, compression, laceration, and transaction.*

PATHOPHYSIOLOGY OF SPINAL INJURY

[OBJECTIVES 3, 5, 14]

Through a good understanding of the mechanism of injury, the knowledgeable paramedic can understand how the spinal cord and column become injured. The mechanism of injury reveals if a spinal column injury, SCI, or both should be anticipated.

Direct Trauma

Direct trauma affects the spinal column and potentially the spinal cord by fracture and injury. Depending on the type of trauma, the spinal cord may swell or sustain a laceration, complete transection, or puncture. Examples of these mechanisms include stabbings (cord lacerations and transections), gunshot wounds (cord puncture), and blunt trauma (cord swelling and compression from bleeding). Furthermore, the cord also may be injured by fragmented vertebral fracture—bone pieces can lacerate or pierce the spinal cord.

Exaggerated Movements

Exaggerated movements of the head, neck, and back can result in vertebral fracture, dislocation, or disk herniation and bruising, tearing, or elongation of the spinal cord.

Flexion and Extension

Spinal flexion and *extension* refer to the normal forward (flexion) and backward (extension) movement of the spine. The degree of natural movement is different for the head and cervical vertebrae, thoracic vertebrae, and the lumbar vertebrae. Abnormal flexion and extension are likely to cause muscle and other soft tissue injury but unlikely to injure the spine. This changes however, when the movement is extreme.

Hyperflexion and Hyperextension

Extreme forward or backward movement is known as **hyperflexion** and **hyperextension.** Such movement can rupture the tendons and ligaments that stabilize the vertebrae and stretch the spinal cord. Stretching the spinal cord can cause it to tear or swell. A common hyperflexion injury occurs when the neck hyperflexes during an MVC and you find lip prints on the patient's shirt. Do not disregard lateral bending. Extreme lateral bending can cause the same injury as hyperflexion and hyperextension.

Rotation

Rotational forces can abnormally twist the spinal column beyond its normal rotating range. This is most likely to affect the cervical spine when the head is twisted from a direct blow. However, a rotational injury also can occur to the lumbar and thoracic areas. One example of this type of injury is a football player who is planted or moving in one direction and his torso is tackled and twisted to the opposite direction.

Axial Loading (Vertical Compression)

Axial loading occurs when significant compression forces squeeze the vertebrae together. This often crushes one or more vertebra and squeezes the intervertebral disks, which can cause them to herniate or rupture (Figure 48-17, *A*). This type of injury can occur as a chronic problem when a patient frequently lifts heavy loads improperly and causes undo pressure on the lumbar spine; this leads to chronic lower back pain, often from slipped disks.

Axial loading also occurs when a patient falls from a significant height and lands on the feet. The top half of the body (head and thorax) continues to move downward as the lower half of the body stops. The result is

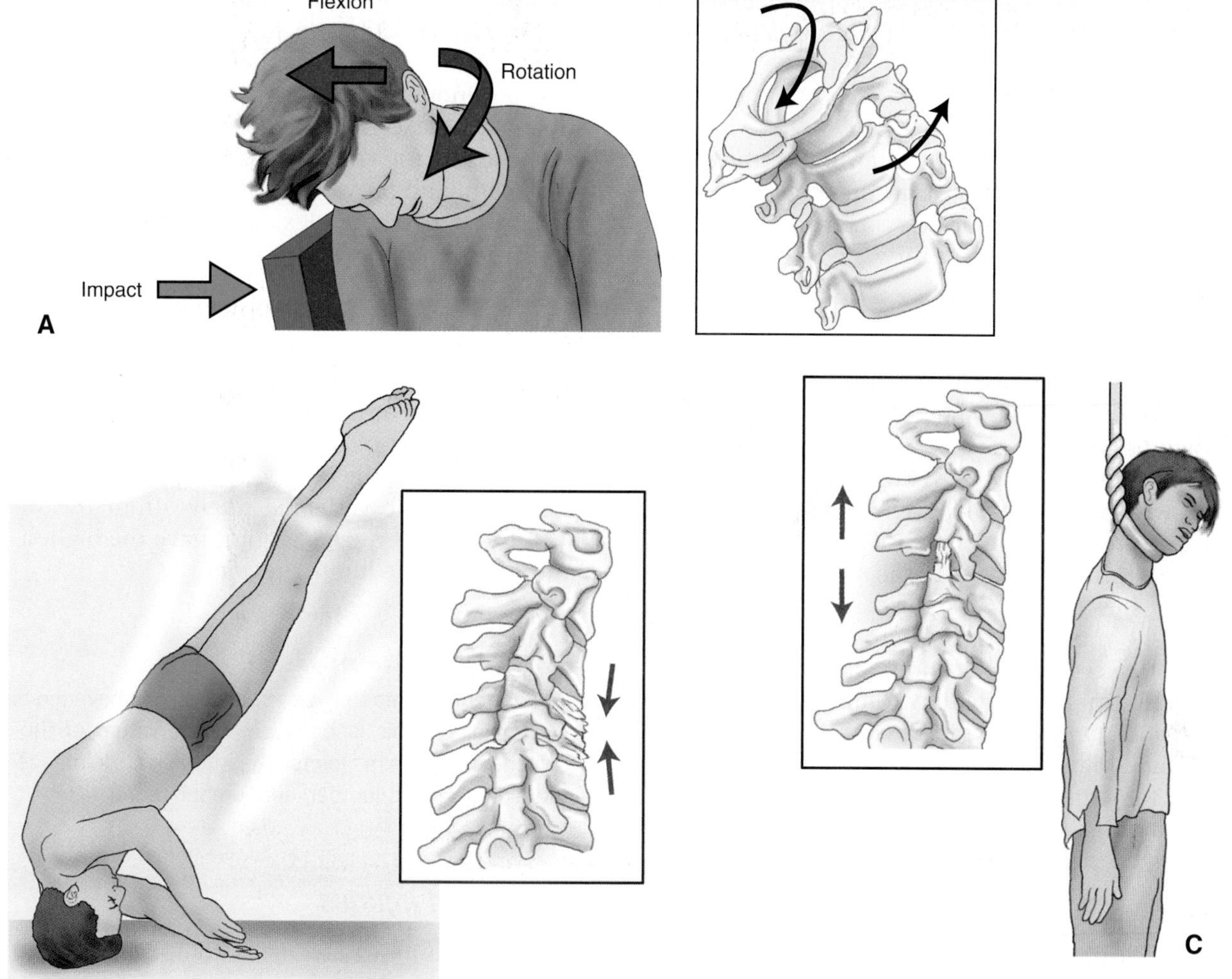

Figure 48-17 **A,** Rotational spine injury. **B,** Axial loading spine injury. **C,** Distraction spine injury.

compression of vertebrae T12 through L2. Individuals who dive into shallow water and strike the head (shallow water diving injury) on the bottom also undergo axial loading and compress the cervical spine as the weight of the body presses down on the cervical area. Another example of cervical axial loading is when a patient's head strikes the windshield during an MVC.

Understanding the mechanism of injury leads to a better understanding of injury patterns and locations. Recognition of axial loading is critical. Although the spine does not receive direct trauma, risk for injury is quite high. Perform a spine assessment on any patient who may have undergone axial loading.

Distraction

Distraction forces are the opposite mechanism of compression (axial) forces. This occurs when the body is pulled in opposite directions (Figure 48-17, *B*). Consider a bungee jumper and someone who is hung. In both cases the patient is moving and is jerked to a stop at one point while gravity pulls the rest of the body away from the fixed end. The result is stretching and separation of the spinal column, its ligaments and supporting muscles, and tearing of the spinal cord. Although the type of distraction force determines exactly how the injury occurs, the cervical region is most vulnerable to distraction forces because it has the least support and protection.

The most classic distraction injury is a **hangman's fracture,** which, as its name implies, occurs during a judicial hanging. The rope and knot are set to the lateral side of the neck. In addition to distraction forces as the rope pulls tight, the rope causes a severe lateral force, snapping the head sideways as the spine stretches. This causes bending and fractures at the C1-C2 region, which quickly tears the spinal cord.

Neither distraction nor compression mechanisms often occur alone. Mixed mechanisms with some sort of rotational, flexion, or extension forces usually occur. Carefully examine what occurred and determine the forces that may have been involved. This will allow you to understand better what type of injuries the patient may have sustained.

Other Mechanisms

Many accidents inflict forces that can injure the spine. You are responsible for evaluating these accidents and determining whether a spine assessment is appropriate and spinal stabilization is necessary.

- *Blast injuries*. Three impacts occur during a blast: (1) flying debris, which can strike and penetrate the spine; (2) a wave of heat and energy that causes a concussive force; and (3) blunt trauma if the patient is blown to the ground.
- *Swift water and severe weather*. Swift water during floods, whitewater sporting events, and in marinas during severe weather can twist a patient's body and spine and throw the patient against fixed objects (e. g., trees, poles, rocks). Crashing waves, such as in tsunamis, can bear down on victims, causing blunt trauma. However, spinal column and cord injuries rarely occur in deep water environments.
- *Electrocution*. Only in rare instances will electrocution cause spine injuries. Alternating current can cause damage to peripheral nerves, but it rarely reaches the spinal cord. If the current does reach the spinal cord, it is likely to cause swelling and symptoms often do not manifest until after the patient is delivered to the emergency department.
- *Lightning strike*. Lightning strikes also do not automatically mean the patient has a mechanism for a spine injury. The energy itself is not enough to injure the spine. However, if the patient is blown to the ground, blunt trauma may be a mechanism if an object struck the spine.

TYPES OF SPINE INJURY

[OBJECTIVE 14]

Many mechanisms can injure the spinal column and spinal cord. The two can be injured together or independently. With a thorough spine assessment you can recognize which is injured, and if either is, immobilize the patient. Column injuries may involve the bone, ligaments, tendons, or muscles. The loss of this structural support places the spinal cord at a higher risk for injury; thus spinal stabilization is indicated.

Spinal Column Injuries

Spinal column injuries are relatively easy to recognize. Look for deformity, dislocation, spine tenderness, or spine pain. Because of the impressive amount of musculature around the vertebrae, vertebral structures are rarely unstable—but they can happen. The type of column injury does not matter. Making a field diagnosis of a fracture, subluxation (partial dislocation), dislocation, or bone contusion is nearly impossible. Remember that a fracture can occur on any portion of the vertebra: the body, a spinous process, pedicles, or the laminae. Do not attempt to make this diagnosis. Instead, recognize the injury, assess for cord damage by completing a spine assessment, and provide spinal stabilization.

Maintain a higher index of suspicion for injuries along specific places on the spinal column. The cervical region, particularly the C1-C2 joint and C7, is most prone to injury because the cervical spine supports the head and has the least amount of spinal cord protection. The cervical bones are the smallest on the spinal column and protect the cord at its widest. The lumbar region has the next highest risk of injury; although the bones are the largest, they lack the additional support and protection that the thoracic vertebrae receive from the ribs. The T12-L1 joint and the L5-S1 joint have the highest risk of injury among the lumbar region.

PARAMEDIC*Pearl*

The vertebral joints between spinal regions have the highest risk of injury. This is because the curvature of the spine switches at these joints: head/cervical joint, cervical/thoracic, thoracic/lumbar, and lumbar/sacral.

Spinal Cord Injuries

Spinal *cord* injuries are more complicated than spinal *column* injuries. Not all spinal cord injuries involve a complete cord transaction (a severed spinal cord). The paramedic must understand how the injury occurred and look for signs of specific SCI. This allows recognition of the difference between numbness and tingling as a result of a primary cord injury or as a result of cord swelling after a contusion. When cord injuries are evaluated, the difference between problems associated with the primary injury and problems associated with a secondary injury must be understood.

Primary Injury

Primary cord injuries directly result from the insult that the spinal column and cord sustained. They cause immediate mechanical disruption, distraction, or transection of the cord. A spinal column injury usually occurs as well (Schreiber, 2006). This may be a puncture from a knife or bone fragment, laceration, cord compression from a crush injury, or a stretching or tear. Primary injuries cause certain signs and symptoms to appear immediately. The symptoms depend on the part of the cord injured.

Secondary Injury

Often limited damage is caused by a primary injury. During transport, you may notice the patient's symptoms begin to worsen. This is a sign of a **secondary cord**

injury, often caused by bleeding, swelling, and ischemia. The primary injury has damaged tissue, and any damaged tissue swells. As the swelling worsens, it will impair the function of the cord. If a blood vessel is affected or damaged, it will worsen the swelling and may lead to cord ischemia. Rapid transport and care at a hospital can help reduce these symptoms.

PARAMEDIC*Pearl*

No research studies have demonstrated rescuer-induced cord injury. It is extremely rare. Worsening symptoms of cord injury after stabilization are most commonly caused by **secondary cord injury.**

A variety of injuries can occur as both primary and secondary injuries. Through proper evaluation and care, you can recognize when symptoms are caused by a primary injury and try to minimize spine movement to reduce the risk of secondary injuries.

Cord Concussion. Spinal cord concussions are similar to brain concussions in mechanism and manifestation. This type of injury can occur with some penetrating injuries (e.g., a gunshot wound) and as a result of a direct blow in sports or hand-to-hand combat (e.g., a knife-edge hand strike to the neck). They cause a transient (temporary) neurologic deficit, usually as a result of blunt trauma, in which the cord is "stunned" for a period of time. No structural damage (column or cord) or permanent damage usually occurs.

Cord Contusion. A contusion is soft tissue bruising. Thus a cord contusion is bruising of the spinal cord. This injury presents similarly to a cord concussion, but symptoms persist for a longer period. Cord contusions indicate a more significant mechanism of injury and suggest some capillary bleeding within the spinal cord. Long-term residual effects usually do not occur.

Cord Compression. Both primary and secondary injuries can lead to spinal cord compression. Primary cord compression can occur with a crushed vertebra or intervertebral disk. Secondary cord compression occurs when soft tissues around the cord swell after an injury and compress the cord within the spinal column. Both mechanisms can cause ischemia to the compressed portion of the cord. If not corrected, this can lead to permanent damage.

Laceration. Any puncture wound, bone fragment, or knife wound can cause a cord laceration. Lacerations cut the cord's nerve bundles and can also cause significant bleeding and swelling—all within the spinal foramen. Even small lacerations can cause significant bleeding. These effects of the laceration can cause significant cord impairment. Small lacerations can lead to some recovery, especially when most damage is associated with swelling and bleeding. Large lacerations often lead to permanent cord damage and nervous system impairment.

Complete Cord Transection

An injury that completely cuts across the spinal cord is known as a complete cord **transection.** This injury completely eliminates the body's ability to send or receive nervous system impulses distal to the injury site. Complete cord transections are permanent, irreparable injuries that lead to paralysis. Complete transections occurring above T1 lead to **quadriplegia** (paralysis of all extremities). Quadriplegia, now known as *tetraplegia,* paralyzes the extremities as well as the abdominal and thoracic muscles that aid breathing. Be prepared to assist these patients with positive-pressure ventilation. **Paraplegia** occurs with cord transections below T1. Paraplegics have full use of their upper extremities and no use of their lower extremities. The location of the transection determines whether the patient maintains use of abdominal and thoracic muscles. Table 48-2 summarizes the level of expected function and region of transection.

Incomplete Cord Transection

When only a portion of the cord is damaged at a given point and some nervous bundles remain intact, the condition is known as an **incomplete cord transection.** Recall the earlier description of the tracts of the spinal cord. It is for this reason that incomplete cord transections only affect part of the cord and leave open the potential for some neurologic recovery. Three important types of incomplete cord transactions are discussed in the following sections.

Anterior Cord Syndrome. The death or transection of the anterior portion of the spinal cord leads to **anterior cord syndrome.** This most often occurs when the anterior spinal artery is disrupted and anterior cord infarction occurs. Anterior cord syndrome leads to some paralysis with the loss of pain and temperature sensation below the lesion site. The posterior column remains intact, so the patient maintains some sense of touch, sense of vibration, and proprioception.

Central Cord Syndrome. Many conditions can cause **central cord syndrome;** however, EMS professionals are most likely to see it as a result of trauma. In general it is caused by a hemorrhage in the central portion of the spinal cord or central cord necrosis. Neck hyperextension is the most common mechanism. As a result, central cord syndrome most commonly occurs in the cervical region, and the central motor neurons are destroyed. Classic symptoms of central cord syndrome are initial quadriplegia followed by a return of lower extremity function (within minutes), a slower increase in distal upper extremity function, and bladder dysfunction. Patients maintain a sense of proprioception and vibration; however, they lose their ability to sense pain and temperature. Some patients also report a burning sensation in their extremities (Gondim, 2006; Schreiber, 2006).

Brown-Séquard Syndrome. Brown-Séquard syndrome commonly results from penetrating trauma or disk herniation in which one half of the spinal cord is affected, essentially creating a hemicordectomy. Other

TABLE 48-2 Level of Function after Complete Cord Transection

Location of Transection	Extremities and Movement	Respiratory System	Communication and Other Functions
C1-C3	Limited head and neck movement, complete paralysis of limbs and body	Loss of chest muscle and diaphragm use, will require ventilator	Requires complete assistance for daily functions, potentially can speak depending on fracture
C4-C5	Full head and neck movement; limited shoulder use; no hand wrist, or forearm use; no lower extremity function	Diaphragmatic breathing only, no cough reflex, assistance needed clearing airway	Can speak, may use a computer with voice recognition; requires complete assistance with daily functions
C5	Full head, neck, and shoulder movement; can flex elbows but no extension; no finger or wrist movement	Same as C4	Same as C4
C6	Full head, neck, and shoulder use; can flex elbow and extend wrist; no finger movement	Same as C4	May be able to grip some objects passively, but grip will be weak; able to speak; needs regular assistance for daily functions
C7-C8	Gains movement of the thumb, partial finger movement, full elbow and wrist use	Can breathe without ventilator, but stamina is low	Some management of bowel and bladder, independent upper body cleaning and dressing
T1-T4	Full head, neck, and upper extremity use; gains chest muscle use as injury lowers	Can breath normally at rest, abdominal accessory muscles compromised	Can clean self, feed independently, and communicate normally
T5-T9	Full upper body use above injury, strength dependent on injury site, complete paralysis of lower legs	Able to breathe normally, some decreased endurance	Relatively independent
T10-L1	Partial paralysis of lower body and legs, ability to transfer independently	Normal respiratory system	Often lives independently
L2-S5	Full upper body control and balance; some hip, knee, and foot movement; use increases as injury site lowers	Normal respiratory system	Lives independently

Data from Miami/Jackson Memorial Medical Center. (1998). *Rehab team site.* Retrieved December 1, 2006, from http://www.calder.med.miami.edu.

causes include spinal cord tumors and spinal epidural hematomas. The classic signs and symptoms of Brown-Séquard syndrome are a loss of motor control, proprioception, and vibratory sensation on one side of the body—the same (ipsilateral) side as the affected cord half. Patients experience a loss of pain and temperature sensation on the opposite (contralateral) side (Gondim, 2006). It is important to note that many patients do not exhibit the classic presentation and may only have partial motor and sensory impairment. Recall that the impulses for light touch and crude touch travel on opposite sides of the spinal cord. Therefore complete loss of the sensation of touch is uncommon in partial cord transections.

Other Cord Injuries and Conditions

Conus Medullaris Syndrome and Cauda Equina Syndrome. The adult patient's spinal cord ends roughly between L2 and L3 at a point known as the *conus medul-*

laris, a group of nerve roots that continue down the remainder of the spinal column known as the *cauda equina.* An injury to the lower lumbar region can injure either of these structures and result in symptoms ranging from back pain to leg pain, numbness in the perineum, and possibly incontinence of bowel and/or bladder. Asymmetric leg weakness often is present (Gondim, 2006).

Conus medullaris syndrome occurs when the conus medullaris is injured. This syndrome results in a rapid onset of symptoms mimicking SCI: bilateral weakness, numbness and tingling, or motor deficit. A cauda equina injury, known as **cauda equina syndrome,** occurs when the spinal nerves below the conus medullaris are injured. Symptoms typically develop gradually and most often include lumbosacral lower back pain, unilateral weakness or numbness and tingling, or unilateral motor deficit.

Both syndromes may occur concurrently or independently, depending on the injury location. Tables 48-3 and 48-4 summarize the differences in signs and symptoms of these two syndromes.

Spinal Cord Injuries without Radiologic Abnormality. The spinal cord can be injured with no evidence of injury visible on radiographs. An **SCI without radiologic abnormality (SCIWORA)** is most commonly seen in the pediatric patient but can occur in other patients. The elastic nature of the pediatric cervical spine can allow a spine injury to occur that cannot be seen on radiographs. The paramedic will not be able to determine the presence of SCIWORA; however, you will still be able to detect an abnormality or deficit during the spine assessment, indicating the presence of an injury.

Shock in Spinal Cord Injury. Spinal shock occurs when the blood vessels distal to a spinal cord transection dilate, causing the vasculature to be much larger than the blood supply is capable of filling. Because of the cord transection, the vessels cannot constrict. The result is profound hypotension with moist, warm, flushed skin distal to the transection, possible bradycardia, and all the other symptoms of cord injury. Bradycardia results if cervical or thoracic outflow to the heart has been altered. Spinal shock is temporary and the symptoms generally correct themselves within 24 hours. A more long-term condition is **neurogenic shock,** which presents similarly to spinal shock but does not correct itself over time. Additionally, neurogenic shock is associated with other symptoms, including loss of bladder and bowel control and **priapism.** Because neurogenic shock is rare, many paramedics work in systems with frequent major traumas and never see neurogenic shock.

During neurogenic shock, distal vasodilation reduces preload, which reduces cardiac output. The autonomic nervous system often is affected and the body loses its ability to release epinephrine and norepinephrine. Signs from the sympathetic division of the autonomic nervous system cannot be sent to the adrenal medulla. Without the release of epinephrine and norepinephrine, the heart rate does not increase in response to the hypotension.

Autonomic Dysreflexia Syndrome. Once a patient's reflexes return after spinal shock, a patient is at risk for **autonomic dysreflexia (AD) syndrome**, a true medical emergency. AD develops as intact sensory nerves distal to the SCI transmit signals back to the sympathetic

TABLE 48-3 Symptoms of Cauda Equina

Symptoms	Cauda Equina Syndrome
Presentation	Gradual onset, generally only one side affected
Motor function	Noticeable paraplegia, atrophy may develop
Pain	Significant radicular (nerve root) pain, less-severe lower back pain
Reflexes	Decreased ankle reflex
Sensory signs and symptoms	Numbness in saddle region, no sensory dissociation, loss of sensation in lower extremity specific dermatomes, pubic numbness
Other	Erectile dysfunction, genital numbness, urinary retention (late)

Data from Dawodu, S. T., & Lorenzo, N. (2007). *Cauda equina and conus medullaris syndromes.* Retrieved March 28, 2008, from http://www.emedicine.com.

TABLE 48-4 Conus Medullaris Syndrome

Symptoms	Conus Medullaris Syndrome
Presentation	Sudden onset, affects both sides of the body
Motor function	Symmetric strength, mild distal extremity paresis
Pain	Significant lower back pain, mild radicular pain
Reflexes	Decreased ankle and knee reflex
Sensory signs and symptoms	Numbness in perianal region, symmetric and bilateral sensory dissociation
Other	Impotence common, incontinence common

Data from Dawodu, S. T., & Lorenzo, N. (2007). *Cauda equina and conus medullaris syndromes.* Retrieved March 28, 2008, from http://www.emedicine.com.

nervous system (Campagnolo, 2006). Sympathetic overstimulation develops as the body tries to send vasoconstriction signals distal to the injury, but they cannot be transmitted. Massive vasoconstriction and hypertension above the injury site occur as a result. It is estimated that between 48% and 90% of patients with an SCI above T6 experience autonomic dysreflexia syndrome, especially when the patient sustains spinal shock. Complications from the hypertension include seizures, retinal and cerebral hemorrhage, and acute myocardial infarction. Other symptoms of AD include pallor, piloerection, headache, diaphoresis, and visual disturbances. AD requires hospital care. Prehospital management focuses on supporting the critical systems (Campangolo, 2006). Insertion of a foley catheter, if authorized, can be lifesaving.

GENERAL MANAGEMENT OF SPINAL INJURIES

[OBJECTIVE 12]

Management of patients who have a mechanism of injury for a spine injury begins in the scene size-up with mechanism recognition. Once recognized, you must take control of the patient's spine during the initial assessment and maintain control until a full spine assessment is completed. Controlling the patient's spine does not mean immediate stabilization of the spine. Rather, it means minimizing any unnecessary spine movement by maintaining manual stabilization of the cervical spine and keeping the patient from moving any of the three weight centers that lead to spine movement: the head, shoulders, and hips.

Complete patient assessment, moving the patient only when absolutely necessary, such as for safety, to complete an assessment, or to manage a distracting injury. Once you have completed the patient assessment, calmed the patient, and managed any distracting injuries, perform a spine assessment. Remember that the physical examination component of the spine assessment is a specific examination and is not included as part of your rapid or focused trauma assessment. If any positive findings arise during the spine assessment, or if the patient is unreliable, he or she must be immobilized. Remember: when in doubt, immobilize.

Spinal Stabilization and Immobilization Techniques

Once a determination has been made by the paramedic to immobilize a patient, the specific device to accomplish that action should be chosen and efficiently applied. Regardless of the device chosen, certain principles should guide the paramedic's treatment of the patient (Box 48-4). Correct spinal immobilization is best accomplished with several EMS professionals, preferably with more than two rescuers.

BOX 48-4 Guiding Principles to Spine Immobilization

- Stabilize the head and weight centers (shoulders and hips).
- The person at the head calls all movements.
- Apply an appropriately sized cervical collar early.
- Move in small increments.
- Axial movements are safer than lateral movements.
- Bring the spine into a neutral in-line position as soon as safely possible.
- Properly fill in any voids with an appropriate amount of padding.

Begin by manually controlling the head and cervical spine in a neutral in-line position. Once the provider has assumed control of the head and cervical spine, he or she cannot release the patient's head until the patient is completely secured to a long spine board for transport or control is transferred to another rescuer. Because this provider will remain at the head throughout the immobilization of the patient, he or she should closely monitor the patient's level of consciousness, airway status, and ventilatory rate, depth, and quality. This provider should not use a bag-mask device or manually maintain an airway because those tasks would require releasing the patient's head. Another EMS professional should be assigned this task. When moving the patient becomes necessary, the provider maintaining manual stabilization directs the move.

The patient's torso must be securely fastened to the device, with voids filled and padded before securing the patient's head. In the event the patient vomits, turning the backboard to turn the patient's head is easier than controlling the patient's torso. To secure the patient to the backboard properly, the shoulders, hips, and legs must be secured. The straps must eliminate possible movement (e.g., axial, lateral, rotational). This is why padding becomes so important. A minimum of five straps are needed to secure a patient properly to a spine board. Use two straps to create an X over the chest, two straps to create an X over the pelvis, and one strap to secure the legs. Using straps straight across the body does not limit the movement of the weight centers described. A commonly used strapping system is spider straps (Figure 48-18). Once placed on a stretcher, secure the patient with the stretcher straps, including shoulder straps, to reduce the likelihood of the backboard and patient sliding on the stretcher in the event the ambulance brakes or accelerates suddenly or is involved in a collision.

Spinal Alignment

The ultimate goal of any spinal stabilization process is to return the spine to its natural anatomic in-line position. This allows the spinal foramen to have its largest opening,

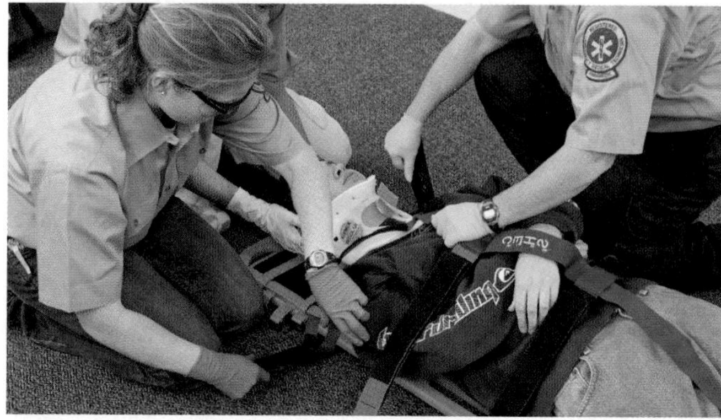

Figure 48-18 Spider straps are an excellent way to secure a patient to a long board for immobilization.

allowing the spinal cord the maximal amount of space possible to swell after an injury. When moving a patient into an in-line position, remember that the spine is not one bone. It is 33 fairly small and relatively fragile bones.

PARAMEDIC*Pearl*

Think of the spine as a chain. Dragging the chain sideways (lateral movements) will cause the chain to curve—as when the spine moves laterally. However, dragging the chain toward an end (axial movement) keeps all the chain links in line—hence the spine stays in line.

Proper spine alignment requires alignment of the three weight centers connected to the spine: the head, shoulders, and hips (Isaac & Johnson, 2006). Picture a straight line running through the hips and shoulders. When you align the spine, these two lines must be parallel to each other and perpendicular to the spine. Both shoulders also should be directly over both hips. Aligning the shoulders and hips before aligning the head is often a better choice because it eliminates unnecessary head movement. Return the head to its neutral in-line position by supporting the head's weight, not by pulling traction (this could be fatal in a C1-C2 fracture).

PARAMEDIC*Pearl*

In most patients, you know the head is in line when the eyes and nipples are parallel to each other and in line with the navel. However, landmarks may be altered as a result of surgical enhancement or the effects of gravity, age, and weight.

Spinal alignment can be performed at any time during the patient assessment and management process. The only time spinal alignment is contraindicated is when the patient reports a marked increase in pain when attempting to straighten the spine or dramatic resistance is noted when doing so. If this occurs, immobilize the patient in his or her present position. This often is easiest performed with the patient on his or her side with lots of padding. Document your reasons for not aligning the spine.

Manual In-Line Stabilization

Manual in-line stabilization is applied during the initial assessment and occurs when the paramedic grasps the patient's head firmly between his or her hands with the fingers and thumbs extended to avoid any extension, flexion, lateral bending, or rotation of the head (see Chapter 24). This stabilizing move should be done with no traction exerted on the patient's head. Manual in-line stabilization can be maintained from the front, rear, or side of the patient. The only difference is how you position your hands. Stabilization from the rear requires thumb placement behind the ears with the fingers spread across the cheeks and jaw (Figure 48-19). Generally, manual stabilization from the front causes less patient anxiety because the patient can see who is touching him or her.

PARAMEDIC*Pearl*

If your patient is prone, position your hands so that your right hand is on the right side of the patient's head and your left hand is on the patient's left. You will need to cross your arms to do this, making an X. Think about how you cross your arms initially; cross them in that manner so that as you log roll the patient into a supine position, your arms uncross. This eliminates the need to release manual stabilization to adjust your hands.

In some rare cases, moving the patient's head into a neutral in-line position is not possible. Movement of the patient's head and neck should not be attempted if neck movement compromises airway or ventilation or initiates or increases spasms in the neck, pain, or neurologic deficit. The risks associated with moving these patients exceed the risks of transporting the patient immobilized onto a spine board in the position found. Cervical collars cannot be adjusted to immobilize these patients, so the paramedic should not attempt to apply one. When this situation occurs, stabilize the head and neck with bulky padding and document completely. The SAM Splint (SAM Medical Products, Portland, Ore.), a flexible splint that can be formed into nearly any position, can be used as an improvised cervical collar if approved by medical direction.

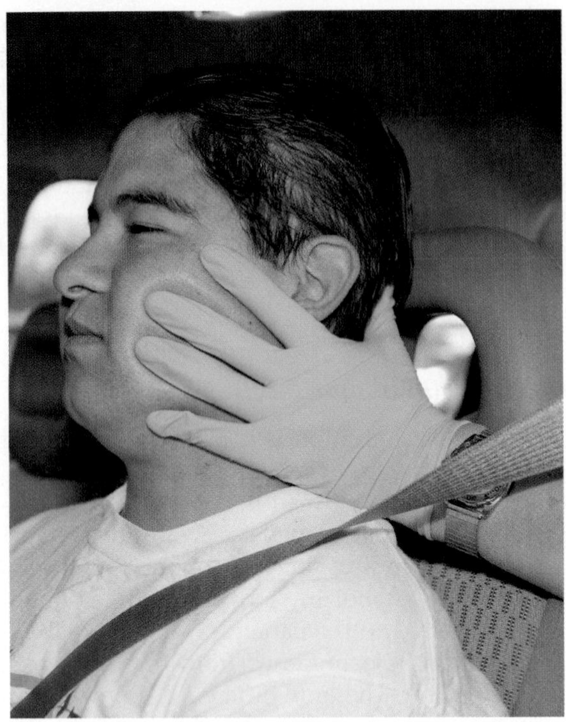

Figure 48-19 Manual in-line stabilization from behind the patient requires thumb placement behind the ears with the fingers spread across the cheeks and jaw.

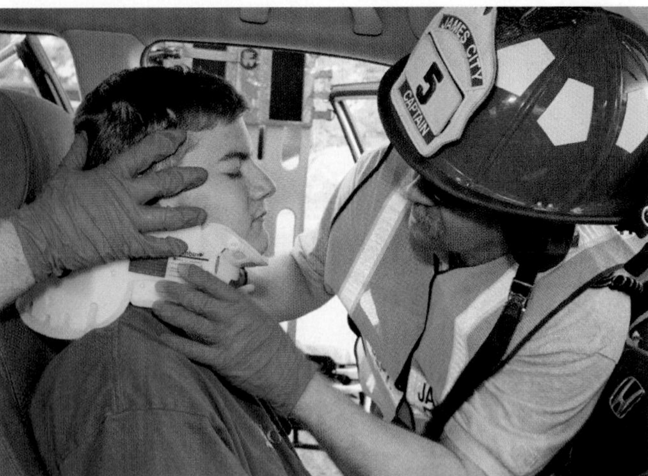

Figure 48-20 A properly applied cervical collar allows the head to remain in a neutral in-line position.

Measuring and Applying the Rigid Cervical Collar

A cervical collar is not designed to immobilize the patient's head. Rather, it is intended to reduce flexion and extension of the neck. The cervical collar does not prevent a patient from turning the head sideways. This is just one reason why you must continue to maintain manual stabilization until the patient is fully immobilized.

A properly applied cervical collar allows the head to remain in a neutral in-line position (Figure 48-20). A cervical collar that is too large will cause the patient's neck to extend. Conversely, a cervical collar that is too small will not eliminate neck flexion. A properly sized collar supports the head in the neutral position by resting on the chest and the jaw without applying pressure on the jaw. Once the collar is in place, make sure that the patient can still speak easily. If the patient pulls down on the collar to speak, it likely is too large.

Application of Half Board and Vest Devices

Half spine boards and extrication vests are excellent tools for immobilizing the cervical spine and upper thoracic column. They do not effectively immobilize the lumbar spine. Keep this in mind when using these pieces of equipment. Although application of the vest device is specific to the model, a few principles remain the same for all devices. Half spine boards and extrication vests are intended for patients who are stable and in a seated position—generally inside a vehicle after an MVC. They are particularly useful for the management of patients with a suspected cervical spine injury. Use of a short board or vest device is contraindicated in unstable patients or patients in an unsafe situation. If either of these situations is present, perform a rapid extrication straight to a long board. Skill 48-1 shows the steps for spinal immobilization of a seated patient.

Rapid Extrication

Rapid extrication is the process of manually stabilizing and moving a patient from a sitting position onto an immobilization device without the use of a short backboard or a vest-type device. Rapid extrication is indicated only if the following are true:

- The patient has a life-threatening problem.
- The scene is hazardous and imminently dangerous for the patient or rescuers.
- The patient must be moved quickly to access more critically injured patients.

Rapid extrication should only be used when life-threatening conditions exist and no time is available to apply a vest-type extrication device. Rapid extrication is not an ideal procedure because it does not allow complete spine protection during the process. It is appropriate when you can only do the best you can for the situation.

The goals of rapid extrication are to (1) move the patient as quickly as possible to a safer, more spine-stable position (long board) and (2) maintain control over the spine's three heavy weight centers: the head, shoulders, and hips. Doing the latter will allow you to maximize patient movement while minimizing spine movement. Skill 48-2 shows the steps for rapid extrication.

SKILL 48-1 SEATED SPINAL IMMOBILIZATION

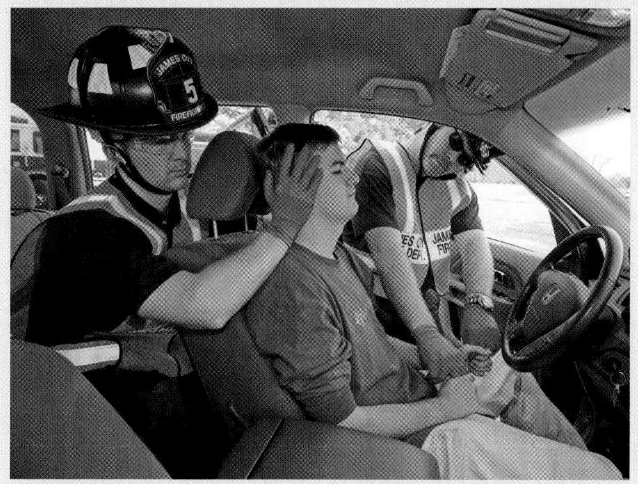

Step 1 Take appropriate standard precautions. Direct an assistant to place and maintain manual in-line stabilization of the patient's head. Assess distal pulses, movement, and sensation in each of the patient's extremities.

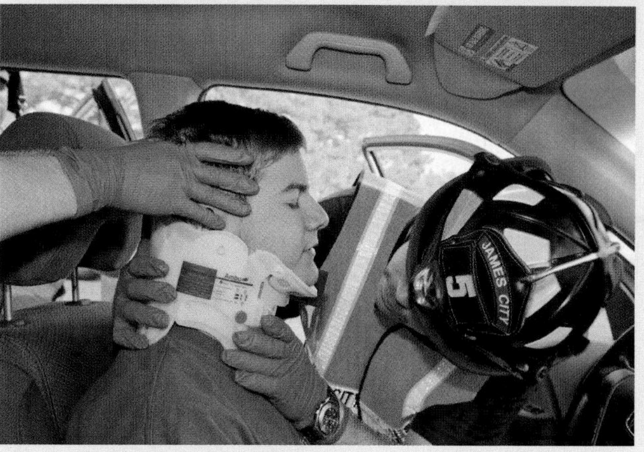

Step 2 Apply a rigid cervical collar of appropriate size.

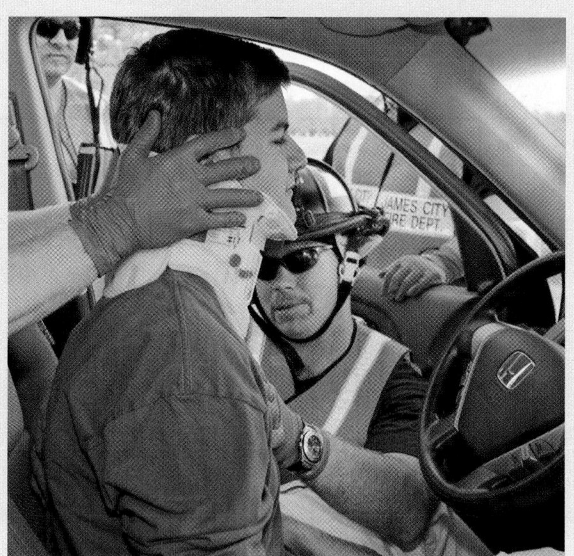

Step 3 As a unit, lean the patient forward to create a void between his or her back and the seat.

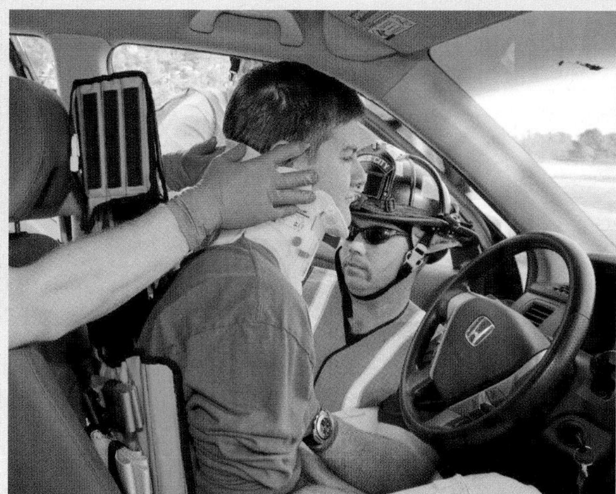

Step 4 Slide the vest device into the void, placing its base near the patient's waistline so that its torso flaps are just beneath the patient's armpits. When positioning the device behind the patient, make sure the patient is centered.

Continued

SKILL 48-1 SEATED SPINAL IMMOBILIZATION—continued

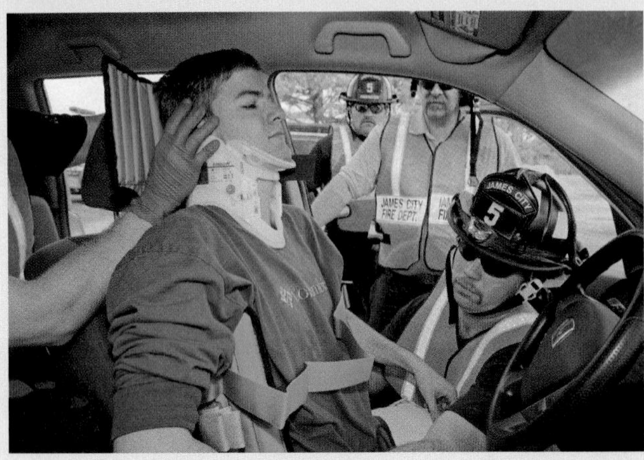

Step 5 While maintaining control over the patient's head, shoulders, and torso, lean the patient back against the vest and seat. Begin securing the device to the patient. The torso is secured first. Secure the torso straps per the manufacturer's recommendations.

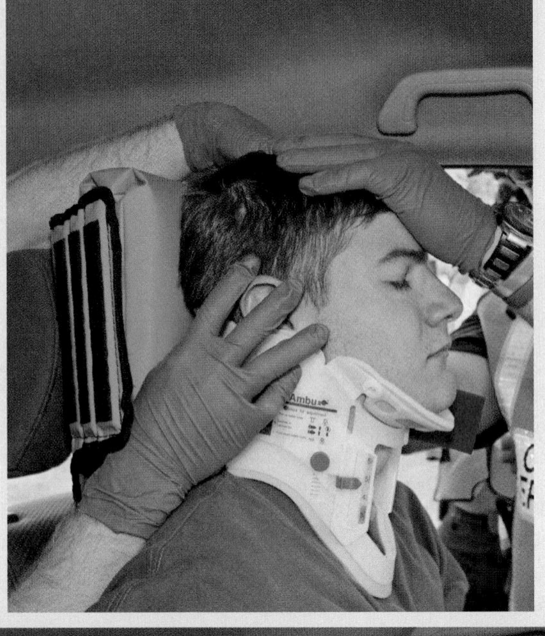

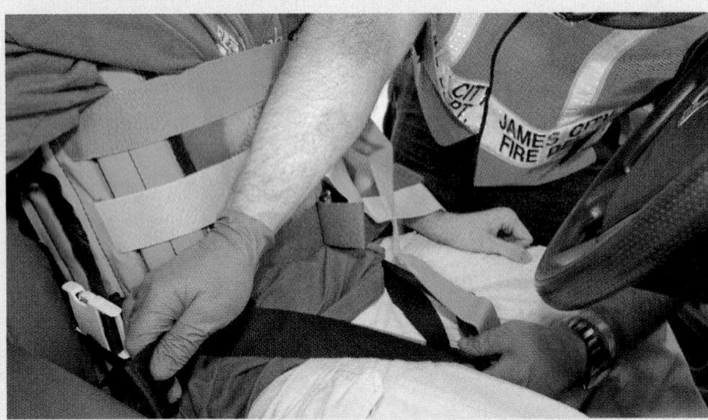

Step 6 Secure the patient's legs next. Fasten and tighten the leg straps. Evaluate how the patient's torso is fixed to the device and adjust as necessary.

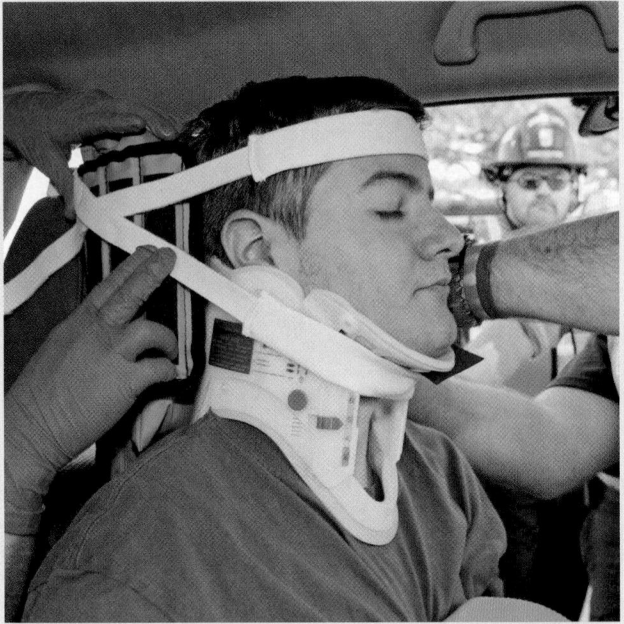

Step 7 Secure the patient's head to the device last. *Do not* bring the patient's head to the board. Bring the board to the patient's head. Pad behind the head as necessary. A common mistake made by many EMS professionals is failure to provide enough padding between the back of the device and the patient's head. This results in neck extension.

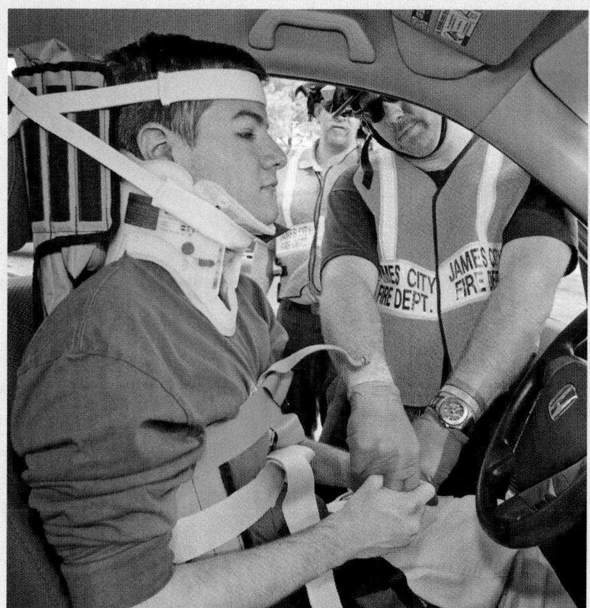

Step 8 Reassess distal pulses, movement, and sensation in the patient's extremities.

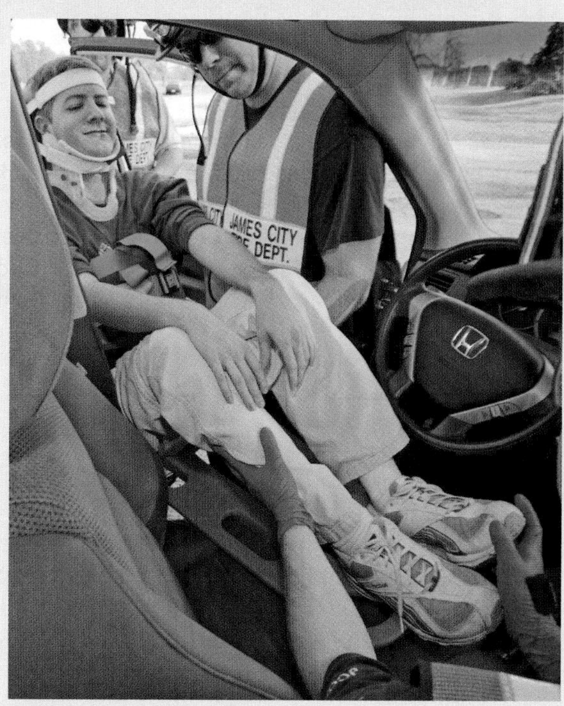

Step 9 Once completely secure, safely transfer the patient to a long board with proper lifting and moving procedures. Extricating the patient's head first often is easier. However, if the patient is in a vehicle with a large center console, then extrication head first would require moving the patient's legs over the console. Such a move would manipulate the patient's hips and thus the lumbar spine. In these instances extricate the patient feet first onto the long spine board and finish spinal stabilization.

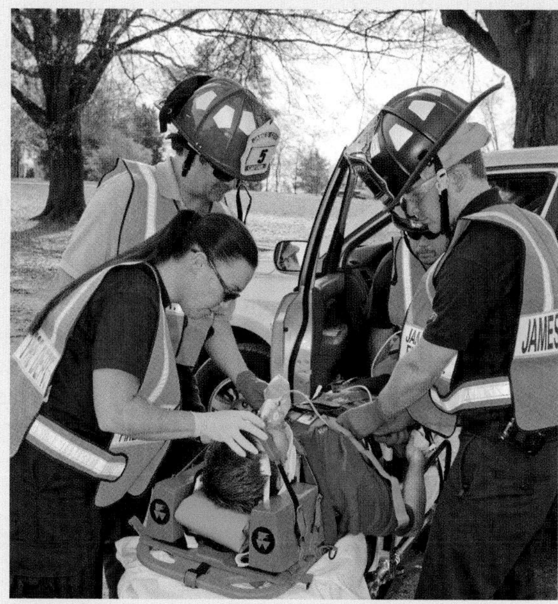

Step 10 Loosen the top chest strap, secure the patient to the long board, then secure the patient and board to the stretcher.

BOX 48-5 Traditional Long Board Straps

Traditional long board strapping places one strap over the chest, one over the hips, and one over the legs. This is ineffective at eliminating patient movement for several reasons. First, most patients are not as wide as the board in all places, yet straps are secured to the outer edge of long boards. Second, three simple straps do not eliminate axial or lateral movement. Place yourself on a board with three straps and try to move around; see how much movement you actually have.

Immobilization with a Long Spine Board

A long spine board is nothing more than a flat, rigid surface. It can be used to immobilize legs, the pelvis, hips, or the spine (Box 48-5). Supine immobilization is the most common and simplest form of immobilization for the stable spine-injured patient.

PARAMEDIC*Pearl*

Reasons to immobilize a patient on the side include late-term pregnancy, vomiting, impaled objects, patient comfort, pelvic fracture, flail chest, or hemothorax (must lay on affected side). Attempts to straighten the spine will be met with resistance and increased pain.

Spine boards are long, rigid, hard, and quite uncomfortable. For this reason, consider laying a blanket down on top of the board before placing a patient on it. The blanket will not reduce the board's effectiveness but will greatly improve patient comfort. Also, the board is flat, and patients are not. Laying the patient flat places the patient in an unnatural position. For proper spinal stabilization, the patient's natural contours must be maintained. Adult patients require 1 to 2 inches of padding beneath the head. Pad the small of the back and under the patient's knees to place the knees and hips in a more natural position. Skill 48-3 shows the steps for long board immobilization.

An effective method of strapping patients onto long boards is the X method. Bring two straps, one over the top of each shoulder, and cross them over the sternum. Attach the straps to the side of the board opposite the shoulder they crossed. This will secure the shoulders. Next bring the straps over the top of each iliac crest, cross them over the pelvis, and secure them near the opposite hip—creating an X over the hips. Legs can be secured with straight straps over the thigh and ankles. Because many patients are not as wide as spine boards, securing straps to the outside edge of the board creates a space between the patient and where the straps are secured. This void is known as a *terrible triangle* and allows patient movement.

BOX 48-6 Immobilization in the Lateral Position

Immobilizing a patient in a lateral position is no more difficult than traditional immobilization; it simply takes a little more practice. Once you have placed the patient in either the right or left lateral recumbent position, look to see what voids you need to fill. Use the lower arm and a few towels to fill the void between the side of the head and the board. You will need to provide padding between the legs to maintain the hips in a somewhat neutral position. Then provide padding to fill the terrible triangles alongside the chest, pelvis, and legs. The triangles will be a bit wider and taller than in supine patient immobilization, but they can be filled with rolled-up blankets. With proper padding, lateral immobilization is as effective as supine immobilization, often is more comfortable for the patient long term, and also impresses the emergency department staff as you demonstrate your patient advocate skills.

To eliminate terrible triangles, place a towel or blanket roll along the patient's side. The roll will fill the void and thereby eliminate excess lateral patient movement.

Immobilization of a patient in a lateral position is sometimes necessary. This procedure is discussed in Box 48-6.

PARAMEDIC*Pearl*

Make a concerted effort to minimize unnecessary patient movement. When the patient is rolled onto his or her side to check for unseen trauma, quickly cut the patient's clothing straight down the back, from the collar or neck line through the waistband of pants or skirts worn by the patient. This will protect the patient's modesty once he or she is placed onto the spine board and permit the paramedic to remove the clothing quickly with minimal movement.

The Standing Takedown

EMS professionals often arrive on scenes of MVCs and known falls to find patients walking around. This does not mean they do not have a spine injury, and a mechanism for a spinal injury still might have occurred. You can perform a complete patient assessment and spine assessment on the standing patient. If after performing a spine assessment you determine that spinal stabilization is indicated, perform a standing takedown to place the patient safely onto a spine board. Skill 48-4 explains how to perform this procedure.

Immobilizing Pediatric Patients

When immobilizing a pediatric patient, remember that children have their own unique anatomy. One of the most important anatomic differences in young children

Text continued on p. 456.

SKILL 48-2 RAPID EXTRICATION

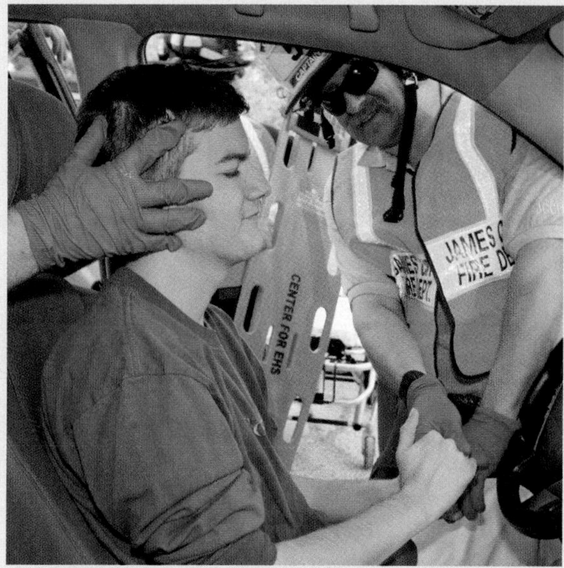

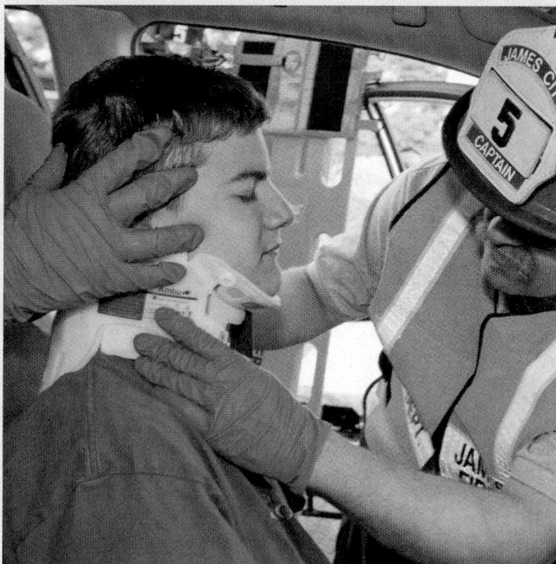

Step 1 Take appropriate standard precautions. Direct an assistant (Rescuer 1) to place and maintain manual in-line stabilization of the patient's head. Assess distal pulses, movement, and sensation in each of the patient's extremities and apply a rigid cervical collar of appropriate size.

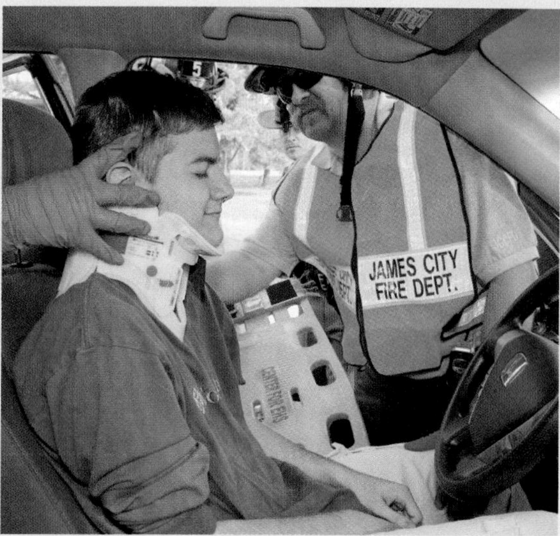

Step 2 Plan extrication moves carefully. Ask Rescuer 2 to position an ambulance stretcher with a long backboard next to the open vehicle door so that it is ready to receive the patient.

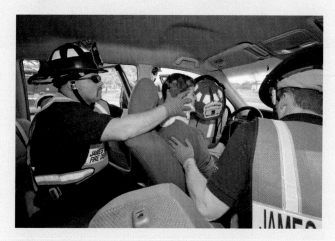

Step 3 While maintaining manual stabilization, rotate the patient in a series of short, controlled moves so that his or her back faces the open doorway of the vehicle. Support and control the patient's torso and legs during each move. The series of short moves continues until Rescuer 1 can no longer maintain manual stabilization of the patient's head and neck.

Continued

SKILL 48-2 RAPID EXTRICATION—continued

Step 4 Carefully transfer manual stabilization of the patient's head and neck to the rescuer in the doorway of the vehicle.

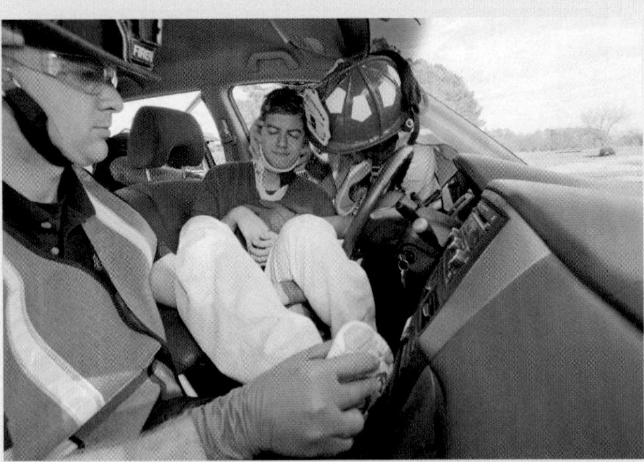

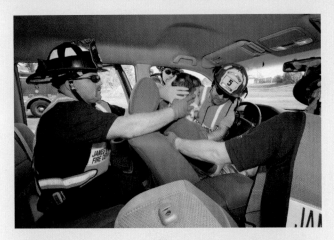

Step 5 Rescuer 1 positions the foot end of a long backboard onto the vehicle seat. The head end of the board is positioned on the ambulance stretcher. Rotation of the patient is continued until he or she can be lowered out of the vehicle door opening and onto the long backboard.

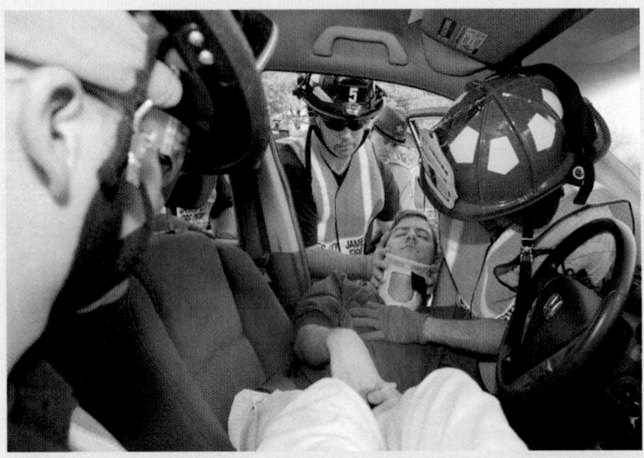

Step 6 While Rescuer 2 supports the patient's head and neck, the patient is carefully lowered onto the backboard.

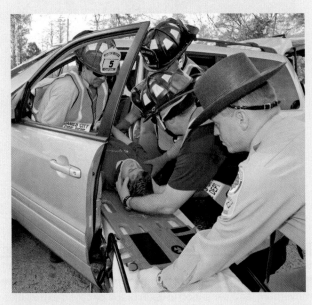

Step 7 While controlling the patient's pelvis and legs, the patient is moved upward onto the long backboard.

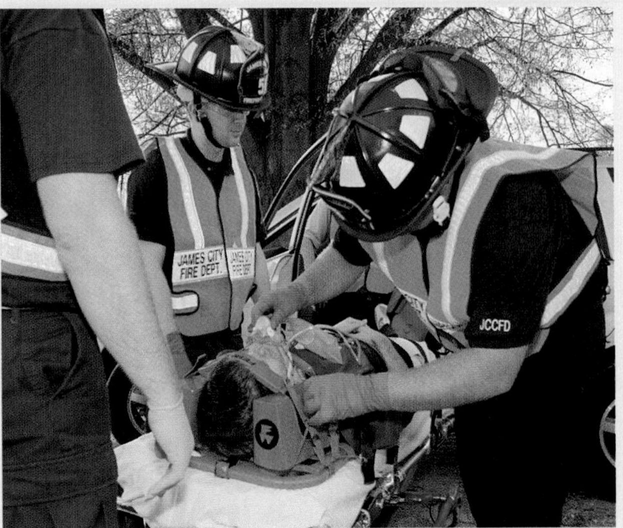

Step 8 If the scene is safe, secure the patient to the board and the board to the stretcher. Reassess distal pulses, movement, and sensation in the patient's extremities. If the scene is unsafe, move the patient to a safe area and then secure the board and stretcher.

SKILL 48-3 LONG BOARD IMMOBILIZATION

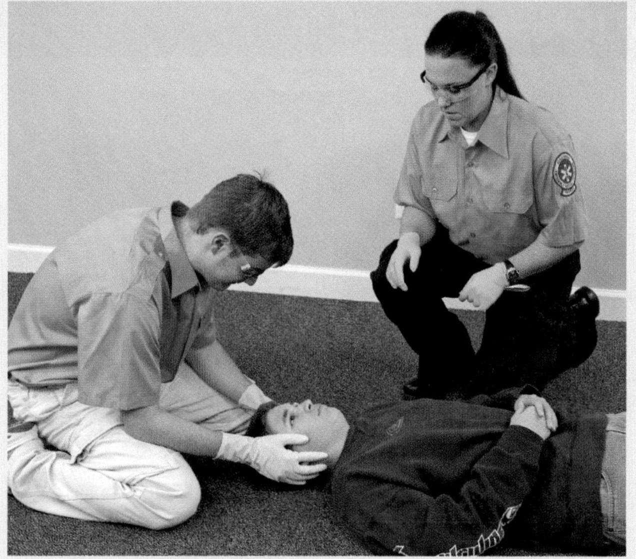

Step 1 Take appropriate standard precautions. Direct an assistant to place and maintain the patient's head in an in-line position.

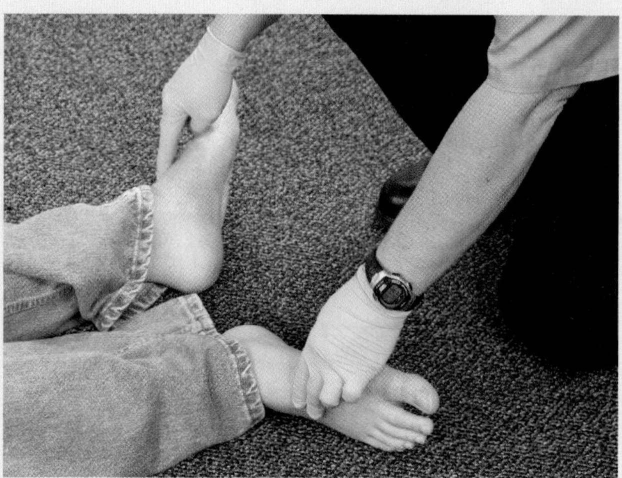

Step 2 Assess distal pulses, movement, and sensation in each of the patient's extremities.

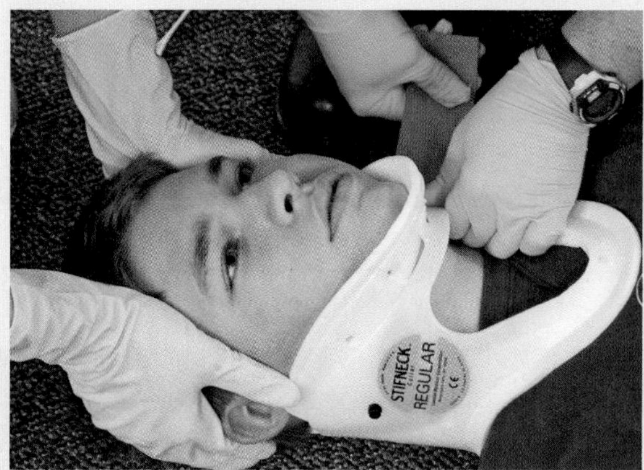

Step 3 Apply a rigid cervical collar of appropriate size.

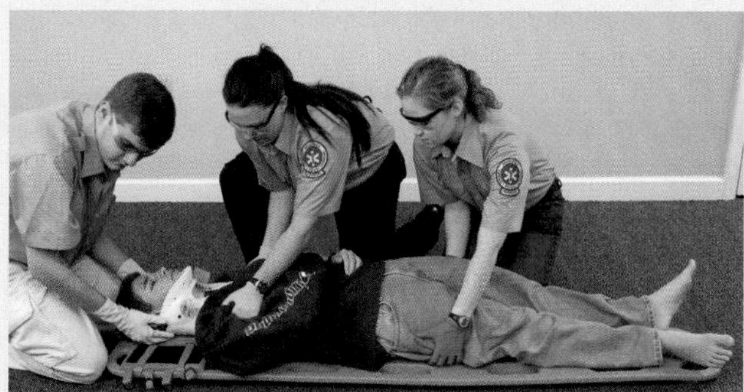

Step 4 Position the long board and then move the patient onto it without compromising the integrity of the spine. Ensure the patient is centered on the board. Apply padding to voids between the patient's torso and the board as necessary.

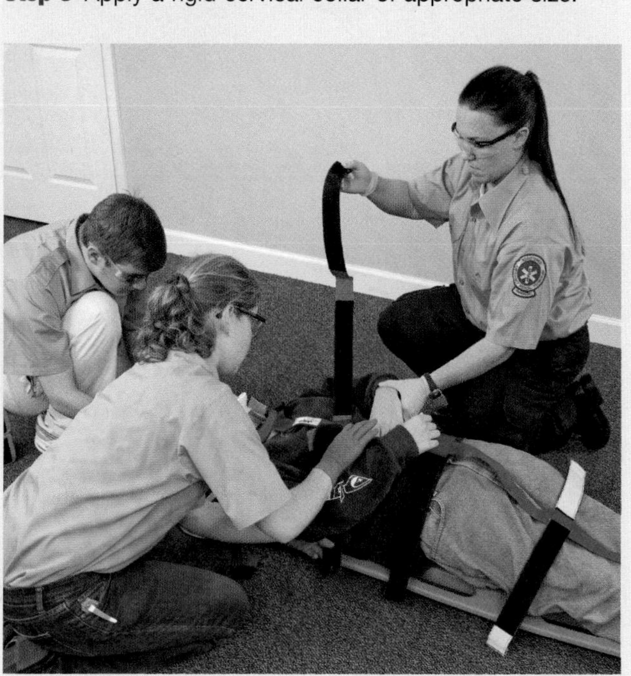

Step 5 Secure the patient's torso to the board.

Continued

SKILL 48-3 LONG BOARD IMMOBILIZATION—continued

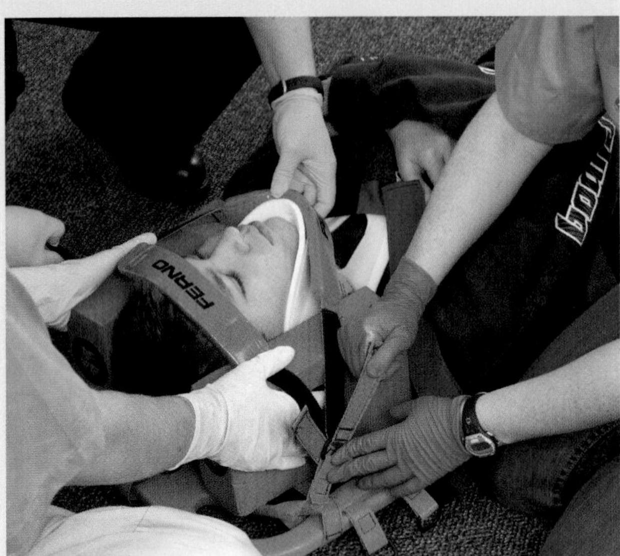

Step 6 Secure the patient's head to the board with a combination of straps and head blocks to fill the voids between the head and the edge of the long board. Place a head block device on either side of the patient's head to prevent lateral movement. Then place two straps across the patient's forehead in an X formation with a low-to-high strapping pattern. Straps traditionally placed across a cervical collar provide no additional protection and do nothing to reduce movement.

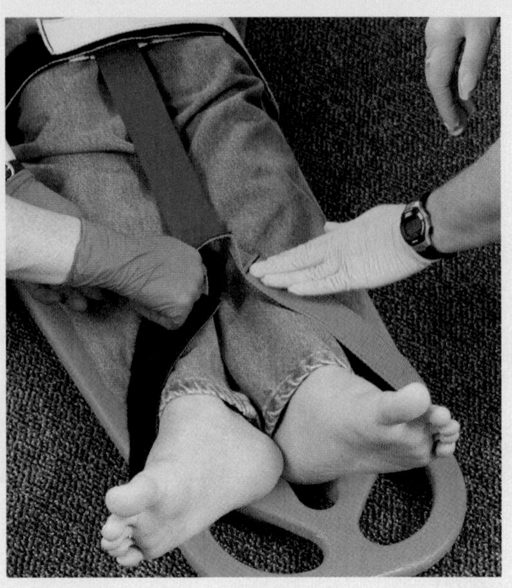

Step 7 Secure the patient's legs to the board.

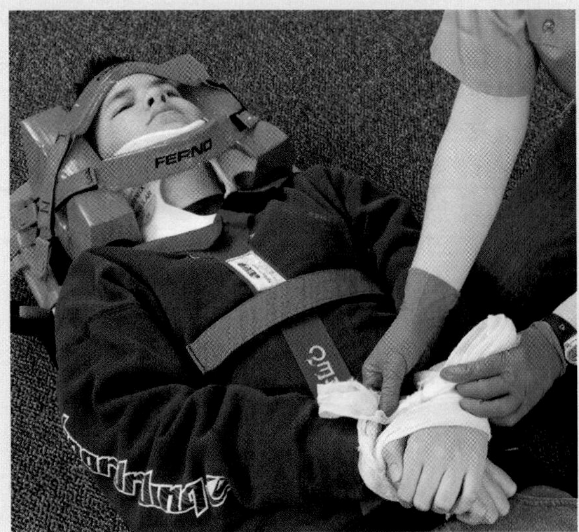

Step 8 Secure the patient's arms.

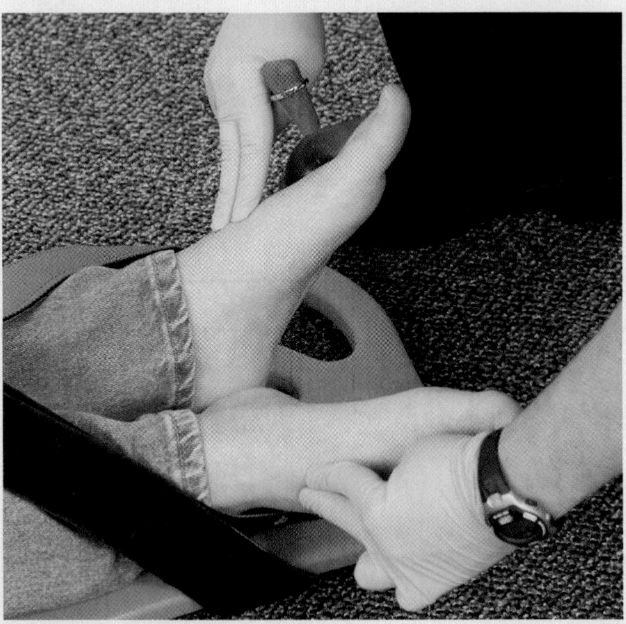

Step 9 Reassess distal pulses, movement, and sensation in the patient's extremities.

SKILL 48-4 STANDING TAKEDOWN

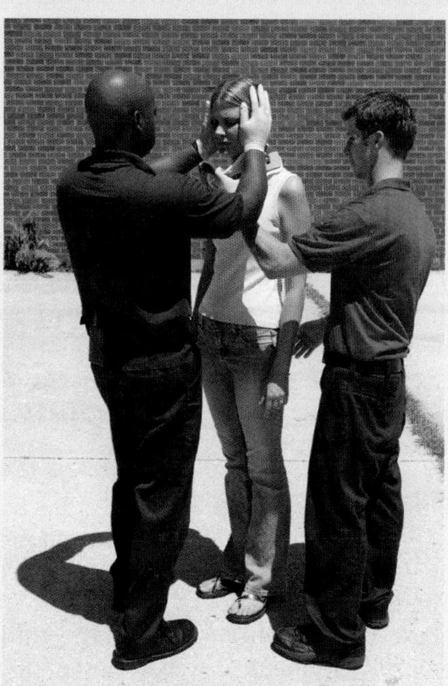

Step 1 Wear appropriate personal protective equipment. Approach the patient from the front. Apply manual inline stabilization by placing your hands on each side of her head.

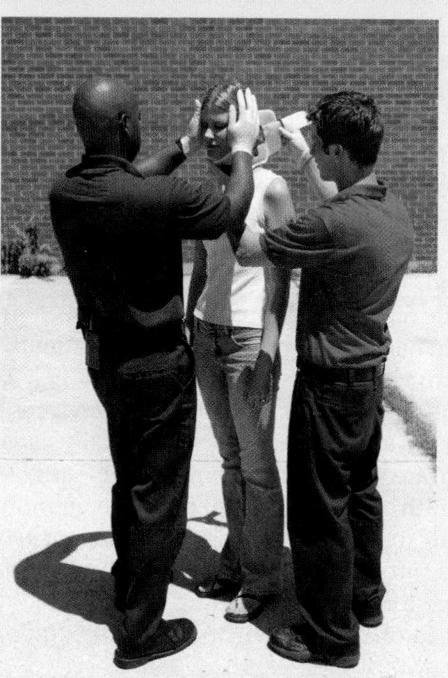

Step 2 Ask a second rescuer to assess the patient's pulse, motor function, and sensation in all extremities. Have the second rescuer size the patient for a cervical collar, assess her neck and spine for injury, and then apply the collar.

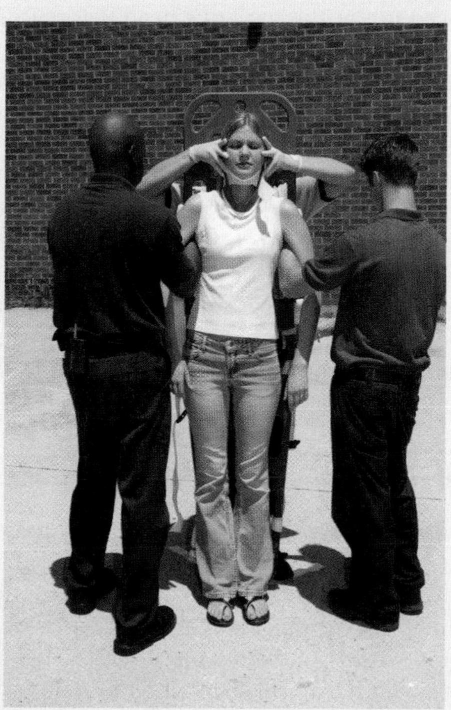

Step 3 While the first rescuer continues holding manual inline stabilization of the patient's head and neck, ask a second rescuer to position a long backboard behind the patient, between the arms of the first rescuer. Ask another rescuer to place his arms under the patient's armpits and grasp the backboard. The backboard is then placed against the patient's back.

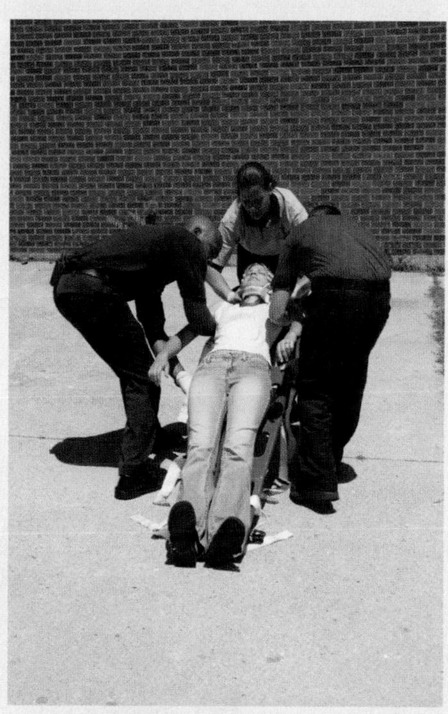

Step 4 Inform the patient that you will be lowering her backward. Once all are ready, the rescuer in back gives the order to lean the patient toward him and onto the ground. Once on the ground, reasess the patient's pulse, motor function, and sensation in all extremities, and then secure patient to the long board.

is that the back of their head sticks out further than their shoulders. This means that if you lay them flat you will force the neck to flex forward. Avoid this by placing padding between the long spine board and the patient's upper back. The terrible triangles also will be much wider for pediatric patients; more padding will be needed between the patient and the edge of the board. Because young patients often are scared, be sure to explain what is going to happen in terms the child can understand.

Pediatric immobilization devices have been developed to help manage these problems and are useful for children up to 5 to 6 years of age (Figure 48-21). The head support of a pediatric immobilization device is recessed backward to allow for the proportionally larger head. They also are narrow to comply more easily with the child's width. Used properly, pediatric immobilization devices are stand-alone systems and do not have to be integrated into a long spine board. However, if the child is too large for the pediatric system, he or she will need to be placed on a long spine board with extra padding.

Immobilizing Older Adults

Older adults may have many orthopedic disorders that can alter the shape and strength of their spine, hips, and shoulders. Be prepared to provide extra padding typically not needed for the average adult patient. Also, geriatric patients often have a decreased sense of pain and may not be able to feel the discomfort from ischemia developing if they are lying on a bare spine board for an extended period. To combat this, be sure to lay a blanket down the length of the spine board to provide a general padding layer.

Immobilizing the Pregnant Patient

Immobilizing a pregnant patient may bring about **supine hypotensive syndrome** from pressure on the inferior vena cava and possibly impair adequate ventilation as the developing fetus and uterus press against the diaphragm. Once the patient has been fully immobilized onto the spine board, it should be tipped up onto its side approximately 15 degrees (roughly 6 inches). This will shift the fetus to the side and off the inferior vena cava. Keep in mind that this position and the weight shift as the ambulance accelerates and decelerates is disconcerting to the patient. Therefore the paramedic should never be out of the view of the patient. When tipping the backboard, remember to tip the board to the left, elevating the right side of the board. Most ambulance vehicles in the United States have the stretcher mounted to the left, or driver's side wall. Elevating the right side of the board gives the paramedic unencumbered access to the full anterior surface of the patient.

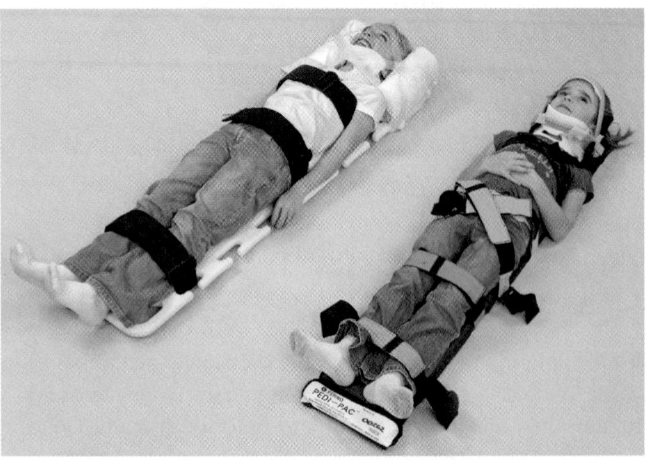

Figure 48-21 Pediatric immobilizers are excellent devices for appropriately sized children.

Immobilizing the Obese Patient

Spinal stabilization of an obese patient poses a unique challenge because cervical collars and rigid backboards are not designed to immobilize a large patient.

An obese patient lying supine may ventilate poorly because of displacement of weight and abdominal mass against the diaphragm. Obese individuals routinely use several pillows to elevate the head and torso while sleeping.

Maintaining neutral alignment of the head and spine in an obese patient necessitates the use of blankets, towels, or trauma padding stacked several inches high and placed under the patient's head before immobilizing the head. Carefully pad the void created between the neck and backboard. Adequately elevating the head to maintain neutral alignment will prevent hyperextension of the head and neck.

Do not force an obese patient onto a spine board that is too small for the patient. This poses a risk to both the rescuers and the patient. If the patient will not fit on the spine board, place him or her on an appropriately sized stretcher and eliminate as much spine movement as possible. Be sure to document the modified treatment plan in this situation; the diagnosis has not changed, just your treatment.

Helmet Removal

Helmet styles vary widely in size, configuration, and design, ranging from light head protection, such as a helmet worn by a bicyclist, to a motorcycle helmet, and to a helmet for a football player, which provides full facial protection with a solid cross piece at the level of the chin. Deciding whether to remove a helmet (along with other protective gear) can be a difficult decision. Removal can require quite a bit of head movement, especially if the helmet fits snugly. At the same time, many helmets force the patient's head and neck to flex forward if left in place while the patient lays supine.

Removing a helmet provides the ability to maintain neutral head position and easily gain access to the airway.

At times a helmet should obviously not be removed, such as in the case of an impaled object passing through both the helmet and the skull or an injured athlete wearing shoulder pads and a helmet. A generally accepted rule is that helmets worn without shoulder pads or other protective gear should be removed on scene before immobilization.

During the late 1990s the National Association of Athletic Trainers met with many groups, including the National Registry of Emergency Medical Technicians, to develop a list of recommended treatments for athletes who are spine injured and wearing helmets in addition to other protective gear (including shoulder pads). They developed the following list of recommendations (National Youth Sports Safety Foundation, 1998):

- All face masks should be removed before transport, regardless of current respiratory status.
- EMS systems regularly caring for helmeted athletes should have face mask removal equipment, heavy duty shears, and/or screwdrivers.
- Only remove the helmet and chin strap of a shoulder padded athlete when the following are true:
    - The helmet does not hold the head securely.
    - The airway cannot be controlled after face mask removal.
    - The face mask cannot be removed.
    - The helmet prevents transport in an appropriate position.
- If you will be removing helmets, practice the skill regularly.
- When possible, remove cheek padding or deflate air padding before removal.

To safely remove any helmet, one rescuer must assume manual stabilization of the patient's cervical spine. A second rescuer should pull the edges of the helmet away from the patient's head and slide the helmet so that the base follows the skull's natural curve until it can be pulled straight off (Figure 48-22). Avoid putting excess traction on the helmet because doing so may put traction on the head and neck. Once removed, apply a cervical collar and continue immobilization (Box 48-7).

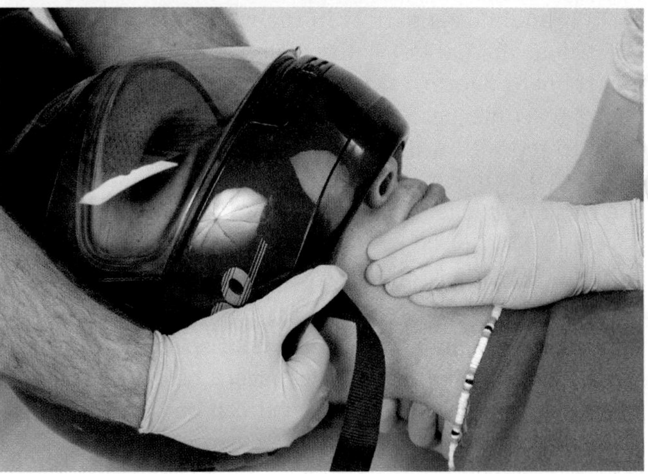

Figure 48-22 To safely remove a helmet, one rescuer must assume manual stabilization of the patient's cervical spine. A second rescuer should pull the edges of the helmet away from the patient's head and slide the helmet so that the base of the helmet follows the skull's natural curve until it can be pulled straight off.

BOX 48-7 Managing a Firefighter's Helmet

A potentially spine-injured firefighter wearing a breathing apparatus and full protective gear can be a challenge when removing the helmet, the face piece, and any protective hood. The helmet chin strap ordinarily is fastened last; therefore it should be unfastened first. If the firefighter is found prone, the "bill" on the back of the helmet will cause the head and neck to rotate either left or right and necessitates manual stabilization of the head until the helmet can be removed.

A regulator or pressure-reduction device fastens into the front of the face mask and must be disconnected to remove the mask. Most regulators trigger airflow when the pressure inside the mask changes negatively, causing a valve to open air to flow freely. Once the regulator is removed, expect air to escape forcibly and loudly until either the bottle is emptied or the regulator is set.

The straps of the mask will need to be loosened before removing the mask. The mask is designed to be worn snugly over the face, forming an airtight seal. Lift the mask slowly over the chin first, across the forehead, and away from the top of the head.

A Nomex hood often is worn over the head, under the straps of the mask and is easily removed, much like a ski mask.

Spinal Immobilization in Water

Immobilization in water should only be performed by rescuers specifically trained in the procedure. This includes professionals such as swift water rescue specialists, lifeguards, those trained in wilderness water safety, and water rescue teams. When you respond to a public pool–related injury, be prepared to find the patient already on a backboard. Since 2000 the American Red Cross has been teaching lifeguards to remove all patients from the water on a backboard—although not necessarily fully immobilized. If you do immobilize the patient in the water, pay close attention to his or her safety; if you drop the patient, he or she will sink with the board. Also remember that the patient will be wet and cold; be sure to dry him or her to the best of your ability and then cover the patient with blankets to maintain warmth. Simply covering the wet patient with blankets will not stop heat loss. Monitor for signs of mild hypothermia.

To immobilize a patient in the water, have several rescuers float the patient flat on the surface while you sink a backboard beneath the patient. Slowly allow the backboard to come up flat under the patient's back. If you need to reposition the board, sink it again. Do not slide the patient. Once properly positioned, completely secure the torso and legs to the long board and then the head.

PARAMEDIC*Pearl*

If immobilizing in the water, perform full spinal stabilization. Only partially immobilizing the patient before extrication from the water is a disservice and can be harmful to the patient because it allows excess movement.

ASSESSMENT AND MANAGEMENT OF NONTRAUMATIC SPINAL CONDITIONS

[OBJECTIVES 15 TO 21]

Back pain is one of the most common chief complaints EMS providers receive. A variety of conditions and diseases cause back pain; management of these problems focuses on providing comfort and reassurance and, when necessary, pain management.

Lower Back Pain

Acute and chronic lower back pain is a major problem in today's society. Lower back pain is responsible for more than 6 million annual emergency department visits (Perina, 2006). It affects nearly two thirds of the adult population and is one of the leading causes, and most expensive reasons, for missed days of work—especially for EMS providers. Unfortunately, less than 20% of lower back pain cases can be given a precise diagnosis. Frequently, though, it is caused by a musculoskeletal injury, ligament or tendon injury, or nerve root inflammation. Other more serious cases of lower back pain are cauda equina syndrome, metastasis of cancer (especially prostate cancer), and meningitis.

When evaluating nontraumatic lower back pain, be sure to obtain a thorough history. Determine when the pain started and how. Try to determine whether any sort of injury did occur. Ask what makes the pain better or worse. Stretching often relieves musculoskeletal pain. Establish the onset type and determine if it was gradual or sudden. Have the patient describe the pain. Examine the back and look for swelling, warmth, and signs of inflammation. Try to have the patient pinpoint one specific point of discomfort, if possible.

If no recent trauma caused the back pain, no immobilization is needed. Position the patient in as comfortable a position as possible and consider pharmaceutical management. Often a combination of pain relievers and muscle relaxants or sedatives provides the best relief. Spastic muscle pain may be relieved with medications such as diazepam. Always document vital signs and a pain scale rating before and after medication administration.

Degenerative Disk Disease

Among the leading causes for chronic lower back pain is degenerative disk disease, which is a combination of natural aging and degeneration of the intervertebral disks. Over time the degenerating disks go through three stages: dysfunction, instability, and restabilization. During the dysfunction stage the outer disk layers tear slightly, the disk loses some of its watery padding, and the disk may separate from the vertebrae. This presents with muscle contraction, tenderness, localized inflammation, and pain extending through the injured area (primarily the lumbar or cervical spines).

The instability stage develops as disk space decreases from fluid loss and reabsorption begins. Patients may report the sensation of their back "catching" and accessory bone movements. Back flexion often is quite difficult. Soon, however, restabilization begins as the disk hardens and stenosis sets in. Although pain substantially subsides, the back will become stiff, reduced movement will be noted, and scoliosis may be diagnosed (Kishner, 2006).

Prehospital management at any stage of degenerative disk disease is supportive. Consider pain management if the patient is in severe pain. Also spend time teaching patients proper body mechanics to help slow the disease process and prevent further injury.

Spondylosis

Spondylosis is the development of bony overgrowths along the anterior, lateral, and foramen sides of the vertebrae. In the lumbar and thoracic regions, spondylosis is generally asymptomatic; however, in the cervical region it can cause a variety of painful symptoms. As patients age, spondylosis develops in multiple intervertebral spaces and can cause neurologic dysfunction. It fact, it is the leading cause of atraumatic spinal cord dysfunction in patients older than 55 years old. As the bony growths develop, primarily where disk degeneration has occurred, they compress spinal nerves and the spinal cord. This leads to significant cervical neck pain and eventually can lead to peripheral sensory and motor dysfunction—particularly in the upper extremities. Patients often complain of occipital head pain radiating into the shoulders with a significant increase in pain on neck flexion and extension. Lhermitte's sign occurs when the patient also reports the sensation of electrical shooting in the neck on neck extension. Little can be done out of the hospital for spondylosis. In-hospital care focuses on comfort, rehabilitation, and potentially surgery. Many patients with chronic spondylosis are given antiinflammatory medications such as acetaminophen, corticosteroids, and analgesics (Galhom, 2005).

Herniated Intervertebral Disk

Disk herniation occurs when the inner nuclear materials of an intervertebral disk protrude out through the fibrous outer disk layers. This is typically caused by traumatic events, be it a single traumatic event or repeated abuse, such as from improper lifting. Herniated disks can be extremely painful and render patients nearly immobile. Patients often know they have this problem and receive treatment for it. When disk herniation occurs from a new traumatic event, it should be treated as a spine injury until proven otherwise; it is impossible to diagnose the difference in the prehospital setting (Ramachandran, 2006).

Patients often report extreme pain that may follow dermatomes (affected spinal nerve). The pain is often exacerbated by movement, spine flexion and extension, sneezing and coughing, and potentially leg movement.

Prehospital care is supportive. Provide pain management and transport in a position of comfort. Patients may be more comfortable seated, on the side, or supine.

Spinal Tumors

Spinal tumors (neoplasms) are an abnormal, rapid growth in the spinal foramen. If unrecognized, the patient can sustain devastating permanent damage. Cancerous tumors can originate within the spinal foramen; however, more than 85% of spinal neoplasms originate from metastatic cancers. Cancers known to metastasize to the spinal column include breast, prostate, renal, lung, lymphoma, and sarcoma (Huff, 2005).

As the neoplasm grows and begins to compress the spinal cord, slowly developing pain is the first symptom. As it continues to grow symptoms begin to mimic compression injuries, although the associated motor and sensory weakness often is unilateral. The neoplasm's location within the spinal foramen determines what kinds of specific symptoms develop. Brown-Séquard syndrome can develop. Other signs of neoplastic cord compression include bowel and bladder dysfunction, leg weakness, and a rapid loss in sensory skills (Huff, 2005).

Anticipate a spinal tumor whenever a patient has had gradually worsening atraumatic back pain and now has signs of cord injury, particularly when the patient has a cancer history. Provide supportive care and monitor the critical systems carefully. If the neoplasm is in the cervical column it could affect the respiratory drive (Huff, 2005).

MEDICATIONS USED IN SPINAL CORD INJURY MANAGEMENT

A variety of medications are used to provide long-term care for spinal cord injuries. Unfortunately, many of these medications are not intended for use by EMS professionals. However, at times medications may be indicated for SCI patients.

Steroids for Spinal Cord Injury

Corticosteroids have been beneficial in reducing swelling after an SCI and may help promote early healing. Some of the most commonly used corticosteroids include methylprednisolone (Solu-Medrol) and dexamethasone (Decadron, Hexadrol). In some areas early administration of high-dose methylprednisolone is used to reduce the severity of spinal cord injuries. Dexamethasone also is commonly used to help reduce morbidity after SCI and is preferred by some neurologists. When a corticosteroid is used, it must be initiated within 8 hours of the injury; in general, the earlier the administration the better.

Medications for Neurogenic and Spinal Shock

During both neurogenic and spinal shock, the patient loses control of sympathetic nervous system responses. This can cause profound hypotension and is further complicated by the patient's inability to compensate for the loss of blood pressure. Thus the patient will have hypotension and a normal to bradycardic heart rate. Pneumatic antishock garments and military antishock trousers have remained controversial at best; they are best accepted for the management of unstable pelvis fractures. Instead, initiate large-bore intravenous access and begin infusions of normal saline and/or Ringer's lactate. After a fluid bolus, recheck lung sounds and blood pressure. If the patient remains hypotensive and you believe no internal bleeding to be present, consider the use of vasopressors.

The most commonly used prehospital vasopressor is dopamine. A naturally occurring catecholamine, dopamine has its own effects and also causes the release of norepinephrine—one of the chemicals the body cannot release on its own after an SCI. Dopamine will increase cardiac contractility, cardiac output and, at high enough doses, can increase peripheral vascular resistance by causing vasoconstriction.

Controlling the Combative Patient

You have likely heard that if the patient is combative, then it is better to not immobilize than to try and force the combative patient onto a long spine board. This is a particularly common situation with the intoxicated patient as well as the patient who also has a traumatic brain injury. If you have reason to believe that the combative patient would greatly benefit from immobilization, consider obtaining medical control orders for intramuscular sedative medications. Intramuscular medications are indicated because generally the patient refusing immobilization will also refuse an intravenous line. Some effective intramuscular sedatives are midazolam (Versed), diazepam (Valium), haloperidol, and droperidol. Avoid using paralytics unless you plan to proceed to rapid-sequence intubation. Either way, only perform sedation for immobilization under orders from medical direction, if required in your system.

Case Scenario CONCLUSION

You begin to immobilize the patient. You roll the patient appropriately to the backboard. You notice that he has pain on palpation of the middle thoracic spinous processes. No obvious laceration is present. Once in the back of the ambulance, you prepare for transport to the receiving facility. During transportation you perform an extended secondary survey. The patient is able to move his arms. He has good flexion and extension of his elbows and wrists. Movement of his hands and fingers appears normal. The patient cannot move his legs. He is breathing regularly and his vital signs remain stable.

Questions

8. *What is important in the treatment of this patient?*
9. *What should be done for patient comfort?*
10. *More specifically, where do you think his injury is located with this added information?*

DOCUMENTING YOUR ASSESSMENT AND CARE OF THE SPINE-INJURED PATIENT

How you document the assessments and care for a patient with a spine injury and the mechanism for a spine injury is important. Your report must be thorough. Write your reports for all patients in a consistent manner; this will help prevent errors in documentation. Record initial assessment findings, vital signs, and routine physical examination findings. Document repeated vital signs measurements every 5 to 15 minutes based on patient stability.

Begin documenting the spine assessment by identifying the mechanism of injury; how the patient was found; and any history of the patient being ambulatory, moving, or being moved before EMS arrival. Clearly record that your patient was reliable (A&O×4, calm, sober, willing to cooperate, no distracting injuries). State in writing that the patient has a history clear of numbness, tingling, electrical shooting sensations, and spinal column pain. Document your specific spine examination and that no spine tenderness was present, how you assessed motor and sensory skills, and that they were both normal.

Anytime a patient fails the spine assessment and an injury is found, document whether you suspect a column injury, cord injury, or both. Expand on the extent of injury with associated findings (e.g., Babinski's sign, priapism). Document what tools were used in immobilization. The processes of immobilization do not need documentation because they are standard and assumed to be properly performed. In cases of obese patients, or when you immobilize in an atypical fashion, be sure to state clearly your reasons for doing so in writing.

If a patient refuses a spine assessment and immobilization, be sure to document thoroughly and have the patient sign all refusal forms. Even when patients accept transport, they need to state in writing that they refused a portion of standard care. Put this in writing and report it to the receiving facility's staff.

Case Scenario SUMMARY

1. *What are your initial thoughts regarding this patient?* This patient has fallen from a ladder. He is reporting pain in his back and an inability to move his legs. This patient should be treated seriously. In treating this patient, rapid assessment, treatment of injuries, and careful immobilization should not be delayed.
2. *What is your impression of the mechanism of injury?* This patient has fallen from a distance of approximately 20 feet. Even for a very tall man this is greater than three times his height. Any mechanism that delivers significant force should indicate suspected trauma, including SCI. Other injuries associated with SCI include the following:
   - An MVC with significant damage to either or any of the vehicles, intrusion into the driver or passenger compartment, engine displacement, bending of the vehicle frame, or vehicle rollover with ejection
   - An MVC in which the patient's head strikes the windshield
   - Ejection from a moving vehicle
   - A pedestrian struck by an automobile
   - Any motorcycle crash
   - In adults, a fall from greater than three times the patient's height
   - Contact sports injuries, such as in football, wrestling, or boxing
   - Shallow water diving injury
3. *What should be done for initial treatment?* Initial treatment should include cervical spine immobilization, oxygen supplementation, and treatment of

life-threatening injuries. With the patient's report of inability to move his legs, stabilization of his cervical spine as quickly as possible is important.

4. *Is this a primary or secondary cord injury?* Primary cord injuries directly result from the insult that the spinal column and cord experienced. They cause immediate mechanical disruption, distraction, or transection of the cord. Often limited damage is caused by a primary injury. During transport, you may notice the patient's symptoms begin to worsen. This is a sign of a secondary cord injury, often caused by bleeding, swelling, and ischemia. This patient obviously has a primary injury. This injury could become worse if secondary injury occurs. This will become apparent over the next hours to days.

5. *Discuss the significance of the left femur deformity.* Patients who sustain spinal cord trauma may lose sensation of other parts of the body. A primary and secondary survey must be conducted to detect any life-threatening injuries. On initial examination this patient has suffered a fall with loss of feeling in his legs. This does not preclude injury to the chest, abdomen, head, neck, or extremities. A femur fracture can result in significant blood loss, and identifying, treating, and monitoring this patient for signs of shock are vital.

6. *Where is his injury most likely located?* Typically a patient who has paraplegia has a lesion distal to T1, and a patient who has tetraplegia has a lesion above T1. Further description of injury location occurs after an investigation into motor function.

7. *Describe the differences between cord contusion, concussion, compression, laceration, and transaction.* Spinal cord concussions are similar to brain concussions in mechanism and manifestation. This type of injury can occur with some penetrating injuries (e.g., a gunshot wound) or as a result of a direct blow in sports or hand-to-hand combat (e.g., a knife-edge hand strike to the neck). They cause a transient (temporary) neurologic deficit, usually as a result of blunt trauma, in which the cord is stunned for a period. In general, no structural damage (column or cord) or permanent damage occurs. A contusion is soft tissue bruising. Thus a cord contusion is bruising of the spinal cord. This injury presents similarly to a cord concussion but symptoms persist for a longer period. Cord contusions indicate a more significant mechanism of injury and suggest some capillary bleeding within the spinal cord. Long-term residual effects usually do not occur. Both primary and secondary injuries can lead to spinal cord compression. Primary cord compression can occur with a crushed vertebra or intervertebral disk. Secondary cord compression occurs when soft tissues around the cord swell after an injury and compress the cord within the spinal column. Both mechanisms can cause ischemia to the compressed portion of the cord. If not corrected, this can lead to permanent damage. Any puncture wound, bone fragment, or knife wound can cause a cord laceration. Lacerations cut the cord's nerve bundles and also can cause significant bleeding and swelling—all within the spinal foramen. Even small lacerations can cause significant bleeding. The effects of the laceration can cause significant cord impairment. Small lacerations can lead to some recovery, especially when most damage is associated with swelling and bleeding. Large lacerations often lead to permanent cord damage and nervous system impairment. Hence, rolling the patient to check the back for signs of penetrating trauma is important. Injuries that completely cut across the spinal cord are known as complete cord transections. This injury completely eliminates the body's ability to send or receive nervous system impulses distal to the injury site. Complete cord transections are permanent, irreparable injuries that lead to paralysis.

8. *What is important in the treatment of this patient?* This patient should be appropriately immobilized, rolled for examination of his back, and readied for delivery to the emergency department. The femur fracture should be splinted. Pulses should be assessed at distal extremities. Supplemental oxygen should be supplied. Continual reassessment of vitals signs with careful attention to any signs of shock should be done. The patient should be in full spinal cord immobilization. The patient also should be protected for hypothermia.

9. *What should be done for patient comfort?* The patient should be given pain medication. The patient is not reporting pain from his femur fracture but is reporting back pain. With careful monitoring of blood pressure, morphine sulfate may be an appropriate choice for pain control. Local protocols must be followed. The patient also should be kept warm.

10. *More specifically, where do you think his injury is located with this added information?* See Table 48-2 for help locating the patient's injury. This patient has full movement of his arms, with good flexion and extension of the elbow and hands. He has no sensation or movement in his legs. His respiratory function appears to be intact and he does not mention fatigue. His injury is most likely located at T5-T9.

Chapter Summary

- The spinal column is composed of 33 vertebrae: seven cervical, 12 thoracic, five lumbar, five sacral, and four coccygeal.
- The spinal cord runs through the spinal foramen, beginning at the base of the skull and terminating between vertebrae L2 and L3 in adults at the conus medullaris.
- Many mechanisms can potentially injure a spinal column and cord; the EMS professional is responsible for determining when a mechanism is significant enough to cause injury and when it is not.
- Any patient who has a mechanism of injury for a spine injury must undergo a thorough spine assessment. If a spine assessment cannot be performed, fully immobilize the patient.
- A complete spine assessment includes determining patient reliability; evaluating the history for spine pain, numbness, tingling, or electrical shooting sensations; and performing a specific examination, evaluating for spine tenderness and specific motor and sensory skills.
- If a patient fails the spine assessment, immobilize the patient and document the findings; spine pain and tenderness indicate a column injury, whereas numbness, tingling, electrical shooting sensations, and impaired motor or sensory skills all indicate a cord injury.
- PMS (***p***ulses, ***m***ovement, and ***s***ensation) best evaluates musculoskeletal injuries, not spine injuries.
- When immobilizing a pediatric patient, remember to pad beneath the shoulders, not the head.
- Do not hesitate to place a patient in a lateral recumbent position while on the long board. You can safely immobilize a patient in that position; it simply takes additional padding.
- Provide ample padding to eliminate all terrible triangles.
- Secure the patient to a long board with Xs across the shoulders and chest, hips, and head and straps across the legs.
- Not all spine injuries are trauma related. If no trauma has occurred, immobilization is not indicated; look for and identify another cause.

REFERENCES

Campagnolo, D. I. (2006). *Autonomic dysreflexia in spinal cord injury*. Retrieved December 1, 2006, from http://www.emedicine.com.

Drake, R., Vogl, W., & Mitchell, A. (2005). *Gray's anatomy for students*. St. Louis: Elsevier.

Galhom, A. (2005). *Cervical spondylosis*. Retrieved December 4, 2006, from http://www.emedicine.com.

Gondim, F. de A. A. (2006). *Spinal cord trauma and related diseases*. Retrieved November 2, 2006, from http://www.emedicine.com.

Huff, J. S. (2005). *Spinal cord neoplasms*. Retrieved December 4, 2006, from http://www.emedicine.com.

Isaac, J., & Johnson, D. (2006). *Wilderness and rescue medicine*. Portland, ME: Wilderness Medical Associates.

Kahn, J. (2005). Spinal trauma. *Journal of Emergency Medical Services, 30,* 78-95.

Kishner, S. (2006). *Degenerative disk disease*. Retrieved December 4, 2006, from http://www.emedicine.com.

The National SCI Statistical Center. (2006). *Spinal cord injury: Facts and figures at a glance*. Retrieved June 8, 2006, from http://www.spinalcord.uab.edu.

National Youth Sports Safety Foundation. (1998). *Inter-association task force for appropriate care of the spine-injured athlete*. Retrieved December 1, 2006, from http://www.nyssf.org.

Perina, D. (2006). *Mechanical back pain*. Retrieved December 4, 2006, from http://www.emedicine.com.

Ramachandran, T. S. (2006). *Disk herniation*. Retrieved December 4, 2006, from http://www.emedicine.com.

Russell, S., & Triola, M. (2006). *The precise neurological exam*. Retrieved March 26, 2008, from http://www.edinfo.med.nyu.edu.

Sanders, M., & McKenna, K. (2005). *Mosby's paramedic textbook* (3rd ed.). St: Louis: Elsevier.

Schreiber, D. (2006). *Spinal cord injuries*. Retrieved November 15, 2006, from http://www.emedicine.com.

SUGGESTED RESOURCES

Butman, A., Martin, S., Vomacka, R., & McSwain, N. Jr. (1996). *Comprehensive guide to pre-hospital skills: A skills manual for EMT-Basic, EMT-Intermediate, EMT-Paramedic*. St. Louis: Mosby.

Haskell, G., & Vokshoor, A. (2006). Primum non nocere—First, do no harm: The importance of neutral spinal alignment for patients of all sizes. *Journal of Emergency Medical Services, 31,* 77-81.

National Association of Emergency Medical Technicians. (2006). *PHTLS: Basic and advanced life support* (6th ed.). St. Louis: Mosby.

Maine Emergency Medical Services Spine Assessment Program (2002). Retrieved March 28, 2008, from http://mainegov-images.informe.org.

U.S. Department of Transportation. (1998). *EMT-Paramedic national standard curriculum*. Washington, DC: National Highway Traffic Safety Administration.

Chapter Quiz

1. You arrive at the scene of an MVC on a state highway to find a 29-year-old man partially ejected onto the hood of a car. He is prone on the hood and his lower torso is entangled in wreckage. You should ________.
   - **a.** manually stabilize the head and neck in the position found
   - **b.** begin a rapid extrication sequence
   - **c.** attempt to turn the patient to the supine position
   - **d.** apply a cervical collar

2. You are called to an alley where a 35-year-old man has fallen 40 feet from a scaffold. During assessment you note he has no sensation from the nipple line down. An SCI has most likely occurred in what area of the spine?
   - **a.** C3
   - **b.** C7
   - **c.** T4
   - **d.** L1

3. When palpating the spinal column along a patient's back, you are palpating which part of the vertebrae?
   - **a.** The vertebral body
   - **b.** The spinous process
   - **c.** The vertebral foramen
   - **d.** The intravertebral disk

4. C2 is also known as the ________.
   - **a.** atlas
   - **b.** atlantis
   - **c.** tailbone
   - **d.** axis

5. C2 is a unique vertebra because it ________.
   - **a.** has an odontoid process that allows the head to pivot in any direction
   - **b.** has an abnormally large vertebral body to protect the spinal cord because it is at the base of the skull
   - **c.** lies just below the end of the spinal cord
   - **d.** is the first true vertebra in the spinal column

6. You are on scene managing a patient with a suspected cervical spine injury with cord involvement. The patient is reporting numbness and tingling in all four extremities with pain and tenderness in C4 and C5 after a head-first fall off a 15-foot roof. The patient is supine with the head facing the right shoulder. Which is the appropriate first step in treating this patient?
   - **a.** You should immobilize the head in place because straightening the neck decreases the vertebral foramen diameter, which could worsen the cord injury.
   - **b.** You do not need to provide any immobilization because less than 2% of column injuries are unstable and you risk further injury.
   - **c.** You should straighten the head and neck, which maximizes the vertebral foramen space and gives the spinal cord room to swell.

7. In the adult patient you would expect to find the conus medullaris ________.
   - **a.** between T12 and L1
   - **b.** between L1 and L2
   - **c.** between L4 and L5
   - **d.** between L5 and S1

8. Dermatomes are ________.
   - **a.** areas of skin innervated by a single spinal nerve
   - **b.** areas of skin innervated by a group of spinal nerves
   - **c.** areas of muscle innervated by a single spinal nerve
   - **d.** groups of skin, muscle, vessels, and fat innervated by a single spinal nerve

9. When evaluating nerve endings in a specific dermatome you should evaluate ________.
   - **a.** numbness, tingling, sensation of sharp and soft, and motor skill
   - **b.** numbness, tingling, and motor skills
   - **c.** sensation of sharp and soft
   - **d.** sensation of vibration and deep pressure

10. If you cannot decide if a patient's injury mechanism was significant enough to injure the spine, you should ________.
    - **a.** decide that the spine is likely uninjured, only if the patient is ambulatory
    - **b.** decide that the spine is likely injured, even if the patient is ambulatory
    - **c.** decide that the spine is likely uninjured, regardless of patient position
    - **d.** perform a full spine assessment

11. True or False: Evaluating PMS is an important component in the detailed spine assessment.

12. While performing a spine assessment on a 10-year-old boy who fell from his bike, the patient begins reporting pain along the right side of his neck. You have already determined that he has no spine pain or tenderness and no numbness or tingling. At this point, you ________.
    - **a.** continue to test motor and sensory skills in all extremities, and if they are normal, clear the spine
    - **b.** stop your assessment and declare he has a spine injury
    - **c.** stop your assessment after checking PMS and clearing his spine
    - **d.** complete the assessment and completely immobilize the patient regardless of findings

13. You should perform a spine assessment ________.
    - **a.** after managing all other immediate life threats
    - **b.** during your physical examination to save time
    - **c.** during transport to the hospital
    - **d.** after completing the physical examination and managing any distracting injuries

Chapter Quiz—continued

14. Which of the following patients does not pass the spine assessment and needs immobilization?

a. A 19-year-old man involved in a driving while intoxicated MVC with no complaints, no spine tenderness, and intact motor sensory skills.

b. A 94-year-old man with a history of two previous spinal fractures. The patient reports right flank pain after a fall down a flight of stairs. He has no spine pain or tenderness and no numbness or tingling. Motor skills are intact and he can differentiate sharp and soft sensations in all extremities except for his right foot, which he says is a normal finding since his last spine injury.

c. A 37-year-old woman, 8.5 months pregnant, reporting severe right knee pain after an MVC. A deformity to the knee is obvious, with a loss of PMS distal to the injury site.

d. A 22-year-old woman with mild dizziness after striking her head against a desk with loss of consciousness after tripping on a rug. The patient is A&O×4, has a clear history, and a clear physical examination.

15. An example of a distraction injury is ________.

a. a head-first fall down a flight of stairs

b. a hanging

c. having the head snap sideways as it strikes the corner of a desk during a fall

d. having a steel pole fall against the cervical spine

16. Spinal cord injuries developing some time after the initial traumatic event are called ________.

a. primary cord injuries

b. delayed-onset cord injuries

c. secondary cord injuries

d. swelling

Terminology

Anterior cord syndrome Collection of symptoms seen after the compression, death, or transection of the anterior portion of the spinal cord.

Atlas First cervical vertebra.

Autonomic dysreflexia syndrome A condition characterized by hypertension superior to an SCI site caused by overstimulation of the sympathetic nervous system.

Axial loading Application of excessive pressure or weight along the vertical axis of the spine.

Axis Second cervical vertebrae.

Babinski's sign An abnormal finding indicated by the presence of great toe extension with the fanning of all other toes on stimulation of the sole of the foot when it is stroked with a semi-sharp object from the heel to the ball of the foot.

Brown-Séquard syndrome Group of symptoms that develop after the herniation or transection of half of the spinal cord manifested with unilateral damage.

Cauda equina Peripheral nerve bundles descending through the spinal column distal to the conus medullaris. Cauda equina are not spinal nerves.

Cauda equina syndrome Complications, such as back pain, resulting from injury to the cauda equina.

Central cord syndrome Collection of symptoms seen after the death of the central portion of the spinal cord.

Cervical vertebrae First seven vertebrae in descending order from the base of the skull.

CNS-PAD An acronym for central nervous system padding: ***p***ia mater, ***a***rachnid mater, ***d***ura mater.

Coccyx (coccygeal vertebrae) Terminal end of the spinal column; a tail-like bone composed of three to five vertebra. No nerve roots travel through the coccyx.

Conus medullaris Terminal end of the spinal cord.

Conus medullaris syndrome Complications resulting from injury to the conus medullaris.

Dermatome An area of skin innervated by a given spinal nerve to give that skin sensory capabilities.

Distracting injury An injury that occupies the patient's attention and focus. The injury causes significant enough pain that the patient may not feel pain from other injuries, particular spine injuries.

Free nerve endings Most common type of dermal nerve ending; responsible for sensing pain, temperature, and pressure.

Hangman's fracture A fracture of the axis, the second cervical vertebra. This may occur with or without axis dislocation.

Hyperextension Extension beyond a joint's normal range of motion.

Hyperflexion Flexion beyond a joint's normal range of motion.

Incomplete cord transection A partial cutting (severing) of the spinal cord in which some cord function remains distal to the injury site.

Lumbar vertebrae Vertebrae of the lower back that do not attach to any ribs and are superior to the pelvis.

Meissner corpuscle Encapsulated nerve endings in the superficial dermis responsible for sensing vibrations and light touch.

Myotome A muscle group innervated by a single spinal nerve, giving it the ability to flex and extend; similar to a dermatome.

Neurogenic shock Shock with hypotension caused by a sudden loss of control over the sympathetic nervous system. Loss can be caused by a variety of mechanisms from traumatic injury to disease and infection.

Paraplegia Paralysis of the lower extremities. The injury can either be complete (a complete loss of muscle control and sensation below the injury site) or incomplete (a partial loss of muscle control or sensation below the injury site).

Priapism A persistent, painful erection associated with injury of the spinal cord caused by lack of inhibition of parasympathetic stimulation from the loss of sympathetic tone and not associated with sexual arousal.

Primary cord injury An SCI caused by a direct traumatic blow.

Proprioception Ability to sense the orientation, location, and movement of the body's parts relative to other body parts.

Quadriplegia See *Tetraplegia*.

Sacrum (sacral vertebrae) A heavy, large bone at the base of the spinal cord between the lumbar vertebrae and the coccyx. Roughly triangular in shape, it comprises the back of the pelvis and is made of the five sacral vertebrae fused together.

Secondary cord injury An SCI that develops over time after a traumatic injury to the spinal column or the blood vessels that supply the spinal cord with blood. Generally caused by ischemia, swelling, or compression.

Spinal cord injury (SCI) An injury to the spinal cord that results from trauma; usually a permanent injury.

Spinal cord injury without radiological abnormality (SCIWORA) An SCI not detected on a standard radiograph.

Spinal nerves A total of 31 pairs of nerves that leave the spinal column that affect specific dermatomes and myotomes throughout the body.

Spinal shock Shock with hypotension caused by an injury to the spinal cord.

Supine hypotensive syndrome A fall in the pregnant patient's blood pressure when she is placed supine; caused by the developing fetus and uterus pressing against the inferior vena cava.

Tetraplegia Paralysis to all four extremities as a result of an SCI high in the spine. The injury can either be complete (a complete loss of muscle control and sensation below the injury site) or incomplete (a partial loss of muscle control or sensation below the injury site).

Thoracic vertebrae A group of 12 vertebrae in the middle of the spinal column that connect to ribs.

Transection A complete cutting (severing) across the spinal cord.

Vertebrae Specialized bones comprising the spinal column.

Vertebral foramen Open space in the middle of vertebra.

CHAPTER 49

Thoracic Trauma

Objectives

After completing this chapter, you will be able to:

1. Explain the relevance of thoracic injuries as a part of overall mortality rate from major trauma.
2. List the thoracic injuries that may result in early death if left untreated in the prehospital setting.
3. Describe the incidence, morbidity, and mortality rates of thoracic injuries in the trauma patient.
4. Discuss the types of thoracic injuries.
5. Discuss the anatomy and physiology of the organs and structures related to thoracic injuries.
6. Discuss the pathophysiology of thoracic injuries.
7. Discuss the assessment findings associated with thoracic injuries.
8. Discuss the management of thoracic injuries.
9. Identify the need for rapid intervention and transport of the patient with thoracic injuries.
10. Discuss the management of chest wall injuries.
11. Describe the impact of rib fractures on oxygenation and ventilation.
12. Predict thoracic injuries on the basis of mechanism of injury.
13. Discuss the pathophysiology of specific chest wall injuries, including the following:
    - Rib fracture
    - Flail segment
    - Sternal fracture
14. Discuss the management of lung injuries.
15. Explain the physiologic consequences of flail chest.
16. Discuss the assessment findings associated with chest wall injuries.
17. Identify the need for rapid intervention and transport of the patient with lung injuries.
18. Discuss the pathophysiology of traumatic asphyxia.
19. Discuss the assessment findings associated with traumatic asphyxia.
20. Discuss the management of traumatic asphyxia.
21. Identify the need for rapid intervention and transport of the patient with traumatic asphyxia.
22. Discuss the assessment findings associated with lung injuries.
23. Discuss the pathophysiology of injury to the lung, including the following:
    - Simple pneumothorax
    - Open pneumothorax
    - Tension pneumothorax
    - Hemothorax
    - Hemopneumothorax
    - Pulmonary contusion
24. Define *pneumothorax* and *hemothorax*.
25. List the signs and symptoms of a tension pneumothorax.
26. Identify the need for rapid intervention and transport of the patient with chest wall injuries.
27. Discuss the pathophysiology of tracheobronchial injuries.
28. Discuss the assessment findings associated with tracheobronchial injuries.
29. Discuss the management of tracheobronchial injuries.
30. Identify the need for rapid intervention and transport of the patient with tracheobronchial injuries.
31. Discuss the pathophysiology of myocardial injuries, including the following:
    - Pericardial tamponade
    - Myocardial contusion
    - Myocardial rupture
32. Discuss the assessment findings associated with myocardial injuries.
33. Discuss the management of myocardial injuries.
34. Define *Beck's triad.*
35. Identify the need for rapid intervention and transport of the patient with myocardial injuries.
36. Describe the pathophysiology of aortic rupture.
37. Discuss the pathophysiology of vascular injuries, including injuries to the following:
    - Aorta
    - Venae cavae
    - Pulmonary arteries and veins
38. Discuss the assessment findings associated with vascular injuries.
39. Discuss the management of vascular injuries.
40. Identify the need for rapid intervention and transport of the patient with vascular injuries.
41. Discuss the pathophysiology of diaphragmatic injuries.
42. Discuss the assessment findings associated with diaphragmatic injuries.
43. Discuss the management of diaphragmatic injuries.
44. Identify the need for rapid intervention and transport of the patient with diaphragmatic injuries.
45. Discuss the pathophysiology of esophageal injuries.
46. Discuss the assessment findings associated with esophageal injuries.
47. Discuss the management of esophageal injuries.
48. Identify the need for rapid intervention and transport of the patient with esophageal injuries.

Chapter Outline

Case Scenario

You are called to an apartment complex for a cardiac arrest. When you arrive, you find fire department EMTs performing cardiopulmonary resuscitation (CPR) on a man who looks to be approximately 25 years old. According to fire department personnel and bystanders, the man was working under his car when the jacks failed, causing the car to pin the patient to the ground. He called for help. His neighbors responded and somehow got the car back on the jacks. Before the man could get out from under the car, it fell a second time, rendering him unresponsive. He was unresponsive when the fire department arrived and was in cardiac arrest when they extricated him.

Questions

1. *What potential causes of cardiac arrest can you think of in this case?*
2. *What physical assessment findings would be most useful to differentiate these causes?*
3. *What treatment should be immediately initiated?*

[OBJECTIVES 1, 2, 3, 4]

Thoracic injuries directly account for 20% to 25% of deaths from trauma, resulting in more than 16,000 deaths annually in the United States (LoCicero & Mattox, 1989). The most common cause of injuries leading to accidental deaths in the United States is motor vehicle crashes (MVCs). In these crashes, immediate deaths are usually attributable to a rupture of the heart or the thoracic aorta. Early deaths (within the first 30 minutes to 3 hours) from thoracic trauma often are preventable. These early deaths occur from tension pneumothorax, cardiac tamponade, airway obstruction, and continued uncontrolled hemorrhage. In the prehospital setting these problems often are reversible or may be temporized. Therefore you must be able to recognize and treat them in the field.

Among the victims sustaining thoracic trauma, approximately 50% will have chest wall injury: 10% minor, 35% major, and 5% flail chest injuries (LoCicero & Mattox, 1989). Injuries to the lung tissue are reported in 25% of patients. These injuries include contusion, laceration, or hematoma. Hemothorax and pneumothorax also are common injuries in patients with thoracic trauma.

CHEST WALL INJURY

[OBJECTIVES 5 TO 10]

An intact chest wall is necessary for normal ventilation. However, it is the most commonly injured area of the thorax. Because chest wall injuries are not always obvious, you can easily overlook them. Chest trauma, particularly blunt trauma, can severely disturb the physiology of respiration. Fortunately, most individuals have substantial respiratory reserve and can tolerate significant chest wall injury with adequate support.

Older patients or those with preexisting respiratory problems (e.g., chronic obstructive pulmonary disease) are sometimes unable to compensate for even minor chest wall trauma. Therefore you will need to monitor these patients closely and consider transporting them to a trauma center.

Observing the patient's respiratory effort and calculating the respiratory rate, the adequacy of his or her tidal volume, and the overall work of breathing are important tasks. Many chest wall injuries can only be detected by carefully palpating the chest wall, noting any areas of deformity, tenderness, or crepitus.

Rib Fracture

[OBJECTIVES 11, 12, 13]

Description and Definition

Simple rib fractures are the most common form of significant chest injury. They account for more than half of the cases of blunt chest trauma. The importance of this injury is not the fracture itself but the associated potential complications.

Epidemiology and Demographics

Rib fractures occur more commonly in adults than in children. This is attributed to the relative inelasticity of the older chest wall compared with the more compliant nature of the chest wall in children. The true danger of rib fracture involves not the rib itself, but the potential for penetrating injury to the pleura, lung, liver, or spleen. Parenchymal injuries, such as pulmonary lacerations, can be caused by fractured ribs and possibly rapid deceleration (Sawyer & Sawyer, 2006).

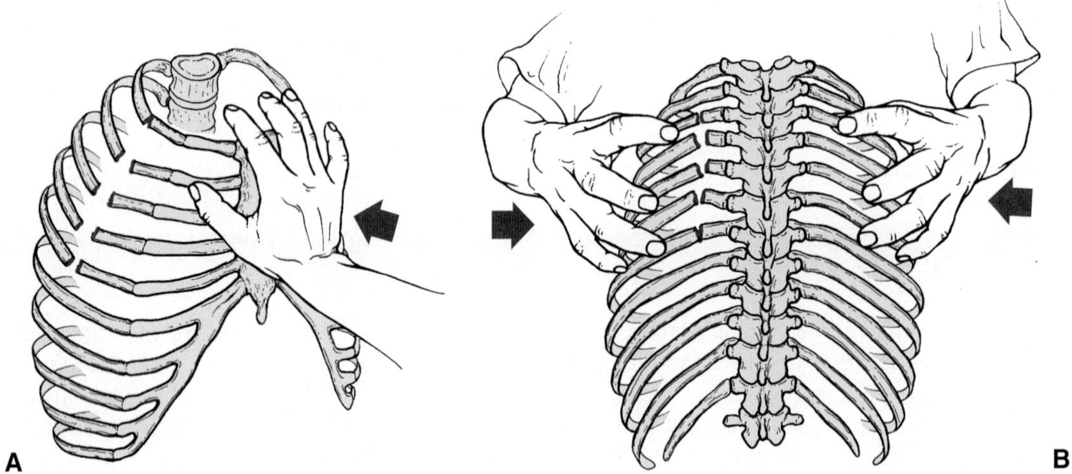

Figure 49-1 Mechanisms of injury that produce rib fractures. **A,** Anteroposterior compression of the chest most commonly results in fractures of the ribs laterally. **B,** Compression of the ribs from the side, however, produces posterior rib fractures. This mechanism of injury is most commonly seen in infants who have been grasped and shaken with side-to-side compression of the infant by an adult's hands.

Ribs usually break at the point of impact or at the posterior angle, which is structurally the weakest area (Figure 49-1). The fourth through ninth ribs are most commonly fractured because they are thin and poorly protected.

Fractures of the first to third ribs suggest high-velocity trauma because they are mostly protected by the clavicle, scapula, and muscles of the upper chest wall (Miller, 2006). Fractures of these ribs may indicate severe intrathoracic injury, such as rupture of the aorta, tracheobronchial tree injury, injury to the brachial plexus, and subclavian vessel injury (Figure 49-2).

Fractures of the lower ribs (ninth, tenth, and eleventh ribs) suggest an associated intraabdominal injury. A left lower rib injury has an increased probability of associated splenic injury. A right lower rib injury has an increased probability of liver injury. When posterior rib fractures occur, the fifth through ninth ribs are most frequently injured. Lower posterior rib fractures are associated with spleen and kidney injury.

An open rib fracture may be associated with visceral injury. The presence of two or more rib fractures at any level is associated with a higher incidence of internal injuries. Multiple rib fractures may result in atelectasis, hypoventilation, inadequate cough, and/or pneumonia.

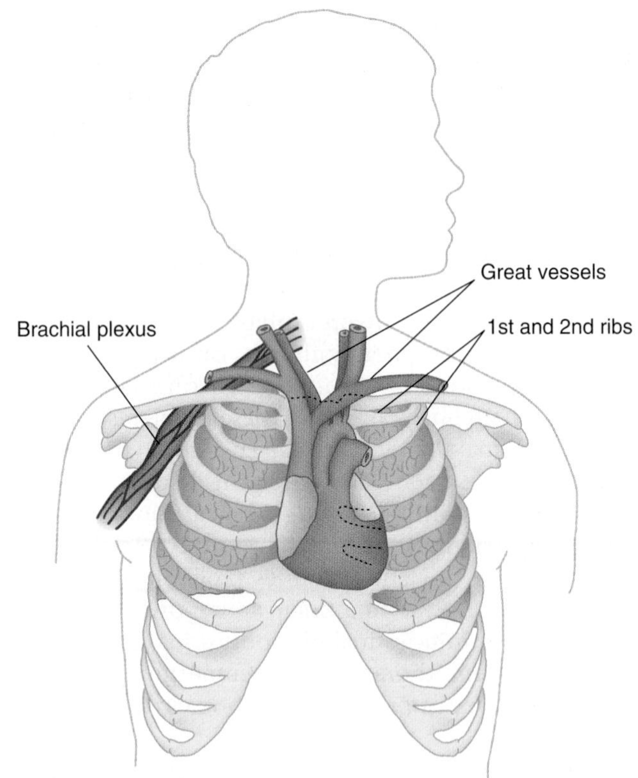

Figure 49-2 The relation of the first through third ribs to the brachial plexus, great vessels, heart, and lungs.

History and Physical Findings

Suspect the presence of rib fractures if you note the presence of tenderness, bony crepitus, ecchymosis, and muscle spasm over the ribs. Also, the compression of the involved rib remote from the site of injury usually produces pain at the site of fracture. Box 49-1 lists other assessment findings associated with rib fractures.

Therapeutic Interventions

When you suspect a rib fracture, strongly consider transporting the patient to a trauma center. Because pain and decreased ventilatory function occur with even minor chest wall trauma, pay careful attention to

BOX 49-1 Rib Fractures: Assessment Findings

- Localized pain
- Pain that worsens with movement, deep breathing, or coughing
- Point tenderness
- Crepitus or audible crunching
- Splinting on respiration
- Anteroposterior pressure that elicits pain

the patient's respiratory status while he or she is in your care.

The prehospital treatment of patients with a simple acute rib fracture is based on providing adequate pain relief and maintaining pulmonary function. Administer oxygen, apply a pulse oximeter, and provide positive-pressure ventilation if needed. Capnography should be used if available. Encourage coughing and deep breathing. Do not use binders, belts, or other restrictive devices. Although they can decrease pain, they also promote hypoventilation, with subsequent atelectasis and pneumonia. You may give opiate analgesics, such as morphine, intravenously (refer to local protocols). Take particular care to avoid oversedation, especially in older patients. Also be aware of the potential for opiates to cause hypoventilation and/or hypotension, which typically responds to a fluid challenge of normal saline. The administration of opiates also may mask other signs and symptoms.

Sternal Fracture and Dislocation

[OBJECTIVES 13, 14]

Description and Definition

Sternal fractures and dislocations are caused by anterior blunt chest trauma. Examples of such trauma include a blow to the chest, severe hyperflexion of the thoracic cage, and deceleration compression injury (as in an automobile crash when the chest strikes the steering wheel or dashboard). During rapid deceleration from a frontal impact, the forward thrust of the body against the fixed seatbelt across the sternum results in a fracture at that location. The location of the sternal fracture can vary. It depends on the position of the belt, patient size, magnitude of the impact, and vector of the forces (Eckstein & Henderson, 2006) (Figure 49-3).

Epidemiology and Demographics

The mortality rate associated with sternal fractures has been reported to be as high as 25% to 45%. The deaths largely result from myocardial or lung injury, such as myocardial contusion, myocardial rupture, or pulmonary contusion. Associated injuries that can cause morbidity and mortality include the following:

- Pulmonary and myocardial contusion
- Flail chest
- Vascular disruption of thoracic vessels

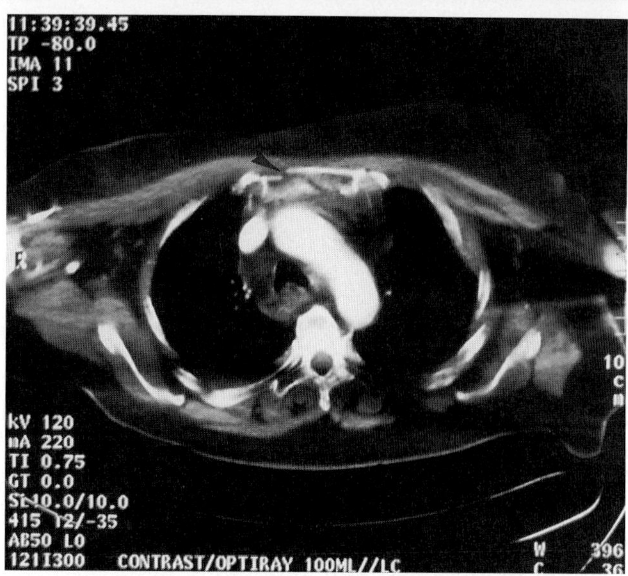

Figure 49-3 Computed tomography of sternal fracture *(arrowhead).*

BOX 49-2 Sternal Fracture: Assessment Findings

- History of blunt anterior chest trauma
- Localized anterior chest pain
- Point tenderness over the sternum
- Soft tissue swelling
- Palpable deformity
- Crepitus
- Tachypnea
- ECG changes associated with myocardial contusion

- Intraabdominal injuries
- Head injuries

Restrained passengers are more likely than unrestrained passengers to sustain a sternal fracture. The occurrence of sternal fractures has increased threefold since the use of across-the-shoulder seatbelts became widespread (Eckstein & Henderson, 2006). However, the risks of not using shoulder belts far outweigh the risks associated with them.

History and Physical Findings

The chief concern for sternal injury is not for the fracture itself but for the possibility of myocardial contusion, cardiac rupture, tamponade, or pulmonary injury. Point tenderness, crepitus, deformity, and pain over the sternum, in combination with an appropriate history, should lead you to suspect a sternal fracture. Box 49-2 lists other signs and symptoms of a sternal fracture.

Therapeutic Interventions

All patients with a suspected sternal fracture should be evaluated in a trauma center to identify and treat any potentially serious associated underlying injuries. You should administer oxygen, apply a pulse oximeter, and provide positive-pressure ventilation if needed. Capnography should be used if available. Because of the possibility of a myocardial contusion, place the patient on a cardiac monitor. You may give opiate analgesics, such as morphine, by intravenous (IV) administration as needed for pain, in consultation with medical direction.

Flail Chest

[OBJECTIVES 13, 15]

Description and Definition

Flail chest results when two or more adjacent ribs are fractured at two points, allowing a freely moving segment of the chest wall to move in paradoxic motion (Figure 49-4). It is one of the most commonly overlooked injuries resulting from blunt chest trauma. Because of its common association with pulmonary contusion, it also is one of the most serious chest wall injuries.

The physiologic functions of respiration are adversely affected in a number of ways by flail chest. The flail segment paradoxically moves inward with inspiration and outward with expiration. This is because of the lack of bony support and in response to the changes of intrathoracic pressures relative to atmospheric pressure during the respiratory cycle (Figure 49-5). This pathologic motion has a compound effect on ventilation. The inward movement of the segment compresses the lung beneath it. This creates decreased ventilation on the side of the injury and a shift of the mediastinum to the opposite side. This, in turn, compresses the normal (uninjured) side, decreasing ventilation and reducing venous return to the heart.

Epidemiology and Demographics

The mortality rate of flail chest is reported to be between 8% and 35%. Moreover, death is directly related to the underlying and associated injuries. Those who recover may develop long-term disability with dyspnea, chronic thoracic pain, and exercise intolerance.

History and Physical Findings

Flail chest may be recognized on physical examination. This requires you to expose the patient's chest and examine the chest wall closely for paradoxic motion, which is the hallmark of this condition. In addition, the pain of the injury causes muscular splinting, reduced chest expansion, and subsequent hypoventilation. Muscular splinting of the chest early in the postinjury period may mask the paradoxic motion until the flail becomes apparent hours later with the development of fatigue (Wanek & Mayberry, 2004). Underlying pulmonary contusion (bruising of the lung) is considered the major cause of respiratory insufficiency with flail chest. Other signs and symptoms of flail chest are given in Box 49-3.

Therapeutic Interventions

The prehospital stabilization of the flail segment by positioning the person with the injured side down or by placing a sandbag on the affected segment has been

BOX 49-3 Flail Chest: Assessment Findings

- Chest wall contusion
- Respiratory distress
- Paradoxic chest wall movement
- Pleuritic chest pain
- Crepitus
- Pain and splinting of affected side
- Tachypnea
- Tachycardia

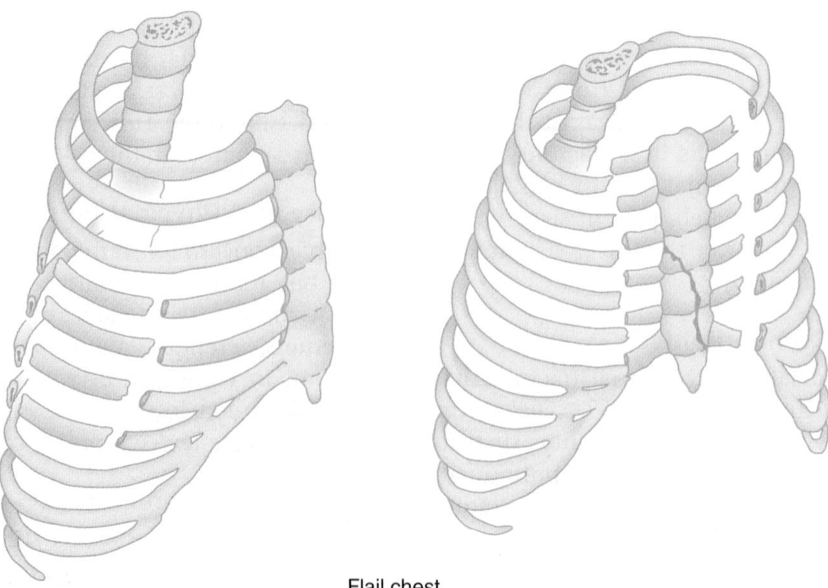

Figure 49-4 Fracture of several adjacent ribs in two places with lateral flail or central flail segments.

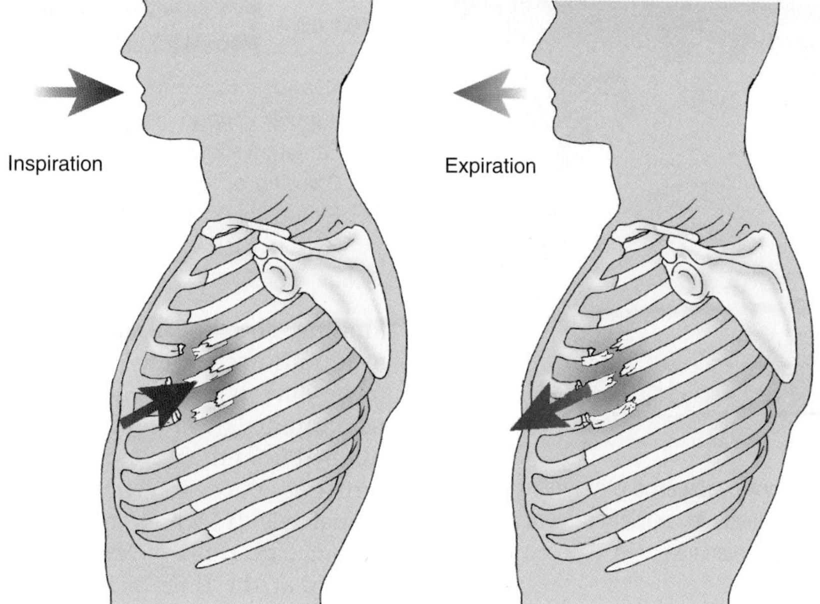

Figure 49-5 During inhalation, the flail segment is pulled inward by negative intrathoracic pressure. With exhalation, positive pressure forces the segment to protrude outward, impairing the ability to exhale.

abandoned (Pepe & Eckstein, 1998). These interventions actually inhibit expansion of the chest. They also increase atelectasis of the injured lung (Eckstein & Henderson, 2006). Administer high-flow oxygen and perform continuous cardiac monitoring and pulse oximetry. Furthermore, closely observe the patient for rapid deterioration in the field as a result of respiratory failure or an associated injury, such as a tension pneumothorax. Respiratory failure is the primary indication for endotracheal intubation for patients with suspected flail chest. For those EMS systems where it is available, continuous positive airway pressure by mask may avert the need for intubation in the awake and cooperative patient.

Nonpenetrating Ballistic Injury

[OBJECTIVE 10]

Description and Definition

Many law enforcement officers, prehospital professionals, and private security guards now wear lightweight synthetic body armor to protect themselves against gunshot injury. These vests are bullet resistant rather than bulletproof, depending on the weapon being used. They are made of many different combinations of synthetic fibers, such as Kevlar. These vests are usually capable of stopping penetration by the low-velocity missiles of most handguns. However, the kinetic energy of the missile can still be transmitted through the layers of protective cloth or armor and produce significant injury without penetration. Although bullet penetration is prevented, the heart, liver, spleen, lung, and spinal cord are vulnerable to nonpenetrating ballistic injury that may occur, despite innocent-appearing skin lesions.

History and Physical Findings

Patients who have been shot with nonlethal projectiles (e.g., rubber bullets, beanbag shotgun shells) or with standard bullets while wearing bullet-resistant vests usually present with redness, bruising, and marked tenderness to palpation over the impacted area (Eckstein & Henderson, 2006). Carefully palpate the area of tenderness and surrounding structures to identify any subcutaneous emphysema, crepitus, or bony step-offs.

Therapeutic Interventions

Transport all victims of nonpenetrating ballistic injury to a hospital for close observation and monitoring. Protective body armor has significantly improved survival rates and has dramatically decreased the need for surgical intervention in those wearing it. However, do not underestimate the possibility of an underlying injury resulting from this new form of nonpenetrating ballistic injury.

Traumatic Asphyxia

[OBJECTIVES 16 TO 21]

Description and Definition

Traumatic asphyxia is a syndrome characterized by a deep purple color of the skin of the head and neck, bilateral subconjunctival hemorrhage, petechiae, and facial edema.

Etiology

Traumatic asphyxia is caused by severe compression of the chest by an extremely heavy object. The compressive forces cause a marked increase in pressure in the chest and the superior vena cava. This results in the backflow

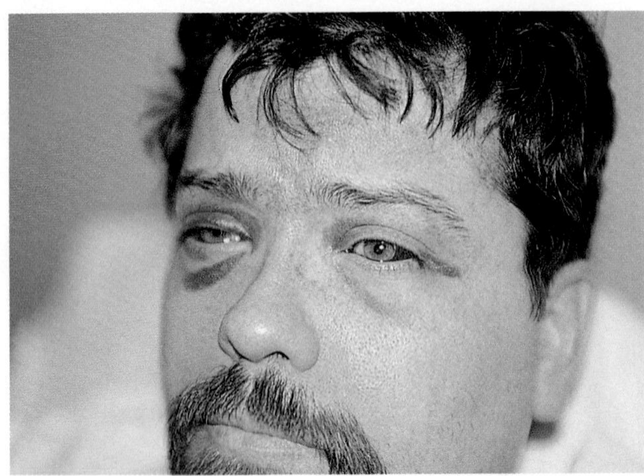

Figure 49-6 In traumatic asphyxia, increased pressure in the capillaries of the head and neck leads to capillary rupture and the characteristic facial swelling and petechiae.

of blood from the right heart into the great veins of the head and neck. The venae cavae and large veins of the head and neck are without valves. This allows pressure to be transmitted to the capillaries of the head and neck, which become engorged with blood (Figure 49-6). The blood begins to stagnate. As the blood decreases in oxygen content, the skin becomes purplish in discoloration.

History and Physical Findings

Although the appearance of these patients can be quite dramatic, the condition itself is usually benign and self-limiting. The clinical significance lies with the possibility of intrathoracic injury from the violent force necessary to produce traumatic asphyxia. Chest wall and pulmonary injuries are most common. Visual disturbances have resulted from these conditions, usually from retinal hemorrhage, which is generally a permanent injury, and retinal edema, which may cause transient changes in vision. One third of these patients lose consciousness, usually at the time of injury. Intracranial hemorrhages are rare. The signs and symptoms of traumatic asphyxia are shown in Box 49-4.

BOX 49-4 Traumatic Asphyxia: Assessment Findings

- Cyanosis to the face and upper neck
- Jugular venous distention
- Facial swelling
- Swelling or hemorrhage of the conjunctiva
- Skin below compressed area remains pink
- Hypotension when compressive force released

Therapeutic Interventions

A patient with traumatic asphyxia should be evaluated in a trauma center to identify and treat any potentially serious associated underlying injuries. Administer high-flow oxygen with continuous cardiac monitoring and pulse oximetry. Establish IV access. Expect hypotension once the compressive force is released. Determine the rate of fluid administration in consultation with medical direction.

Case Scenario—continued

Your assessment confirms that the patient is apneic and pulseless. You note that the skin is splotchy in appearance on the upper chest, neck, and face. No visible trauma is evident, with the exception of some abrasions. The cardiac monitor reveals a slow, wide QRS rhythm that does not produce a pulse. The patient's pupils are fixed and dilated. You direct the fire department to continue CPR as your partner establishes an IV and you prepare to intubate the patient. After approximately 1 minute of additional CPR, the cardiac rhythm changes to sinus tachycardia and the patient has a palpable pulse. At this time his pulse is 98 beats/min, blood pressure is 90/P mm Hg, and respiratory rate is 0. The patient remains unresponsive.

Questions

4. *What could explain the patient's splotchy skin or the spontaneous return of the pulse?*
5. *What is the clinical significance of the fixed and dilated pupils? Does this finding have any influence on your treatment plan? Why or why not?*
6. *Should this patient's spine be immobilized? Why or why not?*
7. *What additional treatment should be provided?*

PULMONARY INJURIES

Subcutaneous Emphysema

[OBJECTIVES 17, 22]

Description and Definition

Subcutaneous emphysema is the presence of air in the soft tissue space. It may extend up to the neck and down to the groin.

History and Physical Findings

The presence of localized subcutaneous emphysema over the chest wall in the presence of blunt trauma usually indicates the presence of a traumatic pneumothorax. Subcutaneous emphysema is usually detected by noting the presence of a "crunching" sensation on palpation of the chest wall. Although the presence of air itself in the tissues is a benign condition, in cases of chest trauma it usually represents serious injury to any air-containing structure within the thorax. An esophageal tear from a penetrating injury also may produce a pneumomediastinum manifested by subcutaneous emphysema over the supraclavicular area and anterior neck.

Although subcutaneous emphysema is a benign condition, massive accumulations can be uncomfortable for the patient.

Therapeutic Interventions

Subcutaneous emphysema is an important physical finding to detect. Its presence should prompt you to consider transporting the patient to a trauma center. There is generally no prehospital treatment for subcutaneous emphysema, and hospital treatment is directed at the underlying cause.

Pulmonary Contusion

[OBJECTIVE 25]

Description and Definition

Pulmonary contusion is a direct bruise of the lung tissue, followed by bleeding and edema in the alveolar spaces. This is much like when a bruise forms on the skin as a result of direct trauma. However, the damage is more serious when the lung is involved. The buildup of blood, fluid, and inflammatory components can impair oxygenation and cause respiratory distress. In some aspects, it is very similar to pneumonia that develops over a period of a few hours or minutes, without the infectious component.

Great force is required to produce pulmonary contusion, such as a fall from a significant height, high-speed auto crashes, and other forms of significant trauma. Although only 5% to 16% of patients with an isolated pulmonary contusion will die, the mortality rate of those with even one associated extrathoracic injury is five times greater (Richardson & Spain, 2000).

Etiology

Pulmonary contusion is reported to be present in 30% to 75% of patients with significant blunt chest trauma. It is most often caused by automobile crashes with rapid deceleration (LoCicero & Mattox, 1989). It also can be caused by the high-energy shock waves of an explosion in air or water.

Pulmonary contusion is the most common significant chest injury in children. Furthermore, it is most commonly caused by an automobile or pedestrian-impact accident (Roux & Fisher, 1992). One theory holds that the more elastic chest wall, as in younger individuals, transmits increased force to the thoracic contents (Eckstein & Henderson, 2006).

History and Physical Findings

The assessment findings of pulmonary contusions depend on the severity of the injury. Moreover, they may present with varying degrees of dyspnea. You may note crackles (rales), diminished breath sounds, or absent breath on auscultation over the affected area. You may or may not see rib fractures. However, blunt trauma often leaves telltale injuries, such as hematomas, ecchymoses, tenderness, abrasions, or lacerations. If you discover flail chest, pulmonary contusion is commonly present. Surprisingly, many of the worst contusions occur in patients without rib fractures. Up to half of patients with a pulmonary contusion cough up blood **(hemoptysis).** Other assessment findings are listed in Box 49-5.

BOX 49-5 Pulmonary Contusion: Assessment Findings

- Tachypnea
- Tachycardia
- Cough
- Hemoptysis
- Apprehension
- Respiratory distress
- Dyspnea
- Cyanosis
- Chest wall bruising

Therapeutic Interventions

Take care not to focus on more dramatic injuries while failing to recognize the evolving pulmonary contusion. Most patients with significant pulmonary contusions will be hypoxic on your prehospital evaluation. Consequently, treat them with high-flow oxygen. Apply a pulse oximeter and cardiac monitor. Use capnography if available. Establish IV access but do not be overly aggressive with the administration of IV fluids. In a patient with a suspected pulmonary contusion, excess fluid will worsen patient outcome. You must rapidly transport the patient because the rapid development of pulmonary edema can require aggressive treatment to prevent death.

Pneumothorax

[OBJECTIVES 23, 24]

Description and Definition

A **pneumothorax** is an accumulation of air in the pleural space. This condition is a common complication of chest trauma. It is reported to be present in 15% to 50% of patients with penetrating chest trauma. Pneumothorax has three main classifications depending on whether air has direct access to the pleural cavity: simple, open, and tension (Eckstein & Henderson, 2006).

PARAMEDIC*Pearl*

The most common presenting symptoms of pneumothorax are shortness of breath and chest pain. The patient's appearance is highly variable. It can range from acutely ill with cyanosis and tachypnea to misleadingly stable. The physical examination may show decreased or absent breath sounds on the affected side, or it may be deceptively normal.

Simple Pneumothorax

Description and Definition. A pneumothorax is considered simple when no communication with the atmosphere exists and the mediastinum or diaphragm has not shifted as a result of the accumulation of air (Eckstein & Henderson, 2006) (Figure 49-7).

History and Physical Findings. The signs and symptoms vary depending on the size of the pneumothorax. Small tears may resolve on their own. The patient may not have difficulty breathing or other signs of respiratory distress. You may not be able to detect the pneumothorax on physical examination, and pulse oximetry readings may remain in the normal range. Larger tears may result in signs and symptoms of respiratory distress. Possible assessment findings are shown in Box 49-6.

Therapeutic Interventions. Your treatment of pneumothorax involves the basics: providing oxygenation and ventilation, applying a pulse oximeter and cardiac monitor, and obtaining IV access. Capnography should be used if available. Perform spinal stabilization if warranted. Rarely intubation may be necessary. However, when combined with aggressive ventilation, intubation can cause an increase in the size of the pneumothorax.

Open Pneumothorax

Description. In an open pneumothorax, an injury, such as a stab wound, penetrates the chest wall and pleura. This allows air to enter the pleural cavity (Figure 49-8). This entry of environmental air allows the lung to collapse, creating a pneumothorax. More importantly, an open connection exists between the pleural space and the environment.

History and Physical Findings. In a large open pneumothorax, movement of air through the chest wall often causes a sucking sound with respirations. The loss of chest wall integrity causes the involved lung to paradoxically collapse on inspiration and expand slightly on expiration. This forces air in and out of the wound. As a result, the wound associated with an open pneumothorax is called a *sucking chest wound.* This injury is most commonly caused by shotgun wounds. Large open wounds in the chest are a concern because air travels the route of least resistance. If the hole in the chest is large (compared with the size of the trachea), less air will go through the trachea and to the uninjured lung. Possible assessment findings are shown in Box 49-7.

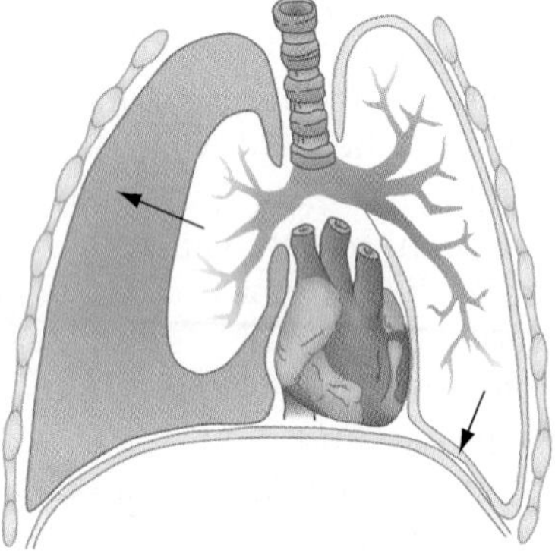

Figure 49-7 A simple pneumothorax is shown in the right lung with air in the pleural cavity and collapse of the right lung.

BOX 49-6 Simple Pneumothorax: Assessment Findings

- Tachypnea
- Tachycardia
- Respiratory distress
- Absent or decreased breath sounds on affected side
- Hyperresonance
- Decreased chest wall movement
- Dyspnea
- Chest pain referred to shoulder or arm on affected side
- Slight pleuritic chest pain

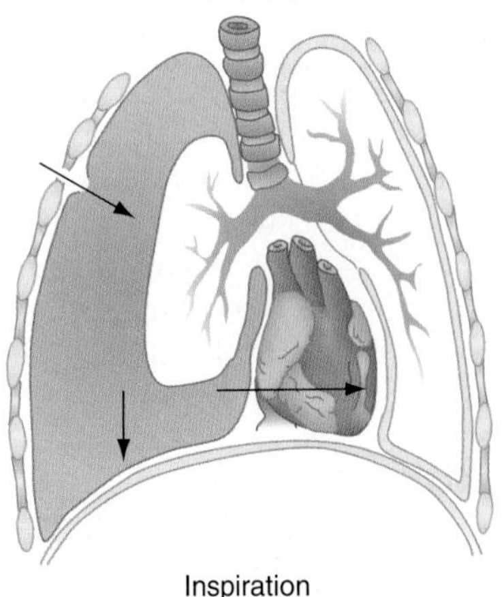

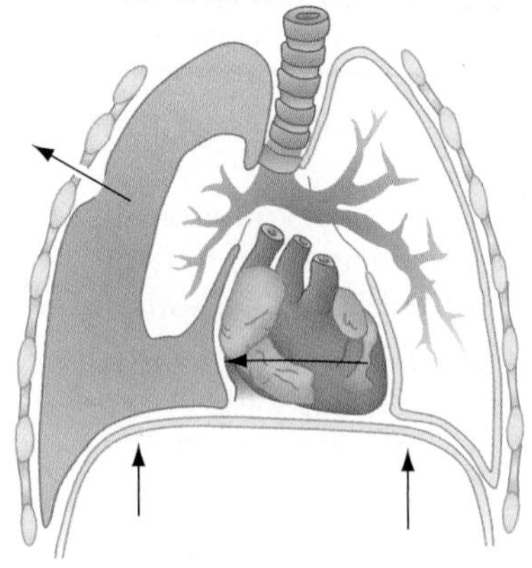

Figure 49-8 Open pneumothorax. Collapse of the right lung and air in the pleural cavity are shown, with communication to the outside through a defect in the chest wall. In a sucking chest wound, lung volume is greater with expiration.

Therapeutic Interventions. Recognition of an open pneumothorax is critical. Cover the open wound with an occlusive dressing as soon as possible. Never pack the wound because the negative pressure during inspiration can suck the dressing into the chest cavity. Covering the wound with an occlusive dressing converts an open pneumothorax to a closed pneumothorax, prevents further extension of the pneumothorax, and allows restoration of the normal respiratory mechanics. Be sure to tape the dressing on only three sides. Commercial dressings, such as petroleum gauze, exist for this purpose. Alternative dressings include the use of aluminum foil, a defibrillation pad, plastic wrap, or a VeniGuard (Figure 49-9). Additional treatment includes providing oxygenation and ventilation, applying a pulse oximeter and cardiac monitor, and obtaining IV access. Use capnography if available. Perform spinal stabilization if warranted.

When placing an occlusive dressing on an open chest wound, be sure to observe the patient closely for any signs of developing tension pneumothorax (described below). This is especially the case for patients who are intubated and receiving positive-pressure ventilation by a bag-mask device. This is the reason for taping the dressing on only three sides, not four. If such signs develop, you can release any pressure in the pleural space by temporarily removing a corner of the dressing and replacing it when the pressure is relieved (Buchman et al., 2004). The possibility of a **tension pneumothorax** with an open wound should prompt you to transport the patient rapidly. In addition, you must inform the receiving staff of this possibility.

BOX 49-7 Open Pneumothorax: Assessment Findings

- Defect in the chest wall
- To-and-fro air motion out of defect
- Penetrating injury to the chest that does not seal itself
- Sucking sound on inhalation
- Tachycardia
- Tachypnea
- Respiratory distress
- Subcutaneous emphysema
- Decreased breath sounds on affected side

Tension Pneumothorax

[OBJECTIVES 23, 25]

Description. **Tension pneumothorax** is the progressive accumulation of air under pressure within the pleural cavity, with shift of the chest contents (mediastinum) to the opposite side and resultant compression of the opposite lung and great vessels (Figure 49-10). It can occur from blunt or penetrating trauma or as a complication of treatment of an open pneumothorax.

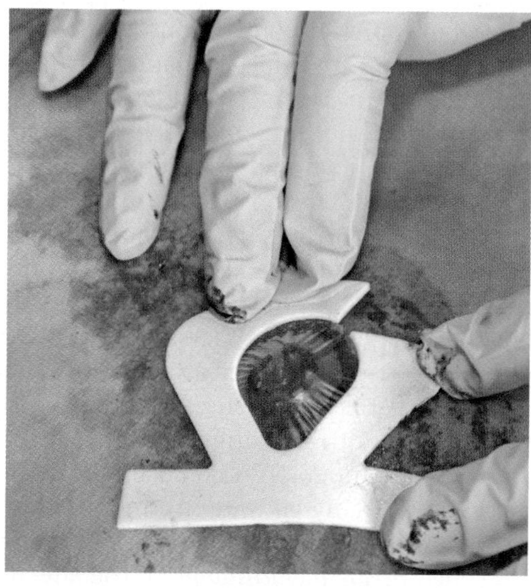

Figure 49-9 Cover an open chest wound with an occlusive dressing that is secured on only three sides.

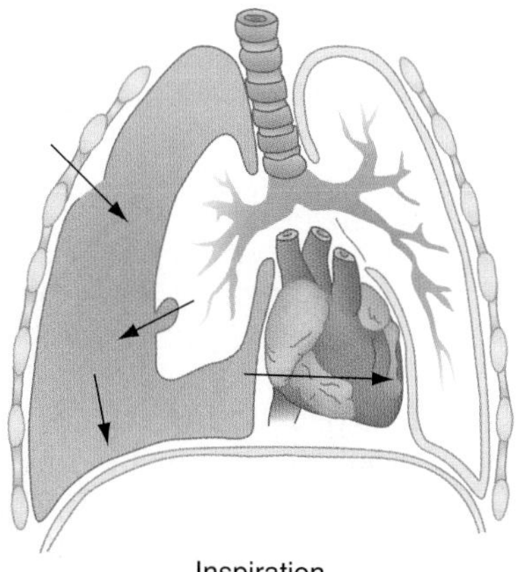

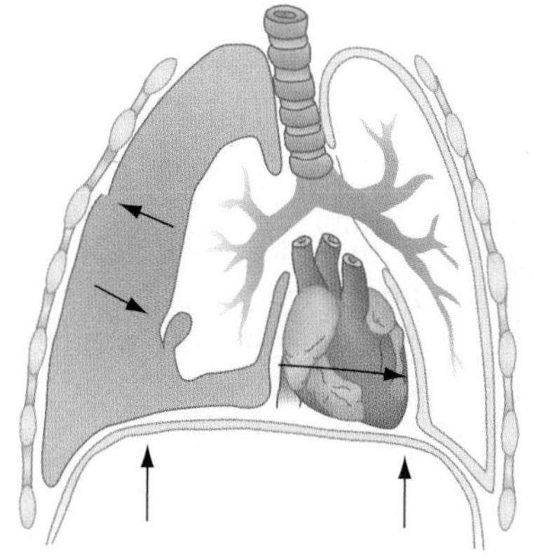

Figure 49-10 Tension pneumothorax. Note the pressure with which the right pneumothorax under tension pushes against the heart and opposite lung, preventing effective heart contraction and full inspiration of the opposite lung. The mediastinal structures shift to the side opposite the injury.

In a tension pneumothorax, the injury acts as a one-way valve, preventing free bilateral communication with the atmosphere. This leads to a progressive increase of intrapleural pressure. Air enters on inspiration but cannot exit with expiration. This, in turn, compresses the venae cavae, leading to decreased filling of the heart and decreased cardiac output. These changes result in the onset of hypoxia, respiratory distress, and shock within minutes. If allowed to progress, a tension pneumothorax can compress the heart and opposite lung to the point that it prevents the heart from contracting or the opposite lung from moving air. This results in the patient literally suffocating (Rosen et al., 1991). The mechanical ventilation of a patient with a preexisting pneumothorax is a significant risk for tension pneumothorax.

History and Physical Findings. A patient with a tension pneumothorax is typically tachypneic and tachycardic. Signs of air hunger are usually present. You may see cyanosis. If the patient is not hypovolemic, jugular venous distention often is present. Breath sounds are diminished or absent on the affected side. Palpation of the trachea may reveal deviation toward the unaffected side, but often it is not felt or not present. Tracheal deviation is a late sign of tension pneumothorax; do not rely on it as a consistent sign of a tension pneumothorax. Hypotension will not occur as early as hypoxia and may represent a preterminal event. Additional assessment findings are shown in Box 49-8.

BOX 49-8 Tension Pneumothorax: Assessment Findings

- Hyperinflation of the affected side
- Poor ventilation despite an open airway
- Restlessness, agitation, extreme anxiety
- Increased airway resistance on ventilating patient
- Respiratory distress (severe dyspnea, tachypnea, air hunger in conscious patient)
- Neck vein distention (may not be visible in the presence of hypovolemia)
- Decreased or absent breath sounds on the affected side
- Tympany (hyperresonance) to percussion on the affected side
- Tachycardia
- Signs of shock
- Tracheal deviation away from side of injury (may or may not be present)
- Cyanosis
- Bulging of intercostal muscles
- Narrow pulse pressure
- Subcutaneous emphysema

Therapeutic Interventions. When you suspect a tension pneumothorax, do not delay treatment until arrival at the hospital. The treatment should include providing high-flow oxygen and applying a pulse oximeter and cardiac monitor. Capnography should also be used. Establish IV access, preferably en route to the hospital.

The patient will require emergent needle decompression (also called *needle thoracostomy*) of the affected lung (Skill 49-1). You perform decompression by inserting a large-bore catheter through the second or third intercostal space in the midclavicular line on the affected side. Make sure that you insert the needle directly above the rib, because blood vessels are attached to the bottom of the ribs. A number of commercially available needle thoracostomy kits are available. Most of these also have a "flutter valve" attachment. This attachment prevents additional air from accumulating in the pleural space and the tension pneumothorax from reoccurring. Current trauma guidelines recommend not wasting time to apply a one-way valve. Needle decompression can suddenly and dramatically improve the patient's condition and improve the patient's dyspnea.

Hemothorax

[OBJECTIVES 23, 25, 26]

Description and Definition

The term **hemothorax** refers to a collection of blood within the pleural cavity. One of the most frequent causes is blunt or penetrating trauma to the chest. The injury allows capillaries or small blood vessels to bleed into the pleural cavity. This may occur with or without bone fractures. Blood displaces the lung and reduces air space available for oxygenation (Sawyer & Sawyer, 2006) (Figure 49-11). Because the pleural space can accommodate between 2500 and 3000 mL of blood, a hemothorax may produce hypovolemic shock and dangerously compromise ventilation.

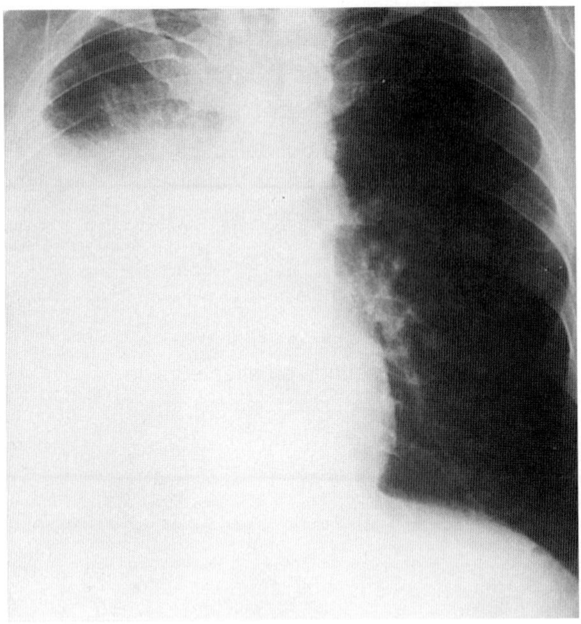

Figure 49-11 This chest radiograph shows a right hemothorax.

SKILL 49-1 NEEDLE DECOMPRESSION

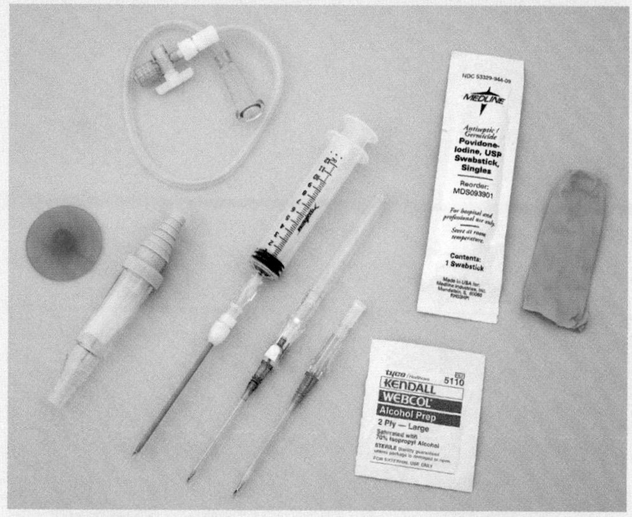

Step 1 Take appropriate standard precautions. After ensuring that the patient's signs and symptoms are consistent with a tension pneumothorax, prepare the necessary equipment to perform a needle thoracostomy. If necessary, obtain approval from medical direction to perform the procedure.

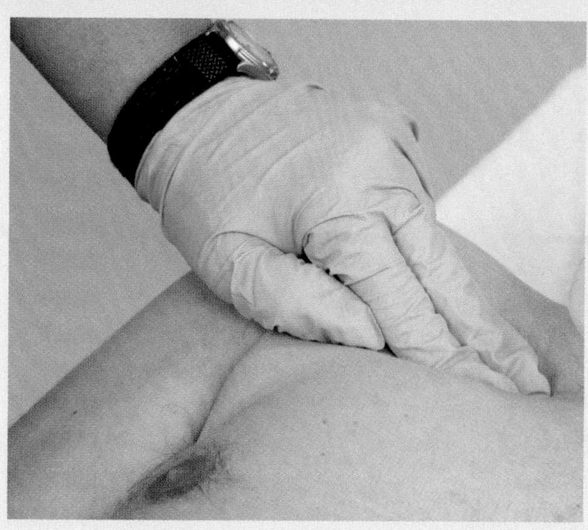

Step 2 Expose the patient's chest and identify landmarks on the affected side. Landmarks include the midclavicular line, clavicle, suprasternal notch, angle of Louis, and the second intercostal space. Palpate from the angle of Louis across the second rib and locate the third rib at the midclavicular line on the affected side.

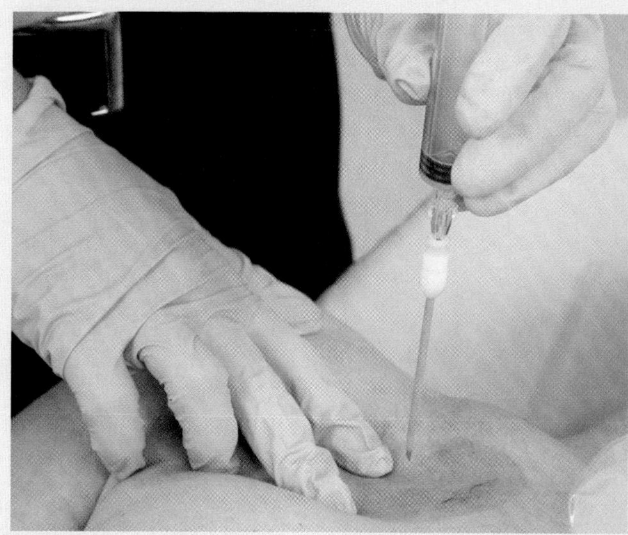

Step 3 After cleansing the site, insert a 14- or 16-gauge over-the-needle catheter perpendicular to the skin over the top of the third rib and into the second intercostal space, midclavicular line on the affected side. Insert the catheter approximately 2 to 3 cm or until a rush of air is heard. In a tension pneumothorax, a rush of air similar to bursting a balloon is heard. A small puff of air may be heard in a normal lung. Holding the catheter in place, remove the needle (leaving the catheter in place).

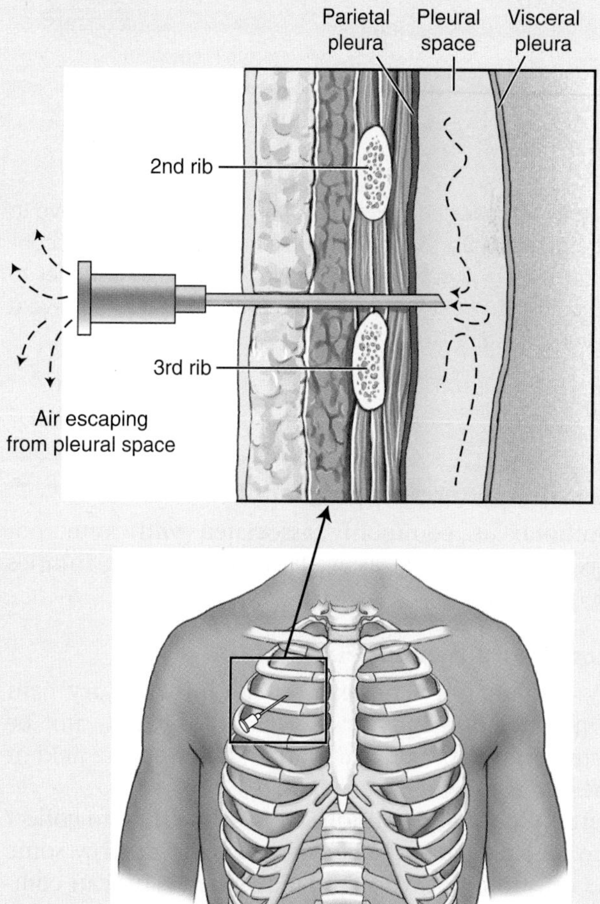

Continued

SKILL 49-1 NEEDLE DECOMPRESSION—continued

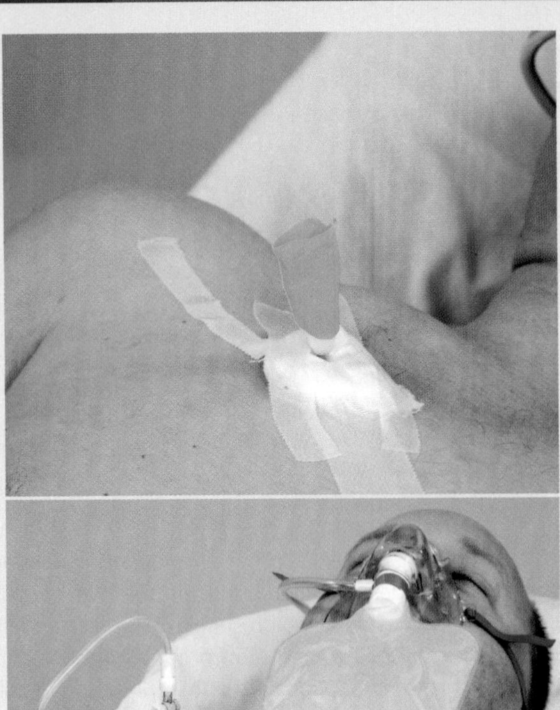

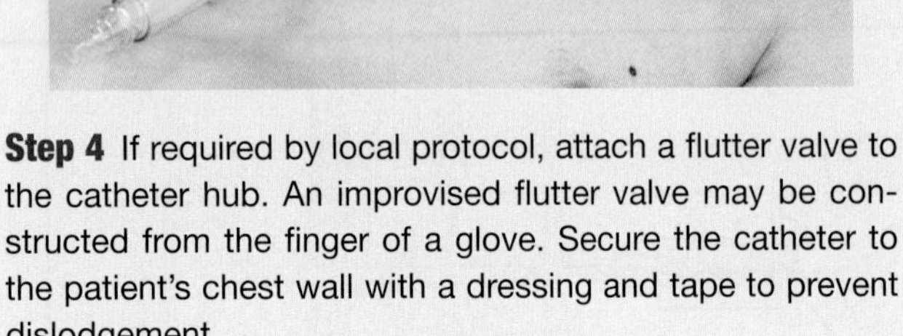

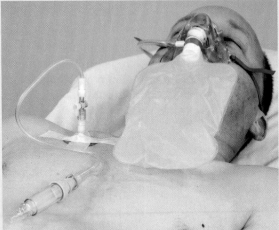

Step 4 If required by local protocol, attach a flutter valve to the catheter hub. An improvised flutter valve may be constructed from the finger of a glove. Secure the catheter to the patient's chest wall with a dressing and tape to prevent dislodgement.

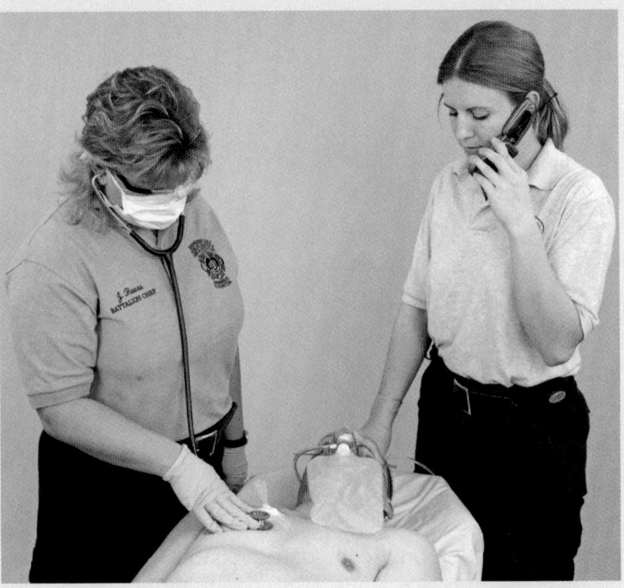

Step 5 Reassess the patient's breath sounds, respiratory status, and vital signs. Notify medical direction of the procedure.

Epidemiology and Demographics

Hemothorax is commonly associated with pneumothorax (25% of cases) as well as extrathoracic injuries (73% of cases).

History and Physical Findings

Many patients only complain of the initial injury pain and may not notice dyspnea. Hemothorax may not be detected on the initial examination, either in the field or in the emergency department.

Certain medical conditions allow tissue fluid to collect in the pleural space. These conditions often allow some blood cells to follow this fluid movement. This can complicate the diagnosis of hemothorax because it is not pure blood that collects in the pleural space. Nontraumatic hemothorax is a relatively uncommon occurrence. However, it may result from cancer, pulmonary embolism, spontaneous rupture of blood vessels, emphysema, infections, or vascular malformations (Mancini & Eggerstedt, 2006).

On your physical examination of the patient, auscultation may reveal decreased breath sounds in the lower lobes when the patient is sitting up. When the patient is supine, the blood may distribute over the posterior surface of the lung. This may make it much more difficult to hear decreased breath sounds.

Therapeutic Interventions

Management of a patient with a hemothorax includes ensuring adequate oxygenation and ventilation, applying a pulse oximeter, establishing IV access, using capnography, and monitoring by ECG. Minimize the administration of IV fluids. Aggressive IV fluid administration may increase the rate of bleeding. Your management of initial traumatic insults should follow traditional trauma care guidelines. Unnecessarily placing the patient with a suspected hemothorax in full spinal immobilization may increase his or her respiratory distress. Therefore perform spinal immobilization only when necessary.

Hemopneumothorax

[OBJECTIVE 23]

Description

A **hemopneumothorax** is a pneumothorax with bleeding in the pleural space. It is usually the result of penetrating trauma, such as a gunshot wound or stab. An initial injury allows air to enter the pleural cavity and create a pneumothorax. Bleeding caused by the trauma allows blood to collect in the pleural space along with the air, creating a hemopneumothorax. The bleeding can originate from an injured blood vessel, bruising of the lung or chest wall components, or even rapid deceleration (Sawyer & Sawyer, 2006).

History and Physical Findings

Hemopneumothorax has similar symptoms and clinical findings as hemothorax, including dyspnea, tachypnea, and tachycardia. Patients also may exhibit obvious chest trauma, have possible hypotension, and be in shock. Physical examination of the patient may reveal rib crepitus, possible flail segments, subcutaneous emphysema, or hematoma. Auscultation of the lungs will reveal decreased or absent breath sounds from the affected lung and hyperresonance on percussion.

Therapeutic Interventions

Treatment involves aggressive airway control and oxygenation. Apply 100% oxygen by nonrebreather mask, establish IV access, and apply a pulse oximeter and cardiac monitor. Use capnography if available. You must pay careful attention to the possible development of a tension pneumothorax. Watch for signs of increasing distress, dropping blood pressure, increasing tachycardia, or dropping oxygen saturations. Rapid transport is key because many of these severe injuries require surgical evaluation.

Tracheobronchial Injury

[OBJECTIVES 27, 28, 29, 30]

Description and Definition

Injuries to the respiratory tree (tracheobronchial injuries) may occur with either blunt or penetrating injuries of the neck or chest. A direct blow to the neck may crush the cervical trachea against the vertebral bodies and transect the tracheal rings or cricoid cartilage. Penetrating injuries tend to be more obvious because of their immediate symptoms and location of the wounds. In contrast, blunt injuries can be subtle. Respiratory distress, hypoxia, hemoptysis, and subcutaneous emphysema should suggest the presence of a major airway injury.

Epidemiology and Demographics

Although the occurrence of tracheobronchial disruption has increased, it is still a relatively rare injury, occurring in fewer than 3% of patients with significant chest injury. However, it carries an overall mortality rate of 30%; 50% of those patients will die within the first hour.

History and Physical Findings

Patients with tracheobronchial disruption have one of two distinct clinical pictures. In the first group the wound opens into the pleural space, producing a large pneumothorax. These patients often have hemoptysis, dyspnea, subcutaneous emphysema, unequal breath sounds, and cyanosis. Auscultation of the heart may reveal a crunching sound with each heartbeat **(Hamman's sign).**

The second group has a complete transection of the tracheobronchial tree but little or no communication with the pleural space. A pneumothorax is not usually present. These patients are relatively free of symptoms at the time of injury but become symptomatic days to weeks later.

Therapeutic Interventions

If you suspect a tracheobronchial injury, rapidly transport the patient to a trauma center because the definitive diagnosis and treatment of these injuries is complex. You must take extreme care when attempting blind intubation in the field so as not to place the endotracheal tube through a transected airway into the soft tissue or a false passage. In most cases surgical repair of the disrupted airway should be performed as soon as possible, with placement of a tracheostomy performed in the controlled setting of the operating room.

CARDIOVASCULAR TRAUMA

Blunt cardiac injury usually results from high-speed MVCs in which the chest wall strikes the steering wheel. Other causes, such as falls from heights, crushing injuries, blast injuries, and direct blows, are less common. The importance of suspecting blunt cardiac injury lies in recognizing the associated potentially fatal complications. Life-threatening dysrhythmias, conduction abnormalities, congestive heart failure (CHF), cardiogenic shock, cardiac tamponade, cardiac rupture, and rupture of heart valves have all been reported as complications.

Cardiac Contusion

[OBJECTIVES 31, 32, 33]

Description and Definition

A cardiac contusion typically occurs when a large force is applied to the chest wall. The sternum is displaced posteriorly and the heart is compressed between the sternum and the chest. High-speed deceleration injuries are the most common cause of myocardial contusion. However, MVCs that occur at slow to moderate speeds also may result in cardiac injury. In one study an automobile collision speed of only 20 to 35 mph resulted in myocardial contusion in several patients, without external evidence of chest trauma (Eckstein & Henderson, 2006).

PARAMEDIC*Pearl*

Commotio cordis (ventricular fibrillation caused by a blunt, nonpenetrating blow to the chest, most commonly from a baseball) is an underappreciated cause of sudden cardiac death in young patients. It most frequently occurs in males at a mean age of 14 years. Although once thought rare, an increasing number of these events have been reported. Prompt CPR and early defibrillation are associated with a favorable outcome.

History and Physical Findings

The clinical picture of myocardial contusion is varied and nonspecific. It may involve excruciating pain and shock. On the other hand, it may be a benign condition with only subtle ECG changes and no clinical symptoms. Patients may have dysrhythmias or ST wave changes caused by other injuries, such as significant hypoxia as a result of pulmonary injuries or blood loss, which are reversed once the hypoxemia or blood loss is corrected.

A patient with a blunt cardiac injury likely has additional abdominal, skeletal, or central nervous system injury. This additional injury may mask the signs and symptoms of cardiac injury. However, certain findings provide significant clues to the possible presence of cardiac trauma. Up to 73% of patients with cardiac contusion have been reported to demonstrate external signs of thoracic trauma (e.g., contusions, abrasions, palpable crepitus, rib fractures, visible flail segments).

Other associated injuries include pulmonary contusion, pneumothorax, hemothorax, external fracture, and great vessel injury. A reduction in cardiac output, which can be clinically insignificant or manifest as pronounced cardiogenic shock, may occur in patients with significant cardiac contusion.

Because of its anterior position in the thorax and proximity to the sternum, the right ventricle is far more likely to be injured than the left ventricle. A cardiac contusion usually results in moderate right ventricular damage with only minor electrical changes, which can be missed easily on a standard 12-lead ECG (Eckstein & Henderson, 2006). Right-sided ECGs (see Chapter 22) have not been found to be of any benefit (Walsh et al., 2001). The most sensitive but least specific sign of myocardial contusion is sinus tachycardia. It is present in approximately 70% of patients with documented myocardial contusion (Eckstein & Henderson, 2006). A 12-lead ECG obtained in the field may reveal a right bundle branch block.

Observe and relay information to the receiving facility concerning mechanism of injury, status of the motor vehicle, steering wheel and dashboard damage, use of seatbelts, deployment of air bags, estimated speed of the vehicle before the crash (if known), and position of the patient when found.

Therapeutic Interventions

Your treatment of any patient who sustains significant blunt chest trauma should include rapid transport to a trauma center. The treatment of a suspected myocardial contusion should be similar to that of a myocardial infarction (heart attack): administering high-flow oxygen, continuous cardiac monitoring, establishing an IV line while en route to the hospital, and administering analgesic agents. Treat dysrhythmias with appropriate medications, as per current advanced cardiac life support guidelines. Fibrinolytic agents and aspirin are contraindicated in the setting of acute trauma.

Pericardial Tamponade

[OBJECTIVES 31, 34, 35]

Description and Definition

Pericardial tamponade is the accumulation of fluid (blood) in the pericardial space that impedes cardiac filling and cardiac output. As the volume of the pericardial fluid increases, the ventricles are restricted and unable to fill adequately. This results in decreased cardiac output and ultimately decreased systolic blood pressure. The pulse pressure, which is the difference between the systolic and diastolic blood pressures, is decreased.

Suspect pericardial tamponade in any patient who has sustained a penetrating wound or blunt trauma to the chest or upper abdomen. You can never be certain of the trajectory of the bullet or the length, force, and direction of a knife thrust. Obviously wounds directly over the anterior chest wall and epigastric area are more likely to produce a cardiac injury resulting in tamponade than are those in the posterior or lateral sides of the chest. Nevertheless, assume that a penetrating wound, particularly a stab wound, anywhere in the thorax or upper abdomen may have injured the heart.

Epidemiology and Demographics

The reported incidence of acute pericardial tamponade is approximately 2% in patients with penetrating trauma to the chest and lower abdomen. It is rarely seen after blunt chest trauma. Patients with acute pericardial tamponade can deteriorate in minutes. However, many of these patients can be saved if you take the proper steps.

History and Physical Findings

The physical findings of pericardial tamponade are hypotension, distended neck veins **(jugular venous distension [JVD])** and, rarely, distant muffled heart tones. This so-called Beck's triad is often difficult to detect clinically, especially in the prehospital setting. Furthermore, the presence of significant blood loss from other injuries may preclude the development of JVD. The most reliable signs of pericardial tamponade are the presence of JVD in association with hypotension and tachycardia. When this triad is present in the setting of chest trauma, consider the presence of acute pericardial tamponade as well as tension pneumothorax.

Pulsus paradoxus is defined as an excessive drop (more than 10 mm Hg) in systolic blood pressure during the inspiratory phase of the normal respiratory cycle. This sign may be an additional clue to the presence of pericardial tamponade. Measure it by careful auscultation while the pressure in the blood pressure cuff is slowly lowered. The first reading on a sphygmomanometer is recorded at the point at which some beats become audible during expiration. The second reading is taken when every beat becomes audible. If the difference between these two readings is greater than 10 mm Hg, pulsus paradoxus is present. At times it may be possible to diagnose pulsus paradoxus by palpation alone, when the pulse either disappears or markedly diminishes during inspiration. It is commonly present in patients with many other conditions, including chronic obstructive pulmonary disease, acute bronchial asthma, pneumothorax, pulmonary edema, and any other condition that results in respiratory distress.

Therapeutic Interventions

The prehospital treatment for cases of pericardial tamponade is essentially the same as outlined for any victim of major trauma. Tension pneumothorax, which is much more common, may mimic acute pericardial tamponade. If the patient presents in extremis (extremely critical condition, with death imminent if untreated) or his or her clinical condition rapidly deteriorates, consider performing a needle thoracostomy (in consultation with medical direction). If this procedure is not therapeutic, it may be diagnostic for pericardial tamponade under the appropriate clinical presentation. You must rapidly transport this patient to the nearest trauma center. Furthermore, a high suspicion of pericardial tamponade mandates that you aggressively administer IV fluids in the field as long as on-scene time is not prolonged. This is because cardiac output in the setting of pericardial tamponade depends on maintaining an adequate preload. This condition is one of the few clinical entities in which IV fluid administration may help the major trauma patient. Cardiac tamponade is examined in more detail in Chapter 22.

PARAMEDIC*Pearl*

The absence of field vital signs in patients with blunt trauma appears to be incompatible with survival. However, the absence of field vital signs in patients with penetrating trauma has been reported to carry a 4% survival rate with patients who are neurologically intact. For this reason, rapidly transport patients with penetrating chest trauma, particularly when you suspect tamponade, to the nearest trauma center for emergent thoracotomy.

Cardiac Rupture

[OBJECTIVE 31]

Description and Definition

Cardiac rupture refers to an acute traumatic perforation of the ventricles or atria. High-speed MVCs are responsible for most cases of traumatic myocardial rupture. Cardiac rupture is the most common cause of death in cases of nonpenetrating cardiac injuries. Approximately one third of these patients have multiple-chamber rupture, and one fourth have an associated ascending aortic rupture.

Epidemiology and Demographics

Cardiac rupture is nearly always immediately fatal. It accounts for 15% of fatal thoracic injuries. Blunt cardiac rupture is estimated to account for 5% of the 50,000 annual highway deaths in the United States (Brown & Grover, 1997). In various studies the incidence of cardiac rupture in cases of blunt chest trauma ranges from 0.5% to 2%.

Only a small number of survivors of ventricular rupture have been reported. Most survivors of cardiac rupture are patients with atrial rupture. Because of the nature of the mechanisms involved in cardiac rupture, associated multisystem injuries are common. More than 70% of reported survivors of myocardial rupture had other major associated injuries. These injuries included pulmonary contusions, liver and spleen lacerations, closed head injuries, and major fractures.

History and Physical Findings

In a review of survivors of myocardial rupture, the common signs and symptoms included hypotension (100%); tachycardia (89%); distended neck veins (80%); cyanosis of the head, neck, arms, and upper chest (76%); unresponsiveness (74%); distant heart sounds (61%); and associated chest injuries (50%) (Eckstein & Henderson, 2006).

Therapeutic Interventions

The treatment for a patient with suspected cardiac rupture includes ensuring adequate oxygenation and ventilation, applying a pulse oximeter, using capnography, establishing IV access, and monitoring by ECG. When caring for a patient who has sustained blunt chest trauma, concentrate on rapid transport and pay attention for any signs of pericardial tamponade. En route to the hospital, consider the possibility of a tension pneumothorax.

Case Scenario CONCLUSION

The patient's spine is immobilized and his lungs are ventilated with a bag-mask device connected to 100% oxygen. You are unable to intubate the patient and his teeth clench after the second attempt. You insert an oral airway and your partner continues positive-pressure ventilation. On arrival at the emergency department, approximately 200 mL of IV fluid has been administered. The patient's mental status is unchanged and his pulse is 98 beats/min, blood pressure is 118/65 mm Hg, and respiratory rate is 0.

In the emergency department the patient's pupils are slowly reactive and he begins to exhibit decorticate posturing (abnormal flexion). The patient is sedated, paralyzed, intubated, and admitted to the intensive care unit with a diagnosis of thoracic compression syndrome (traumatic asphyxia). He awakens on the second day and is transferred to a rehabilitation facility, where he recovers completely.

Looking back

8. *What is thoracic compression syndrome or traumatic asphyxia?*
9. *Given the patient's final diagnoses and disposition, was your treatment appropriate? Why or why not?*

INJURY TO THE GREAT VESSELS

Aortic Rupture

[OBJECTIVES 36, 37, 38, 39, 40]

Description and Definition

The thoracic aorta is the most common vessel injured by blunt trauma. The descending thoracic aorta is relatively fixed and immobile. With sudden deceleration, a shearing force or whiplash effect on the aorta is produced. Eighty percent to 90% of aortic tears occur in the descending aorta just distal to the left subclavian artery. Lethal cardiac injuries often are associated with aortic tears. These include pericardial tamponade, aortic valve tears, myocardial contusion, and coronary artery injuries. Passenger ejection, pedestrian impact, severe falls, and crush injuries commonly result in ascending thoracic aortic ruptures. Patients who sustain an ascending aortic rupture rarely survive long enough to be evaluated in the emergency department.

Epidemiology and Demographics

The mortality rate from aortic rupture has risen dramatically from less than 1% in 1947 to as high as 15% in recent years. This suggests a strong association with high-speed automobile transportation. A significant number of accident victims sustain this injury without immediately dying. Ten percent to 20% survive, at least temporarily, because of tamponade of aortic blood by the adventitia. The mean age of patients sustaining aortic rupture is 33 years; more than 70% of these patients are men. Because these patients are usually healthy, almost 85% can survive if diagnosis and surgical intervention are prompt (Kram et al., 1989).

History and Physical Findings

Aortic rupture most commonly occurs from high-speed MVC deceleration. Vertical deceleration injuries resulting from falls can cause a rupture of the ascending aorta by producing an acute lengthening of the ascending aorta. This is the likely mechanism responsible for aortic rupture in airplane and elevator accidents. Other reported causes of aortic rupture include direct kicks by animals, crush injuries, sudden burial by landslide, and airbag deployment.

Consider the possibility of aortic disruption in every patient who sustains a severe deceleration injury. This is especially true if the automobile was moving in excess of 45 mph or if evidence of severe blunt forces to the chest (such as from a damaged steering wheel) exists. In the case of any moderate- or high-speed MVC, you must carefully evaluate the extent of damage to the vehicle, the complaints of the victims, and the physical manifestations of blunt chest trauma. Promptly relay this information to the receiving hospital or to online medical control.

Despite the severe nature of the injury, the signs and symptoms of an aortic rupture often are lacking. Associated pulmonary, neurologic, orthopedic, facial, and abdominal injuries are commonly present. Coexisting injuries can mask the signs and symptoms of an aortic injury or divert your attention away from the more lethal aortic rupture. An aortic tear can be present without any external evidence of a chest injury. One third to half of patients reported in the literature have no external signs of chest trauma.

The most common symptom is interscapular or retrosternal pain. This often is found in nontraumatic aortic dissection. However, it is present in only 25% of patients with a traumatic aortic disruption. Other symptoms described in the literature but that are not commonly seen include dyspnea resulting from tracheal compression and deviation, stridor or hoarseness caused by compression of the laryngeal nerve, dysphagia caused by esophageal compression, and extremity pain caused by ischemia from decreased arterial flow.

Clinical signs are uncommon and nonspecific. Generalized hypertension, when present, is an important clinical sign. A less-common clinical finding is the acute onset of upper extremity hypertension, along with absent or diminished femoral pulses. This "pseudocoarctation syndrome" has been reported to occur in up to one third of these patients. It is attributed to compression of the aortic lumen by a surrounding hematoma.

Therapeutic Interventions

Evaluation for possible aortic rupture should concentrate on identifying a mechanism of injury compatible with aortic rupture. It also should include treating hypotension, tension pneumothorax, and pericardial tamponade. Immediately relay the patient's condition and expeditiously transport him or her to a trauma center to increase the patient's chance for survival.

Injury to the Venae Cavae or Pulmonary Vessels

[OBJECTIVE 37]

Description and Definition

Injuries of the great vessels are usually associated with injuries to the chest, abdomen, or neck. These areas contain several large blood vessels: the superior **vena cava,** the inferior vena cava, the **pulmonary arteries,** and the four main **pulmonary veins.** Injuries to any of these vessels may be accompanied by massive hemothorax, hypovolemic shock, and cardiac tamponade. Frequently blood loss is not obvious because it remains within the chest cavity.

Therapeutic Interventions

You must immediately transport the patient with injury to the great vessels to a trauma center.

DIAPHRAGMATIC INJURIES

[OBJECTIVES 41, 42, 43, 44]

Description and Definition

Traumatic diaphragmatic injuries may result from direct penetration of the diaphragm or blunt forces to the chest or abdomen, leading to rupture of the diaphragm. The mechanism of injury in penetrating trauma is direct violation of the diaphragm by the penetrating object or missile. In blunt trauma, increased intraabdominal or intrathoracic pressure is transmitted to the diaphragm, leading to rupture. Most cases involve left-sided diaphragmatic rupture because the right hemidiaphragm is protected by the liver.

Etiology

Diaphragmatic injuries not diagnosed and surgically repaired acutely may not become clinically evident until months to years later, when herniation of abdominal contents into the chest leads to delayed but potentially life-threatening complications.

Epidemiology and Demographics

The incidence of diaphragmatic injury is estimated to be 1% to 6% of all patients sustaining multiple trauma. Approximately half of the cases of diaphragmatic injury are from penetrating trauma, and the other half are from blunt trauma, of which approximately 85% are attributable to MVCs.

History and Physical Findings

The signs and symptoms of traumatic diaphragmatic hernia vary. In the prehospital setting, they commonly are overshadowed by the associated injuries. The physical findings may reveal tachypnea, hypotension, absence of breath sounds, abdominal distension, or bowel sounds in the chest (Troop et al., 1985).

Therapeutic Interventions

Although you will probably not be able to identify diaphragmatic rupture, you should be aware of patients who are at risk for this injury and need transport to a trauma center.

ESOPHAGEAL INJURIES

[OBJECTIVES 45, 46, 47, 48]

Description and Definition

Because of its well-protected position posteriorly, esophageal trauma occurs in approximately 5% of patients with injuries to the neck but only 1% of blunt trauma victims. It usually is not an isolated injury. Cervical esophageal injuries are the most common because of a lack of protection by the bony thorax, and the trachea is the most common associated site of injury. In some cases the esophageal injury may initially be overlooked because of the dramatic presentation of a patient with a tracheal injury.

History and Physical Findings

Typical symptoms seen in cervical esophageal injuries include neck pain, difficulty swallowing, cough, voice changes, and hematemesis (bloody vomitus). Physical findings may include neck tenderness, resistance to flexion, crepitus, and stridor. In one large study the most common life-threatening problem in the emergency setting was airway compromise.

Therapeutic Interventions

You can manage the airway of most patients with eso-phageal trauma by rapid-sequence intubation. However, a significant number (12%) require a surgical airway (cricothyrotomy) (Hatzitheofilou & Strahlendorf, 1993).

Operative repair is indicated in almost all traumatic esophageal injuries (more than 90%). Thus you must rapidly transport this patient to a trauma center. The transport should occur as quickly as possible to avoid any delayed complications, such as the development of fistulas, infection, or abscesses. Blunt traumatic injuries to the esophagus occur much less often than penetrating injuries.

Case Scenario SUMMARY

1. *What potential causes of cardiac arrest can you think of in this case?* Causes of traumatic cardiac arrest are different than those in medical cases. Myocardial concussion, profound hypotension, tension pneumothorax, pericardial tamponade, and traumatic asphyxia are all potential causes of traumatic cardiac arrest in this case.
2. *What physical assessment findings would be most useful to differentiate these causes?* Evidence of blunt chest trauma, although pertinent, does not help differentiate the causes above. Evidence of significant blood loss, such as visible hemorrhage, pelvic fracture, or a distended abdomen, may suggest hypotension as the cause. Condition of the jugular veins also may be useful. JVD is suggestive of a tension pneumothorax, pericardial tamponade, or traumatic asphyxia, whereas flat vessels may indicate hypovolemia. Unequal breath sounds may indicate a tension pneumothorax, whereas a petechial rash is strongly suggestive of traumatic asphyxia.
3. *What treatment should be immediately initiated?* Airway control, ventilation, and chest compressions. CPR has already been initiated.
4. *What could explain the patient's splotchy skin or the spontaneous return of the pulse?* The spontaneous return of pulse is consistent with either myocardial concussion or traumatic asphyxia. Given the mechanism and other physical findings, the splotchy skin virtually confirms that this patient has traumatic asphyxia, also known as thoracic compression syndrome.
5. *What is the clinical significance of the fixed and dilated pupils? Does this finding have any influence on your treatment plan? Why or why not?* Fixed and dilated pupils indicate the presence of cerebral hypoxia. Although not predictive of the patient's final outcome, these signs signal the need for rapid and definitive restoration of cerebral circulation. Continue CPR and take steps to oxygenate, ventilate, and restore normal cardiac output.
6. *Should this patient's spine be immobilized? Why or why not?* Yes, but it should not delay treatment or transport. The patient had almost 1 ton fall on him. That is a significant mechanism of injury and justifies spinal stabilization.
7. *What additional treatment should be provided?* Given the return of a spontaneous pulse and acceptable blood pressure, your focus should be directed at securing the airway and providing assisted ventilation with high-flow oxygen. The cardiac monitor and pulse should be carefully monitored to detect any changes that might warrant starting chest compressions.
8. *What is thoracic compression syndrome or traumatic asphyxia?* Thoracic compression syndrome occurs when the thoracic cavity is compressed, resulting in a dramatic increase in intrathoracic pressure. Once this pressure exceeds the venous pressure of blood returning to the heart, cardiac output ceases and the patient is in cardiac arrest. The high intrathoracic pressure often forces blood back through the venae cavae into the venous system, causing capillary rupture and the classic petechial rash found with the condition. Normal blood flow typically spontaneously returns once the pressure is removed from the thorax, except in cases of long duration.
9. *Given the patient's final diagnoses and disposition, was your treatment appropriate? Why or why not?* Yes. Successful intubation would have been optimal, but this case—and the patient's outcome—demonstrates that adequate ventilation and oxygenation can be provided in patients who are not intubated if good basic life support airway and ventilation skills are used.

Chapter Summary

- Thoracic trauma includes a wide range of injuries, many of which may result in death if not recognized early. You must take into account the mechanism of injury to suspect potential injury to the heart, lungs, or great vessels.
- You must suspect and treat certain injuries, such as tension pneumothorax, in the field.
- You must be able to identify and treat these injuries rapidly to provide potentially lifesaving care.

REFERENCES

Brown, J., & Grover, F. L. (1997). Trauma to the heart. *Chest Surgery Clinics of North America, 7,* 325.

Buchman, T. G. (2004). Thoracic trauma. In J. E. Tintinalli, G. D. Kelen, J. S. Stapczynski, O. J. Ma, & D. M. Cline (Eds.), *Emergency medicine: A comprehensive study guide* (6th ed.). New York: McGraw-Hill.

Eckstein, M., & Henderson, S. (2006). Thoracic trauma. In J. Marx, R. Hockberger, & R. Walls (Eds.). *Rosen's emergency medicine: Concepts and clinical practice* (6th ed.). St. Louis: Mosby.

Hatzitheofilou, C., & Strahlendorf, C. (1993). Penetrating external injuries of the esophagus and pharynx. *British Journal of Surgery, 80,* 1147.

Kram, H. B., Appel, P. L., Wohlmuth, D. A., & Shoemaker, W. C. (1989). Diagnosis of traumatic aortic rupture: A 10-year retrospective analysis, *Annals of Thoracic Surgery, 47,* 282.

LoCicero, J., & Mattox, K. L. (1989). Epidemiology of chest trauma. *Surgery Clinics of North America, 69,* 15.

Mancini, M. C., & Eggerstedt, J. M. (2006). *Hemothorax.* Retrieved June 20, 2006, from http://www.emedicine.com.

Miller, L. M. (2006). Chest wall, lung, and pleural space trauma. *Radiologic Clinics of North America, 44,* 213-224.

Pepe, P., & Eckstein, M. (1998). Re-appraising the prehospital care of the patient with major trauma. *Emergency Medicine Clinics of North America, 16,* 1-15.

Richardson, J. D., & Spain, D. A. (2000). Injury to the lung and pleura. In K. L. Mattox, D. V. Feliciano, & E. E. Moore (Eds.). *Trauma.* New York: McGraw-Hill.

Rosen, P., Barkin, R. M., & Sternbach, G. L. (1991). *Essentials of emergency medicine.* St. Louis: Mosby–Year Book.

Roux, P., & Fisher, R. M. (1992). Chest injuries in children: An analysis of 100 cases of blunt chest trauma from motor vehicle accidents. *Journal of Pediatric Surgery, 27,* 551.

Sawyer, M. A., & Sawyer, E. M. (2006). *Blunt chest trauma.* Retrieved September 21, 2006, from http://www.emedicine.com.

Troop, B., Myers, R. M., & Agarwal, N. N. (1985). Early recognition of diaphragmatic injuries from blunt trauma. *Annals of Emergency Medicine, 14,* 97.

Walsh, P., Marks, G., Aranguri, C., Williams, J., Rothenberg, S. J., Dang, C., et al. (2001). Use of V4R in patients who sustain blunt chest trauma. *Journal of Trauma, 51,* 60.

Wanek, S., & Mayberry, J. C. (2004). Blunt thoracic trauma: Flail chest, pulmonary contusion, and blast injury. *Critical Care Clinics, 20,* 71-81.

SUGGESTED RESOURCE

Cogbill, T. H., & Landercasper, J. (2000). Injury to the chest wall. In K. L. Mattox, D. V. Feliciano, & E. E. Moore (Eds.). *Trauma.* New York: McGraw-Hill.

Chapter Quiz

1. What are the signs and symptoms of tension pneumothorax?

2. What is Beck's triad?

3. What mechanism of injury is most closely associated with aortic rupture?

4. What is a flail chest?

5. What is Hamman's sign?

6. What is a sucking chest wound?

7. What is pulsus paradoxus?

8. What is traumatic asphyxia?

Chapter Quiz—continued

9. What is the prehospital treatment for a sucking chest wound?

____

____

10. True or False: The prehospital treatment of a flail chest includes stabilization of the flail segment with the use of a sandbag.

Terminology

Cardiac rupture An acute traumatic perforation of the ventricles or atria.

Hamman's sign A crunching sound with each heartbeat.

Hemoptysis The coughing up of blood.

Hemothorax Blood within the thoracic cavity; a potentially life-threatening injury.

Jugular venous distension (JVD) The presence of visually enlarged external jugular neck veins.

Pericardial tamponade Life-threatening injury in which blood collects within the pericardium until the increasing pressure prevents the heart from filling with blood, causing death.

Pneumothorax A collection of air in the pleural space; usually from either a hole in the lung or a hole in the chest wall.

Pulmonary arteries Left and right pulmonary arteries supplying the lungs.

Pulmonary veins Vessels that return blood from the lungs to the left atrium of the heart.

Pulsus paradoxus A fall in systolic blood pressure of more than 10 mm Hg during inspiration (also called *paradoxic pulse*).

Subcutaneous emphysema Air trapped beneath the skin that feels like crackling when palpated.

Tension pneumothorax Life-threatening injury in which air enters the space between the lungs and the chest wall but cannot exit. With each breath, the pressure increases until it prevents ventilation and causes death.

Vena cava One of two large veins returning blood from the peripheral circulation to the right atrium of the heart.

CHAPTER 50

Abdominal Trauma

Objectives *After completing this chapter, you will be able to:*

1. Describe the epidemiology, including the morbidity and mortality rates and prevention strategies, for a patient with abdominal trauma.
2. Describe the anatomy and physiology of the organs and structures related to abdominal injuries.
3. Predict abdominal injuries on the basis of blunt and penetrating mechanisms of injury.
4. Describe open and closed abdominal injuries.
5. Explain the pathophysiology of abdominal injuries.
6. Describe the assessment findings associated with abdominal injuries.
7. Identify the need for rapid intervention and transport of the patient with abdominal injuries based on the assessment findings.
8. Integrate pathophysiologic principles into the assessment of a patient who has abdominal injury.
9. Differentiate abdominal injuries on the basis of assessment of the patient and his or her history.
10. Formulate a field impression for patients with abdominal trauma on the basis of assessment findings.
11. Apply the epidemiologic principles to develop prevention strategies for abdominal injuries.
12. Integrate pathophysiologic principles into the assessment of a patient with abdominal injuries.
13. Describe the management of abdominal injuries.
14. Develop a management plan for patients with abdominal trauma on the basis of field impression.
15. Describe the epidemiology, including the morbidity and mortality rates and prevention strategies, for hollow organ injuries.
16. Explain the pathophysiology of hollow organ injuries.
17. Describe the assessment findings associated with hollow organ injuries.
18. Describe the treatment plan and management of patients with hollow organ injuries.
19. Describe the epidemiology, including the morbidity and mortality rates and prevention strategies, for solid organ injuries.
20. Explain the pathophysiology of solid organ injuries.
21. Describe the assessment findings associated with solid organ injuries.
22. Describe the treatment plan and management of patients with solid organ injuries.
23. Describe the epidemiology, including the morbidity and mortality rates and prevention strategies, for abdominal vascular injuries.
24. Explain the pathophysiology of abdominal vascular injuries.
25. Describe the assessment findings associated with abdominal vascular injuries.
26. Describe the treatment plan and management of patients with abdominal vascular injuries.
27. Describe the epidemiology, including the morbidity and mortality rates and prevention strategies, for pelvic fractures.
28. Explain the pathophysiology of pelvic fractures.
29. Describe the assessment findings associated with pelvic fractures.
30. Describe the treatment plan and management of patients with pelvic fractures.
31. Describe the epidemiology, including the morbidity and mortality rates and prevention strategies, for other related abdominal injuries.
32. Explain the pathophysiology of other related abdominal injuries.
33. Describe the assessment findings associated with other related abdominal injuries.
34. Describe the treatment plan and management of patients with other related abdominal injuries.
35. Describe the epidemiology, including the morbidity and mortality rates and prevention strategies, for diaphragmatic injuries.
36. Explain the pathophysiology of diaphragmatic injuries.
37. Describe the assessment findings associated with diaphragmatic injuries.
38. Describe the treatment plan and management of patients with diaphragmatic injuries.
39. Describe the epidemiology, including the morbidity and mortality rates and prevention strategies, for retroperitoneal injuries.
40. Explain the pathophysiology of retroperitoneal injuries.
41. Describe the assessment findings associated with retroperitoneal injuries.
42. Describe the treatment plan and management of patients with retroperitoneal injuries.
43. Describe the epidemiology, including the morbidity and mortality rates and prevention strategies, for penetrating abdominal injuries.
44. Explain the pathophysiology of penetrating abdominal injuries.
45. Describe the assessment findings associated with penetrating abdominal injuries.
46. Describe the treatment plan and management of patients with penetrating abdominal injuries.

Objectives—continued

47. Describe the epidemiology, including the morbidity and mortality rates and prevention strategies, for trauma in pregnancy.
48. Explain the pathophysiology of trauma in pregnancy.
49. Describe the assessment findings associated with trauma in pregnancy.
50. Describe the treatment plan and management of a pregnant patient with trauma.
51. Describe the epidemiology, including the morbidity and mortality rates and prevention strategies, for genitourinary trauma.
52. Explain the pathophysiology of genitourinary trauma.
53. Describe the assessment findings associated with genitourinary trauma.
54. Describe the treatment plan and management of a patient with genitourinary trauma.

Chapter Outline

Case Scenario

You and your paramedic engine company respond to a "stab wound" at an apartment complex downtown. When you arrive, you are met by a police officer who informs you that an 8- to 10-inch kitchen knife was found near the patient. The patient is an approximately 30-year-old man who is unresponsive, sitting upright in a chair. He is pale and cold to the touch. His carotid pulse is rapid and thready, and he is breathing five to six times per minute. A minimal amount of blood can be seen on the patient's shirt over the right side of the patient's abdomen.

Questions

1. *What is your general impression of this patient?*
2. *What additional assessment will be important in the evaluation of this patient?*
3. *What intervention should you initiate at this time?*

[OBJECTIVE 1]

Abdominal trauma is associated with high rates of morbidity and mortality despite improvements in both vehicle safety and advancements in the medical care of injured patients. In fact, blunt abdominal trauma accounts for approximately two thirds of all trauma cases seen at some centers (Ong et al., 1994). The critical nature of abdominal trauma primarily relates to hemorrhage. Consequently, any delay to surgical intervention and control of hemorrhage increases the chances of morbidity and mortality. This is the case whether the abdominal trauma is blunt or penetrating or affects a **solid organ, hollow organ,** or vascular structure. Examples of solid organs include the liver, spleen, pancreas, kidneys, adrenal glands, and ovaries (female). Hollow organs include the stomach, intestines, gallbladder, urinary bladder, and uterus (female). Even in the case of pelvic fractures, considered by some to be more of an abdominal injury than an orthopedic injury, the major cause of death is still hemorrhage. Therefore in all cases of abdominal trauma, your main goal as a prehospital professional is to prevent or control hemorrhage when possible and get the patient rapidly to a facility capable of surgical intervention and hemorrhage control.

Hemorrhage presents the major challenge in abdominal trauma. This understanding can help guide prevention strategies. Certain factors may worsen hemorrhage in abdominal trauma, including medications that worsen hemorrhage, such as warfarin (Coumadin). In addition, alcohol is cited as a cause or contributing factor in approximately half of all motor vehicle crashes (MVCs) (Demetriades et al., 2004). Therefore any interventions that decrease the incidence of alcohol-related crashes also can decrease the incidence of abdominal trauma and improve the survival rate from such crashes. Continued improvements in vehicle design and safety also can help decrease both the incidence and severity of abdominal trauma. The most important role you will play as an EMS professional in cases of abdominal trauma is to provide a rapid response and rapid transport to a trauma center.

Although abdominal trauma occurs with other mechanisms of injury, it is commonly associated with MVCs. In this chapter, MVCs are frequently cited as an example because they are the most common mechanism of injury you will encounter as a paramedic.

ANATOMY AND PHYSIOLOGY

[OBJECTIVE 2]

The abdomen is bordered superiorly by the diaphragm, inferiorly by the skeletal structures and supporting ligaments of the pelvis, posteriorly by the vertebral column, anteriorly by the anterior abdominal wall, and laterally by the muscles of the abdomen and flanks (Figure 50-1).

To describe and document an abdominal injury accurately and recognize the structures that may be involved, you must understand the surface anatomy of the abdomen. You also must understand how that surface anatomy corresponds to the location of the underlying abdominal organs. Although other delineations have been made, the abdomen most often is described as being divided into four quadrants. These quadrants are the right and left upper quadrants and the right and left lower quadrants. The right upper quadrant (RUQ) contains the liver, gallbladder, part of the stomach, right kidney, ascending colon, transverse colon, and major blood vessels. The left upper quadrant (LUQ) contains the stomach, spleen, pancreas, transverse colon, descending colon, and left kidney. The right lower quadrant (RLQ) contains the appendix, ascending colon, right ovary (female), and right fallopian tube (female). The left lower quadrant (LLQ) contains the descending colon, sigmoid colon, left ovary (female), and left fallopian tube (female). Also helpful to know are the locations of the xiphoid process, symphysis pubis, and umbilicus as well as their relations to the underlying abdominal structures (Figure 50-2).

The abdomen also includes a variety of structures that lie beyond the posterior aspect of the peritoneum but in front of the back muscles and vertebral column. These so-called **retroperitoneal** structures include parts of the duodenum and pancreas as well as the kidneys and ureters, parts of the colon, and several vascular structures. Many pelvic structures such as the rectum, ureters, and reproductive organs, as well as their associated nerves and blood vessels, are also located retroperitoneally (Figure 50-3).

In general, abdominal injuries are described as being either open, if the abdominal contents are exposed to the outside environment, or closed if they are not. Injuries also are often described as being either blunt or penetrating. Note that all penetrating injuries also are open ones, whereas blunt trauma may be either open or closed. The pathophysiologic features of specific abdominal organ injuries are covered in more detail later in this chapter.

An **index of suspicion** is the anticipation of potential injuries on the basis of the patient's chief complaint, mechanism of injury, and the assessment findings. Abdominal injuries, particularly closed ones, may be subtle. Therefore you must maintain a high index of

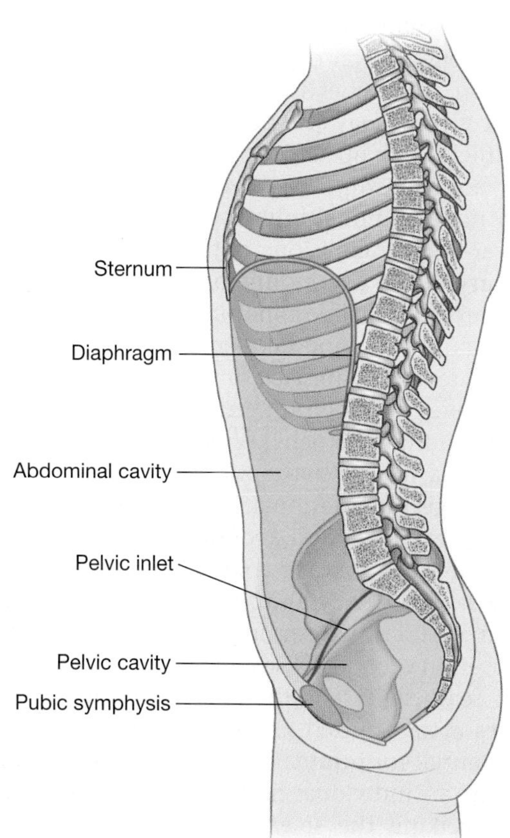

Figure 50-1 Boundaries of the abdomen.

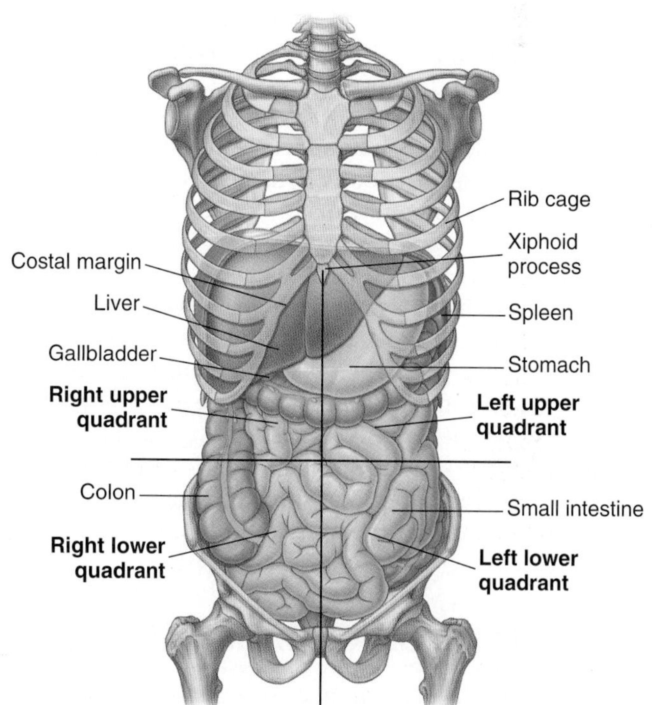

Figure 50-2 Surface anatomy of the abdomen. Note the division into quadrants.

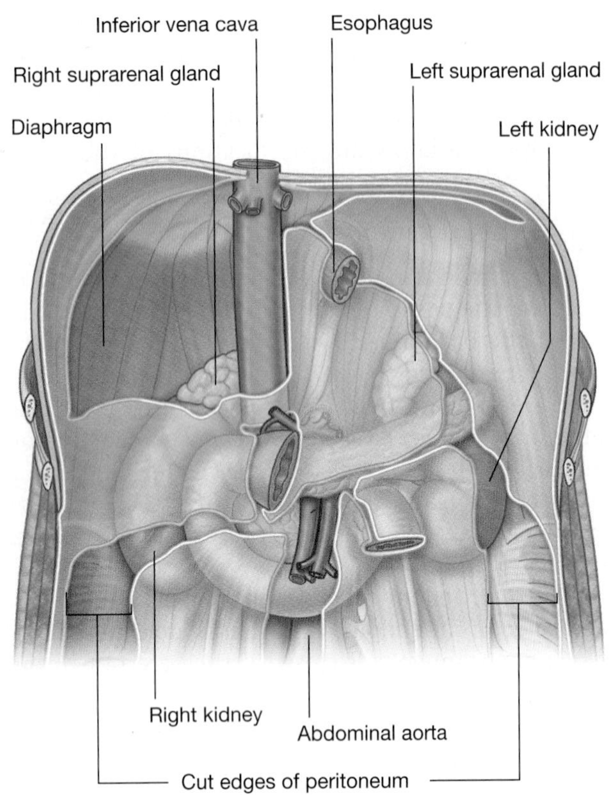

Figure 50-3 Retroperitoneal structures.

suspicion to recognize and properly treat these injuries. As previously emphasized, hemorrhage is the major cause of death in abdominal trauma. However, the patient may have a significant closed intraabdominal hemorrhage without signs of peritonitis. This is particularly dangerous because patients can bleed quite rapidly from closed intraabdominal injuries without displaying any external signs and develop hemorrhagic shock.

Hemorrhage is not the only pathophysiologic factor involved in abdominal trauma. The spillage of abdominal contents also can be seriously detrimental to the patient's condition. The hollow organs of the abdomen (e.g., the large and small intestines) contain enzymes, acids, and bacteria involved in digestion. If these substances escape the lumen of the intestines, they can lead to localized infection, progressing to sepsis and death. Although this takes longer to develop than the hemorrhagic shock associated with abdominal trauma, it can be easier for you to recognize once it exists. Because these substances are quite irritating to the peritoneum, signs of **peritonitis** may develop. These signs may include localized pain and a rigid abdomen from the muscle spasm associated with peritonitis.

MECHANISMS OF ABDOMINAL INJURY

[OBJECTIVES 3, 4, 5]

As previously emphasized, you must maintain a high index of suspicion in your assessment of patients with potential abdominal trauma. You can better anticipate the injuries sustained by a patient if you possess an understanding of the differing mechanisms of injury in abdominal trauma. You will need to conduct a thorough scene survey and gather a thorough history from the patient and bystanders to determine the forces involved and the injuries you will likely encounter.

Two basic forces are involved in blunt abdominal trauma: compression forces and shear, or deceleration, forces. Compression forces result, for example, from an MVC when the anterior portion of the abdomen ceases forward motion as the car comes to a stop. Meanwhile, the internal organs continue moving forward, eventually being compressed from behind between the anterior abdominal wall and the posterior abdominal wall and spinal column.

Deceleration forces occur when part of an internal structure is fixed and part of it is mobile. In the previous example of the MVC, the aortic arch may be sheared off as it continues forward while the descending aorta remains stationary. Similar injuries can occur at the pedicles of the spleen and kidneys and in the liver as the right and left lobes move around a stationary ligamentum teres.

Because the most common example of blunt abdominal trauma is an MVC, an understanding of the forces just outlined is important. Any or all of these forces may come into play depending on the specifics of the collision. In addition, as a prehospital care provider, you should note that specific types of collisions yield specific injury patterns.

In a head-on or other frontal impact, the patient, especially an unbelted driver or front-seat passenger, often is pushed down and under the dashboard. On the other hand, these victims may also be thrown forward through the windshield and up and over the hood of the car. Traumatic aortic disruptions, liver and spleen injuries, and many nonabdominal injuries can result.

In a rear-impact collision, different injury patterns result. Injury most commonly occurs to the cervical spine. However, intraabdominal injuries also can occur from the compression and deceleration forces identified above. In a lateral, side-impact, or "T-bone" collision, the diaphragm, liver or spleen (depending on which side of the patient was hit), and pelvis often are injured. In some circumstances a vehicle may spin out of control, exposing the passengers to rotational forces. These forces often result in cervical spine and abdominal visceral injuries. Patients involved in rollover collisions and ejections are at greater risk of virtually all injury mechanisms.

Whether a patient is restrained may alter the pattern of injury seen in each of these circumstances. In general, wearing a seatbelt lessens the degree to which any of these forces is transmitted to the body, thereby decreasing the potential for injury. Importantly, wearing a seatbelt prevents an individual from being ejected from the vehicle or striking the steering wheel. Steering wheel injuries themselves create a specific pattern of abdominal injury, mostly involving the upper, anterior abdominal, and anterior thoracic contents. However, seatbelt use (especially improper seat belt use) is associated with a typical injury pattern. This pattern includes compression injuries to the pancreas, liver, spleen, small bowel, and kidneys. Despite this, wearing seat belts is vital and should be routine whenever a person is driving or riding in a vehicle. The specific injury pattern seen with seatbelt use is uncommon if the seatbelt is properly worn. Moreover, this injury pattern is far less serious than the injuries associated with not wearing a seatbelt.

Other mechanisms are also associated with specific injury patterns. For example, motorcycle or bicycle riders may be involved in frontal or lateral impact and ejections, or they may "lay the bike down." In a frontal impact the cyclist's head, chest, or abdomen may strike the handlebars. If he or she is ejected over the bars, a secondary collision with the ground occurs, with associated injuries that depend on the site of impact and the kinetic energy imparted. Similar secondary collisions occur if the cyclist is ejected after a lateral impact. Even if he or she is not ejected, the cyclist may injure the same anatomic regions as the victim of a side-impact MVC. However, in the cyclist's case, he or she does not have the protection of the passenger compartment to reduce the kinetic energy transferred to the body. "Laying the bike down," or deliberately letting go of the motorcycle when losing control, is not avoiding a crash—it *is* a crash. Significant soft tissue injury (in addition to any of the previously described injuries) often results as the rider's body strikes and even slides along the pavement.

Pedestrians struck by cars are injured in specific and predictable ways. This injury pattern often is described as occurring in three phases. In the first phase, the car's bumper hits the victim. This often results in leg, knee, or pelvis injuries depending on the height of the bumper in relation to the height of the victim. In the second phase, head and abdominal or torso injuries occur as the victim is thrown onto the hood and/or windshield of the car. In the third phase, the victim hits the ground, often resulting in abdominal organ compression injuries as well as head and spine injuries.

Of course, an MVC is not the only mechanism associated with blunt abdominal trauma. Falls are the second leading cause of nonfatal injury in the United States. They often result in significant deceleration injuries. Patients also may be injured when they are struck, intentionally or accidentally, by a blunt object. The resulting compression forces will injure whichever structures lie under the affected area. Finally, although fortunately rare, blast injuries create specific injury patterns. These patterns may include abdominal injuries depending on the specific circumstances involved (Box 50-1).

Penetrating injuries to the abdomen are less common than blunt ones. Also, at least from a prehospital perspective, they may be more straightforward. The two major factors that determine the nature and extent of injury in penetrating abdominal trauma are the region(s) of the abdomen involved and the amount of energy transferred to the body.

BOX 50-1 Blast Injuries

Primary: Result from the direct effects of the pressure wave. Gas-containing organs such as the intestines are at greatest risk.

Secondary: Result from flying objects striking the body. Injuries are similar to other penetrating trauma.

Tertiary: Result when the patient is thrown against a stationary object or the ground. Injuries are similar to other blunt trauma.

Penetrating injuries are often described as being low-velocity, medium-velocity, or high-velocity injuries. Low velocity typically includes knife and other stab wounds. Medium velocity includes most civilian handguns and some rifles. Military and hunting rifles may enter the high-velocity range.

The main determinant of injury from penetrating trauma is the region of the abdomen involved. However, this is not 100% reliable in all circumstances. For example, a person who is stabbed with a knife in the RUQ likely has a liver injury and not a splenic injury; however, this is not necessarily true for other forms of penetrating injury. Gunshot wounds that appear to enter in one area and exit another may in fact not have taken a direct path. As a result, the nature and extent of injuries cannot be reliably determined from the apparent path of the projectile. The same can be true for other forms of penetrating injury, such as a projectile propelled by blast forces.

Gunshot wounds to the abdomen deserve further special attention. For gunshot wounds, the amount of impacted energy can be described by the following formula:

$$\text{Kinetic energy} = \tfrac{1}{2}M \times V^2$$

where M is mass and V is velocity. (Technically, this formula applies for all forms of energy transfer, including both blunt and penetrating trauma. However, the mass or velocity of most energy-producing objects is usually not as well known as it is in the case of gunshot wounds.) Thus the velocity of the projectile is the important determinant of the amount of kinetic energy transferred to the body and therefore the amount of damage sustained by the patient. The shape, tumble, and physical factors of the actual projectile also are quite important.

Note that this is independent of the cosmetic appearance of the wound, the number of bullets a weapon can fire without reloading, or other similar aspects of the nature of the weapon or of the bullet itself. Shotguns are capable of delivering multiple projectiles to the target at the same time. However, the kinetic energy of each individual pellet (one or more of which may have hit the patient) is still described by the above formula. Likewise, so-called assault weapons may or may not lead to multiple wounds in the same patient, but the nature and characteristics of each individual wound are still described by the same kinetic energy formula. Also, "dum dum" or other specialty bullets are designed to impart the maximal amount of their kinetic energy to the target, unlike standard bullets, which may lose a large percentage of their potential energy traveling through tissue. However, no bullet, specially designed or otherwise, can impart more kinetic energy than described by the formula.

Velocity, and therefore delivered energy, is usually measured as the bullet leaves the barrel of the weapon. It falls off rapidly with increasing distance. Therefore the distance of the patient from the muzzle of the gun at the time of injury is an important factor in determining the likely amount of injury sustained in a gunshot wound victim. Additional significant factors pertaining to wounding potential include the path the bullet takes and the type of tissue struck, among others.

ASSESSMENT

[OBJECTIVES 6 TO 12]

You will not be able to provide the main beneficial therapies for abdominal trauma in the field as with commonly encountered prehospital scenarios such as cardiac arrest. Instead, most significant abdominal injuries require definitive care in the hospital. Therefore your main goal in assessing victims of abdominal trauma is determining which patients need rapid transport to the hospital, perhaps to a designated trauma facility. Failure to do this rapidly and effectively can lead to increased morbidity and mortality rates from unrecognized abdominal injury.

This process of rapidly determining who needs immediate transport can be facilitated by a staged assessment process in which you first look for critical findings as provided in Box 50-2. If you note any of these critical findings, treat immediate life threats (airway compromise, respiratory compromise, significant external hemorrhage) and transport the patient without delay. This is often described as a "load and go" situation. You can defer any further assessment or conduct it en route to the hospital. At the same time you perform this rapid assessment, you should begin rapid treatment of these critical findings, such as the treatment of hypovolemic shock.

If you do not identify any of these critical findings, then you can conduct a more thorough assessment and make appropriate transportation and destination decisions on the basis of the result of that assessment. Regardless of the findings during the primary survey, all seriously ill or injured patients should have ongoing assessments while they are in your care.

Although this chapter primarily concerns victims of abdominal trauma, you must remember that patients may sustain more than one injury, the true nature of the injury may not be immediately apparent, and injuries may change over time. Therefore you still must perform an overall assessment of the patient with an apparent abdominal injury. Of note, head injury or the presence of intoxicants such as drugs or alcohol can mask the signs and symptoms of shock from abdominal trauma. Likewise, hemoperitoneum from either a solid organ or vascular injury may not immediately be apparent on abdominal examination alone. In fact, this condition often is associated with an initially normal abdominal examination and is then identified by the presence of unexplained shock or shock out of proportion to the known injuries. Obviously you can make this determination only after a thorough examination that includes all other areas, not simply the abdomen.

Visible wounds and/or the mechanism of injury may suggest intraabdominal injury; however, a focused but complete abdominal examination for the victim of abdominal injury still is warranted. For example, peritonitis from a hollow organ injury may be present with a subjective complaint of abdominal pain as well as the objective finding of tenderness on palpation or percussion of the abdomen. You also may note the presence of guarding, rigidity, or distention, although the latter is a late finding and should not be relied on to determine the absence of peritonitis or significant abdominal pathology. In fact, more subtle clues such as ecchymosis or abrasions may be the only clues to significant intraabdominal injury, particularly when the mechanism of injury or the presence of unexplained shock also suggests that intraabdominal injury may have occurred.

After you have conducted the primary survey, regardless of whether critical findings are identified, a more comprehensive assessment is warranted. In most cases, you should perform it en route to the hospital. This comprehensive assessment (the secondary survey) includes obtaining vital signs, which may be the best or earliest indicators of hemorrhagic shock.

The secondary survey should include inspection, or looking for abrasions and bruising, although you probably already took a quick look for these findings during the primary survey. You may not have noticed a seatbelt sign or other specific injury pattern during the primary survey because of your search for life-threatening injuries. Other findings to look for during the secondary survey include distention, obvious external blood loss,

BOX 50-2 Critical Findings in Abdominal Trauma

- Altered mental status (Glasgow Coma Scale score less than 14)
- Airway compromise
- Respiratory distress (respiratory rate less than 10 or more than 29 breaths/min)
- Shock (systolic blood pressure less than 90 mm Hg)
- Signs of peritonitis

wounds, eviscerations, and the presence of impaled objects. A complete inspection of the abdomen also includes inspecting the back.

Although often described as not useful in the prehospital environment, auscultation for the presence or absence and character of bowel sounds is part of the standard medical assessment of patients with abdominal trauma in the hospital. The main problem is that auscultation in the often loud and uncontrolled prehospital environment is unreliable. Even if it is technically possible to perform, the findings often are unreliable and of little value because decreased or absent bowel sounds is a nonspecific finding. Moreover, bowel sounds may still be present even in the face of significant intraabdominal injury.

Likewise, **percussion** is not always taught or recommended as a prehospital skill. However, you can easily learn the technique, although it requires some practice (Rathe, 2000). It also is more sensitive than palpation alone for peritonitis, which may occur with hollow organ injury. For percussion, take the following steps:

1. First, hyperextend the middle finger of one hand and place the distal interphalangeal joint firmly against the patient's abdomen (Figure 50-4).
2. With the end (not the pad) of the opposite middle finger, use a quick flick of the wrist to strike the first finger.
3. Categorize what you hear as normal, dull, or hyperresonant.
4. Practice your technique until you can consistently produce a "normal" percussion note on your (presumably normal) partner before you work with patients.

Palpation can elicit signs of tenderness associated with any abdominal injury as well as the guarding or rebound tenderness associated with peritoneal irritation. Palpation also includes assessing extraabdominal structures, such as checking for pelvic stability and tenderness as well as checking for tenderness in the back that may indicate retroperitoneal injury.

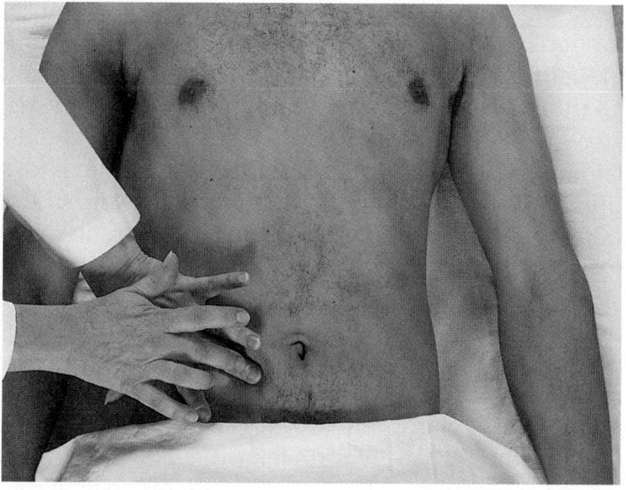

Figure 50-4 Abdominal percussion.

Remember, your goal is not to diagnose any specific abdominal injury. Indeed, the absence of significant findings on a thorough abdominal assessment cannot completely rule out intraabdominal injury, as it has already been noted that morbidity (and the symptoms associated with it) can be delayed in abdominal trauma. Instead, the goal is for you to recognize who *might* have a significant abdominal injury based on history, mechanism of injury, and physical examination, and then develop a field impression, a list of likely injuries (differential diagnosis), and an appropriate destination and treatment plan based on these findings.

MANAGEMENT

[OBJECTIVES 13, 14]

As previously identified, surgical intervention is the only effective therapy for significant abdominal injury. No definitive therapy is possible in the field. In fact, the opposite is true because bleeding continues until the time of surgery and survival is determined by the length of time from the injury to definitive surgical control of hemorrhage. Thus any delay in the field negatively affects survival from abdominal trauma. Therefore your focus must be rapid evaluation and evacuation of patients with abdominal trauma to an appropriate receiving facility. Rapid transport is of limited value if the receiving facility cannot provide immediate surgical capability.

Not all victims of abdominal trauma have *serious* abdominal injuries. However, critical findings during the primary survey, such as unexplained shock, and physical signs of significant abdominal injury necessitate rapid transport to a facility with immediate surgical capability. However, some patients may be appropriately transported to other facilities or even not transported at all. Your local protocols should address this and identify the closest *appropriate* facility for victims of abdominal injury.

However, your prehospital care for patients with abdominal trauma does not solely consist of driving fast to the hospital. You should pay careful attention to the patient's airway, breathing, and circulation (ABCs) in all cases of trauma—and abdominal trauma is no exception. Airway and breathing are seldom affected by isolated abdominal injury. But many patients have more than one injury; therefore you must address the ABCs in all cases to avoid missing potentially life-threatening injuries.

Because the major cause of morbidity and mortality in abdominal trauma is hemorrhagic shock, begin shock resuscitation immediately and continue it during transport. This usually consists of intravenous (IV) fluids, usually normal saline or lactated Ringer's solution, administered through a large-bore (14- or 16-gauge) peripheral IV.

In some EMS systems the pneumatic antishock garment (PASG) may be used for patients with decompensated shock and suspected intraperitoneal or retroperitoneal hemorrhage or a pelvic fracture. Do not inflate the abdominal compartment in patients with obvious respiratory compromise, presence of an evisceration, or suspected diaphragmatic hernia and in pregnant patients. Check with your medical director and local EMS protocols about the use of the PASG in your area.

SPECIFIC ABDOMINAL INJURIES

Hollow Organ Injuries

[OBJECTIVES 15, 16, 17, 18]

The classic hollow organ injury is that of duodenal rupture. The typical patient with this injury is an unrestrained driver involved in a head-on MVC. Alternatively, this type of injury also may occur with a direct blow to the abdomen.

Hollow organ injuries are associated with morbidity and mortality from two main causes: blood loss (hemorrhage) and the spillage of intraluminal contents into the peritoneum (contamination). In the latter case, peritonitis develops as gastric juices, partially digested food, bacteria, and/or fecal matter leave the damaged hollow organ to surround the nearby intraabdominal structures.

Although any hollow intraabdominal structure can be injured from any mechanism, some general patterns exist. The small and large intestines are most frequently injured, for example, from penetrating injuries or from blunt force deceleration injuries. Meanwhile, the stomach is most often injured as a result of blunt trauma. A full stomach during the trauma further increases the risk of gastric injury. The duodenum also is most often injured because of blunt trauma. Importantly, this injury often is difficult to detect and recognition often is delayed.

As with all abdominal trauma, evaluation begins with a careful assessment of the ABCs. Critical findings include the presence of shock in association with a mechanism of injury consistent with potential hollow organ damage. Although external signs of abdominal trauma (e.g., impaled objects, gunshot wounds, bruises) may be present, you must look for unexplained shock or shock out of proportion to the known injuries because this often indicates intraabdominal injury. Likewise, obvious signs of intraabdominal pathology, such as distention, guarding, and rigidity, may be present. However, their absence does not rule out significant injury, especially in the setting of unexplained shock. In the case of known or suspected significant intraabdominal trauma with shock, rapid transport to an appropriate trauma facility is indicated. You should perform a more thorough assessment, as well as ongoing assessments, en route to the hospital.

Your management of hollow organ injuries is similar to that for all abdominal trauma. It includes support of the ABCs, rapid treatment of the patient, and transportation to an appropriate receiving facility. You should continually reevaluate en route and attempt to recognize and treat hemorrhagic shock for all victims of abdominal trauma, regardless of whether hollow organs, solid organs, or both are injured.

Solid Organ Injuries

[OBJECTIVES 19, 20, 21, 22]

Solid organ injuries can result from either blunt or penetrating trauma. In either case, the major cause of morbidity and mortality is hemorrhagic shock as a result of blood loss. For injuries to the liver alone, this perhaps is obvious and anticipated. Splenic injures (the spleen is the most commonly injured solid organ), however, may be more difficult to recognize. They are commonly associated with other intraabdominal injuries (usually injury to another solid organ or blood vessel; concomitant solid and hollow organ injury is uncommon). In addition, they may present as left shoulder, rather than abdominal, pain because of diaphragmatic irritation associated with the splenic injury. **Kehr's sign** is the name given to the occurrence of acute left shoulder pain due to the presence of blood or other irritants in the peritoneal cavity. Kehr's sign is an example of referred pain (pain that occurs in a localized area separate from the site of the causative injury). Although commonly associated with splenic rupture, Kehr's sign is also associated with a ruptured ectopic pregnancy.

The reason that solid organ injuries so often lead to hemorrhage and shock is that both the liver and spleen are vascular structures surrounded by a fibrous capsule. They fill large portions of their respective right and left upper quadrants; therefore they frequently are injured when projectiles penetrate these areas. In blunt trauma, their firm but vascular nature means that both direct and deceleration forces tend to fracture the organ. If that force is significant enough to rupture the fibrous capsule as well, then blood flows freely into the peritoneal cavity. Without the tamponading effect of the capsule, this bleeding can be brisk and severe and hemorrhagic shock may result.

Assessing the potential victim of a solid organ injury is similar to assessing any patient for possible hemorrhagic shock. In addition to the primary survey, you also must look for obvious external signs of abdominal trauma, especially in the right upper and left upper quadrants, and other evidence of a mechanism of injury consistent with solid organ injury. Shock itself, especially unexplained shock or shock out of proportion to the known injuries, is also an important finding. Specific critical findings involving abdominal trauma include a distended or rigid abdomen or a patient who exhibits guarding on palpation of the abdomen. Even in the absence of critical findings during the primary survey, a secondary survey and ongoing assessments while en route to the hospital are indicated.

One goal of the secondary survey is to identify noncritical findings that may still alter the patient's destination or clinical course. These include abnormal vital signs as well as significant abnormalities on inspection, percussion, or palpation of the abdomen. This more complete examination also may help you develop a differential diagnosis and treatment plan for the victim of a solid organ injury. The fundamentals of that treatment plan are the same as for all victims of abdominal trauma: prompt attention to the ABCs, especially circulatory support; careful treatment; and rapid transport to an appropriate receiving facility.

Case Scenario—continued

You and your partner quickly move the patient to the ground. On examination you find a 1-inch stab wound in the right upper quadrant with minimal blood loss. The abdomen is soft and moderately distended. The patient's pupils are midpoint and nonreactive. He has no peripheral pulses. The remainder of the examination is normal. Vital signs are pulse, 130 beats/min (carotid pulse only), blood pressure is not able to be auscultated or palpated, and respirations are 5 breaths/min.

Questions

4. *Is this patient high priority? Why or why not?*
5. *What stage of shock is this patient in? Should you infuse IV fluids? How much?*
6. *What additional treatment should be initiated?*
7. *What destination is most appropriate for this patient? Should you transport to the hospital with lights and siren? Why or why not?*

Vascular Injuries

[OBJECTIVES 23, 24, 25, 26]

Vascular injuries often result from MVCs, frequently as a result of improperly worn lap and/or shoulder belts. For example, compression from an improperly fitted lap belt can lead to thrombosis of the iliac artery or abdominal aorta.

Similar to other intraabdominal injuries, the major cause of morbidity and mortality from vascular injuries is hemorrhagic shock. This should come as no surprise given the obvious potential for brisk bleeding from the vascular structures found in the abdominal cavity, such as the inferior vena cava and the descending aorta.

As with other intraabdominal injuries, your goal is to find and address signs of such hemorrhage and shock on an initial assessment, focused history, and physical examination. If you do not identify any critical findings, conduct a more detailed and ongoing assessment as previously described. If you initially identify critical findings or they develop later, then initiate aggressive resuscitation from hemorrhagic shock—including rapid transportation to an appropriate receiving facility—in line with local protocols.

Pelvic Fractures

[OBJECTIVES 27, 28, 29, 30]

The pelvis consists of several bones (sacrum, ilium, ischium, and pubis). These bones are strong, solid, and well protected in the body. Fractures of the pelvis imply that a large amount of force has been transmitted to the body. These fractures usually result from auto/pedestrian collisions, MVCs, and motorcycle crashes.

Because they represent high-energy events, pelvic fractures are associated with injuries to intraabdominal structures, retroperitoneal structures, and blood vessels. Specifically, the incidence of tears in the thoracic aorta is significantly increased in association with pelvic fractures.

As with abdominal trauma, the key to identifying a pelvic fracture is a primary survey in which you look for critical findings and then a secondary survey and ongoing assessment. The latter two ideally should be performed en route to a designated trauma facility if you note critical findings. In the case of pelvic fractures, the major cause of morbidity and mortality is hemorrhagic shock. This may be caused by blood loss from the bone itself, from the pelvic veins or arteries, or from associated injury to structures outside the pelvis. You can best determine hemorrhage and shock by the standard assessment of vital signs, mental status, and so forth. Also, you should palpate the pelvis to check for pain or instability that may indicate a fracture and source of significant bleeding.

Treat hemorrhagic shock from a pelvic fracture the same as hemorrhagic shock from any other source. This includes providing airway and breathing support as well as circulatory support with IV fluids per local protocol. In addition, in the case of pelvic fracture, an important prehospital intervention is to stabilize the bony injury to slow or stop the bleeding. This should be part of routine care and treatment for patients with a suspected pelvic fracture. This is commonly accomplished with the PASG. Other commercially available or locally improvised devices to stabilize pelvic fractures also may be authorized by local protocol.

Injuries to the urethra and bladder also are associated with pelvic fracture. You should look for these during the secondary survey. This includes checking the perineum for ecchymosis and blood as well as checking the penile meatus (opening) for blood.

Abdominal Wall Injuries

[OBJECTIVES 31, 32, 33, 34]

In abdominal trauma the abdominal wall that covers and protects the intraabdominal structures also can be injured. This can result from either blunt or penetrating trauma. Fortunately, most abdominal wall injuries are not the cause of significant morbidity and mortality. However, their presence can indicate more severe or even occult abdominal injuries that might otherwise be missed. Therefore you should carefully assess for these injuries.

An abdominal wall contusion is not usually difficult to recognize, even with a brief inspection of the abdomen. Alone, an abdominal wall contusion may be impressive, but it is not a critical finding. However, it can indicate that significant blunt force trauma has been applied to the underlying structures. Therefore, especially in the presence of otherwise unexplained shock, consider an abdominal wall contusion a valuable clue to possible hemorrhagic shock.

When present, abdominal wall contusions and hematomas may be clues to underlying injuries. However, as with all such bruises, the distinct color and appearance of these abdominal wall injuries is from the presence of blood visible under the skin. This blood can result from a variety of sources, ranging from the rupture of capillaries to lacerations of solid organs, such as the liver or spleen. For example, local trauma from the seatbelt is a common cause of injury to the abdominal wall muscles, with an associated contusion. A ruptured spleen may lead to intraabdominal hemorrhage that eventually becomes visible as ecchymosis around the umbilicus (Cullen's sign) (Figure 50-5). Depending on the briskness and severity of hemorrhage, visible ecchymosis may be delayed for several hours from the time of initial injury. Therefore the absence of a visible bruise does not indicate a lack of intraabdominal injury.

Penetrating trauma to the abdominal wall may be easier to recognize, and it more obviously indicates significant intraabdominal injury. You must assume that any penetration of the abdominal wall has penetrated the peritoneum and entered the peritoneal cavity until proven otherwise at the hospital. The presence of any penetration of the abdominal wall therefore is a critical finding on assessment and indicates the need for rapid transport to an appropriate receiving facility.

You should begin treatment for shock, if present, en route. If the penetrating object is still present in the wound, do not remove it. Rather, stabilize an impaled object in place.

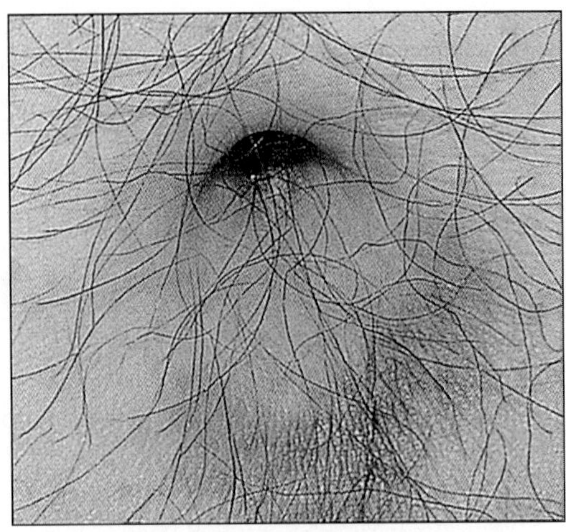

Figure 50-5 Cullen's sign.

An impressive associated abdominal injury is an abdominal evisceration. In these circumstances, an object has penetrated the peritoneum and created a large enough hole that the intraabdominal contents (most commonly the intestines) have begun to protrude. In such cases you should not push the protruding contents back into the abdomen. Infection and peritonitis would be the inevitable result. Instead, cover protruding contents with a clean, or ideally sterile, dressing moistened with normal saline. Then immediately transport the patient to an appropriate receiving facility.

Diaphragmatic Injuries

[OBJECTIVES 35, 36, 37, 38]

Another injury often associated with abdominal trauma is injury to the diaphragm. The diaphragm is the large, dome-shaped muscle that separates the thorax from the abdomen and plays a crucial role in respiration. This injury usually occurs from significant blunt trauma that ruptures the diaphragm, although penetrating injuries can injure the muscle as well. In either case, the injury to the diaphragm itself is seldom severe enough to impair respiration. Instead, the real danger is the herniation of the abdominal contents upward into the chest cavity. This can be severe enough to impair respiration. However, the degree of diaphragmatic injury and associated herniation is frequently small at first and extends over time. Therefore this injury often is subtle and not appreciated on initial field, or even emergency department, examination. Because of the presence of the liver in the right upper quadrant, the left (especially the left posterolateral) hemidiaphragm is the most frequently injured. When a diaphragmatic injury is known or suspected, administer supplemental oxygen and support ventilation as necessary. Transport the patient to an appropriate trauma facility while paying careful attention to his or her respiratory status. Use of a PASG is contraindicated in patients with diaphragmatic rupture.

Retroperitoneal Injuries

[OBJECTIVES 39, 40, 41, 42]

Retroperitoneal structures include parts of the duodenum and aorta, the kidneys, and the pancreas. Injuries to the pancreas deserve specific attention. Pancreatic injuries most commonly occur from penetrating injuries. However, they also may occur from blunt trauma as the pancreas is compressed against the vertebral column, such as by the handlebars in a bicycle crash or the steering wheel in an MVC.

When the pancreas is injured from either blunt or penetrating trauma, the enzymes it normally produces to aid digestion are released into the peritoneum instead. These chemicals have an irritating effect on the peritoneum and intraabdominal structures. Because these are digestive enzymes, they start to break down the internal organs and tissue with which they have come in contact. This process often is described as autodigestion because the pancreatic enzymes literally start to digest the patient's own tissues.

Although this enzymatic breakdown leads to chemical peritonitis, the assessment of patients with potential retroperitoneal injuries such as pancreatic trauma can be difficult. As previously stated, peritonitis from this irritation and autodigestion may be readily recognized on physical examination by findings such as abdominal rigidity, guarding, and rebound tenderness. However, because the posterior peritoneum separates the pancreas from the true abdomen, these findings may be significantly delayed. When you suspect pancreatic injury, treatment of the patient should include careful attention to the ABCs, especially resuscitation from shock.

Penetrating Injuries

[OBJECTIVES 43, 44, 45, 46]

The importance of kinetic injury transfer in penetrating injuries has already been covered. These types of injuries are relatively common, accounting for more than 40% of fatal traumatic injuries in one study (Sauaia et al., 1995). Assessment of a patient with a potential penetrating abdominal injury is usually straightforward. Conscious patients usually provide the history of being shot or stabbed (although estimates regarding the size of the knife or the specifics of the gun are notoriously inaccurate). Beyond the history, the physical examination of the patient with a penetrating abdominal injury also is usually straightforward. One or more wounds are typically apparent. Do not attempt to determine or describe entrance versus exit wounds because this information also is notoriously inaccurate. Instead, simply describe wounds by size and location.

The location of stab wounds and impaled objects can reliably provide clues regarding the potential injury to underlying structures. However, gunshot wounds, even those that appear through and through, often take an indirect path and can injure structures far removed from the apparent site of injury.

Depending on which intraabdominal structures are injured in penetrating trauma, assessment of the patient may show any of the signs and symptoms of hollow organ and/or solid organ injury. The treatment plan for penetrating abdominal injury includes paying careful attention to the ABCs, stabilizing any impaled objects, and aggressively treating hemorrhagic shock because the latter is usually the cause of death in penetrating abdominal trauma.

Case Scenario CONCLUSION

You intubate the patient and begin assisting his ventilations with 100% oxygen. Breath sounds are clear, although slightly diminished on the right side. Your partner tells you that ventilating the patient's lungs is easy. No tracheal deviation or subcutaneous emphysema is noted. En route to the trauma center, you and your partner are unable to place an IV despite several attempts. The cardiac rhythm is sinus tachycardia without ectopy.

On arrival in the emergency department the patient's pulse remains unchanged and his blood pressure is 48/36 mm Hg (measured by Doppler). The patient is rapidly taken to surgery for repair of lacerations to the liver, portal vein, and hepatic vein. Despite multiple postoperative complications, the patient was ultimately discharged from the hospital with a good prognosis for long-term recovery.

Looking Back

8. *Given the patient's final disposition, was your treatment appropriate? Why or why not?*

9. *How important was IV therapy in this patient's case? How could you have established vascular access after your inability to initiate an IV?*

Trauma in Pregnancy

[OBJECTIVES 47, 48, 49, 50]

Abruptio Placentae

One of the more difficult problems in caring for the pregnant patient with abdominal trauma is that of **abruptio placentae** (also called *placental abruption*). This condition occurs when the placenta separates from the uterine wall after the twentieth week of gestation. This typically occurs spontaneously, but approximately 2% to 10% of cases occur as a result of trauma, usually MVCs, assaults, or falls (Gaufberg, 2006).

As the placenta separates from the uterine wall it bleeds, leading to hematoma formation and further separation. This compresses both structures and may compromise the blood supply to the fetus. Signs and symptoms of abruptio placentae include abdominal pain or cramping, uterine pain, uterine tenderness, uterine contractions, and vaginal bleeding (absent in up to 30% of cases).

Although fortunately not common, abruptio placentae can be life threatening for both the fetus and the mother. In addition, pregnant women should be instructed to wear their lap and shoulder belts at all times while in a car despite the potential discomfort, and perhaps paradoxic nature, of this advice. A properly fitting lap belt (low on the hips) is far less likely to induce placental abruption than is the force transmitted to the mother's abdomen by the steering wheel, dashboard, or other surface she may encounter if improperly restrained.

When you recognize placental abruption, you can best treat it by paying careful attention to the ABCs and treating hemorrhagic shock, if present, in the mother. In general, transport a woman in the later stages of pregnancy on her left side to avoid having the gravid uterus compress the vena cava and decrease blood return to the heart.

Premature Labor

A fall, MVC, or other blunt trauma also may trigger premature labor in a pregnant patient. Although uterine contractions after trauma are common, premature delivery caused by preterm labor is not. Actual preterm delivery resulting from premature labor (in the absence of abruption) probably occurs no more frequently among traumatized women than in the general population (Hughey, 2005).

As in all cases of trauma to pregnant women, the best care for the fetus is proper care for the mother. Therefore perform the standard assessment of the ABCs and treatment of shock and other problems identified during the primary survey.

Uterine Rupture

The last specific problem related to abdominal trauma in pregnancy that you should consider is uterine rupture. An improperly worn lap belt, especially one worn too high over the uterus, is a risk factor for this rare condition. Your assessment and treatment strategies are similar to those for placental abruption.

Genitourinary Trauma

[OBJECTIVES 51, 52, 53, 54]

Bladder

The genitourinary system is commonly injured in conjunction with abdominal trauma. For example, the bladder is frequently injured in association with lower abdominal and pelvic injuries, especially blunt force trauma. This is even more likely if the bladder is full at the time of the injury.

This fact is relatively simple to understand. The bladder is similar to a water-filled balloon in these circumstances, and a significant enough force will cause the bladder to rupture into the abdominal cavity or pelvic cavity. When this occurs, shock and/or peritonitis may result. No specific prehospital treatment is possible for bladder injuries; rather, provide supportive care and treatment for hemorrhagic shock if it develops.

External Genitalia

Given their relatively unprotected location outside the body, external genitalia, especially in men, are frequently injured in abdominal trauma. The external genitalia can be burned, lacerated, penetrated by a projectile, or contused, as can any other exposed body part. Specific assessment findings will correspond to the injured anatomy and to the type of trauma sustained. For example, the anterior urethra may be injured during a straddle impact. In this case, you may note local pain, swelling, bruising, and possibly hematuria. Direct injuries to the external genitalia can be impressive and are therefore seldom overlooked, at least in the hospital setting, once the patient can be fully undressed. However impressive, they are rarely life threatening and should not distract you from performing a good primary and secondary survey.

The signs of *internal* injury are of greater importance than the obvious external genitalia trauma. These signs are sometimes obvious only through an examination of the *external* genitalia. One of the best-known examples is looking for blood at the urethral meatus of a male patient as a marker of pelvic fracture and therefore a contraindication to urethral catheter insertion.

If you encounter a significant external genitalia injury, control hemorrhage with direct pressure. Little other specific prehospital treatment is possible for these injuries beyond paying careful attention to the ABCs and treating hemorrhagic shock, if it exists.

Kidneys and Ureters

The kidneys and ureters can be injured in association with abdominal trauma, often as a result of direct trauma (blunt or penetrating) to the back or flank. Such injuries can result in contusions, hematomas, and disruptions of the collecting system (ureters). When this occurs, the patient may present with back pain, especially with a direct renal injury. You may note ecchymosis at the site of injury. Ecchymosis involving the flanks is called *Grey-Turner's sign*. If the patient has urinated since the injury, he or she may also report blood in the urine (hematuria). As with many abdominal and associated injuries, no specific field treatment is available for these injuries beyond the ABCs and treatment of shock.

Case Scenario SUMMARY

1. *What is your general impression of this patient?* This patient is clearly high priority given his level of consciousness, color, skin temperature, slow respirations, and thready and slow carotid pulse.
2. *What additional assessment will be important in the evaluation of this patient?* The primary survey suggested that the patient is in shock (based on skin color and temperature as well as mental status). Further evaluation of the skin and vital signs will be important to establish the degree of shock. A rapid trauma assessment also will be important to identify the cause of the shock.
3. *What intervention should you initiate at this time?* This patient appears to be in severe shock, potentially caused by a stab injury. The airway should be controlled, ventilation with high-flow oxygen provided, and a rapid trauma assessment performed to understand better the cause of the patient's condition. IV access also should be established but not until transport to definitive care has begun.
4. *Is this patient high priority? Why or why not?* Yes. He is tachycardic, he has no apparent blood pressure, and his respiratory rate has slowed. He is in imminent danger of going into respiratory arrest and possibly cardiac arrest.
5. *What stage of shock is this patient in? Should you infuse IV fluids? How much?* Because his blood pressure has dropped, this patient is in the decompensated stage of shock. Aggressive therapy is required to restore cellular perfusion and prevent further organ damage. Although IV fluid infusion remains controversial for individuals in hemorrhagic shock, it is appropriate for this patient because of his profound hypotension. Typical fluid guidelines range from 10 to 20 mL/kg of body weight. Although local protocols vary, this patient typically would receive 750 to 1000 mL of an isotonic solution such as normal saline or lactated Ringer's solution.
6. *What additional treatment should be initiated?* Once the airway is controlled and positive-pressure ventilation provided, the patient should be prepared for transport. IV access can be established en route. Bleeding from the abdominal wound, although minimal, should be monitored and direct pressure provided if it increases.
7. *What destination is most appropriate for this patient? Should you transport to the hospital with lights and siren? Why or why not?* This patient is extremely unstable and should be rapidly transported to a designated trauma center. In many systems a "lights and siren" transport would be warranted.
8. *Given the patient's final disposition, was your treatment appropriate? Why or why not?* Yes. Rapid airway control, ventilation, administration of oxygen, and transport to the trauma center are appropriate in this case. Although IV access is the obvious appropriate course of treatment, it may be difficult to obtain access in decompensated shock. Obtaining IV access should *never* delay rapid transport.
9. *How important was IV therapy in this patient's case? How could you have established vascular access after your inability to initiate an IV?* Administration of IV fluids, although controversial, is important in this case. As previously noted, delaying transport of a critical patient to secure an IV is never appropriate. Depending on local protocols, this patient may be an excellent candidate for adult intraosseous infusion.

Chapter Summary

- Morbidity and mortality from abdominal trauma are primarily related to hemorrhage.
- The goal of prehospital care for abdominal trauma is to prevent or control hemorrhage when possible and rapidly transport the patient to a facility capable of surgical intervention when necessary.
- Abdominal trauma may involve solid organs, hollow organs, and vascular structures in any combination.
- The spillage of abdominal contents from the rupture of hollow organs leads to peritonitis, the second leading cause of morbidity and mortality.
- You should maintain a high index of suspicion in the assessment of patients with potential abdominal injuries.
- Your assessment of a patient with abdominal trauma should proceed in a staged fashion, beginning with a search for critical findings.

Chapter Summary—continued

- You should rapidly transport patients with critical findings on a primary survey to an appropriate receiving facility.
- For victims of significant abdominal trauma, conduct further assessment and initial treatment for shock while en route to the hospital.

REFERENCES

Demetriades, D., Gkiokas, G., Velmahos, G. C., Brown, C., Murray, J., & Noguchi, T. (2004). Alcohol and illicit drugs in traumatic death: Prevalence and association with type and severity of injuries. *Journal of the American College of Surgeons, 199*(5):687-692.

Gaufberg, S. V. (2006). *Abruptio placentae.* Retrieved December 20, 2007, from http://www.emedicine.com.

Hughey, M. J. (2005). *Trauma during pregnancy,* Military Obstetrics & Gynecology. Winnetka, IL: Brookside Associates.

Ong, C. L., Png, D. J., & Chan, S. T. (1994). Abdominal trauma—A review. *Singapore Medical Journal, 35*(3), 269-270.

Rathe, R. (2000). *Examination of the chest and lungs.* Retrieved December 12, 2006, from http://www.medinfo.ufl.edu.

Sauaia, A., Moore, F. A., Moore, E. E., Moser, K. S., Brennan, R., Read, R. A., et al. (1995). Epidemiology of trauma deaths: A reassessment. *Journal of Trauma: Injury Infection & Critical Care, 38*(2), 185-193.

SUGGESTED RESOURCES

Borden Institute. (2004). *Emergency war surgery* (3rd ed.). Washington, DC: Walter Reed Army Medical Center.

Campbell, J. E. (Ed.) (1995). *Basic trauma life support for paramedics and advanced EMS providers* (3rd ed.). Englewood Cliffs, NJ: American College of Emergency Physicians.

Committee on Trauma. (2004). *Advanced trauma life support course manual* (7th ed.). Chicago: American College of Surgeons.

Chapter Quiz

1. True or False: The main cause of morbidity and mortality in abdominal trauma is hemorrhage.
2. True or False: The two main goals of prehospital care for abdominal trauma patients are to control hemorrhage and transport the patient rapidly to an appropriate receiving facility.
3. True or False: Important host factors that may worsen hemorrhage in abdominal trauma patients include alcohol and medications such as warfarin (Coumadin).
4. True or False: The superior border of the abdomen is the diaphragm.
5. True or False: The kidneys, as well as parts of the duodenum, pancreas, and colon, are located retroperitoneally.
6. True or False: Injuries are described as open if the abdominal contents are exposed to the external environment.
7. True or False: Abdominal injuries may be subtle, so a high index of suspicion is important when assessing patients with abdominal trauma.
8. True or False: If the contents of hollow organs spill into the abdominal cavity, peritonitis may result.
9. True or False: In a car crash, the internal organs may continue to move forward after the car has stopped and may be squeezed between the anterior abdominal wall and the spinal column. This is an example of compression force.
10. True or False: In a car crash, the aortic arch may be sheared off as it continues forward while the descending aorta remains fixed and stationary. This is an example of shear, or deceleration, force.
11. True or False: A pedestrian struck by a moving car may be injured in three phases. First, the car's bumper strikes the patient; second, the patient is thrown onto the hood; and third, the patient hits the ground. As a result knee, head, and abdominal injuries often occur.
12. True or False: Flying objects striking the body from a nearby explosion are considered secondary blast injuries, and these injuries are similar to other penetrating injuries.
13. True or False: The two major factors determining the severity of penetrating abdominal injuries are the region of the abdomen involved and the amount of energy striking the body.
14. True or False: A gunshot wound to the RUQ of the abdomen that exits the right back can reliably be predicted to have injured the liver with little risk of injuring other intraabdominal structures.

15. True or False: For gunshot wounds, the maximal amount of energy that could be applied to the body is the kinetic energy of the projectile, described as mass multiplied by half of the velocity squared.

16. True or False: Critical findings in the assessment of the victim of abdominal trauma include altered mental status, airway compromise, and shock.

17. True or False: If critical findings are noted on the initial assessment, the patient should be transported without delay.

18. True or False: The four parts of the abdominal trauma assessment are described as inspection, auscultation, palpation, and percussion.

19. True or False: Signs to look for during the inspection phase of the abdominal assessment include bruising, bleeding, distention, evisceration, and the presence of impaled objects.

20. True or False: The goal of the complete abdominal assessment is to diagnose which specific organ or organs have been injured as a result of abdominal trauma.

21. True or False: The only effective therapy for most abdominal injuries is surgical intervention. Thus rapid transport to a facility capable of providing this is the main prehospital treatment for most victims of abdominal trauma.

22. True or False: While the patient is being transported, treatment for shock with IV fluids often is indicated.

23. True or False: The PASG may have a role in controlling abdominal hemorrhage and stabilizing pelvic fracture. Local protocol should guide their use.

24. True or False: Hollow organ injuries result in morbidity and mortality from two causes, hemorrhage and contamination.

25. True or False: The spleen is the most commonly injured solid organ.

26. True or False: Improperly worn lap and/or shoulder belts increase the risk of vascular injuries.

27. True or False: Substantial force is required to fracture the pelvis. Therefore these injuries often are associated with injuries to the intraabdominal contents and vascular structures as well.

28. True or False: All penetrating abdominal injuries are critical findings and require rapid transportation to an appropriate receiving facility.

29. True or False: Impaled objects should be removed and the wound covered to prevent contamination.

30. True or False: In abdominal evisceration, the protruding contents should be covered with a moistened sterile dressing and the patient immediately transported to the hospital.

31. True or False: The major cause of death in diaphragmatic rupture is severe damage to the diaphragm muscle, impeding respiration.

32. True or False: Striking the handlebars in a bicycle crash may cause injury to the pancreas as this retroperitoneal structure is compressed against the spinal column.

33. True or False: Trauma in pregnancy can lead to several problems for both the mother and the fetus, including placental abruption and premature labor.

34. True or False: Women in the later stages of pregnancy should be transported on their left side to avoid having the gravid uterus compress the vena cava.

35. True or False: Pregnant women should not wear seatbelts because it would increase the risk of uterine rupture or placental abruption if they are involved in a car crash.

36. True or False: Injuries to the genitourinary system often occur in association with abdominal trauma.

Terminology

Abruptio placentae Separation of the placenta from the uterine wall after the twentieth week of gestation.

Hollow organ An organ (a part of the body or group of tissues that performs a specific function) that contains a channel or cavity within it, such as the large and small intestines.

Index of suspicion Expectation that certain injuries or patterns of injuries have resulted to a body part, organ, or system based on the mechanism of injury and the force of impact to the patient.

Kehr's sign Acute left shoulder pain due to the presence of blood or other irritants in the peritoneal cavity.

Kinetic energy $\frac{1}{2} M \times V^2$, where M is mass and V is velocity; also called the *energy of motion.*

Percussion A diagnostic technique that uses tapping on the body to differentiate air, solids, and fluids.

Terminology—continued

Peritonitis Inflammation of the peritoneum typically caused by infection or in response to contact with blood or digestive fluids.

Retroperitoneal Abdominopelvic organs found behind the peritoneum.

Solid organ An organ (a part of the body or group of tissues that performs a specific function) without any channel or cavity within it; examples include the kidneys, pancreas, liver, and spleen.

CHAPTER 51

Musculoskeletal Trauma

Objectives

After completing this chapter, you will be able to:

1. Describe the incidence, morbidity, and mortality rates of musculoskeletal injuries.
2. Predict injuries on the basis of mechanism of injury, including the following:
   - Direct
   - Indirect
   - Pathologic
3. Discuss the anatomy and physiology of the musculoskeletal system.
4. Describe changes in bones associated with age.
5. Discuss the following types of musculoskeletal injuries:
   - Fracture (open and closed)
   - Dislocation and fracture
   - Sprain
   - Strain
   - Compartment syndrome
6. Discuss the pathophysiology of musculoskeletal injuries, including the following:
   - Fracture (open and closed)
   - Dislocation and fracture
   - Sprain
   - Strain
   - Compartment syndrome
7. Discuss the usefulness of the pneumatic antishock garment in managing fractures.
8. Discuss the relation between the volume of hemorrhage and open or closed fractures.
9. Discuss the assessment findings associated with the following musculoskeletal injuries:
   - Fracture (open and closed)
   - Dislocation and fracture
   - Sprain
   - Strain
   - Compartment syndrome
10. List the "six *P*'s" of assessing a musculoskeletal injury.
11. Identify the need for rapid intervention and transport when dealing with musculoskeletal injuries.
12. Discuss how to manage the following musculoskeletal injuries:
    - Fracture (open and closed)
    - Dislocation and fracture
    - Sprain
    - Strain
    - Compartment syndrome
13. Discuss why you need to assess pulses, movement, and sensation before and after splinting.
14. Discuss the general guidelines for splinting.
15. Explain the benefits of cold application for musculoskeletal injury.
16. Explain the benefits of heat application for musculoskeletal injury.
17. Discuss the prehospital management of dislocation/fractures, including splinting and realignment.
18. Describe the special considerations involved in managing femur fracture.
19. Describe the procedure for the reduction of a shoulder, finger, or ankle dislocation and fracture.
20. Explain the importance of manipulating a knee dislocation and fracture with an absent distal pulse.

Chapter Outline

Case Scenario

You and your partner are called to a "bike accident." On arrival you find a 26-year-old male competitive cyclist who informs you that he was on a 51-mile training ride when he was struck head on by a large station wagon. The impact rolled him over the hood and roof of the car, and he came to rest 20 feet behind the car. He was not wearing a helmet. His skin is sweaty and flushed. He is awake but disoriented to time. He does not know whether he had a loss of consciousness. His chief complaints include pain to the right forearm (with obvious deformity), lower lumbar pain, and a tender left hip. According to a physician on the scene, the accident happened 10 to 15 minutes before your arrival.

Questions

1. *What is your general impression of this patient?*
2. *Given the mechanism of injury and initial presentation, what injuries might you suspect?*
3. *What treatment should be immediately initiated?*

[OBJECTIVE 1]

Despite the advances in medicine and public education, people still injure themselves in avoidable traumatic events. Often these events result in injuries to the musculoskeletal system.

The musculoskeletal system is a complex system that consists of bones, nerves, vessels, muscles, tendons, ligaments, and joints. These are all subject to injuries. Furthermore, the injuries can vary from minor to severe. Some of the more common injuries examined in this chapter are sprains, strains, open and closed fractures, and joint dislocations.

Musculoskeletal injuries are commonly found in polytrauma patients. Although sometimes distracting to the paramedic, fractures and related musculoskeletal injuries are seldom life threatening. They are, however, life changing for the patient. Extremity trauma often presents with extreme pain and psychological anguish. Patients may live with chronic pain and limited range of motion and function for the remainder of their lives as a result of the injury.

In addition to these problems, several other concerns are associated with musculoskeletal injuries. Hemorrhage, tissue damage, contamination of an open fracture, and vascular and nerve damage are all concerns with musculoskeletal trauma. You must be aware of the possible associated injuries with musculoskeletal trauma. In addition, you must be prepared to treat the patient appropriately and be diligent in your treatment; mishandling an extremity injury can exacerbate or cause further injury.

MECHANISMS OF MUSCULOSKELETAL INJURIES

[OBJECTIVE 2]

As society progresses and advances, people find more ways to injure themselves. For instance, cars and bikes are faster. Sports are more extreme. The "staples" of injury mechanisms that medical professionals have come to understand are still predictive of injuries. As a paramedic, you must continually evaluate and consider additional **mechanisms of injury (MOI).**

Mechanisms that result in musculoskeletal injury include direct, indirect, twisting, penetrating, and pathologic conditions. By understanding how the injuries have occurred, you will be prepared to find and treat those injuries.

Direct Injury

Direct injury to the musculoskeletal system can occur when blunt or penetrating force is applied to a bone or group of bones in the body. The resulting injury occurs at the point of impact. An example of a direct injury is the victim of an automobile/pedestrian accident. The victim is walking across an intersection when struck by a motor vehicle. The impact of the vehicle on the patient's femur causes a fracture to the long bone at the site of impact. This creates a direct injury to the musculoskeletal system (Figure 51-1).

Indirect Injury

An indirect injury occurs away from the point of impact. Mechanisms for indirect injuries are similar to those for direct injuries in that a direct impact occurs to a bone or group of bones. The difference with indirect injuries is that the impact sends a wave of energy through the body and leaves the patient with an injury at an area away from the point of impact. An example of an indirect injury is the patient who falls while riding a bicycle down a mountain path. The patient extends his arm and hand to ease his fall to the ground. In doing so, the patient lands with most or all of his weight on his hand. This sends a shock wave up the arm into the shoulder girdle. The force of the impact causes the humerus to dislocate from the acromioclavicular joint. The point of impact was the hand on the ground. The injury was found at the proximal humerus. The transfer of the energy from one area to another is the cause of the indirect injury (Figure 51-2).

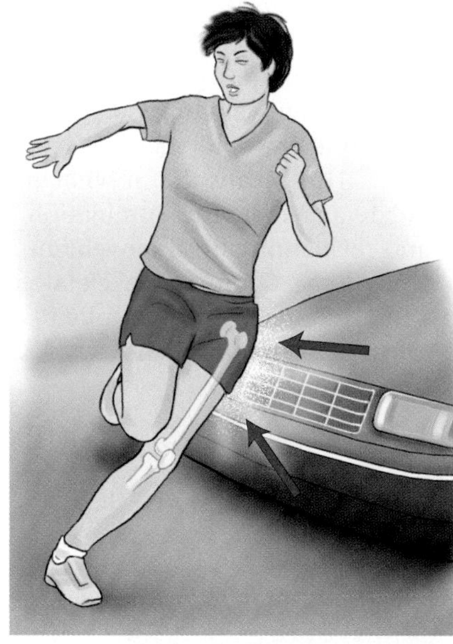

Figure 51-1 Direct injuries occur at the point of impact.

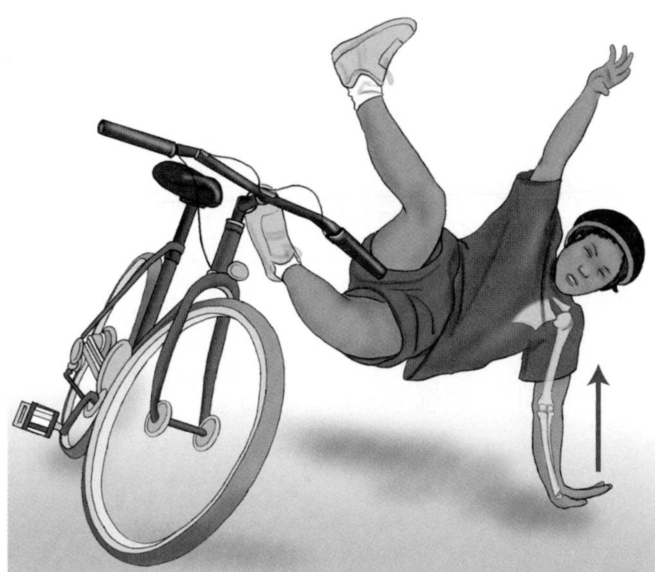

Figure 51-2 Indirect injuries occur away from the point of impact.

Twisting Injuries

Twisting injuries are common lower extremity injuries for snow skiers. This type of injury occurs when the bones or ligaments are taken beyond their natural position and twisted into an abnormal state. For instance, a downhill snow skier makes a sudden direction change with his upper body, but his feet are lodged in the snow and unable to keep up with the turning motion. In most cases the skis become separated from the patient, causing no damage. However, if the feet remain locked in the skis, a twisting injury can occur at the top of the ski boot. This is known as a *boot top injury*. It is a common type of twisting mechanism of injury (Figure 51-3).

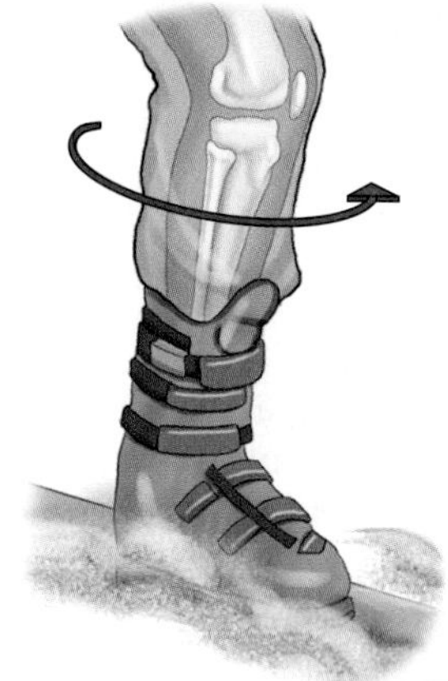

Figure 51-3 Twisting injury to the leg.

Penetrating Injuries

Penetrating injuries are becoming more common because of violence on the streets, in homes, and in schools. This makes understanding this mechanism of injury all the more important. Penetrating injuries can be caused by firearms, knives, construction equipment, and any other item capable of breaking the skin and exposing the bones, joints, and muscles to destructive forces.

An example of a penetrating injury is the patient who accidentally discharges his or her own weapon. The bullet leaves the barrel of the weapon and travels through the soft tissue of the forearm, penetrating the radius. This penetration causes the radius to shatter and an open wound is created on both sides of the forearm. As the projectile travels through the soft tissue, cavitation occurs. This causes internal tissue damage surrounding the projectile's path. In large muscles, the damage created by cavitation may not be obvious. Additional information regarding the effects of this type of injury is provided in Chapter 43.

Pathologic Injuries

Pathologic mechanisms of injury are found in patients with long-term illness or as part of the degenerative processes associated with aging. Two common conditions found with pathologic injuries are arthritis and osteoporosis. These conditions make the patient more susceptible to inflammation, fractures, and discomfort. This can make your assessment difficult. Painful, swollen, deformed joints may not be fractured or dislocated but may be normal for the patient with a pathologic condition. In addition, an older adult who falls while walking and is found with a fractured femur may have sustained the fracture while walking and then fell to the floor as a result of the fracture. The underlying cause of the fracture is a weakening of the bone tissue in the femur rather than the direct force associated with the fall. In these situations, an in-depth physical examination will help differentiate the injury. More details regarding these specific conditions are covered later in this chapter.

RISK FACTORS

Some patients have factors that put them at higher risk for musculoskeletal injuries. Not all these risks can be eliminated. However, some can be mitigated with proper planning and education. Some common risks include the following:

- Participating in contact sports
- Operating or riding in motor vehicles
- Operating heavy machinery and farm equipment
- Operating off-road vehicles
- Falling from a height
- Participating in outdoor activities such as hiking, climbing, horseback riding, snow skiing, water-skiing
- Running and participating in other noncontact sports
- Age
- Diet
- Genetic predisposition

Your role in helping prevent these mechanisms of injury can be as important as the treatment you provide to those who eventually injure themselves. By participating in injury prevention programs, you will accomplish the true goal of EMS—public safety. Some preventative steps that you can encourage the public to take include the following:

- Proper sports training and protective equipment
- Seatbelt use
- Child safety seat use
- Airbags in all vehicles
- Gun safety and education programs
- Motorcycle education for both on-road and off-road users
- Boater education
- Fall prevention, including:
  - Parent education related to childproofing homes and fall prevention
  - High-rise window guards
- Bicycle education programs
  - Healthy living

REVIEW OF MUSCULOSKELETAL ANATOMY

[OBJECTIVE 3]

The musculoskeletal system plays an integral role in the body. The muscles and skeleton provide form to the body and make movement possible. They protect internal structures and take part in metabolic functions. A strong understanding of the anatomy and physiology of the musculoskeletal system will promote better diagnosis and treatment of injuries in the field. This will help you better treat injuries.

Skeletal Muscles

Skeletal muscles are composed of striated muscle cells (Figure 51-4) and connective tissue. These muscles are attached to bone by tendons. Skeletal muscle is a voluntary muscle. This means that it will contract when stimulated and relax when the stimulation ends. This contraction and relaxation afford movement of the skeletal system and body. Groups of skeletal muscles are wrapped in a thick connective tissue called *fascia* (Figure 51-5). These muscle groups are then named according to their location and function.

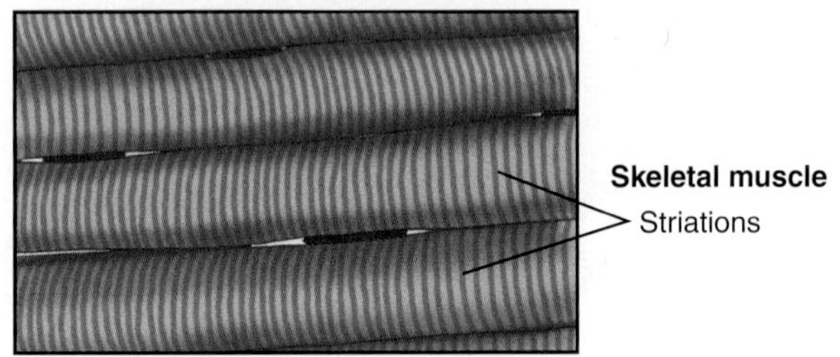

Figure 51-4 Striated muscle cells.

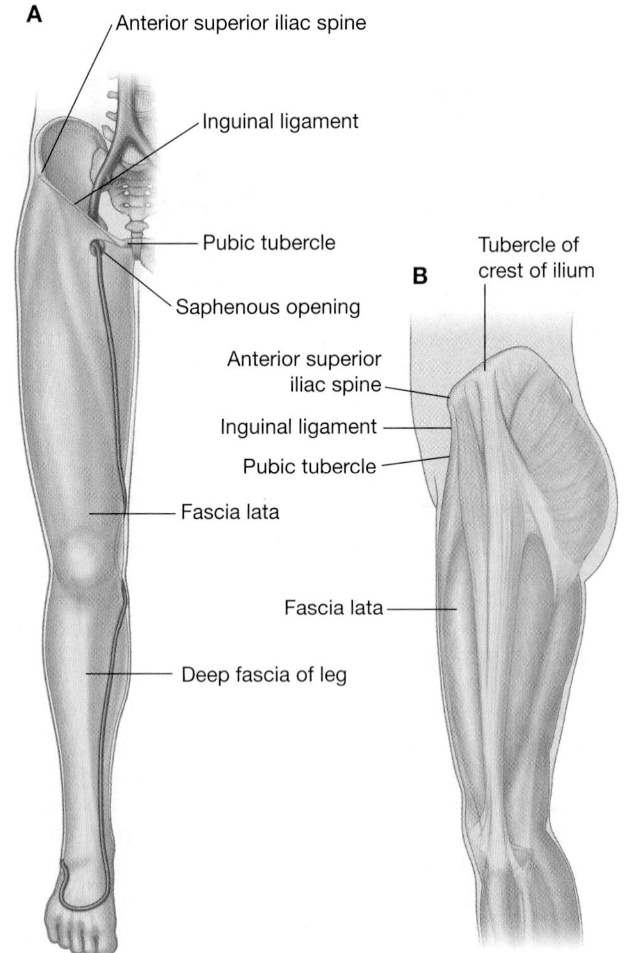

Figure 51-5 Fascia lata. **A,** Right limb. Anterior view. **B,** Lateral view.

Bones

Bones are the basis for the skeletal system (Figure 51-6). They contain a variety of tissues, such as nervous tissue, blood vessels, bone tissue, and connective tissue. The skeletal system has 206 bones that provide support, movement, protection, and blood cell production. The ends of a bone are called the *epiphyses* (singular, epiphysis). The shaft of the bone is called the *diaphysis.* Bones are covered with a thick membrane called the *periosteum.* The blood vessels and nerves are woven through the bone structure. The marrow is in the center of the bone, which is known as the *medullary cavity.* Bones articulate with other bones to create joints and are connected with ligaments. Bones are attached to skeletal muscle by tendons.

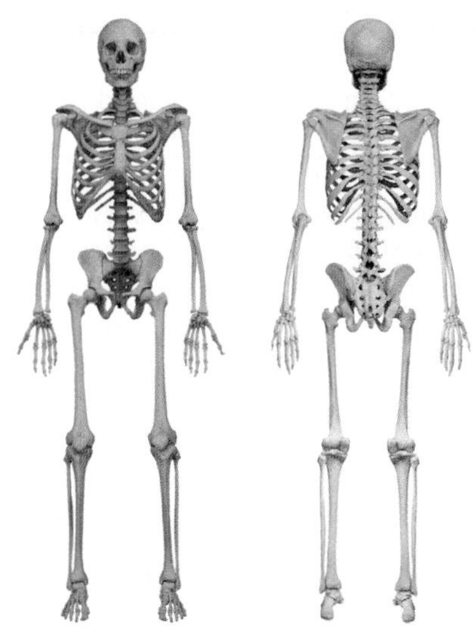

Figure 51-6 The skeletal system.

Ligaments

Ligaments are thick connective tissue that connects bone to bone at joints. This tissue is composed of an abundant amount of collagenous fibers. This type of tissue is known as *dense connective tissue.*

Tendons

Tendons are thick connective tissue that connects muscle to bone. Like ligaments, this tissue is composed of an abundant amount of collagenous fibers. This type of tissue is also known as *dense connective tissue.* Tendons are a continuation of the fascia that covers the skeletal muscle groups.

Case Scenario—continued

You have the first responders apply manual spinal stabilization and oxygen (6 L by nasal cannula). Your partner starts an intravenous (IV) line. Additional examination reveals a 3-inch laceration to the forehead, a 1-inch laceration to the chin, a 3-inch laceration on the left shin, and a puncture over the left wrist. He has abrasions over the right chest. Lung sounds are clear and equal. He also has an abrasion over the left hip, and his abdomen is tender in both lower quadrants. The patient denies head or neck pain, chest pain, or difficulty breathing. Vital signs are pulse, 110 beats/min; blood pressure, 120/92 mm Hg; and respirations, 32 breaths/min.

Questions

4. *Has your general impression of this patient changed after a more thorough examination? Why or why not?*
5. *Given the available information, what are this patient's potential injuries?*
6. *Which of these injuries are the highest priority and why?*
7. *Imagine yourself as this patient, alert and oriented and aware of your condition. What would you be afraid of? What could someone do to comfort you at this point?*
8. *What additional treatment should be provided?*

AGE-ASSOCIATED CHANGES

[OBJECTIVE 4]

As the human body ages, it changes. At first these changes are positive. They make the body stronger and larger to handle the daily activities of life. However, as a person continues to age, the body becomes slower to heal and more susceptible to injury.

At birth, the musculoskeletal system is not fully developed. Muscles are not yet strong and developed. Bones are not hardened and have not grown to full length. The cartilage, ligaments, and tendons have yet to expand fully and grow. This developmental stage in children has both good and bad implications. Because bone and muscle tissue are not fully developed, they are more pliable. In other words, when confronted with a traumatic force, a child's bones tend not to break, but rather flex or bend with the force. This is a protective mechanism because children tend to fall frequently. The flexibility of their bones helps avoid frequent breaks.

However, some concerns exist regarding tissue being so pliable. For instance, if a bone is damaged, the damage may not be obvious to you, the paramedic. In addition, bones help protect organs. When bones flex with impact, the force of the impact is borne by the internal organs. This can create internal injuries with minimal to no external signs. You must have a high level of suspicion when assessing a child with a traumatic injury. Be aware that damage to young bones could alter future growth and development of those bones.

Similarly, older adults have unique issues related to the musculoskeletal system. The muscles of older adults have less elasticity and strength. Plus, their bones have become weaker and more brittle. This is partly caused by the aging process and partly from lack of use. Regardless, this weakness predisposes the body to injury that may not have been a concern earlier in life.

The bones of the older adult are prone to fracture because they are more porous and brittle. The body also is prone to pathologic disorders of the skeletal system that may predispose the older adult to skeletal injuries. Specifically, osteoporosis is related to a higher incidence of fractures.

The aging process also puts the older adult patient at higher risk for spinal injuries because of a reduced water content of the intervertebral disks, an arc shape of the vertebral column called *kyphosis,* and the increased risk of disk herniation. The thoracic region also is more prone to injury with age. As the bones of this region harden and lose spring, they may fracture on impact. The ossification of the costal cartilage also means the older adult may have hypoventilation when the thoracic region is injured. This is caused by the rigidity of the bones and articulating cartilage.

INJURIES TO THE MUSCULOSKELETAL SYSTEM

[OBJECTIVES 5, 6]

As previously described, injuries to the musculoskeletal system occur in a variety of ways. The mechanisms of injury include direct, indirect, penetrating, and pathologic conditions. Specific injuries examined in this chapter include the following:

- Fractures
  - Open
  - Closed
- Sprains
- Strains
- Joint dislocations
- Muscle contusions
- Muscle fatigue, cramps, and spasm
- Compartment syndrome

Fractures

[OBJECTIVES 7, 8]

Fractures involve a break in the cortex of a bone. They can occur anywhere on the skeletal system. Moreover, they can be either open or closed. Fractures that have bone ends exposed to the outside of the body or that have broken the skin are considered **open fractures.** The fracture that does not break the skin is called a **closed fracture.** You must remember that regardless of whether they are open or closed, fractures can be extremely painful and can cause blood loss and shock.

In addition to the possibility of blood loss, open fractures have a risk of infection. Once the skin opens and exposes the bones and underlying tissue to pathogens, the possibility of infection greatly increases. As with any wound, an open fracture must be protected from these pathogens and external bleeding controlled. Closed fractures have not broken the skin, but this does not mean that they will not. Proper handling of the fracture prevents a closed fracture from becoming an open fracture. Isolated fractures are typically not life threatening. However, the patient with a fracture should still be handled rapidly and carefully. Patients can have a life-changing outcome if they are improperly handled. More information on the treatment of the skeletal injury is covered below.

Depending on the mechanisms involved, bones break in different ways. Other factors involved in determining how a bone will break are the age of the patient and the overall health of the bone. The types of fractures beyond open and closed are shown in Figure 51-7.

Other types include the following:

- *Comminuted fracture.* A break that involves several breaks in the bone, causing bone fragment damage; consider the combined blood loss and potential for other injuries.
- *Greenstick fracture.* A bone break in which the bone is bent but only broken on the outside of the bend; children are most likely to have these because the bones are softer.
- *Spiral fracture.* A bone break caused by a twisting motion.
- *Oblique fracture.* A bone break occuring at a slanting angle across the bone.
- *Transverse fracture.* A bone break that occurs at right angles to the long part of the bone involved.
- *Stress fracture.* A bone break, especially one or more of the foot bones, that can be caused by repeated, long-term, or abnormal stress.

PARAMEDIC*Pearl*

Stress fractures usually occur in weight-bearing bones. They are also called *hairline fractures.*

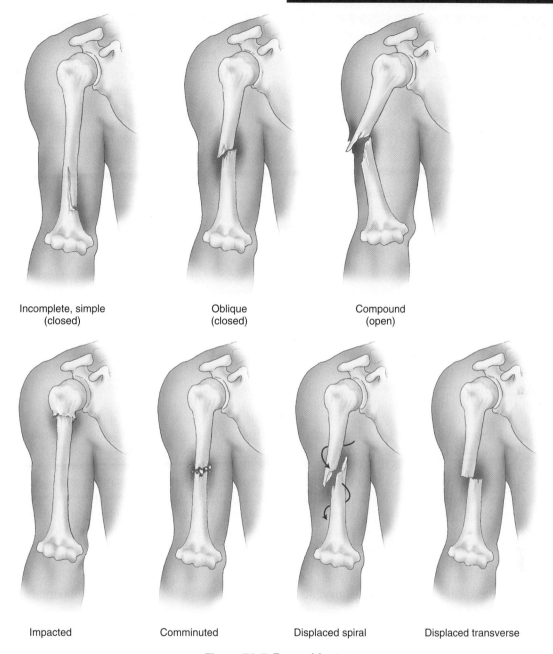

Incomplete, simple (closed)

Oblique (closed)

Compound (open)

Impacted

Comminuted

Displaced spiral

Displaced transverse

Figure 51-7 Types of fractures.

Pediatric patients are susceptible to fractures of the long bones in the area of the **epiphyseal plate.** These injuries can be serious. In most cases these injuries need the attention of a specialist. The epiphyseal plate fracture involves the area of the bone responsible for the growth of the bone. These growth plate injuries occur when the bones of the body are still growing. They may result in the separation or fragmentation of the area, which may prevent proper growth of the bone. Furthermore, an injury to this area may cause unusual deformity to joints or an unnatural bending (Figure 51-8).

Hemorrhage is common with fractures. The amount of blood loss depends on the size of the bone and the type of injury sustained. Table 51-1 shows the amount of possible blood loss with each of the major bones.

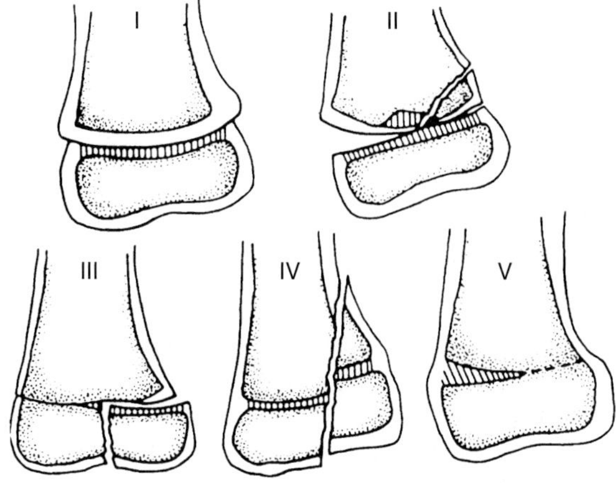

Figure 51-8 Epiphyseal plate.

TABLE 51-1 Possible Blood Loss from Fractures

Bone Injured	Approximate Internal Blood Loss (mL)
Rib	125
Radius or ulna	251-500
Humerus	500-750
Tibia or fibula	500-1000
Femur	1000-2000
Pelvis	1000 to massive

Reprinted from the National Association of Emergency Medical Technicians. (2007). *PHTLS: Basic and advanced prehospital trauma life support* (6th ed.), St. Louis: Mosby/JEMS.

You will see fractures in all ages and in both male and female patients. You must obtain a thorough history of a patient with a possible fracture. The history of the event can help you predict potential injuries. The patient may at first identify only the injury that hurts the most. If you can determine the mechanism of injury, you are more likely to discover all injuries.

Assessment of the fracture site should include evaluating for swelling, redness, and deformity. Note whether an open wound is present at the site that may suggest either a penetrating wound causing the fracture or an open fracture caused by broken bone ends. Evaluate distal pulses, movement, and sensation (PMS). Check for distal pulses in the injured extremity. Ask the patient to wiggle the distal phalanges. Touch an area distal to the fracture and ask the patient if he or she can feel the touch.

Diagnosing the exact type of fracture is not crucial in the prehospital setting. Care for a fracture or possible fracture should include immobilization, the dressing of any open wounds, application of ice to the injury, and pain control. Methods of immobilization and possible pharmacologic interventions are examined later in this chapter.

PARAMEDIC*Pearl*

Do not place an ice pack directly on the skin. Place gauze between the ice pack and the skin to avoid any localized tissue damage from the cold source.

Sprains

Sprains are injuries that occur when ligaments are stretched beyond their normal range of motion, sometimes resulting in tearing of the ligament. Sprains, particularly of the knees and ankles, are common injuries. This can be attributed to the tremendous forces placed on these areas with activities such as running, climbing, and biking. Many individuals with sprains never seek medical attention. When evaluating a patient with a possible sprain, do not jump to conclusions and assume the patient's injury is "just a sprain." You must consider the possibility of other injuries, such as fractures and dislocations. If the patient is not transported, your patient education should include instructing the patient to watch for any increased pain, decreased mobility, or increased swelling. These could be signs and symptoms of a worsening condition, such as compartment syndrome.

TABLE 51-2 Description of Sprains

Type of Sprain	Description
Grade I	No joint instability; swelling and hemorrhage are minimal. Frequent grade I sprains can result in permanent stretching of the ligaments and long-term disability.
Grade II	Joint is normally intact; swelling and bruising are increased, as is internal bleeding. Ligament is partially torn or incurs many very small tears; may present as a fracture, with limited range of motion.
Grade III	Ligaments are completely torn; may be accompanied by dislocation, have nerve and blood vessel damage and disruption, and present like a fracture with loss of mobility and function of extremity.

Reprinted from Marx, J. A., Hockberger, R. S., Walls, R. M., et al. (Eds.) (2002). *Rosen's emergency medicine: Concepts and clinical practice* (6th ed.). Philadelphia: Elsevier.

Sprains can be classified into three categories or grades: grade I, grade II, and grade III. A grade I sprain is the least serious type of sprain; it also is the most common. This injury involves stretching of the ligaments and presents with immediate pain. Some swelling may be immediate, but more commonly the swelling progresses over days, with increasing pain and limited use. A grade II sprain occurs when the ligament has been partially torn. This injury presents with immediate pain and swelling. The patient commonly describes hearing or feeling a pop. In addition, the patient will have limited range of motion. A grade III sprain is the worst type of sprain. It is identified by complete tearing of the ligament. The patient will experience immediate pain and swelling and will lose function of the extremity. The extremity commonly appears deformed (Table 51-2). Grade III sprains often occur with dislocation of the joint.

Differentiating a sprain from a fracture in the field is difficult. Make sure to gather a good history of the event. This is crucial to finding and treating all injuries. Remember that a patient may have a fracture *and* a sprain.

As with fractures, identifying the exact degree of a sprain is not crucial. Treatment should be focused on reducing the swelling and any associated pain. You can accomplish this with immobilization and ice during the first 24 hours. After that time, a combination of heat soaks and ice will help repair the joint through increased circulation. Unless contraindications exist (e.g., hypotension), medication for pain control would also be indicated.

Strains

A **strain** is damage to muscles and/or tendons caused by excessive use or forcible stretching. Recall that tendons attach bones to the muscles, which allows movement of the skeletal system. Strains are common injuries. Typical mechanisms for this injury are overexertion, overextension, and a lack of stretching before beginning exercise. Areas commonly injured include the back, arms, and legs.

Strains can cause significant loss of function and swelling to the affected area. In some cases, the strain can be so severe that it causes an avulsion of the bone from the tendon. In these cases the patient may present with an unusual deformity where you would expect to find a muscle. The pain experienced from this type of strain may vary from minimal to extreme depending on the patient. The patient may indicate that the affected area felt like "something just popped."

The care you provide for strains should include immobilization and medication for pain control if no contraindications exist. In cases of a back strain, the patient should be allowed to assume a position of comfort unless the mechanism of injury warrants full spinal stabilization.

Dislocations

Joint dislocations occur when the articulating bones of a joint are displaced from their natural position of function (Figure 51-9).

The joints of the body are held in place by ligaments that connect the bones meeting at the joint. When these ligaments are unable to continue to hold the joint or the bones are taken beyond their normal range of motion, the joint can become dislocated. Dislocations are often associated with sprains. Common areas of dislocations include the following:

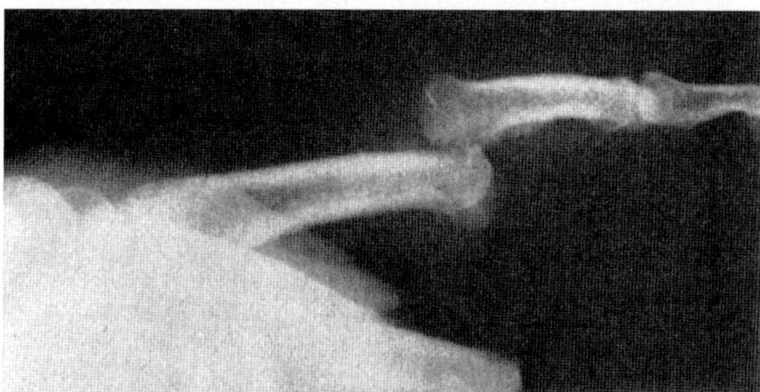

Figure 51-9 Dislocation.

- Shoulders
- Elbows
- Fingers
- Hips
- Knees
- Ankles

Suspect a dislocation when a joint is not moving appropriately, has **false motion,** or is deformed. Dislocations can result in joint instability, nerve damage, and vascular compromise if they are not treated properly. In addition, dislocations can involve sprains as well as fractures of the distal and proximal ends of the bones. These factors may further complicate recovery.

For these reasons, all patients with a dislocation should receive immediate definitive care. The prehospital management is similar to that described with fractures. Immobilize the joint in the position of function if possible. Do not force a dislocation into an anatomic position. If it cannot be easily placed in an anatomic position, then immobilize the joint as found. You can apply ice to the injured joint. Analgesic medications are also appropriate.

Muscle Contusions

A contusion is damage to tissue without disrupting the skin. A muscle contusion can occur as a result of blunt force trauma to the muscle. The same blunt trauma also may have injured the bone, resulting in a fracture. If you are not careful, the patient's pain and more obvious injury from the muscle contusion may cause you to miss the fracture. Always consider the possibility of a fracture when evaluating a contusion.

A muscle contusion may result from a variety of mechanisms of injury, including crushing of the muscle, blunt object impact, blast injuries, and falls. When any of these forces is at work, the muscle is crushed below the skin and over the bone. Crushing damages the blood vessels and muscle cells, resulting in bleeding and swelling in and around the muscle tissue. A muscle contusion is painful. Pain will be present at the site of injury and associated with redness and swelling. Crush syndrome is discussed in more detail in Chapter 45.

All muscles are subject to contusion, including the large muscles of the body. Take the presentation of a large muscle injury seriously. The bleeding and swelling associated with a contusion may occlude circulation to the area itself and tissue distal to the injury. As previously explained, skeletal injury and other masked internal injuries may be associated with a muscle contusion. Perform a complete assessment of the injured area, noting all signs and symptoms. Assessment should include the evaluation of a possible disruption or fracture to the bone. When in doubt, splint it. Applying ice to the area may decrease swelling and pain. Remember to assess distal PMS before and after treatment. Be sure to consider pain management as well.

Compartment Syndrome

Compartment syndrome refers to any condition in which structures, such as nerves and blood vessels, are constricted within a space. This syndrome can be caused by any of the mechanisms or injuries already identified. In addition, this condition can be caused by nontraumatic events, such as infection.

Remember that muscle groups are surrounded by fascia. Fascia divides each muscle group into compartments. Within these compartments, capillary perfusion pressures must be great enough to perfuse the tissue within the compartment. If the muscles within a compartment are damaged, resulting in bleeding or swelling, the capillary perfusion pressure may not be great enough to perfuse the tissue. This can result in tissue ischemia and further muscle damage. The muscle will continue to swell with the body's inflammatory response, further limiting capillary perfusion. To save the muscle, the pressure within the compartment must be released. This can only be done with an emergent surgical procedure known as a **fasciotomy.** A fasciotomy involves making a surgical incision into the muscle compartment under pressure. This allows the release of pressure and reperfusion of the tissue. If the pressure is not relieved, the muscle will die and must be surgically removed.

You must be able to recognize conditions that predispose to compartment syndrome and transport the patient to the closest, most appropriate facility. The signs and symptoms of compartment syndrome can be subtle (Box 51-1). One of the most identifiable symptoms is pain that is out of proportion to the injury. In addition, the pain is usually unresponsive to typical analgesic therapy. Compartment syndrome can be misdiagnosed as a sprain or strain. Failure to identify this condition can result in the patient losing muscle tissue.

BOX 51-1 Signs and Symptoms of Compartment Syndrome

- Pain out of proportion with the injury
- Tension of a muscle during a relaxed state
- Loss of distal sensation, initially found in the fingers and toes
- Extreme pain on extension of the injured extremity
- Pulse deficit in the injured extremity; even though this is a late sign, assess this early and often

SIGNS AND SYMPTOMS OF MUSCULOSKELETAL INJURIES

The signs and symptoms found in patients with musculoskeletal trauma vary and range from minor pain to exposed bone fragments and deformity. In the field, identifying the exact injury or combination of injuries can be difficult. You can remember the signs of musculoskeletal injury by using the mnemonic DCAP-BTLS, which stands for the following:

Deformity
Contusion
Abrasion
Punctures/penetration
Burns
Tenderness
Lacerations
Swelling

Other signs and symptoms of musculoskeletal trauma are shown in Box 51-2. You must maintain a high level of suspicion for the possibility of unseen injuries. Furthermore, you must treat all suspected fractures as just that—a fracture until proven otherwise.

BOX 51-2 Signs and Symptoms of Musculoskeletal Trauma

- Diffuse pain
- Point tenderness on palpation
- Painful movement
- Swelling and skin tension
- Deformity
- Crepitus
- Decreased range of motion
- Inability to use or move extremity
- Difficulty breathing (with rib and thoracic injuries)
- False movement
- Loss of pulse distal to injury
- Loss of sensation distal to the injury
- Position limb is found in
- Hematoma
- Cyanosis of extremity
- Guarding or self-splinting

INFLAMMATORY CONDITIONS

A few inflammatory conditions should be considered when evaluating a patient with musculoskeletal pain. Inflammatory conditions can present with pain, swelling, and decreased range of motion. The difference in these conditions is that they do not have an acute onset associated with a single event, such as a fracture or dislocation might. These conditions, bursitis and tendonitis, are caused by long-term repetitive use and overuse.

Bursitis

Bursitis is the inflammation of the bursa sacs of the joints. It is a long-term problem that can be caused by repetitive motion. It also has been linked to gout and infection. Patients may experience pain on a daily basis.

A bursa is a small fluid-filled sac that acts as a cushion at the pressure point of or near a joint. When this sac becomes inflamed, pain and a lack of ability of the bursa to complete its job result. The condition is typically caused by long-term use and abuse of the affected area. This injury also can be caused by an injury to the joint or friction within the joint from kneeling on hard surfaces.

Typically, bursitis is not treated in the prehospital setting, but rather on an outpatient basis. The treatment includes rest, ice on the affected area, analgesics, and nonsteroidal antiinflammatory drugs. The treatment for this condition is designed to reduce pain and inflammation of the bursa and related joint.

The physical examination will reveal pain with movement of the joint. The range of motion initially may be limited because of pain, and muscle atrophy occurs in chronic cases. Distal circulation is not usually compromised. The patient will describe the pain as increasing over several weeks. In addition, the patient often has a history of repetitive activity. If the patient does not have a history of repetitive motion (e.g., a carpenter using a hammer), then inform the patient that other medical conditions may be causing the pain, such as gout, and that he or she should be evaluated by a physician. Always consider the possibility of an underlying condition such as fracture, strain, or compartment syndrome. Consider immobilization, pain control, and transport.

Tendonitis

Tendonitis is inflammation of a tendon caused by trauma or excessive use of the extremity. The inflammation causes tenderness, pain, and possible restricted movement of the muscle attached to the tendon. This restriction may result in limited extremity movement. You may notice some swelling to the area. Distal circulation is not affected. However, distal function and range of motion may be limited. The pain increases over several days or weeks. It is usually not precipitated by a single event, but rather a long history of repetitive function. Prehospital treatment of this patient is identical to that of the patient with bursitis. Consider possible more serious causes, such as fracture. Gathering a thorough history of recent events can help determine the underlying cause of the pain. Consider immobilization, pain management, and transport. The typical long-term treatment for tendonitis includes nonsteroidal antiinflammatory drugs and the possible use of corticosteroids injected around the injured area.

Arthritis

When a joint becomes inflamed, the condition is called **arthritis.** Arthritis is characterized by pain, swelling, stiffness, and redness. Although the condition is simply called *arthritis,* the term relates to joint inflammation and destruction that may have one of a number of causes. These causes include osteoarthritis, rheumatoid arthritis, and gouty arthritis, to name a few (see Chapter 28). Evaluating a painful, swollen, deformed extremity may be difficult in a patient with arthritis. It can mimic fractures and dislocations, and it can hide fractures and dislocations. Your physical assessment will reveal joints that are swollen, painful, and deformed and have a limited range of motion. Patients with arthritis, regardless of the cause, live with this limited function and pain daily. You must evaluate the possibility of new injury. However, doing so in the field may be difficult, if not impossible. As with the previously described inflammatory conditions, you should consider other underlying causes of pain and deformity. Furthermore, consider immobilization and pain control. Remember that many patients diagnosed with arthritis may be taking pain medication and may require higher than normal doses of analgesics. Consult medical direction for guidance in these situations.

ASSESSMENT AND TREATMENT OF MUSCULOSKELETAL INJURIES

[OBJECTIVES 9, 10, 11, 12]

Your assessment and treatment of the patient with a musculoskeletal injury will vary on the basis of severity of the mechanism of injury. By themselves, musculoskeletal injuries are rarely life threatening. However, these injuries are commonly associated with other injuries that *can* be life threatening. If you determine that the musculoskeletal injury is an isolated injury, then you can perform a focused assessment. If the musculoskeletal injury is part of several injuries in a multisystem trauma patient, then complete a head-to-toe physical examination after treating any life threats associated with the patient's airway, breathing, and circulation.

Patients with musculoskeletal injuries can fit into one of the following four categories that can help determine the urgency of the treatment and transport:

1. Patients with life- or limb-threatening injuries or conditions, including life- or limb-threatening musculoskeletal trauma
2. Patients with other life- or limb-threatening injuries and only simple musculoskeletal trauma
3. Patients with life- or limb-threatening musculoskeletal trauma and no other life- or limb-threatening injuries
4. Patients with only isolated injuries that are not life or limb threatening

Evaluate and ensure scene safety, including conducting a comprehensive scene size-up. Once you complete the scene size-up, move to the primary survey. With the primary survey, evaluate the patient's airway, breathing, and circulation. After you have evaluated life threats and have determined the patient is stable, perform a focused assessment on the injured extremity. You can remember

BOX 51-3 Six *P*'s of Musculoskeletal Injury Assessment

- Pain or tenderness
- Pallor (pale skin of injured extremity)
- Paresthesia (numbness and tingling sensation)
- Pulses (diminished or absent distal pulses)
- Paralysis (inability to move the injured extremity)
- Pressure (a feeing of tension within the extremity)

the evaluation points by using the "six *P*'s" listed in Box 51-3.

Begin by visualizing the extremity, looking for DCAP-BTLS as previously described. Avoid excessive movement of the extremity, which could cause additional injury. Next, feel the extremity. Evaluate the injury site as well as areas proximal and distal to the injury. Feel for skin temperature, distal pulses, and **crepitus.** Ask the patient to move his or her distal phalanges. Touch the extremity distal to the injured area and ask the patient if he or she can feel your touch. Ask the patient if he or she feels numbness or tingling in the extremity. Determine if the extremity feels tight to the patient. This could suggest bleeding and/or swelling.

In addition to the physical assessment of the injured extremity, question the patient about the events surrounding the injury. Determining if the pain developed suddenly or gradually over time will help isolate the cause. If a traumatic event surrounds the injured extremity, such as a fall, question the patient about the event. Many traumatic events such as falls and MVCs can be brought on by medical events. What may initially appear to be a simple fractured arm may actually be a myocardial infarction with a syncope episode, which resulted in a fall and fractured extremity.

Evaluate the injured extremity several times while the patient is in your care. If the presentation of the injured extremity changes, such as a distal pulse no longer present, you may need to reassess the treatment rendered or provide additional interventions. You must rapidly recognize and treat musculoskeletal injuries. These injuries commonly are not life threatening but they definitely can be life altering. Your ability to recognize the injury and properly treat it and transport the patient to the closest, most appropriate facility will lessen the possibility of the patient losing use of the injured area.

SPLINTING AND OTHER SPECIFIC TREATMENTS

[OBJECTIVES 3, 13, 14, 15, 16]

Your treatment goals are first to do no harm to the injured patient and next allow the patient to recover fully from the incident. You can accomplish these goals for the patient who has sustained a musculoskeletal injury by limiting movement of the injured site with immobilization while reducing the associated pain and swelling.

BOX 51-4 RICE Acronym for Musculoskeletal Treatment

- ***R**est*
- ***I**ce*
- ***C**ompression*
- ***E**levation*

Treatment of the injury should follow the acronym RICE (***r**est*, ***i**ce*, ***c**ompression*, and ***e**levation*) (Box 51-4). You can achieve this by splinting, applying ice (as available), wrapping the injury snugly, and then elevating the injury to reduce swelling. Elevation is contraindicated if compartment syndrome is suspected.

PARAMEDIC*Pearl*

In some EMS systems the use of a compression bandage in the treatment of a musculoskeletal injury is controversial. Follow your local protocols.

Applying ice to the injured extremity can relieve pain and decrease swelling. Do not place an ice pack directly on the skin because this can result in local tissue damage. Wrap the ice pack in gauze and then place it on the injury. Heat is used to treat some musculoskeletal injuries, such as spasms and arthritis. However, it is not commonly used as an emergency treatment in the prehospital setting.

Immobilizing the injured site can greatly help reduce pain and swelling and prevent further injury. Immobilization with a splint slows the bleeding associated with fractures while decreasing the chances for further tissue damage. When you follow the general rules of splinting, the goal of immobilization is accomplished (Box 51-5).

Types of Splints

Splints come in a variety of shapes, sizes, and materials. Something as simple as a magazine can be used to splint a forearm. Splints are generally categorized as rigid, soft, and traction.

Rigid splints do not always conform to the extremity. They may need padding to conform to the patient. In addition, rigid splints must be the correct size initially to immobilize the extremity. Rigid splints include board splints, cardboard splints, wire ladder splints, plastic splints, padded arm board splints, and contoured metal splints. Regardless of the type of rigid splint you use, you must fit the splint to the extremity before applying it.

Soft, or flexible, splints are pliable and adjustable for the specific injured extremity. Once adjusted and applied, however, the soft splint may become rigid to help immobilize the extremity. Examples of soft splints include pillows, blankets, air splints, vacuum splints, SAM splints

BOX 51-5 General Rules of Splinting

- Assess pulses, movement, and sensation before and after splinting.
- Expose the injured site before attempting to apply the splint.
- Immobilize above and below.
  - In joint injuries, this includes the bones above and below the injured site.
  - In bone injuries, this includes the joints above and below the injured site.
- Cover all open wounds and control bleeding before applying the splint.
- Do not place exposed bones into the skin.
- Immobilize extremities in anatomic position and in a position of comfort.
- To move injuries back to normal anatomic position, use in-line traction. This may require analgesia (in consultation with medical direction) before attempting. Stop if resistance is met or a change in sensation occurs.
- Pad all splints before applying.
- Apply cold to the injured area.
- Elevate the extremity after splinting is complete (if not contraindicated).
- Align the injured area if the extremity is severely deformed, pulseless, or cyanotic.
- Whenever possible, splint the patient before moving.
- When in doubt, splint it.

(SAM Medical Devices, Portland, Ore.), padded flexible aluminum splints, slings, and swathes. The objective of these splints is to immobilize the extremity while limiting the possibility of tissue necrosis from pressure being applied improperly to the extremity. A pneumatic antishock garment (PASG) (sometimes called *military antishock trousers* [MAST]) can be used as a soft splint for femur fractures and pelvic injuries. Once applied and inflated, these pants function as an air splint. They immobilize the injury while providing cushioning for comfort during transport.

Traction splints are a specialized splint designed for midshaft closed femur fractures. The traction splint is designed to limit tissue damage and pain by aligning and stabilizing the fracture site. The traction splint is not designed to reduce the femur fracture. However, by helping relax the large muscles surrounding the femur, the patient usually experiences a reduction in pain.

In addition, you may reduce the significant amount of bleeding associated with a femur fracture by applying the traction splint. When applying a traction splint, remember that the patient also must be placed on a backboard to help stabilize the femur. Traction splints available include the Hare traction splint, the Kendrick Traction Device, and the Sager traction splint.

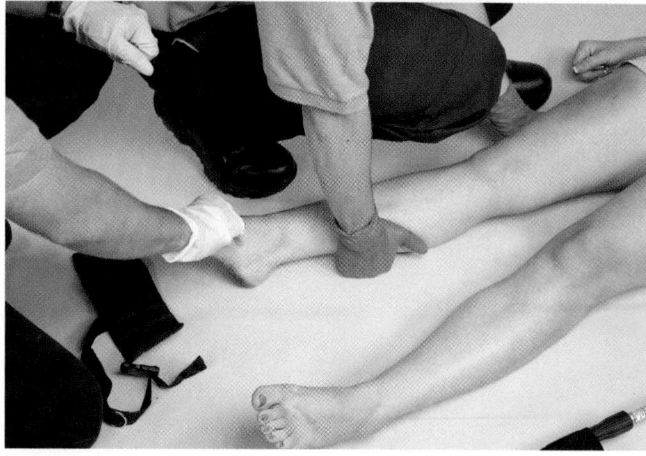

Figure 51-10 Application of a splint begins with manual stabilization of the injured extremity followed by assessment of distal pulses, movement, and sensation.

PARAMEDIC*Pearl*

Regardless of the type of splint you choose, remember to follow the general principles and rules of splinting. Avoid delaying the transport of the polytrauma patient to apply a splint. In most cases the backboard can act to splint most injuries in an emergency. Also be mindful that not all splints fit all patients. Therefore you must be flexible when choosing a splint and pick a splint that is correct for the injury at hand.

Application of Splints

Rigid and Flexible Splints

[OBJECTIVE 17]

When applying a splint, begin by manually stabilizing the injured extremity (Figure 51-10). Your partner or the patient can do this. Then assess distal PMS. Next, slowly place the extremity in the position of function. This may require the judicious use of morphine or fentanyl first (consult medical direction). Traction should then be applied while gently straightening. If you meet resistance or an increase in pain or neurologic symptoms when you move the extremity, splint the extremity as it is found.

Once you select the desired splint, you must size it to the length of the extremity. The splint should be long enough to pass above and below the injured site, as previously described. You may need to cut or bend rigid splints (Figure 51-11). You can mold flexible splints to the desired form (Figure 51-12).

Form the flexible splint to the contour of the extremity. When using a rigid splint, you will have to use gauze, towels, or other padding to fill the voids between the patient and the splint. Place the splint against the injured extremity. Have your partner or patient hold the splint. With roller gauze, wrap the splint and the extremity snugly. Make sure to wrap above and below the injury. For example, with a fractured radius, the splint and gauze

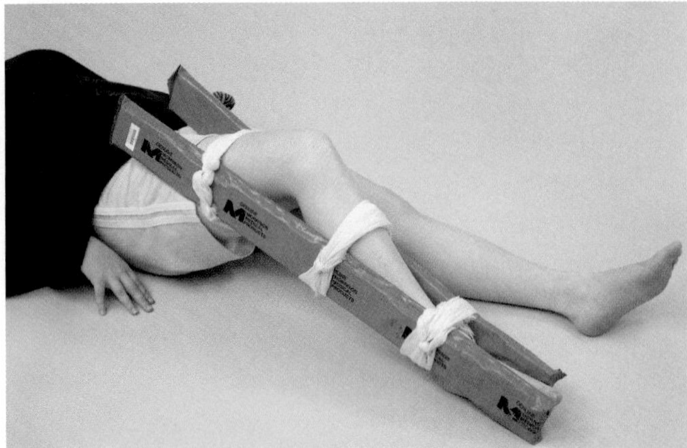

Figure 51-11 Rigid splint.

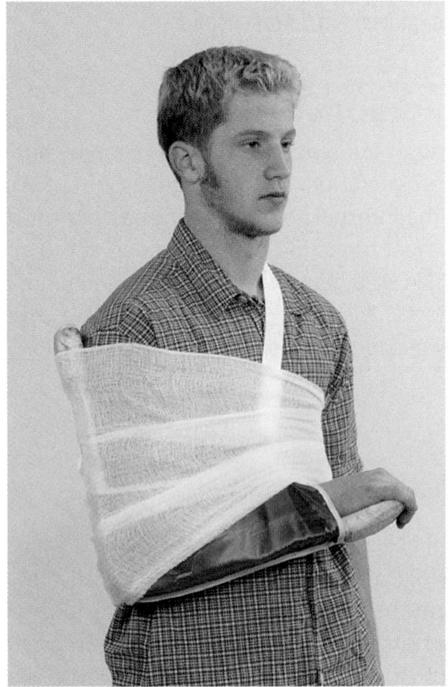

Figure 51-12 Flexible (or formable) splint.

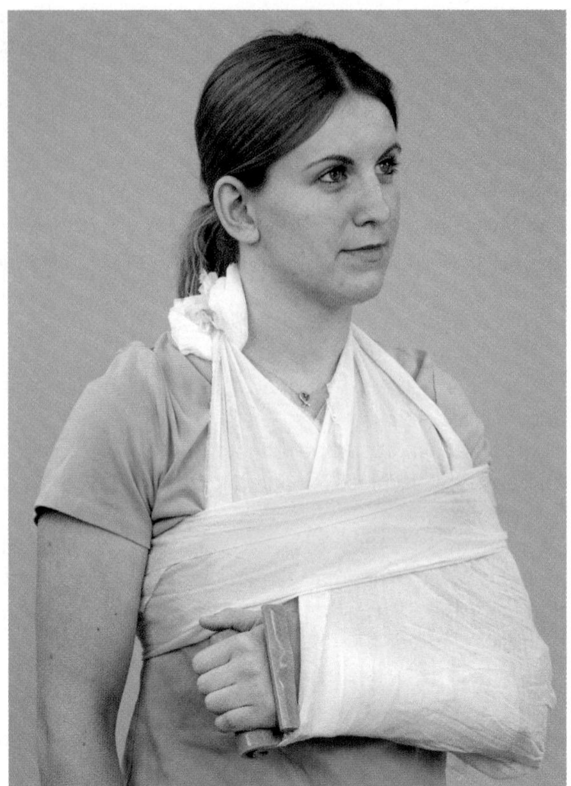

Figure 51-13 A sling and swathe.

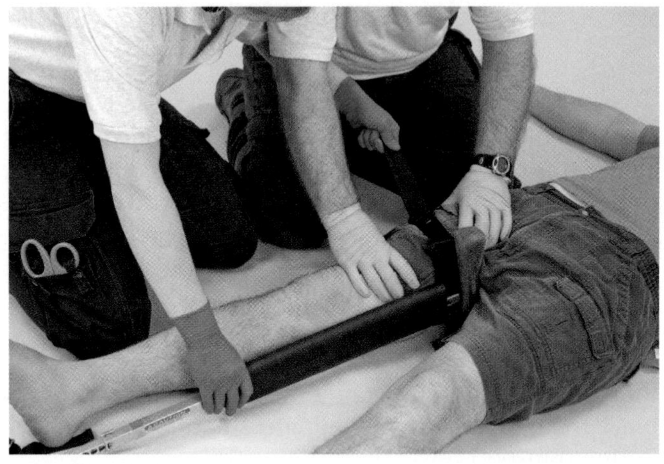

Figure 51-14 A unipolar traction splint (e.g., Sager splint) has one pole that provides external support for the injured leg.

would be wrapped from the hand to the mid-humerus. Tape or tie the gauze in place. To add further support to an injured arm, apply a sling and swathe (Figure 51-13). Immobilize the joint above and below the injury, or immobilize the bone above and below the injury.

After you have applied the splint, you must reevaluate distal pulses, movement, and sensation. If distal pulses are no longer present, the splint may have been applied too tightly. Reevaluate the splint, adjusting the tightness of the gauze wraps as needed. Then apply an ice pack to the injured area.

Traction Splints

[OBJECTIVE 18]

When applying a traction splint, begin by manually immobilizing the injured leg. Evaluate distal pulses, movement, and sensation. A unipolar traction splint (e.g., the Sager splint) has one pole that provides external support for the injured leg (Figure 51-14). A bipolar traction splint (e.g., the Hare splint) uses two external poles, one on each side of the injured leg, to provide external support (Figure 51-15). Select the traction splint of your choice. You may need to adjust a bipolar traction splint for length before applying it to the patient. This measurement should be made against the uninjured leg. The injured leg often will be shorter because of the injury. The splint should be measured from the ischium and extend 6 to 8 inches beyond the extremity. A unipolar

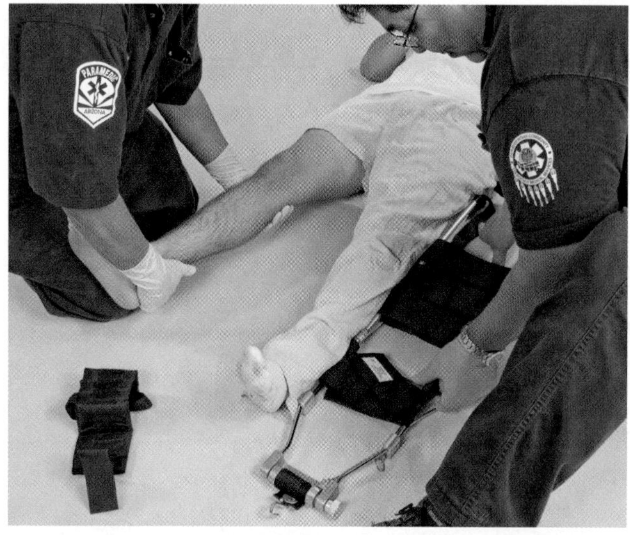

Figure 51-15 A bipolar traction splint (e.g., Hare splint) uses two external poles, one on each side of the injured leg, to provide external support.

traction splint, such as the Sager, does not need to be premeasured.

After the splint is in place, secure the ischial strap. Next secure the traction hook at the distal extremity and then apply mechanical traction. After you have applied traction, position the additional securing straps. Be careful not to cover the injury site. At this time, reassess distal PMS. You can then place ice on the injury site.

SPECIFIC INJURIES

Upper Extremity Injuries

Typical injuries to the upper extremities include both fractures and dislocations to the shoulder, humerus, elbow, radius, ulna, wrist, hand, and finger. In most cases you can easily immobilize upper extremity injuries with a sling and swathe.

Shoulder Injury

[OBJECTIVE 19]

Shoulder injuries can occur in persons of any age, but they are more prevalent in older adults. The weaker bone structure of older adults makes them prone to shoulder injuries. This injury often occurs when the patient extends his or her arm in an effort to break a fall. The patient sustains an injury to the shoulder in the form of a fracture or dislocation.

Approximately 90% of patients with a shoulder injury present with an anterior dislocation or fracture (Figure 51-16). The patient typically presents with the injured arm held close to the chest and body. The head of the humerus can be palpated as a golf ball–sized lump anterior to the clavicle. This injury also makes the shoulder appear to be flat instead of typically rounded. The shoulder also may appear as "hollow," indicating the head of the humerus has been dislodged from its socket. When a posterior dislocation or fracture occurs, the patient often presents holding the affected arm above his or her head.

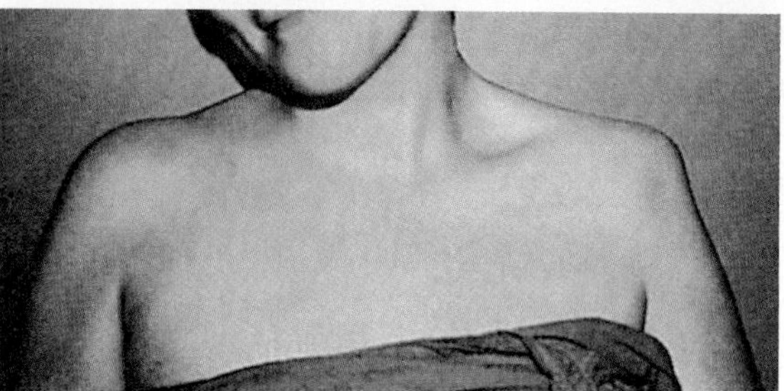

Figure 51-16 Anterior shoulder dislocation.

The management of shoulder injuries includes the following (Skill 51-1):

- Assessment of distal pulses, movement, and sensation in the injured extremity
- Application of a sling and swathe; the use of padding under the sling may improve patient comfort and stabilize the injury.
- If you are not able to immobilize the injury with a sling and swathe, use a splint that keeps the affected extremity stabilized
- Application of ice to the affected area to reduce swelling
- Pain medication

When evaluating a shoulder injury, consider the possibility of other injuries, such as a humeral fracture and/or vessel injury. Depending on the mechanism of injury, consider and evaluate damage to the chest wall. Broken ribs and injury to lung tissue also can exist with a shoulder injury.

Humeral Injury

Trauma to the humerus can result in a fracture of that bone. An injury to the humerus is difficult to stabilize. Furthermore, it has the potential for severe circulatory problems. The most common patients with humeral injuries are children and the elderly. When the middle or distal portion of the humeral shaft is fractured, radial nerve damage is a risk. Fractures of the humeral neck may cause axillary nerve damage in addition to the fracture. When evaluating a patient with an injury to the humerus, consider that deformity may or may not exist with a fracture. If you are unsure whether a fracture exists, apply a splint. Evaluate distal pulses, movement, and sensation before and after you apply the splint. Always consider the presence of additional injuries. Soft tissue injuries, shoulder injuries, and injuries to the thoracic cage may exist. Compartment syndrome also can exist after the injury and treatment.

SKILL 51-1 IMMOBILIZING A SHOULDER INJURY

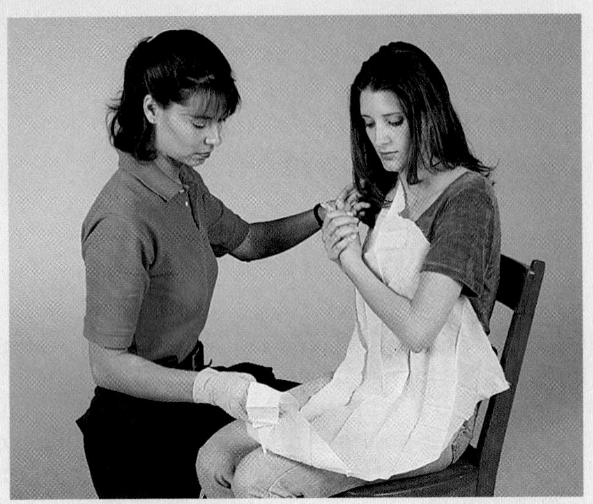

Step 1 Position a triangular bandage over the patient's chest. One point of the triangle should be behind the elbow, one point over the shoulder, and the third point across the patient's lap.

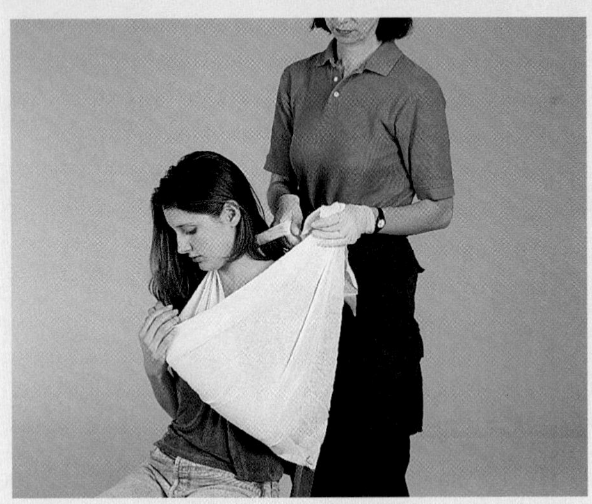

Step 2 Bring the bottom point over the patient's arm and over the injured shoulder.

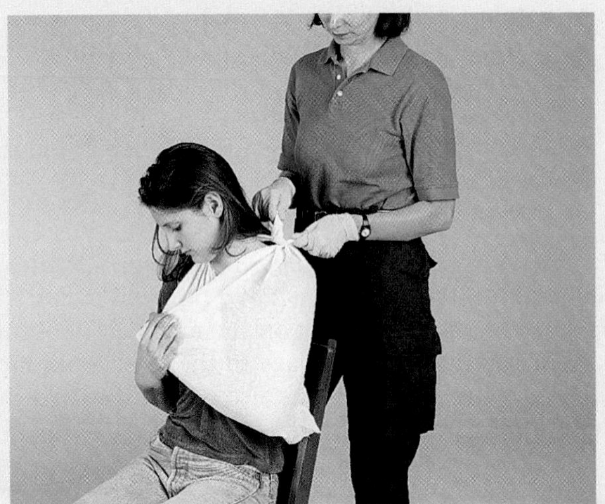

Step 3 Tie the two ends of the sling together. Adjust the height of the sling by moving the position of the knot. Place a 4×4 gauze under the knot for patient comfort.

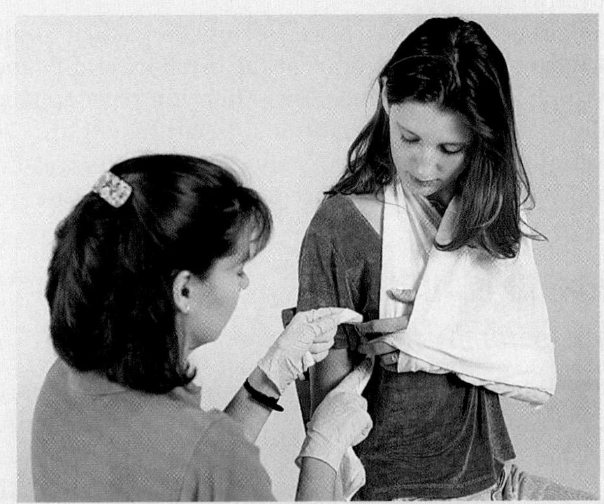

Step 4 Secure the arm in place with a swathe.

Aim treatment of this injury at reducing internal bleeding and immobilizing the fracture site. You can accomplish this by using a sling and swathe with splints surrounding the humerus or by splinting with the extremity extended.

The management of a humeral injury includes the following:

- Assessment of distal pulses, movement, and sensation in the injured extremity
- Realignment of the fractured extremity if neurovascular compromise is present
- Application of a rigid splint with a sling and swathe; the body also can be used as a splint with this injury.
- Application of ice to reduce swelling
- Pain medication

PARAMEDIC*Pearl*

If the patient has a potential neck injury, do not tie a sling around his or her neck.

Elbow Injury

Injuries to the elbow are commonly dislocations. Children and athletes frequently sustain elbow injuries. The typical mechanism of injury occurs with hyperextension or falls from a variety of heights, with the patient landing on an outstretched or bent elbow. In small children, an injury referred to as *nursemaid's elbow* can occur. This happens when the caregiver lifts the child from the ground by holding his or her wrist, dislocating the radius. An elbow injury carries the risk of damage to the brachial artery and radial nerve. In children, an elbow injury may lead to a **Volkmann contracture.**

Physical examination of this patient should include evaluating distal pulses, movement, and sensation. The distal extremity may present with numbness and tingling. If an artery has been disrupted, distal pulses may be weak or absent and the extremity may appear pale and feel cool. Mechanisms resulting in damage to the elbow also can cause damage to the shoulder, such as dislocations, as well as fractures to the humerus, wrists, radius, and ulna. Assess for injury to these areas as well.

The management of an elbow injury includes the following:

- Neurovascular assessment by checks of distal pulses, movement, and sensation
- Splinting the extremity in the position found; splinting can be accomplished with a padded wire splint (Figure 51-17) supplemented with a sling and swathe
- Ice applied to reduce swelling
- Elevation with caution to avoid pain or discomfort to the patient
- Pain medication as appropriate

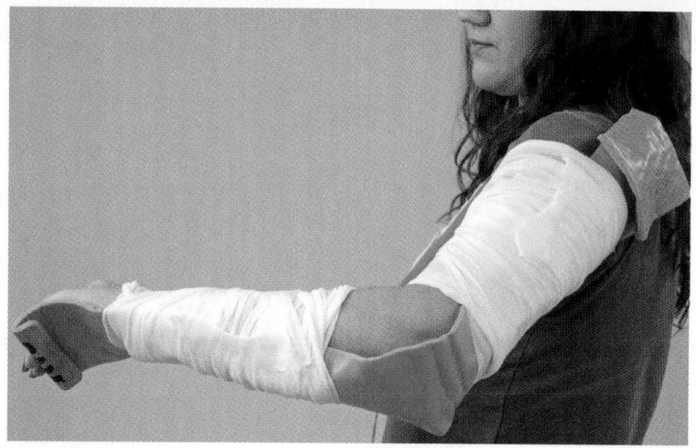

Figure 51-17 Splinting an elbow injury can be accomplished with a padded wire splint. This can be supplemented with a sling and swathe.

Radial, Ulnar, and Wrist Injuries

Radial, ulnar, and wrist injuries are not age specific. These injuries consist of fractures, sprains, and strains. The typical mechanism of injury for these injuries is a fall in which the patient extends his or her arm out, causing a fracture. You will see injuries to the radius, ulna, and wrist with mountain biking, football, skateboarding, roller skating, and other sports.

Wrist injuries typically involve the distal radius, ulna, or any of the eight carpal bones. A Colles fracture of the radius appears with the wrist in a "silver fork" position (Figure 51-18). When assessing injuries such as these, be sure to assess all adjacent structures. Evaluate the distal ulna and radius; evaluate the range of motion of the wrist and the bones of the hand. Assess the range of motion and sensation of all fingers and the thumb.

The management of injuries to the radius, ulna, and wrist includes the following:

- Assessment of distal pulses, movement, and sensation in the injured extremity
- Splinting the extremity in the position found; splinting should include the use of a padded board splint with the hand in a position of function and a sling and swathe (Figure 51-19)
- Application of ice to the affected area
- Elevation of the injured extremity to reduce swelling
- Administration of analgesics as needed

Hand (Metacarpal) Injuries

Injuries to the hand include soft tissue injuries such as bruising, lacerations, and strains as well as fractures to the metacarpal bones. Mechanisms of injury involving the hand include sports, fighting, and work-related injuries, including crushing injuries. One common hand injury is known as a *boxer's fracture*. This injury is sustained when the victim hits an object with a closed fist and damages the fifth metacarpal bone (Figure

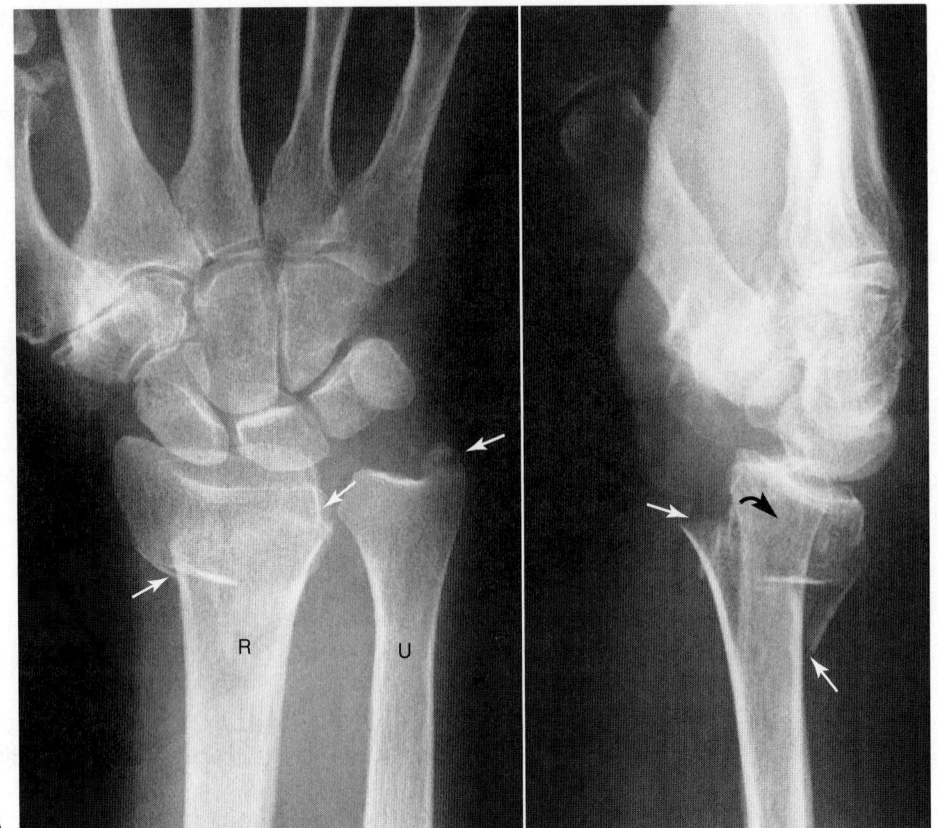

Figure 51-18 Colles fracture. **A,** An impacted distal radial fracture and a fracture of the ulnar styloid are identified on the posteroanterior view in this patient who fell on the outstretched hand. **B,** The lateral view of the wrist shows dorsal displacement and angulation as well as some impaction of the distal radius. If the fracture of the distal radius extended into the joint, it would be termed a *Barton's fracture.*

51-20). Contrary to its name, it is not often seen in professional boxers. Despite the regularity of the fifth metacarpal being injured on the hand, other areas may be injured as well. Persons working with heavy machinery, such as presses, can sustain crush injuries. Lacerations and hematomas also are common with hand injuries. Physical examination of this patient should include assessing the anterior and posterior regions of the hand. Evaluate distal movement, sensation, and capillary refill in all fingers.

The management of injuries to the hand includes the following:

- Splinting the hand in a position of function (Figure 51-21)
- Applying ice and elevating the injured hand to limit swelling and pain
- Administering pain medication as appropriate

Finger (Phalangeal) Injuries

Injuries to the fingers can include fractures, soft tissue injuries, and amputations. Although a finger injury is not usually considered life threatening, some injuries to the fingers can involve long-term disability if they are not initially treated in an appropriate manner. Any open fractures of the hand are at risk of infection. Consider comminuted fractures of the hand or fingers serious. They may need to be surgically repaired by a specialist. Assessment of injured fingers should include evaluating complete range of motion and sensation. Evaluate each joint for pain, deformity, range of motion, and swelling.

You can splint fingers by taping the injured finger to an adjacent finger. This technique is known as *buddy splinting* (Figure 51-22). An important technique in splinting fingers is to always splint in anatomic position. Fingers that are splinted flat may develop long-term disability. If amputated, the missing fingers should be located, if possible. However, transport should not be delayed to look for missing digits. If located, the amputated parts should be wrapped in gauze, kept cool (not frozen), and transported to the hospital for possible reattachment.

The management of injuries to the fingers includes the following:

- Splint the injured finger in the position of function or anatomic position.
- Transport amputated fingers.
- Use ice and elevation to limit swelling and pain.
- Administer pain medication as appropriate.

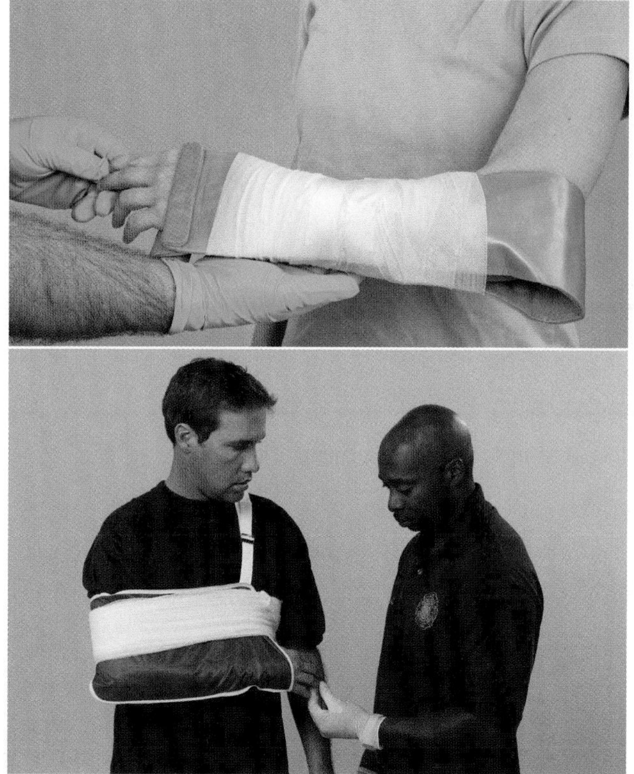

Figure 51-19 Management of an injury to the radius, ulna, or wrist should include the use of a padded board splint with the hand in a position of function and a sling and swathe.

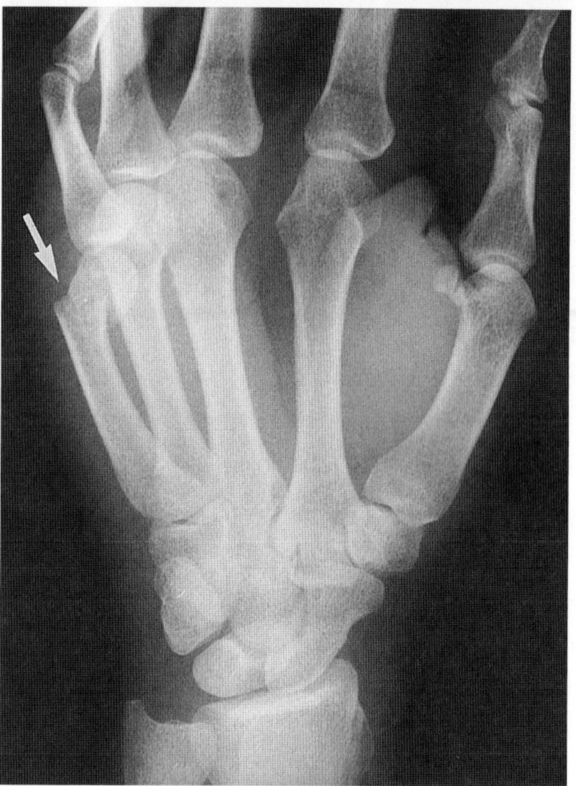

Figure 51-20 Boxer's fracture. This hand radiograph was obtained on a teenager who had hand pain after punching a wall. The fracture usually occurs at the neck of the fifth metacarpal bone.

Lower Extremity Injuries

Injuries to the lower extremities of the body can be challenging to treat because of their size and muscular mass. The lower extremities have a rich blood supply. As a result, an injury may cause extensive internal bleeding. Challenges include managing associated pain while controlling bleeding at the same time.

Common lower extremity injuries include those to the pelvis, hip, femur, knee, tibia, and fibula. Field treatment of these injuries is the beginning of recovery for the patient. Therefore your handling of the injury on scene is critical.

Pelvis Injuries

The pelvis is one of the most vascular skeletal areas of the body. As a result, injury to this area carries the possibility of large blood loss, leading to shock. When the pelvis is fractured, a tremendous amount of force has been exerted regardless of the area affected. Figure 51-23 shows fractures of individual pelvic bones. Iliac crest injuries are normally stable and do not pose a large threat to the patient despite the amount of force exerted.

Injury to the pelvic ring is considered serious. It can result in severe bleeding, leading to death if not aggressively treated. The pelvic ring provides strength to the structure of the pelvis. It typically fractures in at least two locations. When a fracture to this area of the pelvis occurs, a massive amount of force has been exerted. This same force may cause injury to the underlying organs that are vascular and bleed easily when injured. As the hemorrhaging continues in the pelvic cavity, the patient presents with abdominal distention, rigidity, and tenderness.

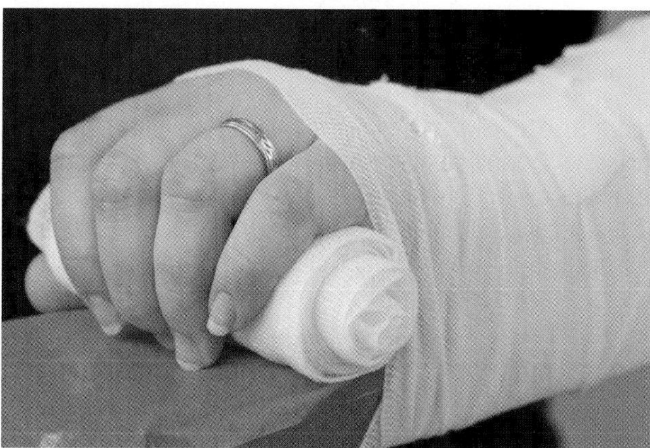

Figure 51-21 Splinting the hand in the position of function.

The goal of treatment for a pelvic injury is to stabilize the pelvis before moving the patient. This stabilization

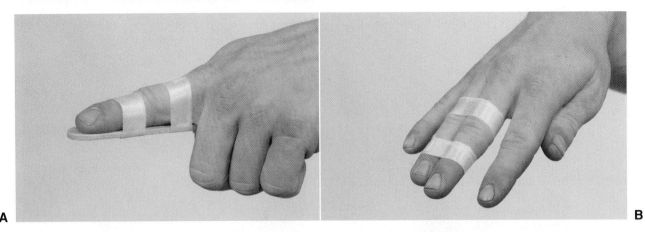

Figure 51-22 Finger immobilization. **A,** Immobilization of a single finger. **B,** Splinting of an injury to two fingers.

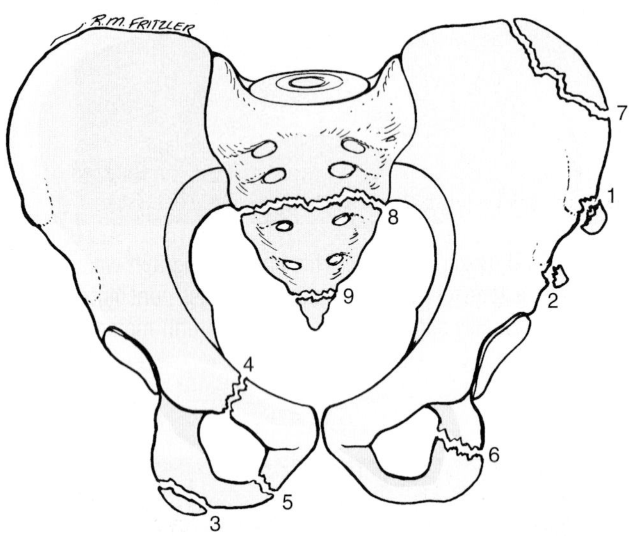

Figure 51-23 Pelvic bone fractures. *1,* Avulsion of anterosuperior iliac spine. *2,* Avulsion of anteroinferior iliac spine. *3,* Avulsion of ischial tuberosity. *4,* Fracture of superior pubic ramus. *5,* Fracture of inferior pubic ramus. *6,* Fracture of ischial ramus. *7,* Fracture of iliac wing. *8,* Transverse fracture of sacrum. *9,* Fracture of coccyx.

limits hemorrhaging from the pelvis. Additional treatment should focus on hemodynamic stabilization and rapid transport to the closest trauma center for definitive care.

Evaluate the pelvis for structural integrity. You can do this by first visualizing the pelvis and legs. Some fractures to the pelvic ring can be seen by noting deformity to the pelvic area. In addition, when a pelvic fracture exists, the legs are commonly shortened, elongated, or abnormally rotated. Assess for pain and crepitation. Assess distal pulses, movement, and sensation in the feet.

You can stabilize fractures of the pelvis with a variety of methods and devices (Figure 51-24), including the PASG, which has long been the mainstay of treatment and stabilization for pelvic fractures. When inflated around an injured pelvis, the PASG acts as an air splint,

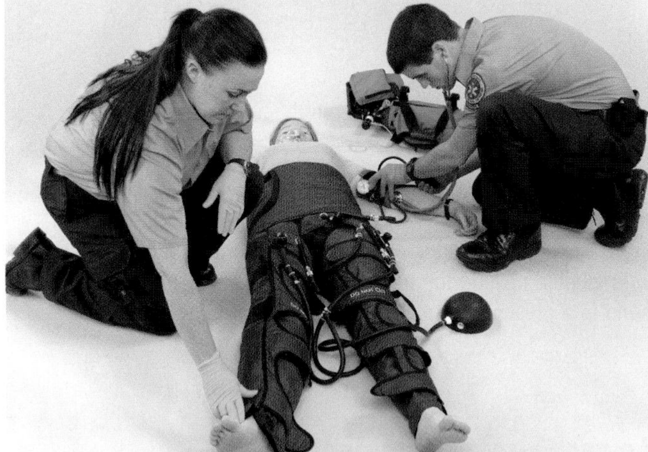

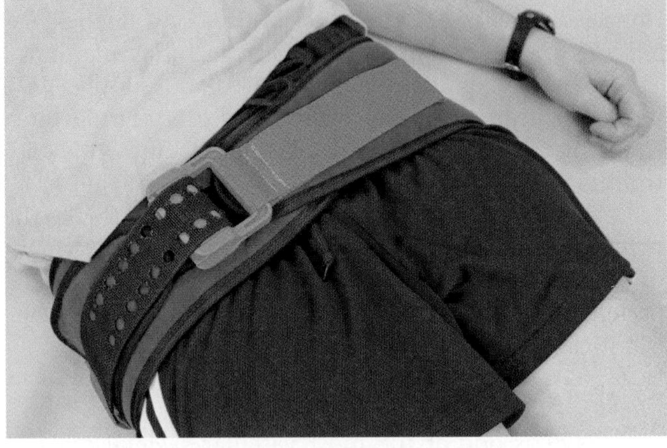

Figure 51-24 The pneumatic antishock garment (PASG) and SAM Sling (SAM Medical Devices, Portland, Ore.) are two devices that may be used to stabilize a pelvic fracture.

immobilizing and cushioning. A bed sheet can also be used to stabilize the pelvis, although the amount of pressure exerted is more difficult to control with a bed sheet. Proper placement of a SAM Sling (SAM Medical Devices) also stabilizes the pelvis while applying the appropriate amount of pressure to the pelvis. The SAM Sling applies the needed pressure to control internal bleeding and is easy to use.

The management of injuries to the pelvis includes the following:

- Perform neurovascular assessment with distal pulse, movement, and sensation checks.
- Splint the injured pelvis with a PASG, SAM Sling, or bed sheet.
- Use a backboard to complete the splinting process.
- Start at least one large-bore IV of an isotonic solution. If major trauma is suspected, start two large-bore IVs with isotonic solution. Consult medical direction to determine the infusion rate appropriate for the patient.
- Give pain medication as needed if no contraindications (e.g., hypotension) exist.
- Transport the patient to the closest appropriate facility for definitive care.

Hip Injuries

Hip injuries most commonly occur in older adults. They are associated with either an anterior or a posterior dislocation of the femur. Hip injuries also can occur from a fracture of the proximal end of the femur. Evaluate the mechanism of injury involved. Remember that, as with pelvic fractures, tremendous force is needed to displace or fracture this area of the body in younger patients. For this reason, be sure to assess the patient for other hidden injuries. Because of the proximity of nerves and blood vessels to the hip, always assess neurovascular function in the injured extremity before and after movement or splinting of the area.

Obtain a thorough history to determine the exact mechanism of injury. In situations involving a fall injury, find out how long the patient has been on the ground and try to determine the cause of the fall. Often an underlying medical condition, such as a stroke or cardiac event, can cause a transient loss of consciousness resulting in a fall. Although the patient's chief complaint may be related to an injured hip, you must be aware that a serious underlying medical condition also may be present.

Assessment of the area should include evaluating which way the patient's foot is pointing. The most common displacement of the hip is posterior, presenting with a flexed knee and the foot rotated internally. In this case the head of the femur is buried in the muscles of the buttocks. When the femur is dislocated to an anterior position or the head and neck of the femur are fractured, the foot will be turned laterally or outward and the affected leg will appear lengthened. In the case of the anterior dislocation, the head of the femur will be palpable in the inguinal area.

The treatment of hip injuries should include the following:

- Neurovascular assessment with distal PMS checks
- Splinting the injured hip with ample padding, including pillows and blankets between and under the legs
- Use of a backboard to complete the splinting process
- At least one large-bore IV of an isotonic solution; if major trauma is suspected, start two large-bore IVs with isotonic solution
- Pain medication as appropriate (if no contraindications)
- Monitoring of vital signs at least every 5 minutes for signs and symptoms of shock

Case Scenario CONCLUSION

The patient's spine is immobilized and an IV has been established. You continue oxygen at 6 L/min and run the IV at a to-keep-open rate. You also splint the right forearm and place sterile dressings over the lacerations. The patient's condition remains unchanged during transport with the exception of the left lower extremity. The patient complains of tingling in the left foot, which has become paler than the right.

On arrival at the emergency department, the patient's condition is largely unchanged, although his skin has become paler. His pulse rate and blood pressure remain in the same range. Emergency department evaluation reveals a severe fracture and dislocation of the pelvis in addition to a fractured right arm. In the operating room, the patient had more than 1000 mL of blood in his abdominal cavity related to the pelvic fracture. Surgery went well and he was discharged from the hospital 24 days after his injury. Despite surgical intervention and rigorous physical therapy, the patient had a pronounced limp and was unable to continue his career as a competitive cyclist.

Looking Back

9. *This patient had substantial blood loss associated with his pelvic fracture. Why did he not develop any "typical" signs of shock, such as tachycardia, hypotension, or pallor?*

10. *Given the patient's final diagnoses and disposition, was your treatment appropriate? Why or why not?*

Femur Injuries

Femur fractures occur as a result of massive force being exerted on the bone. They can occur as a result of an MVC or when a pedestrian is struck by a vehicle. This is a common injury in motorcycle accidents when riders are thrown over the handlebars or are crushed between other vehicles. As described for hip injuries, the head and neck of the femur also may be fractured because of aging and bone deterioration.

The femur is a vascular bone and, when fractured, carries a risk of severing the femoral artery, vein, and nerve. A fractured femur can result in blood loss of 1000 to 2000 mL when coupled with a laceration to the femoral artery. The patient may present with signs of shock early in the assessment process.

As with all extremity injuries, assess distal pulses, movement, and sensation in the injured extremity. If the femoral artery has been damaged, perfusion to the ankle and foot will be affected. Injury to the femoral artery often reveals a cool, pale extremity with weak or absent distal pulses. Compare the injured leg with the uninjured leg. Femur fractures can result in the injured leg being shorter than the uninjured leg. During assessment, keep in mind that femur injuries commonly are associated with pelvic injuries.

The treatment of femur fractures includes immobilizing the injured area, controlling bleeding, and treating the associated hypoperfusion. Administering an isotonic IV solution will help with fluid replacement and, when combined with oxygen treatment, hypoperfusion will be improved. You can stabilize a midshaft femur fracture with a traction splint. The traction splint immobilizes the femur (when used with a backboard) and reduces hemorrhaging, pain, and muscle spasm.

Traction splints are contraindicated when an injury to the knee or the distal or proximal end of the femur is involved or a lower leg or foot injury is present. Traction splints, regardless of the brand, are designed to treat midshaft femur injuries. For other femur injuries or when injuries are present elsewhere on the leg, use a long rigid splint or a backboard with lots of padding to immobilize the fracture site.

The treatment of femur injuries should include the following:

- Assess distal PMS in the injured extremity.
- Control the femur as soon as practical with manual stabilization and traction.
- Splint the injured femur with a commercially available traction splint.
- Use a backboard to complete the splinting process.
- Start at least one large-bore IV of an isotonic crystalloid solution. If major trauma is suspected, start two large-bore IVs with isotonic crystalloid solution to maintain the systolic blood pressure in the range of 80 to 90 mm Hg.
- Give pain medication as appropriate (if no contraindications).
- Monitor vital signs at least every 5 minutes for signs and symptoms of shock.

Skill 51-2 shows the steps for applying a unipolar traction splint. Skill 51-3 shows the steps for applying a bipolar traction splint.

Knee Injuries

[OBJECTIVE 20]

Injuries to the knee may involve a fractured femur, a fracture of the tibia and/or fibula, or a fracture of the patella. Other knee injuries can include dislocation of the joint or patella and ligament damage. Damage to the knee also can involve the often stationary popliteal artery. This artery is the major blood vessel traversing the area. Because of its limited movement, the popliteal artery can be injured or lacerated during a proximal injury. Incidents of popliteal disruption associated with knee dislocation can be as high as 60% (Viswanath & Rogers, 1999).

The mechanisms of injury for the knee include MVCs, automobile/pedestrian accidents, contact sports such as a clipping injury in football, and mountain biking and horseback riding when the rider falls on a flexed knee. Care of this injury can affect the patient's ability to walk after treatment.

Obtain a thorough history to determine the potential severity of the injury as well as other associated injuries. Physical examination should include evaluating the knee. Flexion and extension can be limited with a knee injury. Evaluate pedal pulses and popliteal pulses for presence and strength.

When the patella is dislocated, it can present as a lump to the side of the knee. Examine the distal femur and proximal tibia for swelling and deformity. Expect limited range of motion with a dislocated patella. If the patella relocates itself, range of motion may return to normal but pain may remain. Distal pulses should not be lost with an isolated patella dislocation. If a patient has decreased pedal pulses with a patella dislocation, consider an additional injury.

The typical signs and symptoms of a knee injury include swelling, loss of movement, and pain. Knee injuries can produce extreme pain for the victim and a fear of not being able to walk again. Regardless of the type of injury to the knee, care should include immobilization of the knee, pain control, and psychological support. You can splint the knee with soft or rigid splints in the position the kneee was found.

The treatment of knee injuries should include the following:

- Neurovascular assessment by use of distal PMS checks
- Immobilization of the area with rigid or soft splints; confirm the immobilization of knee, ankle, and hip when splinting
- Pain management as needed
- Application of ice (as available) and elevation

Text continued on p. 529.

SKILL 51-2 APPLYING A UNIPOLAR TRACTION SPLINT

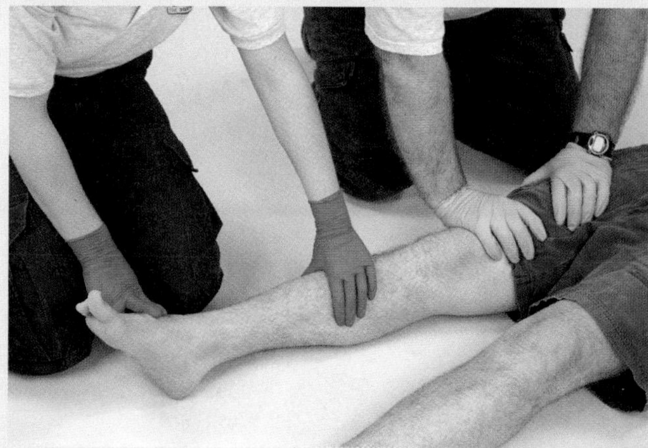

Step 1 While wearing appropriate personal protective equipment, expose the injured site. Remove the patient's shoe and sock. Ask your partner to apply direct manual stabilization of the injured leg to minimize movement of the fracture site. Assess distal pulses, movement, and sensation in the injured leg. Compare your findings with the uninjured leg.

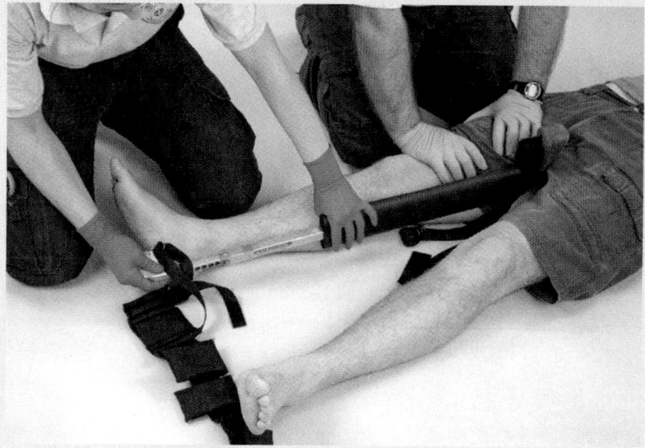

Step 2 Place the splint between the patient's legs. Position the perineal cushion against the groin and ischial tuberosity.

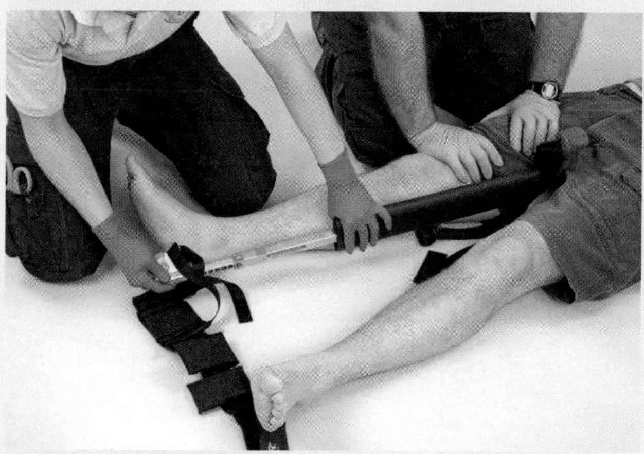

Step 3 Extend the inner shaft of the splint until the pulley wheel or crossbars are even with the patient's heel.

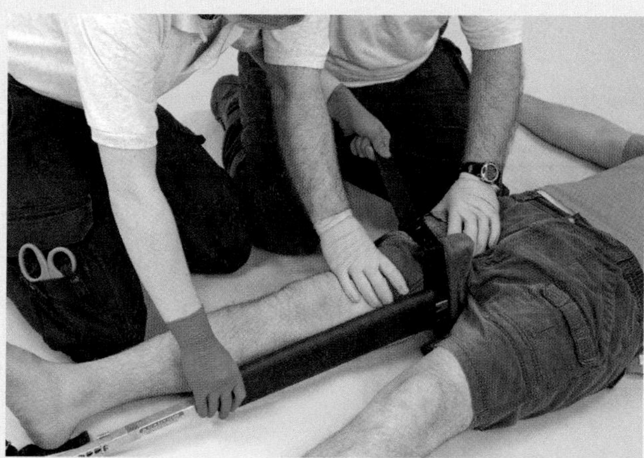

Step 4 Apply the thigh strap snugly around the thigh of the injured leg.

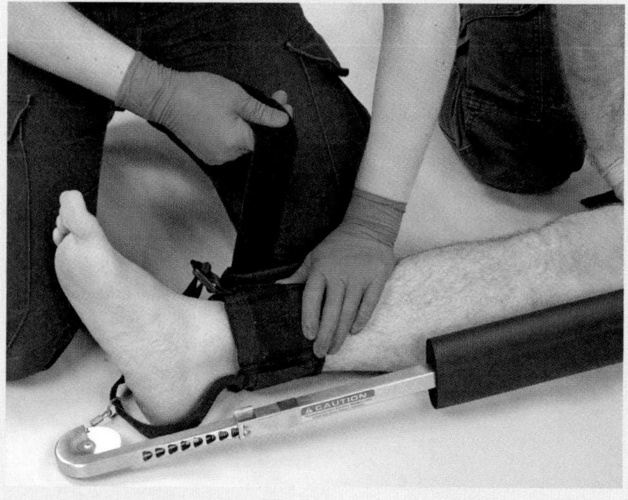

Step 5 Apply the ankle harness firmly around the patient's ankle, above the medial and lateral malleoli. Pull the control tabs on the ankle harness to shorten the ankle sling, pulling it up against the sole of the foot.

Continued

SKILL 51-2 APPLYING A UNIPOLAR TRACTION SPLINT—continued

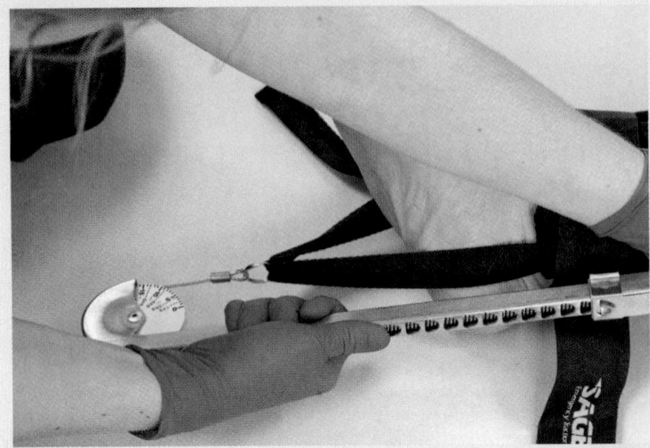

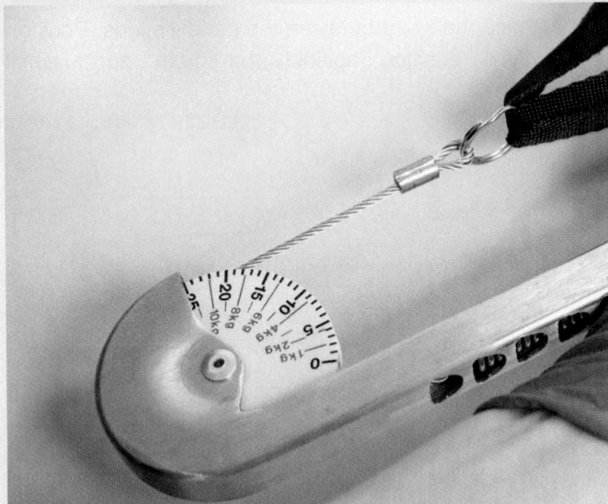

Step 6 Pull out the inner shaft of the splint. Extend the splint shaft to achieve the desired traction while observing the amount registered on the traction scale. Reassess the thigh strap and ensure that it is snug.

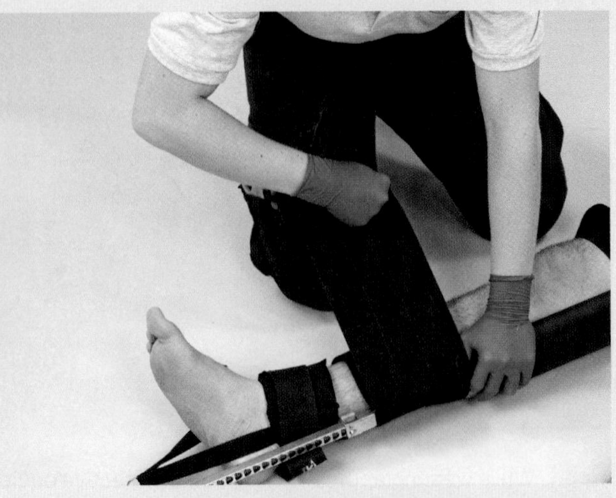

Step 7 Open and secure the hook-and-eye closure support straps around the injured leg. Reassess proximal and distal securing devices.

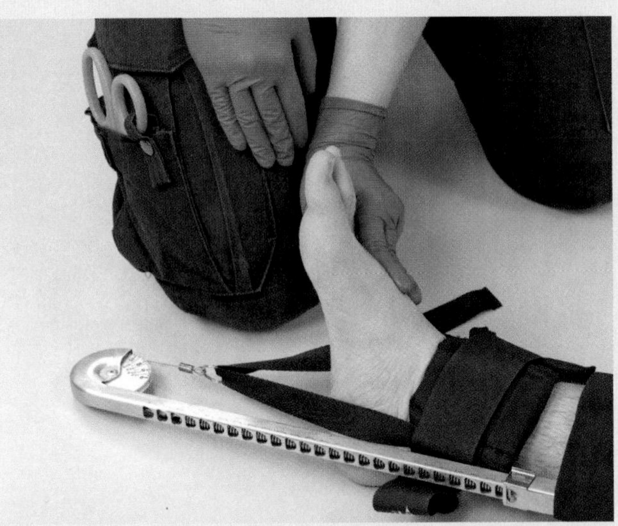

Step 8 Reassess distal pulses, movement, and sensation. Secure the patient to a long backboard.

SKILL 51-3 APPLYING A BIPOLAR TRACTION SPLINT

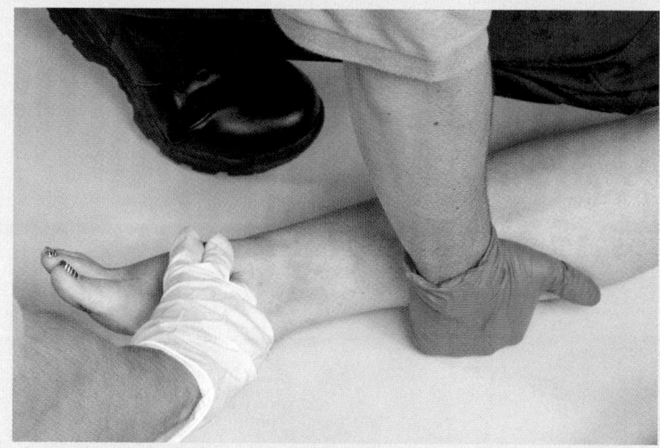

Step 1 While wearing appropriate personal protective equipment, expose the injured site. Remove the patient's shoe and sock. Ask your partner to apply direct manual stabilization of the injured leg to minimize movement of the fracture site. Assess distal pulses, movement, and sensation in the injured leg. Compare your findings with the uninjured leg.

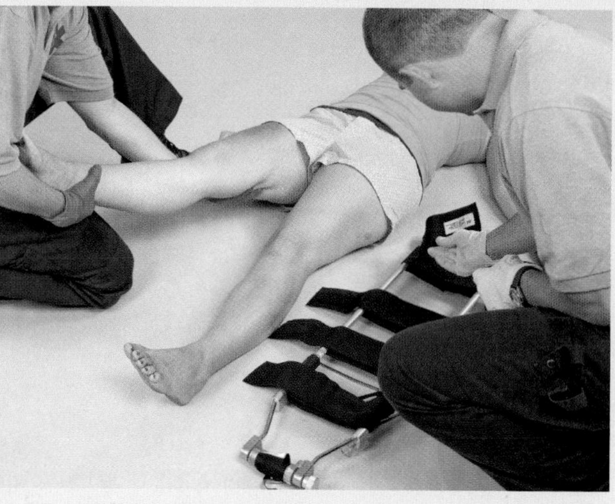

Step 2 Ask your partner to apply manual traction to the patient's injured leg. This action may provide some pain relief. An alternate method is to support the fracture site while the leg is on the ground, apply the ankle hitch, and then apply manual traction before elevating the leg to insert the splint.

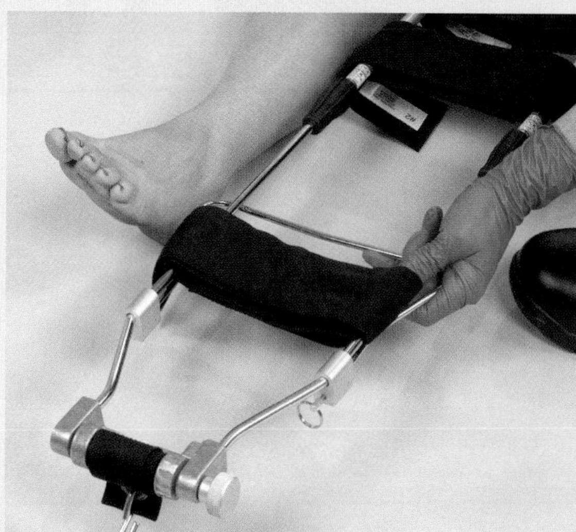

Step 3 Position the splint parallel to the patient's uninjured leg. With the ischial tuberosity as a landmark, extend the splint 8 to 12 inches beyond the patient's uninjured heel. Lock the splint in position.

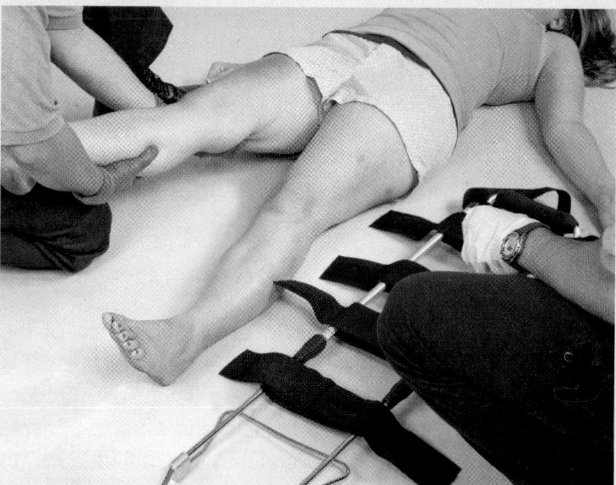

Step 4 Open the hook-and-eye closure support straps and fasten them under the splint. Slide the straps so that two will be above the patient's knee and two will be below.

Continued

SKILL 51-3 APPLYING A BIPOLAR TRACTION SPLINT—continued

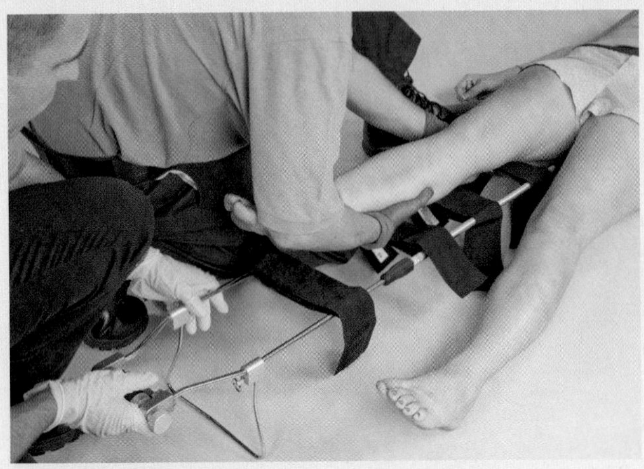

Step 5 While your partner lifts the injured leg, slide the splint under the patient's injured limb so that the ischial pad is seated firmly against the patient's ischial tuberosity. Gently lower the leg.

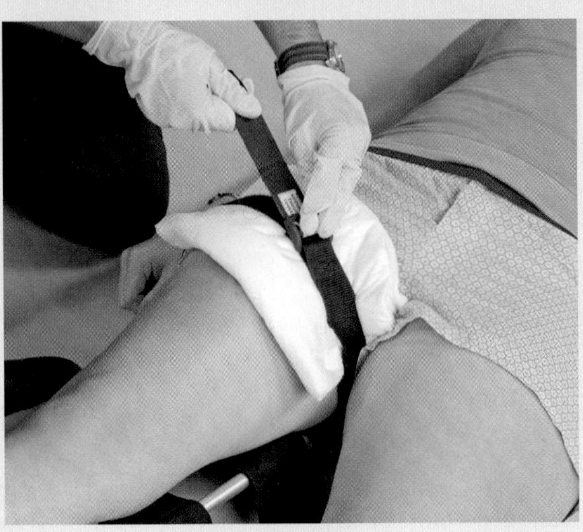

Step 6 Apply the proximal securing strap (ischial strap). Recheck the distal pulse.

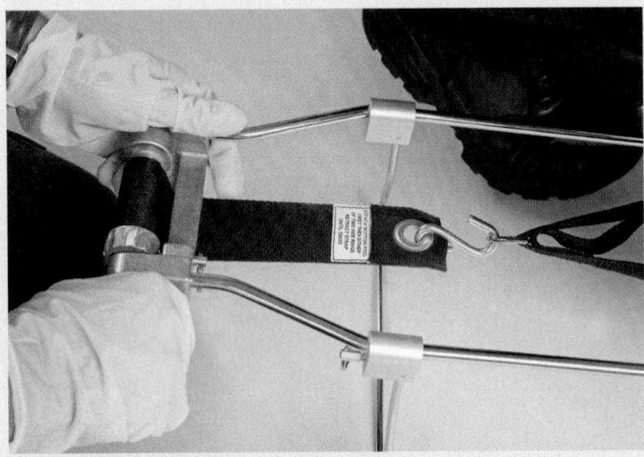

Step 7 Apply the ankle hitch. Connect the S hook of the ratchet mechanism of the splint to the loops of the ankle hitch. Wind the mechanism to apply mechanical traction. Apply traction until the patient's pain and muscle spasms are relieved or, if the patient is unconscious, until the length of the injured leg equals that of the uninjured leg. Release manual traction once mechanical traction is adequate.

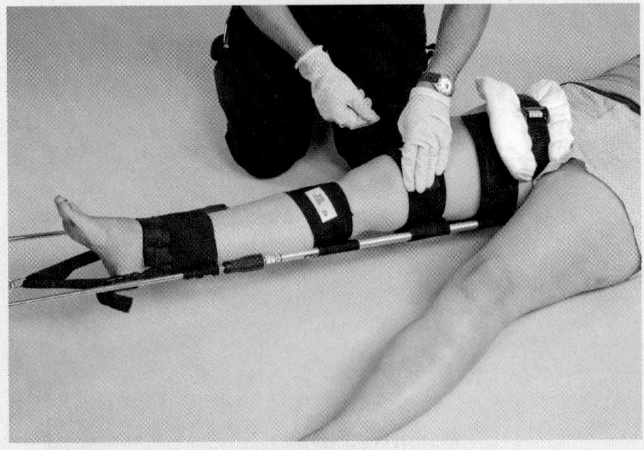

Step 8 Secure the support straps around the injured leg.

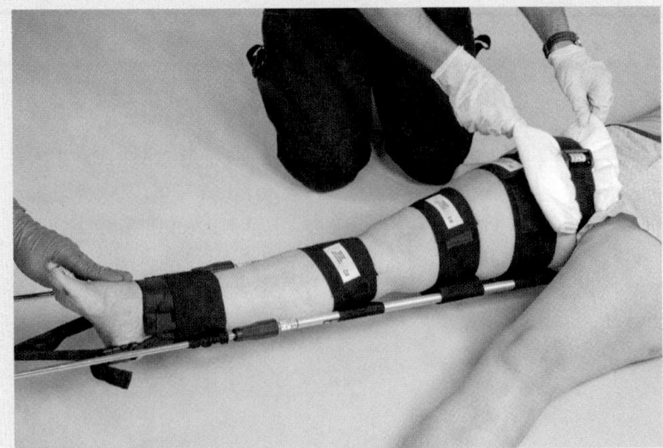

Step 9 Reassess distal pulses, movement, and sensation. Secure the patient and splint to a long backboard.

Tibia and Fibula Injuries

Injuries to the tibia and/or fibula can occur from both contact and noncontact sports, MVCs, and stress to the bones. Stress fractures can occur to the fibula when the victim has overused the bone and caused a weakening of the bone mass. Other forces that can cause tibia and fibula injuries are twisting, crushing, and direct force. Spiral fractures are a common skiing injury. In many instances, both the tibia and fibula will be broken, as in the case of a boot top fracture. The treatment of lower leg injuries includes immobilization of the injured area, consideration of pain management, neurovascular evaluation, and reduction of swelling.

Obtain a thorough history to determine the exact mechanism of injury. Physical examination of the extremity should include assessing the tibia for deformity, swelling, and angulation. The anterior muscle compartment is a common muscle group afflicted with compartment syndrome. Transport a patient with no obvious deformity but extreme pain for evaluation of compartment syndrome. Assess the foot for sensation and numbness as a clue to the presence of this condition.

The treatment of tibia and fibula injuries should include the following:

- Neurovascular assessment with distal PMS checks
- Splinting of the area with a rigid or soft splint
- An IV of an isotonic crystalloid solution
- Application of ice (as available) and elevation
- Pain medication as appropriate

Foot and Ankle Injuries

Patients who sustain ankle and/or foot injuries often have mechanism of injury that involves falls from heights, rotational forces, and crushing forces. A common foot injury occurs to the calcaneus, or heel. It is most often caused by a fall or jump from a height with the person landing on his or her heel. Bilateral calcaneal fractures from a jump from a height are commonly referred to as *Don Juan fractures*. Sprains are the most common injury to the ankle. However, without radiologic confirmation, you must assume a fracture is present until proven otherwise.

Sports can cause many injuries to the foot and ankle, including fractures of the toes and metatarsals from fatigue and impact. Fractures also can present after a patient has bent a toe beyond its normal range of motion.

Obtain a complete history to try to determine the exact mechanism of injury. Physical examination should include evaluating distal PMS. Also consider the presence of other injuries, such as sprains and dislocations. Injury to the distal tibia can be associated with ankle injuries.

The treatment includes the cooling of the affected area, immobilization to assist with pain reduction and swelling, and neurovascular assessment of the extremity. The treatment of foot and ankle injuries should include the following:

- Neurovascular assessment with distal pulses, movement, and sensation checks
- Splinting of the area with rigid or soft splinting material; splinting material can be a blanket, pillow, air splint, vacuum splint, or other rigid splint
- IV administration of an isotonic crystalloid solution
- Application of ice and elevation to reduce swelling
- Pain medication as appropriate

PAIN MANAGEMENT

Splinting musculoskeletal injuries immobilizes them and helps prevent further injury to bone and tissue. Splinting may offer some pain relief as well. In addition, applying ice to the injury can help relieve some of the discomfort associated with a musculoskeletal injury. Depending on the severity of the injury and pain tolerance of the patient, additional pain relief may be necessary. However, in the polytrauma patient or in patients who are hemodynamically unstable, the administration of narcotics may be contraindicated. This should not preclude you from evaluating the need and availability of analgesics on scene or en route to the hospital. In some cases, you may want to consider administering pain medication before immobilizing to make the procedure more tolerable for the patient.

FLUID REPLACEMENT

Patients with a musculoskeletal injury may have lost a significant amount of blood both internally and externally. To compensate for this initial and potential continued loss of fluid and impending shock, begin fluid replacement as soon as practical. The treatment of injuries and transport should not be delayed in order to start an IV. However, venous access is needed in nearly all patients with significant traumatic injuries.

Venous access with an isotonic solution is recommended with all fractures. This will enable both fluid replacement and the administration of pain relievers and possible sedatives for definitive care at the hospital.

FIELD REDUCTIONS

Whether or not you are allowed by medical direction to perform field reductions of dislocations and angulated fractures depends on several factors, such as the distance of the patient to an appropriate treatment center and the assessment findings, which must include a lack of distal pulses, movement, and sensation to the extremity and the possibility of extremity loss if reduction is delayed. Another situation that may call for reduction is to allow more time for patient extrication from entrapment. In this case, the possible hazards of field reduction would be overshadowed by the need to remove the patient and transport.

The techniques to reduce fractures and dislocations are similar from area to area of the skeleton. However, you must use care in the reduction of any area because of the amount of nerve and vessel damage that can occur during and after the reduction. Common areas that require reduction are the dislocation of the fingers, shoulder, ankle, patella, and knee. Hip reductions are not as commonly required. Furthermore, you should not perform a hip reduction in the field. It is both time consuming and may result in severe damage to the surrounding arteries, veins, and nerves.

The general care of any musculoskeletal injury should include the appropriate assessment and basic care before any reduction attempt. Another key factor to remember is that a paramedic is generally given only one attempt to reduce the injured area. This is another that reason hip reductions should not be attempted in the field, because it may take more than two attempts to secure the hip reduction.

As a general rule, reductions are performed only after an IV has been established and pain control and muscle-relaxing medications have been given. You can complete reductions without administering narcotics, but it is not advised because of the pain and discomfort associated with a fracture or dislocation reduction. Narcotics and benzodiazepines also help relax the muscles and surrounding tissues, which aids greatly in the success of the reduction.

General rules regarding reduction in the field include the following:

- Perform only if a delay in reduction of the angulated fracture or dislocation would be harmful to the patient's outcome.
- Perform only if reduction can be accomplished without delay in transport to an appropriate care facility.
- An IV of isotonic crystalloid solution should be placed before reduction. The use of a muscle relaxant, such as a benzodiazepine, may help.
- Grasp the injured extremity firmly and apply traction to the extremity along the normal long axis.
- Allow time for the surrounding muscles to relax; this will allow the bones to realign without unneeded force.
- Once the muscles have relaxed, continue to apply traction along the long axis of the extremity until it is reduced or put back in the anatomically correct position.
- If undue resistance is felt, immediately stop the attempt and transport without delay.
- Splint the injury after the reduction and transport the patient to an appropriate care facility.
- Evaluate distal pulses, movement, and sensation before and after all reductions and after the splint has been applied.
- Indications that a joint dislocation is reduced include the following:
  - A "pop" heard and felt
  - Relief of pain and tension by the patient
  - Reduction of deformity
  - Increased mobility

Case Scenario SUMMARY

1. *What is your general impression of this patient?* He is high priority. Although he appears remarkably stable for a patient who was hit by a car, his altered mental status, unknown loss of consciousness, and multiple complaints make him high priority.
2. *Given the mechanism of injury and initial presentation, what injuries might you suspect?* His mechanism of injury makes almost any injury possible. His disorientation suggests a head injury or cerebral hypoxia. He has an obvious fracture of the right forearm, is at risk of a vertebral injury, and his hip tenderness elevates the index of suspicion for a pelvic fracture, an injury that often causes significant blood loss.
3. *What treatment should be immediately initiated?* Spinal stabilization, high-flow oxygen, and preparation for treatment and transport.
4. *Has your general impression of this patient changed after a more thorough examination? Why or why not?* No. He is still high priority given his multiple injuries. His abdominal tenderness adds to the initial concerns and his vital signs suggest he may be compensating for occult blood loss.
5. *Given the available information, what are this patient's potential injuries?* Multiple soft tissue injuries, fractures of the forearm and possibly pelvis, possible head injury, potential intraabdominal injury and/or bleeding, potential for shock, potential for vertebral injury.
6. *Which of these injuries are the highest priority and why?* Intraabdominal injury and bleeding and pelvic fracture are highest priority because of their potential to cause significant blood loss and shock. A closed head injury with rising intracranial pressure also may be considered a high priority.
7. *Imagine yourself as this patient, alert and oriented and aware of your condition. What would you be afraid of? What could someone do to comfort you at this point?*

This is a young, extremely healthy individual who has been injured and is being confined to a spine board and stretcher. In addition, he is disoriented to time, which can be terrifying because—in addition to being injured and in pain—he may not know what day it is. Like most adults, his greatest fear is uncertainty: "Where am I? What happened? Will I be ok? Where am I going? Can I call my family?" The best comfort to offer this patient is information about what has happened and what will happen. Keep him informed about what you are doing, what will happen next, and when and where he will be transported. *Keep in mind, patients with head injuries may have some difficulty remembering what you have told them, so you may have to repeat yourself a number of times.*

8. *What additional treatment should be provided?* Maintain high-flow oxygen, provide spinal stabilization, start an IV and infuse 250 to 500 mL of isotonic fluid, establish ECG monitoring, begin transport to a trauma center, splint the fracture, and dress wounds.
9. *This patient experienced substantial blood loss associated with his pelvic fracture. Why did he not develop any "typical" signs of shock, such as tachycardia, hypotension, or pallor?* His conditioning as an athlete enabled his body to compensate effectively for the blood loss. As a competitive cyclist, this patient's resting pulse rate is probably 45 to 55 beats/min. His pulse rate of 110 represents a *doubling* of his pulse rate, equivalent to 120 to 140 beats/min in a less-fit individual. In this case, it was easy to be fooled by the apparently normal vitals; this patient was in compensatory shock.
10. *Given the patient's final diagnoses and disposition, was your treatment appropriate? Why or why not?* Oxygen administration was too low, as was the IV fluid infusion. Both errors were probably related to the patient's relatively normal vital signs. Vital sign readings always need to be taken in the context of the patient's baseline.

Chapter Summary

- Musculoskeletal injuries are seldom life threatening; however, they do need prompt medical attention to prevent permanent damage.
- Blood loss is probable with fractured bones and injured muscles.
- The care you provide in the field will depend on the patient's overall condition and other presenting injuries, and it may determine if the patient incurs a long-term disability or regains full use of the injured area.
- Musculoskeletal injuries can be distracting. You must focus on life threats before treating injuries to bones and muscles.
- You must also provide for the psychological support of the patient and give reassurance as you treat and transport the patient to a care facility.
- You must be complete and thorough in your assessment to avoid missing hidden injuries or underlying illnesses.
- The reassessment of injuries is crucial.
- Aggressive pain control benefits the patient and helps facilitate procedures.
- When in doubt, splint it.

REFERENCE

Viswanath, Y. K. S., & Rogers, I. M. (1999). A non-contact complete knee dislocation with popliteal artery disruption, a rare martial arts injury. *Postgraduate Medical Journal, 75,* 552-554.

SUGGESTED RESOURCES

Bone and Joint Decade: http://www.usbjd.org.

National Association of Emergency Medical Technicians (2006). *PHTLS: Basic and advanced life support* (6th ed.). St. Louis: Mosby.

Chapter Quiz

1. When a patient presents with pain out of proportion to obvious injury, you should suspect which of the following?
a. Sprain
b. Strain
c. Dislocation
d. Compartment syndrome

2. A fracture to the radius can result in a blood loss of _________.
a. 250 to 500 mL
b. 500 to 750 mL
c. 750 to 1000 mL
d. 1000 to 2000 mL

3. When splinting an extremity, when should you evaluate distal pulses and sensation?
a. Before splinting
b. After splinting
c. Before and after splinting
d. Only if the extremity becomes pale

4. Which of the following would be an indication to apply a traction splint?
a. Mid-shaft closed femur fracture
b. Femur open fracture with hip dislocation
c. Tibia or fibula closed fracture
d. Open femoral head fracture

5. A 10-year-old boy has fallen from his skateboard onto his outstretched arm. Which of the following injuries would most likely be seen?
a. Colles fracture
b. Humerus fracture
c. Rib fracture
d. Hip dislocation

6. True or False: You can consider administering analgesic medication before applying a splint.

7. In a patient with multisystem trauma, which of the following would take priority in the sequence of care?
a. Femur fracture
b. Shoulder dislocation
c. Venous bleeding
d. Shallow respirations

8. After splinting a fractured radius, you notice that distal pulses to the extremity cannot be found. Which of the following would be the most appropriate course of action?
a. Reevaluate the splint and bandage to see if it is limiting circulation.
b. IV fluid bolus to increase pressure to the extremity.
c. Notify receiving hospital of change and transport rapidly.
d. Do nothing. This is a common finding after splinting.

9. Which of the following can most closely mimic a fracture?
a. Compartment syndrome
b. Tendonitis
c. Rheumatoid arthritis
d. Strain

10. What injury results in a stretched ligament?
a. Strain
b. Sprain
c. Rotation
d. Dislocation

Terminology

Arthritis Inflammation of a joint that results in pain, stiffness, swelling, and redness.

Bursitis Chronic or acute inflammation of the small synovial sacs known as *bursa*.

Closed fracture Fracture of the bone tissue that has not broken the skin tissue.

Crepitus A medical term to describe the grating, crackling, or popping sounds and sensations felt under skin and joints.

Epiphyseal plate Found in children who are still generating bone growth; also known as the growth plate.

False motion Abnormal movement of a bone or joint typically associated with a fracture or dislocation.

Fasciotomy A surgical incision into the muscle fascia to relieve intracompartmental pressures. It is the emergency treatment for compartment syndrome.

Joint dislocation Disruption of articulating bones from their normal location.

Mechanism of injury The way an injury occurs on the body.

Open fracture Fracture of the bone tissue that breaks the skin and may or may not still be exposed.

Sprain An injury to a ligament that results when the ligament is overstretched, leading to tearing or complete disruption of the ligament.

Strain An injury to a muscle that results when the muscle is overstretched, leading to tearing of the individual muscle fibers.

Tendonitis Inflammation of a tendon, often the result of overuse.

Volkmann contracture A deformity of the hand, fingers, and wrist caused by injury to the muscles of the forearm; also known as *ischemic contracture*.

CHAPTER 52

Environmental Conditions

Objectives

After completing this chapter, you will be able to:

1. Define *environmental emergency.*
2. Describe the incidence, morbidity, and mortality rates associated with environmental emergencies.
3. Identify risk factors most predisposing to environmental emergencies.
4. Identify environmental factors that may cause illness or exacerbate a preexisting illness.
5. Identify environmental factors that may complicate treatment or transport decisions.
6. List the principal types of environmental illnesses.
7. Define *homeostasis* and relate the concept to environmental influences.
8. Identify normal, critically high, and critically low body temperatures.
9. Describe several methods of temperature monitoring.
10. Identify the components of the body's thermoregulatory mechanism.
11. Describe the general process of thermal regulation, including substances used and wastes generated.
12. Describe the body's compensatory process for overheating.
13. Describe the body's compensatory process for excess heat loss.
14. List the common forms of heat and cold disorders.
15. List the common predisposing factors associated with heat and cold disorders.
16. List the common preventative measures associated with heat and cold disorders.
17. Integrate the pathophysiologic principles and complicating factors common to environmental emergencies and discuss differentiating features between emergent and urgent presentations.
18. Define *heat illness.*
19. Describe the pathophysiology of heat illness.
20. Identify signs and symptoms of heat illness.
21. List the predisposing factors for heat illness.
22. List measures to prevent heat illness.
23. Discuss the symptomatic variations presented in progressive heat disorders.
24. Relate symptomatic findings to the commonly used terms of heat cramps, heat exhaustion, and heat stroke.
25. Correlate the abnormal findings in assessment with their clinical significance in the patient with heat illness.
26. Describe the contribution of dehydration to the development of heat disorders.
27. Describe the differences between classic and exertional heat stroke.
28. Define *fever* and discuss its pathophysiologic mechanism.
29. Identify the fundamental thermoregulatory difference between fever and heat stroke.
30. Discuss how to differentiate fever and heat stroke.
31. Discuss the role of fluid therapy in the treatment of heat disorders.
32. Differentiate the various treatments and interventions in the management of heat disorders.
33. Integrate the pathophysiologic principles and the assessment findings to formulate a field impression and implement a treatment plan for the patient who has dehydration, heat exhaustion, or heat stroke.
34. Define *hypothermia.*
35. Describe the pathophysiology of hypothermia.
36. List predisposing factors for hypothermia.
37. List measures to prevent hypothermia.
38. Identify differences between mild and severe hypothermia.
39. Describe differences between chronic and acute hypothermia.
40. List signs and symptoms of hypothermia.
41. Correlate abnormal findings in assessment with their clinical significance in the patient with hypothermia.
42. Discuss the impact of severe hypothermia on standard basic and advanced life support algorithms and transport considerations.
43. Integrate pathophysiologic principles and the assessment findings to formulate a field impression and implement a treatment plan for the patient who has either mild or severe hypothermia.
44. Define *frostbite.*
45. Define *superficial frostbite* (frostnip).
46. Differentiate superficial frostbite and deep frostbite.
47. List predisposing factors for frostbite.
48. List measures to prevent frostbite.
49. Correlate abnormal findings in assessment with their clinical significance in the patient with frostbite.
50. Differentiate the various treatments and interventions in the management of frostbite.
51. Integrate pathophysiologic principles and the assessment findings to formulate a field impression and implement a treatment plan for the patient with superficial or deep frostbite.
52. Define *drowning.*
53. Describe the pathophysiology of drowning.
54. List signs and symptoms of drowning.
55. Describe the lack of significance of fresh versus saltwater immersion in relation to drowning.

Objectives—continued

56. Discuss the incidence of wet versus dry drownings and the differences in their management.
57. Discuss the complications and protective role of hypothermia in the context of drowning.
58. Correlate the abnormal findings in assessment with the clinical significance in the patient with drowning.
59. Differentiate the various treatments and interventions in the management of drowning.
60. Integrate pathophysiologic principles and assessment findings to formulate a field impression and implement a treatment plan for the drowning patient.
61. Define *self-contained underwater breathing apparatus.*
62. Describe the laws of gasses and relate them to diving emergencies.
63. Describe the pathophysiology of diving emergencies.
64. Define *decompression illness.*
65. Identify the various forms of decompression illness.
66. Identify the various conditions that may result from pulmonary overpressure accidents.
67. Differentiate the various diving emergencies.
68. List signs and symptoms of diving emergencies.
69. Correlate abnormal findings in assessment with their clinical significance in the patient with a diving-related illness.
70. Describe the function of the Divers Alert Network and how its members may aid in the management of diving-related illnesses.
71. Differentiate the various treatments and interventions for the management of diving accidents.
72. Describe the specific function and benefit of hyperbaric oxygen therapy for the management of diving accidents.
73. Integrate pathophysiologic principles and assessment findings to formulate a field impression and implement a management plan for the patient who has had a diving accident.
74. Define *altitude illness.*
75. Describe the application of gas laws to altitude illness.
76. Describe the etiology and epidemiology of altitude illness.
77. List predisposing factors for altitude illness.
78. List measures to prevent altitude illness.
79. Define *acute mountain sickness.*
80. Define *high-altitude pulmonary edema.*
81. Define *high-altitude cerebral edema.*
82. Discuss the symptomatic variations presented in progressive altitude illnesses.
83. List signs and symptoms of altitude illnesses.
84. Correlate abnormal findings in assessment with their clinical significance in the patient with altitude illness.
85. Discuss the pharmacology appropriate for the treatment of altitude illnesses.
86. Differentiate the various treatments and interventions for the management of altitude illness.
87. Integrate pathophysiologic principles and assessment findings to formulate a field impression and implement a treatment plan for the patient who has altitude illness.
88. Integrate the pathophysiologic principles of the patient affected by an environmental emergency.
89. Differentiate environmental emergencies on the basis of assessment findings.
90. Correlate abnormal findings in the assessment with their clinical significance in the patient affected by an environmental emergency.
91. Develop a patient management plan based on the field impression of the patient affected by an environmental emergency.
92. Describe the etiology, signs and symptoms, and management of a patient struck by lightning.
93. Describe the etiology, signs and symptoms, and management of patients with envenomations.

CHAPTER OUTLINE

Wilderness EMS
Anatomy and Physiology Review
Heat Emergencies (Hyperthermia)
Cold Emergencies
Submersion Injuries: Drowning and Associated Conditions
Diving Emergencies
Altitude-Related Illness
Lightning Injury
Envenomated Animal Bites
Chapter Summary

Case Scenario

You are taking a class on environmental emergencies. The class is being held on a mountain in the West at approximately 10,000 feet. As the class is in progress, a man runs into the room stating he needs help and that his friend is sick. The class instructor meets the man at the door. He is complaining of headache, nausea, vomiting, weakness, and dizziness. The instructor brings the man into the classroom.

Questions

1. *What condition does this man most likely have?*
2. *What is the cause of this condition?*
3. *What are some considerations in the differential diagnosis of this patient?*
4. *List symptoms commonly experienced with this condition.*

[OBJECTIVES 1 TO 9]

Nature can be unforgiving to those who are unprepared for the hazards that are encountered during an outdoor excursion. The extremes that the environment presents include heat, cold, humidity, water, and altitude, each of which can cause illness or injury. Medical or traumatic conditions resulting from these extremes are termed **environmental emergencies** or **environmental illness.** Principal types of environmental illness are caused by these extremes as well as exposure to more specific environmental agents of injury, such as lightning and envenomations. In each case the body will attempt to mitigate the associated negative effects. Unfortunately not all extremes or agents of injury can be handled by the patient's body alone, and often paramedics will need to become involved in environmental emergencies. These environmental emergencies are not uncommon and can lead to significant morbidity and mortality.

Paramedics must know what environmental extremes, environmental risk factors, and agents of injury exist in their service area. This will greatly help in understanding the unique problems that may be caused by those environmental factors. An example of this is the paramedic who works in Hawaii, who may not see patients with frostbite on a regular basis. This same paramedic's patients, however, are very much at risk of heat exhaustion from the combination of heat and humidity present in Hawaii. Understanding the effects of heat and humidity on the body will help in the initial and long-term treatment of these patients.

For this paramedic to not know how to diagnose frostbite would be a mistake, however. The signs and symptoms of frostbite may not be an everyday event, but when encountered it must be recognized and treated properly. For this reason paramedics must be experts in the hazards of their local area while remaining knowledgeable of all types of environmental hazards and emergencies.

In addition to unique environmental risk factors of a community or region, other general risk factors for environmental emergencies exist, including extremes of age, poor preparation for outdoor activities, comorbidities, and lack of specialized or sufficient clothing or gear. The remainder of this chapter discusses more specific environmental conditions as well as their risk factors and management. Environmental factors represent risk for an environmental emergency to develop, and features such as distance from comprehensive care, weather conditions, and fixed obstacles (e.g., snow, glaciers, bodies of water) can complicate treatment or transport decisions.

WILDERNESS EMS

Some paramedics obtain additional training to care for environmental injuries and exposure. Wilderness EMT certifications now exist to adapt street EMS training to wilderness environments, although no standardization or national consensus exists regarding content or appearance of these courses (Johnson, 2004). Specialized teams also have formed within EMS to provide backcountry, wilderness, extended, and technical rescue care (Russell, 2004). Lacking national standards or systemization, these teams tend to be innovative, driven by local needs and environmental challenges, and often are volunteer driven or combinations of various service agencies.

Significant differences exist between wilderness and traditional (street) models of EMS. Most importantly, wilderness EMS models presuppose much longer periods of EMS care and do not assume that all patients will be rapidly—or, in some cases, ever—transported to a definitive medical center. The discussions within this chapter assume traditional EMS protocols. Wilderness EMS and wilderness EMS systems are discussed in more detail in Chapter 54.

ANATOMY AND PHYSIOLOGY REVIEW

[OBJECTIVE 10]

One feature that makes the human body special is its ability to adapt to the extremes of the outside environment. The body strives to stay at constant temperature to provide **homeostasis,** or a state of equilibrium. In the context of environmental influences, homeostatic mechanisms permit the body to remain in equilibrium with its environment. For example, the body adapts to the environmental ambient temperature over the long term by adding or losing fat to adapt for the hot or cold environments. A short-term adaptive mechanism of the body is metabolism, which adjusts to maintain the core temperature. Other short-term adaptive mechanisms include increasing muscle activity (shivering) for heat gain, shunting of blood to the body shell to radiate heat away, and shunting blood from the shell to the core to decrease heat loss. The body also adapts by dilating or constricting blood vessels to allow for regulation of heat loss or gain. Other features of the body protect us against environmental hazards. The skin serves as a physical barrier to materials such as water and pathogens present in the natural environment. It also is a barrier to ambient radiation present from sunlight (although it is limited in this role and can be burned when exposed to excessive radiation). The skin also can absorb heat (when the ambient temperature is above 37° C [98.6° F]) and radiate heat (when the ambient temperature is below 37° C [98.6° F]). It allows the body to cool through sweating but retains water as well.

Homeotherm

[OBJECTIVE 11]

The human body is a **homeotherm,** meaning that it strives to maintain a constant body core temperature. This homeostasis ideally remains within 1° of 37° C (98.6° F). Body temperatures are considered physiologically normal when within 1.5° of 37° C. When the body is at this temperature, chemical reactions are able to occur normally. These reactions assist with a variety of body functions, including the production of heat by the muscles.

Thermoregulation

[OBJECTIVES 12, 13, 14, 15]

The temperature regulator of the brain adjusts body temperature on the basis of input from sources outside the brain. Once the posterior hypothalamus, the **thermoreceptor** of the brain, receives information from these areas of the body, it decides whether the body needs to create heat or eliminate excessive heat. Peripheral thermoreceptors are found in the skin and relay information back to the brain on the basis of the presence of heat or cold receptors. The posterior hypothalamus responds to this input by sending signals back to the affected area to reduce or increase heat loss.

Another set of thermoreceptors are central thermoreceptors found in certain deep tissues of the body. These receptors are mainly in the area of the spinal cord and abdominal viscera and around or in the great vessels. These receptors primarily track temperature changes in the blood and most often react to drops in temperature. The response in this case is to send messages to the skeletal muscle through the central nervous system (CNS). The end result is alteration of vasomotor tone, sweating, and metabolic rate.

Metabolism

[OBJECTIVES 13, 14, 15, 16]

One of the mechanisms at play in maintaining homeostasis when the body is at rest is the metabolic rate. The metabolic rate at rest helps maintain brain function, circulation, and cell stability. This metabolic rate changes to accommodate body needs when active. Such adjustment comes in the form of increased use of nutrients and an increase in the production of calories or units of heat.

As the internal organs sense cooling, metabolism increases; certain blood vessels dilate and others constrict, allowing the warmed blood to circulate around the central organs of the body and warm them. This process takes nutrients, fluid, and oxygen and uses these materials to allow the body to warm. In return carbon dioxide, urine, and other waste products are created. When any part of these elements is missing, metabolism may not process appropriately and changes in body temperature can occur.

During heat exposure or exercise, this same process occurs with different results. The blood vessels allow warmed blood to circulate near the skin and expel the heat generated to the environment.

External Mechanisms of Heat and Cold Response

[OBJECTIVES 13, 14, 15]

In addition to the internal mechanisms affecting the body temperature, other factors also are at work. These factors work from inside and outside the body to affect its surface and core temperature. Although **thermolysis** and **thermogenesis** are the normal means of heat loss and gain to the body, respectively, other outside factors also work to regulate body temperature. These methods involve the transfer of heat from the body to the environment or from the environment to the body.

When the body is in a cold environment it loses heat to the environment. In a hot environment the body gains heat from the surrounding environment. This process is the result of four factors: radiation, convection, conduction, and evaporation. When all these factors are at work, the body gains or loses heat on the basis of the conditions found outside the body.

Radiation

In the mechanism of radiation, the body exchanges heat with the surrounding area by infrared rays. When the body is hotter than its surroundings, it emits these rays and contributes to warming of the immediate environment. When the body is colder than its surroundings, it absorbs the rays from the sun, contributing to heating of the body. Radiation is one of the reasons a cool room full of people quickly heats up. The bodies are radiating heat waves throughout the room, causing the temperature to rise. Many examples of radiation not involving the human body are already familiar, such as baked goods cooling when taken out of the oven and objects heating in a sauna.

Convection

Convection works by a combination of wind, body temperature, and the surrounding environment. During convection of heat from the body, radiated heat is followed by a wind that is cool or cold and helps exchange the heat from the body to the environment. When the breeze is changed from cool to hot, the body is warmed instead of cooled. This is the case in a home heated by forced air; as the warm air is circulated the environment warms along with the human beings inside the environment. The wind chill chart is an example of how the environment can change from warm and friendly to cold and uninhabitable simple by a combination of temperature change and cool breeze (Figure 52-1).

Conduction

Conduction occurs when an object comes in direct contact with another object and heat is transferred. This is the case when a warm body comes in contact with a cool park bench. During this process the body and the object seek to become equal in temperature; thus heat is transferred from the body to the cool park bench. This thermal exchange occurs because the concentration gradient desires to go from hot to cold or high to low.

Evaporation

When the body sweats, it is using the process of evaporation to cool itself. Sweat is excreted from the body onto the skin and absorbs the body heat. As the fluid evaporates, it takes with it heat collected from the body. This process greatly depends on the humidity of the environment; if the environment is full of moisture the fluid on the skin still absorbs the body's heat but is not able to evaporate, thus keeping the body warm. In a desert climate, the evaporative process works quite well and is able to cool the body. In fact, you may not even notice you are sweating because evaporation happens so quickly. This process can be enhanced by spraying cool water onto the skin and thus adding to the evaporation of heat from the body. Maintaining good hydration is important to help with sweating. If the body is dehydrated, sweating is impaired.

Heat Transfer Mechanisms in Tandem

When all four factors—radiation, convection, conduction, and evaporation—are put together appropriately, the body is able to cool or warm itself effectively. For

Wind Chill Chart

Wind (MPH)	Temperature (ºF)																	
Calm	40	35	30	25	20	15	10	5	0	-5	-10	-15	-20	-25	-30	-35	-40	-45
5	36	31	25	19	13	7	1	-5	-11	-16	-22	-28	-34	-40	-46	-52	-57	-63
10	34	27	21	15	9	3	-4	-10	-16	-22	-28	-35	-41	-47	-53	-59	-66	-72
15	32	25	19	13	6	0	-7	-13	-19	-26	-32	-39	-45	-51	-58	-64	-71	-77
20	30	24	17	11	4	-2	-9	-15	-22	-29	-35	-42	-48	-55	-61	-68	-74	-81
25	29	23	16	9	3	-4	-11	-17	-24	-31	-37	-44	-51	-58	-64	-71	-78	-84
30	28	22	15	8	1	-5	-12	-19	-26	-33	-39	-46	-53	-60	-67	-73	-80	-87
35	28	21	14	7	0	-7	-14	-21	-27	-34	-41	-48	-55	-62	-69	-76	-82	-89
40	27	20	13	6	-1	-8	-15	-22	-29	-36	-43	-50	-57	-64	-71	-78	-84	-91
45	26	19	12	5	-2	-9	-16	-23	-30	-37	-44	-51	-58	-65	-72	-79	-86	-93
50	26	19	12	4	-3	-10	-17	-24	-31	-38	-45	-52	-60	-67	-74	-81	-88	-95
55	25	18	11	4	-3	-11	-18	-25	-32	-39	-46	-54	-61	-68	-75	-82	-89	-97
60	25	17	10	3	-4	-11	-19	-26	-33	-40	-48	-55	-62	-69	-76	-84	-91	-98

Frostbite Times: ☐ 30 minutes ☐ 10 minutes ☐ 5 minutes

$$\text{Wind Chill (˚F)} = 35.74 + 0.6215T - 35.75(V^{0.16}) + 0.4275T(V^{0.16})$$

Where, T = Air temperature (˚F) V = Wind speed (mph)

Figure 52-1 A wind chill chart can be used to determine the resultant temperature on the basis of the speed of the wind and the measured temperature.

instance, consider a person who is boating on a 100° F day in the direct sunlight. The relative humidity is a low 25%, with a mild breeze blowing. The body is gaining heat from the environment by sun rays (radiation), the warm breeze (convection), and the air temperature, which is warmer than the body (conduction). Evaporation begins to cool the body as sweat begins to accumulate on the skin; as the breeze blows by the skin, the heated fluid of sweat is taken away. What the person does involuntarily affects how the gained heat is dissipated or kept.

People usually get out of the direct sunlight, use the breeze to help evaporation and convection cool the body, and ultimately move to a cooler environment. These methods use conduction, evaporation, convection, and radiation to reduce heat.

Involuntary Responses

When the brain and hypothalamus sense that the body needs to gain or add heat, they process the message and instruct the body to perform several tasks. These tasks all focus on keeping the main body functions working and in a state of homeostasis. This includes using the shell as a thermal barrier, changing the perspiration levels, shunting blood from the core to the shell or from the shell to the core, and changing the body surface area.

The shell of the body acts as a barrier to many things, including heat and cold. As the temperature drops, the shell protects the internal organs and is the first line of defense. When heat is placed on the shell, it takes the brunt of temperature change, protecting the internal organs from severe heat changes. The shell also acts as an insulator to the environment by having a layer of subcutaneous tissue or fat. This fat layer helps reduce the internal changes experienced from heat and cold environments, similar to insulation in the home.

Perspiration increases in response to the temperature changes that are sensed. On a cold day the body does not sweat as it does when the ambient temperature rises. During a hot day the body sweats in an effort to remove heat by evaporation. As previously discussed, this mechanism can be enhanced by a spray of cool water onto the exposed body to whisk the heat away with evaporation and convection.

In addition, respiratory rate can be increased to eliminate heat; this is a form of evaporation. This form can work against the body in a cold environment because the body removes heat by respiration as stated above, yet on a cold day the goal of the body is to retain heat. (This effect is seen on a cold day when you breathe and create a fog or cloud with the breath; this is the product of a combination of heat from the body and humidity created by the airway.)

Another involuntary response is the restriction of or addition of circulation to the skin. The body maintains or eliminates heat from the core through peripheral vasodilation or constriction.

Metabolism also has an effect on the body temperature. Through an increase or decrease in the rate of metabolism, the body can internally control the amount of heat produced. This production uses nutrients (glucose and oxygen), so if these are missing or low the body will not be able to use metabolism to its fullest. This places diabetic patients at an increased risk of heat and cold emergencies due to their underlying dysfunction in glucose control. Additionally the peripheral neuropathies that can develop in diabetic patients can result in a lack of sensation of heat and cold thereby reducing autonomic responses to these conditions. The autonomic neuropathies that can occur will result in a reduction of the autonomic response even if environmental changes are sensed by the periphery.

In terms of immediate reaction, the body can adapt to hot or cold environments through immediate changes in the skin. A familiar example of this is piloerection, or goose bumps, which appear when the skin is cold and traps air between the hair and skin. The trapped air is then heated by the body, creating an insulating layer.

Body changes can further reduce or add heat by increasing or decreasing the amount of body surface exposed. The size and shape of the body affects how it is able to handle differing temperatures. Tall, slender persons may be better equipped to withstand a hot environment, whereas a shorter, round person will be able to tolerate the cold better. The tall, slender person will be able to dissipate the heat better and lacks the fat layers to insulate from a cold environment. Shorter persons with more fat endure a cold environment better because of their layers of insulation.

Voluntary Responses

Several things come into play during exposure to heat and cold, not the least of which is the human body's ability to evaluate a situation and make changes to adapt (Box 52-1).

In a cold environment the first line of defense is to get out of the cold. Seeking shelter from the cold fulfills a basic need and may have strong psychological benefit. Physiologically, by exposing less skin surface, the shell is protected and the amount of unpleasant exposure to which the shell must submit is limited. Reducing skin surface also is accomplished by the position of the body. During cold exposure, adding insulation also is a good way to stay warm. This added insulation comes in the form of layered dry clothing.

In a warm environment, the voluntary methods to reduce heat also are simple. Initially an individual seeks

BOX 52-1 Voluntary Responses

- Seek shelter
- Expose more skin to the environment
- Expose less skin to the environment
- Layer clothing
- Keep moving

shelter from the heat, such as shade or an air-conditioned environment. The body also does not need the layers of clothing that protect it from the cold. Shedding layers of clothing helps the body eliminate the insulation it needed to stay warm and thus enables the body to eliminate stored or created heat. Eliminating the layers of clothing exposes more surface area to the warm environment. Surface area is increased by not balling up the body but rather by laying open or by sitting with less body surfaces touching each other.

Exercise can help create heat. When the body is sedentary, it still creates heat. When the body is in a heated environment, we tend not to want to exercise or work the muscles. However, to make heat the body can use the muscles. Exercising or moving the body creates needed heat to stay warm in a cold environment.

Outside Contributors

[OBJECTIVES 3, 4]

The body usually does a good job of mitigating the effects of the environment. When dealing with heat, cold, and other environmental concerns, the environment must be evaluated for the contributions it has on the situation at hand and the risk factors for environmental emergencies. Factors to consider include wind velocity, air temperature, terrain, humidity, time of year, likelihood of weather changes, relation to large bodies of water, and distance from shelter.

Wind velocity, as shown in Figure 52-1, can have a detrimental effect on the body and air temperature. As the wind increases in speed it increases convection. If the patient is already cooling improperly and a strong, cold wind is present, his or her condition will become worse.

Extremes of heat or cold can adversely affect the body by forcing it to react. Conduction cools or heats the body, as previously mentioned. As the air temperature becomes extreme, the body often cannot adapt, which causes heat or cold injuries.

Terrain in the mountains, valleys, and deserts affects both the victim and rescuer. Mountainous regions tend to produce afternoon summer storms that can catch a victim unprepared for the onslaught of water and wind. Deserts conversely begin hot in the morning, then often change to piercing cold in the night hours, with varying winds. The victim of an environmental emergency often has been caught in one of these weather extremes and was unprepared for the outcome. The rescuer must be ready to adapt as well or become a victim of the environment in addition to the patient.

Humidity is not often found in the deserts of the Southwest United States, but it is an everyday occurrence during the summers of much of the rest of the nation. A warm, humid environment does not allow evaporation as a heat reduction method. This trapping of heat must be eliminated; thus the paramedic must evaluate other methods of heat loss for the patient. The heat index chart combines ambient temperature and humidity to determine the perceived temperature, much like the wind chill chart combines ambient temperature and wind speed (Figure 52-2).

When patients fail to anticipate the changes in the weather based on reports or the season at hand, a disaster is not only possible but often probable. This lack of planning contributes greatly to the number of victims caught in the environment each year. Each season brings with it a unique problem for the victim and the rescuer; an understanding of weather patterns and prevailing storm activity can save both the rescuer and the victim from hardship.

Location of large bodies of water affects everything from air temperature to rain patterns. Lake effect storms are common in many areas of the country and can contribute to the emergency at hand. When large bodies of water are encountered the paramedic must remember the hazards involved, including lightning. Additional caution must be taken if attempting a rescue from the water. Knowledge of currents, water temperature, and the possibility of wind are imperative to the survival of paramedic and victim.

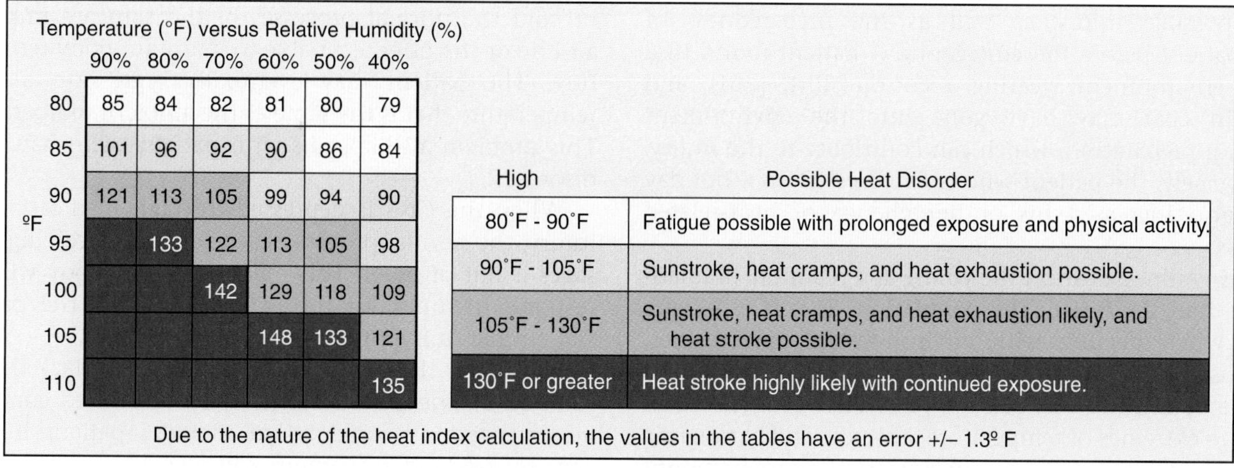

Temperature (°F) versus Relative Humidity (%)

ºF	90%	80%	70%	60%	50%	40%
80	85	84	82	81	80	79
85	101	96	92	90	86	84
90	121	113	105	99	94	90
95		133	122	113	105	98
100			142	129	118	109
105				148	133	121
110						135

High	Possible Heat Disorder
80˚F - 90˚F	Fatigue possible with prolonged exposure and physical activity.
90˚F - 105˚F	Sunstroke, heat cramps, and heat exhaustion possible.
105˚F - 130˚F	Sunstroke, heat cramps, and heat exhaustion likely, and heat stroke possible.
130˚F or greater	Heat stroke highly likely with continued exposure.

Due to the nature of the heat index calculation, the values in the tables have an error +/– 1.3º F

Figure 52-2 Heat stress index.

Shelter location is important for the rescuer and victim if they are both to survive the ordeal. When left with no shelter in extreme environments, the victims may easily perish. Shelter can provide refuge from wind, water, and other hazards the environment can present. The paramedic must consider where shelter can be found in an emergency. It can come in many forms, from a tent to a building to the ambulance and even a cave.

Not all environmental emergencies involve adventures into the high country, but when they do altitude can play a large part in the situation. Altitude can affect the patient's ability to compensate for shock, breathe, and even process simple commands. Altitude also affects the ambient temperature and can make rescue of a victim risky.

The overall health and age of the patient in an environmental emergency may contribute to the situation. In the case of emergencies involving the environment, both the age and general health of the patient can exacerbate the presenting signs and symptoms.

Predisposing Factors

[OBJECTIVES 3, 7, 8, 9, 17]

Some people enjoy outdoor sports and the challenges they present to the athletic body; others who have medical conditions and other issues may find the outdoors both unpleasant and life threatening. In these cases obtaining a good patient history will be of utmost importance to the paramedic's care plan.

Predisposing factors for the paramedic to consider include age, health, medical history, shock, CNS insult, burns, medications, skin disorders, clothing choice, and mental condition of the patient. Young children have underdeveloped thermoregulation systems, and older adult patients have malfunctioning ones that cannot compensate well for temperature extremes. These and other factors may adversely affect the treatment and outcome of the patient in need. Therefore the paramedic should take into account all factors during the assessment process and try to anticipate problems before they occur.

Clothing worn by the victim can be an indicator of the possible injury as well as the preparedness of the patient before the emergency. A patient found in a cold environment wearing a cotton shirt, jeans, and a thin coat may have gone into the environment lacking preparation, which can contribute to the injury. Conversely, the patient who is overdressed on a hot day has also increased his or her chance of heat-related illness.

Many illnesses affect the young and old more dramatically than the rest of the population. This is especially true when dealing with environmental emergencies. Because of the lack of compensatory mechanisms found in the young and old, these populations become susceptible to extremes of temperature, altitude, and barometric pressure. Older adults do not possess the same amount of insulation or subcutaneous tissue as young adults, thereby making them vulnerable to heat and cold extremes. An additional problem with older adult patients is their typical lack of hydration, which also directly affects their ability to dissipate or conserve heat. Couple this with a lack of muscle tissue, and the older adult who is exposed to environmental extremes may succumb earlier than a younger patient.

Pediatric patients are similar to geriatric patients in that they also do not compensate well and lack muscle development capable of producing heat. Their body surface area is large compared with both their fluid volume and overall mass, making them more susceptible to temperature changes. The pediatric patient also is susceptible to the hazards of the environment because of their lack of judgment and inability to perceive the dangers of nature. Children also are at risk for dehydration because they often do not drink enough fluids.

Underlying medical problems that patients possess before they enter an outdoor experience also can play a part in the body's reaction to the hazards presented by the environment. A few of the medical problems that can complicate or contribute to environmental injuries and illnesses include epilepsy, autoimmune disorders, congestive heart failure, strokes, diabetes, hypertension, hypotension, and hyperthyroidism. Each of these diseases affects how body systems—frequently the circulatory system—can deal with environmental extremes.

Another medical problem that affects the patient's ability to endure the environment is the presence of senility, psychosis, or other illness of the brain. These patients may be unable to recognize the presence of hazards. The medications these patients may be taking also can adversely affect their coping mechanisms with the environment.

Many over-the-counter and prescribed medications affect the patient's ability to adjust to the changes presented by the environment. Diuretics mixed with extreme heat, for example, can make a deadly mix, causing dehydration and the possibility of cardiac dysrhythmias.

When a burn patient is exposed to extremes of heat or cold the normal processes of the skin are impaired and he or she often is unable to maintain body temperature. The patient may eventually regress to a body temperature that is the same as the ambient temperature. This problem also appears with patients who have skin disorders.

When the CNS is depressed through medications or injury, the normal process of sending and receiving messages is out of order. This means that the body will not respond to input for the exterior, making the patient susceptible to hypothermia or hyperthermia.

No matter the predisposing condition or lack thereof (Box 52-2), the paramedic must remember to complete an extensive assessment that includes patient history. This history and assessment will reveal many clues that will help determine the optimal treatment.

BOX 52-2 Predisposing Factors of Environmental Emergencies

- Age (very young or old)
- Widespread skin disorders
- Burns
- Central nervous system insult or disease
- Drug use
- Malnutrition and anemia
- Diet
- Heart disease and coronary artery disease
- Shock
- Fluid intake and dehydration
- Alcohol intake
- Diabetes and endocrine disorders

BOX 52-3 Methods to Prevent Cold Emergencies

- Avoid long periods of exposure.
- Drink plenty of clear fluids.
- Eat adequate amounts of carbohydrates, proteins, and nutrients.
- Cover exposed body surfaces.
- Layer clothing:
  - Clothing should be polypropylene or other wicking fabric.
  - The outer layer of clothing should be waterproof and breathable.
  - Avoid use of cotton layers, which increase heat loss when wet.
- Keep clothing and body dry if possible.
- Wear comfortable and loose clothing.
- Add heat from an external source.
- Increase heat production of the body through exercise.
- Get plenty of sleep and rest to allow the body to replenish energy supplies.

BOX 52-4 Methods to Prevent Heat Emergencies

- Avoid long periods of exposure.
- Drink plenty of clear fluids.
- Use time as an advantage; acclimatize to the heat to allow the body a chance to sweat without losing needed salts.
- Avoid exercise and strenuous activities during peak heat hours.
- Use shade to reduce heat.
- Use sunscreen.
- Choose loose clothing that breathes.
- Avoid using diuretics in a heated environment.
- Avoid using amphetamines in a heated environment.
- Limit alcohol intake.

BOX 52-5 Methods to Prevent Other Environmental Emergencies

- Acclimatize to altitudes.
  - After reaching 9000 feet in altitude, rest for at least 2 days.
  - Climb 1000 feet in altitude per day and set camp, then advance 1000 feet and retreat back to camp.
  - Every 3000-foot increase after 9000 feet, rest for 2 to 3 days.
  - If any signs or symptoms of acute mountain sickness are present, descend in altitude.
- Drink plenty of clear fluids.
- Avoid or limit alcohol at altitude.
- Consume plenty of carbohydrates at altitude.
- Use acetazolamide (Diamox) prophylactically with caution because of dehydration side effects.
- Know the side effects of all medications at altitude.

Measures to Prevent Heat and Cold Injury

[OBJECTIVES 18, 19, 20, 21]

Environmental injuries and illnesses are preventable in most cases. In an ideal world, everyone would avoid all hazards around them. Unfortunately this is impossible, so other methods must be evaluated to help mitigate the effects of environmental extremes (Boxes 52-3 to 52-5).

HEAT EMERGENCIES (HYPERTHERMIA)

[OBJECTIVES 8, 17, 22 TO 31]

Heat emergencies, also known as *hyperthermia* or *heat illness,* can manifest for a variety of reasons and in many different forms. These forms include heat cramps, heat exhaustion, and heat stroke. The underlying causes of these emergencies are similar and include lack of clear fluid intake, exposure to the heat, inadequate planning, improper clothing, and poor health. Following is an overview of heat emergencies and associated treatments.

Heat Cramps

Description and Definition

Heat cramps are a common occurrence in the extremes of the environment and in everyday life. They are muscle spasms that occur in conjunction with a hot ambient environment; however, they are caused by physiologic conditions in the patient rather than the heat itself.

Etiology

Heat cramps occur from a combination of poor fluid levels of the body and overexertion with fatigue. As the body sweats, it also loses sodium and other electrolytes. This loss, along with fatigue and dehydration, can bring on acute muscle cramps. Muscles need sodium and other electrolytes to move, which is why insufficient quantities of these electrolytes can cause cramping. Although this pain is rarely a life threat, it is uncomfortable. If untreated, it can progress to other heat emergencies or may be a part of other heat-related illnesses. For example, heat cramps occur in approximately 60% of heat exhaustion cases (Gaffin, 2001).

Epidemiology

Heat cramps are more likely to occur in individuals exerting themselves for several hours in hot environments with heavy sweating, such as industrial workers or athletes. Heat-acclimated individuals appear to be less likely to experience heat cramps.

The most susceptible individuals to heat cramps are those who do not prevent them. This prevention comes in the form of clear fluid or water intake coupled with a well-balanced diet that includes sodium. Unfortunately, most victims of heat cramps do not drink an adequate amount of fluid needed to maintain sufficient levels in the body, and they do not consume a balanced diet.

Physical Findings

[OBJECTIVE 20]

The patient with heat cramps often has cramps in several muscles, typically the fingers, arms, legs, and abdominals. The patient is normally alert and oriented. Body temperature can be normal or slightly elevated, and profuse sweating and warm to hot skin temperature are present. The vital signs of the patient with heat cramps are often within normal limits.

Differential Diagnosis

A patient thought to have heat cramps also may have tetany, a more serious heat illness (heat exhaustion or stroke), or simple muscle cramps.

Therapeutic Interventions

[OBJECTIVES 31, 32, 33]

Oral hydration with electrolyte-containing fluids is usually adequate to treat heat cramps. Treatment with oral salt tablets is contraindicated in all heat emergencies because of the inability of the patient to digest the salt, which may bring about vomiting and further electrolyte imbalances. Instead, salt should be added to water, or commercial salt-containing fluids should be used. Oral hydration formulae are included in Box 52-6.

BOX 52-6 Oral Rehydration

- Basic formula: 1 tsp of salt in 1 L of water; add sugar or honey to taste
- Commercial sports drink: dilute to 50% concentration with water because of heavy concentration of electrolytes that may cause further nausea and vomiting

If oral hydration is not possible because of circumstances or condition of the patient, then intravenous (IV) solutions should be used. Depending on local protocols and guidelines, the fluid choice may vary, with most agencies using an isotonic solution such as normal saline or lactated Ringer's solution. Normal saline is the first fluid of choice in cases of heat cramps.

Further treatment includes removing the victim from the hot environment. The paramedic may take the victim into an air-conditioned area, to the shade, or even the back of an air-conditioned ambulance. Once the patient is cooled and allowed to rest, the paramedic may find the patient does not want any further treatment. This dilemma is up to local guidelines and local medical control.

Heat Exhaustion

Description and Definition

Heat exhaustion is dehydration plus compensated hypovolemic shock in a hot environment. It is more severe than heat cramps and is a common illness in all ages. Heat exhaustion, like heat cramps, is associated with extended exposure to a hot environment and is characterized by nonspecific symptoms such as fatigue, nausea, cramping, and dehydration. Heat exhaustion may manifest with an elevated core body temperature of up to 39° C (103° F).

Etiology

Heat exhaustion has the same underlying causes as heat cramps—sweating and a loss of body fluid, which includes sodium and other electrolytes. A thorough history should be obtained from the patient with suspected heat exhaustion. This will help differentiate the heat illness from fever and malaise associated with infection.

Once again, remember that the patient who has been working in even a 72° F environment is going to lose 1 to 2 L of water from the body. Accompanying this fluid loss is an estimated 20 to 50 mEq of sodium. This combination can affect everything from cardiac output to breathing patterns. In addition to fluid and electrolyte losses, the body also is vasodilating to eliminate heat. This vasodilation has an end result of a decrease in circulating blood volume and preload. The venous pooling that occurs with heat also further enhances this lowered volume and ultimately reduces cardiac output. The body must now battle compensating for the hot environment and the compensated volume shock. Thus the patient quickly becomes fatigued.

Epidemiology

Like heat cramps, heat exhaustion is usually found in athletes and unacclimated laborers working for extended periods in extremely hot environments. The extremes of age are also risk factors for heat exhaustion because of reduced physiologic resources and electrolyte management controls. In some cases the very old and the very young also have trouble hydrating themselves independently.

Physical Findings

[OBJECTIVE 10]

The assessment of a patient with heat exhaustion should include an evaluation of the scene to determine the mechanism of injury and nature of illness. The patient with heat exhaustion normally has been exposed to a heat source over a long period, causing the patient to exhibit signs and symptoms related to heat illness and dehydration. Once the source of the problem has been identified treatment will be much easier to determine and execute.

Assessment of the heat-exhausted patient includes a baseline vital signs check, history of any predisposing factors, and mental status evaluation.

The paramedic should expect the patient to present with an increased body temperature; rapid, shallow breathing; weak or thready, rapid pulse; skin color that is slightly flushed or pale; and skin temperature that is cool and clammy, with heavy sweating. The patient may have a core body temperature close to normal because the body is still compensating for heat gain. In some cases the patient's temperature may be above 100° F but below 105° F. The patient may have nausea and vomiting, fatigue, dizziness, fainting, heat cramps in the large muscle groups, and thirst associated with a decreased urine output. Constant monitoring of the patient for deterioration of level of consciousness is needed to confirm that the patient's condition is not changing to heat stroke.

The paramedic should expect the patient with any heat-related illness to be dehydrated. This dehydration will exhibit the previously mentioned excessive thirst, poor urine output, urine that is dark in color, poor skin turgor, and other signs and symptoms of hypoperfusion.

One study of a running race suggested four risk factors for heat exhaustion in athletes: motivation to exceed previous performance targets, failure to drink fluids during the run, failure of a trained runner to acclimatize for the race, and previous history of heat exhaustion (Lyle et al., 1995).

Differential Diagnosis

The differential diagnosis of heat exhaustion includes uncomplicated dehydration, hypoglycemia, infection, intoxication, and fatigue.

Therapeutic Interventions

[OBJECTIVES 7, 49, 50]

Treatment for the patient with heat exhaustion is similar to the treatment for heat cramps. However, the patient with heat exhaustion needs to be more rapidly treated to reverse the effects of core heating and dehydration.

This treatment includes moving the patient to a cooler area away from the heat source. In the outdoors this may only be to a shaded area, but remember that temperatures from direct sunlight to the shade can change by 15° to 20° F, which can make real changes in the patient's condition. The patient also should be encouraged to rest in an effort to retain remaining fluids and electrolytes. Because this patient may have mild hypovolemic shock, placement in a supine position can help relieve dizziness and lack of core fluids. Loosen any constricting clothing and try to increase convective heat loss.

Replacement of fluids is imperative to protect the patient from further dehydration. This can be accomplished by using oral fluids if the patient will tolerate them or IV fluids. If the patient is able to tolerate oral hydration, the same solutions for heat cramps are once again the appropriate technique (see Box 52-6). IV fluids can be of great assistance in rapid hydration of the patient with heat exhaustion. In most instances isotonic solutions should be used. These solutions include Ringer's lactate and normal saline, with the latter being the fluid of choice. The paramedic should not be surprised to find that a patient may require upwards of 7 L of fluid to restore hydration. In many cases the heat-exhausted patient has spent 8 hours or more in a hot environment and has only drunk minimally during that period.

Other methods to drop body core temperature should be used with the heat-exhausted patient. One of these methods is to spray the victim with cool water and then fan the skin. This will use both evaporation and convection to cool the victim; when coupled with a change in the ambient temperature, the victim should show some immediate improvement. The heat-exhausted patient will be warm (fever) but may develop chills during the cooling process. Although this is normally associated with an infection, it can develop in this situation without infection. It is important that the patient not be cooled so quickly that he or she develops chills or shivering. This would cause thermogenesis, which is exactly what the patient does not need.

As with heat cramps, reduction of the layers of clothing the patient is wearing also helps reduce the core temperature. Be sure to inform the patient of your intentions to remove clothing layers and the reason for your actions. When removal of clothing and fanning the patient brings about chilling, the paramedic may need to slow the cooling process down and even add a layer of clothing. Remember, the goal of treatment is to reduce the core temperature while replacing fluids and ceasing the process of heat gain.

PARAMEDIC*Pearl*

Not all victims of heat exhaustion want or need to be transported to the emergency department. Consult medical direction and determine if the patient is critical enough that his or her condition may progress to heat stroke.

Heat Stroke

Definition and Description

The worst possible environmental injury caused by heat is heat stroke (Box 52-7). This often-fatal condition represents the state in which the body is no longer able to continue reducing heat production. Profound effects occur, especially to the CNS. Heat stroke is associated with a core body temperature greater than 105° F and/or a decreased level of responsiveness secondary to the hyperthermia. It is important that the paramedic realize heat exhaustion and heat stroke are not necessarily progressive. In other words, the patient does not need to first experience heat exhaustion to suffer from heat stroke.

Etiology

[OBJECTIVES 28, 29, 30, 31]

With heat stroke the body's hypothalamic temperature regulation is lost, as is the ability to regulate the internal temperature of the body. This loss of control triggers a chain reaction within the tissues, causing cellular death to the brain, liver, and kidneys. Heat stroke is typically thought to occur at a body temperature of 105° F and above, considered a critically high body temperature. However, the hallmark of heat stroke is an alteration of mental status. This can occur in some patients at body temperatures of less than 105° F.

This lack of control regarding overheating may cause metabolic acidosis from an accumulation of lactic acid. Hyperkalemia often develops as a result of injured muscle cells releasing potassium. Additional causes of hyperkalemia may be from renal failure or metabolic acidosis. Once again, when on the scene of a potentially heat-injured patient, care must be given to both underlying causes and the resulting effects of the heat injury.

BOX 52-7 Differentiating Heat Stroke from Fever

Temperature rise alone should not be confused with an increase of body temperature from fever. Fever represents one response of the body to infection and is intended to create an inhospitable environment for the infecting agent. However, it can be quite uncomfortable and sometimes dangerous for the patient, especially in a wilderness setting, where it may impair performance and be difficult to control. The cause of fever during the inflammatory and infection response is from endogenous **pyrogens** being released. This release of pyrogens by the phagocytic leukocytes causes a fever that may be reduced with antipyretic medications. **Antipyretic medications** work to bring the hypothalamus back to normal operating conditions. In effect antipyretics operate as a reset button for the hypothalamus. Differentiation between heat stroke and fever caused by pyrogens can be accomplished by taking a complete patient history.

Epidemiology and Demographics

[OBJECTIVE 27]

Heat stroke manifests in two forms: classic and exertional. These two similar yet varied illnesses present similarly with a different history and in different populations. The underlying causes are different; a careful history and physical examination may help the paramedic treat both the heat stroke and the underlying illness or injury.

Classic heat stroke appears during long periods of exposure to heat and humidity. Those most commonly affected by classic heat stroke are the very young and old; patients with diabetes, alcoholism, or a cardiac history; and others who are unable to regulate adequately both the ambient temperature and their own body temperature.

Others who may succumb to classic heat stroke include those taking diuretics, psychotropics (antipsychotics, antihistamines, phenothiazines), and anticholinergics. These drugs further alter the ability of the patient to regulate heat and fluid within the body. Many of these medications also alter the ability of the body to regulate vasodilation and heart rate and to compensate for a loss of fluid. One late sign of classic heat stroke is hot, red, dry skin. This is different from exertional heat stroke, which may appear with hot, red, wet skin. The classic heat stroke patient has progressed through heat exhaustion and thus is in decompensated hypovolemic shock.

In **exertional heat stroke,** a sudden rise in core temperature during exercise or extreme stress causes an overwhelming heat stress on the body. The underlying cause of this type of heat stroke is exertion during high ambient temperatures. This exertion can be as simple as working in the yard on a hot, humid day. One example is a firefighter fighting a forest fire. Although well hydrated and in protective gear, the firefighter is exposed to an extremely hot environment while working hard to fight the fire. The space inside the gear becomes, in effect, a sauna, and the firefighter begins to "cook" inside. The body cannot keep up with the sudden surge of heat gain. The longer the body is exposed to the extreme temperature with a lack of cooling, the higher the risk of exertional heat stroke.

All age groups are susceptible to exertional heat stroke. Common to this type of heat stroke are athletes and military personnel, who often have little choice regarding when exercise and activity can take place. As with classic heat stroke, the combination of heat and humidity can produce deadly results. The body, in this case, must deal with ambient temperatures and humidity as well as a body producing heat itself. One big difference between exertional and classic heat stroke is that the patient with exertional heat stroke is not fluid deprived. This patient is well hydrated but his or her body cannot eliminate heat as fast as it is gained. Thermoregulation is thus rapidly overwhelmed.

Physical Findings

[OBJECTIVE 20]

Heat stroke victims have many similar symptoms to heat illnesses previously discussed, but their condition is usually much more advanced and serious. For some time the absence of sweating was considered a major difference between heat exhaustion and heat stroke. This is mostly correct. An estimated 25% of patients with heat stroke still sweat, however. Many of those who are not sweating still have wet skin because of recent sweating. Sweating is impaired because the body is fluid deprived (dehydrated) and needs to conserve fluid in the core to maintain an adequate pressure.

As stated previously, an altered level of consciousness is another hallmark of heat stroke compared with heat exhaustion. Assume that any significantly confused, combative, irritable, or disoriented patient with a heat illness has heat stroke until proven otherwise.

The effects on the cardiovascular system include peripheral vasodilation, resulting in reduced vascular resistance. In classic heat stroke, hypovolemia is present as a result of excessive sweating and fluid loss from the body's attempt to reduce core body temperature through evaporation and convection.

The following signs and symptoms are typical of the patient with heat stroke:

- Altered level of consciousness, including disorientation, combativeness, and irritability
- Unconsciousness in severe cases
- Hallucinations
- Seizures in severe cases
- Extreme body temperature above 40.6° C (105° F)
- Ataxia
- Tachycardia; full pulse that slows late in the process (slows near death)
- Tachypnea; deep at first then progressing the bradypnea and shallow
- Hypotension often lacking diastolic reading
- Red, hot, and dry or wet skin; may be pale if extremely fluid deprived (decompensated hypovolemic shock)
- Lack of sweating (usually)

Differential Diagnosis

Differential diagnosis of heat stroke includes cerebrovascular accident, hypoglycemia, infection, uncomplicated dehydration, intoxication, and neuroleptic malignant syndrome.

Therapeutic Interventions

[OBJECTIVES 17, 31, 32, 33]

Treatment of heat stroke is the same regardless of whether it is classic or exertional. The paramedic must remember the goal of treatment for the patient is based in rapidly cooling the body core temperature and replenishing fluids to the body. Unlike heat cramps and heat exhaustion, rehydration of the patient with heat stroke must be accomplished with aggressive IV fluid resuscitation and very rapid cooling. Other advanced life support treatments required to supplement basic life support treatment may include advanced airway management and cardiac monitoring (Box 52-8).

The treatment of the patient with heat stroke may be intense or mild depending on the severity of the patient's condition. Differentiating the patient with heat stroke from one with febrile issues must be accomplished early in the treatment phase.

BOX 52-8 Specific Treatments for Heat Stroke

- Removal of the patient from the environment
- Rapid cooling of the victim, but avoid shivering
- Fluid resuscitation
  - Typically by IV because the gastrointestinal tract is acidic and may produce vomiting.
  - A fluid challenge and bilateral IVs may be indicated if patient has obvious hypovolemia.
- Administration of high-concentration oxygen by nonrebreather mask
  - Bag-mask device with supplemental oxygen may be needed if respirations are inadequate to maintain perfusion.
  - Consider intubation if the patient is unable to maintain a patent airway or breathing difficulties continue after bag-mask treatment.
- Constant vital signs monitoring
  - Pulse
  - Respirations
  - Blood pressure
  - Oxygen saturation levels
  - Skin color, temperature, and condition
  - Core body temperature
- ECG monitoring for abnormalities throughout treatment process
  - As the body begins to recover from severe heat stroke, dysrhythmias may present at any time.
  - Common dysrhythmias include:
    - ST-segment depression
    - Nonspecific T-wave changes
    - Occasional premature ventricular contractions
    - Supraventricular tachycardias
- Avoidance of vasopressors and anticholinergic medications
  - May cause a hypermetabolic state
  - May potentate heat stroke by inhibiting sweating
- Administration of specific medications may be indicated on a case-by-case basis
  - Diazepam or lorazepam for sedation and seizure control
  - Mannitol to promote renal blood flow and diuresis
  - Glucose if hypoglycemia is present

COLD EMERGENCIES

[OBJECTIVES 88, 89, 90, 91]

Cold emergencies are thought by most to occur in the winter months in cold environments. This is only partially true. Hypothermia can occur during any season and in any climate. Other cold emergencies are common to cold and wet environments often found in the outdoors.

Hypothermia

[OBJECTIVES 34, 35, 36]

Description and Definition

Hypothermia is a core temperature below 35°C (95° F). The drop in body core temperature is a result of excessive exposure to cold environment, a lack of heat production (thermogenesis), or a combination of both.

Etiology

[OBJECTIVES 8, 38, 39, 40, 41]

Hypothermia can be divided into a number of categories based on etiology. It is most commonly categorized as primary (accidental or homicidal or suicidal) or secondary (from natural complications of conditions such as sepsis, trauma, or carcinoma). Other categorizations exist, including acute (short-term loss of temperature control) and chronic (long-term loss of temperature control) as well as immersion and nonimmersion (Danzl, 2001).

Exposure to the cold produces some predictable compensatory mechanisms that seek to limit the exposure of the body to the environment. These limiting measures include piloerection (hair standing on end or goose bumps), shivering, increased muscle tone, peripheral vasoconstriction, increased cardiac output, and increased respiratory rate. When these basic safety mechanisms fail to keep the body warm the body temperature drops. As the body core temperature drops, so does the metabolic rate and cardiac output, further worsening the event and causing even more heat loss.

Hypothermia is categorized in three levels: mild, moderate, and severe. Each level brings a worsening condition that can eventually result in death unless corrected. Temperatures below 86° F are considered critically low. Following are the breakpoints of the three levels of hypothermia:

- Mild (34° to 36° C [93.3° to 96.8° F])
- Moderate (30° to 34° C [86° to 93.2° F])
- Severe (less than 30° C [86° F])

With mild hypothermia the patient may have a variety of signs and symptoms, including the following:

- Normal heart rate
- Adequate blood pressure
- Pale, dry, or wet skin
- Slurred speech
- Shivering
- Uncoordinated movement
- Impaired judgment
- Impaired fine motor skills
- Sluggishness

Patients with moderate hypothermia initially show the signs and symptoms listed above with progressive deterioration over time. This deterioration has the following signs and symptoms:

- Decreased respiratory rate
- Normal heart rate or bradycardia, atrial fibrillation, premature ventricular contractions
- Adequate blood pressure or hypotension (difficult to obtain)
- Pale, cyanotic, or mottled skin
- Confusion to decreased responsiveness
- Stiffening muscles
- Decreased shivering (which stops below 86° to 89.6° F)
- Ataxia
- Respiratory depression
- Muscular rigidity
- Jerky body movements
- Myocardial irritability
- Dilated pupils

Once the patient's core body temperature drops below 30° C (86° F), all compensatory mechanisms have failed and the patient becomes **poikilothermic.** The patient with this low level of core body temperature is in a deteriorated condition that will lead to death if not reversed. Signs and symptoms of this stage include the following:

- Decreased cardiac output, metabolic rate, and cerebral blood flow
- Fixed and dilated pupils
- Compromised airway
- Slow, shallow, or absent respirations; pulmonary edema may develop
- Slowed heart rate
- Possible Osborne waves on ECG (Figure 52-3)
- Cyanotic or mottled skin; lifeless-appearing body
- Eventual ventricular fibrillation or asystole
- Extreme disorientation
- Loss of deep tendon reflexes
- Stiff, rigid muscles
- Cessation of shivering

PARAMEDIC*Pearl*

The severely hypothermic patient experiences a buildup of toxins and metabolic wastes in the core and extremities. Rewarming too fast and without a way to aid in toxin removal can be lethal to the patient.

Epidemiology and Demographics

Predisposing factors to hypothermia include alcoholism (and Wernicke's disease, often associated with alcoholism), burns, hypothyroidism, and extremes of age. In the United States approximately 700 deaths per year are from

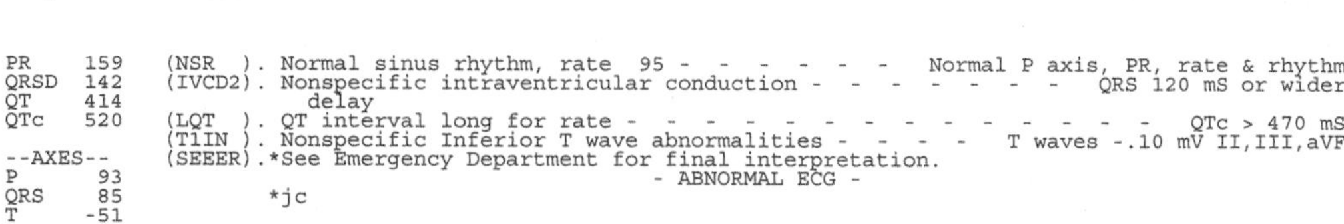

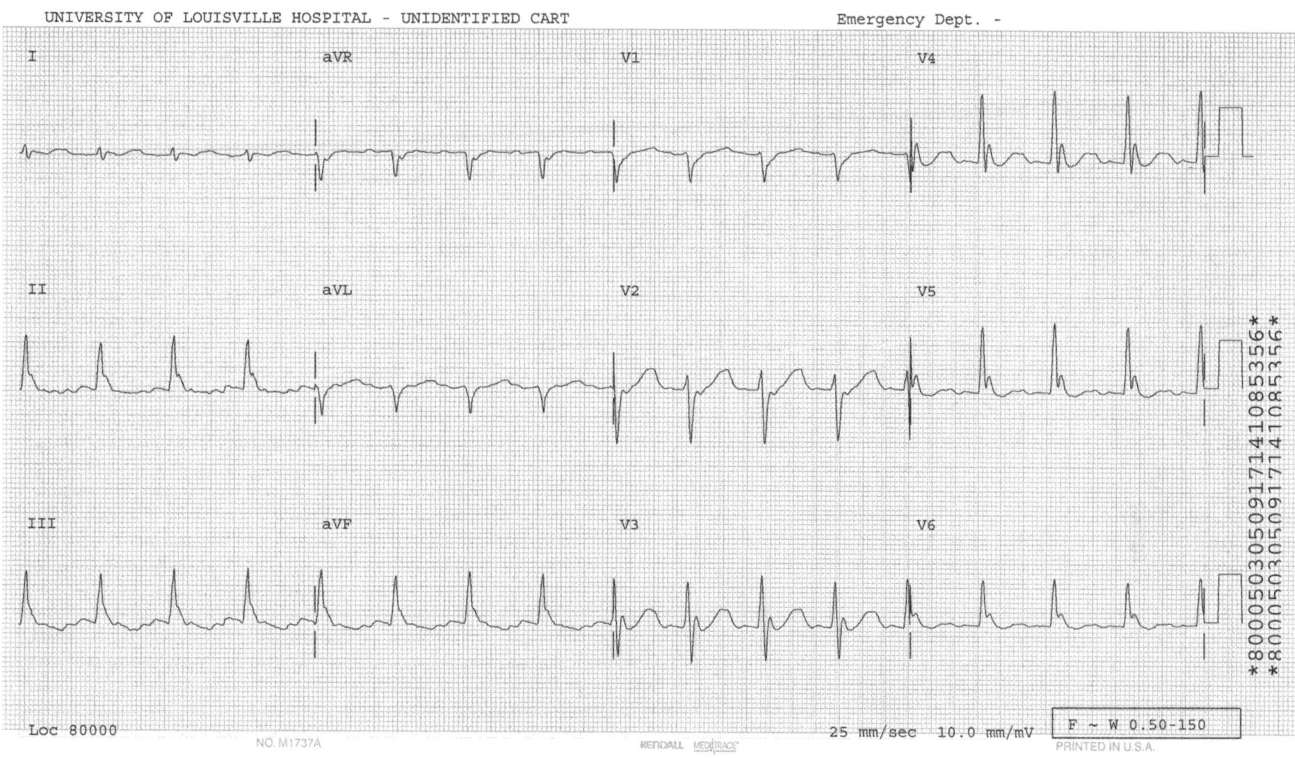

Figure 52-3 Osborn waves.

hypothermia, and more than half occur in patients older than 65 years (Centers for Disease Control and Prevention, 1996). Hypothermia is often assumed to occur only in individuals recreating in or unable to avoid extremely cold ambient temperatures, usually in wilderness settings. However, urban settings account for the majority of cases in industrialized countries, and it is a condition of all seasons and environments (Danzl, 2001). Hypothermia is especially lethal in wartime, and its prevention is a major element in military medicine.

Physical Findings

[OBJECTIVES 9, 40, 41]

The assessment of the hypothermic patient begins with an evaluation of the environment surrounding the patient. Completing this initial evaluation of the scene and the events surrounding the call allows the paramedic insight into the causes of the hypothermia. Once the scene is surveyed and the mechanism of the hypothermia determined, the paramedic should get a general impression of the patient.

PARAMEDIC*Pearl*

The hypothermic patient often demonstrates "the umbles":

- Stumbles
- Mumbles
- Fumbles
- Grumbles
- Bumbles

A general impression coupled with a rapid check of the patient's airway, breathing, and circulation help guide the paramedic in the treatment and remaining assessment of the patient. This process of the initial assessment must begin as quickly as possible and while the paramedic first sees the patient (Box 52-9). The questions paramedics should ask themselves while approaching the patient include the following:

- What caused the state the patient is in?
- What is the location of the cold hazard, and am I at risk?

BOX 52-9 Initial Assessment Reminders for Hypothermia

- Breathing may be slow because of cold injury.
- Breathing and pulse checks may take up to 30 to 45 seconds because of the slowing of body functions.
- Injuries in the cold environment will bring on hypothermia and hypoperfusion more rapidly and in many cases make them worse.
- Evaluate the patient for level of consciousness and remember to look for "the umbles."
- Treat any and all life threats found before moving on to the focused examination.

- Does the patient have an open airway?
- Is the patient breathing?
- Is the breathing adequate, or does it need to be assisted?
- Does the patient have a pulse?
- What is the patient's level of consciousness?
- Are any injuries exacerbating the hypothermia or vice versa?
- Does this patient have any predispositions to hypothermia?
- Is this a high-priority patient?

Once you have completed the initial assessment of the hypothermic patient and treated any life threats found, perform a focused examination to determine any underlying illnesses or injuries. The focused examination also will provide valuable information relating to predisposition to hypothermia. During the focused examination, be careful not to move the patient too abruptly or roughly because this may precipitate further patient injury. Obtain a full set of vital signs, including a core (rectal) temperature. Many field professionals have come to depend on a tympanic thermometer to determine patient body temperature. If a hypothermic thermometer or rectal temperature is not available, an oral thermometer is preferable to a tympanic thermometer. Tympanic and oral thermometers are both inaccurate methods of determining the core temperature of the hyperthermic or hypothermic patient, but they can be used if no other method is available.

Evaluation of the patient's level of consciousness should continue from the time first contact is made to the transfer of care to the emergency department staff. The questions asked to determine level of consciousness and level of hypothermia can begin as simple ones, such as person, place, time, age, and other common knowledge questions. Once these questions have been asked, begin asking questions that require a higher level of reasoning. These questions will evaluate the function of the brain at a level that, if affected by cold injury, will be slow to respond.

During the examination of the patient with a cold injury, inspection will help determine whether any underlying injuries are present. Changes in mental status from hypothermia and cold, stunned peripheral sensation may impair the patient's ability to feel or sense injuries. Locating hidden injuries will be hard to determine without inspection because of the unreliability of the hypothermic patient. You should have a high level of suspicion on the basis of mechanism of injury and what is palpated and inspected on the patient.

Differential Diagnosis

Differential diagnosis of hypothermia includes intoxication, hypoglycemia, cerebrovascular accident, head injury, and hypothyroidism.

Therapeutic Interventions

[OBJECTIVES 42, 43]

Treatment of hypothermia has no quick fix or medication that can reverse it. Instead the paramedic must show patience and use techniques to allow the patient to regain the heat needed to survive. Emergency care of the cold-injured patient depends on the degree of heat loss. It begins with an evaluation of the environment and mechanism of injury. Once this has been determined, you can begin to treat the underlying causes and overt problems. This treatment normally begins with getting the patient out of the environment causing the problem. At the same time, begin measures to stop further heat loss while treating any airway, breathing, and circulation difficulties.

The process of preventing further heat loss involves removing wet clothing, eliminating the wind, and attempting to place insulation below the patient. These important measures will prevent further heat loss by stopping or slowing the processes of convection, conduction, evaporation, and radiation previously discussed. Passive external rewarming (appropriate for all types of hypothermia) includes moving the patient to a warm environment and applying warm, dry clothing and blankets. Insulate the patient above and below the body in a layered manner. Wool blankets typically work best because these materials handle extremes efficiently and tend not to absorb moisture. When wrapping the patient, take care to also cover the head to minimize heat loss.

Active external rewarming includes application of radiant heat, warm air, or heat packs. External heat sources also can be applied when covering and wrapping the patient. The most common of these are heat packs found at most sporting goods stores. If used these heat packs should be wrapped in a towel or other cloth item to avoid burning the patient's skin. To gain optimal warming from the hot packs, place them in the armpits, groin, and around the neck. These areas are highly vascular, containing major arteries that rapidly and efficiently transmit heat. An alternative to commercial heat packs are warmed IV bags or plastic bottles filled with warm water. Extreme care must be taken not to burn the patient.

Active internal rewarming includes warm IV fluids (normal saline) and warm, humidified oxygen. Perform endotracheal intubation if the hypothermic patient is unresponsive or if ventilation is inadequate. If IV fluids are not available and the patient is responsive, oral hydration with sugary foods or warm, sweet liquids is an option that should be used if extended transport time is necessary (in consultation with medical direction). The patient needs sugar and energy to support shivering, which is the best means of heat production. The liquid mixture used may be warm water with sugar or a solution of diluted gelatin and warm water. Either mixture will be rapidly absorbed by the bloodstream and provide needed calories to generate heat. Sugar-containing drinks are preferable to hot drinks such as coffee or tea; both together are best.

Continuously monitor the patient's core temperature, heart and respiratory rates, and blood pressure. Use low-reading thermometers to measure core temperature at 5-minute intervals.

Because of **cold diuresis,** the patient will want to urinate. The bladder fills with fluid when cold is sensed. Once the bladder is full, it is a location for heat loss. If you do not suspect any spinal compromise, allow the patient to urinate if possible. By allowing and assisting the patient to urinate, one source of heat loss will be removed.

Begin cardiopulmonary resuscitation (CPR) if the patient is found to be apneic and pulseless after checking vital signs for 30 to 45 seconds. The heart will slow and circulate adequate oxygenated blood to the body with very slow heart rates (sometimes slower than 10 beats/min). This is especially true in cold water immersions (immersion hypothermia). A heart slowed by metabolic adaptation to cold is sensitive to movement. As the underlying cause of cardiac arrest, hypothermia must be treated and reversed to make resuscitation successful. If the hypothermic patient is in cardiac arrest and ventricular tachycardia or fibrillation is present, attempt defibrillation. Deliver one shock. If no response occurs, focus on CPR and rewarming. Postpone additional defibrillation attempts until the core temperature rises above 30° C (86° F). IV medications are often withheld if the patient's core body temperature is less than this benchmark. If the core temperature is or rises above 30° C, give IV drugs but spaced at longer than standard intervals.

PARAMEDIC*Pearl*

Sometimes patients who appear dead may unexpectedly survive if carefully treated when hypothermia is a result of submersion in cold water. The lowest recorded core temperature of a near-drowning patient who subsequently survived is 14.4° C (58° F) (Gilbert et al., 2000). Remember: Hypothermic patients are not dead until warm and dead.

Frostbite

Clinical Characteristics

[OBJECTIVES 44 TO 49]

Frostbite is a common injury among outdoor enthusiasts working or recreating in the subfreezing environment. **Frostbite** is the freezing of body tissue and can occur during core shunting in a cold environment. This freezing of tissue causes the formation of ice crystals, which draws additional water from the cells into the extracellular space. These ice crystals then expand, which causes destruction of the surrounding cells. As the process continues intracellular electrolyte concentrations increase, which destroys even more cells. **Frostnip** is more superficial and reversible than frostbite. Ice crystals form with severe vasoconstriction (causing some of the pain), but no extracellular freezing or progressive tissue loss occurs.

Frostbite and frostnip typically occur to fingers, toes, ears, and cheeks. Because of their location on the body, low circulation of blood in the cold environment, and likelihood of exposure or wetness during time outside, these extremities and body parts are at risk. Another contributor to frostbite and frostnip is tight clothing. Tight clothing restricts blood flow and thus the ability of the body to keep the extremities warm and blood circulating to them. Eliminating any of these predisposing factors helps prevent frostbite.

Frostbite can be categorized as superficial or deep. The consequence of mistreating frostbite is loss of digits or functional capacity, so an appreciation of appropriate treatment techniques is critical.

Superficial Frostbite. Superficial frostbite or frostnip can be sustained by the skin but may not involve deep tissue. Superficial frostbite involves the epidermis and subcutaneous tissue. The surrounding area is reddened, with a white or yellowish, firm plaque in the area of injury. The skin is soft and resilient below the surface when gently depressed. Superficial frostbite is generally painful because the free nerve endings are still intact.

While gathering patient history, you may find that a previous event of frostbite has occurred. If this is the case, be aware that the patient who has had superficial frostbite in the past is more susceptible to a recurrence if exposed to the cold.

PARAMEDIC*Pearl*

In the past, frostbite, like burns, was classified into degrees of injury. Studies have shown that classification by degrees often is incorrect in relation to the actual severity of the frostbite. Some experts now recommend classifying frostbite into two simple categories: superficial (mild) and deep (severe). Superficial frostbite does not involve eventual tissue loss, whereas deep or severe frostbite does result in tissue loss.

Deep Frostbite. The patient who has deep frostbite also may be suffering from hypothermia. Deep frostbite is the freezing of the epidermis and subcutaneous tissues that may involve muscles, nerves, tendons, and bones. The patient with deep frostbite presents with skin that appears white and hard or frozen to the touch. The patient reports a loss of feeling in the affected area, which feels frozen and hard. The patient also cannot move or bend the affected digit, extremity, or part of the body.

The patient affected by deep frostbite may not initially feel the pain, but this injury will eventually cause significant pain during rewarming. Depending on the depth of the frostbite, long-term care may include amputation of the affected body part. Treatment on scene is aimed at mitigating the long-term effects of frostbite.

Epidemiology and Demographics

[OBJECTIVE 47]

Frostbite is known to be a particular hazard for mountaineers, explorers, tobacco abusers, fatigued or malnourished individuals, and soldiers (McCauley et al., 2001).

Differential Diagnosis

Differential diagnosis of frostbite or frostnip includes chilblains (subcutaneous vesicles caused by long-term exposure to moisture and cold in an extremity), pernio (painful eschar that result from longer exposure than chilblains), trench foot (also known as *immersion foot*), cold urticaria, uncomplicated hypothermia, Raynaud's phenomenon, local infection, ischemic injuries, or blunt trauma.

Therapeutic Interventions

[OBJECTIVES 50, 51]

Regardless of the degree of frostbite, treatment by prehospital providers is aimed at limiting further exposure and injury (Box 52-10). This means that any thawing of the affected areas must be deferred if any chance of refreezing exists. Because of this, thawing is usually best done when a patient is in a controlled environment in or en route to a medical center or other definitive care. Treatments also should minimize movement; do not massage any of the frostbitten areas. Rubbing or massaging the area may cause the ice crystals to move, causing further injury to the patient.

An exception to this rule exists if the patient needs to walk out of a remote or hazardous area on feet that have been frozen. In this case, treatment will not begin until after patient extraction from the area.

BOX 52-10 Proactive Treatment of Frostbite Injuries

- Limit further exposure of the injured area to the environment.
- Elevate and immobilize the injured area during and after thawing.
- Gain IV access for pain management.
- Thawing of injured area by submersion normally takes place at the hospital.
- Consider thawing of injured area if transport time is delayed or prolonged and refreezing is not an anticipated risk.
  - Thawing of area is completed by submersion in 102° to 104° F water.
  - When injured area is immersed, the water temperature will fall greatly, which requires additional warm water to be on hand and added as needed.
- Before thawing of injured area, administer analgesics.
- Once thawed, cover the injured area with loose, sterile, dry dressings.

PARAMEDIC*Pearl*

Remember, the goal of treatment is to limit further injury and attempt to reverse the effects of the potential damage to the patient.

Trench Foot

Clinical Characteristics

During World War I, soldiers were subjected to long periods of standing in cold water found in military trenches. No opportunity was available to dry or warm the feet. The term *trench foot* comes from this unfortunate period in history. Today the condition is more often known as *immersion foot* and is more often found in civilian outdoor enthusiasts or civilians in wet, cold environments who are poorly equipped.

Physical Findings

Trench foot symptoms are similar to those associated with frostbite; however, the injury normally occurs at temperatures above freezing. Also differing from frostbite, the patient with trench foot normally describes symptoms that occurred over days. The extremity initially feels cold and numb and appears blanched.

Differential Diagnosis

Differential diagnosis of trench foot includes chilblains, pernio, frostbite, frostnip, cold urticaria, Raynaud's phenomenon, ischemic or blunt trauma, and local infection.

Therapeutic Interventions

The best treatment for trench foot is prevention and early recognition of symptoms. The feet often are neglected during outdoor excursions. Preventative measures include keeping the feet warm, dry, aerated, and elevated when possible. Change wet socks frequently; avoid sleeping while wearing wet socks and/or boots; and avoid prolonged periods in standing water, mud, and wet environments.

Immediate treatment of the patient with trench foot should include drying of the affected area and removal from the offending environment. While drying the area, begin the warming process along with aeration of the feet. The feet will also benefit from elevation during the drying and warming process. Establish IV access and administer analgesics (if no contraindications are found) to relieve pain.

Recognition and treatment of trench foot are important to the long-term outcome for the patient. Trench foot often leads to tissue sloughing or gangrene of the feet and legs. The treatment the paramedic provides will help alleviate these long-term problems.

SUBMERSION INJURIES: DROWNING AND ASSOCIATED CONDITIONS

Definition and Description

[OBJECTIVE 52]

Several disorders are considered submersion injuries. **Immersion** means "to be covered in water or other fluid. Submersion implies that the entire body, including the airway, is under the water or other fluid" (Soar et al., 2005). **Drowning** is "a process resulting in primary respiratory impairment from submersion/immersion in a liquid medium. Implicit in this definition is that a liquid/air interface is present at the entrance of the victim's airway, preventing the victim from breathing air" (American Heart Association, 2005). Some authorities consider any event of this sort a drowning incident whether the patient lives or dies. Others define *drowning* to mean death by this process and *near-drowning* to indicate this process but without the result of death within the first 24 hours. For drowning to occur, at least the face and airway usually must be immersed. Associated conditions include the following:

- **Immersion syndrome:** sudden cardiac arrest caused by massive vagal stimulation after sudden exposure to cold water.
- **Postimmersion syndrome:** delayed deterioration of a previously asymptomatic or minimally symptomatic patient.
- **Shallow water blackout:** unconsciousness after submersion as a result of intentional hyperventilation before water sports such as competitive swimming or underwater breath-holding contests. A common example of this is a group of children hyperventilating before seeing how far they can swim underwater.

PARAMEDIC*Pearl*

For purposes of uniformity of research, The International Liaison Committee on Resuscitation recommends that the following terms should no longer be used: dry and wet drowning, near-drowning, active and passive drowning, silent drowning, secondary drowning, and drowned versus near-drowned (Idris et al., 2003). However, many of these terms, such as dry and wet drowning and near-drowning, are still in frequent use in clinical care.

Epidemiology and Demographics

In the United States approximately 9000 people die each year from drowning. Drowning is the second leading cause of accidental death in the United States and is the leading cause of accidental pediatric death in states with seat belt laws. Children younger than 5 years account for 40% of the deaths associated with drowning. Teenagers are the second major age group of those who die from drowning, and the third highest group is the elderly. In older adults the most common type of drowning is a result of bathtub incidents. Black children have an approximately threefold higher risk of drowning compared with white children. Interestingly, less swimming ability is *not* a clear risk factor for drowning. A male/female predominance of approximately 5:1 exists for drowning not attributed to boating activities; this risk is more than doubled to 12:1 for boating-related drownings.

Swimming pools and fresh-water drowning account for the majority of drownings. Alcohol use is a common denominator of the victim or the supervising adult in many drownings. The paramedic should be wary of signs of abuse or neglect in pediatric drownings and near-drownings. This is especially true of pediatric incidents involving bathtubs; 67% have been found to be attributable to abuse or neglect.

Etiology

[OBJECTIVES 53, 54, 55, 56, 57]

The classic sequence of drowning starts with panic. One of the following two events takes place:

- When the victim can no longer hold the breath, he or she reflexively takes a breath, which causes water to enter the mouth.
- The victim may make take several violent intakes of air and water while flailing in the water.

In either case, the water intake hits the posterior portion of the oropharynx, causing laryngospasm and bronchospasm. This results in severe hypoxia. In a small percentage of drownings, laryngospasm does not allow any further water to enter the lungs. However, most drownings involve a significant amount of water entering the lungs. This occurs in 85% to 90% of drowning incidents (Newman, 2001). Aspiration of water and laryngospasm are the main contributors to the hypoxia that occurs within the patient. As this condition continues, hypoxemia and acidosis occur, causing cardiac disturbances. Long-term lack of oxygenation of the drowning victim produces central nervous system anoxia and coma.

Patients can drown in fresh water, salt water, tap water, sewer or contaminated water, or pool water. The pathophysiologic characteristics of drowning do not significantly change with different water types. Although the body may react in slightly different ways, the on-scene treatment of drowning victims does not change with the type of water. The paramedic should treat all drowning and near-drowning victims similarly; any consideration to type of water involved will be handled by the receiving facility. With this in mind the paramedic should relay the mechanism of drowning and type of water involved in the drowning to the emergency department (Box 52-11).

BOX 52-11 Mammalian Diving Reflex

The mammalian diving reflex is a complex cardiovascular reflex that is triggered by submersion; it constricts blood flow everywhere except the brain.

PARAMEDIC*Pearl*

The major physiologic consequences of submersion are hypoxia, acidosis, and pulmonary edema. Of these, hypoxia is the most important. Factors affecting patient outcome include water temperature, duration and degree of hypothermia, the diving reflex, the victim's age, water contamination, duration of cardiac arrest, the promptness and effectiveness of initial treatment, and cerebral resuscitation (Feldhaus, 2002).

Physical Findings

[OBJECTIVES 58, 60]

A drowning incident often is associated with other emergencies. Therefore evaluation for spinal trauma and hidden injuries is an essential part of the patient evaluation. If the cause of drowning is unknown, consider spinal trauma as an underlying problem and treat accordingly.

Assessment of the drowning patient begins with a good scene evaluation and evaluation of where and how the victim drowned. This should be followed by a quick check of airway, breathing, and circulation. Be mindful during the assessment process that the victim may have hypoxia as well as injuries sustained before or during the drowning. Assessment of the patient for spinal injury, cardiac disturbances, and hypothermia should be common practice for drowning patients.

With many submersion injuries taking place in cold water environments, hypothermia becomes a factor in both the death and the ability of EMS personnel to resuscitate the victim. During hypothermic states the body processes slow, including the need for oxygen. The lack of oxygen contributes to the death of the patient, whereas the mammalian diving reflex allows the body to tolerate long periods of being under water and apneic. The longest case of submersion with subsequent survival is 66 minutes (Bolte et al., 1988). Most authorities agree that after more than 30 minutes of submersion in warm water, the operation should be considered a body recovery, not a rescue. However, resuscitation should be attempted in all patients submerged in cold water, even for long periods, unless other signs of obvious death are present (postmortem lividity, rigor mortis, or injuries incompatible with life).

PARAMEDIC*Pearl*

Suspect hypothermia in any drowning incident.

Differential Diagnosis

As previously discussed, the differential diagnosis includes trauma, spinal injury, cardiac disturbances, and other comorbidities, including hypothermia, hypoglycemia, CNS disturbances, and other metabolic abnormalities.

Therapeutic Interventions

[OBJECTIVES 57, 58, 59, 60]

As you arrive on scene, your first concern must be personal safety and the safety of the responding crew. Recognition of where the patient is and how the drowning occurred should be at the forefront of treatment.

The most important factors that determine patient outcome are the duration and severity of hypoxia. Reversal of the hypoxic state requires that patient resuscitation begin immediately on contact (Box 52-12).

If *any* type of resuscitation is required for a drowning victim, transport the patient to the hospital for evaluation. Delay at the scene will only complicate the resuscitation of the patient. Consider air medical transport in remote locations. Many complications from a drowning incident do not appear for 24 hours. Complications include sudden respiratory arrest and **adult respiratory distress syndrome (ARDS).** ARDS is a serious complication that brings with it an alarming number of fatalities. The physiologic stress of near-drowning manifests in a variety of ways, one of which is the release or leaking of fluid into the alveoli. This release causes inflammation of the alveolar and lung tissues coupled with respiratory system failure. Other factors are a loss of surfactant, atelectasis, aspiration pneumonia and, in some cases, pneumothorax. All of these affect the ability of the body to regain oxygen and release carbon dioxide, making respiratory and metabolic acidosis a concern for patient survival (Box 52-13).

DIVING EMERGENCIES

[OBJECTIVES 61, 67, 73, 88, 89, 90, 91]

Diving was revolutionized with the development of the ***s**elf-**c**ontained **u**nderwater **b**reathing **a**pparatus* (scuba), a tool that provides divers with oxygen and permits deeper and longer dives than would be possible through normal breath holding. Throughout the world, scuba diving is gaining popularity, with training and certification easily attained. Some of this increase in popularity can be attributed to an increase in those vacationing on cruise ships, where certification is easy to obtain. The low

BOX 52-12 Care and Treatment of the Drowning Victim

- Gain access to the patient, taking precautions not to put your safety at risk.
- Once you have reached the patient, remove the patient from the water as quickly as possible.
- Ventilation is the most important treatment for a drowning victim. Start rescue breathing as soon as the victim's airway can be opened and your safety can be ensured (usually when the victim is in shallow water or out of the water). You do not need to clear the airway of aspirated water because the body quickly absorbs the water aspirated into the bloodstream, and any remaining water is pushed into the bloodstream by positive-pressure ventilation. However, debris, gastric contents, or other foreign material may need to be removed. Routine use of abdominal thrusts is not recommended. These procedures can cause injury, vomiting, and aspiration and delay cardiopulmonary resuscitation.
- Cervical spine stabilization is unnecessary unless the history includes shallow water diving, use of a water slide, signs of injury, or signs of alcohol intoxication (American Heart Association, 2005). If the incident was not witnessed, assume cervical spine injury and provide in-line stabilization.
- After removal from the water, begin cardiopulmonary resuscitation at once if a pulse cannot be felt. Feeling a pulse may be difficult because of peripheral vasoconstriction and decreased cardiac output. Attach a cardiac monitor and defibrillator and attempt defibrillation if a shockable rhythm is identified.
- Give high-flow oxygen. Continuous positive airway pressure may be necessary to improve oxygenation. Be prepared to suction the airway during the resuscitation effort.
- Early endotracheal intubation may be necessary. "The decision to intubate a spontaneously breathing patient should be based on the degree of respiratory distress, the presence or absence of protective airway reflexes, the ability to maintain adequate tissue oxygenation based on pulse oximetry, and the presence of associated head or chest injuries" (Feldhaus, 2002).
- If the patient is in cardiac arrest, consider endotracheal intubation early in the resuscitation effort. Treat cardiac arrest rhythms according to the appropriate advanced cardiac life support algorithm.
- Establish vascular access. Avoid excessive fluid administration, which may cause pulmonary edema.
- Dry and warm the patient, especially if the drowning occurred in cold water. This warming may include respiratory warming, if available.

From American Heart Association. (2005). AHA guidelines for cardiopulmonary resuscitation and emergency cardiovascular care, part 10.3: Drowning. *Circulation, 112*(suppl IV), IV-133; Feldhaus, K. M. (2002). Submersion. In J. A. Marx (Ed.). *Rosen's emergency medicine: Concepts and clinical practice* (5th ed.) (p. 2051). St. Louis: Mosby.

BOX 52-13 Factors Affecting Outcome of the Drowning Patient

The most important factor to survival is rapidity of rescue and time to initiation of cardiopulmonary resuscitation in cases of cardiopulmonary arrest. Several other specific factors can affect prognosis:

- *Water temperature.* Despite long time periods of submersion some patients will recover if the water is cold. As with hypothermia treatment, patients in cold water submersion are not dead until warm and dead.
- *Duration of submersion.* The longer a patient is apneic and submerged, the less the chance of survival. In warm water patients may not be viable after 30 minutes; cold water drowning has documented cases of complete recovery.
- *Water condition.* Dirty or contaminated water that is aspirated is more likely to cause alveolar damage and limit gas exchange at the alveolar level.
- *Age of victim.* The younger the patient, the better the recovery from apnea. The young are resilient and have a better chance of survival with aggressive resuscitation efforts. Most authorities consider patient age less than 3 years to be a favorable factor to ultimate outcome (Dickison, 1999; NAEMT, 2007).

From Dickison, A. E. (1999). Near-drowning, predictors of survival. *Wilderness Medicine Letter, 16*(2); NAEMT. (2007). Environmental trauma II: Drowning, lightning, diving, and altitude. In *Prehospital trauma life support* (6th ed.) (p. 446). St. Louis: Mosby.

incidence of problems may be linked with strict training requirements associated with diving. The paramedic should be aware of the problems that may occur as a result of diving. The injuries that the paramedic may encounter include barotraumas of descent and ascent, air embolisms, decompression sickness, and nitrogen narcosis.

Physics of Diving Emergencies

[OBJECTIVES 62, 63]

The body works under constant pressure from the atmosphere. This mixture of gases exerts a pressure of 760 mm Hg, or 1 atmosphere. This pressure can change depending on the environment, as found with ascent to high altitudes, where the pressure drops approximately 17% at roughly 4600 feet. Descent into water also affects this pressure and depends on the type of water, salt or fresh. Fresh water is less dense and therefore exerts less pressure than salt water.

As the diver enters the water, its density will exert additional pressure against the organs and body of the diver. Because the body is composed primarily of water and water is not compressible, the body is not affected negatively. Many organs are filled with gases, however, which are compressible and thus affected.

Three laws are in play when the diver enters the water: Boyle's law (Box 52-14), Dalton's law (Box 52-15), and Henry's law (Box 52-16). These laws also are meaningful when individuals ascend to high altitudes. For the paramedic to fully understand diving emergencies and how gases are affected during diving, a brief description of each law is provided below.

Barotrauma

[OBJECTIVES 66, 68]

Description and Definition

Barotrauma is physical damage to the body tissue caused by changes in pressure between inside the body and the air or liquid surrounding the body.

Etiology

Barotrauma typically occurs within the body when it moves from a high-pressure environment to one with lower pressure, as a diver would when ascending. Climbers may also experience similar difficulties during ascent to high altitudes. Although not as common, barotrauma can occur when descending, or moving from an area of low pressure to an area of high pressure.

As the diver stays under water, the damage occurs in surrounding tissues of the body's air spaces. This is attributable to the fact that gases are compressible and tissues are not. As the ambient pressure increases, the internal air space provides little or no support to resist the higher external pressure. When the ambient pressure decreases, the higher pressure of gas inside the air spaces causes damage to the surrounding tissues if that gas is trapped.

Two types of barotraumas can occur: barotrauma of descent and barotrauma of ascent. The type of barotrauma is based in the mechanism of the injury. Barotrauma of descent, or the squeeze, occurs as a result of the inability to equalize the pressure between the nasopharynx and the middle ear through the eustachian tube. The problems associated with the barotrauma of descent include the following:

- Middle ear pain
- Ringing in the ears
- Dizziness
- Hearing loss
- Rupture of the eardrum (extreme cases)
- Frontal headaches
- Pain beneath the eye in the maxillary sinuses

Barotrauma of ascent most often occurs as a result of rapid ascent and failure of the diver to clear equilibrate

BOX 52-14 Boyle's Law

Boyle's law states that if the temperature remains constant, the volume of a given mass of gas is inversely proportional to the absolute pressure.

- At sea level, lungs of average size and capacity are under 14.7 pounds of pressure.
- At a depth of 99 feet, with the same amount of air present, the lungs size is one fourth of normal and the air is compressed.
- If additional air enters the lungs at depth, it will expand as the diver ascends, causing expansion injury to the lung tissue.
- **Diver's rule: Do not hold your breath while scuba diving.**

BOX 52-15 Dalton's Law

Dalton's law states that the total pressure of a mixture of gases is equal to the sum of the partial pressures of the individual gases.

- Air is composed of 21% oxygen, 78% nitrogen, and 1% other gases.
- People who fly in unpressurized planes subject themselves to a decrease in air pressure as they ascend and an increase as they descend.
- Breathing is comfortable below 8000 feet.
- The air pressure is increased as the diver descends and decreased as the diver ascends.
- The natural body reaction at altitude is to hyperventilate, a reaction dangerous to divers.
- **Diver's rule: Control breathing at all times while scuba diving.**

BOX 52-16 Henry's Law

Henry's law states that, at a constant temperature, the amount of a given gas dissolved in a given type and volume of liquid is directly proportional to the partial pressure of that gas in equilibrium with that liquid.

- As the pressure of any gas increases, more of that gas will dissolve into any solution with which it is in free contact.
- When ambient pressure is lowered with ascent to altitude, the partial pressure of oxygen and nitrogen in the body must fall, and fewer molecules of each gas will be dissolved in the blood and tissue.
- When ambient pressure is raised during diving, the partial pressure of oxygen and nitrogen in the body must rise, and more molecules of each gas will be dissolved in the blood and tissues.
- The gases that comprise the atmosphere tend to dissolve in the blood plasma and other body liquids during diving.
- As the pressure from diving occurs the air needed is dissolved, and on ascent the nitrogen is released, causing a variety of problems.
- **Diver's rule: Avoid long periods and repetitive dives to deep areas.**

inner ear and nasopharyngeal pressure. During ascent Boyle's law is at work; if air is not allowed to escape because of obstruction, the expanding gases distend surrounding tissues and cause lung injuries. Obstructions can include holding of the breath, bronchospasm, or mucus plug. The most common of these is breath holding as a result of diver panic or the diver running out of scuba tank air.

The most serious injuries from ascent involving the lungs are caused by pulmonary overpressurization syndrome. This is a result of expansion of trapped air within the lungs from breath holding on ascent. It occurs in both shallow and deep dives from expanding air in the lungs. When air is not exhaled during ascent the air within the lungs expands and structural damage to the lung tissue occurs. Other injuries that may occur include arterial gas embolism, air bubbles, or an air embolism. Air entering the circulatory system from the lung may have long-term and devastating effects on the patient.

Two other injuries that may occur include pneumomediastinum and pneumothorax. A pneumomediastinum is the presence of air in the mediastinum, pericardial sac, and tissues around the neck. A pneumothorax may occur if the alveolar sacs rupture in the lungs and cause the collapse of a lung. This is a rare occurrence but one that may require immediate attention by the paramedic.

Epidemiology

Barotrauma is the most common medical complication of scuba diving (Kizer, 2001).

Physical Findings

Physical examination must center on the areas described for barotraumatic injury, particularly the lungs and the ears.

Differential Diagnosis

The differential diagnosis for barotraumatic injury includes infection, decompression sickness, and trauma.

Therapeutic Interventions

[OBJECTIVE 71]

The basis for treatment of most diving injuries is to determine the cause of the injury. While completing this evaluation you must determine if the scene is safe and if the patient is accessible. Treatment should be basic, with airway, breathing, and circulation needs being addressed first. Administer high-flow oxygen to the patient early; this can be the greatest benefit to the victim of any diving injury. Also begin IV therapy for fluid resuscitation and possible medication administration, coupled with blood draws at the time the IV is started. These blood samples will help the emergency department determine the type and cause of diving injury. Specific injuries (e.g., pneumothorax) should be treated with standard techniques.

Nitrogen Narcosis

[OBJECTIVES 68, 69]

Description and Definition

Nitrogen narcosis occurs while the victim is diving and is considered a diving emergency. Nitrogen narcosis is commonly called *raptures of the deep* because it causes a state of stupor and affects cerebral function. The affected diver appears to be intoxicated and acts in an unfamiliar manner. Nitrogen narcosis can be exacerbated or induced when the diver panics. This panic may cause the diver to use more air and produce more carbon dioxide.

Etiology

While breathing compressed air, nitrogen (used as the inert gas) becomes more soluble and can produce an anesthetic and intoxicating effect in divers as they descend to high-pressure depths. Nitrogen narcosis can develop at depths between 70 and 100 feet of sea water (fsw).

Epidemiology

Nitrogen narcosis has historically caused many deaths in divers. In commercial diving and low-depth diving (below 100 fsw) divers generally use heliox (a mixture of helium and oxygen) as the inert gas, which eliminates the risk of nitrogen narcosis. Individual variability exists in terms of susceptibility, and acclimatization appears to reduce risk of developing this condition.

Physical Findings

Nitrogen narcosis causes euphoria and poor thinking. Subsequent errors in judgment and/or technique result in the many deaths from this condition. Focus the physical examination on mental status and judgment of a patient, either by history or observed on the scene.

Differential Diagnosis

Nitrogen narcosis differential diagnosis includes intoxication from drugs or alcohol, hypoglycemia, and CNS infection.

Therapeutic Interventions

[OBJECTIVE 71]

Nitrogen narcosis requires ascent to shallower depths, at which time symptoms should resolve. Treatment is the same as for barotrauma.

Decompression Sickness

[OBJECTIVES 64, 65, 69, 71]

Description and Definition

Decompression sickness, also called *decompression illness,* or *the bends,* is caused by the formation of nitrogen bubbles in the bloodstream and tissues of the body.

Etiology

These bubbles occur if the diver moves from deep water toward the surface too rapidly. Another factor in development of the bends is the exposure divers have to compressed air while below the surface. The bubbles cause excessive pressure in various body areas and occlude circulation in the small blood vessels. This condition shows in the joints, tendons, the spinal cord, skin, brain, and inner ear. These symptoms are typically confined to dives that exceed 33 feet or dives that are prolonged in length, causing excessive nitrogen to be formed within the bloodstream.

Epidemiology and Demographics

According to the Divers Alert Network (DAN) (Box 52-17), 1132 cases of barotrauma related to diving occurred in the United States in 1995 (Marks, 2001).

Physical Findings

Decompression sickness signs and symptoms are normally not visible until after diving. These signs and symptoms vary in location, as does the location of the nitrogen bubbles. Principle areas affected are joints and the abdominal region, with fatigue, paresthesias, and CNS disturbances also occurring. Complete an extensive patient history to determine if decompression sickness is present because the patient may not have shown any difficulties for up to 24 hours after the dive.

Differential Diagnosis

Differential diagnosis of decompression sickness includes fatigue, cerebrovascular accident, intoxication, and infection.

Therapeutic Interventions

[OBJECTIVES 71 ,72]

The basis for treatment is the same as for barotrauma.

BOX 52-17 Divers Alert Network

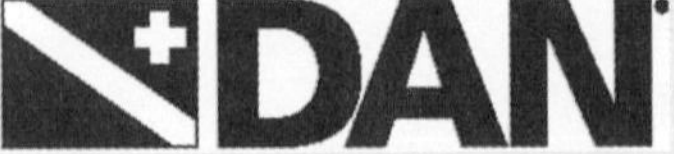

Founded in 1980 and associated with Duke University Medical Center, the Divers Alert Network (DAN) has operated the only 24-hour emergency diving hotline, a lifesaving service for injured divers. Additionally, DAN operates a diving medical information line, conducts vital diving medical research, and develops and provides a number of educational programs for beginning divers to medical professionals. It is the largest association of recreational divers in the world.

DAN's mission statement: DAN helps divers in need with medical emergency assistance and promotes diving safety through research, education, products, and services.

PARAMEDIC*Pearl*

Remember: The most important care for diving injuries is early high-flow oxygen and rapid transport to the appropriate facility.

The long-term care of some compression injuries is **recompression** with a hyperbaric oxygen chamber. Hyperbaric oxygen chambers are designed to subject the patient to oxygen under greater than atmospheric pressure. The force from this pressure causes the nitrogen in the body to redissolve, gradually decompressing and escaping without forming bubbles.

Diving Injury Prevention

Ultimately the best treatment for diving injuries is prevention and education. Prevention includes the following:

- Do not hold the breath while diving.
- Control breathing while underwater.
- Avoid long periods of diving at depth.
- Get plenty of rest between dives.
- Ensure proper hydration.
- Avoid alcohol use when diving.
- Make ascents slowly and allow ample time to surface at the conclusion of a dive.

ALTITUDE-RELATED ILLNESS

[OBJECTIVES 74 TO 79, 88 TO 91]

High-altitude illnesses are similar to diving emergencies in how the body reacts to differing environmental pressures. The difference between altitude and diving is that diving injuries are sustained from high atmospheric pressures and altitude injuries are sustained from a decrease in pressure. High-altitude illnesses are caused by a reduction in the barometric pressure and lowering partial pressure of oxygen. To understand this problem fully, refer to Dalton's law and remember that oxygen concentration remains constant at 21%, but as a person ascends in elevation the partial pressure decreases. This lowering of pressure means less oxygen is available at higher altitudes.

High-altitude illnesses can present in anyone who flies in unpressurized aircraft, travels to the mountains, or participates in hot air balloon rides or glider flights. The most common of these events is travel to mountainous regions with elevations greater than 8000 feet. Predicting which healthy individual will become ill at high altitude is impossible. Patients with certain chronic medical conditions, including angina pectoris, congestive heart failure, chronic obstructive pulmonary disease, and hypertension, should avoid altitude exposure.

Although altitude illness typically appears in patients who are at an elevation of 8000 feet some patients may show minor signs and symptoms as low as 4000 feet.

People travel to the mountains for recreation during all times of year, typically from a sea level environment to elevations well above 8000 feet, without thought of acclimation to high altitude. These patients may not have serious signs and symptoms; however, their trip can be cut short as a result of feeling ill. Ski resorts are most familiar with these patients.

High-altitude illnesses worsen the higher the victim goes and can cause death if not treated properly. With the easiest treatment of these illnesses being descent from altitude, why do so many people continue to suffer from this life-threatening illness? The answer is simple: "I just paid a lot of money to climb Mt. Everest, go skiing in Utah, or travel to Machu Picchu" and the person wants the experience. Unfortunately, the experience is not what was planned.

As previously discussed, some patients are more prone to altitude illness because of preexisting conditions. What is not fully understood is that some people are prone to altitude illnesses with no prior exposure or illnesses. Altitude illnesses also are more likely to occur in patients with previous altitude illness presentations. High-altitude illnesses discussed below are acute mountain sickness, high-altitude pulmonary edema, and high-altitude cerebral edema. These generally exist along a continuum, may be progressive, and may have an overlap of symptoms.

Acute Mountain Sickness

[OBJECTIVE 79]

Description and Definition

Acute mountain sickness (AMS) is the most common of the altitude illnesses and typically manifests at elevations above 8000 feet. Some patients may have mild to moderate symptoms at elevations as low as 6000 feet. Experienced guides and climbers know that acclimation is the best medicine to avoid AMS and other altitude illnesses; the novice or person in a hurry often suffers the worst.

Etiology

The fundamental etiology of AMS is hypoxia from reduced oxygen pressure. Other causes include fluid redistribution, sympathetic activity, inadequate oxygen exchange from hypoventilation, and interstitial fluid. Moderate to severe cases of AMS may involve cerebral edema, overlapping with high-altitude cerebral edema, discussed below.

Epidemiology

AMS is common, but exact rates of incidence depend on rate of ascent, altitude attained (or at which the patient sleeps), length of exposure to altitude, and level of exertion. A physiologic predisposition to developing AMS also may exist (Hackett & Roach, 2001).

Physical Findings

AMS can either be mild or severe. Mild AMS exhibit the following signs and symptoms:

- Headache
- Lightheadedness and dizziness
- Difficulty sleeping
- Loss of appetite
- Breathlessness
- Fatigue
- Nausea and vomiting

These signs and symptoms normally develop within 6 to 24 hours of ascent. If the person refuses to recognize these indications of AMS, more serious ones may present. Severe AMS signs and symptoms include all or any of the above coupled with the following:

- Severe weakness
- Severe, protracted vomiting
- Decreased urine output
- Shortness of breath at rest
- Altered level of consciousness
- Cough and congestion
- Inability to walk a straight line or ataxia
- Pale or changing skin color

Differential Diagnosis

AMS often is confused with a viral infection because the symptoms are similar. Key factors in the history (recent ascent to altitude) differentiate the two. Dehydration, hypoglycemia and other metabolic derangements, intoxication or hangover, and fatigue are other differential diagnoses.

Therapeutic Interventions

If any symptoms of mild to moderate AMS are present and are not relieved by rest and typical methods, descent is the proper treatment.

If signs and symptoms of severe AMS present in the patient, the only answer is immediate descent to prevent further damage to the body. If the patient does not descend, conditions can deteriorate to high-altitude pulmonary edema and/or high-altitude cerebral edema.

High-Altitude Pulmonary Edema

[OBJECTIVES 80, 82, 83, 84]

Description and Definition

High-altitude pulmonary edema (HAPE) represents fluid buildup in the lungs caused by altitude exposure.

Etiology

This fluid buildup prevents effective oxygen and carbon dioxide exchange. As pulmonary pressure increases and hypertension occurs in response to hypoxia and blood flow changes at altitude, edema develops in the lungs. As this condition progresses the level of oxygen in the bloodstream is lowered, leading to hypoperfusion and impairment of cerebral function. The end result can be death if the condition is not recognized and treated.

Epidemiology

HAPE is the most common cause of death from altitude exposure (Hackett & Roach, 2001). Signs and symptoms typically show between 24 and 72 hours at altitude and are preceded by AMS signs and symptoms. Patients will have exerted themselves before the incident, with males and children being the most susceptible.

Physical Findings

In addition to the signs and symptoms of severe AMS, the following symptoms also will be present in a patient with HAPE:

- Persistent wet cough
- Cough that produces a white, watery, or frothy fluid
- Crackles when listening to lung sounds
- Inability to sleep
- Inability to lay supine without the feeling of suffocation
- Dyspnea
- Hyperpnea
- Lethargy
- Irritability
- Confusion
- Coma
- Disorientation

Differential Diagnosis

Differential diagnosis includes pneumonia, other infections, fatigue, other causes of noncardiogenic and cardiogenic pulmonary edema, uncomplicated hypoxia, hypoglycemia, and metabolic disorders.

Therapeutic Interventions

[OBJECTIVES 85, 86, 87]

The primary treatment for HAPE is descent. If the patient is not evacuated and treated rapidly, death can occur.

Administer oxygen to all patients with HAPE. This may immediately reduce some symptoms as arterial hypoxia is corrected. Other specialized equipment and medications may be used, although they often are not routinely available to standard EMS providers. **Gamow bags** (hyperbaric bags) can simulate descent if immediate evacuation is not possible. Nifedipine may be a useful pharmacologic adjunct but cannot replace oxygen and rapid descent, which remain the most important interventions. Recent research suggests that dexamethasone may be helpful for HAPE, although currently it is only formally recommended for high-altitude cerebral edema.

High-Altitude Cerebral Edema

Description and Definition

[OBJECTIVE 81]

High-altitude cerebral edema (HACE) is the most severe of the altitude illnesses. Although all climbers demonstrate brain swelling on magnetic resonance imaging studies, some develop increased intracranial pressure and resulting symptoms, which indicate HACE.

Etiology

HACE results from excessive fluid leakage and swelling of brain tissue. This additional rise in fluid in the cranium causes an increase in intracranial pressure. HACE often is associated with a progression from AMS and/or HAPE. This progression can be as rapid as 12 hours but takes 1 to 3 days of high-altitude exposure to occur. In general HACE occurs at altitudes above 12,000 feet, whereas HAPE can occur in the 8000 to 12,000 range.

Epidemiology

HACE causes and is characterized by increased intracranial pressure. HACE shares characteristics with severe AMS, and the two probably represent different extremes of the same pathophysiologic continuum. Similarly, the two conditions share the same epidemiology and demographics.

Physical Findings

Signs and symptoms of HACE include those found in AMS and may involve those found in HAPE. Additional signs and symptoms include the following:

- Disorientation
- Severe headache
- Ataxia
- Decreased level of consciousness
- Drowsiness not relieved by rest
- Hallucinations
- Confusion
- Stupor
- Coma

HACE may have a rapid onset that progresses to stupor, coma, and death without warning.

Differential Diagnosis

Differential diagnosis for HACE includes cerebrovascular accident, hypoglycemia, other metabolic derangements, intoxication, fatigue, and AMS.

Therapeutic Interventions

[OBJECTIVES 85, 86, 87]

As with HAPE, rapid descent is imperative to patient survival. Administer oxygen to all patients with HACE. Establish an IV in all patients with suspected HACE, and draw blood for later analysis at the receiving medical facility.

Dexamethasone has been found to reduce symptoms, although its efficacy depends on early administration.

Diuretics such as furosemide may be helpful, although their use is controversial because adequate intravascular volume and hydration also are crucial to managing this condition appropriately and may be impaired by diuretics.

If immediate descent is not possible, treatment may include a Gamow bag (hyperbaric bag). Treks into high-altitude camps often have these available; teams that specialize in high-altitude recoveries also have them. The typical paramedic agency will not have these available; therefore treatment should follow local protocols.

Prevention of High-Altitude Illnesses

Prevention is possible in high-altitude illnesses, eliminating the need for costly and difficult descents and disruption of activities. Plan slow ascents with plenty of rest. The typical trek to extreme altitudes involves an initial acclimation to moderate altitudes for 1 week or longer. This is followed by time spent at approximately 8000 feet for 3 days to 1 week. Ascents are then planned for up to 11,000 feet. However, the ascent above 11,000 feet involves 3 to 7 days of rest or sleeping at 11,000 feet, with daily excursions going above that altitude to prepare for future ascent. Further ascent is done in increments of 1000 feet per day and 3000 feet between rest days. Teams attempting climbs such as Mt. Everest may spend up to 1 month acclimatizing before ascent to extreme altitudes. Other prevention methods include the following:

- When possible, drive or walk to high altitude.
- Start below 10,000 feet and walk up.
- If the only option is to fly into altitude, rest and do not overexert for at least 24 hours.
- Once 11,000 feet is attained, limit climbs each day to 1000 feet.
- For every 3000 feet ascended, at least one rest day should be taken.
- Follow the dogma of "climb high, sleep low"; each day that 1000 feet is attained should include a climb to a higher altitude, then descent for the night. This will prepare the climber for the day ahead.
- If symptoms of AMS present, do not proceed until symptoms have subsided.
- If symptoms worsen or do not subside, descent is the only answer.
- Stay hydrated; as ascent is accomplished, the drive to hydrate decreases. This decrease, combined with the dehydration common with altitude, are detrimental to life. Consume at least 4 to 6 L of fluid per day.
- Rest is good when accompanied by light activity because a slowed respiratory rate exacerbates the symptoms of AMS.
- Avoid tobacco, alcohol, and drugs.
- Eat high-calorie foods while at altitude.

The most common medication taken for the prevention of AMS is acetazolamide (Diamox). It works by increasing the amount of alkali excreted in the urine, making the blood more acidic. This condition in the blood drives ventilation, setting a new level of saturation earlier. The improved ventilation and oxygen transport means less alkalosis and ultimately avoidance of sudden drops in oxygen levels at high altitude. Acetazolamide does have a detrimental side effect of dehydration; therefore patients taking this prophylactic medication need to hydrate constantly.

Acetazolamide, dexamethasone, and nifedipine are used to treat the symptoms of AMS as well. The paramedic rarely uses these medications in the field and instead relies on typical EMS treatments.

PARAMEDIC*Pearl*

Remember: Acclimatization is inhibited by overexertion, dehydration, and alcohol.

Case Scenario—continued

The patient is placed on a stretcher. The instructor begins to take a history. The patient states he is in excellent physical health. He is 34 years old and has no past medical history. He denies smoking, drinking, or any recreational drugs. He and his team began hiking up the mountain 2 days earlier. He is a triathlete but has no high-altitude training. His vital signs are pulse, 110 beats/min; respirations, 24 breaths/min; blood pressure, 120/80 mm Hg; and pulse oximetry, 93% on room air.

Questions

5. *What is the appropriate treatment for this patient?*
6. *What could occur if this patient had continued up the mountain to higher altitude?*
7. *What are the signs and symptoms of HAPE and HACE?*

LIGHTNING INJURY

[OBJECTIVES 88, 89, 90, 91, 92]

Description and Definition

Lightning is a dramatic weather phenomenon involving transmission of electricity between the sky and ground.

Epidemiology and Demographics

Lightning strikes occur approximately 20 million times per year in the United States (Huffines & Orville, 1999). Current data suggest that in the United States these strikes injure approximately 500 to 1000 people a year and cause 100 deaths (Cooper et al., 2001). There is a significant geographic propensity to injury and death, with central Florida consistently leading in both each year. The other two states consistently in the top 10 for both casualties and casualty rates (controlled for population) are Colorado and North Carolina. Lightning strikes are most common in the summer months (although in the southeastern states they are common year round), and more than half occur between 3 PM and 6 PM local standard time.

Etiology

The simplest, most common form of lightning occurs when the negative charge on the bottom of thunderstorm clouds induces a positive charge on the surface of the earth (which tends to collect on the tips of tall objects or people). If the induced current between these two charges becomes strong enough, a lightning bolt may form between the two charged objects.

Injury from lightning strikes occurs by a number of mechanisms (Box 52-18).

BOX 52-18 Mechanisms of Lightning Injury

- *Direct strike injury.* A direct strike occurs when the positive charge drawing the strike is located on an individual, and the lightning bolt generated communicates between the individual and the cloud.
- *Splash injury.* In splash injuries the direct strike occurs on an object near the victim. The current seeks the path of least resistance, which may cause it to jump from that object to people or objects nearby if they offer less electrical resistance.
- *Contact injury.* This type of injury occurs when a victim is in direct contact with an object (such as a pole) that is struck or splashed by a lightning bolt.
- *Step voltage injury* (also known as *stride voltage* or *ground current*). Unlike splash injury, in which the current travels through the air, in this type of injury the current travels through the ground as it dissipates from the object directly struck. Because human beings are composed primarily of salt water, they represent less resistance than the ground and a current traveling underneath them can travel up one leg and down the other, following the path of least resistance.
- *Blunt injury.* Patients can be thrown up to 10 yards simply from the concussive force of a lightning strike's shock wave. Any stationary object struck can cause blunt trauma or penetrating trauma. These concussive forces also can cause tympanic membrane rupture and tissue contusions.
- *Streamer injury.* A streamer is the upward leader of the charge combination. Typically it must make contact with the downward leader to cause electrical injury; however, recent reports have suggested that simply being the conduit for a streamer may cause injury (Cooper, 2002).

From Cooper, M. A. (2002). A fifth mechanism of lightning injury. *Academic Emergency Medicine, 9,* 172-174.

Physical Findings

The most consistent feature of lightning behavior and its consequent injuries is unpredictability. However, patient injuries are typically categorized into one of three groups, which are generally useful for predicting outcome: minor, moderate, and severe injury (Cooper et al., 2001).

Minor Injury

Symptoms of minor injury including tympanic membrane rupture, confusion, amnesia, brief unconsciousness, temporary deafness, blindness, paresthesia or dysesthesias in affected extremities, and myalgia. Neurocognitive damage can be permanent even in minor injuries. Vital signs are usually within the patient's normal range, although temporary mild hypertension can be seen.

Moderate Injury

Symptoms of moderate injury include disorientation, combativeness, and coma. Motor paralysis is frequent. Pulses may be absent because of arterial spasm, sympathetic instability, hypotension, or vascular trauma. Although rare, spinal shock may be present. Seizures and superficial or partial-thickness burns are not unusual. Hemotympanum may be present and suggests basilar skull fracture in the setting of lightning injury. Moderate acute injuries tend to cause long-term complications, including sleep disorders, irritability, psychomotor dysfunction and fine motor control impairment, neurologic dysfunction (especially in sympathetic tone), and posttraumatic stress disorder.

Severe Injury

Severely injured patients are in cardiac arrest or arrhythmia when examined. Direct brain damage also can be present. If immediate resuscitation does not result in functional cardiac and respiratory activity, the prognosis is poor for these patients. However, cardiac arrest of a heart injured by lightning but otherwise healthy can often be reversed if CPR and airway maneuvering are rapid, meaning that traditional triage principles involving cardiac arrest should be reversed in lightning strikes, and apneic, pulseless patients should be treated first and most aggressively. Pulmonary edema, pulmonary contusion with hemoptysis, and tympanic membrane rupture also are possible.

Myths of lightning strikes are exposed in Box 52-19.

Differential Diagnosis

Differential diagnosis of lightning strikes includes high-voltage injury from manmade power lines, primary cardiac or respiratory arrest, and burns from other electrical or thermal sources.

Therapeutic Interventions

As noted, traditional triage principles are reversed in known lightning strike and apneic, pulseless patients should be treated first. If their condition is not rapidly corrected, follow traditional triage principles. Otherwise, immediate field treatment of lightning strike patients is largely symptomatic. It is critical to recognize that lightning strike patients do *not* retain a charge and may be handled immediately. Delay of treatment because of this misunderstanding can lead to tragic, unnecessary morbidity and mortality, especially in ischemia from reversible cardiopulmonary arrest.

Complete exposure of the patient (followed by adequate protection from the elements) is necessary. Particularly important examinations in a patient suspected to be have sustained a lightning strike are complete eye examinations, skin examinations, neurologic examinations, and mental status examinations.

All lightning strike patients, regardless of severity, must seek medical care. In many cases delayed, chronic sequelae have more significance for patients than initial symptoms. Pain syndromes such as autonomic dystrophy, sympathetic dystrophy, reflex sympathetic dystrophy, and causalgia are not uncommon, and all cause phantom pains and altered sensations that can be quite debilitating. Posttraumatic headaches are common, and more than half of all lightning strike patients eventually

BOX 52-19 Lightning Strike Myths

The following are myths about lightning and are incorrect.

- *Lightning strikes are always fatal.*
  Truth: Current mortality rate is approximately 5% to 10%
- *Most lightning strike deaths are caused by burns.*
  Truth: A minority of lightning strikes cause deep thermal burns.
- *Patients struck by lightning remain "electrified" and should not be touched.*
  Truth: Patients do not retain a charge and can be treated immediately.
- *Lightning only strikes when clouds are overhead or visible, or when it is raining.*
  Truth: The most dangerous time for a fatal strike is the time before a storm is visible. Lightning can strike more than 10 miles in front of a storm, hence the cliché "out of a clear blue sky."
- *Being inside a building eliminates the possibility of lightning strike.*
  Truth: Many lightning injuries have occurred inside homes and workplaces with plumbing fixtures, telephone lines, and other appliances with metal attachments susceptible to side flashes. Small, unsubstantial shelters also can increase risk of injury.
- *Lightning never strikes the same place twice.*
  Truth: High points such as skyscrapers and radio towers are struck many times each year.
- *Patients who survive an initial lighting strike have not been injured.*
  Truth: Many chronic and subacute conditions can result from nonlethal strikes.
- *Lightning victims who undergo resuscitation for several hours may still recover.*
  Truth: Classic triage should be reversed for multicasualty incidents involving lightning strikes. Immediate cardiac massage and, more importantly, airway positioning may result in rapid return of cardiac activity and breathing. However, no benefit is gained from unusually prolonged resuscitation if response is not immediate.
- *The rubber on car tires or shoe soles protects against lightning strikes.*
  Truth: Millimeters of rubber are a far less significant insulator than air. If the lightning has sufficient charge to travel miles of air, it will overcome these tiny pads of insulation. Cars protect against lightning strikes because of the metal car frame, which conducts current along its body and into the ground by rainwater or off the axles or bumper.
- *Wearing metal on the body or cleated shoes attracts lightning and increases strike risk.*
  Truth: No evidence shows that such objects increase risk of strike unless they significantly increase a person's height (e.g., a long umbrella held very high). Objects against the skin may increase the risk or severity of thermal injury by burns in case of a strike.
- *Lightning always hits the highest object.*
  Truth: Extensive evidence has shown lightning striking mountain gullies, the middle of flagpoles, and even the bottom of the NASA space shuttle gantry.

Modified from Gatewood, M. O., & Zane, R. D. (2004). Lightning injuries. *Emergency Medical Clinics of North America, 22(2),* 369-403.

develop eye injuries. Cataracts are especially common and may occur as late as 2 years after the lightning strike. Transient deafness is common and usually clears, but initial internal ear damage may develop into more chronic conditions such as permanent deafness, vertigo (dizziness), tinnitus (ringing in ears), and ataxia (unsteady gait). Psychological consequences also have been frequently described. Because of this high rate of compli-cations after initial care, an important therapeutic intervention in the field is ensuring adequate follow-up care.

Prevention

Some basic principles can help prevent lightning strikes, although many of the most common myths and misconceptions about lightning behavior and injury also revolve around preventive measures.

Managers of events involving groups should have prearranged plans for reducing lightning risk and, if possible, should have mechanisms to be made aware of threatening weather. Some organizations promote the 30-30 rule: if the time between seeing lightning and hearing thunder is 30 seconds or less, events should be cancelled and individuals should seek shelter for 30 minutes. In general, every 5 seconds of delay indicates the storm is an additional mile away (because of the difference between the speed of light and sound), so the 30-30 rule would mean preventive measures would begin with storms 6 miles away. Although this is a reasonable rule, it is problematic for being both too strict (in many areas essentially eliminating activity when there is a thunderstorm) and too lenient (lightning can travel 10 miles or more in front of a storm front). If activities are on open water, individuals should immediately head for shore. Sailboats and powerboats should include a lightning rod and grounding equipment as part of their standard operating apparatus.

Ground shelter ideally consists of a substantial building or all-metal vehicle (soft-top convertibles and Jeeps are less ideal). Small buildings such as golf shelters, bus shelters, tents, or rain shelters are actually believed to increase strike risk (Gatewood, 2004). If shelter is not available individuals should spread out several yards apart from each other and assume the lightning position. This position involves squatting with both feet together and ears covered by hands. Some authorities suggest that kneeling or sitting cross-legged is acceptable if the position is to be maintained for a long period (Gatewood, 2004).

Case Scenario CONCLUSION

The instructor helps arrange transport for this patient down to a lower altitude. The patient is stabilized and the course resumes.

Question

8. *What are some of the specific actions that will prevent AMS, HAPE, and HACE?*

ENVENOMATED ANIMAL BITES

[OBJECTIVES 88, 89, 90, 91, 93]

Snakes

Clinical Characteristics

Snakes are common in wilderness and suburban settings. However, only a few species have a venomous bite. Of the 3000 species identified worldwide, approximately 15% are considered dangerous to human beings (Gold et al., 2004).

The United States is home to two categories of venomous snakes: the crotalids, or pit vipers (Viperidae family, Crotalinae subfamily), which include rattlesnakes, cottonmouths, and copperheads; and coral snakes, which are in the Elapidae family. Every state in the United States has at least one indigenous venomous land snake, with the exception of Alaska and Maine. The yellow-bellied sea snake, which is a venomous snake, can be found in the waters around Hawaii.

Three types of coral snakes are found in the United States. The Arizona or Sonoran coral snake *(Micruroides euryxanthus)* is found predominantly in Arizona and New Mexico. The eastern coral snake *(Micrurus fulvius fulvius)* and the Texas coral snake *(Micrurus fulvius tenere)* are found as far north as North Carolina, as far west as Texas, and as far south as Florida. Coral snakes are easily identified by their distinctive coloration: dramatic, bright bands of red, black, and cream/yellow. Many harmless snakes have similar color combinations, but true coral snakes (with the exception of rare albino specimens) always have contiguous red and yellow bands. This has generated a helpful mnemonic: "red on yellow, kill a fellow; red on black, venom lack." This mnemonic only applies to coral snakes indigenous to the United States (see Figure 52-4).

The majority of venomous snakes in the United States are pit vipers. Sixteen species of rattlesnake live in the United States, found in the genera *Crotalus* (including the eastern and western diamondback rattlesnakes, the prairie and Pacific rattlesnakes, and the timber rattlesnake) and the genera *Sistrurus* (which are generally smaller and include the pygmy rattlesnake). The majority of U.S. snakebite deaths are caused by diamondback rattlesnake envenomations (Gold et al., 2004). Moccasins (genus *Agkistrodon*) in the United States include the cottonmouth and the copperhead. The cottonmouth lives in semiaquatic habitats, has dark-olive to black coloring, and has a pale white oral mucosa (hence, cottonmouth). The copperhead has markings resembling an hourglass, or an inverted Y. It is generally considered to cause less-severe envenomations than other species but is also more likely than other species to be found in urban environments (Norris & Bush, 2001). Pit vipers in general can be identified by their triangular head shape (versus round), their elliptical pupils (versus round), the heat-sensing pits anterior to the eyes (not present in non-pit vipers), retractable fangs (versus no fangs), and the presence of a single row of subcaudal plates on the tail (versus a double row in non-pit vipers).

Coral snakebites are particularly rare, accounting for only 20 to 60 bites annually in the United States (Norris & Bush, 2001). Only five to six deaths occur each year in the United States from all snakebites (Gold et al., 2004). Two factors may account for this low mortality rate. First, 25% of pit viper bites and 50% of coral snake bites are unvenomated for a variety of reasons (Gold, 2000). Second, although snake venoms are complex toxins with many local and systemic effects, they most often are lethal only in children, the elderly, or those for whom treatment is delayed or who are treated with inappropriate and dangerous modalities (electrical shock, incision), which themselves contribute to death. Most patients survive and the majority also fully recover without long-term complications; nonetheless, careful follow-up is critical and its absence can result in long-term disabilities (Norris & Bush, 2001).

Epidemiologic data and appropriate treatment are hampered by difficulty in accurate identification of snake species. Retrospective studies show that the offending species are listed as "unidentified" in more than 25% of cases during routine care. During the recovery mission in New Orleans after Hurricane Katrina, more than 60% of snakes brought to shelter facilities were misidentified; this is particularly unfortunate because areas struck by severe tropical storms and hurricanes have historically exhibited a corresponding increase in envenomation incidence (Wozniak et al., 2006). The relevance of this for EMS professionals, who have access to more scene information than hospital providers during routine care and who also disproportionately serve as disaster response providers, should be obvious. Also, snakes and other exotic animals are sometimes kept as pets and may be found outside their typical ranges. All EMS providers should be familiar with snake identification principles regardless of where they typically work.

Physical Findings

EMS field management should include careful evaluation of airway, breathing, and circulatory status. Envenomation can cause precipitous deterioration in victims with comorbidities. Carefully examine the wound and document distal neurovascular status. Document the extent of swelling with a marker to delineate the edge of swollen tissue. As swelling progresses, track the edge during transport. Marking the edge of swelling at 15- to 20-minute intervals with a marker can help the accepting facility make valuable conclusions about the severity of the bite.

Differential Diagnosis

Differential diagnosis includes nonvenomous snakebite, bites from other animals, and local nonzoological trauma.

Therapeutic Interventions

Field management of bites from venomous species must assume that the wound is envenomated despite evidence that most are not. Differentiating envenomated from nonenvenomated wounds is difficult, and in the case of coral snakes, once symptoms of envenomation are present they may be much more difficult to reverse. Immobilize the injured area at a level below the heart. Keep the victim calm and warm, and instruct the patient to avoid movement as much as possible once away from striking distance of the snake or snake habitat. Any constricting jewelry, clothing, or tools should be removed. Immediate transportation to a medical facility is required. Despite numerous anecdotal field therapies for snakebite, the most appropriate treatment remains "car keys or diesel fuel" (i.e., rapid transportation). Contraindicated treatment modalities that are not helpful and may be harmful include incision and suction, tourniquets, cryotherapy, and electrical shock. Topical ice has not been well studied but is generally discouraged, including in policy statements by organizations such as the American Red Cross (Norris & Bush, 2001). Commercial extractor devices such as the Sawyer Extractor (Sawyer Products, Safety Harbor, Fla.) were initially thought to offer a benefit in reducing venom exposure, but more recent studies have suggested they do not help and may promote tissue damage. Their use is now controversial and cannot routinely be recommended (Norris & Bush, 2001). All patients with snakebites suspected to be from venomous species should have IV access established and be rapidly transported to a medical center. Antivenin is available for snake envenomations and can have significant improve morbidity and mortality rates.

Prevention

EMS personnel deployed in snakebite-prone areas (including areas recently disrupted by hurricanes or other phenomena) should familiarize themselves with the indigenous species and their characteristics.

In general, individuals should not put unprotected hands or feet into dark, tight, enclosed areas that have not been previously investigated for venomous animals. Appropriate protective clothing includes loose-fitting pants with bloused cuffs, long-sleeved shirts, and boots. If a snake is encountered, individuals should slowly move out of its striking range; this is generally believed to be half the snake's body length, so a distance of 1 body length or more is recommended. Because pit viper antivenin is the same for all species, catching and killing the pit viper is unnecessary.

Arachnids

Clinical Characteristics

Arachnids, or the class Arachnida, includes scorpions (the order Scorpiones) and spiders (the order Araneae). Although this is a vast class that includes approximately 70,000 species, only two spiders and one scorpion genus account for the majority of clinically severe arachnid envenomations in the United States: the *Centruroides* scorpions, the *Loxosceles reclusa* (brown recluse) spiders, and *Latrodectus* (black widow) spiders (see Figure 52-5).

Scorpions inject venom with a portion of their tail (actually part of the abdomen) known as the **telson,** which pierces the victim's skin and injects venom by muscular contractions. This venom is designed to paralyze prey so that it can be consumed. Human beings are obviously not suitable prey, but they may be stung if the scorpion feels threatened. The majority of severe envenomations in the United States are caused by the bark scorpion *Centruroides exilicauda,* whose range is limited to southern Arizona, the bottom of the Grand Canyon, and the area surrounding Las Vegas and western New Mexico. Stings are not rare in these areas; 5000 scorpion stings per year occur in Arizona alone (Saucier, 2004).

Brown recluse spiders are frequently implicated in skin lesions, although some suspicion exists that in endemic areas diverse cellulitic or ulcerated lesions may be indiscriminately assigned to the brown recluse (Saucier, 2004). Brown recluse spiders are night stalkers and are often found in clothing when dressing or in bedding; they bite defensively when this fabric is moved.

Black widow spiders are worldwide in distribution and are found in every state in the United States except Alaska (Boyer et al., 2001). The hallmark of black widow bites is widespread, sustained muscle spasms with an absence of dramatic local tissue injury. Severe abdominal pain and rigidity may be present and has been mistaken for an acute abdomen (a surgical emergency such as appendicitis or perforated bowel). The worst pain is generally present for 8 to 12 hours and then subsides, but symptoms may remain severe for several days.

Physical Findings

The hallmark of a scorpion sting is significant local pain that increases with palpation or light tapping but that has minimal to no erythema or edema. Systemic symptoms generally occur in only 5% of stings (Saucier, 2004).

Brown recluse spider bites can cause serious ulcerated cutaneous damage and necrosis, which may evolve into loxoscelism, a systemic syndrome involving symptoms such as hemolysis, coagulopathy, renal failure, and rarely death. Vital signs are typically normal, although hypertension or hypotension in loxoscelism can be present and may be severe and refractory to initial treatment.

As noted, muscle spasms in black widow spider bites can be so severe that they can be mistaken for surgical emergencies, but aside from rigidity, physical examination is rarely remarkable aside from the possibility of pronounced hypertension.

Differential Diagnosis

Differential diagnosis of arachnid envenomation includes envenomation by other species such as arthropods or snakes, infections of nonvenomous etiology, other forms of dermatitis, and other types of toxicologic exposure.

Therapeutic Interventions

Patients with suspected scorpion stings, as with snake bites, should be kept warm and calm (teaching the patient that 95% of stings result in only local symptoms may help in calming efforts). If possible—while avoiding further injury to others—the scorpion involved should be identified by killing and transporting it or taking photographs. Local cold application, immobilization, and analgesics are indicated as treatment while en route to a medical facility.

Black widow spider bites may require IV opioids, benzodiazepines, and calcium to counter the extreme pain and muscle spasms. Manage the hypertension with the assistance of medical control; nitroprusside or nifedipine is usually considered the antihypertensive of choice by physicians. Antivenin is available but rarely used because of reported deaths and the low mortality rate of the black widow venom itself (approximately three to four deaths per year). In general it is only considered for patients who are very young, very old, pregnant, or who have persistent morbid hypertension.

Brown recluse spider bites are treated locally with ice and immobilization. No commercially available antivenin exists for loxoscelism.

Case Scenario SUMMARY

1. *What condition does this man most likely have?* The patient displays symptoms of AMS, the most common of the altitude illnesses. It typically manifests at elevations above 8000 feet. Some patients may have mild to moderate symptoms at elevations as low as 6000 feet. Experienced guides and climbers know that acclimation is the best way to avoid AMS and other altitude illnesses; the person in a hurry often suffers the worst.
2. *What is the cause of this condition?* The fundamental etiology of AMS is hypoxia caused by reduced oxygen pressure. Other causes include fluid redistribution, sympathetic activity, and inadequate oxygen exchange from hypoventilation and interstitial fluid. The higher the elevation, the lower the oxygen pressure, which can lead to worse symptoms if the patient does not descend or continues to ascend.
3. *What are some considerations in the differential diagnosis of this patient?* The patient may have any of the following conditions:
   - Cardiovascular illness
   - Pulmonary illness
   - Infection
   - Gastroenteritis
   - Hypoglycemia
   - Intoxication
   - Metabolic conditions

   The symptoms of AMS are vague and generalized. Therefore consider other etiologies for the patient's symptoms. AMS also can cause other conditions.
4. *List symptoms that are commonly found in this condition.* AMS can be mild or severe. Mild AMS manifests with the following signs and symptoms:
   - Headache
   - Lightheadedness and dizziness
   - Difficulty sleeping
   - Loss of appetite
   - Breathlessness
   - Fatigue
   - Nausea and vomiting

   These signs and symptoms normally develop within 6 to 24 hours of ascent. If the person refuses to recognize these indications of AMS, more serious ones may present. Severe AMS signs and symptoms include all or any of the above coupled with the following:
   - Severe weakness
   - Severe, protracted vomiting
   - Decreased urine output
   - Shortness of breath at rest
   - Altered level of consciousness
   - Cough and congestion
   - Inability to walk a straight line or ataxia
   - Pale or changing skin color
5. *What is the appropriate treatment for this patient?* Descent.
6. *What could occur if this patient had continued up the mountain to a higher altitude?* HAPE represents fluid buildup in the lungs from altitude exposure. This fluid buildup prevents effective oxygen and carbon dioxide exchange. As pulmonary pressure increases and hypertension occurs in response to hypoxia and blood flow changes at altitude, edema develops in the lungs. As this condition progresses, the level of oxygen in the bloodstream is lowered, leading to hypoperfusion and impairment of cerebral function. The end result can be death if the condition is not recognized and treated. HACE is the most severe of the altitude illnesses. Although all climbers demonstrate brain swelling on magnetic resonance imaging studies, some develop increased intracranial pressure and resulting symptoms, which indicate HACE.

   HACE results from excessive fluid leakage and swelling of brain tissue. This additional rise in fluid in the cranium causes an increase in intracranial pressure. HACE often is associated with a progression from AMS and/or HAPE. This progression can be as rapid as 12 hours but takes 1 to 3 days of high-altitude exposure to occur.
7. *What are the signs and symptoms of HAPE and HACE?* Signs and symptoms of severe AMS and the following symptoms occur in a patient with HAPE:
   - Persistent, wet cough
   - Cough that produces a white, watery, or frothy fluid
   - Crackles when listening to lung sounds
   - Inability to sleep
   - Inability to lay supine without the feeling of suffocation
   - Dyspnea
   - Hyperpnea
   - Lethargy
   - Irritability
   - Confusion
   - Coma
   - Disorientation

   Signs and symptoms of HACE include those found in AMS and may involve those found in HAPE. Additional signs and symptoms include the following:
   - Disorientation
   - Severe headache
   - Ataxia
   - Decreased level of consciousness
   - Drowsiness not relieved by rest
   - Hallucinations
   - Confusion
   - Stupor
   - Coma

Continued

Case Scenario SUMMARY—continued

8. *What are some of the specific actions that will prevent AMS, HAPE, and HACE?* The key to altitude illness is prevention. Prevention is especially possible in high-altitude illnesses, eliminating the need for costly and difficult descents and disruption of activities. Plan slow ascents with plenty of rest. The typical trek to extreme altitudes involves an initial acclimation to moderate altitudes for 1 week or more. This is followed by time spent at approximately 8000 feet for 3 days to 1 week. Ascents are then planned for up to 11,000 feet. However, the ascent above 11,000 feet involves 3 to 7 days of rest or sleeping at 11,000 feet with daily excursions going above that altitude to prepare for future ascent. Further ascent is done in increments of 1000 feet per day and 3000 feet between rest days. Teams attempting climbs such as Mt. Everest may spend up to 1 month acclimatizing before ascent to extreme altitudes. Other prevention methods include the following:

- When possible, drive or walk to high altitude.
- Start below 10,000 feet and walk up.
- If the only option is to fly into altitude, rest and do not overexert for at least 24 hours.
- Once 11,000 feet is attained, limit climbs each day to 1000 feet.
- For every 3000 feet ascended, at least one rest day should be taken.
- Follow the dogma of "climb high, sleep low"; each day that 1000 feet is attained should include a climb to a higher altitude, then descent for the night. This will prepare the climber for the day ahead.
- If symptoms of AMS occur, do not proceed until symptoms have subsided.
- If symptoms worsen or do not subside, descent is the only answer.
- Stay hydrated; as ascent is accomplished the drive to hydrate decreases. This decrease, combined with the dehydration common with altitude, are detrimental to life. At least 4 to 6 L of fluid should be drunk per day.
- Rest is good when accompanied by light activity because a slowed respiratory rate exacerbates the symptoms of AMS.
- Avoid tobacco, alcohol, and drugs.
- Eat high-calorie foods while at altitude

Chapter Summary

- Management of environmental emergencies requires integration of pathophysiologic principles. Key to this is an understanding of anatomy, physiology, and metabolic mechanisms the body uses to maintain homeostasis. When these mechanisms are overwhelmed, a careful history and physical examination should allow the paramedic to differentiate environmental emergencies based on assessment findings and develop a patient management plan. Abnormal findings in the assessment should be correlated with their clinical significance as detailed in the individual sections of this chapter.
- The differentiation between urgent and emergent conditions may be different in remote or austere areas than in "street" paramedicine. In remote or rugged environments conditions that may only be urgent in urban medicine may need to be managed emergently because of difficulties in adequately treating and transporting patients in a timely fashion. On the other hand, truly emergent conditions may need to be managed for longer periods than would be typically allowed in traditional EMS systems, making them take on more features of urgent medical management rather than emergent medical management.
- As with most injuries and illnesses, many preventive measures can be taken in advance of a trip. Unfortunately many victims of environmental injuries do not prepare properly and subsequently suffer dire consequences.
- Basic knowledge of how the environment can affect the human body is helpful to the paramedic attempting to reverse the events that have occurred within the patient. Paramedics may not encounter primary injuries and illnesses from the environment on a regular basis. This should not preclude the paramedic from suspecting environmental disorders in patients.
- Paramedics encounter a wide variety of calls in their careers—all carry with them the risk of personal injury. The paramedic must remember when dealing with environmental incidents not to act hastily. This will keep the paramedic from becoming another victim or part of the problem. Scene safety is always important to the paramedic, and never more so in the environment. Consider, for example, the paramedic who approaches the home of an elderly patient on a cold winter day for a report of a fall victim. Consideration must be given to the overt reason for the call, a fall, but consideration must also be given to the location of the incident and the fact that the environment plays a role in the condition of the patient. Will you be able to look beyond the obvious and search for circumstances that exacerbate patient conditions? A good paramedic will.

REFERENCES

American Heart Association. (2005). AHA guidelines for cardiopulmonary resuscitation and emergency cardiovascular care, part 10.3: Drowning. *Circulation, 112*(suppl IV), IV-133.

Bolte, R. G., Black, P. G., & Bowers, R. S. (1988). The use of extracorporeal rewarming in a child submerged for 66 minutes. *Journal of the American Medical Association, 260,* 377.

Boyer, L. V., McNally, J. T., & Binford, G. J. (2001). Spider bites. In P. Auerbach (Ed.). *Wilderness medicine* (4th ed.). St. Louis: Mosby.

Centers for Disease Control and Prevention. (1996). Hypothermia-related deaths. *Morbidity and Mortality Weekly Report, 45,* 1093.

Cooper, M. A. (2002). A fifth mechanism of lightning injury. *Academic Emergency Medicine, 9,* 172-174.

Cooper, M. A., Andrews, C. J., Holle, R. L., & Lopez, R. E. (2001). Lightning injuries. In P. Auerbach (Ed.). *Wilderness medicine* (4th ed.). St. Louis: Mosby.

Danzl, D. (2001). Accidental hypothermia. In P. Auerbach (Ed.). *Wilderness medicine (*4th ed.). St. Louis: Mosby.

Dickison, A. E. (1999). Near-drowning, predictors of survival. *Wilderness Medicine Letter, 16*(2).

Feldhaus, K. M. (2002). Submersion. In J. A. Marx (Ed.). *Rosen's emergency medicine: Concepts and clinical practice* (5th ed.) (p. 2051). St. Louis: Mosby.

Gaffin, S. L. (2001). Pathophysiology of heat-related illness. In P. Auerbach (Ed.). *Wilderness medicine* (4th ed.). St. Louis: Mosby.

Gatewood, M. O., & Zane, R. D. (2004). Lightning injuries. *Emergency Medicine Clinics of North America, 22*(2), 369–403.

Gilbert, M., Busund, R., & Skagseth, A. (2000). Resuscitation from accidental hypothermia of 13.7° with circulatory arrest. *The Lancet, 355,* 375.

Gold, B. S. (2000). Snake venom poisoning. In R. Rakel (Ed.). *Conn's current therapy, 2000* (pp. 1152-1141). Philadelphia: W.B. Saunders.

Gold, B. S., Barish, R. A., & Dart, R. C. (2004). North American snake envenomation: Diagnosis, treatment and management. *Emergency Medicine Clinics of North America 22*(2), 423–443.

Hackett, P. H., & Roach, R. C. (2001). High-altitude medicine. In P. Auerbach (Ed.). *Wilderness medicine* (4th ed.). St. Louis: Mosby.

Huffines, G. R., & Orville, R. E. (1999). Lightning ground flash density and thunderstorm duration in the contiguous United States. *Journal of Applied Meteorology, 38,* 1013.

Idris, A. H., Berg, R. A., Bierens, J., Bossaert, L., Branche, C. M., Gabrielli, A., et al. (2003). Recommended guidelines for uniform reporting of data from drowning: the "Utstein style." *Resuscitation, 59,* 45-57.

Johnson, D. E. (2004). Wilderness EMS. *Emergency Medicine Clinics of North America 22,* 2.

Kizer, K. W. (2001). Diving medicine. In P. Auerbach (Ed.). *Wilderness medicine* (4th ed.). St. Louis: Mosby.

Lyle, D. M., Lewis, P. R., Richards, D. A., Richards, R., Bauman, A. E., Sutton, J. R., et al. (1995). Heat exhaustion in *The Sun-Herald City to Surf* fun run. *Medical Journal of Australia, 162*(2), 112.

Marks, A. D. (2001). Wilderness injury prevention. In P. Auerbach (Ed.). *Wilderness medicine* (4th ed.). St. Louis: Mosby.

McCauley, R. L., Smith, D. J., Robson, M. C., & Heggers, J. P. (2001). Frostbite. In P. Auerbach (Ed.). *Wilderness medicine* (4th ed.). St. Louis: Mosby.

National Association of Emergency Medical Technicians. (2007). Environmental trauma II: drowning, lightning, diving, and altitude. In *Prehospital trauma life support* (6th ed.) (p. 446). St. Louis: Mosby.

Newman, A. B. (2001). Submersion incidents. In P. Auerbach (Ed.). *Wilderness medicine* (4th ed.). St. Louis: Mosby.

Norris, R. L., & Bush, S. P. (2001). North American venomous reptile bites. In P. Auerbach (Ed.). *Wilderness medicine* (4th ed.). St. Louis: Mosby.

Parrish, H. M. (1966). Incidence of treated snakebites in the United States. *Public Health Report, 81,* 269.

Russell, M. F. (2004). Wilderness EMS systems. *Emergency Medicine Clinics of North America, 22*(2), 561.

Saucier, J. R. (2004). Arachnid envenomations. *Emergency Medicine Clinics of North America 22*(2), 405.

Soar, J., Deakin, C. D., Nolan, J. P., Abbas, G., Alfonzo, A., Handley, A. J., et al. (2005). European Resuscitation Council guidelines for resuscitation 2005. Section 7. Cardiac arrest in special circumstances. *Resuscitation, 67*(suppl 1), S135-S170.

Wozniak, E. J., Wisser, J., & Schwartz, M. (2006). Venomous adversaries: A reference to snake identification, field safety, and bite-victim first aid for disaster-response personnel deploying into the hurricane-prone regions of North America. *Wilderness & Environmental Medicine, 17*(2), 246-266.

SUGGESTED RESOURCES

Advanced Wilderness Life Support: http://www.awls.org
American Red Cross: http://www.arc.org
Appalachian Center for Wilderness Medicine
507 Lenoir St.
Morganton, NC 28655
Website: http://www.paws.wcu.edu/kwells/index.html
Divers Alert Network: http://www.diversalertnetwork.org
Laboratory for Exercise and Environmental Medicine: http://www.umanitoba.ca/faculties/physed/research/labs_offices/exercise_environment/index.shtml
Landmark Learning: http://www.landmarklearning.org
Starfish Aquatics Institute: http://www.starfishaquatics.org
Stonehearth Outdoor Learning Opportunities: http://www.soloschools.com
Wilderness EMS Institute: http://www.wemsi.org
Wilderness Medical Associates: http://www.wildmed.com
Wilderness Medical Society: http://www.wms.org
Wilderness Medicine Institute of the National Outdoor Leadership School: http://www.nols.edu/wmi
Wilderness Medicine Outfitters: http://www.wildernessmedicine.com

Lightning Position Statements

National Athletic Trainers' Association: http://www.nata.org/publications/otherpub/lightning.pdf
National Collegiate Athletic Association: http://www.siue.edu/ATHLETIC/SPMED/lightning.pdf
National Oceanic and Atmospheric Association: http://www.lightningsafety.noaa.gov

Chapter Quiz

1. In cases of lightning strike, _______.
  a. victims must not be touched for 1 full minute to ensure any residual charge has cleared
  b. most victims sustain deep thermal burns
  c. lightning may strike a person or object even if it is surrounded by higher objects
  d. resuscitation should be carried out longer in lightning-related cardiac arrests than in other causes

2. The external mechanism of heat/cold response involving direct contact between objects is _______.
  a. radiation
  b. conduction
  c. convection
  d. evaporation

3. The mnemonic "red on yellow, kill a fellow" refers to _______.
  a. scorpions
  b. coral snakes
  c. cottonmouths
  d. black widow spiders

4. True or False: Fit athletes and military personnel are less likely to be victims of exertional hyperthermia.

5. The medication most commonly taken for prevention of AMS is ____________.
  a. acetazolamide (Diamox)
  b. aspirin
  c. nifedipine
  d. dexamethasone (Decadron)

6. *The bends* is another term for _______.
  a. barotrauma of descent
  b. barotrauma of ascent
  c. decompression sickness
  d. nitrogen narcosis

7. Methods to prevent cold emergencies include _______.
  a. reducing intake of water because it cools the core
  b. telling the person to keep warm
  c. avoiding long periods of exposure to cold environments
  d. rapidly cooling the victim

8. A patient with a rigid, painful abdomen but an unremarkable skin examination has likely sustained a _______.
  a. scorpion sting
  b. rattlesnake bite
  c. coral snake bite
  d. black widow spider bite

9. In cases of drowning cardiac arrest:
  a. CPR should be started in the water and should not be interrupted to remove the patient from the water until pulses return, 30 minutes have passed, or the provider is too tired to continue.
  b. The Heimlich maneuver is a useful tool to remove water from the lungs.
  c. The presence of hypothermia may change how resuscitation drugs should be used.
  d. No patient has ever survived being submersed for longer than 1 hour.

10. *Hypothermia* is defined as _______.
  a. a core body temperature less than 95° F
  b. a core body temperature less than 98.6° F
  d. a core body temperature greater than 98.6° F
  c. a core body temperature greater than 100.3° F

Terminology

Adult respiratory distress syndrome (ARDS) A life-threatening condition that causes lung swelling and fluid buildup in the air sacs.

Altitude illness A syndrome associated with the relatively low partial pressure of oxygen in the atmosphere at altitudes encountered during mountain climbing or travel in unpressurized aircraft.

Antipyretic medication A medication that reduces or eliminates a fever.

Ataxia Inability to control voluntary muscle movements; unsteady movements and staggering gait.

Classic heat stroke Heat stroke caused by environmental exposure and results in core hyperthermia greater than 40° C. (104° F).

Cold diuresis The occurrence of increased urine production on exposure to cold.

Decompression sickness An illness occurring during or after a diving ascent that results when nitrogen in compressed air converts back from solution to gas, forming bubbles in tissues and blood.

Drowning A process resulting in primary respiratory impairment from submersion or immersion in a liquid medium.

Environmental emergency A medical condition caused or exacerbated by weather, terrain, atmospheric pressure, or other local environmental factors.
Exertional heat stroke A condition primarily affecting younger, active persons characterized by rapid onset (developing in hours) and frequently associated with high core temperatures.
Frostbite A condition in which the skin and underlying tissue freeze.
Frostnip Reversible freezing of superficial skin layer marked by numbness and whiteness of the skin.
Gamow bag Portable hyperbaric chamber that can help with altitude sickness emergencies.
Heat emergencies Conditions in which the body's thermoregulation mechanisms begin to fail in response to ambient heat, causing illness.
High-altitude cerebral edema (HACE) The most severe high-altitude illness, characterized by increased intracranial pressure.
High-altitude pulmonary edema (HAPE) A high-altitude illness characterized by increased pulmonary artery pressures and edema, leading to cough and fluid in the lungs (pulmonary edema).
Homeotherm Organism with stable independent body temperature; an organism whose stable body temperature is generally independent of the surrounding environment.
Immersion To be covered in water or other fluid.
Poikilothermic An organism whose temperature matches the ambient temperature.
Pyrogens Substances, such as endotoxins from certain bacteria, that stimulate the body to produce a fever, increasing body temperature.
Recompression A method used to treat divers with certain diving disorders, such as decompression sickness.
Telson Venom-containing portion of a scorpion's abdomen that is capable of venomous injection into human beings.
Thermogenesis The process of heat generation.
Thermolysis A chemical process by which heat is dissipated from the body; sometimes results in chemical decomposition.
Thermoreceptor A sensory receptor that responds to heat and cold.

CHAPTER 53

Farm Response

Objectives *After completing this chapter, you will be able to:*

1. Discuss common mechanisms of injury in the farm setting.
2. Explain the differences in approach to a patient with crush injury compared with a laceration injury.
3. Discuss the causes and management of compartment syndrome.
4. Explain the urgency of caring for a patient who has received a hydraulic injection injury.
5. Describe how to recognize organophosphate poisoning.
6. Identify the hazards associated with farm confined spaces and risks posed to potential rescuers.

Chapter Outline

Case Scenario

It is just after dinner on a warm, late summer evening and your crew is dispatched to a "possible heart attack" on a farm. You are greeted by a woman who tells you that she thinks her husband is having a heart attack. She is worried that he is working too hard since she and her husband just bought the farm early in the spring. The woman states that her husband came to dinner after working on the farm all day and said he was not feeling well. He had been harvesting corn in the "back 20" and had just finished when he heard the dinner bell. After washing his hands and sitting at the table, he started looking pale and said he was having trouble breathing. You find the patient, a 42-year-old man, sitting in an overstuffed chair. His shirt is untucked and his belt unfastened. He states that he cannot catch his breath. The man speaks in two- to three-word phrases between breaths. The man has assumed a tripod position to help him breathe. He denies any chest pain, discomfort, or pressure.

Questions

1. *What is your initial impression of the patient?*
2. *What additional information do you need to complete your assessment?*
3. *What may be causing the man's respiratory distress?*

[OBJECTIVE 1]

Managing a farm trauma patient can test all the skills and abilities of the best-trained paramedic. It takes call volume to become proficient in patient care skills and techniques. Managing a trauma patient in an urban setting is different than managing a trauma patient in a rural setting. If there was ever a need for emergency responders to be able to understand a patient's condition and decide which protocol was appropriate, a farm trauma patient is it. This chapter discusses many of the trauma and hazardous conditions emergency responders could face while managing an emergency on the farm. The chapter is not meant to be all inclusive, but rather to raise awareness to the fact that if farms exist in an EMS response area, farm emergency preplanning should be undertaken.

More than 2 million farms in the United States exist on slightly less than half (41%) the total acreage in the country. The economic effect of agriculture is tremendous. The total value of agricultural production in 2002 was more than $200 billion. In most rural communities and in many states, agriculture is the largest industry and the industry with the highest economic impact. From an economic standpoint, farm deaths and disabling injuries can cripple a community. According to the National Safety Council, every time a farm death occurs, the community incurs an $800,000 loss. Often the farm will be sold or taken out of production. When this happens, local inputs are not purchased, local people are not employed, and local taxes are not paid.

Emergency responders in rural communities can have a two-pronged effect on the local farm community. First, they can better prepare to manage farm emergencies by taking specialized training geared toward farm-related trauma and hazards on local farms. Second, they can teach farmers and their families what to do and what not to do when they discover emergencies on their farms. Often those who discover the incident are injured or killed by the same hazards that caused injury or death to their loved one or employee. Emergency responders are superb examples at approaching emergency scenes. Teaching these skills to the farm population builds goodwill and can result in better care to patients (Figure 53-1).

PARAMEDIC*Pearl*

As large an industry as agriculture is, few calls are made for emergency response. Farm residents are extremely independent. If they can remove themselves from a dangerous situation, they often will. They may even transport serious injuries to the hospital themselves because they believe, sometimes inappropriately, that the time required for EMS professionals to arrive could be better spent driving to the medical center. In general, if a farmer summons EMS assistance, the responders should expect a serious situation.

Other challenges facing emergency responders relate to a host of other hazards to which farmers are exposed on a regular basis. These hazards include a variety of chemicals and hazardous materials, toxic environments and confined spaces, injuries involving animals, and health conditions caused by dusts, molds, and animal diseases. Paramedics must understand these various conditions and begin to question how they intersect and affect initial patient care procedures.

PARAMEDIC*Pearl*

Preplanning and incident command may be needed more often than not at the scene of an agricultural emergency. In addition, many agencies may be needed, including fire service, trench rescue, and possibly excavation equipment or off-road equipment. Getting to the patient with an ambulance may be impossible depending on the season. Weather can make extrication and scene safety dangerous. In late winter and spring, the moisture from the ground and from rain or snow adds challenges. The responding paramedic must be familiar with farming practices in the local area.

TRACTOR EMERGENCIES

Tractors and machinery are involved in most deaths and serious injuries on farms (Figure 53-2). This is a direct relation to the amount of use and exposure to various hazards involving tractors and machinery. Few farms operate without at least one tractor and machine that is used daily. Tractor overturns result in half of all farm deaths. One of the inherent attributes of farm work is its remoteness. Many incidents are not discovered until well after the entrapment occurred, typically when the operator did not show up when expected. By this time the body's compensatory mechanisms may be exhausted. Determining how many farm deaths could be avoided if

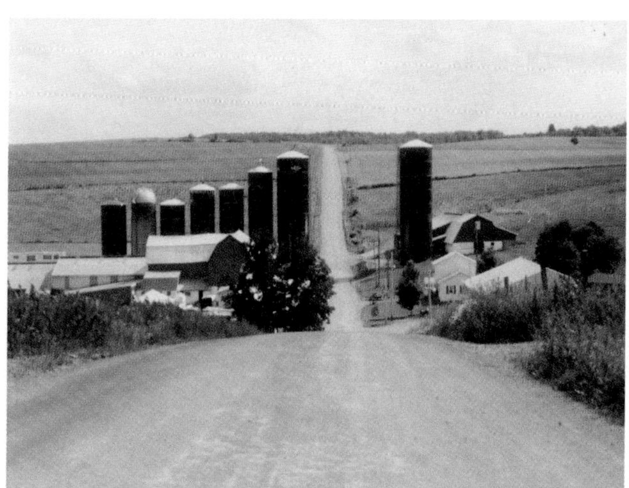

Figure 53-1 A normal farm hosts numerous hazards that can lead to serious injury and death. Because of the rural nature of farming, injury incidents often are not discovered until several hours after they occur.

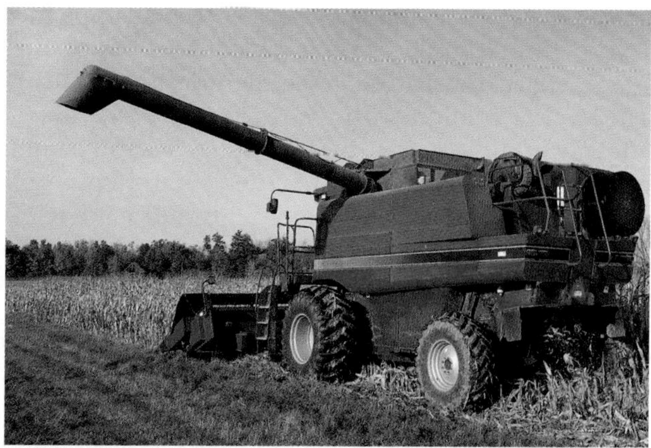

Figure 53-2 Tractors and machinery are involved in more than 50% of fatalities and disabling injuries on the farm. Emergency responders should learn how to manage emergencies involving farm tractors and machines.

trauma incidents were witnessed or discovered early, as is the case of many other types of trauma incidents, simply is not possible. Presumably, if trauma care were delivered quickly, lives would be saved.

PARAMEDIC*Pearl*

For the most part, trauma protocols are written to help field personnel make decisions within the golden hour. Farm trauma patients often need treatment that extends beyond normal protocols. Paramedics who can recognize this are valuable.

Overturned tractors pose some of the biggest challenges for emergency responders. Emergency responders need to be creative in stabilizing the vehicle under poor conditions. They also need to be creative in caring for a patient who may have been trapped for several hours. Assessing the scene of an overturned tractor incident identifies several serious hazards to the responders. First among these are stability issues. A tractor on its side can be extremely hazardous to the emergency crew. Methods to stabilize a tractor and attached implement may be similar to those for stabilizing a motor vehicle, but the amount of resources (cribbing and tools) might be extremely limited. Another big difference responders must address involves the tractor fluids (e.g., fuel, oil, engine coolant) that may interfere with the patient. When an automobile overturns, the fluids are usually far away from the patient. When a tractor overturns and an operator is pinned near the operator's station of the tractor, he or she can be exposed to many of the machine's fluids. Significant burns can occur to a victim's skin from hot and/or caustic fluids. Another major consideration is how to shut off the tractor's engine. Tractors do not have standard shut-off procedures or controls. Finally, if the tractor has an implement attached to the power take-off (PTO) that is suddenly stopped, significant energy and torque can be retained. Once released, this becomes a source of potential injury, as the attached implement may go through one or more revolutions. Once these hazards are acknowledged, responders need to determine their level of comfort with the response.

Teamwork is crucial in managing a farm trauma patient. Responders must divide the various responsibilities. At any trauma scene are hazards and patient care issues that need to be identified and managed. Everyone on the scene must understand the hazards present. However, only those personnel who are trained to deal with the hazards need to be involved in managing them. Likewise, everyone on the scene should understand the condition of the patient, but only EMS professionals who are appropriately trained in farm-related emergencies should render care. Teamwork is critical at any trauma incident but especially at a trauma incident where the patient has been entrapped for an extended period. Without proper teamwork, extrication activities might proceed before proper patient care treatments are in place, which could compromise the patient's condition.

Crush Syndrome

[OBJECTIVE 2]

Crush syndrome can be defined as the multiple systemic complications of soft tissue injury and the disruption of muscle integrity following a crush injury or compartment syndrome. This is one of the biggest considerations paramedics must think about when dealing with a patient who has been entrapped by an overturned tractor (Figure 53-3). A tractor operator may be trapped under a tractor for several hours with a compromised airway or serious internal bleeding. For these patients, great care needs to be taken to not lift the tractor from them too quickly.

Description and Definition

Crush syndrome is a condition caused by a severe compressive injury to muscles that may result in muscle cell death. Peripheral tissues can survive for up to 6 hours, especially in cold conditions in which metabolism is slowed. When blood flow is halted, oxygen is not carried to the cells. Without oxygen, the cells die. As the muscle cells die, toxins such as myoglobin and potassium are released from the cells. Myoglobin is a large molecule that damages and obstructs the renal tubules. Further disturbances occur as extracellular electrolytes move into the cell, causing a shift of fluid into the intracellular compartment. This worsens preexisting hypotension and shock and further decreases renal output. In addition, levels of serum creatine phosphokinase (CPK), lactic acid, phosphate, and creatinine are elevated. Finally, disseminated intravascular coagulation (or coagulopathy) (DIC) can occur. Once the load causing the compression is lifted, these toxins can begin to circulate with the restored

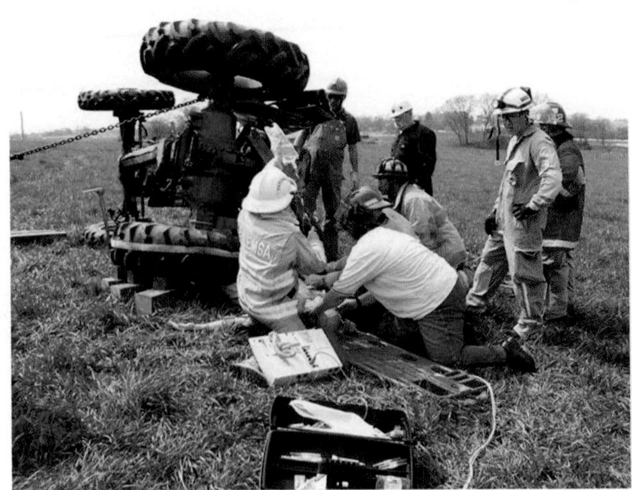

Figure 53-3 An operator trapped under a tractor for several hours could develop crush syndrome, a condition that can be extremely challenging to treat in the farm community.

blood flow. These toxins can have a fatal effect when they reach the heart and kidneys, which is referred to as *reperfusion injury*.

Crush syndrome can develop when a person has become trapped under a heavy object for an extended period. A tractor overturning and pinning the operator by the pelvis and lower extremities can lead to this condition.

Epidemiology and Demographics

Few data are available on how often crush syndrome does or could occur in the agricultural setting. Investigations are rarely conducted for any injury on a farm. Farm deaths are often only reported through a coroner's report. One significant unknown is how many tractor overturn victims who were rescued and later died from their injuries may have survived if treated differently.

A total of 4082 work-related deaths occurred in agricultural production from 1992 to 1998. The largest identifiable source of fatal traumatic injury tractors (37%), followed by trucks and harvesting machines. Together these three sources of injury accounted for more than half of the fatalities in agricultural production. The most common injury events were "overturning vehicles/machines" with more than one quarter of the deaths attributable to this category (Hard et al., 2002). With these statistics, an estimated 1000 overturns occurred on the farm during this period. A number of those victims were likely alive during rescue activities. If emergency personnel on the scene understood and treated for crush syndrome, perhaps these numbers would have been lower. However, determining this is impossible.

History and Physical Findings

EMS personnel need to look beyond the obvious to determine whether crush syndrome is a possibility. A patient who has had a large muscle mass compressed for more than 1 hour warrants suspicion for this injury. If a patient is found to have been trapped for 4 to 6 hours with compromised blood circulation, crush syndrome should certainly be considered and appropriate treatment given.

Because of the entrapment, few signs and symptoms point to crush syndrome. When a patient is entrapped, looking for tissue injury or determining distal pulses is difficult if not impossible. The patient may present as alert and oriented, perhaps with little or no feeling beyond the entrapment. Treatment for crush syndrome should be administered before releasing the patient. This is due to the fact that injury occurs when the entrapped limb is reperfused. Responders must resist the urge to immediately lift the tractor off the patient. This is to allow treatment for crush syndrome to take place. Because most farm extrications take time to perform, treatment can begin while the rescue team makes preparations to perform the lift. Working in conjunction with the rescue team, the paramedic must coordinate the administration of medications for crush syndrome before the lift is made so that they may exert their effect in avoiding reperfusion injury. As long as medications are administered before the actual lifting takes place, they will exert their effect. It is possible, however, that in the setting of prolonged rescue situations you may need to delay the administration of certain medications until 20 minutes before the lifting event. This avoids the situation where specific medications are continually given over a prolonged period when they are only needed at the time of release. However, other medications may be infused during the entire extrication process. These treatments are discussed in the following section. This care needs to be explained to the family, who will be anxious to know why you are not rapidly extricating the patient.

Differential Diagnosis

Crush syndrome may be one of the few instances in which a victim of a tractor rollover with entrapment can survive. Mechanism of injury will clearly show multisystem trauma. Victims often do not survive unless this trauma is quickly discovered and properly trained individuals arrive in a timely manner and render appropriate care. Chest injuries and internal bleeding are common causes of tractor-related death. These conditions must be rapidly discovered and treated if the victim is to survive. If a trauma patient is discovered and crush injury syndrome is not an issue, a more rapid extrication can proceed. This may still be difficult because tractor stability issues can become a concern for the crew. Care must be taken to ensure the safety of the crew and the patient when extrication activities progress.

Therapeutic Interventions

Approaching the scene of a tractor overturn incident is similar to approaching any incident. Rescuers first need to evaluate the scene. What specific hazards can be observed that can cause injury and complications to the crew, bystanders, and the victim? Once these hazards are identified, they must be secured. If this cannot be done, secure the scene from anyone else becoming a victim until more experienced personnel arrive.

Determine the mechanism of injury. Develop an index of suspicion for potential injuries or conditions based on the mechanism of injury. Based on what appears to have happened, what injuries or conditions could the patient have? Develop a team and assign duties.

As soon as is practical, patient assessment and care must take place. This *must* be done while preparation for extrication is taking place and during the extrication process. If crush syndrome is suspected, appropriate medications must be administered before releasing the patient. Disastrous results can occur if the victim is extricated before being treated, especially if crush syndrome is a factor. Caring for a patient with crush syndrome in the farm setting differs from most other trauma incidents in a rural setting (e.g., motor vehicle trauma). Most seriously injured patients involved in motor vehicle trauma are rapidly extricated. However, in a farm incident involving possible crush syndrome, the length of time the victim has been trapped must first be determined. Sometimes this may require using the best guess possible. The incident was most likely discovered by the family or neighbors. In many cases, the family and neighbors provided initial care for the patient before emergency services arrived. When EMS personnel arrive, the family and others at the scene may put considerable pressure on the responders to move quickly. As in any rescue situation, it is not in the rescuer's or patient's best interest to simply rush in and remove the patient. As a general rule, if the victim has been trapped for less than 1 hour, a rapid extrication (if warranted) can be performed. However, if the victim has been trapped for more than 1 hour, crush syndrome must be considered and appropriate treatment must take place before releasing the patient. This may be done in consultation with medical control. The first priority is that of scene safety and stabilization to prevent injury to responders or further injury to the patient. If the patient can simply be removed from the scene without specialized rescue techniques the likelihood of crush syndrome is extremely low, although crush injury may be present. In all other situations the paramedic should work closely with the rescue crew to ensure treatment is provided during the rescue evolution and the patient is treated for crush syndrome before release.

PARAMEDIC*Pearl*

If crush syndrome is suspected, paramedics on scene should make early contact with medical direction. In most cases the paramedic will contact medical direction at the trauma center where the patient will be transported.

Perform a rapid trauma assessment, stopping only to correct any life-threatening conditions observed. Spinal stabilization will most likely be needed. Assess and manage the patient's airway and breathing. Airway and breathing problems lead to death more quickly than any other problem. If this is an issue when initial assessment is taking place, any treatments must take place immediately. If the weight of the load on the patient is determined to be causing severe breathing difficulty, the load must be at least partially relieved. Securing the airway by intubation will not be effective because too much pressure will be exerted on the chest cavity to allow effective lung expansion.

You may be limited in effectively determining circulatory status. At least identify and control any obvious major bleeding you can see and assess pulses (carotid and radial if possible). Determine if internal bleeding and/or compartment syndrome might be present. Keep in mind that most people trapped under the weight of a tractor probably have some amount of fluid tamponade. In other words, the tractor is acting as a tourniquet.

The mainstay of treatment for crush syndrome is intravenous (IV) fluid to prevent kidney failure secondary to the presence of myoglobin, hypotension, and free oxygen radicals. Establish at least one large-bore IV line as soon as the patient is safely accessible. Multiple IV lines are appropriate due to the amount of fluid the patient will require and the possibility of dislodgement during the extrication event. This is particularly true if the patient has been trapped for an extended period (longer than 1 hour). Initially any preexisting dehydration or fluid loss should be corrected. Patients may need up to 21 L of fluid in the first 24 hours after their injury. In the prehospital setting, 1 to 1.5 L of fluid per hour should be administered, maintaining the urine output at 300 mL per hour. Normal saline is the fluid of choice, and fluids containing potassium should be avoided due to the preexisting hyperkalemia. To help maintain kidney function, mannitol may be administered. The use of furosemide in patients with crush syndrome is controversial at best. Some feel that in the absence of mannitol it is acceptable, while many others believe the side effects associated with the medication outweigh its benefits. Consult with your local medical director regarding the use of furosemide before encountering a situation such as this (Box 53-1).

Sodium bicarbonate may be considered for the patient with crush syndrome. Sodium bicarbonate has several useful actions, including reversing the preexisting acidosis that often is present. It is one of the first steps in treating hyperkalemia, as it promotes the movement of potassium into the intracellular space in exchange for hydrogen ions. Sodium bicarbonate also increases urine pH, decreasing the amount of myoglobin precipitated in the kidneys. Depending on the severity of injury, 50 to 100 mEq of bicarbonate may be ordered for the patient before release from compression (James, 1994). The onset of action of sodium bicarbonate is almost immediate and its duration is about 45 minutes. Therefore the paramedic should work closely with the rescue crew to coordinate the timing of the administration of sodium bicarbonate. Although saline and mannitol may be administered

BOX 53-1 Treatment for Crush Syndrome

Treatment for crush syndrome must take place before the release of the crushing load. Everyone on scene must understand what the potential condition of the patient is. Early contact with medical direction is important. Perform the following before releasing the load:

- Secure airway and breathing with oxygen administration.
- Aggressively treat for shock.
- Apply a cardiac monitor.
- Evaluate and treat for bronchoconstriction.
- Secure IV access and give fluid resuscitation.
- Administer medication for pain control and hyperkalemia.

Courtesy from David Oliver, Emergency Services Rescue Training.

throughout the rescue evolution, sodium bicarbonate should only be administered before release and not continuously. In general, administering the medication 20 minutes before release is acceptable as this provides a margin of error on each side of the rescue crew's estimated time of release.

Other interventions that may be considered include the following:

- Albuterol, as it promotes the movement of potassium to the intracellular space.
- Glucose, as it also promotes the movement of potassium into the intracellular space. However, in the absence of co-administration of insulin, this procedure is controversial. Check with your medical director regarding this matter prior to being in a situation where it is needed.
- Morphine sulfate for pain management.
- Insulin to promote the movement of glucose (and ultimately potassium) into the intracellular space. This is normally a hospital treatment; however, in prolonged rescue evolutions it is not uncommon for physicians or nurses to come to the scene from the hospital. In this situation they may choose to administer insulin at the scene.
- Calcium is a traditional treatment for medically induced hyperkalemia. However, due to the associated electrolyte abnormalities associated with crush syndrome, the prophylactic use of calcium is not recommended. Calcium may be considered if there are signs of cardiotoxicity secondary to hyperkalemia, such as a widening of the QRS complex by more than 50%. Unlike other medications, calcium does not promote the movement of potassium into the intracellular space, but rather antagonizes the cardiotoxic effects of potassium by restoring the resting membrane potential.

PARAMEDIC*Pearl*

The ECG monitor can be an important tool when trying to determine whether crush syndrome is a factor. The only signs of crush injury syndrome a paramedic in the field might see are from the ECG. These are consistent with the findings of hyperkalemia and include peaked T waves and widened QRS complexes.

By now, the paramedic should have determined the patient care priorities and how and when the patient will be transported. This needs to be discussed with the incident commander as well as medical direction at the receiving facility. Everyone on the scene must be aware of the condition of the patient and the priority of treatment. The patient's condition dictates the quickness of extrication as much as the skills and resources available to conduct extrication activities.

PARAMEDIC*Pearl*

In the prehospital setting complications to the three main body systems may cause the patient to deteriorate rapidly, leading to death: the respiratory, cardiovascular, and nervous systems. Concentrated attention on these systems (in the order listed) makes the priority of care issues easier to manage.

Complete Extrication. Once extrication activities begin, they must continue until the victim is completely extricated. Nothing could be worse for the patient than to have the load lifted halfway off and then stopped to reset the tools. Stress this to the incident commander. Once the patient is removed and secured to the long board, quickly move him or her to the transport vehicle.

Managing a trauma patient who has been involved in a tractor overturn can be an overwhelming challenge. You need to assess and treat potential injuries and conditions while dealing with tremendous emotion by the family and neighbors. This is why developing and using a standard approach to all trauma patients is imperative, even the ones with minor injuries. Practicing an effective trauma assessment and care procedure will ensure you have the skills when they are needed. Paramedics who understand how to recognize and treat crush can have a positive effect in saving farmers' lives. The nature of tractor overturns can provide rural paramedics an opportunity to confront this condition.

Patient and Family Education

Rural EMS personnel have a tremendous opportunity to help reduce the potential for agricultural deaths and injuries in their regions. Conducting educational programs for farmer groups dealing with how to manage various emergency situations on their farms can lead into a discussion on how to prevent such incidents. For example, a sure way to avoid crushing injuries and death from tractor overturns would be to ensure each tractor has a **rollover protective structure (ROPS)** and each operator wears a seat belt whenever operating the tractor. The tractor may still turn over, but the operator will be protected by the rollover structure. Programs such as this are available through many farm safety organizations and agricultural universities. Teaching farm families how to treat and care for certain injuries tends to put farm safety in a different light. They are more apt to adopt measures to reduce the likelihood of an injury emergency when they learn the types of injuries that can occur.

MACHINERY EMERGENCIES

Farm machines pose an extreme number of hazards, and many farm workers are regularly exposed to these hazards. Common machinery hazards include **pinch points, wrap points, shear points, crush points,** and **pull-in points**. Pinch points and crush points cause blunt trauma injuries (Figure 53-4). Shear points, as the name indicates, lead to lacerations and severed limbs. Pull-in points and wrap points can cause severe twisting and crushing entrapments and, in some cases, amputations (Figure 53-5). Many farm machines also have considerable amounts of **stored energy** in them that can cause injury if this energy is released. Because most farm machines are used in rough conditions, if the machine breaks down during operation the farmer may attempt to analyze or fix the problem while the machine is running. They may be caught by any one of these hazards. Few statistics exist regarding how many injuries occur from farm machinery. Unless the farmer becomes entrapped, emergency services often are not summoned. When entrapment does occur, emergency responders must be methodical in their approach to extrication strategies. In all likelihood the victim will not be free when emergency services personnel arrive on the scene. If members of the farm family or other workers can disentangle the victim, they often will before the arrival of emergency responders. Once disentangled and extricated, they may even drive the patient to the local medical facility themselves. This is why emergency responders should expect a serious situation exists if they are summoned to a farm machinery entanglement.

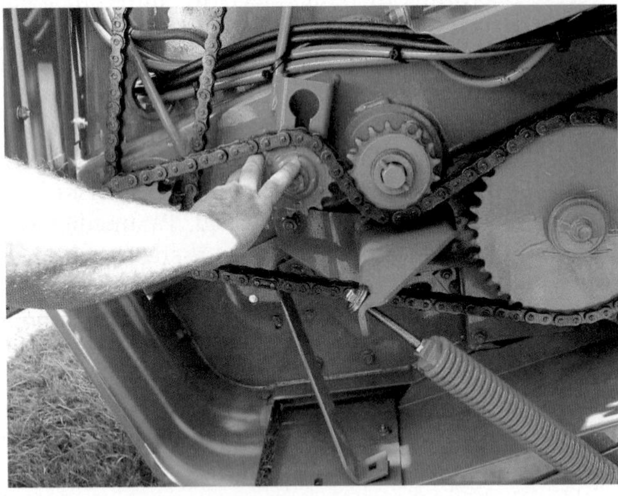

Figure 53-4 Farm machines have many parts that can lead to serious injury and death.

Most farm machinery is powered by one of three ways: mechanically through the PTO from the tractor, by its own motor (either gas or electric), or by hydraulics. The PTO transfers power from the tractor to an implement (machine) at either 540 or 1000 rpm. Normally this shaft is guarded by a safety shield, but if that shield is damaged or removed, entanglement can easily occur (Figure 53-6). If a person becomes entangled in this wrap point, serious consequences can occur. If the victim is lucky, clothing is ripped from his or her body, resulting in blunt trauma injuries as the clothing is pulled off (Figure 53-7). If the victim is less fortunate, one or more limbs are pulled off in a traumatic amputation. If neither of these happens, the victim is pulled into the shaft and wrapped around it, resulting in instant death (Figure 53-8).

Compartment Syndrome

[OBJECTIVE 3]

Another condition as important as crush syndrome in tractor overturn injuries is compartment syndrome, which can result from a crushing entrapment.

Description and Definition

Compartment syndrome occurs when pressure within a closed muscle compartment exceeds the perfu-

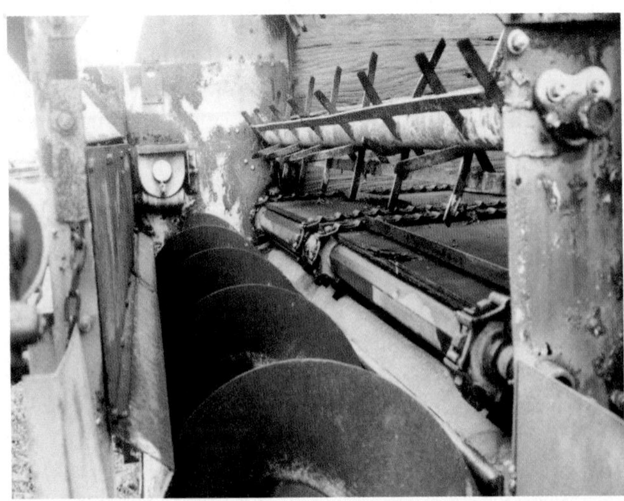

Figure 53-5 An operator often works near machines that are running. A simple auger is one of the most dangerous tools on a farm.

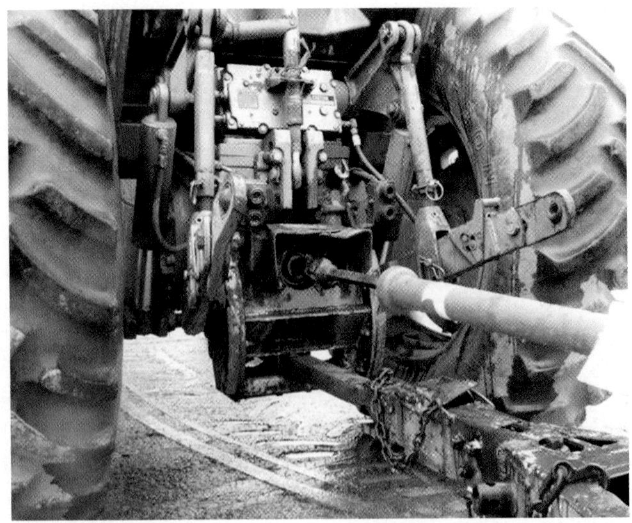

Figure 53-6 A power take-off connects the tractor to a driveshaft that powers an implement (machine). An unshielded shaft is a disaster waiting to happen. It only takes a second to become hopelessly trapped by this rotating shaft.

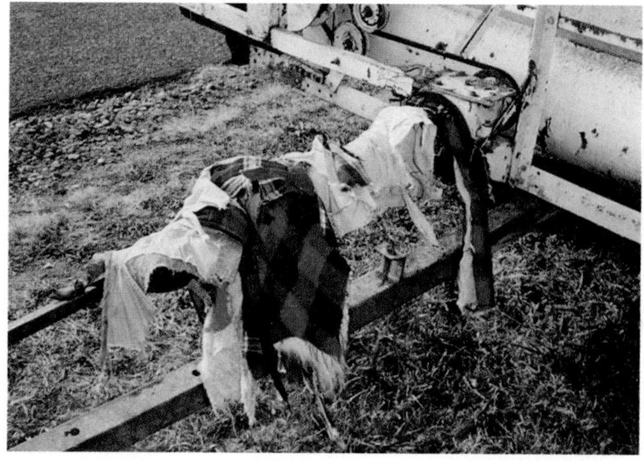

Figure 53-7 If a person is lucky, his or her clothing will be ripped from the body by a rotating shaft.

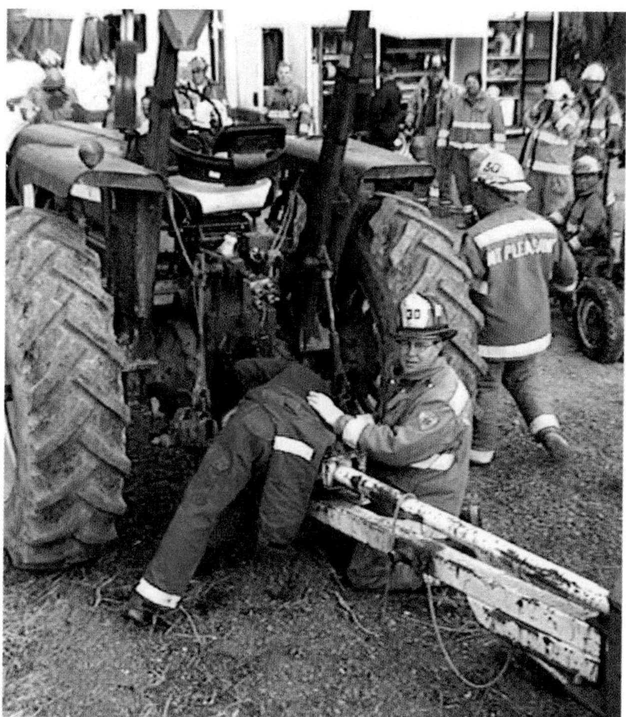

Figure 53-8 If a person becomes entrapped in the power take-off, paramedics must develop a strong index of suspicion for a host of potential injuries.

sion pressure and blood flow, impairing nerve signals. This results in ischemia to all distal tissues, including the nerves. Muscle groups are surrounded by tough layers of fascia that form compartments. During blunt trauma these muscle groups can be damaged and begin to swell. The fascia often remains intact, however. Because the fascia is tough, it has a limited elasticity. As the muscles within the fascia swell, the pressure inside the compartment increases. Most commonly swelling occurs because of irritated tissues filling with fluid; however, in significant trauma capillaries and blood vessels can be ruptured. Ruptured blood vessels result in swelling, thus causing compartment syndrome to develop much more rapidly. When this happens, oxygenated blood cannot enter the muscles and waste products do not exit. This results in extreme pain as well as muscle damage. This also can cause damage to the neurovascular bundle within the compartment if it compresses against a bone.

Epidemiology and Demographics

Compartment syndrome can be prevalent with many machinery entanglement scenarios because usually one limb becomes entangled as the operator performs a function near the operating machine. The compartments of the lower leg, the foot, and the forearm are particularly prone to developing compartment syndrome (Wallace & Smith, 2003). Many machinery entanglements occur because the operator attempted to adjust the mechanism while it was running (thus the hand or arm becomes entrapped) or tried to unclog the machine while it is running (using either the hands and arms or feet and legs). Entrapment occurs so quickly that the victim is unable to react fast enough to pull away to safety.

History and Physical Findings

Compartment syndrome can occur in a timeframe of 15 minutes to 6 days after an injury. However, the peak incidence is 12 hours after the injury. When swelling develops because of bleeding, the onset is much more rapid. The classic sign is extreme pain—often described as disproportionate to the apparent injury, especially if the muscle is stretched. The skin appears taut and may be shiny. The patient may also report tingling or burning sensations in the affected muscle. The muscle may feel tight. When compartment syndrome occurs in the forearm or lower leg, the distal tissues often are cyanotic, numb, and cold, with impaired movement.

Differential Diagnosis

Suspect acute compartment syndrome whenever a traumatic injury has occurred, such as a fracture or especially an entanglement. Likewise, suspect it with any crushing injury or a badly bruised muscle.

Therapeutic Interventions

Recognition of the presence of, or the potential for, compartment syndrome is the key factor in the prehospital treatment of compartment syndrome. All associated injuries should be treated with standard basic life support or advanced life support therapy. The injured extremity should be kept at heart level. Elevation is contraindicated because it will decrease blood flow, thereby increasing ischemia. If the extremity is dependent in relationship to the heart, venous engorgement will occur. This increases hydrostatic pressure, causing more fluid to enter the interstitial space and resulting in a further increase in compartmental pressures. Because compartment syndrome can lead to crush syndrome, the paramedic should be alert for the development of this condition. Treatment as described previously should be administered if crush syndrome is suspected. The definitive treatment for compartment syndrome is a fasciotomy. Therefore early notification of the hospital is crucial.

Patient and Family Education

Paramedics have a good opportunity to explain to farmers the importance of prompt medical attention for any potential fractures and crushing injuries. Rural EMS personnel have a tremendous opportunity to help reduce the potential for agricultural deaths and injuries in their regions. Conducting educational programs for farmer groups dealing with how to manage various emergency situations on their farms can lead into a discussion on how to prevent such incidents. For example, two ways to avoid a machinery entanglement injury are to keep the machine guards in place and not go near machines while they are running.

Hydraulic Injection Injuries

Description and Definition

Hydraulic oil pressures on farm machines equal 1000 to 3000 psi (Figure 53-9). Pressures of 100 psi can break the skin. A pinhole leak in a hydraulic line that contains 2000 psi of pressure is estimated to exceed 7000 psi. The velocity of fluid forced through such a system (or through a pinhole break in the line) can be in excess of 600 ft/sec. This speed is close to the muzzle velocity of a rifle and is sufficient to drive fluids through gloves and coveralls. Skin penetration has been recorded at distances of 4 inches from the fluid source to the skin (Flotre, 1992). Farmers who have sustained a hydraulic fluid injection have stated feeling little pain when the injury occurred, almost like a bee sting. Because of this, few individuals stop what they are doing to seek medical care. However, 1 to 3 hours after the initial injection the affected area becomes swollen and painful.

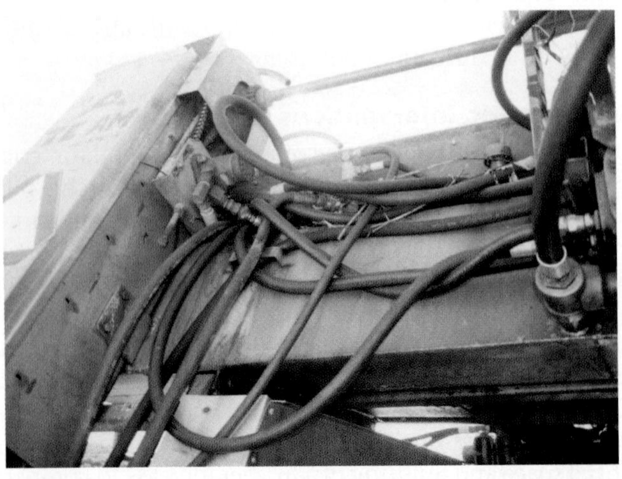

Figure 53-9 Hydraulic hoses transfer fluid under high pressure. On most farm machines pressures of 1000 to 3000 psi are typical.

Epidemiology and Demographics

[OBJECTIVE 4]

Three main factors figure in the pathophysiology of **hydraulic injection injury:** (1) physical distention of the tissues by the injected fluid, which results in vascular compression and leads to ischemic necrosis and gangrene; (2) chemical irritation of the tissues, which leads to inflammation, inflammatory edema, and further vascular compromise; and (3) secondary bacterial infection, which leads to septic inflammation and tissue necrosis (Flotre, 1992). Hydraulic injection injuries often result in tissue necrosis that is so severe that amputation is the only treatment. A successful outcome always depends on the interval between injury and removal of the injected material.

How frequently farmers receive high-pressure injection injuries is unknown. Because they often do not result in entrapping injury, EMS personnel may never see them on a farm response. Nonetheless, if this injury is ever encountered, medical personnel must treat it as a true surgical emergency.

History and Physical Findings

A common cause of hydraulic injection injury among farmers occurs when a farmer notices a leak in a hydraulic line and attempts to stop the leak by holding a rag or gloved hand over the leak. In addition, noticing a leak in a hydraulic line as the machine is operating outside is difficult, so an operator or bystander can be injected by simply walking near the leaking hose.

Suspicion of a hydraulic injection injury is raised by the history of the incident because the injury site itself will appear minimal. An injection site may be seen, especially if swelling occurs around the site. As time progresses swelling and signs of inflammation increase.

Therapeutic Interventions

Before approaching the patient, paramedics should determine the mechanism of injury and develop a strong index of suspicion and an initial plan of action. Then, once the power to the machine has been controlled and any stored energy has been addressed, patient assessment can begin. Give careful attention to the mechanism of injury. Was the patient entrapped by a wrap point, a pull-in point, or a crush point? Will spinal immobilization be necessary or simply immobilization of the entrapped part? Complications to the respiratory, cardiovascular, and nervous systems can rapidly lead to death. Concentrating emergency care efforts on these critical systems makes caring for a trauma patient much easier.

With machinery entanglements, clothing becomes wrapped around a shaft so tightly that the airway often becomes compromised. This clothing may need to be cut to relieve the pressure. This is an important point to stress to farm workers in a **"First on the Scene" program**. If the airway is compromised by a machinery entanglement, it will have to be relieved before emergency responders arrive on the scene if the victim is to live. Trauma can occur to the upper airway as well as the chest, which can cause airway obstruction.

Machinery entanglement may or may not cause considerable bleeding. The entrapment itself may control bleeding, or the clothing that is wrapped tightly may act as a tourniquet. With acute amputations blood vessels often constrict, which limits blood loss.

The appropriate treatment of a hydraulic injection injury is decompression and debridement in a surgical unit. Field treatment would involve cold compresses at the injection site and elevation of the limb to prevent or decrease swelling. Transport the patient to a facility that has experience treating this type of injury.

Patient and Family Education

A patient and his or her family members may not understand the urgency of treatment of hydraulic injection injuries. EMS personnel need to stress the importance of seeking medical attention for this type of injury.

General Considerations

Each of the methods of power transfer can create injuries through energy that is stored and released unexpectedly. Emergency responders must recognize how a machine is powered and how to secure that power before any patient care activities can take place. Never assume that the machine will be secured on arrival, as would be the case in most other industrial settings. Many family members who would potentially locate the entrapped victim may not know how to shut off and secure all the machines on the farm. Emergency responders in rural areas should learn how to secure power sources on the farm.

After the main power source is secured and locked out, rescuers need to anticipate any stored energy. This is energy that is trapped as a result of the entrapment of the victim. For example, if the patient is wound around a shaft, pressure (energy) on the shaft may cause unwanted movement if one end of the shaft is released. Rescuers must isolate the entanglement site by securing any anticipated stored energy source. Once the hazards have been secured, patient care efforts can proceed. Once the patient care needs have been identified and begun, extrication efforts can begin.

Teamwork is critical in any trauma incident, especially farm trauma incidents. Because of the length of entrapment time involved, the utmost attention must be focused on caring for the patient as well as managing the extrication and disentanglement. Rarely will an entrapment in a farm machine be minor enough to warrant turning the machine in reverse to remove an entrapped patient. In many instances, especially with wrap-type injuries, dismantling or even cutting a piece of the machinery away from the patient, not trying to remove the piece from the patient, may be the best option.

Where serious entrapment has occurred and the patient's condition is compromised or drastically deteriorates, field amputation may be a viable alternative. Emergency personnel may never consider field amputation in any other situations, but several instances on the farm may lead to this option. Paramedics in rural farm communities should consider preplanning field amputations. Proper preplanning will help paramedics on scene identify the source(s) of assistance. If field amputation is a viable option, the request should be made early in the incident response because securing the necessary personnel and equipment takes time.

Case Scenario—continued

Your assessment reveals an alert, oriented man in acute respiratory distress. The patient's skin is pale, cool, and clammy. Lung sounds indicate bilateral crackles in the lung bases extending one third up the thoracic cavity. The patient occasionally produces frothy, pink sputum. Vital signs are blood pressure, 90/60 mm Hg; pulse, 120 beats/min and regular; and respirations, 28 breaths/min and labored. The patient denies medications other than a baby aspirin and vitamin supplement daily. He states he has no known drug allergies. The man's wife states he has not seen a doctor in "too many years" and the patient reluctantly nods his head. The patient's ECG reveals sinus tachycardia with no ectopy or ST segment changes. His skin is cool and diaphoretic, with peripheral cyanosis. While you assess the patient, your partner administers supplemental oxygen at 15 L/min by nonrebreather mask.

Questions

4. *Has your first impression changed?*
5. *What conditions might cause delayed-onset pulmonary edema in this patient?*
6. *What additional assessment and treatment options for the man should be considered?*

CHEMICAL EMERGENCIES

On most farms a variety of products are found that can cause both acute and chronic reactions (Figure 53-10). Rural emergency responders must understand that these products exist and how farmers, their families, and employees can become exposed to them. Also, with this understanding responders can realize how these same products can be involved in incidents off the farm, whether deliberate or unintentional. Understanding what products exist enables responders to select the appropriate personal protective equipment (PPE) if they need to enter a potentially contaminated site to remove and/or treat an injured or exposed patient.

Types of Farm Chemicals

Most people associate the word *chemical* with a material used to control a pest **(pesticide),** such as an insecticide (material that controls insects), herbicide (material that controls weeds), fungicide (material that controls fungus), or rodenticide (material that controls rodents). These are members of only one class of chemicals often found on farms. Besides these products, fertilizers, seeds treated with chemical products, cleaners, disinfectants, sanitizers, fuels, and other fluids can cause acute or chronic reactions. Responders should review ways people can become poisoned and be suspicious whenever dealing with general malaise or sickness calls involving farmers. Rural paramedics should visit farms in their response areas to learn about the various chemical products found on farms and what kind of exposures farmers face to those products. Only with this understanding can paramedics effectively prepare for treating exposed patients.

Many of the more potent pesticides found on farms are insecticides. Many of these are derivatives of nerve agents developed during wars. Although many of the most toxic insecticides have been banned and taken out of circulation in the United States, some less-toxic ones are still in use and have similar properties to the original materials. These families of pesticides are known as **cholinesterase inhibitors.** The neurotransmitter acetylcholine acts as a messenger that carries a signal for a nerve, muscle, or gland to work. The enzyme **acetylcholinesterase** terminates the action of the acetylcholine, which stops the nerve, muscle, or gland from continuing to fire. A cholinesterase inhibitor blocks the acetylcholinesterase activity, which allows the muscles, nerves, and glands to continue to receive signals (Figure 53-11). This is seen by the various signs exhibited by the patient, which are noted by the mnemonic SLUDGE-BBM: ***s***alivation, ***l***acrimation, ***u***rination, ***d***iarrhea, ***g***astrointestinal upset, ***e***mesis, ***b***radycardia, ***b***ronchoconstriction, and ***m***iosis (Box 53-2). Suspect exposure to organophosphate or carbamate pesticides if a patient exhibits these signs.

Routes of Exposure

Pesticides on farms are an obvious hazard. Although fewer and fewer farmers purchase and apply pesticides themselves (more are hiring professionals), many farmers still store and apply pesticide materials. A review of routes of exposure is important (Figure 53-12). Poisons can typically enter the body through inhalation, ingestion, absorption, and injection. Not all materials poison a person the same way. For example, product A readily passes through the skin (dermal absorption), whereas product B does not pass through the skin. However, product B is highly toxic if inhaled, whereas product A has low inhalation toxicity.

The fastest route of exposure is inhalation. When fine particulates are inhaled, they can quickly move into the bloodstream and into the cells to affect the body's pathophysiology. Highly toxic materials often have a

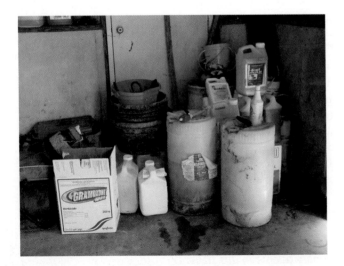

Figure 53-10 Farms have a variety of poisonous materials accessible.

BOX 53-2

The mnemonic SLUDGE-BBM is a good way to remember the symptoms of organophosphate and carbamate poisoning; two popular families of pesticides used on farms.

Salivation
Lacrimation
Urination
Diarrhea
Gastrointestinal upset
Emesis
Bradycardia
Bronchoconstriction
Miosis

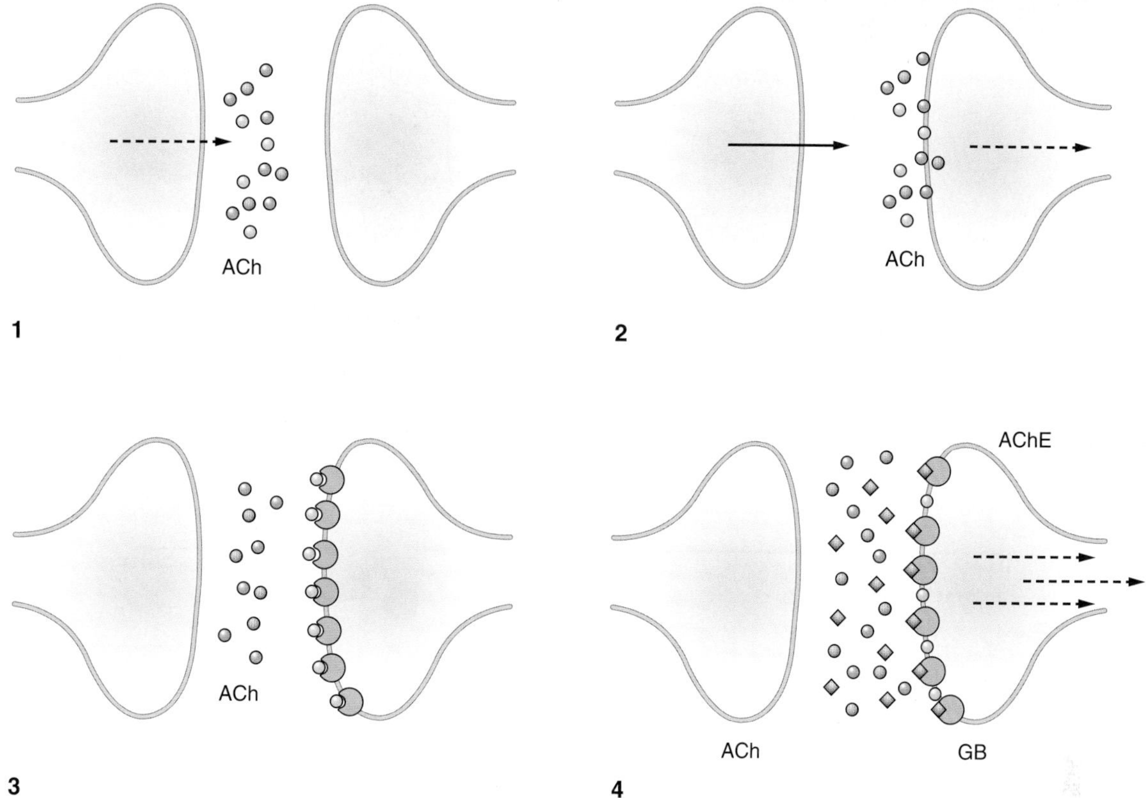

Figure 53-11 *1,* Nerve signals must pass between nerve synapses. *2,* Acetylcholine (ACh) is a neurotransmitter that allows nerve signals to travel across nerve synapses. *3,* Acetylcholinesterase *(AChE)* is another neurotransmitter that blocks acetylcholine, which in turn stops the nerve signals from crossing. *4,* Nerve agents (cholinesterase inhibitors such as sarin [GB]) block the ability of acetylcholinesterase to stop the nerve signals. Nerves continue to innervate target organs, muscles, and so forth.

high inhalation hazard, meaning that those handling this material should wear respiratory protection.

If a material is ingested, it must pass through the gastrointestinal tract before it is absorbed, often leaving enough time to reverse the potential effects as long as action is taken early. Do not wait for symptoms to occur before trying to reverse the effects; the effort will most likely be too late. Ingestion can occur when an applicator does not wash his or her hands properly after handling the material and then eats something that passes the residue from the hands to the food and to the mouth. Another source of ingestion is attempted suicide by purposely consuming a product. Children can become poisoned on a farm by playing around chemical storage areas and getting residue on their hands. Another common childhood ingestion is drinking a product that looks like either milk or a soft drink.

Approximately 90% of pesticide exposure is from dermal exposure. Lack of appropriate PPE (e.g., gloves, chemical-resistant clothing, face shields and goggles, boots) and inadequate washing are the reasons for this exposure. If PPE is used, often it is saved for reuse and not disposed of or washed (decontaminated) between uses. If PPE is not used (especially chemical-resistant suits), pesticide residue stays on the clothing and can continue to expose the individual and possibly family members. Dermal absorption involves the skin, mucous membranes, and the eyes. Applicators may wear gloves, boots, and coveralls but not eye protection and still be poisoned if they get splashed on the face. Injection exposure is caused when a chemical enters the bloodstream through a break in the skin. This may result from high air pressure injection or trauma situations with lacerations, punctures, or abrasions.

Organophosphates and Carbamates

[OBJECTIVE 4]

Description and Definition

The largest group of older nerve agents is the organophosphates. These products attack the nervous system by inhibiting a victim's cholinesterase. Most organophosphates are easily absorbed through the skin, the mucous membranes, and the gastrointestinal tract as well as by inhalation of mists and dusts. Excessive stimulation of

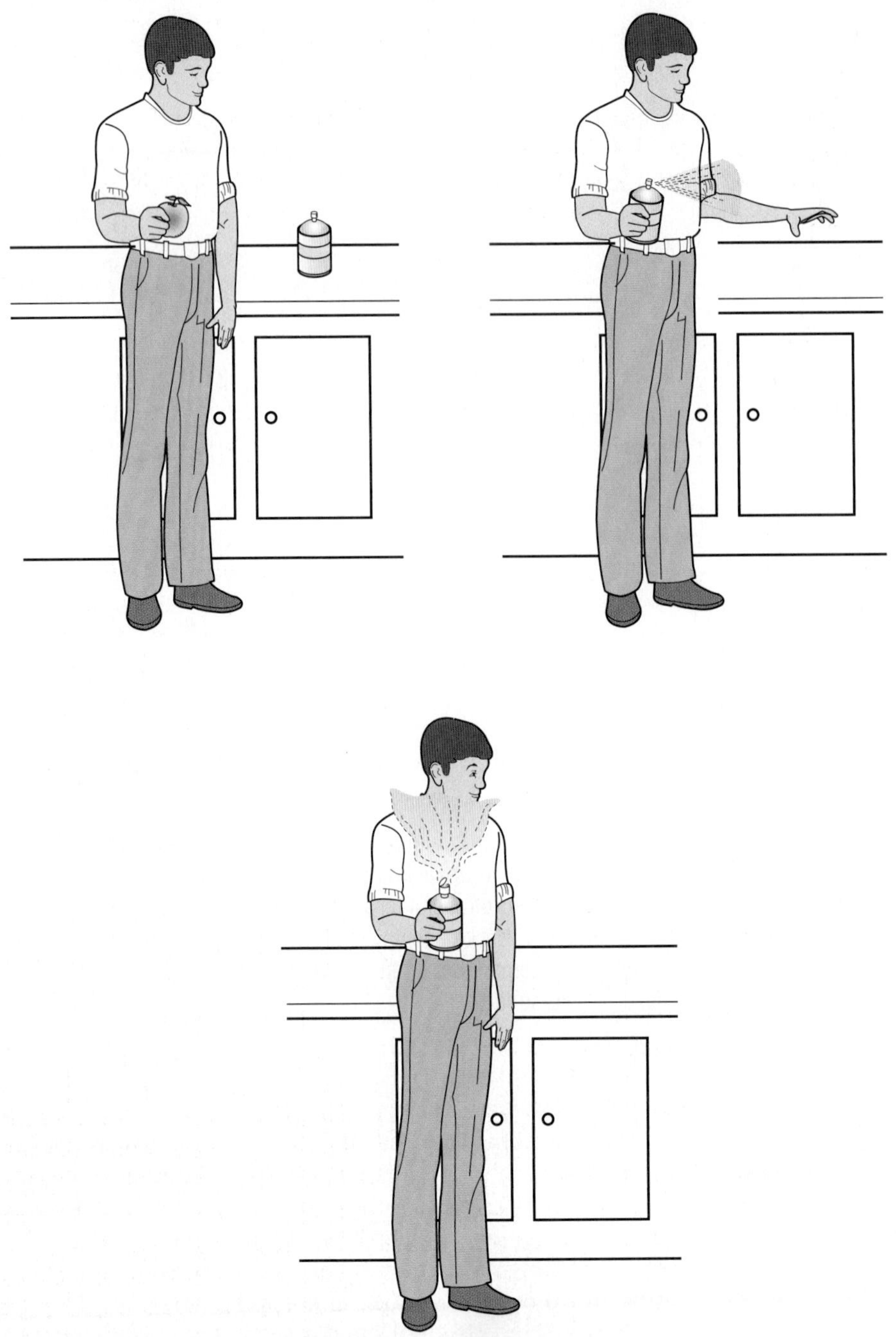

Figure 53-12 Routes of exposure.

certain receptors can cause patients exposed to organophosphates to have a runny nose, salivation, and wheezes as early signs. When possible the paramedic should attempt to obtain the name of the chemical the patient was exposed to, or the label of the chemical, as this information can help guide emergency department care.

Therapeutic Interventions

After ensuring personal protection and avoidance of becoming contaminated, airway management is crucial in patients exposed to these agents. Secretions should be immediately suctioned and the airway controlled as necessary. Intubation may be required if secretions are copious or secondary to laryngospasm, bronchospasm, or respiratory failure. If rapid sequence intubation is an option, the paramedic should avoid the use of succinylcholine. Recall that this medication is degraded by acetylcholinesterase, and because of the lack of this the effects of succinylcholine are significantly prolonged. Seizures, although uncommon, can occur and represent severe toxicity. They are treated with standard therapy including benzodiazepines. Patients should be decontaminated as soon as is reasonably possible, including the removal of contaminated clothing. Time is of the essence in treating these patients because the effects on the cholinesterase are irreversible if not stopped in time with appropriate antidotes. Administration of atropine is the main treatment in organophosphate exposures. Additionally, pralidoxime (2-PAM) can be administered if available. However, in a 1992 study it was shown that the administration of 2-PAM provided no additional benefits compared with treatment with atropine alone (de Silva et al., 1992). The role of 2-PAM remains controversial, and some authors feel that atropine alone is not effective. As a result, 2-PAM remains a standard treatment in the treatment of these patients and is considered the definitive treatment because it reactivates acetylcholinesterase by uncoupling the organophosphate molecule from it.

Another family of pesticides closely related to organophosphates is the carbamate family. A patient with carbamate poisoning presents the same way as with organophosphates. The difference in the treatment of patients exposed to carbamates is that they will respond better to atropine alone. This is an important distinction because in most cases atropine is the first drug of choice (e.g., with an insecticide poisoning). If the patient improves with this treatment, 2-PAM administration is not necessary.

Organochlorines

Description and Definition

Another popular family of pesticides are the organochlorines. This family involves a wide range of chemicals that contain carbon, chlorine, and sometimes several other elements. A range of organochlorine compounds are produced, including many herbicides, insecticides, fungicides, and industrial chemicals (e.g., polychlorinated biphenyl). The compounds are characteristically stable and fat soluble and will bioaccumulate. Organochlorines pose a range of adverse human health risks, with some being carcinogenic. These materials contribute to many acute and chronic illnesses.

History and Physical Findings

Symptoms of acute poisoning with organochlorines are abrupt and affect the central nervous system. These can include tremors, headache, dermal irritation, respiratory problems, dizziness, nausea, confusion, paresthesia of the face, seizures, and coma. Death can occur 4 to 8 hours after exposure secondary to respiratory failure as well as metabolic acidosis from prolonged seizures.

Therapeutic Interventions

No specific antidote is available for organochlorine poisoning. Treatment focuses on the management of life threats identified in the primary survey. The initiation of pain, such as a sternal rub, should be avoided as this can cause seizures. Airway protection is paramount as the patient is susceptible to both vomiting and an altered mental status. If the patient is alert and has ingested the material, consider the administration of activated charcoal. Ideally the activated charcoal should not contain sorbitol, as this can cause vomiting. However, if there is any indication the patient will experience an alteration in mental status, this must be avoided. The patient should be decontaminated if possible prior to arrival at the hospital. These chemicals can sensitize the myocardium and cause dysrhythmias; therefore cardiac monitoring should be initiated.

Bipyridil Herbicides

Description and Definition

Another family of pesticides are called *bipyridil herbicides*. An example of this is the herbicide Paraquat (Syngenta, Basel, Switzerland). Paraquat poisoning is worth separate mentioning because of its high toxicity and use as a poisoning agent. Suicidal use of Paraquat has been common.

This material is a widely used herbicide on many farms because it has few environmental hazards. Most symptoms of Paraquat poisoning do not occur for several hours, so paramedics typically diagnose Paraquat poisoning on circumstantial evidence. It does not usually result in rapid death, but the patient often experiences a prolonged and painful progressive toxicity resulting in death from respiratory failure. The most important fact paramedics must understand about treating a patient with suspected Paraquat poisoning is to not administer oxygen. In human beings Paraquat builds up in surfactant-producing cells in the lung and kidneys. Oxygen perpetuates the damage caused by pathologic processes in the lungs. Once Paraquat has entered the pulmonary cells, no treatment for toxicity is effective. Even though a patient is asymptomatic, do not delay care. Once symptoms of Paraquat poisoning develop, reversing the effects is not possible.

Epidemiology and Demographics

Ingestion is the most common route of poisoning with Paraquat. It can be easily mixed with food, water, or other beverages. Eating or drinking Paraquat-contaminated food or beverage can be poisonous. Paraquat poisoning also is possible after skin exposure. Poisoning is more likely to occur if the skin exposure lasts a long time, involves a concentrated version of Paraquat, or occurs through skin that is not intact (skin with sores, cuts, or a severe rash). If it is inhaled, Paraquat can cause poisoning leading to lung damage (Centers for Disease Control and Prevention [CDC], 2003).

History and Physical Findings

Because Paraquat is highly poisonous, the form marketed in the United States has a blue dye to keep it from being confused with beverages such as coffee, a sharp odor to serve as a warning, and an added agent to cause vomiting if consumed.

After a person ingests a large amount of Paraquat, he or she is likely to have pain and swelling of the mouth and throat immediately. The next signs of illness after ingestion are gastrointestinal symptoms such as nausea, vomiting, abdominal pain, and diarrhea (which may become bloody). Severe gastrointestinal symptoms may result in dehydration, electrolyte abnormalities, and low blood pressure (CDC, 2003).

Differential Diagnosis

The signs and symptoms above do not absolutely mean Paraquat exposure; however, erring on the side of caution is best. Assume that the patient has had an acute exposure and treat accordingly.

Therapeutic Interventions

Treatment consists of removing the Paraquat from the body through decontamination and providing supportive prehospital medical care. This includes administering IV fluids to help counteract potential dehydration. Withhold oxygen unless the patient is having breathing difficulties. As mentioned above, Paraquat accumulates in surfactant-producing cells in the lungs and kidneys. Oxygen perpetuates the damage caused by pathologic processes in the lungs.

Patient and Family Education

In the United States, Paraquat is classified as a restricted-use pesticide, which means that it can be used only by licensed applicators. However, prehospital personnel should reinforce the fact that all pesticides can be extremely toxic, and anyone who works in areas where chemicals are stored, mixed, or applied should wear the appropriate PPE. This information is found on the container's label. Paramedics also can discuss various signs and symptoms of pesticide poisoning and relate them to the need to seek medical treatment.

Patient Assessment

[OBJECTIVE 5]

A critical component of dealing with a patient who has potentially been exposed to any hazardous material is to remove the patient from the chemical and the chemical from the patient while avoiding any cross contamination (uncontaminated people becoming contaminated in the treatment process). To achieve this, the scene must be broken into three distinct zones (Figure 53-13). A hot

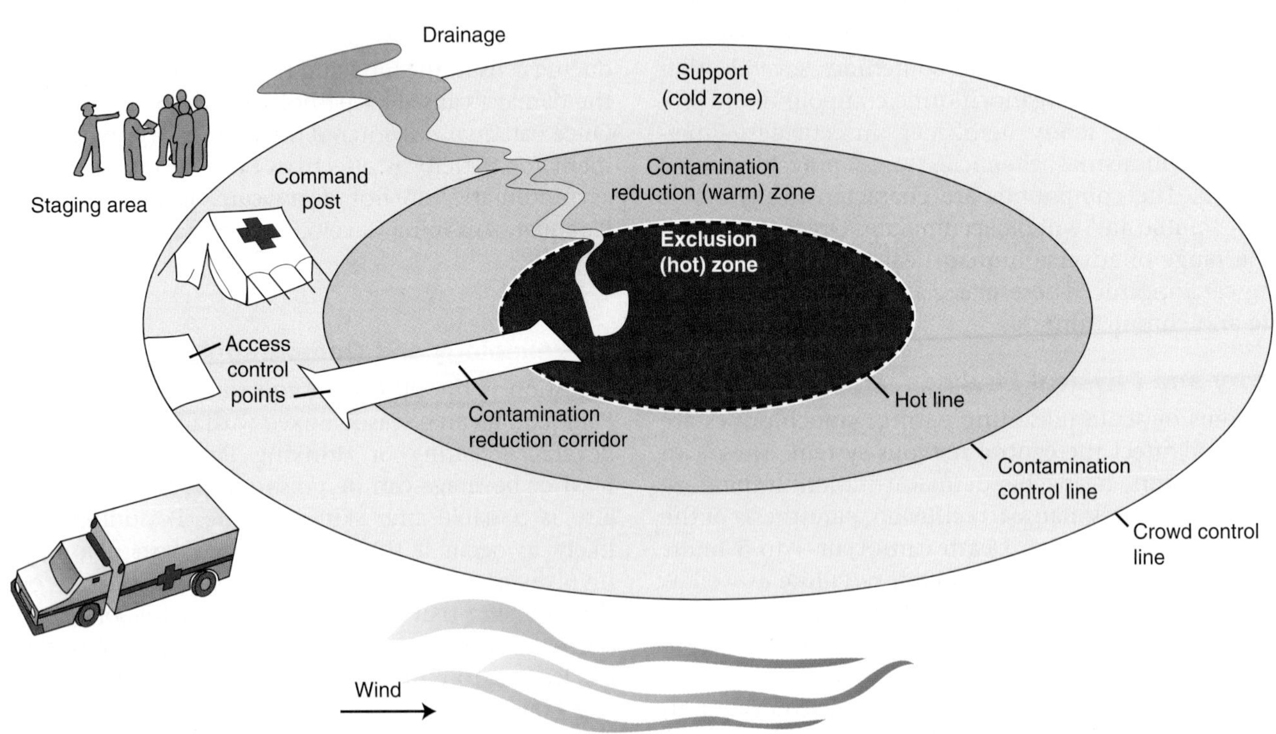

Figure 53-13 With any emergency involving any hazardous material, define the three zones (hot zone, warm zone, and cold zone) to manage potential contamination. A contaminated patient must be brought (either with assistance or by himself or herself) out of the hot zone to be decontaminated in the warm zone, then medically treated in the cold zone.

zone is an area large enough to ensure that anyone outside the zone is not going to be contaminated. A warm zone is an area just outside the hot zone where decontamination is conducted. The only patient care normally conducted inside the warm zone is opening the airway, cervical spine stabilization, and placement on a backboard. Only properly attired personnel (in appropriate PPE for the incident) are allowed in the hot and warm zones. A cold zone is the area outside the warm zone where patient care is conducted, resources (personnel and equipment) are staged, and the incident commander is stationed. Primary and secondary surveys and treatment are conducted in the cold zone.

Removing the patient from the poison means moving the patient (either physically or having the patient move himself or herself) from the hot zone to the warm zone. Removing the poison from the patient means removing clothing that may have been contaminated. For a person overcome from fumes inside an enclosed space, perhaps all that is needed is to move the person from the hot zone to the cold zone. Rarely will full decontamination be necessary for a patient who has been exposed to fumes. If the patient was exposed to solids or liquids, remove the patient's clothing and wash his or her body with water and mild liquid detergent. Brush off any dry material before washing. To avoid cross contamination, only personnel in appropriate PPE (chemical resistant) should come in contact with the patient at this point. The only patient care during this phase would be opening an airway and providing cervical spine stability if appropriate. Also, if appropriate, the patient can be secured to a long board. Pay particular attention to the patient's eyes if they were exposed. Constantly irrigate the eyes if possible.

Patient assessment and treatment are conducted in the cold zone after the patient has been decontaminated. Treatment of a patient exposed to farm chemicals is no different from treating any other patient in that a methodical process is used. The goal of prehospital care is to determine whether the patient is experiencing any complications from the poisoning. If the poisoning is determined to be affecting the patient's respiratory, cardiovascular, or nervous systems, you must act to reverse the situation. The goal to treating poisoning patients is to create a way to reverse the effects by slowing or reversing the absorption or speeding its elimination from the body. Not all pesticides or poisons have an antidote, so paramedics must develop a systematic approach to treating what they find, especially regarding the airway, breathing, and cardiovascular and nervous system disorders. Rely on the product labels to help determine what the product is and how to treat exposure. With the label in hand, contact a poison control center for additional information.

Ensure an open airway. Some materials cause progressive reactions, so a patient's airway may deteriorate over time. Ensure adequate breathing. Not every patient who has been exposed to farm chemicals needs or should receive supplemental oxygen, however. Keep in mind this can be detrimental to patients who have been poisoned by Paraquat. If the patient is not breathing or is not adequately breathing, begin positive-pressure ventilations and then intubate. If the patient is breathing at a stable rate but shows signs of cardiopulmonary or neurologic deficit, do not withhold oxygen.

Assess circulation and begin cardiopulmonary resuscitation if necessary. Follow advanced cardiac life support protocols, noting any modifications for poisonings. Control obvious bleeding, assess pulses and blood pressure, and establish IV access for any patient with signs and symptoms of cardiopulmonary or neurologic deficit. Make sure that the IV site has been thoroughly decontaminated before venipuncture. Poisoning by injection can occur if any residue is present at the IV site.

Assess neurologic status. Many farm chemicals have an effect on neurologic status. If the patient's status improves after being brought out of the hot zone, assume that he or she was exposed to an asphyxiant. If the patient's neurologic status deteriorates, suspect exposure to a nerve agent.

Examine for associated injuries. These can be related to trauma or thermal or chemical burns or reactions.

Conducting a sound patient history is crucial when dealing with a patient who has been exposed to farm chemicals. Whatever mnemonic used should enable the paramedic to ascertain the medical history of the patient and the events that led up to the potential exposure. Some conditions such as allergies, preexisting illness, and certain medications can exacerbate chemicals exposure symptoms. The effects of many chemicals do not present immediately, so EMS personnel must be detectives to pinpoint the cause of the symptoms and signs. A thorough assessment process must be in place and practiced on a regular basis.

PARAMEDIC*Pearl*

Many poisonings initially appear similar to flu symptoms, with fatigue, headache, dizziness, blurred vision, and nausea. Exposed individuals also may be sweating excessively, salivating, and experiencing diarrhea. Paramedics must keep in mind the early and later signs and symptoms of chemical poisoning when dealing with farm workers and always remember to ask about exposure to chemicals. Remember, some of the materials found on farms are less toxic and might not affect a person immediately. Moderate signs and symptoms include the inability to walk, chest discomfort, and constriction of the pupils. Signs and symptoms of advanced poisoning are unconsciousness, muscle twitching, mouth and nose secretions, coma, and ultimately death.

Case Scenario CONCLUSION

The patient tells you that he was working on the hatch to the corn silo that had been broken by a recent storm. He says that the silo had just been filled the day before and he "didn't want the birds to get into the silo and eat all the corn." The patient noticed some mold on the silage and a slight odor of bleach, but he did not use any respiratory precautions because he was in open air for the majority of the time. He claims to have been in the silo for approximately 10 minutes.

Looking back

7. *What is your final impression of the patient?*
8. *What treatment options are available for this patient?*
9. *What patient and family education should be provided?*

CONFINED SPACE EMERGENCIES

[OBJECTIVE 6]

Farmers work in a considerable number of spaces that would be considered confined according to the Occupational Safety and Health Administration (OSHA). However, the majority of farmers are exempt from OSHA inspection requirements; thus they are not apt to follow confined space entry procedures when they enter and/or work around these spaces. In contrast, although farmers are not required to follow proper procedures, emergency responders performing rescue functions are obliged to follow them.

According to OSHA, a confined space is large enough for someone to enter, has limited access and egress, and is not designed for continuous occupancy. OSHA further defines a permit-required confined space as having the same characteristics as above in addition to (1) a hazardous atmosphere, or (2) containing a material that can engulf an entrant, or (3) be configured in such a way that an entrant can be trapped or asphyxiated by inwardly converging walls or a floor that slopes downward and tapers to a smaller cross section, or (4) contains any other recognized serious safety or health hazard. Most of the common spaces that OSHA would consider a confined space that farmers normally enter would be considered a permit-required confined space. These include silos, grain bins, and manure storage vessels.

Silos

A variety of structures are used to ferment feeds for later use by the farmer. Forages (hay crops and corn silage crops) are normally stored in a silo, but other forages and some grains are stored and fermented in silos as well. For the fermentation process to take place, bacterial action is necessary. This action causes heat and releases a variety of gases, some of which can be harmful and even fatal to the farmer or rescuer. Any production of gases in an enclosed space leads to a lower concentration of oxygen, which leads to an environment that will not support life without some sort of supplemental breathing protection. Once this fermentation process ends, heat and gas production ceases and dissipates.

Farms may have horizontal silos, vertical silos, or both. Horizontal silos usually pose fewer immediate dangers than vertical silos because they are not considered confined spaces. Horizontal silos have an easy way to get out or get rescuers in if trouble is encountered. One of the biggest concerns involving horizontal silos is equipment turnover, with collapsing material potentially burying the operator. Vertical silos are cylindrical structures and are considered confined spaces. Rescue from farm silos usually involves vertical silos.

Two basic types of vertical silos are used: conventional and oxygen limiting. **Conventional silos** are typically unloaded from the top of the silage by a mechanical unloading machine or by hand. If the silo is unloaded by hand, an operator must enter the space. If this is the case, the environment inside must be adequate to support life. Even if the silo is unloaded by a mechanical unloading machine, an operator must periodically (usually at least once per week) enter the silo to service the unloader and/or the silo itself.

Whenever someone enters the silo the potential for an injury emergency or need for a rescue exists. Typical emergencies are caused by falls climbing up the silo chute or the outside ladder, falling inside the silo, entering the silo and being overcome by silo gas, being entrapped in the unloader, or having a medical emergency. Performing rescue from a silo is a highly technical skill. Depending on the patient's condition, extrication is either down the chute, out the top, or through the side of the silo.

An **oxygen-limiting silo,** as the name suggests, limits the amount of oxygen inside. These structures are typically unloaded from underneath the material. They are designed to keep air out. The normal oxygen level inside these structures is approximately 4%—well below what a human being needs to survive. If a person enters

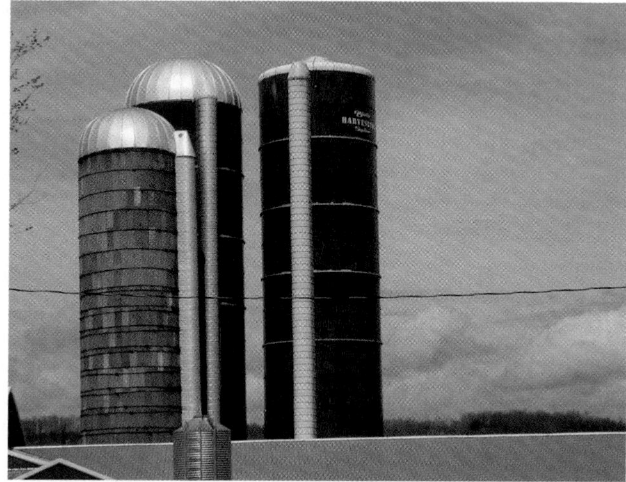

Figure 53-14 Typical farm silos found on many livestock farms. The silo on the *left* is a typical conventional silo. The silo on the *right* is a typical oxygen-limiting silo. The middle silo is a modified oxygen-limiting silo. In most situations a modified silo should be treated as an oxygen-limiting structure. Rescuers must use confined space procedures when dealing with emergencies involving these structures.

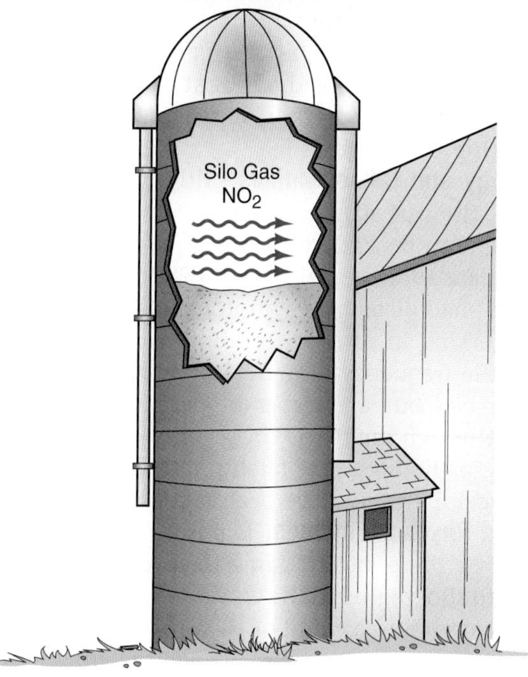

Figure 53-15 Silo gas (nitrogen oxides) is heavier than air, so it settles on the top of the silage. Silo gas is typically present for 2 to 3 weeks after the silo is filled.

this space without breathing protection, rescuers would be focused on body recovery instead of a viable rescue. Following proper confined space entry procedures will keep the rescue personnel safe (Figure 53-14).

Silo Filler's Disease

Description and Definition. Clearly the biggest danger to anyone who enters a silo (either a farm worker or a rescue person) are the gases produced during the normal fermentation or from a fire process. *Silo filler's disease* is the term used when a person has been exposed to **silo gas.** Although more than one type of gas is produced in a silo, the term *silo gas* refers to the most common family of gas produced from the fermentation of silages: nitrogen oxides (NOx). Inhalation of these gases can cause sudden death, pulmonary edema, and/or severe lung scarring. The oxides causing silo filler's disease may persist for 2 to 3 weeks in silos newly filled with green chopped plant material (Figure 53-15). Workers may be exposed when entering a silo, the silo chute, or the adjacent feed room. Workers most commonly inhale low concentrations of NOx and develop minor transient respiratory symptoms. High concentrations of NOx can kill within minutes. Workers may inhale moderate concentrations for extended periods without developing symptoms or detecting danger. Reactions to moderate concentrations (pulmonary edema) can be delayed up to 30 hours, with relapse in 2 to 6 weeks. Relapse can occur even without reexposure and may be caused by the development of bronchiolitis obliterans.

Determination of exposure to NOx followed by proper treatment and monitoring of exposed patients are imperative to prevent death or serious complications. Preventing exposure to silo gas could eliminate this occupational illness.

Of the several forms of NOx, three may be found in silos on the farm: nitric oxide (NO), nitrogen dioxide (NO_2), and nitrogen tetroxide (N_2O_4), collectively referred to as NOx. Nitrous acid (HNO_2) also may be present. Of these compounds, NO_2 and N_2O_4 are medically significant.

NOx is formed through fermentation in conventional silos (i.e., upright silos that are not air tight) freshly filled with green chopped plant material. This chopped corn, alfalfa, oats, or other plant material forms silage, which constitutes a crucial portion of the feed ration for beef and dairy cattle; alfalfa silage also may be fed to sheep. Production of NOx commences within 4 hours after silo filling has begun. Concentrations of NOx reach a maximum in 1 to 2 days, after which production continues at a decreasing rate for 1 week to 10 days. Both NOx and carbon dioxide, which are produced simultaneously, lie at or near the silage surface and in depressions in the silage, where they replace oxygen. Because NOx are heavier than air, they roll down the silo chute like water when a chute door at an appropriate level has been left open and concentrate in the feed room between the barn and silo, at the base of the silo, or in the chute itself.

Presence and concentration of NOx vary widely among different silo towers and also depend on the quality of the chopped plant material. The NOx are produced from inorganic nitrates in plants. Higher NOx production is associated with certain crops, certain soil conditions (those heavily fertilized with nitrates), and certain plant growth conditions (prolonged drought with rain just before ensiling, cloudy weather, damage to leaves or roots, harvesting after a frost).

Epidemiology and Demographics. Although probably not common, the true scope of exposure to NOx on the farm is thought to be underestimated. An unpublished survey in the late 1960s revealed that 4.2% of Wisconsin farm operators had developed symptoms of NOx inhalation when working in or near freshly filled silos. Other statistics on the frequency of agricultural NOx exposure are not available, but a number of deaths have been documented through the years. The severity of the hazard partially rests in the high case fatality rate: 29% of cases cited in medical literature have been fatal.

History and Physical Findings. Exposure to NOx may occur wherever these heavy gases have concentrated: within a closed silo, higher in the chute (when the worker opens a chute door and a cloud of NOx rolls past), at the base of a silo chute (when a door between the chute and silo has been left open), or in the feed room or barn next to the silo (when gases have flowed through open doors into these structures). A worker typically climbs the chute and enters the silo to work at leveling silage or to feed silage to animals. Either one is a potentially fatal task when attempted soon after filling or when the silo has not been adequately ventilated. Because NOx is only mildly irritating to the upper respiratory tract but highly damaging to the alveoli, workers may continue actively working in atmospheres with low to moderate NOx concentrations for hours, inhaling the potent oxides without detecting danger. The high carbon dioxide and low oxygen concentrations induce deep breathing, which speeds penetration of NOx into the alveoli, where the gas does its damage. When NOx concentrations are high, a worker may be too weak to retrace his or her steps. The danger is increased when movement of a worker releases gases trapped in the silage or when a worker enters or falls into a cavity in the silage. Gases concentrated in adjacent buildings or at the base of the silo may be inhaled by workers, children at play, or livestock. The danger from NOx is greatest in summer or early fall, during the 2 weeks after filling. (Hay crop silage is usually harvested in summer, whereas corn silage is harvested in late summer and early to mid autumn.)

Reactions to NOx depend on the concentration of gas inhaled and the length of exposure. Relatively mild exposure to NOx produces ocular irritation and a transient upper respiratory tract syndrome manifests as cough, possibly with dyspnea, fatigue, nausea, cyanosis, vomiting, vertigo, or somnolence (drowsiness). Symptoms may be severe enough to induce workers to leave the silo. However, when reactions to NOx are minimal, workers may stay in the silo and increase the probability of a more severe reaction.

Very high concentrations of NOx induce immediate distress, resulting in collapse and death within minutes. The mechanism of this reaction is not completely understood; death may be caused by airway spasm or laryngospasm, reflex respiratory arrest, or simple asphyxiation from low ambient oxygen concentrations. Persons who collapse in silos and are immediately rescued may survive only to experience the respiratory responses described below.

At somewhat lower concentrations, NOx induces pulmonary edema (normally within 30 hours after exposure), bronchiolitis obliterans (within days to weeks), or both. These reactions typify silo filler's disease. At the time of exposure, patients may have had no or minimal symptoms or the symptoms associated with mild exposure. However, a slowly evolving and progressive inflammation of the lungs results in massive pulmonary edema most commonly from 6 to 12 hours later. Death from asphyxiation may occur within hours, but the majority of patients completely recover with appropriate therapy within days or weeks.

Differential Diagnosis. Silo filler's disease may be confused with a number of illnesses, including **hypersensitivity pneumonitis** or a **toxic organic dust syndrome,** which results from exposure to moldy hay or grain. Exposure to mold typically occurs while uncapping the silo or removing moldy silage from the top silo layers well after the harvest season. Because the initial illness may be mild, patients may present during a relapse 2 to 6 weeks after exposure to NOx. A detailed medical history is crucial to diagnose silo filler's disease correctly. In addition to noting exposure to a recently filled silo, most commonly in late summer or early fall, a patient may recall seeing signs of NOx near the silo or experiencing the transient symptoms previously described. Prompt diagnosis and treatment of patients with acute symptoms are vital to prevent possible death and, in the case of initial illness, to lessen the probability of relapse (National Ag Safety Database, 2002).

Therapeutic Interventions. As in any hazardous environment, the patient must be removed to fresh air. If the patient has been exposed to silo gas, urge the patient to see his or her physician. Any symptomatic patient who has been exposed to NOx should be closely monitored by a physician for 48 hours because of the possibility of sudden pulmonary edema. Prehospital intervention should include oxygen therapy, bronchodilators, and assisted ventilation if necessary. If pulmonary edema is present, treat per protocol.

Patient and Family Education. Farmers need to understand thoroughly the hazards associated with newly filled silos. Once filled, no one should enter the silo for at least 2 weeks. If entrance is imperative during the filling process, the blower should be run for 30 minutes before entering the silo and kept running while anyone is inside. All silo doors should be kept closed during and after filling to prevent NOx from flowing down the chute. The door between the silo room and barn should be kept closed. Children and animals should be kept away from the silo and adjacent feed room during filling and for 2 weeks afterward. A few days before the silo is entered for the first time, the filler opening should be pulled open from the ground (not from the chute) with a rope. The blower should be operated for at least 30 minutes before entrance, and other means of ventilation should be maximized.

Detector tubes (also called *colorimetric tubes*) that measure the concentrations of NO_2 in silos are reasonably priced and reliable if properly used. If the slightest throat irritation or coughing occurs while working with fresh silage, a worker should immediately exit the silo. In any case of symptomatic exposure to silo gas, the worker should immediately report to a physician and be monitored for either immediate or delayed reactions (National Ag Safety Database, 2002).

Other Silo Gases

Carbon monoxide and methane are two other gases produced in small quantities during normal silage fermentation. Both are asphyxiants. Carbon monoxide, carbon dioxide, and nitrogen dioxide are all produced in larger quantities during a silo fire. The goal in dealing with anyone who is inside the silo during or shortly after the fermentation process or during a silo fire is to get him or her to fresh air and administer oxygen as soon as is practical. Ventilating the silo while the person is inside does some good. The ventilation process may push the gases out of the silo and down the silo chute. Rescuers must first use an appropriate gas detection meter to determine the gases present and their levels before any rescue attempts. If necessary, use breathing protection and/or ventilation.

Manure Storage Gases

Two additional gases to which livestock farmers may be exposed are ammonia and hydrogen sulfide **(manure gas).**

Description and Definition

Ammonia is an irritant and, at normal levels, causes such irritation of the upper airway (exhibited by coughing and nose and throat irritation) that any healthy person who can escape will do so. Exposure to high concentrations (or lower concentrations for an extended period) of ammonia causes burning of the eyes, nose, throat, and respiratory tract and can result in blindness, lung damage, or death. Ammonia reacts with water to produce ammonium hydroxide. If this happens inside the body, cells can become damaged.

Hydrogen sulfide, commonly referred to as *manure gas,* is a much more hazardous gas. This gas is produced by the decomposition of organic material. It is prevalent when manure is stored in a liquid form for an extended period. Most livestock farmers store manure for later use as a fertilizer material, and hydrogen sulfide is produced during this process (Figures 53-16 and 53-17). In low concentrations this gas is an irritant much like ammonia, but at high concentrations it can cause systemic poisoning, which can lead to instant death. The first symptom other than the classic rotten egg odor, even in low concentrations, is eye irritation that feels like grains of sand under the eyelids. Before using the stored manure as a fertilizer material, farmers agitate or mix it. Manure pit agitation can result in the sudden release of large quantities of hydrogen sulfide (H_2S). At moderately high concentrations, exposure to this gas causes runny nose, cough, dyspnea, and even pulmonary edema. At higher concentrations (especially when exposed during agitation of the pit) a patient can suddenly collapse as a result of respiratory paralysis and pulmonary edema. At high concentrations a person's ability to smell becomes paralyzed, so the most effective warning mechanism is not functional.

When manure pits constructed under a barn are agitated before emptying, tremendous amounts of manure gas are released. This gas can rise into the barn where animals, farm operators, and employees are located.

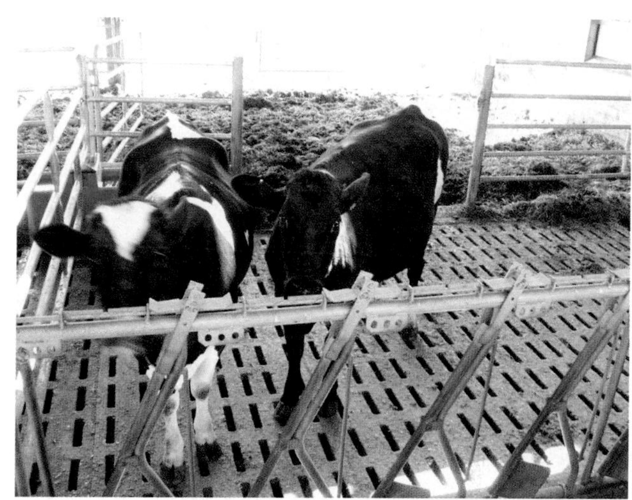

Figure 53-16 Many modern livestock operations have manure storage under their barns.

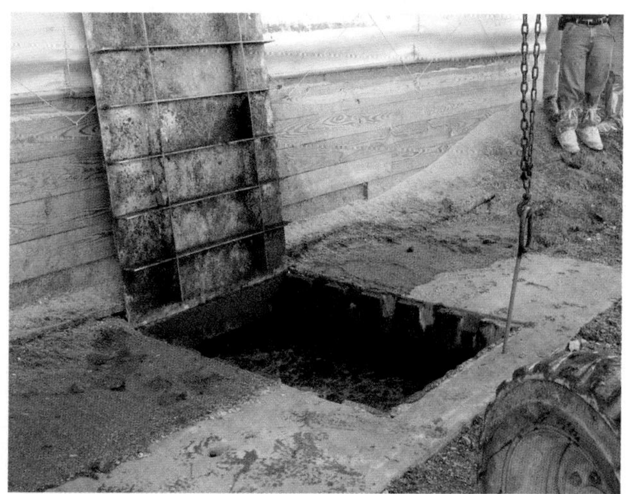

Figure 53-17 A clean-out access point outside the structure often is present to remove the manure from the collection area.

Epidemiology and Demographics

In the United States an estimated 700,000 persons work in confinement operations. The largest group of exposed workers with the most frequent and severe health problems are associated with swine confinement houses. Concentrations of manure gases may exceed levels recommended as safe in industrial occupational settings. Nearly 70% of swine confinement workers have one or more symptoms of respiratory illness or irritation.

History and Physical Findings

Presence of H_2S is usually apparent because of the characteristic rotten egg smell. Concentrations greater than 150 ppm may overwhelm the olfactory nerve so that the victim may have no warning of exposure. Toxicity depends on the level of exposure. Low-level exposure is more chronic in nature. These victims have irritation to the mucous membranes (conjunctivitis) and the respiratory system (wheezing). They also may have headaches and bronchial symptoms. Higher-level exposures result in acute symptoms. Coughing, shortness of breath, pulmonary edema, cyanosis, vertigo with nausea and vomiting, and confusion are typical physical findings. Extremely high concentrations can lead to cardiorespiratory arrest because of brainstem toxicity. The paramedic may see myocardial infarction and seizures (Mandavia, 2005).

Differential Diagnosis

The differential diagnosis of toxic gas exposure typically includes asthma, bronchitis, carbon monoxide toxicity, and cyanide toxicity.

Therapeutic Interventions

Remove the patient from the environment and administer oxygen. Intubation may be necessary for ventilatory support and airway protection. Treat bronchoconstriction if present with a bronchodilator. Treat for pulmonary edema if present per protocol.

Patient and Family Education

Emergency responders are in a unique position to educate local farmers regarding the importance of choosing and wearing appropriate PPE. Emergency workers are required to recognize a hazardous environment, determine what hazards need to be protected against, and how to be protected from those specific hazards. This education is valuable to farmers as well.

Scene Size-Up Considerations

If you are responding to a silo incident, determine the following:

- What is the crop inside the silo?
- When was the last load put into the silo? If within 3 weeks, assume silo gas is present until you can rule it out.
- How full is the silo?
- How long was the victim inside?
- How is the silo unloaded?
- Is the power to the silo unloader shut off? Lock this out or post a person to ensure no one turns it on.
- Can the silo blower be turned on? How long has it been on? The blower will be effective at ventilating the space if the silo is at least two thirds full (Figure 53-18).
- Can the victim be seen from the loading platform at the top of the silo?
- If so, is he or she trapped in the unloading machinery?
- Do we have the training, skills, and equipment to enter this confined space? If not, where will the appropriate responders be dispatched from?

If you are responding to a manure storage incident, determine the following:

- Has the farmer been agitating the manure pit? Many modern livestock facilities have manure storage areas under the barn; thus the inside of the building can technically contain high levels of hydrogen sulfide and/or methane gas. Emergency crews should use a gas detector to ensure the environment is safe before entry.
- Is ventilation of the space possible? If so, use intrinsically safe ventilation equipment. Quantities of methane gas present may be explosive.

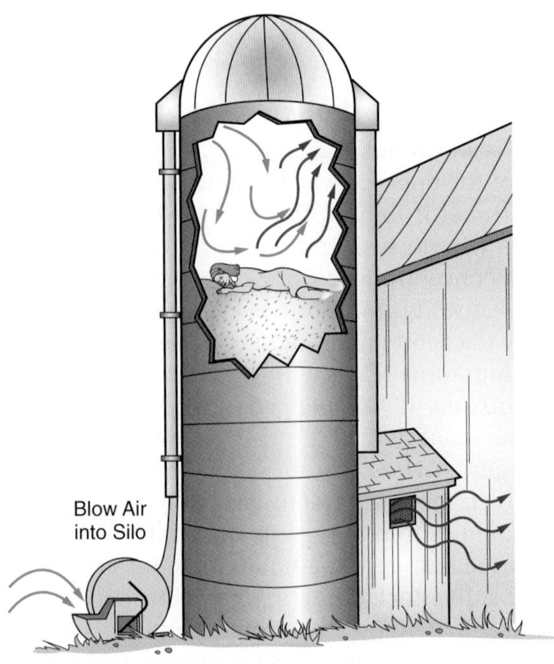

Figure 53-18 Ventilating a confined space may help make the space safer.

- Is the power to any submerged pumps turned off? Lock this power out or station a person to ensure no one turns it on.
- Do we have the training, skills, and equipment to enter this confined space? If not, where will the appropriate responders be dispatched from? Many livestock housing facilities have limited entry and exit doorways and are technically considered confined spaces.

PARAMEDIC*Pearl*

Encourage the patient, especially if he or she is exhibiting mild symptoms and refuses treatment, to seek medical attention. Pulmonary edema can ensue several hours later and, if left untreated, lead to asphyxia and respiratory arrest.

Case Scenario SUMMARY

1. *What is your initial impression of the patient?* Your initial impression may include an acute medical condition leading to pulmonary edema. Differential diagnoses included heart failure, toxic gas inhalation, Paraquat poisoning, pneumonitis, and toxic organic dust syndrome.
2. *What additional information do you need to complete your assessment?* Additional information needed includes a head-to-toe assessment and a detailed SAMPLE history. You should ask about recent exposure to manure, silage, dust, and other toxins, especially any exposure that may have occurred within the last 24 to 90 hours.
3. *What may be causing the man's respiratory distress?* Pulmonary edema may be caused by any number of factors. However, because of the limited information, age of the patient, and occupation, you should suspect inhalation of a toxic agent.
4. *Has your first impression changed?* The initial impression may be changed by the additional information. Ruling out an acute myocardial infarction is possible because of the additional information.
5. *What conditions might cause delayed-onset pulmonary edema in this patient?* Pulmonary edema may have a delayed onset in patients exposed to toxins commonly found in a farm environment. These toxins include NOx from silage, hydrogen sulfide (manure gas), ammonia, carbon monoxide, and cyanide. Detailed questioning of the patient and his activities can identify exposure to such toxins.
6. *What additional assessment and treatment options for the patient should be considered?* Additional information needed includes a detailed history of recent events to identify exposure to toxins and the length of exposure to any toxin. Details should extend back over the past several days (up to 90 or more hours). In addition, if the patient had a recent episode of pulmonary edema or respiratory distress, the current episode may be a relapse.
7. *What is your final impression of the patient?* Based on the detailed recent history of cleaning a silo, the final impression of the man's condition is silo filler's disease.
8. *What treatment options are available for this patient?* Prehospital care consists of ventilatory support, supplemental oxygen, and IV access. Bronchodilators may be needed to enhance the patient's ability to breathe. Be prepared to intubate the patient if needed.
9. *What patient and family education should be provided?* Because the man and his wife recently acquired the farm, they should be advised to understand the hazards associated with farming, including silo filler's disease. If livestock are present, additional hazards may be encountered about which the farmer and his family must be advised.

Chapter Summary

- Managing emergencies on a farm often requires modified procedures and protocols.
- Most farms use at least one tractor daily, and tractor overturns result in half of all farm deaths.
- Crush injury syndrome is a condition that can be seen in farm trauma situations because of the length of time a person often is entrapped.
- Numerous hazard points on farm machines can cause a severe entanglement that can challenge even seasoned rescue technicians.
- Power take-off entanglements can result in severe crushing injuries and acute amputations.
- Hydraulic oil pressure is normally 2000 psi but can exceed 7000 psi through a pinhole leak. Under this

pressure, the fluid can easily penetrate the skin and cause serious complications.

- A host of hazardous materials are present on farms to which farmers, their families, and employees can be exposed. Some of the materials are derivatives of nerve agents.
- Many areas on farms are considered confined spaces by OSHA definition. Although the majority of farmers are exempt from OSHA inspections, emergency responders must recognize confined spaces and follow OSHA confined space standards when managing these emergencies.
- Emergency responders must recognize the potential for deadly gases generated inside silos and manure storage because they may respond to calls involving these aspects of farming.

REFERENCES

Centers for Disease Control and Prevention. (2003). *Facts about Paraquat, CDC chemical emergencies fact sheet,* Atlanta, GA: Centers for Disease Control and Prevention.

de Silva, H. J., Wijewickrema, R., & Senanayake, N. (1992). Does pralidoxime affect outcome of management in acute organophosphorus poisoning? *Lancet 339,* 1136-1138.

Flotre, M. (1992). High-pressure injection injuries of the hand. *American Family Physician, 45*(5), 2230-2234.

Hard, D. L., Myers, J. R., & Gerberich, S. G. (2002). Traumatic injuries in agriculture. *Journal of Agricultural Safety and Health, V8*(1), 51-65.

James, P. B. (1994). Hyperbaric oxygen treatment for crush injury. *British Medical Journal, 309*(6967), 1513.

Mandavia, S. (2005). *Toxicity, hydrogen sulfide.* Retrieved March 15, 2006, from http://www.emedicine.com/EMERG/topic258.htm.

National Ag Safety Database. (2002). *Oxides of nitrogen ("silo gas").* Retrieved February 19, 2007, from http://www.cdc.gov/nasd/docs/d001501-d001600/d001505/d001505.html.

Wallace, S., & Smith, D. G. (2003). *Compartment syndrome, upper extremity.* Retrieved March 15, 2006, from http://www.emedicine.com/orthoped/topic55.htm.

SUGGESTED RESOURCES

Managing Agricultural Emergencies, Penn State University: http://www.farmemergencies.psu.edu

National Ag Safety Database: http://www.cdc.gov/nasd

Chapter Quiz

1. Which of the following are involved in the majority of deaths and serious injuries on farms?
- **a.** Cattle and swine
- **b.** Chemicals and fertilizers
- **c.** Silos and manure storages
- **d.** Tractors and machines

2. A major contributing factor in high death rates from tractor overturns is/are ______.
- **a.** chemicals being involved
- **b.** overturning in muddy conditions
- **c.** size of the implement being towed
- **d.** the overturn not being immediately discovered

3. The condition caused by a severe compressive injury to muscles resulting in muscle cell death is called ______.
- **a.** compartment syndrome
- **b.** compressive cell syndrome
- **c.** crush syndrome
- **d.** myocardial infarction

4. Managing a patient with crushing injuries should be handled ______.
- **a.** always as a rapid extrication
- **b.** never as a rapid extrication
- **c.** as a rapid extrication if entrapment has been less than 1 hour
- **d.** as a rapid extrication if entrapment involves a large muscle mass that has been entrapped for 4 hours

5. The mainstay of treatment for crush syndrome is ______.
- **a.** insulin and glucose
- **b.** IV fluid
- **c.** furosemide
- **d.** rapid extrication

6. Energy is transferred from a tractor to an implement by a rotating shaft called a(n) ______.
- **a.** hydraulic shaft
- **b.** implement driveshaft
- **c.** power take-off shaft
- **d.** tractor driveshaft

7. A pesticide is ______.
- **a.** a chemical that stops or controls the effects of a poison
- **b.** a chemical that neutralizes or counteracts the effects of a harmful substance
- **c.** a material designed to kill every host
- **d.** a substance that prevents, repels, or destroys the growth of an unwanted host.

8. A patient with diarrhea, excessive urination, pinpoint pupils, bronchospasm, emesis, lacrimation, and excessive salivation has most likely been exposed to ______.
- **a.** fertilizer material
- **b.** organophosphate chemicals
- **c.** manure gas
- **d.** Paraquat herbicide

9. True or false: If a farmer is exempt from following OSHA confined space standards when entering a silo, emergency responders also are exempt for entering that same silo for emergency purposes.

10. The condition created when a person has been exposed to silo gas is called ______.
    a. silo filler's disease
    b. silo gas disease
    c. silo unloader's disease
    d. toxic organic syndrome

11. Silo gas is produced from fermenting silage inside a silo and typically is present inside a silo for approximately ______.
    a. 2 hours after the silo is filled
    b. 2 days after the silo is filled
    c. 2 weeks after the silo is filled
    d. 2 months after the silo is filled

12. The gas that smells like rotten eggs is ______.
    a. ammonia
    b. hydrogen sulfide
    c. nitrogen dioxide
    d. methane

Terminology

Acetylcholinesterase A body chemical that stops the action of acetylcholine (a neurotransmitter involved in the stimulation of nerves).

Bronchospasm Constriction or narrowing of the airway.

Cholinesterase inhibitor A chemical that blocks the action of acetylcholinesterase; thus the neurotransmitter acetylcholine is allowed to send its signals continuously to innervate nerve endings.

Compartment syndrome A condition caused by swelling of the muscle tissue inside its fascial tissue compartment; blood flow in or out of the muscle tissues is disrupted, which causes severe pain and muscle damage; can be caused by a machinery entrapment.

Conventional silo A vertical structure used to store ensiled plant material in a aerobic environment.

Crush syndrome Condition that results when entrapment causes muscle cell death from a lack of oxygen.

Crush points Formed when two objects are moving toward each other or when one object is moving toward a stationary object and the gap between the two is decreasing.

Emesis Vomiting.

"First on the Scene" program An educational program that teaches people what to do and what not to do when they come upon an injury emergency.

Hydraulic injection injuries High-pressure fluid that leaks from hydraulic hoses and is injected into the body.

Hydrogen sulfide A hazardous gas produced by the decomposition of organic material prevalent when manure is stored in a liquid form for an extended period.

Hypersensitivity pneumonitis Inflammation in and around the tiny air sacs (alveoli) and smallest airways (bronchioles) of the lung caused by an allergic reaction to inhaled organic dusts or, less commonly, chemicals; also called *extrinsic allergic alveolitis, allergic interstitial pneumonitis,* or *organic dust pneumoconiosis.*

Lacrimation Tearing of the eyes.

Manure gas A name used for several different gases formed by decomposition of manure (methane, carbon dioxide, ammonia, hydrogen sulfide, and hydrogen disulfide); in certain concentrations, all are toxic to animals and human beings.

Miosis Pinpoint pupils.

Oxygen-limiting silo A vertical structure used to store ensiled plant material in an anaerobic environment.

Pesticide A substance that prevents, repels, or destroys an unwanted host.

Pinch points A machinery entanglement hazard formed when two machine parts move together and at least one of the parts moves in a circle.

power take-off (PTO) A tractor component that connects the tractor to a driveshaft that powers an implement.

Pull-in point Machinery entanglement hazard created when an operator attempts to remove material being pulled into a machine.

Rollover protective structure (ROPS) A structure mounted on a tractor designed to support the weight of the tractor if a tractor overturn occurs; if a tractor has a ROPS and the operator wears a seat belt, the

Terminology—continued

operator will stay in the safety zone if the tractor overturns.

Shear points Hazardous machinery locations created when the edges of two objects are moved toward or next to one another closely enough to cut a relatively soft material.

Silo gas The gases (NOx) produced from the fermentation of plant material inside a silo.

Stored energy Any energy (e.g., mechanical, electrical, hydraulic, compressed air) that has the potential of being released either intentionally or inadvertently, causing further injury or problems.

Toxic organic dust syndrome A flulike illness caused by the inhalation of grain dust, with symptoms including fever, chest tightness, cough, and muscle aches; inhalation may occur in an agricultural setting or from covering a floor with a material such as straw.

Wrap point A machinery entanglement hazard formed when any machine component rotates.

CHAPTER 54

Wilderness EMS

Objectives

After completing this chapter, you will be able to:

1. Define and describe wilderness medicine and wilderness EMS.
2. Define and describe a wilderness EMS system.
3. Describe the differences in practice environments between traditional EMS and wilderness EMS.
4. Describe the differences in protocols between traditional EMS and wilderness EMS.
5. Describe the differences in certification and training between traditional EMS and wilderness EMS.
6. Demonstrate techniques used to clear a cervical spine clinically in a wilderness setting.
7. Describe the differences in equipment between traditional EMS and wilderness EMS.
8. Describe the differences in resources between traditional EMS and wilderness EMS.
9. Describe the differences in team interfaces between traditional EMS and wilderness EMS.
10. Identify current wilderness EMS systems in the United States.
11. Identify challenges facing wilderness EMS systems.

Chapter Outline

Case Scenario

A wealthy landowner recently donated hundreds of acres to the state with the intention it would become a state park. The land is now owned by the state, but it has not yet been developed. Signs have been posted stating that the land will become a park but that it is not yet developed or managed by the state. The state has asked that county agencies manage emergencies on the land, and you run the rescue division of the local EMS rescue squad. Until now your operations primarily have involved vehicle rescue, but many of your members have expressed an interest in branching out into other technical rescue and wilderness rescue operations. The acreage includes a prime rock climbing area and a large lake that until now has been inaccessible to the public. Although the area is not yet formally opened, you know that many locals have already begun climbing there.

Questions

1. *What agencies could you contact to discuss management of this area and potential situations there?*
2. *What equipment will your rescue squad need to consider purchasing?*
3. *What additional training should your members consider obtaining?*

WILDERNESS MEDICINE

[OBJECTIVE 1]

Wilderness medicine is a term with a variety of definitions. According to the Wilderness Medical Society (WMS), wilderness medicine "focuses on medical problems and treatment in remote environments . . . [including] aspects of physiology, clinical medicine, preventive medicine, and public health" (WMS, 2007). This statement suggests that wilderness medicine is defined by location. However, other authorities note that medical management in a city after an earthquake or during an ice storm closely resembles management in remote environments (National Association of Emergency Medical Technicians, 2007). Some conditions considered part of wilderness medicine occur more frequently in urban (e.g., hypothermia, heat illness) and suburban (e.g., lightning strikes, submersion injury) locations

(WMS, 2007). Some authors suggest wilderness medical care is defined by time or distance, such as initial care delivered more than 1 hour from comprehensive care. However, the definition of comprehensive care itself is fluid, and what is considered comprehensive care in a developing country might be considered wilderness in a developed country.

Wilderness medicine and *wilderness medical care* therefore are terms that must be used contextually. For the purposes of this text, wilderness medicine is medical management in situations where care and prevention are limited by environmental considerations, prolonged extrication, and/or resource availability.

Note that specifics of wilderness medical techniques and environmental emergencies are addressed in Chapter 52. Specifics of technical wilderness rescue, including high-angle rescue, low-angle rescue, swift water rescue, litter rigging, extrication techniques, and other specific skills and equipment are addressed in Chapter 63.

One categorization scheme applicable to EMS divides clinical wilderness medicine into four categories: (1) recreational, (2) professional, (3) expedition, and (4) disaster medicine (Russell, 2004).

The recreational model applies when a wilderness EMS–trained individual comes upon a patient or is injured himself or herself while recreating and provides care. The considerations for unexpected volunteer care such as this are discussed in more detail in Chapter 52.

The professional model applies when an individual or group plans to administer care in an austere environment and is called on to perform these duties when needed. This is a **wilderness EMS system** and is the main topic of this chapter. Note that providers in the professional model may be paid or volunteer despite the term *professional*.

The expedition model involves the imbedding of a wilderness medical care provider within an expedition and is beyond the scope of this textbook.

The disaster medicine model involves the creation of a wilderness EMS system specifically trained for insertion into a disaster environment to provide care. This topic is covered in more detail in Chapter 66.

Military and tactical field medicine (described in more detail in Chapter 65) also has obvious overlaps with wilderness medicine and operates in a similar environment of austere resources. Ultimately, disaster and military and tactical medicine share enough similarities (out-of-hospital care, prolonged patient care, austere or hostile environment, minimal resources, delay to comprehensive care) to sometimes be considered within a greater wilderness medicine framework, but are different enough in critical ways to deserve their own attention as separate topics (Sholl & Curcio, 2004).

WILDERNESS EMS

Some individuals choose to obtain training in wilderness medical care, whether for reasons of personal education, volunteer service, or professional duties. This training often includes U.S. Department of Transportation (DOT)–endorsed EMS certification with additional wilderness modules, creating certifications such as **wilderness first responder** and **wilderness emergency medical technician.** However, the DOT does not recognize the additional wilderness modules, and no national consensus exists on curriculum or certification standards such as exist for the core first responder and emergency medical technician certificates. Other certifications have appeared that augment other medical degrees and certifications, such as **wilderness first aid** and **wilderness command physician.**

Throughout this process individual organizations, responding to a consumer demand, have created a diverse range of certifications and curricula that can be considered wilderness EMS despite the absence of a widely accepted governing body consensus on content or standards. Some standardization attempts have been made. WMS has developed curriculum guidelines for general prehospital wilderness medical care (Otten et al., 1991) and a suggested minimal level of training for wilderness first aid certification (Lindsey et al., 1999). At least one organization, the Wilderness EMS Institute (WEMSI), has been formed that is solely devoted to wilderness EMS topics. WEMSI created public domain curricula in the 1980s intended to be widely adopted as a standard and are unique in being freely available (Johnson, 2004). However, widespread acceptance has not yet occurred. The Rural Affairs Committee of the National Association of EMS Physicians published guidelines describing wilderness EMS treatments that differed from traditional EMS (Goth & Garnett, 1993). These guidelines addressed cardiopulmonary arrest, dislocations, spine injury, and wounds, and although their recommendations are now widely accepted they represent only a small portion of a comprehensive curriculum. Although each of these sources represents a contribution to an emerging and complex standard of care, so far no comprehensive EMS-specific collection or governing body has emerged. Of note, some authorities suggest that nothing is different about wilderness EMS that requires separate standards or that too much regional variation exists to establish national standards (Johnson, 2004). Others argue that mortality rates would not be expected to change as a result of upgrading wilderness EMS operations (Goodman et al., 2001). These perspectives have been forcefully and directly repudiated by wilderness EMS advocates (Johnson, 2004).

One expected landmark in the evolution of wilderness EMS as a field would be national standardization or collective endorsement of curricula and certifications. Models exist for this on the state level. Alaska has specific state protocols addressing wilderness EMS operations (Johnson, 2004). Maine and Maryland officially recognize wilderness medical certifications in their EMS structure (Maine Emergency Medical Services, 2005; Maryland Institute for Emergency Medical Services Systems, 2007). Other states, including Washington, New Mexico, and

North Carolina, have some level of formal wilderness EMS approval (Johnson, 2004). National standardization might reasonably be expected to develop from individual or collective action of WEMSI, the DOT, WMS, the National Association of EMS Physicians, the National Association of EMTs (NAEMT), or the Wilderness Medicine Section of the American College of Emergency Physicians. In Europe, the Union Internationale des Associations d'Alpinisme (International Union of Alpine Associations) has standardized postgraduate mountain medicine training for physicians, allowing for a standardized European certification in the mountain medicine branch of wilderness medicine. Of note, European wilderness EMS also places a more prominent role on physician participation.

Wilderness EMS involves the training and background of individual providers and also defines a particular subfield of EMS operations. When should an EMS scene be considered a wilderness EMS scene? As previously discussed, the answer is contextual and depends on local protocols and resources. However, NAEMT suggests that the following elements should be considered in defining wilderness EMS activities (NAEMT, 2007):

- Access to the scene
- Weather
- Daylight
- Terrain
- Special transport and handling needs
- Access and transport times
- Available personnel
- Communications

WILDERNESS EMS SYSTEMS

[OBJECTIVE 2]

Some regions, recognizing the prevalence of environmental emergencies and a regular need for wilderness medical care in their area, have developed wilderness EMS systems. A wilderness EMS system is a formally structured organization, integrated into or part of the standard EMS system, that is configured to provide wilderness medical care to a discrete region or activity. Some systems are created by groups of organizations working together; many, if not most, wilderness EMS personnel are volunteers (Russell, 2004).

Wilderness EMS Systems versus Traditional ("Street") Systems

Standards of care and appropriate practice can differ significantly depending on resources, training, and setting. EMS standards of care differ for different levels of training, from a first responder to a physician. However, the standard of care for the same level of training may change in different settings, such as an urban critical care unit, a rural volunteer EMS service, a remote third-world village, or an alpine expedition. Language sometimes hinders the ability to communicate these differences, as does the fact that these differences are contextual and subjective (no strict definition exists regarding when street care ends and wilderness care begins). This becomes problematic when a system tries to implement different practices for different environments. Simply in terms of language, care that uses wilderness protocols may be referred to as *delayed care, prolonged care, backcountry care, remote care, extended care, isolated care, wilderness care, special operations care, atypical care, mountain medicine, rural care, expedition medicine,* or *search and rescue care.* Care not provided in these environments can be termed *street care, traditional care, urban care,* or *standard care.* For the purposes of terminology, the simplest answer is to label the former practice environments *wilderness EMS* and the latter *traditional EMS.* Wilderness EMS also may overlap into other specialty EMS activities, such as disaster care, military care, or tactical EMS care.

Agencies that operate wilderness and traditional protocols in parallel should have clearly defined mechanisms for clarifying if a mission is considered wilderness EMS or traditional EMS because the differences have potential protocol and medicolegal consequences.

A patient care encounter defined as a wilderness EMS operation usually involves one or more of the following differences from traditional EMS operations.

Differences in Practice Environment

[OBJECTIVE 3]

Wilderness EMS operations may require caregivers to operate in austere or dangerous environments. These environmental considerations may alter expected duration of care, type of care, and transport decisions. For example, consider an otherwise healthy patient who fractures her ankle on a winter day at 6 PM after taking a misstep on a city sidewalk curb 10 minutes from a trauma center. Imagine how different the same patient's care would be if she sustained the same fracture at the same time of day and in the same season after a misstep on a trail edge 4 miles into a trail system and rolling 20 feet down a gulley (without further injury). The only characteristic that has changed is the environment, and yet this single feature turns a routine call into a complex EMS operation involving multiple personnel, additional equipment, and high-level medical decision making. It requires the insertion of personnel and limited equipment 4 miles into an austere environment. Personnel must have training to provide low-angle technical rescue, potential extended treatment and prevention of hypothermia, and management of conditions unfamiliar to rapid urban transport such as toileting needs and prevention of pressure sores.

In addition to patient care considerations, differences in practice environment require additional training for the providers to remain safe. The ability to care for themselves and their team, not just patients, is critically important for wilderness EMS providers. EMS providers on a wilderness rescue team must be self-sufficient and safe or they are more of a hindrance than a help. In this example alone, basic survival skills, hypothermia prevention, personal cold weather gear, water and food, map and compass skills, land and water navigation skills, communications equipment capable of remote access (including possibly satellite phone or the ability to operate for prolonged periods without communicability) and possibly **all-terrain vehicle (ATV)** or snowmobile operation skills would be required to keep the providers safe while operating in an austere winter environment. The core survival skills required for wilderness activities (including wilderness EMS response) often are identified as the 10 essentials (Box 54-1). Wilderness EMS providers must never leave the road without these in mind, or they are a danger to themselves and the team's mission success. This example clearly demonstrates that a simple EMS call in a traditional setting can become a complex extended operation simply by changing the practice environment.

Numerous other examples of wilderness EMS practice environments would raise unfamiliar issues for traditional EMS providers and systems. Such activities include caving, mountaineering and alpine sports, scuba diving, boating on open water, swift water sports, climbing, trail activities (e.g., hiking, ATVs, snowmobiling, cross-country skiing, biking, horseback riding), rock climbing in high-angle environments, and countless others. The skills involved in rescue and medical care in any of these environments are a necessary part of a related wilderness EMS operation. In addition, as previously noted, some wilderness EMS activities require training more typically found in disaster EMS, tactical EMS, and military EMS.

Wilderness EMS systems typically prepare their caregivers to perform in these environments by providing alternative protocols and additional training.

BOX 54-1 Ten Essentials for Rescuer Safety

1. Attitude: Positive belief that you can make things better and the will to survive
2. Food: High-carbohydrate foods that require no preparation or can be made into a drink
3. Water: (a) General rule: 2 L/day if not active, up to 3 L/day if active (and more if local climate is hot and dry); (b) ability to purify water
4. Clothing: (a) Warm clothing that retains heat even if wet (usually wool or synthetics, not cotton); (b) waterproof raingear: top, bottom, and shoes
5. Shelter: Commercial shelter on person or ability to improvise shelter with materials at hand
6. Warmth/fire: Ability to boil water and build a fire with materials at hand or on person
7. Navigation: Map and compass skills, route-findings skills, headlamp and flashlight (at least two light sources during night operations)
8. Weather awareness: Basic understanding of weather patterns and knowledge of how to react to severe weather (including lightning and floods)
9. Signaling: Whistle, preferably plastic without ball; possibly a mirror; extra fully charged battery if carrying radio or other two-way communication device
10. First aid kit

Modified from Hubbell, F. C. (2007). Wilderness emergency medical services and response systems. In P. Auerbach (Ed.). *Wilderness medicine* (5th ed.) (pp. 694-707). St. Louis: Mosby.

Differences in Protocols

[OBJECTIVES 4, 5, 6]

Although some wilderness EMS systems provide intensive on-line or scene-based medical direction or allow providers to develop innovative practices, most choose to address the unique challenges of wilderness care by providing additional protocols. Debate exists regarding how to best prepare and supervise wilderness EMS providers. Some authorities argue for implementation of explicit and carefully designed protocols and on-line command, and others contend that well-trained providers can improvise and require on-line command only for consultation (Conover, 2006; Johnson, 2006). The most robust systems prepare caregivers to implement atypical and advanced skills by using offline protocols but also build in a certain degree of flexibility and provide online direction to account for the dynamic nature of wilderness EMS operations. Examples of atypical or advanced skills as well as other differences in wilderness EMS protocols and medical direction are described in the following sections.

Cervical Spine Clearance. One of the hallmark deviations of wilderness EMS from traditional EMS practice is the option to clear a cervical spine of injury. This practice has been advocated by experts and introduced into several wilderness EMS systems (Russell, 2004; Conover, 1992). (Note that some authorities advocate avoiding the term *clearance* because of the provider's inability to rule out cervical injury definitively. They would suggest terms such as *focused spinal examination* or *spinal injury risk assessment.* However, for simplicity of language and because the wilderness EMS provider is in fact clearing the spine of injury for the purposes of prehospital management, the term is used here. Be advised that in some systems other terminology is recommended.)

Avoiding the full spinal immobilization required in a traditional EMS system can dramatically simplify a wilderness EMS operation involving extrication. Most protocols of this sort use the NEXUS (National Emergency X-Radiography Utilization Study) criteria (Panacek et al., 2001), which were developed for hospital-based emergency physicians to clarify when radiographs could be avoided in trauma patients. Many local versions of cervical spine clearance protocols exist, and some states have adopted such protocols even for their traditional EMS providers. An example of a cervical spine clearance protocol is provided in Box 54-2.

Patient Packaging and Waste Elimination. Immobilized trauma patients in traditional EMS systems are rapidly transported to an emergency department. In wilderness EMS systems, patients may require immobilization for

BOX 54-2 Wilderness Cervical Spine Clearance

The following criteria are used to assess if a patient's spine can be clinically cleared in the field. The patient must be assessed for:

Intoxication
Neurologic deficit
Distracting Injury
Altered level of consciousness/mental status
Neck and back pain or tenderness

If none of these conditions is present, the patient has a negative examination result. If one or more of the conditions are present, the patient has a positive examination result. Patients with a mechanism for potential spinal injury and a positive examination result must have their spines immobilized. Spinal immobilization in all other patients is optional.

Spinal stabilization should be considered for severe neck or back pain regardless of mechanism. Environment and extrication factors should be considered in this decision and medical direction consulted if possible.

No spinal clearance practices should be routinely implemented by employees or volunteers in an EMS system unless permitted to do so by on-line or off-line medical direction.

Modified from Hawkins, S. C. (2007). Spinal injury. In *Burke County EMS special operations protocols* (p. 18). Morganton, NC: Burke County Emergency Medical Services.

hours or even days. Many baskets and transport systems are available for wilderness medical applications. Stokes baskets (Figure 54-1) are one of the most common versions currently in use.

Severe pain and pressure ulcers can develop within 90 minutes of unpadded immobilization unless the patient is permitted, and helped, to move from side to side in the litter (NAEMT, 2007; Chan et al., 1994; Linares et al., 1987; Mawson et al., 1988; Delbridge et al., 1993). If a patient is spinally immobilized and significant movement is impossible, a full-body vacuum splint or vacuum mattress is preferable to a long backboard, and leg movement should be permitted to prevent deep venous thrombi (NAEMT, 2007). Padding should be carefully placed to eliminate voids and spaces where skin can rub against the backboard or basket.

The patient should be allowed to urinate and defecate as needed and with dignity. Discussing the management strategy for these needs with the patient early in the extrication process may minimize embarrassment and confusion regarding how such needs should be addressed (and also prevent skin breakdown and ruined insulation layers). If the patient is truly spinally immobilized, pads can be placed underneath the pelvis and careful cleaning will be required. Both men and women can urinate while in a Stokes basket if it is turned upright; women may require a small funnel device available commercially in backpacking supply outlets (Figure 54-2).

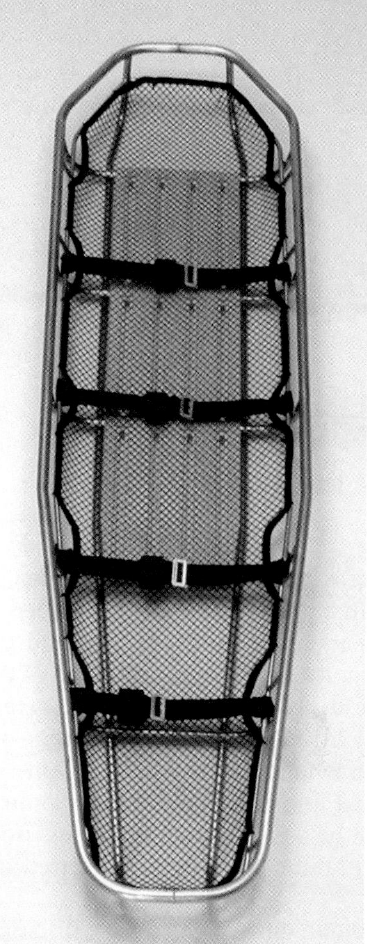

Figure 54-1 When using a basket litter, remember first to stabilize the patient's spine with padding and a long spine board.

Patients who are immobilized should also receive protection from the elements (e.g., insulation against cold, removal of insulating factors in heat, sunscreen and eye protection in direct sun). Extended extrications should also account for food and water needs of the patient (who by virtue of illness or injury may be more susceptible to heat illness, hypothermia, and dehydration) as well as providers.

Chapter 63 more completely describes the rigging and use of baskets and litters in wilderness medical operations.

Scope of Care. In both wilderness EMS and disaster EMS settings, scope of care may be expanded to address the fact that transfer to comprehensive care may be delayed. Expanded scope of care in wilderness settings may include medications (e.g., antibiotics, steroidal medications) and interventions (e.g., reduction of dislocations, suturing) that can temporize or reverse a condition that might otherwise be detrimental to a patient if managed by traditional EMS practices.

Traditional areas of care are sometimes expanded in wilderness EMS. For example, intravenous (IV) access and hydration are core skills for traditional EMS. However,

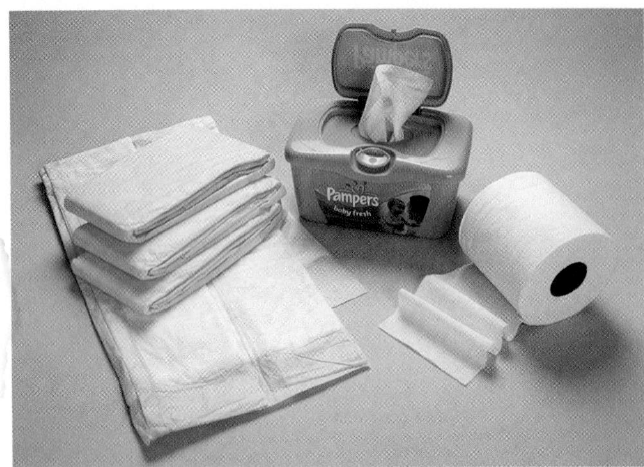

Figure 54-2 Elimination supplies.

little training is provided regarding managing fluids and electrolytes in a patient for a prolonged period. In wilderness EMS operations, which may extend over hours or even days, traditional EMS management of IV fluids could be counterproductive or dangerous in an extended medical care setting. In addition, the mechanics of IV maintenance in the wilderness may be different. Ways to keep fluids warmed and solution flowing, sometimes against gravity, must be considered. Use of pressure bags or fluid bolus with a saline lock may be preferred to continuous infusion.

Medical Direction. As previously discussed, opinions differ regarding medical direction of wilderness EMS providers. Online physician direction is cumbersome, labor intensive for physicians, unavailable for many systems without access to a physician trained in wilderness EMS, and potentially dangerous if operations depend on communication tools that may be unreliable in wilderness settings. Certification as a wilderness command physician is available in annual courses run by WEMSI, which trains physicians to provide online medical direction for wilderness EMS operations. Numerous wilderness medicine electives offered by universities can prepare physicians for the decision making required in wilderness medical settings. Commercially available wilderness medical certifications geared toward mid- and upper-level providers also are available. These include Wilderness Advanced Life Support offered by Wilderness Medical Associates (WMA); Upgrade for Medical Professional, offered by the Wilderness Medicine Institute of the National Outdoor Leadership School (NOLS); and Advanced Wilderness Life Support offered by the University of Utah. Such courses can orient medical control physicians to wilderness EMS care, although none specifically trains them in online wilderness EMS medical direction.

Offline physician and leadership direction (in the form of protocols) ensures uniformity of practice and perhaps medicolegal protection and requires less time commitment for a physician. However, it may not be capable of addressing the dynamic and diverse challenges involved in wilderness EMS operations. More than 95% of rescues are performed without a physician present (Hubbell, 2007b) and the majority are performed without on-line physician direction, making protocolized care the more common approach to wilderness medical direction.

Training wilderness EMS personnel in general principles and skills and then encouraging them to apply these to specific operational challenges permits the innovation and flexibility that is the hallmark of austere medical care, but may raise medicolegal and quality issues. This approach may be most reasonable for systems that draw from multiple organizations or are entirely volunteer-based. Intensive training of a small group of providers and exhaustive postmission reviews can address quality and medicolegal concerns to some extent and provide some needed standardization of approach. Clearly the ideal wilderness EMS system draws from all these models to ensure quality care and medicolegal protection.

Of note, private guiding businesses sometimes individually contract with physicians to act as medical advisors for their guides. Many times the guides are required to have wilderness EMS certifications. These relationships and providers are independent of EMS systems and vary widely regarding quality control and protocols. Several authorities in wilderness EMS publish sample protocols that can prove useful to physicians and organizations considering such relationships.

Differences in Certification and Training

[OBJECTIVE 5]

Providers typically obtain additional training to implement the alternative protocols and interventions that characterize wilderness EMS care. Traditional providers cannot simply be inserted into wilderness EMS settings; they require extensive additional training, equipment, and logistical support.

Much of the additional training is done in-house by wilderness EMS systems, but many encourage or require more formal certification or training. Formal wilderness EMS courses have become more common; currently more than half a million people in the United States are estimated to have some sort of certificate training in wilderness EMS (Hubbell, 2007b). As previously noted, at the governmental regulatory level only a few states recognize any type of wilderness EMS certification.

Stonehearth Outdoor Learning Opportunities (SOLO), founded in 1974, was probably the first commercial school to provide formal wilderness medical training on a regular basis and as their sole focus and the first to build a campus dedicated to this subspecialty (Hubbell, 2007a). WMA was incorporated a short time later, in 1978. The Wilderness Medicine Institute (WMI) originally formed as a western branch of SOLO in Colorado but then became an independent school. More recently, WMI was incorporated into the NOLS and is now WMI of NOLS. Currently, WMA, SOLO, and WMI of NOLS produce the commercial curricula most often used for wilderness EMS certification. Many other organizations offer their own certifications in wilderness medicine.

In another model independent schools—such as Landmark Learning, college training programs, and experiential education schools—offer independently marketed courses that result in certification by WMA, SOLO, or WMI of NOLS. As noted, WEMSI also offers an alternative model of a public domain curriculum that can be used without cost by independent programs and that result in WEMSI certification.

Multiple sources are therefore available for wilderness EMS–related certifications. In the absence of certifying bodies, consumers should carefully look at the quality and reputation of a sponsoring organization before pursuing certification offered by them. Consumers typically obtain certification in one of the following categories:

- Wilderness first aid
- Wilderness first responder
- Wilderness EMT
- Wilderness command physician
- Wilderness advanced life support/advanced wilderness life support
- Basic disaster life support
- Advanced disaster life support

Box 54-3 contains a partial list of vendors and institutions offering wilderness EMS–related certifications and courses. The Suggested Resources at the end of this chapter lists Web sites for these vendors and institutions.

New Opportunities in Wilderness EMS Training and Certification. The Academy of Wilderness Medicine, a WMS project, now offers a fellowship certification in wilderness medicine to all levels of medical providers who meet required criteria (Academy of Wilderness Medicine, 2007). In 2003 Stanford University developed the world's first postresidency wilderness medicine fellowship training program for physicians (Stanford School of Medicine, 2007). A number of family practice residencies, including the Montana Family Medicine Residency (2007), Marshall University Family Practice Residency Program (2007), and the Central Maine Medical Center Family Practice Residency (Freda, 2004) offer formal tracks in wilderness medicine for their residents. Western Carolina University (Cullowhee, NC) is developing a wilderness medicine track within its emergency medical care bachelor of science degree program, which would be the first paramedic-specific wilderness medical training program in the United States and the first wilderness medical training program providing an academic degree for paramedical providers (Hubble, 2006). Landmark Learning, a school that traditionally teaches wilderness EMS, is now offering **relief medic** training and certification to students already certified as wilderness EMTs or wilderness first responders (Landmark Learning, 2007).

BOX 54-3 Institutions Offering Commercial or Public Wilderness Medical Training

- Adirondack Wilderness Medicine
- Aerie Backcountry Medicine
- American Safety & Health Institute (Wilderness Emergency Care Program)
- APT Antincendio
- Argentine Rescue and First Aid School
- CDS Outdoors, Inc.
- Divers Alert Network
- Landmark Learning
- MedicalOfficer.Net, Ltd.
- Medic Response Safety
- Mountain Aid Training International
- National Disaster Life Support Foundation
- National Ski Patrol
- Rescue Specialists
- Stonehearth Open Learning Opportunities
- UCSF-Fresno Parkmedic Program
- University of Utah
- Wilderness Emergency Care
- Wilderness EMS Institute
- Wilderness Medical Associates
- Wilderness Medical Society
- Wilderness Medicine Institute
- Wilderness Medicine Outfitters
- Wilderness Medicine Training Center
- Wilderness Safety Council

Organization web sites are listed in the Suggested Resources section of this chapter.

Differences in Equipment

[OBJECTIVE 7]

Wilderness EMS operations require familiarity with and access to equipment more typically associated with fire or rescue operations rather than traditional EMS care. This may include ATVs and snowmobiles (both operational and rescue training), helicopters, high-angle climbing and safety equipment, technical ropes (with associated knot and rigging training), boats (swift water, open water, and/or maritime), swift water rescue equipment, and hiking equipment (including packs, footwear, clothing, and hydration and nutrition gear and materials). Patient treatment and transport equipment also may be different and include stokes baskets, litter wheels, rescue sleds, and other tools not typically required in traditional EMS operations.

More detailed technical information regarding specialized rescue and wilderness medical equipment is presented in Chapter 63.

Some have suggested that wilderness EMS personnel should consider more aggressively pursuing environmentally low-impact equipment and practices. They argue that this is particularly important given the areas in which wilderness EMS operates and the knowledge that environmental health and human health are fundamentally interlinked. Some specific projects have appeared as a result of this principle. For instance, all National Park Service diesel vehicles in the Great Smoky Mountains now run exclusively on biodiesel (National Park Service, 2007). The Appalachian Center for Wilderness Medicine developed a Green EMS Initiative that has designed a prototype hybrid fuel wilderness EMS response vehicle (Hawkins, 2007b).

However, such equipment discussions become more contentious when, for example, the topic arises of using a motorized rescue vehicle in a wilderness area banning motorized traffic. In general, ethicists have suggested that preservation of wilderness areas is an important goal but preservation of human life is the first priority (Iserson & Morenz, 2007).

Differences in Resources

[OBJECTIVE 8]

A marker of wilderness medicine has been noted to be a state of reduced resources. However, when wilderness EMS is considered, often the difference in resources is more in type than in volume. Wilderness EMS providers rarely have access to ambulances, ambulance-based gear, and on-line medical direction while at the scene of injury or illness. However, wilderness EMS providers may have increased access to other resources, such as helicopter services (air medical and rescue, hospital and military based), rescue gear, specialists in wilderness rescue, volunteer help, and extended care equipment, compared with traditional EMS providers.

Of note, however, is that air evacuations by helicopters or fixed-wing aircraft are dangerous, expensive, and not always available because of weather concerns and should not be relied on as a primary rescue mechanism for most wilderness EMS systems. The majority of rescues result in personnel carrying the patient out on foot (Hubbell, 2007b). Patient carryouts demonstrate another difference in resource availability between traditional and wilderness EMS systems—the potential need for significantly more personnel. On the best of trails, an estimated 30 or more rescuers are required to treat and carry a single patient 2 to 3 miles (Ellozy, 2006). One general formula is that each mile of carryout requires six well-rested litter bearers and takes 1 to 2 hours to complete (Hubbell, 2007b).

Differences in Team Interfaces

[OBJECTIVE 9]

Wilderness EMS providers in some ways must be more adept at interacting and cooperating with multiple teams and types of providers than traditional EMS providers. (This is another way that wilderness EMS closely mirrors disaster care.) Although a traditional EMS provider typically only interacts with an accepting hospital-based team, a wilderness EMS provider may interact and operationally interface with many other providers during the course of patient care. Some interfaces that should be expected by a wilderness EMS provider include the following:

- Air medical personnel
- Law enforcement personnel (e.g., state police, federal or state rangers, game wardens); in many states search and rescue is a law enforcement activity
- Military personnel
- Professional trip leaders and guides
- Search and rescue, mountain rescue, ski patrol teams
- Disaster teams
- Volunteers
- Civil air patrol

Although these individuals and agencies can offer additional resources and services, tension also can develop among multiple providers or multiple agencies. Any cooperative efforts that might be anticipated should be discussed at the leadership level before patient care situations arise and before specific operations if necessary. Protocols and staff interactions developed outside specific missions are helpful in enhancing interagency cooperation. Incident Command System terminology and roles should be implemented to avoid confusion at the management and operational levels. The Incident Command System is discussed in more detail in Chapter 62.

Case Scenario—continued

One evening at 6 PM you get a call that a climber has fallen at the climbing area. You call volunteers in the rescue division and eventually assemble a response team. On your arrival you find a 24-year-old man at the bottom of a climbing route, approximately 2 miles from the nearest road but accessible by a double-track trail. He is wearing a helmet and appears confused. He is bleeding from a scalp laceration and complains of neck pain. His partner says he thinks his harness failed and he fell approximately 20 feet, striking a small tree on the way down. Physical examination reveals a small scalp laceration with no crepitus or step-off and midline tenderness of the cervical and lumbar spine. The patient and his partner deny any recent alcohol or illicit drug use, and no evidence of intoxication or neurologic deficit is present. He states he did not lose consciousness. He is sitting up and asking for help in walking out to the road.

Questions

4. *Should this patient's spine be immobilized? Why or why not?*
5. *What are your transport considerations given the time of day?*
6. *What can be done to reduce patient suffering during transport?*

CURRENT WILDERNESS EMS SYSTEMS

[OBJECTIVE 10]

United States National Park Service

The first U.S. national park, Yellowstone National Park, was established by President Ulysses S. Grant in 1872. The National Park Service (NPS), a bureau of the Department of the Interior, was created by an act signed by President Woodrow Wilson in 1916. As more parks were established and visitors increasingly ventured into remote and rugged terrain within them, the need for wilderness EMS providers grew. In response to this, some NPS rangers became trained as EMTs. These federal employees practiced scopes of care that sometimes exceeded traditional EMTs. For example, NPS basic EMTs were permitted to administer epinephrine long before the 1994 EMT-Basic revision that introduced this skill to traditional EMS systems (Russell, 2004; Fortenberry et al., 1995).

In particularly rugged regions, especially in western parks, the benefit of having an explicit wilderness EMS system became apparent. The **Parkmedic** Program is a wilderness EMS system established in 1975 and was initially built as a local wilderness EMS system to provide care to Sequoia and Kings Canyon National Parks. Since then it has expanded to train NPS rangers in most of the larger western parks as well as Hawaii, the Everglades, and the Shenandoah and Smoky Mountains National Parks. The University of California–San Francisco at Fresno (UCSF-Fresno) emergency medicine residency program and UCSF-Fresno University Medical Center provide medical training for the Parkmedic Program. This training includes a Parkmedic certification course offered every other year to rangers (EMTs) from throughout the NPS, who then return to their sponsoring parks and work within the individual park's EMS system under local medical advisors. The certification course provides more than 200 hours of training and results in traditional Advanced EMT certification augmented by additional pharmacologic and procedural training and skills appropriate for wilderness medical care. This puts the Parkmedic's scope of practice somewhere between the traditional categories of Advanced EMT and Paramedic. UCSF-Fresno also provides annual refresher courses and monthly training as well as online and offline medical direction specifically for Kings Canyon and Sequoia National Parks (UCSF, 2007; Kaufman et al., 1981). One study of 434 patients treated over a 1-year period by Parkmedics found that 10% of patients treated required advanced life support interventions (Johnson et al., 1991).

Approximately 20 to 30 parks have Parkmedic programs. In the remaining national parks, rangers not trained by the specific Parkmedic program also provide limited wilderness medical care at the EMT or emergency medical responder level, with UCSF-Fresno serving as medical consultants to the NPS EMS system as a whole. This program is therefore one of the largest and most ambitious wilderness EMS systems specifically designed for wilderness medical care, providing standardized care to millions of national park visitors and park employees each year (Burelbach et al., 2004). This care is frequently needed. In 2003 alone, 3251 visitors required rescue operations, some of which required emergency medical aid (including advanced life support interventions). Although 124 of these visitors died, authorities estimate an additional 427 "saves"—patients who would have been expected to die but who survived because of NPS intervention (Farabee, 2005). Interventions such as these are among the most compelling arguments for the importance of wilderness EMS systems.

United States Department of Defense

Military medical care is typically considered a separate category of paramedicine; yet military and battlefield medical care clearly meets the definition of wilderness medicine. Considered in this context, the U.S. Department of Defense (DOD) maintains perhaps the largest and most complex wilderness EMS system in the country, including paramedical, nursing, and physician-level providers in the various service branches. Military medical provider involvement in organizations such as WMS has increasingly been reinforcing the similarities between the two practice models. The benefits of cross training and sharing techniques between wilderness and military EMS providers are obvious and represent a fertile source of growth in wilderness EMS. The Coast Guard and Air Force pararescue teams may be the most widely used DOD resources deployed in support of U.S. civilian rescues. Integration of retired military medical providers into civilian wilderness EMS systems represents another important way the DOD contributes to wilderness EMS systems in the United States.

National Certifying and Coordinating Bodies

Many organizations, although they do not field formal teams, can be considered wilderness EMS systems as a result of the degree that they standardize and certify teams and organizations operating within a given subspecialty.

National Ski Patrol

The National Ski Patrol (NSP) is a 26,000-member association that provides training and education programs for emergency rescuers who serve the outdoor recreation community, specifically skiers and snowboarders. The NSP provides many courses in winter safety and rescue, including a wilderness medical certification in Outdoor Emergency Care, a program requiring 80 to 100 hours of class and study time (National Ski Patrol, 2007a). It also coordinates a wilderness first-aid course, Outdoor First Care, involving 6 to 8 hours of class and study time (National Ski Patrol, 2007b). In the past it offered a Winter

Emergency Care certification, which has been discontinued and merged into the other two programs. (The Winter Emergency Care program discontinued by NSP should not be confused with the Winter Emergency Care Program still available through the American Safety & Health Institute.)

The NSP offers wilderness medical training and serves as the professional organization for affiliate local ski patrols, which are present at nearly every major alpine (downhill) and Nordic (cross country and back country) ski area in the United States. These wilderness EMS systems are tasked with prevention and treatment of injuries and illness on ski slopes. Some ski areas include nongroomed backcountry that ski patrollers also serve, and in other areas ski patrollers have formal or informal arrangements to augment local EMS and search-and-rescue operations in regions adjacent to private ski area boundaries.

Mountain Rescue Association

Mountain Rescue Association (MRA), founded in 1958, offers training and certifications to teams involved in mountain rescue operations. Most nonprofit independent rescue groups involved in mountain rescue are or aspire to be affiliated with this organization.

Unlike organizations such as the National Association for Search and Rescue (NASAR) and NSP, MRA interfaces with providers only at the team level and does not train or certify individuals. More than 90 MRA-certified units are now in operation (MRA, 2007). In addition to being a nonprofit organization, MRA has a formal policy that affiliated teams do not charge for their services (Russell, 2004). MRA offers its affiliated member teams extensive training in technical mountain rescue and search-and-rescue operations and the privilege of MRA certification through proficiency testing of the teams. It does not offer formal wilderness medical training of its own.

National Cave Rescue Commission

An umbrella organization with a similar role, in this case overseeing cave rescue teams, is the National Cave Rescue Commission (NCRC). This organization operates under a charter from the National Speleological Society, granted in 1979. The NCRC provides training and development opportunities for persons and organizations engaged in cave rescue activities (NCRC, 2007). In a similar fashion as MRA, NCRC provides technical training and support for technical cave rescue but does not provide specific wilderness medical training certifications or wilderness medical courses.

Divers Alert Network

The Divers Alert Network provides certification courses in medical management of diving conditions, rescue insurance for members, and an emergency medical hotline for divers.

National Association for Search & Rescue

NASAR is a 14,000-member nonprofit organization "dedicated to advancing professional, literary, and scientific knowledge in fields related to search and rescue." NASAR operates a multitude of courses involving technical rescue and search skills, including canine-assisted searches. NASAR developed a wilderness medical certification (search and rescue medical responder), but as of 2002 only 31 students had obtained this certification (NASAR, 2002) and it is no longer listed in the NASAR course catalogue (NASAR, 2007).

Local Wilderness EMS Systems

Although two of the wilderness EMS systems described above are federally supported (NPS and DOD), most wilderness EMS systems are organized locally. Indeed, even the Parkmedic system operates as a local wilderness EMS system for the two national parks it serves, although as a federal program it could be expanded to serve multiple areas. This section describes wilderness EMS systems that operate on a local level. Many operate as affiliates of the organizations previously described as national certifying and organizing bodies.

Search and Rescue Teams

Multiple autonomous search and rescue (SAR) teams exist throughout the country. SAR teams are one of the most prevalent forms of wilderness EMS systems because "lost persons" situations are a common challenge for law enforcement and emergency management throughout the country. These operations often require specialized personnel (usually volunteers) to provide search, rescue, and medical stabilization services in environments that often are austere.

Specific details regarding SAR operation are beyond the scope of this chapter but generally evolve through five stages: awareness, initial action, planning, operations, and conclusion. A U.S. National Search and Rescue Plan directs the organization of SAR operations and agencies in the United States. Searches may be as small as single-municipality, volunteer, ground-based searchers, or they may be complex enough to involve multistate personnel and assets such as aircraft, specially trained human trackers, and dog teams. NASAR offers multiple certification courses that provide more specialized training in SAR principles and practices.

An example of a regional SAR team is the Allegheny Mountain Rescue Group, an all-volunteer nonprofit SAR group providing response within a 4-hour radius from Pittsburgh, including portions of Pennsylvania, Ohio, West Virginia, and Maryland.

Other Wilderness Medical Entities

Some local EMS services have developed divisions that provide wilderness medical care. These fall within county emergency management programs, local EMS programs, and semiprofessional and volunteer rescue squads. These divisions sometimes form specialty teams identified by various names, including technical rescue team, special operations team, special tactical operations response medics, wilderness rescue team, and so forth. Although such formal wilderness EMS teams are a relatively new phenomenon, they are becoming more common throughout the country.

These wilderness EMS systems often maintain atypical vehicles (e.g., ATVs with patient transport adaptations or trailers; snowmobiles and sleds; swift water, open water, and maritime boats; off-road trucks). They may cooperate on a formal (organized before an incident) or informal (ad hoc) basis with local volunteer organizations, guides, experiential education programs and camps, and outdoor enthusiasts who may be present or available during a mission.

An example of this type of wilderness EMS system is the Burke County EMS Special Operations Team (Anthony, 2007), the first such EMS team to be formed in North Carolina. Burke County EMS Special Operations paramedics are on call to provide rescue and wilderness medical care to wilderness environments, including Linville Gorge Wilderness Area (the deepest gorge in the eastern United States), the Table Rock climbing area, multiple remote ATV trail systems, South Mountain State Park, and other remote sites in Burke County, N.C. The team requires at least EMT-Paramedic certification and then provides additional skills and protocols that expand the scope of care, including skills such as reduction of dislocated joints and medications such as antibiotics and steroids.

Nonprofit Rescue Associations and Teams

Some volunteer teams work independently of local EMS services. These often arise as volunteer nonprofit organizations composed of outdoor enthusiasts or off-duty medical professionals with a particular interest in rescue and wilderness medical care. They operate in a similar fashion to the EMS-based systems but may vary in the degree to which they are integrated into the local EMS system.

Examples of this model include the Crag Rats, based in the Hood River region of Oregon, which is the oldest mountain rescue organization in the country. This all-volunteer team provides services to Mount Hood, the Columbia River Gorge, and surrounding areas. The 11,239-foot Mount Hood, one of the most frequently climbed mountains in the world, presents some of the most challenging and frequent mountain rescue and wilderness medical operations in the United States. In the past 25 years more than 35 climbers have died on its slopes. However, since 1923 the Crag Rats have prevented the injury or death of far more climbers and outdoor recreationalists. The Crag Rats are charter members of MRA (Mountain Aid Training International 2007).

Regional Cooperative Ventures

Wilderness EMS systems and operations often benefit from the cooperation of multiple agencies and individuals, both in terms of training and actual mission operations. At least two organizations have developed cooperative ventures to promote the regionalization of wilderness medicine and EMS services.

The Appalachian Center for Wilderness Medicine, based in western North Carolina, is an innovative program designed to promote regional collaboration among researchers, students, practitioners, patients, academicians, EMS personnel, and vendors involved in wilderness medical pursuits and related fields in the southern Appalachian states (Hawkins, 2007b). Its efforts have already resulted in a number of regional collaborations and projects.

Mountain Aid Training International has developed a New England Consortium whose mission includes "teaching wilderness medicine and rescue topics to . . . interested students in New England, to include . . . EMS personnel from each sponsoring hospital in the program" (Mountain Aid Training International, 2005). Gearing programs toward a specific geographic audience could permit students to network together and instructors to focus on regionally relevant topics rather than a national (too broad) or local (too restricted) curriculum.

Disaster Response Providers

Disaster response providers, including both governmental and nongovernmental organizations, are trained to operate in austere environments that meet the definition of wilderness medical care previously discussed. In the sense that these organizations serve as extensions of or replacements for a compromised EMS system, they may be considered wilderness EMS systems. On the other hand, significant differences exist between the provision of disaster and wilderness care (some of which are discussed below). A number of exciting ventures explore the interface between these two types of EMS. At least one author who practices both wilderness and disaster medicine has advanced a forcible argument for why wilderness and SAR EMS providers are ideal candidates for disaster deployment (Conover, 2006). As previously mentioned, Landmark Learning now offers relief medic training and certification to students already certified as wilderness EMTs or wilderness first responders (Landmark Learning, 2007). Merging of wilderness and disaster training might be expected in the future as both disaster medicine and wilderness medicine mature as fields of medical care.

Federal Response Teams

The federal disaster response plan and associated teams have undergone substantial changes after the terrorist attacks of September 11, 2001. The National Disaster

Medical System (NDMS) was developed in 1984 as a public/private partnership between the Federal Emergency Management Agency (FEMA), the Department of Health and Human Services, the DOD, the Department of Veterans Affairs, and civilian hospitals and medical professionals. Originally located in the Department of Health and Human Services and operating under memoranda of understanding, it was codified into law and merged into the new Department of Homeland Security (DHS) in 2002 (Mothershead et al., 2006). In 2007 NDMS returned to the Department of Health and Human Services.

NDMS is a wilderness EMS system capable of fielding large numbers of temporarily self-sufficient teams into disaster areas to provide austere medical care. The bulk of these teams are disaster medical assistance teams (DMATs), of which 85 exist and approximately 24 are considered operational at any given time (Mothershead et al., 2006). Such teams consist of physicians, nurses, paramedics, and other support personnel who receive specialized disaster training and equipment and become federal employees in the event of a disaster deployment. A DMAT is designed to be self-sufficient for 72 hours and be capable of treating approximately 250 patients per day. These activities are supported by accompanying food, water, shelter, latrines, power, and supplies as well as advanced medical equipment such as ventilators, defibrillators, and point-of-service laboratory devices (Russell, 2004).

This massive deployment of resources raises the legitimate question as to whether DMATs actually provide wilderness or austere medical care. Given the definition used in this chapter, the environment in which they work typically qualifies as austere or wilderness. However, disaster management strategies have increasingly moved toward the temporary replication of hospital-based services incapacitated by disaster. In this sense, DMATs and other formal disaster response projects such as Carolina MED-1 attempt to reduce the resource deficiency in the definition of wilderness medicine. Such an approach, which is extremely resource intensive, is functional in disaster settings and probably politically necessary as the American public increasingly expects the rapid return of comprehensive medical care in disasters. Yet to accomplish this goal, this structure sacrifices much of the agility and flexibility typically characteristic of wilderness medicine, thus representing a fundamental way disaster medicine evolving in the United States differs from classic wilderness medicine.

NDMS also maintains multiple other teams, including four disaster veterinary assistance teams, 10 disaster mortuary response teams, and three national medical response teams specially trained to handle chemical, biologic, and radiologic incidents (Mothershead et al., 2006).

FEMA maintains 28 specially equipped and trained urban SAR task forces whose mission is to locate, extricate, and provide initial medical care to victims trapped by collapsed buildings. If needed, FEMA deploys the three closest task forces within 6 hours of notification and additional teams as needed. These teams also are intended to be self-sufficient for 72 hours and are deployed with medical supplies and technical rescue gear designed for urban and structural disasters (Goodman & Hogan, 2002; FEMA, 2007).

When considered as a whole, the NDMS/FEMA system represents one of the most comprehensive and well-funded disaster and austere medical care systems in the world. However, as evidenced by recent disasters such as the hurricane season of 2005 (highlighted by Hurricane Katrina, which devastated the U.S. Gulf Coast), even copious funding does not always prevent weaknesses and controversy in the provision of disaster and wilderness medical care.

EMS disaster care is discussed more completely in Chapter 66, Disaster Response and Domestic Preparedness.

Nongovernmental and Faith-Based Response Teams

In addition to the federal government, numerous nongovernmental organizations and faith-based teams provide disaster relief or remote and/or third-world medical care. These vary in organizational sophistication and services provided; however, some do provide rudimentary medical, dental, and some elective surgical care to remote, impoverished, or disaster-stricken areas. The parameters of their care typically fall within the broad characteristics of wilderness medicine, with the exception of some of the elective surgical procedures.

An example of such a team is Doctors Without Borders (Médecins Sans Frontières; MSF), an "international medical humanitarian organization that delivers emergency aid to people affected by armed conflict, epidemics, natural or manmade disasters, or exclusion from health care in more than 70 countries" (MSF, 2007). Founded in 1971, MSF now performs more than 3800 field operations each year. It is often one of the first humanitarian organizations to appear in an area where local healthcare is not present or is devastated, and its teams are configured with healthcare kits, equipment, and training "custom designed for specific field situations, geographic conditions, and climates." This gear ranges from rudimentary equipment more typical of classic wilderness medicine to equipment more similar to a DMAT, such as a complete operating room or all the supplies needed to treat hundreds of cholera patients (MSF, 2006).

Case Scenario CONCLUSION

Bleeding from the head wound is adequately controlled by direct pressure. The patient's spine is immobilized, and he is transported 2 miles on the rescue division's new ATV. Diagnostic testing reveals that the patient has no skull fracture or brain injury but he does have stable lower cervical and upper thoracic vertebral fractures.

Looking Back

7. *Given the patient's final disposition, was your treatment appropriate? Why or why not?*
8. *What could be done to improve your team's response?*

CHALLENGES FACING WILDERNESS EMS

[OBJECTIVE 11]

As a relatively new area of interest within EMS, wilderness EMS faces many challenges in organizing and providing care in wilderness and austere environments.

Standardization of Certifications and Practice

As previously noted, a major challenge to wilderness EMS systems is the absence of a coordinating or certifying body. Training and practice are regulated only at the local level, even in the states that recognize wilderness EMS certifications. This situation presents many challenges for wilderness EMS systems and providers, including quality assurance, medical control for expanded scope operations, and research and reports that use standardized terminology and care.

Questions Regarding Wilderness Rescue

Some fundamental questions still exist regarding whether wilderness rescue and systematic wilderness EMS are appropriate. Some argue that the absence of formal medical care and rescue operations is part of the appeal of wilderness activities and that individuals venturing in these areas should be self-sufficient and capable of treating and rescuing themselves (Russell, 2004).

Another point of contention is whether beneficiaries of rescue operations should be required to pay for the cost of the rescue or whether collective insurance or fees should be levied on all wilderness users to pay for those who require rescue or medical care. The standard in European wilderness EMS systems is to charge for services rendered; consequently, most individuals and groups purchase rescue insurance (Russell, 2004). Concern exists that, because of fear regarding the cost of rescue, those without insurance may wait so long to call for help that the rescue is complicated or too late. In the United States, rescues and wilderness EMS medical care are usually volunteer based or provided by the government, with no charge applied to those rescued. This partly stems from the philosophical convictions of those providing the rescue, such as the policy of the MRA that no charge be levied by affiliate organizations. Another reason is that governmental bodies, such as the NPS and state providers, are obligated to protect the safety of participants in their regions; thus medical care, and by extension rescue, often are considered an obligation of the state (although some authorities point out that no specific mandated "duty to rescue" exists on the part of state or national parks [Hubbell, 2007b]).

In particularly remote areas, rescue becomes expensive and dangerous in its own right; thus proponents of limiting or charging for rescue services argue that the participant should be responsible to some degree for adequate preparation and the consequences of a complex, high-risk rescue. In most areas where rescue is dangerous, expensive, or frequent, the NPS or other response agency posts warnings and recommends preparation for self-treatment or self-rescue. Nonetheless, most continue to provide rescue and medical care services. Some measures, such as the NPS practice of leasing a helicopter for high-altitude rescues on Mt. McKinley, are expensive and controversial (the American Alpine Club, for example, recommends discontinuing this program) (Russell, 2004). The controversy at this particular wilderness area was compounded by a decision by the NPS in 1995 to levy a $150 fee on Mt. McKinley climbers to defray rescue costs. Although some feel this is appropriate, others argue that this unfairly restricts access to public resources and unfairly and disproportionately singles out climbers. (In 2001 only 5% of rescues involved climbers; the remaining 95% involved in other activities did not pay a fee to defray rescue costs involving their activities [Russell, 2004; Davidson, 1994].)

Finally, disagreement exists among EMS specialists over what level of care wilderness EMS systems should provide. Some argue that wilderness EMS care should be confined to basic life support and first aid, with others promoting the insertion of advanced life support capabilities into the wilderness setting.

Funding and Participation

In addition to funding for specific rescues, numerous other challenges exist for funding the infrastructure for wilderness EMS systems.

Paramedic Shortage

Nationally a perceived shortage of qualified paramedics exists in traditional EMS according to the Committee on the Future of Emergency Care in the United States Health System (Institute of Medicine, 2006). This is controversial because firm national data are lacking, although numerous localities do report unfilled positions. Such a shortage could be from (1) the perception that paramedics are underpaid relative to other public service personnel (e.g., fire and law enforcement); (2) long-term federal underfunding of EMS relative to fire services and law enforcement (e.g., only 4% of first-responder DHS funds went to EMS in 2002 and 2003) (Garza, 2005); (3) frequent local underfunding of EMS; (4) a loss of potential paramedics into more lucrative healthcare fields such as nursing or midlevel practitioners; (5) a loss of actual paramedics who pursue bridge courses, converting their paramedic certification into nursing or midlevel provider licensure; or (6) the emotional and physical difficulties of an EMS career (e.g., shift work, lifting, environmental exposure, job stressors), including lost time and disability from back injuries, which have been shown in recent studies to be nearly epidemic in EMS (Nielsen, 2006). Whatever the cause, if the purported paramedic shortage does exist, the resulting stress on specialty subservices such as wilderness EMS would not be hard to imagine.

Ranger Shortage

Many authorities also believe the country has a critical NPS ranger shortage. The root causes of this differ somewhat from paramedic shortages.

One stressor on rangers and ranger staffing is the increased attention to national security since the terrorist attacks of 2001. The NPS 2003 Annual Report noted that NPS "operational funding will continue to be impacted by the need to improve security. . . . The NPS was forced to use almost $8 million in fee receipts for the increased security requirements demanded by three Code Orange periods in fiscal year 2003. This displacement of lower-priority needs . . . is likely to adversely affect already-strained park budgets, which have been absorbing unfunded increases in operational costs of the past several years" (National Parks Conservation Association, 2007a). Additional rangers and elaborate wilderness EMS systems might both be considered lower-priority needs. The National Parks Conservation Association (NPCA) reports that NPS spends $63,500 each day that the nation is on Orange Alert and points out that ranger diversion can be even more damaging. "When rangers from parks such as Rocky Mountain and Shenandoah are sent to guard dams and icon parks, their positions remain unfilled" (NPCA, 2007b). NPS rangers also are tasked with other unexpected duties, such as helping search for debris from the space shuttle Columbia (Stannard, 2003), creating relative decreases in ranger availability for traditional activities such as rescue and medical care.

Furthermore, outdoor and wilderness activities are one of the fastest-growing recreational activities in the United States; from 1980 to 2001 visitation to NPS parks increased by more than 60 million people. Despite the natural expectation that a corresponding increase in medical and rescue needs would develop, the number of permanently commissioned rangers dropped 16% and the number of seasonal rangers dropped 24% during this same period (NPCA, 2007b). Wilderness EMS might thus already be one of the "unfunded increases in operational costs" referenced by the NPS.

Federal salary funding also is a potential source of ranger shortage. For example, in 2004 NPS received a 1.5% budget increase to cover a 4.1% mandatory pay increase for park staff (NPCA, 2007). These stressors all represent a challenge to building or enhancing federally implemented wilderness EMS systems. President George W. Bush announced the National Park Centennial Initiative in 2006. The initiative proposed a federal Centennial Challenge Matching Fund that would be used to match philanthropic contributions (up to $100 million per year) for the benefit of national parks between now and the 100th anniversary of the National Park Service in 2016. In 2008, Congress appropriated funds for the first round of National Park Centennial Projects to improve parks nationwide. Congress continues to work on legislation to create the President's National Park Centennial Challenge Matching Fund.

Volunteer Dependence

Given the budgetary and operational limitations of EMS-based and federally based wilderness EMS systems, the reason so many wilderness EMS systems rely on volunteer or semivolunteer individuals becomes clear. Although volunteers can provide services equal to or superior to paid personnel, a sustainable model for rapid wilderness EMS growth and sophistication would include some mechanism for compensation in certain areas. In Europe, where at least mountain rescue teams are professional and employ full-time personnel, fees charged can support salaries, equipment, and training (Hubbell, 2007b). This model has strengths and weaknesses but does promote standardization and solves some of the funding and availability problems inherent in a largely volunteer system. The current dependence on volunteerism, although admirable in terms of those volunteering, represents a potential weakness if wilderness EMS operations grow to exceed the capabilities of volunteer service.

Case Scenario SUMMARY

1. *What agencies could you contact to discuss management of this area and potential situations?* As the property transitions into a state park, rangers and other state park service personnel can be expected to take a more active role in rescue and first aid initial medical care. Other resources may be available from the state. The federal government may have National Guard or military equipment available for technical rescues. These resources and their availability should be discussed with military and federal authorities early during general strategic planning and ideally well before an actual rescue becomes necessary. In many jurisdictions law enforcement has a primary role in search and rescue and may be able to offer personnel, funding, or equipment. If the rescue squad here is not formally part of the local EMS system, it should be integrated into any response plans. Some specialized technical response teams operate throughout a region—even multiple states—and may be available. Tertiary care hospitals in the region may operate helicopter air medical services that can be used for nontechnical extrications and rapid transport to trauma centers.
2. *What equipment should your rescue squad consider purchasing?* The area includes backcountry, lake, and high-angle environments. Equipment needs could include high-angle technical gear (ropes, harnesses, rescue and climbing hardware, baskets, and rigging systems), a boat, a mechanism to transport the boat to and from the scene (e.g., trailer, truck), personal flotation devices, wetsuits, an ATV and/or snowmobile, litter wheel, extra radios, and packs suitable for carrying at least BLS equipment and responder gear to a patient. Ideally each responder also should be deployed with the 10 essentials (see Box 54-1).
3. *What additional training should your members consider obtaining?* Members responding to extended or backcountry wilderness rescues in this area might benefit from formal wilderness first responder or wilderness EMT certification from a reputable school. Additional training could include boat rescue (to account for the lake) and swift water rescue if the lake feeds into any moving water. Many schools also teach high-angle rescue, which would be necessary for any technical rescues involving the climbing area. The system's medical director might consider exploring wilderness medical protocols and corresponding in-house training to extend the capability of paramedics operating in extended care situations.
4. *Should this patient's spine be immobilized? Why or why not?* Following traditional EMS operations, the patient's spine should be immobilized on the basis of mechanism of injury alone. However, unless mechanized transport is easily available, in this situation not spinally immobilizing also would be a benefit, especially because of the late hour of the day. Implementing the spinal clearance protocol, the patient would pass the intoxication and neurologic deficit criteria. However, he would fail the altered mental status and neck tenderness criteria. If any one of the criteria is present, the patient's spine must be immobilized, so this patient should not be clinically cleared.
5. *What are your transport considerations given the time of day?* Transport must be expedited given the late hour of the day. If extricating the patient is not feasible by sundown, consider night operation capability versus sheltering with care on-site until daylight. Patient safety and rescue must at all times be balanced with safety considerations for providers.
6. *What can be done to reduce patient suffering during transport?* Adequate padding is critical for backcountry spinal immobilization. Transport times often are longer than in traditional EMS systems, so more pain medications may be needed than are typically used or defined by protocol for traditional EMS operations. Tell the patient early on how bathroom needs will be handled.
7. *Given the patient's final disposition, was your treatment appropriate? Why or why not?* In this scenario an ATV was available, which greatly facilitated rescue and transport. The operation would be much more complicated without this asset.
8. *What could be done to improve your team's response?* Think through your responses to the questions as they were presented and consider in retrospect what could be improved. In the stem of the scenario, response time could have been improved had a paging system or on-call system been in place to contact volunteers who were appropriately trained and available to respond. In terms of prevention, teams can consider hosting sessions where climbing safety and proper harness use are emphasized; this also can be done in conjunction with local climbing clubs or outdoor retailers. Such activities sometimes make for the most efficient response—one that is not needed in the first place.

Chapter Summary

- *Wilderness medicine* is a term that must be understood contextually. In this chapter it is defined as medical management in situations where care and prevention are limited by environmental considerations, prolonged extrication, or resource availability.
- Wilderness EMS systems plan and help implement the provision of wilderness medical care to a discrete region or type of activity and help integrate wilderness medical principles into the greater EMS system. Wilderness EMS systems differ from traditional (street) systems in important ways. Some of these include differences in environment in which the provider delivers care, protocols and online and offline medical direction, certification and training, equipment, resources, and organizations with which the providers are expected to interact. Wilderness EMS systems are currently in place that provide standards and resources for medical care and rescue in certain environments (e.g., MRA, the NCRC). Others provide wilderness medical care for certain regions (e.g., the Parkmedic program, local EMS or nonprofit rescue services) or temporary care in regions with situational austerity (e.g., the NDMS system).
- Wilderness EMS systems may be federally funded, locally funded, or nonprofit. Some wilderness EMS organizations operate as schools or commercial ventures providing wilderness medical training.
- Numerous options are available to the EMS provider interested in obtaining or providing additional training in wilderness EMS and in providing patient care in diverse practice environments.
- Numerous challenges also exist to the growth of wilderness EMS as a field: federal funding, disparities in EMS funding relative to other public service entities, a reliance nationally on volunteer service, and an ongoing debate regarding the appropriateness and source of funding for rescues and wilderness medical care.
- Given the rapid growth of wilderness activities and a corresponding demand for wilderness medical care, these challenges are expected to be addressed and wilderness EMS will continue to grow as an important EMS subspecialty.

REFERENCES

Academy of Wilderness Medicine. (2007). Retrieved February 13, 2007, from http://www.wms.org/academy/default.asp.

Anthony, K. (2007). *Burke County EMS Special Operations Team.* Retrieved February 22, 2007, from http://www.bceoc.org/specialops.htm.

Burelbach, A., Lewin, M. R., Shalit, M., & Stroh, G. (2004). Resident's perspective: The national Parkmedic program. *Annals of Emergency Medicine, 43,* 114-119.

Chan, D., Goldberg, R., Tascone, A., Harmon, S., & Chan, L. (1994). The effect of spinal immobilization on healthy volunteers. *Annals of Emergency Medicine, 23*(1), 48.

Conover, K. (1992). EMTs should be able to clear the cervical spine in the wilderness. *Journal of Wilderness Medicine, 3*(4), 339-343.

Conover, K. (2006). Self-sufficiency, command and control for medical disaster responders: The wilderness search and rescue perspective. *American College of Emergency Physicians Disaster Medicine Section Newsletter, 15*(1).

Davidson, S. (1994). Access: Management and policy. *Climbing, 144,* 30.

Delbridge, T. R., Auble, T. E., Garrison, H. G., & Menegazzi, J. J. (1993). Discomfort in healthy volunteers immobilized on wooden backboards and vacuum mattress splint. *Prehospital Disaster Medicine, 8*(S2).

Ellozy, M. (2006). Accidents. *Appalachia, LVII*(1), 106.

Farabee, C. R. (2005). *Death, daring & disaster: Search and rescue in the national parks (revised edition)* (p. xxvi). Lanham, MD: Taylor Trade Publishing.

Federal Emergency Management Association. (2007). *About US&R: What US&R does.* Retrieved February 20, 2007, from http://www.fema.gov.

Fortenberry, J. E., Lane, J., & Shalit, M. (1995). Use of epinephrine for anaphylaxis by emergency medical technicians in a wilderness setting. *Annals of Emergency Medicine, 25*(6), 785-787.

Freda, J. (2004). *Central Maine Medical Center family practice residency wilderness medicine track.* Retrieved February 22, 2007, from http://www.geocities.com.

Garza, M. (2005). Who's on the mark? Controversy surrounds EMS pursuit of equal resources, priority & focus in Congress. *Journal of Emergency Medical Services, 30*(6), 43.

Goodman, C., & Hogan, D. (2002). Urban search and rescue. In D. Hogan, J. Burstein (Eds.). *Disaster medicine* (pp. 112-122). Philadelphia: Lippincott Williams and Wilkins.

Goodman, T., Iserson, K. V., & Strich, H. (2001). Wilderness mortalities: A 13 year experience. *Annals of Emergency Medicine, 37*(3), 279.

Goth, P., & Garnett, G. (1993). Rural Affairs Committee of the National Association of EMS Physicians: Clinical guidelines for delayed/prolonged transport: I-IV. *Prehospital Disaster Medicine, 8*(3), 77-80, 254-255, 335-340, 369-371.

Hawkins, S. C. (2007). *Appalachian Center for Wilderness Medicine.* Retrieved March 9, 2007, from http://www.appwildmed.org.

Hubbell, F. C. (2007a). 20 Years! And counting . . . *Wilderness Medicine Newsletter: Principles and Practices of Extended Care and Rescue, 20*(1), 2.

Hubbell, F. C. (2007b). Wilderness emergency medical services and response systems. In P. Auerbach (Ed.). *Wilderness medicine* (5th ed.) (pp. 694-707). St. Louis: Mosby.

Hubble, M. (2006). Personal communication, Cullowhee, NC.

Institute of Medicine. (2006). *Emergency medical services at the crossroads* (p. 104). Washington, DC: The National Academies Press.

Iserson, K. V., & Morenz, B. (2007). The ethics of wilderness medicine. In P. Auerbach (Ed.). *Wilderness medicine* (5th ed.) (p. 2181). St. Louis: Mosby.

Johnson, D. E. (2004). Wilderness emergency medical services. *Emergency Medicine Clinics of North America: Wilderness Medicine, 22*(2), 561-573.

Johnson, D. E. (2006). Self-sufficiency, command and control for medical disaster responders [Editorial]. *Wilderness Medicine News E-letter, 6*(11).

Johnson, J., Maertins, M., Shalit, M., Bierbaum, T., Goldman, D., & Lowe, R. (1991). Wilderness emergency medical services: The experiences at Sequoia and Kings Canyon National Parks. *American Journal of Emergency Medicine, 9*(3), 211-216.

Kaufman, T., Knopp, R., & Webster, T. (1981). The Parkmedic program: Prehospital care in the national parks. *Annals of Emergency Medicine, 10*(3), 156-160.

Landmark Learning. (2007). *Relief medic.* Retrieved February 19, 2007, from http://www.landmarklearning.org.

Linares, H. A., Mawson, A. R., & Suarez, E. (1987). Association between pressure sores and immobilization in the immediate post-injury period. *Orthopedics, 10,* 571.

Lindsey, L., Aughton, B., Doherty, N., Gray, M., Hubbell, F., Kerrigan, D., et al. (1999). Wilderness first responder: Recommended minimum. *Wilderness Environmental Medicine, 10*(1), 13-19.

Maine Emergency Medical Services. (2005). *Prehospital treatment protocols.* Retrieved February 13, 2007, from http://www.maine.gov.
Marshall University. (2005). *Marshall University Family Practice Residency Program.* Retrieved June 18, 2007, from http://meb.marshall.edu.
Maryland Institute for Emergency Medical Services Systems. (2007). *Maryland medical protocols for emergency medical service providers. Baltimore: 2007.* Retrieved March 24, 2007, from http://miemss.umaryland.edu.
Mawson, A. R., Bundo, J. J., & Neville, P. (1988). Risk factors for early occurring pressure ulcers following spinal cord injury. *American Journal of Physical Medical Rehabilitation, 67,* 123.
Médecins Sans Frontières. (2007). *About us: What is Doctors Without Borders/Médecins Sans Frontières?* Retrieved February 20, 2007, from http://www.doctorswithoutborders.org.
Montana Family Medicine Residency. (2007). *Wilderness medicine track.* Retrieved February 22, 2007, from http://www.mfmr.org.
Mothershead, J. L., Yeskey, K., & Brewster, P. (2006). Selected federal disaster response agencies and capabilities. In Ciottone, G. (Ed.). *Disaster medicine.* Philadelphia: Mosby Elsevier.
Mountain Aid Training International. (2005). *MATI Wilderness Medical Consortium.* Retrieved February 19, 2007, from http://www.mountainaid.com.
Mountain Aid Training International. (2007). *Mountain search and rescue: Hood River, Oregon.* Retrieved February 19, 2007, from http://www.cragrats.org.
National Association for Search & Rescue. (2002). *Number of students NASAR instructors have taught and coordinators have tested from September 1989 to September 30, 2002 by courses.* Retrieved February 19, 2007, from http://www.nasar.org.
National Association for Search & Rescue. (2007). *NASAR course offerings.* Retrieved February 19, 2007, from http://www.nasar.org.
National Association of Emergency Medical Technicians. (2007). Wilderness trauma care. In *Prehospital trauma life support.* St. Louis: Mosby.
National Cave Rescue Commission. (2007). Retrieved March 24, 2007, from http://www.caves.org.
National Parks Conservation Association. (2007a). *Death by a thousand cuts.* Retrieved March 24, 2007, from http://www.npca.org.
National Parks Conservation Association. (2007b). *Staffing shortages: An erosion of the park ideal.* Retrieved March 24, 2007, from http://www.npca.org.
National Park Service. (2007). *Smokies guide: The official newspaper of Great Smoky Mountain National Park, Spring,* 10.
National Ski Patrol. (2007a). *Outdoor Emergency Care Program.* Retrieved February 19, 2007, from http://www.nsp.org.
National Ski Patrol. (2007b). *Outdoor First Care.* Retrieved February 19, 2007, from http://www.nsp.org.
Nielsen, C. (2006). Pick, pack & carry. *Journal of EMS, 31*(7), 58-61.
Otten, E., Bowman, W., Hackett, P., Spadafora, M., & Tauber, D. (1991). Wilderness prehospital emergency care (WPHEC) curriculum. *Journal of Wilderness Medicine, 2*(2), 80-87.
Panacek, E. A., Mower, W. R., Holmes, J. F., & Hoffman, J. R. (2001). NEXUS Group. Test performance of the individual NEXUS low-risk clinical screening criteria for cervical spine injury. *Annals of Emergency Medicine, 38*(1), 22-25.
Russell, M. F. (2004). Wilderness emergency medical services systems. *Emergency Medicine Clinics of North America: Wilderness Medicine, 22*(2), 561-573.
Sholl, J. M., & Curcio, E. P. III. (2004). An introduction to wilderness medicine. *Emergency Medicine Clinics of North America: Wilderness Medicine, 22*(2), 265.
Stanford School of Medicine. (2007). *Wilderness medicine at Stanford.* Retrieved February 22, 2007, from http://emed.stanford.edu.
Stannard, M. B. (2003). Rangers struggle with staff shortage. *Deseret News (Salt Lake City),* July 14.
Stolber, S. G., & Barringer, F. (2007). White House memo: The president shows his environmentalist colors. *The New York Times,* February 8.
University of California, San Francisco. (2007). *Parkmedic program.* Retrieved February 19, 2007, from http://www.fresno.ucsf.edu.
Wilderness Medical Society. (2007). *Frequently asked questions: What is wilderness medicine?* Retrieved February 12, 2007, from http://www.wms.org.

SUGGESTED RESOURCES

Adirondack Wilderness Medicine: http://www.adkwildmed.com
Aerie Backcountry Medicine: http://www.aeriemed.com
Allegheny Mountain Rescue Group: http://www.amrg.info
American Alpine Club: http://www.americanalpineclub.org
American Medical Response Reach and Treat Team: http://www.summitpost.org/article/172226/amr-reach-and-treat-who-we-are-and-what-we-do.html
American Mountain Guides Association: http://www.amga.com
American Safety & Health Institute: http://www.ashinstitute.org/wilderness.htm
Appalachian Center for Wilderness Medicine: http://www.appwildmed.org
Appalachian Search and Rescue Conference: http://www.asrc.net
APT Antincendio: http://www.aptgroup.it/a_chisiamo_en.htm
Argentine Rescue & First Aid School [in Spanish]: http://www.easpa.com.ar
Burke County (NC) EMS Special Operations Team: http://www.bceoc.org
CDS Outdoor School: http://www.cdsoutdoor.org
Crag Rats: http://www.cragrats.org
Divers Alert Network: http://www.diversalertnetwork.org
Federal Emergency Management Agency: http://www.fema.gov
International Mountaineering and Climbing Federation/Union Internationale des Associations d'Alpinisme: http://www.uiaa.ch
International Society for Mountain Medicine: http://www.ismmed.org
Landmark Learning: http://www.landmarklearning.org
Médecins Sans Frontières/Doctors Without Borders: http://www.doctorswithoutborders.org
MedicalOfficer.Net, Ltd: http://www.medicalofficer.net
Medic Response Health & Safety: http://www.medicresponse.com
Mountain Aid Training International: http://www.mountainaid.com
Mountain Rescue Association: http://www.mra.org
Nantahala Outdoor Center: http://www.noc.com
National Association for Search & Rescue: http://www.nasar.org
National Cave Rescue Commission: http://www.caves.org/io/ncrc
National Disaster Life Support Foundation: http://www.bdls.com
National Disaster Medical System: http://www.hhs.gov/aspr/opeo/ndms/index.html
National Ski Patrol: http://www.nsp.org
North American Rescue Institute: http://www.soloschools.com/nari.html
Rescue 3 International: http://www.rescue3international.com
Rescue Specialists: http://www.rescuespec.com
Rigging for Rescue: http://www.riggingforrescue.com
Stonehearth Open Learning Opportunities: http://www.soloschool.com
UCSF-Fresno Parkmedic Program: http://www.fresno.ucsf.edu/em/parkmedic.htm
U.S. Coast Guard: http://www.uscg.mil
U.S. Department of Defense: http://www.defenselink.mil
U.S. National Park Service: http://www.nps.gov
Wilderness Emergency Care: http://www.wildernessemergencycare.com
Wilderness Emergency Medical Services Institute: http://www.wemsi.org
Wilderness First Aid: http://www.wfa.net
Wilderness Medical Associates: http://www.wildmed.com
Wilderness Medical Society: http://www.wms.org
Wilderness Medicine Institute: http://www.nols.edu/wmi
Wilderness Medicine Outfitters: http://www.wildernessmedicine.com
Wilderness Medicine Training Center: http://www.wildmedcenter.com/home.html
Wilderness Medicine, University of Utah: http://www.awls.org

Chapter Quiz

1. True or False: In the United States, no state recognition of wilderness EMS certification exists.

2. Cervical spine clearance in the wilderness with NEXUS criteria could be accomplished even if the patient has ________.
   a. altered mental status
   b. arm pain
   c. intoxication
   d. neurologic deficit

3. In general terms, a wilderness EMS system is a formally structured organization configured to provide wilderness medical care to ________.
   a. only a national park
   b. only a region or activity
   c. only hikers and climbers
   d. only those individuals who subscribe to special rescue insurance covering such care

4. Advanced protocols for wilderness EMS care often include (select all that apply) ________.
   a. field antibiotics
   b. field appendectomy
   c. field clinical clearance of the cervical spine.
   d. field reduction of dislocations

5. True or False: Although wilderness medicine often is characterized by working in a resource-deficient environment, wilderness EMS providers may have more access to some resources than their counterparts in traditional EMS.

6. True or False: In the United States, consensus exists that those receiving wilderness medical care should pay for this service.

7. Challenges facing systems providing wilderness, austere, and disaster care include the perception that which of the following may be underfunded (select all that apply)?
   a. EMS systems
   b. Individuals participating in nonprofit rescue organizations
   c. NDMS
   d. NPS

8. In the context of this chapter, wilderness medicine is defined as medical management in situations where care and prevention are limited by which of the following? Select all that apply.
   a. Environmental considerations
   b. Prolonged extrication
   c. Provider training
   d. Resource availability

Terminology

All-terrain vehicle (ATV) Any of a number of models of small open motorized vehicles designed for off-road and wilderness use; three-wheeled (all-terrain cycles) and four-wheeled (quads) versions are most often used for personnel insertion; six- and eight-wheel models exist for specialized applications.

Parkmedic A National Park Service ranger who has undergone additional wilderness medical training and who operates in certain parks under the medical direction of emergency physicians from UCSF-Fresno; scope of practice lies between a traditional EMT-Intermediate and EMT-Paramedic, with additional wilderness medical training.

Relief medic Emergency medical technician who has obtained additional training and certification in disaster and relief medical operations.

Wilderness command physician A physician who has received additional training by a WEMSI-endorsed course in wilderness medical care and medical direction of wilderness EMS providers and operations.

Wilderness EMS An individual or group that preplans to administer care in an austere environment and then is called on to perform these duties when needed.

Wilderness EMS system A formally structured organization, integrated into or part of the standard EMS system and configured to provide wilderness medical care to a discrete region.

Wilderness Emergency Medical Technician An emergency medical technician who has obtained EMT certification by DOT criteria and who also completes additional modules in wilderness care; sometimes abbreviated as WEMT, W-EMT, or EMT-W.

Wilderness first aid A level of certification indicating a provider has been trained in traditional first aid with added training in wilderness care and first aid administration in austere environments.

Wilderness first responder A first responder who has obtained certification by DOT criteria and who also completes additional modules in wilderness care.

Wilderness medicine Medical management in situations where care and prevention are limited by environmental considerations, prolonged extrication, or resource availability.

DIVISION 9

PUTTING IT ALL TOGETHER

CHAPTER 55

Assessment-Based Management

Objectives

After completing this chapter, you will be able to:

1. Explain how effectively assessing a patient is critical to making clinical decisions.
2. Explain the general approach, assessment, and management priorities for the following patients or conditions:
   - Chest pain
   - Medical and traumatic cardiac arrest
   - Acute abdominal pain
   - Gastrointestinal bleed
   - Altered mental status
   - Dyspnea
   - Syncope
   - Seizures
   - Environmental or thermal problem
   - Hazardous material or toxic exposure
   - Trauma or multiple-trauma patients
   - Allergic reactions
   - Behavioral problems
   - Obstetric or gynecologic problems
   - Pediatric patients
3. Explain how the paramedic's attitude affects his or her assessment of patients and decision making.
4. Explain how uncooperative patients affect the paramedic's assessment and decision making.
5. Explain strategies the paramedic can use to prevent labeling patients and having tunnel vision.
6. Develop strategies to decrease the distractions in the prehospital environment.
7. Describe how manpower considerations and staffing configurations affect the paramedic's assessment of patients and his or her decision making.
8. Synthesize concepts of scene management and choreography to simulated calls.
9. Explain the roles of the team leader and the patient care person.
10. List and explain the rationale for carrying in the essential patient care items.
11. When given a simulated call, list the appropriate equipment to take to the patient.
12. Explain the general approach to the emergency patient.
13. Describe how to communicate information effectively face to face, over the telephone, by radio, and in writing.

Chapter Outline

Case Scenario

You are called to the scene of a homeless man who is complaining of chest pain. He is in the lobby of a local shelter. He states he has pain radiating to his back between his shoulder blades. The pain is described as a tearing sensation that came on suddenly while at rest. He also has shortness of breath. His initial vital signs are as follows: pulse, 104 beats/min; blood pressure, 166/98 mm Hg; respirations, 18 breaths/min and slightly labored; and pulse oximetry, 100% on room air.

Questions

1. *What is your initial impression of this patient?*
2. *What is tunnel vision, and how could it affect your care of this patient?*
3. *What is labeling, and how could it affect your management of this patient?*
4. *What are possible diagnoses for this patient, and how do they affect your management?*

You have learned that the ability to perform a good patient assessment and obtain a patient's pertinent medical history are some of the more important skills a paramedic can master. In this chapter, you will consider the principles of assessment-based management and how to perform an appropriate assessment and implement a treatment plan for patients with common complaints.

EFFECTIVE ASSESSMENT

[OBJECTIVE 1]

Assessment is the foundation of care. Clearly you cannot treat or report anything that you have not found. Therefore you must gather, evaluate, and integrate information during your patient assessment to make the right patient care decisions. **Assessment-based management** is taking the information you obtain from your patient assessment and using it to treat the patient. You should not use a "cookbook" approach for every patient. Instead, assessment-based management requires you to use the information you have learned about illnesses and injuries and correlate it with the assessment information you gather from a specific patient. You then evaluate that data and pull it all together to create a treatment plan and provide the appropriate emergency care.

Accurate Information

To make decisions you must have accurate information. Often 80% of a medical diagnosis is based on the patient's history. Your knowledge of disease processes and injury patterns and maintaining an index of suspicion affect the quality of the history you acquire from the patient.

The history you obtain from the patient should focus on his or her chief complaint and the associated problems. The patient's ability to describe his or her symptoms and your ability to listen have a great effect on the assessment (Figure 55-1). You can miss important clues if you do not listen carefully.

When performing the physical examination, focus on the body systems associated with the patient's complaint. Do not overlook the importance of the physical examination. In addition, do not perform the examination in a cursory manner. However, the thoroughness with which you are able to perform a physical examination can be affected by field situations, such as an unsafe scene.

PARAMEDIC*Pearl*

As you gain experience, you will develop the ability to multitask. For instance, you will be able to ask questions and listen to the answers while performing skills at the same time. However, until you are experienced you should ask questions and simply listen. Your partner can perform the necessary skills.

Pattern Recognition

As a paramedic, you gather patient information, relate it to your knowledge of pathophysiology and the signs and symptoms of illnesses and injuries, and determine whether the patient's presentation fits a particular pattern

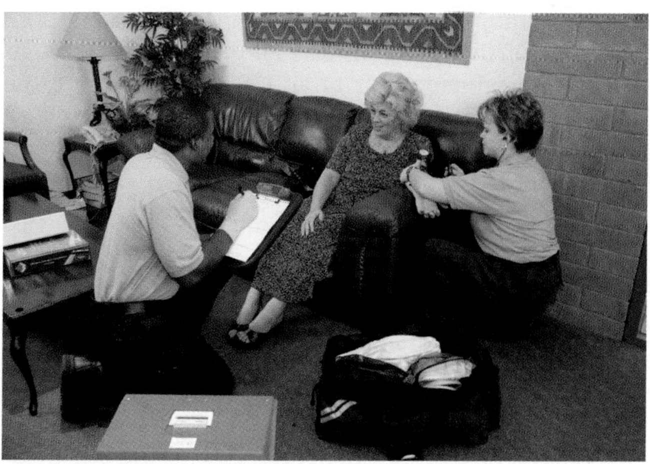

Figure 55-1 The patient's ability to describe symptoms and your ability to listen have a great effect on the assessment. Important clues are lost by not listening.

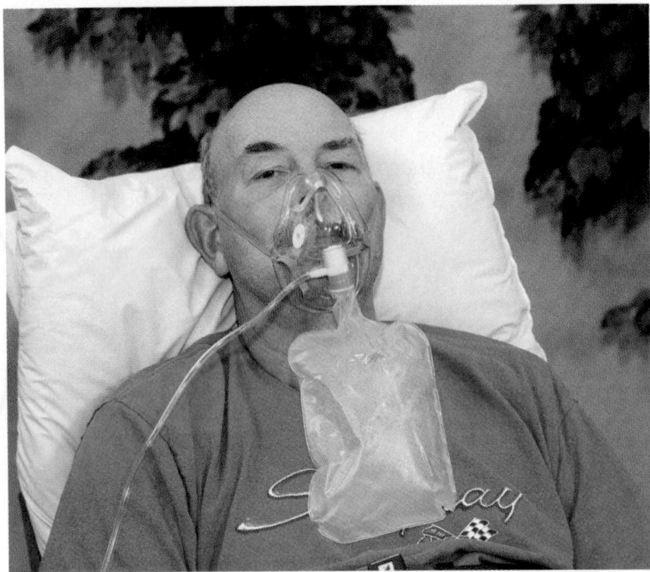

Figure 55-2 The greater your knowledge base, the better the chances of an accurate assessment and accurate patient care decisions.

or not. This process is known as **pattern recognition.** With pattern recognition you consider the patient's chief complaint as well as all the patient's assessments and symptoms. For example, you have been called to a patient who is reporting difficulty breathing (Figure 55-2). Difficulty breathing can result from a variety of illnesses or injuries. Medical conditions associated with difficulty breathing include allergies, congestive heart failure, chronic obstructive pulmonary disease, asthma, pneumonia, pulmonary edema, pulmonary embolism, anxiety, and many others. A chief complaint of difficulty breathing in a trauma patient may be the result of a chest injury, choking, neck injury, shock, head injury, or airway burn, among other causes. The greater your knowledge base, the more likely you will make an accurate assessment and accurate patient care decisions. Convergent thinking, or the "inverted pyramid" approach, is an effective method of approaching patients when using pattern recognition. This style of thought considers all of the patient's complaints and presentations in an effort to determine the most likely cause of the complaints. This avoids the situation where a cause is erroneously determined based on one complaint.

Field Impression

[OBJECTIVE 2]

Paramedics receive training in the general approach, assessment, differential diagnosis, and management priorities for the following patients and conditions:

- Chest pain
- Medical and traumatic cardiac arrest
- Acute abdominal pain
- Gastrointestinal bleeding
- Altered mental status
- Dyspnea
- Syncope
- Seizures
- Environmental or thermal problem
- Hazardous material or toxic exposure
- Trauma or multitrauma patients
- Allergic reactions
- Behavioral problems
- Obstetric or gynecologic problems
- Pediatric patients

Your ability to recognize patterns of illness or injury in these situations enables you to form a field impression and then formulate a treatment plan. Sometimes pattern recognition is a gut instinct based on experience. For example, you are dispatched to a residence for an older adult who is reporting abdominal pain. You notice a distinct odor as you enter the residence, and you immediately know that the patient has gastrointestinal bleeding. This odor is difficult to describe; but once you have experienced it, it is unforgettable.

After forming a field impression, develop a plan of action (treatment plan) based on the patient's condition and environment. Your decision to provide basic life support and advanced life support care will be driven by your treatment protocols and judgment. You must have the right field impression to know which protocol to use.

Treatment protocols provide a sequence of steps to follow when providing patient care for specific conditions. However, a standardized treatment protocol is not always appropriate for every patient with the same complaint (e.g., difficulty breathing). As a result, you must know when and how to apply protocols and when to deviate from them. For instance, you respond to a 57-year-old patient who is reporting shortness of breath. On arrival, you find him sitting in a tripod position. His breathing is labored with audible wheezing. Your auscultation of the lungs reveals crackles and wheezes bilaterally. The patient explains that he was supposed to have dialysis yesterday, but he "didn't feel good," so he did not go. Your assessment of the patient reveals jugular venous distention and pitting edema in both feet. The patient's blood pressure is 160/90 mm Hg. His respiratory rate is 24 breaths/min. Your field impression is that the patient is in need of dialysis and has pulmonary edema. Your protocols indicate that a patient in respiratory distress with wheezing should receive oxygen, an intravenous (IV) line, pulse oximetry, a cardiac monitor, and a breathing treatment of albuterol.

You have applied a pulse oximeter and placed the patient on oxygen by nonrebreather mask at 15 L/min. You have established an IV line and attached a cardiac monitor, which shows sinus tachycardia at a rate of 138 beats/min. Based on your knowledge and the patient's presentation, you believe that the appropriate pharmacologic treatment for this patient should include furosemide (Lasix), not albuterol. Because your treatment plan involves a deviation from your protocols, you realize that you must contact medical direction, request an order for furosemide, and explain why you do not believe albuterol administration is appropriate.

When contacting medical direction, you must paint an accurate verbal picture of the patient so that the physician can clearly see the patient and the situation as you see it. Your ability to accurately paint that verbal picture helps the physician develop trust in your judgment. If the physician cannot trust your judgment, he or she is unlikely to allow you to make patient care decisions based on your own assessment.

Factors Affecting Assessment and Decision Making

A Paramedic's Attitude

[OBJECTIVE 3]

A paramedic's attitude can affect patient assessment and decision making. Your attitude must be nonjudgmental. Otherwise you may short circuit the information-gathering process. This can lead to GIGO, or "***g***arbage ***i***n, ***g***arbage ***o***ut." And, as previously emphasized, without adequate information you may be unable to recognize illness or injury patterns.

> **PARAMEDIC*Pearl***
>
> Patients depend on you for assessment and emergency care, not for your assessment of their social standing or "likability."

Uncooperative Patients

[OBJECTIVE 4]

Uncooperative patients can be a challenge to assess and treat. Keep in mind that uncooperative behavior may be a result of an illness or injury. In all uncooperative, restless, belligerent patients, consider the following as possible causes:

- Hypoxia
- Hypovolemia
- Hypoglycemia
- Head injury or concussion
- Drug or alcohol use, toxins, poisons
- Fever or hyperthermia
- Electrolyte imbalances

Labeling and Tunnel Vision

[OBJECTIVE 5]

Labeling is using a derogatory term when referring to a patient based on an event, habit, or personality trait that may not be accurate. Labeling a patient sets an inappropriate tone, may be distracting, and may result in a biased assessment (Figure 55-3). Examples of labels include "just another drunk," "druggie," and "frequent flyer." Labeling is unprofessional and simply bad practice.

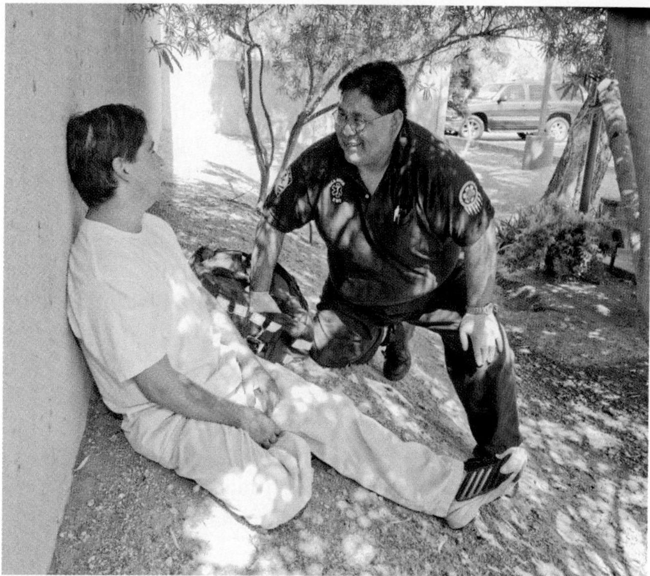

Figure 55-3 When healthcare professionals label a patient, they set an inappropriate tone, create distraction, and may cause a biased assessment.

Having **tunnel vision** means focusing or considering only one aspect of a situation without first taking into account all possibilities. Consider the following real-life situation. Volunteer first responders are dispatched to a private residence for a 65-year-old man reporting chest pain. Equipped with limited medical supplies, the first responders enter the scene with their airway pack and automated external defibrillator. They find the patient lying prone in the doorway of his residence with his cell phone in one hand. As they near the patient, they note that he appears to be unresponsive but they can see his chest rise and fall, and his breathing does not appear to be labored. His skin looks pale. On reaching the patient, they logroll him to continue their assessment and note an overwhelming odor of alcohol and a fresh abrasion on the patient's forehead. Two paramedics from the local EMS agency arrive on the scene, approaching the patient and first responders with only a stretcher. The paramedics immediately assume command of the scene and quickly develop tunnel vision, which subsequently affects the remainder of their patient assessment and decision making.

Much to the amazement of the first responders on the scene, the paramedics determine that the patient is "simply drunk" without any further assessment. They request assistance in moving the patient to the stretcher. This is accomplished under the direction of the paramedics, with two paramedics and two first responders each taking one of the patient's extremities and lifting him onto the gurney. En route to the hospital, the patient is given oxygen by nonrebreather mask and a cardiac monitor is applied. Family members remaining at the scene question the first responders about the care the paramedics provided. While talking with the family, the first responders learn that the patient was diagnosed earlier that same day with advanced leukemia and given 6 months to live. On hearing the news that same day, the patient's wife left him. While absorbing the information from his doctor and dealing with his wife's abrupt departure, the patient began drinking. Hours later, he had a sudden onset of chest pain, which prompted his call to 9-1-1. Worried that he was having a heart attack and that the first responders would not arrive in time to help him, the patient fell in his doorway en route to his car (he planned to drive himself to the hospital). The paramedics missed the patient's chest pain history because of their tunnel vision about the smell of alcohol. The patient was subsequently diagnosed with angina pectoris and given a prescription for nitroglycerin.

PARAMEDIC*Pearl*

When you form a field impression too early, it can result in a biased assessment and an inappropriate treatment plan.

Environment

[OBJECTIVE 6]

Environmental factors can also affect your assessment and decision making. Scene chaos, violent or dangerous situations, crowds of bystanders, crowds of responders, excessive noise, and inclement weather can all be distractions.

In addition, sometimes obvious injuries (e.g., amputation, severe burn) may distract you and take your attention away from more serious problems. You must learn to recognize the seriousness of the injury, move past it, and get yourself in gear to provide the appropriate patient care. This includes performing a primary survey to find all life-threatening conditions. The obvious injuries that are not life threatening can be treated after the patient's life-threatening conditions have been treated. Remember: having tunnel vision may cause you to make an early judgment without all the information you need to provide the appropriate emergency care.

Patient Compliance

The patient's willingness to cooperate can affect your assessment. For example, the physical examination of a cooperative patient is more likely to reveal important information that you can use to form your field impression than an assessment of a patient from a distance. The latter assessment may be all that you can accomplish with a patient who is combative or refusing care. The decisions you make about the patient's treatment plan also may be affected by the patient's compliance. A patient is more likely to be cooperative if he or she has confidence in those providing care. Cultural and ethnic barriers also may affect the patient's compliance.

Manpower Considerations

[OBJECTIVE 7]

Manpower can affect the paramedic's assessment of the patient and decision making. If you are the lone paramedic on the scene, you will need to develop a system with your EMT partner for gathering information so that treatment can begin as quickly as possible. If two paramedics are on scene, information gathering and treatment can be done at the same time. If multiple responders are present, the scene can quickly become confusing and chaotic. This confusion and chaos typically occurs because too many people are asking the same questions of the patient. This results in disorganized information gathering. Therefore you must preplan and designate roles before arrival on the scene.

Assessment and Management Choreography

[OBJECTIVES 8, 9]

During a multiple-tier response, many challenges can occur when gathering the information you need for patient care. Too many people may ask for a patient history, and the noise level may become excessive. This situation can quickly worsen if responders are of the same certification level and have no clear plan. This is often referred to as "assessment by committee" and is not an effective practice because it fragments the clinical picture necessary for pattern recognition and assessment-based management.

When a scene is well choreographed, each person is assigned a role and a chaotic scene becomes quiet and well managed (Figure 55-4). This gives the patient and family a sense of confidence in their rescuers. Before responding to a call, members of the team must have a preplan. A universally understood plan allows others to participate effectively. A basic game plan helps prevent chaos. However, a preplan should not be cast in stone

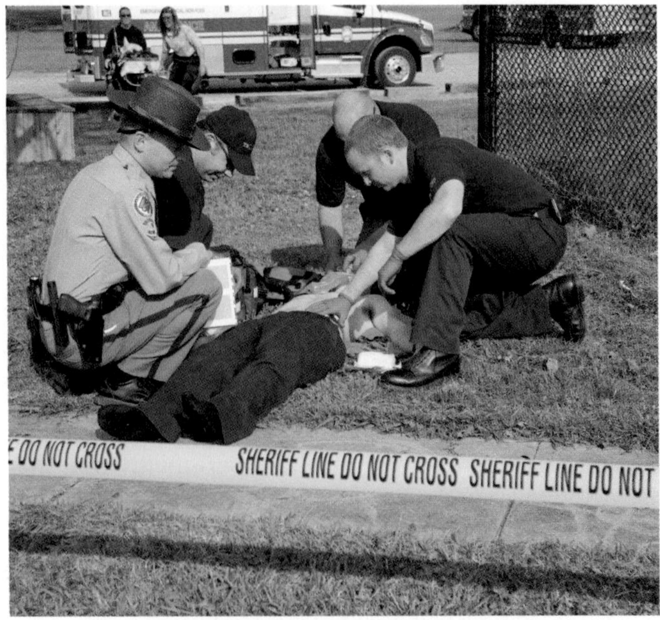

Figure 55-4 When a scene is well choreographed, each person is assigned a role and the scene is well managed.

because field situations are dynamic and can change at any moment. Do not forget to give the first responders who initiated care before your arrival time to let you know what they have found, rather than brushing by them to get to the patient.

The preplan must include designated roles assigned to team members. Paramedics working alone must assume all ALS roles on scene. Two paramedics or crews of multiple paramedics must have a preplan. In other words, you must find a way to designate who is going to do what. This can be simple. The person sitting in the passenger seat can attend the patient and lead the call. After every call, switch roles. Alternately, if you have the same partner all the time, you can trade tasks each shift. Regular partners may develop their own plan and flow.

The team leader is usually the one who stays with the patient through to definitive care. The team leader establishes contact and a dialogue with the patient. He or she obtains the history, performs the physical examination, gives a verbal report over the radio and at the receiving facility, and completes the prehospital care report. The team leader attempts to maintain an overall patient perspective, provide leadership to the team by designating tasks, and coordinate transportation (Figure 55-5). During the resuscitative phase of patient assessment, the team leader actively participates in critical interventions. In multiple-casualty situations, the team leader may act as EMS command. When on the scene of a cardiac emergency, the team leader interprets the patient's ECG, talks on the radio, gives (or relays) drug orders, controls the drug box, and documents the medications given and their effects.

The patient care person performs the following important tasks:

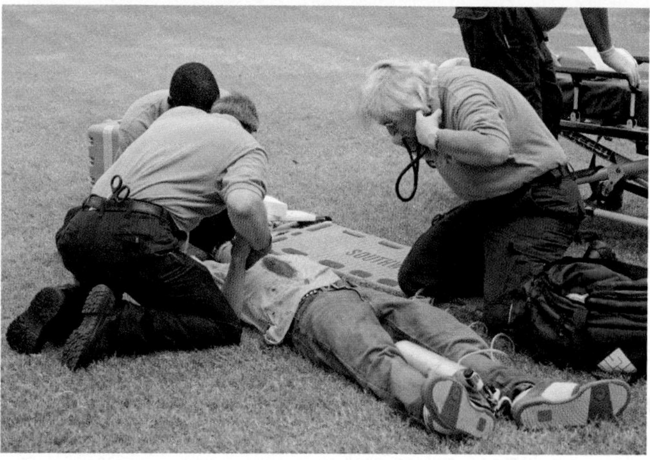

Figure 55-5 The team leader has many roles, including maintaining an overall patient perspective, providing leadership to the team by designating tasks, and coordinating transportation.

- Provides scene cover (watches the team leader's back)
- Gathers scene information, talks to relatives and bystanders
- Attaches monitoring leads
- Administers oxygen
- Establishes vascular access
- Administers medications
- Obtains transportation equipment
- Acts as a triage group leader during multiple-casualty situations
- Administers medications, monitors endotracheal tube placement, and monitors BLS interventions during cardiac emergencies

Case Scenario—continued

You apply supplemental oxygen, obtain a 12-lead ECG, and start an IV. The 12-lead ECG reveals ST segment elevation in leads V_3 and V_4. You complete a physical examination and note that the patient is unkempt. His skin is diaphoretic. Lung sounds reveal bilateral crackles. Heart sounds are normal but tachycardic. The patient's abdomen is soft, nontender, and not distended. His lower extremities have 2+ pitting edema. You administer a sublingual nitroglycerin tablet.

Questions

5. *What does the ECG indicate?*
6. *How do these findings affect your management?*
7. *What is pattern recognition?*
8. *What is pattern response?*

THE "RIGHT STUFF"

The importance of recognizing patterns on the basis of a patient's history and physical examination findings was emphasized at the beginning of this chapter. Pattern recognition brings about the pattern response. A **pattern response** refers to the paramedic anticipating the equipment and emergency care interventions needed on the basis of the patient's history and physical examination findings.

Many EMS professionals make the mistake of going to the patient first (the scene) and then deciding what equipment they need. Then they must return to the emergency vehicle to retrieve it. This costs the patient valuable time and delays care. Paramedics are expected to respond quickly with the equipment they anticipate needing. One of the primary benefits of prehospital care is shortening the time it takes the patient to receive ALS care. Providing appropriate ALS care requires having the "right stuff" within arm's reach; this means carrying the right equipment to the patient's side.

PARAMEDIC*Pearl*

A paramedic must be prepared for the worst. Not having the right equipment immediately available compromises patient care and can cause chaos at the scene.

Following are examples of common pattern responses:

- *Difficulty breathing*. When responding to a patient with a chief complaint of difficulty breathing, the pattern response is a respiratory crisis. You know right away that the patient will need oxygen, an IV, pulse oximeter, and cardiac monitor. Based on your assessment, you will determine what pharmacologic therapy will be appropriate. Equipment that you should take into the scene includes the stretcher, airway pack (including oxygen, suction, bag-mask device, intubation equipment, and Combitube), drug box, pulse oximeter, and cardiac monitor. Taking anything less could delay patient care.
- *Cardiac emergency*. The pattern response to a cardiac call includes taking oxygen and airway supplies, the drug box, pulse oximeter, cardiac monitor, defibrillator, and the stretcher.
- *Possible spinal injury*. The pattern response to calls for suspected spinal injury includes taking spinal stabilization equipment.
- *Altered mental status*. For altered mental status, the pattern response includes an airway pack, IV, drug box, glucometer, pulse oximeter, and cardiac monitor.

Essential Items

[OBJECTIVES 10, 11]

Having the right equipment is similar to backpacking. You should have the items downsized to the essentials that help you move rapidly. You must bring the essential equipment in to *every* patient. This equipment includes anything you will need to manage the ABCDEs (***a***irway, ***b***reathing, ***c***irculation, ***d***isability, ***e***xposure), cardiac monitoring, and defibrillation. Essential equipment is listed in Box 55-1.

BOX 55-1 Essential Equipment

Airway Control

- Oral airways
- Nasal airways
- Suction (electric or manual)
- Suction supplies
- Laryngoscope and blades
- Endotracheal tubes, stylettes, syringes, and tape

Breathing

- Pocket mask
- Bag-mask device
- Spare masks
- Oxygen tank and regulator
- Oxygen masks, cannulas, and extension tubing
- Occlusive dressings
- Large-bore IV catheter for chest decompression

Circulation

- Dressings
- Bandaging and tape
- Infection control supplies
- Blood pressure cuff and stethoscope
- Cardiac monitor and defibrillator
- IV fluids and equipment

Disability

- Rigid collars
- Pen light

Exposure

- Scissors
- Space blanket or something to cover the patient
- Notepad and pen or pencil

PARAMEDIC*Pearl*

Some paramedics choose to take only the stretcher in and "scoop and run" with the patient, preferring to do the assessment and interventions in the ambulance. This type of care is inappropriate. It creates a delay in getting vital lifesaving equipment to the patient. Always anticipate the worst case scenario. Make it a habit to take the essential equipment in with you to the patient—every time. At the same time, keep in mind that time is of the essence—do not dally on the scene. Move quickly and efficiently to complete the essentials on the scene, and then transport the patient to definitive care (completing additional care en route).

Optional Take-In Equipment

The optional equipment you can carry in to the patient depends on your local protocols, the number of paramedics responding, and the difficulty in accessing patients. You may not need to bring optional items for every patient contact. How supplies are carried may depend on how your EMS system is designed. For example, additional supplies may be carried on paramedic ambulances and/or on paramedic nontransport vehicles.

GENERAL APPROACH TO THE PATIENT

[OBJECTIVE 12]

As a paramedic, you set the tone for the call before saying anything. Your demeanor, your clothing, and the tone of your voice contribute to how people perceive you as a medic. Your general approach to the patient should be calm and orderly. Your uniform should be clean and free of tears, holes, or stains. The difference between a wrinkle-free shirt and a wrinkled shirt (as though you just climbed out of bed) could be that bit of confidence in you that the patient desperately needs. Be confident but not arrogant. Be compassionate yet strong. Your bedside manner is extremely important. Patients may not be able to rate your performance, but they can rate your people skills and service.

As emphasized, having a preplan is necessary; it prevents confusion and improves the accuracy of your assessment. In such a plan, one team member (normally the team leader) talks to the patient. Engage in an active, concerned dialogue with the patient and listen to what he or she is saying. Be sure to take notes when you acquire the patient's history. This will help prevent the same questions from being repeatedly asked.

Carry in all the essential equipment so that you are ready to provide resuscitative care if necessary and help prevent chaos because of missing equipment.

Scene Size-Up

Patient assessment begins with the scene size-up. During the scene size-up, take into account the safety of the scene, mechanism of injury, number of patients, and position in which the patient presents. Also take into account the environment and determine if possible hazards exist that may have affected the patient and will affect your ability to provide patient care. Avoid tunnel vision.

Patient Assessment

After the scene size-up, the next part of the patient assessment is forming a general impression and a primary survey. During the primary survey, assess the patient for life-threatening problems. Be systematic and rapidly determine the patient's chief complaint. During the secondary survey, assess the degree of the patient's distress and obtain vital signs as soon as possible.

By the end of the primary survey, you should be able to determine if you have a critical or noncritical patient. Knowing what makes a patient critical is important. Anything that can interfere with a patient's life, senses, or ability to use his or her extremities creates a critical or priority patient. After making this decision in trauma calls, you must have the patient en route to the hospital in less than 10 minutes. For most medical calls, stabilizing on scene is generally appropriate (while limiting scene time) before transport. Exceptions to this guideline include patients who have signs and symptoms consistent with a myocardial infarction or stroke. In these situations scene time must be minimized and the patient transported as quickly as possible to an appropriate receiving facility. A brief description of three general types of approaches to the patient follows.

Resuscitative Approach

The resuscitative approach may be called for if immediate intervention is necessary. It is used when the patient has a life-threatening problem, such as the following:

- Cardiac or respiratory arrest
- Respiratory distress or failure
- Unstable dysrhythmias
- Seizures
- Altered mental status or coma
- Shock or hypotension
- Major trauma
- Possible cervical spine injury

Immediately begin resuscitative measures. Do what you have to on scene and then transport the patient. Acquire more history and details after the immediate resuscitation.

Contemplative Approach

The second type of approach is the contemplative approach. Immediate intervention is not necessary. In general, you conduct the history and physical examination first, then provide the interventions as necessary.

Evacuation

The third approach is immediate evacuation. Immediate evacuation to the ambulance may be necessary if the patient needs life-saving interventions you cannot provide. In other situations the scene also may be un-stable, unsafe, or too chaotic to allow for a rational assessment.

Case Scenario CONCLUSION

You prepare the patient for transport. He is still complaining of chest pain. He rates the pain as a 6 out of 10. His blood pressure is 148/92 mm Hg, pulse is 94 beats/min, respirations are 20 breaths/min, and pulse oximetry is 100%. You administer a second nitroglycerin tablet and contact the receiving facility.

Questions

9. *What can be done to comfort this patient?*
10. *What information should be provided in the report to the receiving facility?*

PRESENTING THE PATIENT

[OBJECTIVE 13]

After you have assessed your patient, provided the appropriate treatment, and initiated transport, you must relay patient information to the receiving facility. You have a responsibility to relay information about your patient accurately to the receiving physician so he or she can visualize the patient who has not yet arrived. For instance, when describing a motor vehicle crash in a radio report, accurately describe the crash in a way that the physician can "see" the crash scene. For example:

"Medic 5 to Region Medical Center."

"Go, ahead Medic 5."

"Region, we are en route to your facility with a 50-year-old male who was involved in a one-car motor vehicle crash. Patient was a restrained driver in a car that had a front-end impact with a tree. Estimated speed 65 miles per hour. Major front-end damage to the vehicle with engine intrusion into the passenger compartment. The patient was found unresponsive, restrained, entrapped in the vehicle, with the steering wheel and dash rolled down onto his legs. The steering wheel was found to be compressing the patient's chest. Patient was still breathing on his own at a rate of 28, very shallow breaths when we arrived."

From this description of the car accident, the physician is able to visualize the vehicle and the accident, providing a better understanding of the mechanism of injury the patient sustained. Without being at the scene, the physician is able to see the crash when you provide a good description.

Effective communication and transfer of patient information is vital to both prehospital and hospital care. Good verbal and written reporting skills are essential in establishing trust and credibility. Good assessment and reporting go hand in hand.

BOX 55-2 Components of a Verbal Report

Patient identification, age, gender, and degree of distress

Subjective findings

- Chief complaint
- Present illness or injury: pertinent details about the present problem, pertinent negatives
- Allergies, medications, and pertinent medical history

Objective findings

- Physical examination findings: vital signs, pertinent positive findings, pertinent negative findings

Assessment: paramedic's field impression (the cause of the patient's symptoms) and anticipated problems (what else may go wrong in the immediate and near future)

Plan: what has been done, orders requested

PARAMEDIC*Pearl*

A good verbal and written report implies that good assessments and good patient care were performed. A poor verbal report and/or documentation imply that the patient was not thoroughly assessed and that the care given was less than adequate.

An effective verbal report is concise and usually takes less than 1 minute to communicate. It is usually free of extensive medical jargon. A verbal report should generally follow the ***s***ubjective, ***o***bjective, ***a***ssessment, ***p***lan (SOAP) format or some variation of it. One possible format for verbal reporting is shown in Box 55-2. The key to developing proficiency in verbal reporting is repetition and understanding the format. Start by using a small preprinted form. With practice, you will eventually depend on the form less and less.

Case Scenario SUMMARY

1. *What is your initial impression of this patient?* This patient has chest pain. The information that he is homeless may be important. What is the patient's nutrition? Has he had medical care? Has he contracted pneumonia? Is he hypothermic? The vital signs indicate a hypertensive patient with tachycardia. Chest pain should always be taken seriously. Pattern recognition tells you that cardiac chest pain most often occurs in middle-age and older adults. Risk factors include smoking, obesity, previous cardiac problems, hypertension, family history, diabetes mellitus, and hypercholesterolemia. In this scenario, none of this information was provided on purpose. Despite the patient's socioeconomic status or personal habits, chest pain should raise concern.

2. *What is tunnel vision, and how could it affect your care of this patient?* Having tunnel vision means focusing or considering only one aspect of a situation without first taking into account all possibilities. Forming an opinion on a patient based on his or her social situation, body habitus, hygiene, race, nationality, skin color, disability, or any other condition other than medical condition can be detrimental to patient care.
3. *What is labeling, and how could it affect your management of this patient?* Labeling is using a derogatory term when referring to a patient based on an event, habit, or personality trait that may not be accurate. Labeling a patient sets an inappropriate tone, may be distracting, and may result in a biased assessment. Avoid labeling. Keeping out all bias is difficult, but it should never cloud clinical judgment.
4. *What are possible diagnoses for this patient and how do they affect your management?* This patient reports chest pain that radiates to the back and has a tearing sensation. He also has hypertension. You should consider the following diagnoses:
   - Aortic dissection
   - Acute myocardial infarction
   - Angina or unstable angina
   - Pneumonia
   - Pneumothorax
   - Pulmonary embolus
   - Pancreatitis
   - Chest wall pain
   - Musculoskeletal chest pain
   - Pleuritic chest pain
5. *What does the ECG indicate?* ST segment elevation in leads V_3 and V_4 is suggestive of an anterior wall myocardial infarction.
6. *How do these findings affect your management?* The patient should receive aspirin, nitroglycerin, and morphine for pain management if no contraindications exist. If beta-blockers are part of your myocardial infarction protocol, consider administration because of the patient's hypertension and his acute pain. Rapidly prepare the patient for transport to the receiving facility. Obtain serial 12-lead ECGs and closely monitor the patient's vital signs.
7. *What is pattern recognition?* Pattern recognition is gathering patient information, relating it to the healthcare professional's knowledge of pathophysiology and the signs and symptoms of illnesses and injuries, and determining whether the patient's presentation fits a particular pattern. In this case the patient has chest pain. He has a tearing sensation in his back. As information from history, physical examination, and diagnostic tests is obtained, formulating a field impression is important. It may be as simple as "very sick" or "not so sick." This patient is having an acute myocardial infarction. The decision that this patient is sick and requires immediate transport is part of pattern recognition.
8. *What is pattern response?* Pattern response is anticipating the equipment and emergency care procedures needed. This allows easier care of the patient. As an example, this patient is reporting chest pain. A pattern response is to grab the pharmacology bag or drug box, supplemental oxygen, and cardiac monitor because they will most likely be needed. If these are not initially carried in, patient care may be delayed. Running back to the ambulance to get equipment is not an effective use of time.
9. *What can be done to comfort this patient?* Despite oxygen and two doses of sublingual nitroglycerin, the patient still has chest pain. Because the nitroglycerin has not resolved his pain and the patient has an adequate blood pressure, administer morphine sulfate for pain control. Also transport the patient in a position of comfort.
10. *What information should be provided in the report to the receiving facility?* Relay the patient's history, physical examination, and diagnostic findings to the receiving facility. This patient initially presented with findings of chest pain radiating to his back with a tearing sensation. Pattern recognition would lead to the belief that this may be a dissection of the thoracic aorta. Provide the receiving facility with the findings on the ECG and the treatment you have provided. Giving a complete report is important. The receiving facility needs maximal information but with good time management.

Chapter Summary

- Assessment-based management requires that you treat the patient and not simply follow the protocol.
- With the information you gathered from your assessment of the scene, the patient's SAMPLE history, and physical examination findings, you must realize that deviation from protocol may be necessary to treat your patient appropriately.
- Use everything at your disposal to help form your assessment: your senses, the patient's signs and symptoms, medical history, and environment. Then treat your patient.
- Do not get tunnel vision. Horrific injuries, children who are sick or injured, and situations that stress your ability to perform can cause you to focus on only one aspect of the patient's care instead of care of the whole patient.
- Learn how to choreograph the scene. Preplan with your partner, practicing what you would do in any situation.
- An accurate verbal report provides the physician and receiving facility staff with a description of what you saw, what you did, and how the patient is at this point in your care.

Chapter Quiz

1. When responding to a motor vehicle crash with major front-end damage, you find an unrestrained driver unresponsive on the ground. How would you classify this patient?
   a. Low priority
   b. Medium priority
   c. High priority
   d. Dead on arrival

2. True or False: Assessment-based management requires that a paramedic must not deviate from established treatment protocols.

3. True or False: A poor verbal report and/or documentation may give an impression that the patient was not thoroughly assessed and that the care given was less than adequate.

4. True or False: Essential equipment includes anything you will need to manage the ABCDEs, cardiac monitoring, and defibrillation.

5. When responding to a patient who has difficulty breathing, you expect the patient's signs and symptoms to present in a certain manner. This is called _______.
   a. case-based management
   b. patient presentation
   c. pattern recognition
   d. pattern response

6. When responding to a chest pain call, the equipment that should be brought to the patient should include _______.
   a. automated external defibrillator, long spine board, and suction unit
   b. bag-mask device, intubation equipment, and cardiac monitor
   c. oxygen, drug box, and cardiac monitor
   d. stretcher, airway bag, drug box, and cardiac monitor

7. You have been called to a shooting. The patient is a 16-year-old male who has been shot in the chest. What equipment would be appropriate to take with you to his side?
   a. Stretcher, airway bag, trauma bag, backboard, spinal immobilization supplies
   b. Stretcher, airway bag, drug box, cardiac monitor, backboard
   c. Stretcher, cardiac monitor, drug box, backboard, spinal immobilization supplies
   d. Stretcher, trauma bag, backboard, spinal immobilization supplies

8. You are called to a patient with a chief complaint of difficulty breathing. The patient states she had a heart attack 2 years ago. Physical examination reveals crackles, bilateral pedal edema, sweaty skin, and jugular venous distention. You suspect ______.
   a. asthma
   b. congestive heart failure
   c. pneumonia
   d. pulmonary embolus

9. On arrival at the scene of a motor vehicle crash, you find a 73-year-old man who was the unrestrained driver of the vehicle. He is complaining of difficulty breathing. Your physical examination reveals absent lung sounds on the right side and bruising on the right chest. You suspect _______.
   a. cardiac tamponade
   b. heart attack
   c. pneumonia
   d. pneumothorax

10. You have been called to the scene of a child who has been injured in a fall from a tree. On arrival, you find a 5-year-old girl with both arms at gross angles with open fractures to both radiuses. She has lost little blood. You should immediately _______.
   a. apply a cervical collar
   b. assess circulation distal to the fractures
   c. assess the airway
   d. try to control bleeding

Terminology

Assessment-based management Taking the information you obtain from your assessment and using it to treat the patient.

Labeling The application of a derogatory term to a patient on the basis of an event, habit, or personality trait that may not be accurate.

Pattern recognition Gathering patient information, relating it to the healthcare professional's knowledge of pathophysiology and the signs and symptoms of illnesses and injuries, and determining whether the patient's presentation fits a particular pattern.

Pattern response Anticipating the equipment and emergency care interventions needed on the basis of the patient's history and physical examination findings.

Tunnel vision Focusing on or considering only one aspect of a situation without first taking into account all possibilities.

CHAPTER 56

Clinical Decision Making

Objectives

After completing this chapter, you will be able to:

1. Compare medical care in the prehospital environment with medical care in other settings.
2. Distinguish critical life-threatening, potentially life-threatening, and non–life-threatening patient presentations and the paramedic's decision-making process for each.
3. Evaluate the benefits and shortfalls of protocols, standing orders, and patient care algorithms.
4. Define the parts, stages, and sequences of the critical thinking process that the paramedic uses.
5. Describe the effects of the "fight or flight" response and the positive and negative effects it has on a paramedic's decision-making process.
6. Summarize the six *R*'s of "putting it all together": ***r***ead the patient, ***r***ead the scene, ***r***eact, ***r***eevaluate, ***r***evise the management plan, and ***r***eview performance.

Chapter Outline

Case Scenario

It is 8:55 AM on a cool fall morning when your crew is dispatched to the intersection of 4th Avenue and Main for a single-car crash. On arriving at the scene, you notice a car has collided with a concrete light pole, with the majority of the impact just behind the front seat on the passenger side of the car. No hazards are noted and the scene appears safe. As you approach the car, a police officer tells you that a truck cut in front of the car and the driver of the car lost control. The officer indicates the driver is complaining of head, neck, and back pain. You approach the driver, who is sitting in the car. He looks pale and sweaty even though the ambient temperature is 56° F. The patient, a 68-year-old man, states that his head and neck hurt and he is having a hard time breathing. The man is still wearing his seat belt. A police officer is sitting in the back seat of the vehicle holding the man's head and neck still. The officer states that the man's breathing seems to be getting worse.

Questions

1. *What is your initial impression of the patient?*
2. *What additional information do you need to complete the assessment?*
3. *What may be causing the man's respiratory distress?*

The cornerstone of effective paramedic practice is clinical decision making. The end result of successful clinical decision making is quality patient care. As a paramedic, you use all your formal and informal education in making clinical decisions. Your formal education includes, for example, physical assessment techniques and knowledge of clinical conditions and mechanism of injury. Your informal education includes, for example, self-learning through continuing education and other educational opportunities.

For paramedics, making clinical decisions begins with the tasks of gathering information, evaluating it, and bringing it all together. You gather information from both the patient and the scene. This information can be quite specific, such as nature of the call, patient history, and physical signs and symptoms. It also includes general information gathered with your senses (what you observe, hear, feel, and smell). You pull all this information together and evaluate it for relevance and appropriateness. Then you synthesize it into a clinical picture of the patient's condition.

Additional subfactors affect the clinical decision-making process. These include the patient's cultural and religious beliefs, background, and attitude. These factors affect the entire clinical decision-making process, making it more than a simple decision without regard for the patient. Rather, it is a multifaceted process, with the patient as the primary focus (Mears & Sweeney, 2000). The multifaceted process of making clinical decisions is challenging but not impossible.

This clinical picture of the patient is used to develop and then implement a plan to best treat his or her condition(s). As a part of this overall process, you must apply appropriate judgment for the best possible patient outcome, and you must exercise independent decision making based on the clinical picture.

Finally, as all the elements of clinical decision making come together, you must think and work effectively under pressure. The pressures on the job come from other providers, the patient, the patient's family, the bystanders, medical control, and the EMS system itself.

THE PREHOSPITAL ENVIRONMENT

[OBJECTIVE 1]

As a paramedic, you are responsible for assessment and care of the same patients as other practitioners, but it must be done in a unique workplace with limited personnel and without the advantage of advanced diagnostic technology. Your workplace involves working in all extremes of weather, from the bitter cold of winter to the hottest days of summer, as well as in rain and snow. It also entails working with difficult situations on the streets, in houses and in buildings away from other resources, as well as with different personnel from other agencies, such as fire or police departments. The focus of the other personnel on the scene is different from your focus.

THE NATURE OF PREHOSPITAL CARE

[OBJECTIVE 2]

Besides dealing with extreme environmental conditions, you may experience calls for assistance that range from emergent to nonemergent issues. These issues may run the gamut. The call may involve an obvious critical life threat, such as a full arrest, a stabbing, or a shooting. On the other hand, the call may involve a potential life threat, such as a motor vehicle crash or a patient with multiple medical conditions. Finally, the call may simply involve a non–life-threatening situation, such as a sick patient with coldlike symptoms.

Each of these types of calls requires you to gather information, implement a patient treatment plan, apply clinical judgment, and exercise independent decision making. Not all calls require you to perform all your technical treatment skills. At times, you may simply need to provide comfort as best as you can (Weinmann, 2003).

Guidance and Authority for Paramedics

[OBJECTIVE 3]

As a paramedic, your clinical decision-making process is generally guided by protocols, standing orders, and patient care algorithms. These guidelines and protocols are typically developed by state regulating bodies, local medical direction, or both. Guidelines and protocols are becoming increasingly evidenced based. As a result, the best possible patient care outcomes are promoted. Moreover, in being increasingly evidence based, guidelines and protocols provide a standardized approach to patient care. When implemented as part of the EMS system, they improve the clinical practice of the system itself and the individual services within that system (Handly et al., 1994; Limmer & Monosky, 2002; Spaite & Criss, 2003; Dunford et al., 2003).

Protocols, standing orders, and patient care algorithms guide the clinical decision-making process. However, you must understand their limitations. These limitations include several factors, such as protocols, guidelines, and algorithms that address only "classic" patient presentations. Nonspecific patient symptoms do not follow a classic model. In addition, protocols, guidelines, and algorithms do not address multiple disease conditions or multiple treatment modalities. Nor do they readily promote critical thinking. Instead, they lead to a linear, or "cookbook," approach to patient care. This type of patient care is not acceptable. Protocols and algorithms are guidelines, but good clinical judgment should always take priority within the bounds of what the individual is approved to do.

THE CRITICAL THINKING PROCESS

The actual process of making clinical decisions involves a series of interconnected information gathering and analyzing points. Together these are used to apply a principle of care. The care that you provide is evaluated during and after the patient care encounter.

Concept Formation

[OBJECTIVE 4]

You begin to form an overall concept of care **(concept formation)** for a patient when you first arrive on the location of an incident. You receive data, such as the mechanism of injury and/or illness, and information from the scene assessment. Next, you conduct an initial assessment and physical examination by using a standardized and logical approach (Limmer & Monosky, 2002). The next general step is to obtain a chief complaint either from the patient or bystanders or as a deductive process if the patient is unable to provide a chief complaint and no bystanders or family members are present. In addition, you gather a pertinent medical history and assess the patient's affect. This includes whether the patient is in pain, whether he or she has an altered mental status, and what is happening to and around the patient at the scene. Affective data may include social or family situations or interactions you may witness at the scene (Luger et al., 2003). Finally, you take the data from the diagnostic tests completed and interpret it into usable information.

Case Scenario—continued

A head-to-toe examination and SAMPLE history reveal an alert, oriented man in acute respiratory distress. No trauma is evident. The head, ears, eyes, nose, and throat appear normal, and no deformity is noticeable or palpable on the face, head, or neck. Some tenderness is noted around the base of the neck (C7 to T1). No injury is present on the chest, abdomen, or extremities. The steering wheel and steering column are intact, with no deformity in either structure. The patient's skin is pale, cool, and clammy. Lung sounds indicate bilateral crackles in the lung bases extending one third up the thoracic cavity. The patient occasionally produces frothy sputum. Vital signs are blood pressure, 170/110 mm Hg; pulse, 128 beats/min and irregular; respirations, 32 breaths/min and labored. The patient states he has congestive heart failure and takes Lasix and "some other things" to help him breathe. He further tells you that he had a rough night and needed three pillows simply to be able to breathe and get some rest. He was on his way to his physician's office when the crash occurred. While you are assessing and questioning the patient, your partner provides the man with supplemental oxygen at 15 L/min by nonrebreather mask. After the oxygen has been started, the man states he is breathing easier. An ECG reveals atrial fibrillation.

Questions

4. *Has your first impression changed?*
5. *Do the man's vital signs suggest shock?*
6. *What extrication, treatment, and transportation options should be considered?*

Data Interpretation

The step of **data interpretation** requires using the data you have gathered in the concept formation stage and integrating it with your knowledge of anatomy, physiology, and pathophysiology. Certain factors can affect your interpretation of the data. These include previous experiences in dealing with patients in general and prior dealings with the particular disease or condition of the current patient.

One area of data interpretation often is overlooked or misunderstood: the paramedic's attitude. Your attitude can have a significant impact on your interpretation of data. Your attitude encompasses any biases you may have based on socioeconomic status and/or other classifications. These biases may cause you to impose your beliefs on the patient care situation. On the other hand, your attitude may be empathetic, and you may show concern for the patient regardless of the differences between you. Both instances have an effect on patient care, one negative and one positive (Clark et al., 1991; Eisenburg, 1979).

Application of Principles

Once you have gathered the data and interpreted them into usable information, the next step is the appropriate **application of principles** to treatment and care of the patient. Initially, you begin this step as you apply critical thinking in a clinical sense and arrive at a field impression, or a working diagnosis (Croskerry, 2000). A working diagnosis is merely an initial formulation of the information at hand that you process into an idea of what is happening to the patient.

After you decide what you think is happening to the patient, the next step in the critical thinking process is for you to apply the appropriate protocol or standing order to the situation. This is where the process moves from the information gathering and interpretation stage to the physical treatment or intervention stage.

Evaluation

Once you have completed any patient procedure or treatment, you must evaluate the effectiveness of that treatment. The **evaluation of treatment** rendered mandates that you reassess the overall patient and, specifically, the body systems affected by that treatment. This evaluation seeks to discover the answers to two critical questions; the first is whether the treatment worked as intended, and the second is the clinical condition of the patient after the treatment (Gallagher, 2003).

After you have evaluated the treatment and any clinical indications of the patient's current status, consider revising your initial impression of the patient's condition. This revision should include whether the protocol or standing order that you used was appropriate and whether the treatment was effective and had the expected and desired physiologic response. If the treatment was effective and the appropriate protocol or standing order was used, then continue the protocol. However, if you find that the treatment or protocol was ineffective during your reassessment evaluation, then apply a subsequent or different treatment or protocol to the patient's situation (Dunford et al., 2003). If another treatment or protocol is needed, then the critical thinking process returns to applying another treatment or protocol to achieve the desired results.

You should apply all your experience and knowledge to provide patient care. However, you should not become so dogmatic in your thoughts and actions that as subsequent reassessments are completed and another treatment or protocol is indicated, you are unwilling to modify your initial treatment or protocol. The appropriate and accepted action is always to modify the treatment or protocol (Dunford et al., 2003).

Reflection on Actions

After you have completed the patient care encounter, the critical thinking process should involve some form of reflection on the call. The purpose of the reflection is to ensure the quality of patient care. This **reflection on actions** may involve a personal reflection, or it may entail a run critique of some sort. In certain instances, this may be done formally or, in most instances, accomplished informally (Denig et al., 2002).

Fundamental Elements of Critical Thinking

[OBJECTIVE 4]

The critical thinking process is composed of several fundamental elements. The first of these essential elements is an adequate fund of knowledge. You have gained this knowledge through your initial and continuing education. This initial element is crucial for applying critical thinking. It also is a base on which subsequent actions are evaluated (Allery et al., 1997; Tomlin et al., 1999). The other essential elements include your ability to focus on specific and multiple elements of data; then gather and organize data into workable concepts; identify and deal with medical ambiguity, such as incomplete histories or nonclassic symptoms; distinguish between the relevant and irrelevant data; analyze and compare similar or contrary situations; and finally provide rational decision-making reasoning and construct logical arguments regarding why you performed treatments.

FIELD APPLICATIONS OF ASSESSMENT-BASED PATIENT MANAGEMENT

[OBJECTIVES 1, 5]

As previously discussed, the spectrum of patient conditions ranges from the emergent acute conditions to the nonemergent, nonacute conditions. In the context of critical thinking, the severity of these conditions relates directly to the general amount of critical thinking you will need. For patients with major emergent and acute conditions, the degree of critical thinking you will need to apply is relatively low. This would appear to be counterintuitive; however, when examined, the most critical patients actually require little critical thinking on your part but immediate and practiced treatment. You will actually apply the greatest amount of critical thinking to the moderate- or minor-acuity patients. For these patients, the symptoms are less dramatic and the need to relate these often confusing symptoms into a cogent treatment plan is greater (Hollander et al., 1995; Hennes et al., 2005).

Another aspect of critical thinking while in the field is the ability to think under pressure. This ability is essential in the out-of-hospital arena. In fact, you may be under pressure from the patient or his or her family, and in many instances you are operating in difficult locations, such as crime scenes. Moreover, the EMS system itself provides pressure, with the need to leave the scene, get to the hospital, and then return to service. In addition, you will feel pressure from the need to communicate significant patient care-related information to the hospital staff, who was not at the scene and often is removed from the confusion of the scene.

When thinking under pressure, your hormones come into play. As the pressure on you increases, the hormonal dump of epinephrine induces the "fight or flight" response. This hormonal response enhances your visual and auditory acuity and improves your reflexes and strength as the epinephrine surges through your body. While this increased epinephrine level heightens the physical abilities, it can also impair the cognitive or thinking processes of the brain as the body goes into survival mode. The surge of epinephrine also can decrease your ability to concentrate and process patient assessments. This physical response can confound your clinical decision-making process, and you should anticipate it.

Mental Preparation

You can anticipate and combat the detrimental effects of the epinephrine surge. One method is to practice your assessment and treatment skills to the near instinctive level. This can be facilitated by using logical, repeatable, and reliable assessment techniques and treatment modalities. This will help produce an automatic response when under pressure.

Another tool you can use to reduce the negative effects of operating under pressure is a mental checklist. The first item on the checklist is *stop and think*. Think about what is happening and what needs to be done next. Then scan the situation to gain an awareness of the overall scene. Then, with knowledge of what is happening and with situational awareness, you can decide what needs to be done and then act to accomplish it. After deciding what to do and then acting to accomplish it, maintain clear and concise control of the scene, including working with other providers, bystanders, or family members. Finally, you need to evaluate your actions and the patient repeatedly and often. This protects the patient and reduces patient care into manageable blocks of care.

Other techniques are available to help you think under pressure. These techniques can help facilitate the behavior you want when treating patients, are easy to learn and perform, and provide a good mindset before encountering a stressful situation. The first technique is to stay calm and not panic. This is easily said, but the ability to not succumb to the situation is essential; take a mental step back, take a breath, and do not panic. The situation confronting you may be chaotic, but the chaos does not need to extend to your treatment and care of the patient in that situation.

The next technique is to assume and plan for the worst case possible. If the situation becomes the worst case possible, then you have already imagined it and mentally prepared for it. However, if the situation is not the worst case, then the reality of the situation has not met your expectations and, therefore, it will be easier to deal with. A second aspect of planning for the worst is always to err on the side of patient safety and optimum care. If you are in doubt regarding whether to perform an assessment or be more aggressive, and it is authorized and the patient's condition warrants it, do it.

Finally, you must balance and process the assessments, the various assessment tools (e.g., cardiac monitor, blood pressure, capnography), and your individual decision-making style. Three general styles exist of balancing and processing the situation and the data and making decisions.

Situational Analysis, Data Processing, and Decision-Making Styles

The first style involves situational analysis. Situational analysis styles range from reflective to impulsive. You must understand the situation and apply the most beneficial technique or procedure for the patient's good. Research has proven that clinicians operate in two modes. One is reflective, or when the clinician thinks before performing an action. The other mode is impulsive, or when the clinician performs an action because a preset idea or condition is present (Gallagher, 2003). Understanding how you handle situational analysis is key to mentally preparing for difficult calls.

The second style involves data processing. Data processing styles vary from divergent to convergent. This concerns the manner in which you process data. A divergent style involves gathering several sources of data, such as medication and drug references, to come to a conclusion. A convergent style involves operating with one source of data, such as one textbook or reference.

The third style involves decision making. Decision-making styles include anticipatory and reactive. This is at the crux of patient care. With an anticipatory style, you see a problem or condition and treat it in the initial symptom stages with an idea of what could occur if it is not treated. With a reactive style, you wait until a patient presents with a clear condition and set of symptoms before initiating treatment.

All three of these styles reveal important characteristics you must be aware of, on an individual basis, before you are confronted with a chaotic and confusing situation. Understanding "why" you as an individual do certain "things" in a certain way mentally prepares you before you have to deal with difficult situations (Croskerry, 2000).

Case Scenario CONCLUSION

You and your partner face a transportation dilemma, and your partner asks you for guidance. You realize that putting the patient in a supine position on a long spine board will only worsen his dyspnea, yet you need to immobilize the patient's head, neck, and spine to prevent any sudden or unnecessary movement. Your partner suggests that you sedate and intubate the patient to facilitate extricating and transporting him on a long spine board. After thinking for a moment, you opt to use the Kendrick Extrication Device (KED) to stabilize and secure the spine. Once the man is stabilized in the KED, he is placed in a sitting position on the gurney. The head, neck, and back are immobilized and the patient is able to remain in a sitting position that allows easier breathing.

Looking back

7. *What is your final impression of the patient?*
8. *Is the patient appropriately immobilized to prevent additional spinal injury?*
9. *Does using the KED and placing the patient in a sitting position violate protocols?*

PUTTING IT ALL TOGETHER: THE SIX *R*'S

[OBJECTIVE 6]

There is a simple mnemonic to remember all the aspects necessary in clinical decision making from a theoretical process to an active process. It is the six *R*'s: ***r***ead the scene, ***r***ead the patient, ***r***eact, ***r***eevaluate, ***r***evise management plan, and ***r***eview performance (Figure 56-1).

Read the scene. You should evaluate the environmental conditions and the immediate scene. You must decide what is happening. You also need to consider what factors such as weather, location, and overall environment will affect care. You should observe the mechanism of injury and identify what may be the primary, secondary, and tertiary injuries based on the scene.

Read the patient. Form a first impression of the patient. Observe the patient's level of consciousness, skin color, gait, posture, position, and location. You should consider what is obvious and what is not, using pertinent negatives. Talk with the patient if possible. Consider whether he or she called for assistance for an existing or worsening condition or for a new problem (Colwell et al., 2003). Touch the patient. Note skin temperature and condition. Check pulses (Are they present?). Check the quality of the pulses in all areas. Auscultate the patient. Listen to the anterior and posterior areas of the lungs, bases, and apices. Listen to the upper and lower airway. Gather a complete and accurate set of vital signs. This helps with patient triage, treatment decisions, and underlying pathologies. In addition, remember to understand the influences of age, medical conditions, and medications (Bray et al., 2005).

React. After taking the patient and scene data into account, you must act. React to life threats in the order they are found. Determine the most probable cause that fits the patient's signs and symptoms. Work toward the most serious possibility and, if a clear condition is not discernable, base your treatment on the presenting signs and symptoms.

Reevaluate, reevaluate, reevaluate. Make sure you conduct focused and detailed examinations. Reevaluate the patient's response to treatments and interventions. Consider whether the patient responded appropriately and as expected. During the revaluation, consider whether you discovered any less-obvious conditions that may or may not be comorbid conditions.

Revise your management plan on the basis of information gathered during the previous phases to determine whether the current management plan is effective or ineffective. If your plan is ineffective, then revise it to be consistent with the patient's signs and symptoms.

Review your performance at a run critique. After you have completed the call, perform a critique of what went right and what went wrong for the patient (a primary concern) and for you (a secondary concern). Just as physicians and EMS systems evaluate performance, you must do so as well (Feldman et al., 2005). This critique is a critical review meant to reinforce positive actions and change negative actions.

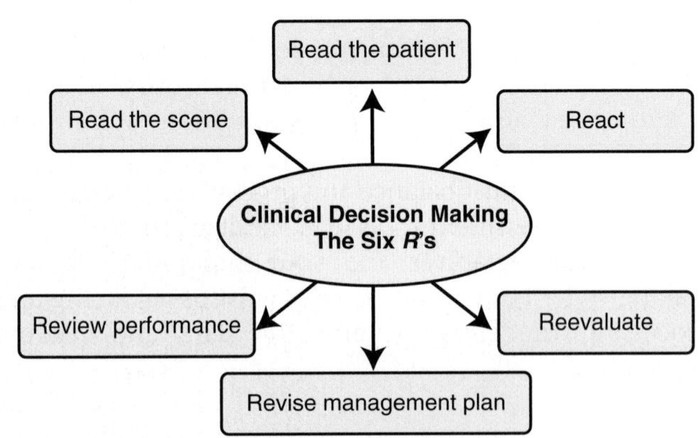

Figure 56-1 Clinical decision making: the six *R*'s.

Case Scenario SUMMARY

1. *What is your initial impression of the patient?* Your initial impression may include trauma associated with signs and symptoms of shock. The patient may also have a head, neck, or back injury.
2. *What additional information do you need to complete the assessment?* Additional information needed includes a head-to-toe evaluation and a detailed SAMPLE history. Last oral intake may be important if the man's injuries require surgical intervention.
3. *What may be causing the man's respiratory distress?* The respiratory distress may be caused by a number of factors, including fractured ribs, pneumothorax, hemothorax, or medical conditions such as pulmonary embolism, chronic obstructive pulmonary disease, acute myocardial infarction, or congestive heart failure.
4. *Has your first impression changed?* The initial impression is changed by the additional information. Evidence of acute trauma is scant; however, the patient's admission of a history of congestive heart failure suggests that condition as the cause of his dyspnea.
5. *Do the man's vital signs suggest shock?* Shock is a condition in which blood flow to the tissues is inadequate. This patient's blood pressure is elevated, eliminating shock as a problem. The patient's pulse is elevated, perhaps because of the stress of the crash or the exacerbation of his congestive heart failure. The

increased rate of breathing is consistent with dyspnea and pulmonary edema as a result of congestive heart failure.

6. *What extrication, treatment, and transportation options should be considered?* The standard protocol for trauma patients reporting head, neck, or back pain requires spinal stabilization, preferably on a long spine board. Given this patient's statement that he needed three pillows to breathe the night before and the presence of crackles in the lung bases, placing the patient in a supine condition may not fully serve his needs. Patients with congestive heart failure prefer to sit fully upright or at least in a semi-Fowler's position. Treatment for the condition includes high-flow oxygen, nitroglycerin, furosemide and, in some cases, morphine. Bronchodilators may be ordered if wheezing accompanies the patient's crackles. Airway and ventilatory support with endotracheal intubation coupled with positive pressure ventilation may be needed.
7. *What is your final impression of the patient?* The patient sustained some injuries as a result of the crash. Because of the limits on diagnostic capabilities, you cannot rule out a head, neck, or back injury. However, his respiratory distress from congestive heart failure poses an urgent problem that needs prompt intervention. Both conditions—potential for head, neck, and back injuries as well as dyspnea—need to be treated.
8. *Is the patient appropriately immobilized to prevent additional spinal injury?* Spinal stabilization included immobilizing the patient from his head to his buttocks. The KED successfully does this and permits the patient to be placed in a position of comfort for transport. EMS protocols typically call for placing the patient supine on a long spine board. Doing so in this case would worsen the patient's dyspnea and perhaps his hypoxia. Unless injured, the man's arms and legs can be allowed to move freely.
9. *Does using the KED and placing the patient in a sitting position violate protocols?* Although using the KED and placing the patient in a sitting position may appear unorthodox and contradictory to protocol, in this case it is appropriate and in the best interests of the patient. Protocols are guidelines and useful in the treatment of most patients. However, some patient conditions do not always fit into the protocols. Thus protocols may need some modification to best serve the individual patient.

Chapter Summary

- Clinical decision making is the cornerstone of effective paramedic practice. It involves all clinical education, both formal and informal.
- The paramedic must work in difficult environments, and under pressure from various sources. You must also deal with patients with acute and emergent life-threatening conditions as well as those with nonacute, nonemergent, and non–life-threatening conditions.
- The paramedic's clinical decision-making process is generally governed by protocols, standing orders, and patient care algorithms either from state regulating bodies or by local medical control or a combination. You must recognize that protocols, standing orders, and patient care algorithms do not address all conditions or multiple conditions that may present in the field.
- Critical thinking involves fundamental elements. These include an adequate fund of knowledge, the ability to focus on specific and multiple elements of data, the ability to gather and organize data into workable concepts, the ability to identify and deal with medical ambiguity, the ability to distinguish relevant from irrelevant data, the ability to analyze and compare similar or contrary situations, and the ability to provide rational decision-making reasoning and construct logical arguments concerning what you have done.
- Clinical decision making mandates that you read the scene and the patient. In addition, you must react and reevaluate the scene, the patient, and his or her reaction. Next, you must revise your treatment plan as necessary. Finally, you must review your performance to ensure quality patient care.

REFERENCES

Allery, L. A., Owen, P. A., & Robling, M. R. (1997). Why general practitioners and consultants change their clinical practice: A critical incident study. *British Medical Journal, 314,* 870-874.

Bray, J. E., Martin, J., Cooper, G., Barger, B., Bernard, S., Bladin, C., et al. (2005). An interventional study to improve paramedic diagnosis of stroke. *Prehospital Emergency Care, 9,* 297-302.

Clark, J. A., Potter, D. A., & McKinlay, J. B. (1991). Bring social structure into clinical decision making. *Social Science Medicine, 32,* 853-866.

Colwell, C. B., Pons, P. T., & Pi, R. (2003). Complaints against an EMS system. *Journal of Emergency Medicine, 25,* 403-408.

Croskerry, P. (2000). The cognitive imperative: Thinking about how we think. *Academy of Emergency Medicine, 7,* 1223-1231.

Denig, P., Wahlstrom, R., deSaintonge, M. C., & Haaijer-Ruskamp, F. (2002). The value of clinical judgment analysis for improving the quality of doctors' prescribing decisions. *Medical Education, 36,* 770-780.

Dunford, J., Davis, D. P., Ochs, M., Doney, M., & Hoyt, D. B. (2003). Incidence of transient hypoxia and pulse rate reactivity during paramedic rapid sequence intubation. *Annals of Emergency Medicine, 42,* 721-728.

Eisenburg, J. M. (1979). Sociologic influences on decision-making by clinicians. *Annals of Internal Medicine, 90,* 957-964.

Feldman, M. J., Lukins, J. L., Verbeek, P. R., Burgess, R. J., Schwartz, B., et al. (2005). Use of treat and release medical directives for paramedics at a mass gathering. *Prehospital Emergency Care, 9,* 213-217.

Gallagher, E. J. (2003). Thinking about thinking. *Annals of Emergency Medicine, 41,* 121-122.

Handly, M. R., Stuart, M. E., & Kirz, H. L. (1994). An evidence-based approach to evaluating and improving clinical practice: Implementing practice guidelines. *HMO Practice, 8,* 75-83.

Hennes, H., Kim, M. K., & Pirrallo, R. G. (2005). Prehospital pain management: A comparison of provider's perceptions and practices. *Prehospital Emergency Care, 9,* 32-39.

Hollander, J. E., Delagi, R., Sciammarella, J., Viccellio, P., Ortiz, J., & Henry, M. C. (1995). On-line telemetry: Prospective assessment of accuracy in an all-volunteer emergency medical service system. *Academy of Emergency Medicine, 2,* 280-286.

Limmer, D., & Monosky, K. (2002). Assessment of the altered mental status patient. *Emergency Medical Services, 31,* 54-58, 81.

Luger, T. J., Lederer, W., Gassner, M., Lockinger, A., Ulmer, H., & Lorenz, I. H. (2003). Acute pain is underassessed in out-of-hospital emergencies. *Academy of Emergency Medicine, 10,* 627-632.

Mears, R., & Sweeny, K. (2000). A preliminary study of the decision-making process within general practice. *Family Practice, 17,* 428-429.

Spaite, W., & Criss, E. (2003). Out of hospital rapid sequence intubation: Are we helping or hurting our patients? *Annals of Emergency Medicine, 42,* 729-730.

Tomlin, Z., Humphrey, C., & Rogers, S. (1999). General practitioner's perception of effective health care. *British Medical Journal, 318,* 1532-1535.

Weinmann, M. (2003). Everyone dies. *Emergency Medical Services, 32,* 40.

SUGGESTED RESOURCES

Department of Transportation. *Emergency Medical Technician Paramedic National Standard Curriculum,* http://www.nhtsa.dot.gov.

NAEMSE. (2006). *Foundations of education: An EMS approach* (Chapter 13). St. Louis: Mosby.

Chapter Quiz

1. A shortfall when using protocols, standing orders, and patient care algorithms is _________.

a. they are developed by state regulatory bodies and medical directors
b. they do not promote paramedic critical thinking
c. they improve the clinical practice of individuals
d. they reflect the latest patient care modalities because they are determined by national professional medical associations

2. An advantage when using protocols, standing orders, and patient care algorithms is _________.

a. they address treating a patient who requires multiple treatment modalities
b. they provide a framework for in-field differential diagnosis
c. they provide a standardized approach to patient care
d. they provide the foundation for creative patient care problem solving

3. A paramedic records each patient care encounter by maintaining a review log that documents the patient assessment, treatment provided, effects of the treatment, and final disposition of the patient. The format of the review log complies with HIPAA requirements. Establishing a patient care log is an example of _______.

a. application of principles
b. concept formation
c. data interpretation
d. obsessive-compulsive disorder
e. reflection on actions

4. List the six *R*'s in decision making.

____
____
____
____
____
____

5. Using the critical thinking model, a paramedic initiates definitive patient care in the _________ phase.

a. application of principle
b. concept formation
c. data interpretation
d. evaluation

6. Data interpretation is based on what areas of study in the paramedic curricula?

____
____
____
____

7. A paramedic has interpreted the data and developed a treatment plan that follows the organization's allergic reaction protocol. After administering the first medication, the patient's vital signs continue to deteriorate. According to the critical thinking model, the paramedic should _______.
   a. consider alternative treatments and protocols to respond to the current patient condition
   b. contact online medical control for advice and instructions
   c. deliver the next medication in the allergic reaction protocol
   d. discontinue the allergic reaction protocol and immediately transport the patient to nearest emergency department as a life-threatening situation

8. What should paramedics do to prepare to operate as a clinical caregiver under a stressful situation?
   ____
   ____
   ____

9. Which patient would require the highest level of critical thinking?
   a. Adult pedestrian struck by a vehicle and suffering from significant life-threatening multisystem injuries
   b. Pediatric drowning patient in respiratory arrest
   c. Sick patient with vital signs that do not present a "classic" clinical condition
   d. Unconscious and unresponsive patient with no available medical history

10. Being impulsive or performing an action because a preset idea or condition is present is an example of ________.
   a. data processing
   b. decision-making style
   c. management plan
   d. situational awareness

Terminology

Application of principles The step at which the paramedic applies critical thinking in a clinical sense and arrives at a field impression or a working diagnosis.

Concept formation The initial formation of an overall concept of care for a particular patient that begins when the paramedic arrives on location of the incident.

Data interpretation The step that uses all the data gathered in the concept formation stage with the paramedic's knowledge of anatomy, physiology, and pathophysiology to continue the decision-making process.

Evaluation of treatment A reassessment of the patient overall and specifically the body system(s) affected by that treatment to answer two critical questions: Did the treatment work as intended? What is the clinical condition of the patient after the treatment?

Reflection on actions A final step that may involve a personal reflection or a run critique; in certain instances this may be done formally, but in most instances it is accomplished informally.

CHAPTER 57

Ground and Air Transport of Critical Patients

Objectives *After completing this chapter, you will be able to:*

1. Describe the role that critical care ground transport plays in the care of critical patients.
2. List the responsibilities of agencies in developing staffing needs.
3. Develop an understanding of who comprises a critical care ground transport team.
4. List some of the equipment needed for critical care ground transport.
5. Describe the advantages and disadvantages of air medical transport.
6. Identify criteria for working as a member of an air medical flight crew.
7. Identify the conditions and situations for which air medical transport should be considered.
8. Describe various considerations for preparing for air medical transport.

CHAPTER OUTLINE

Case Scenario

Your flight medical crew is dispatched to a scene of a motor vehicle crash in a rural setting. The vehicle has major damage, including intrusion into the driver's compartment with prolonged extrication of 30 minutes. Transport time exceeds 50 minutes by ground transport or 20 minutes by air transport. The en-route medical report includes an elderly patient in his 70s who was an unrestrained driver. You arrive and see the fire department still extricating the patient from the entrapment. The patient appears to be unresponsive, with shallow breathing and pale skin. His carotid pulse is rapid and thready.

Questions

1. *What is your general impression of this patient?*
2. *What additional assessment will be important in the evaluation of this patient?*
3. *What intervention should you initiate at this time?*

Although air medical transport for critically ill or injured patients has been common in the out-of-hospital setting since the 1980s, critical care transport by ground is a relatively new specialty in out-of-hospital care by paramedics. This chapter addresses transporting a critical patient by ground or air ambulance.

STAFFING

[OBJECTIVES 1, 2, 3]

Critical care transport by ground ambulance relies on a multidisciplinary team of healthcare professionals. Currently no national standards exist regarding the staffing of critical care ground transport. Several organizations have recommendations on how staffing should occur. The American College of Emergency Physicians "believes that a patient's condition and the potential for complications should dictate the level of services available during interfacility transportation. Critical Care Transport Teams are an important means of providing an appropriate level of care during the transfer of critically ill and injured patients" (2005). The U.S. Department of Health and Human Services defines specialty care transports as "the interfacility transportation of a critically injured or ill beneficiary by a ground ambulance vehicle, including the provision of medically necessary supplies and services, at a level of service beyond the scope of the EMT-Paramedic. [Specialty care transport] is necessary when a beneficiary's condition requires ongoing care that must be furnished by one or more health professionals in an appropriate specialty area, for example, emergency or critical care nursing, emergency medicine, respiratory care, cardiovascular care, or a paramedic with additional training" (2007).

Even though national standards do not apply to the field of paramedics as of yet, professional organizations and governmental agencies share the same message—ensuring that patients are treated by trained healthcare professionals who deliver the highest quality of care possible. All state and local requirements must be met regarding staffing critical care ground units. An agency's responsibilities when staffing critical care ground transports include having written policies that define how the units will be staffed, how they should provide patient care, and treatment protocols. These policies should include infection control procedures, continuing education requirements, and scheduling that includes day/night rotations with strict safety standards for rest.

As previously mentioned, critical care ground transports are conducted by a multidisciplinary team of healthcare professionals. The most common individuals that comprise the critical care team include a critical care paramedic, registered nurse, respiratory therapist, physician's assistant, and nurse practitioner. In some EMS systems paramedics, advanced EMTs, and EMTs also may be part of the critical care ground transport team. The individual in charge of care should be, at a minimum, a critical care paramedic. Numerous critical care paramedic courses are available nationwide. Before attending a critical care transport course, most courses require that participants must have successfully completed training programs in trauma, cardiopulmonary resuscitation, advanced cardiac life support (ACLS), and pediatric advanced life support (PALS). A critical care transport course typically consists of 80 to 100 hours of instruction in topics not usually covered in a traditional paramedic program.

EQUIPMENT

[OBJECTIVE 4]

The cornerstone of the critical care paramedic's success is his or her knowledge and availability of the equipment used in the ambulance. The ambulance must be able to handle the configuration of all needed equipment. Agencies must ensure that the ambulance is licensed in accordance with all applicable state laws, has adequate interior lighting to ensure patient observation, and has the ability for two-way communication with online medical direction. The ambulance should have a minimal fuel capacity for a range of 175 miles and lights visible under normal conditions from a distance of 500 feet from the front of the ambulance. The ambulance siren should be able to be heard under normal conditions from a distance of not less than 500 feet away. The patient compartment should be large enough to provide a workspace that does not compromise the ability to provide adequate care or hinder providers from performing emergency procedures. The patient compartment should be equipped with all standard equipment found on a mobile intensive care unit, including the following:

- Respirators and ventilators (Figure 57-1)
- Cardiac monitor with defibrillator, transcutaneous pacing, cardioversion, and capnography capability (Figure 57-2)
- Pulse oximeter
- A minimum of three intravenous (IV) infusion pumps or a triple-chamber infusion pump for administering multiple IV medications (Figure 57-3)
- Intubation equipment and suction units
- IV poles for inside the unit and a portable pole for transport into facilities
- Medication drug box

Medical directors and clinical directors should define the specific equipment needed for their service areas. The patient compartment also should be large enough to

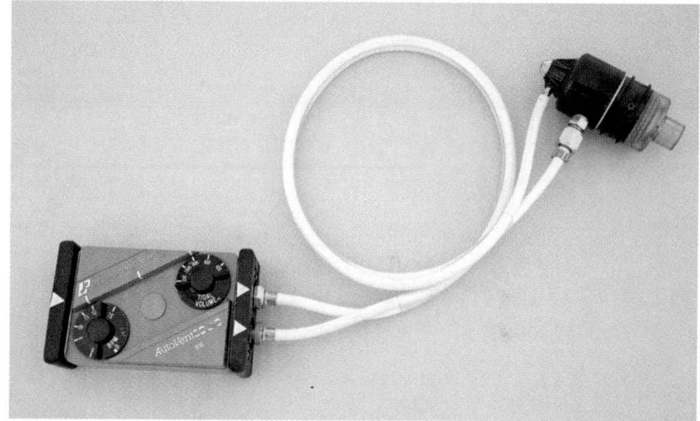

Figure 57-1 Ventilator.

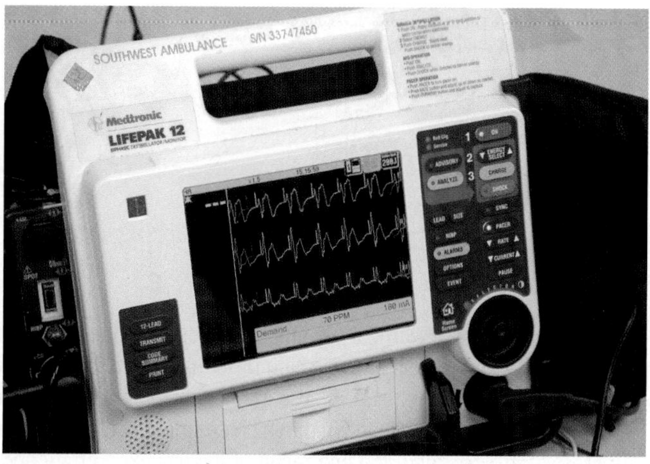

Figure 57-2 Cardiac monitor.

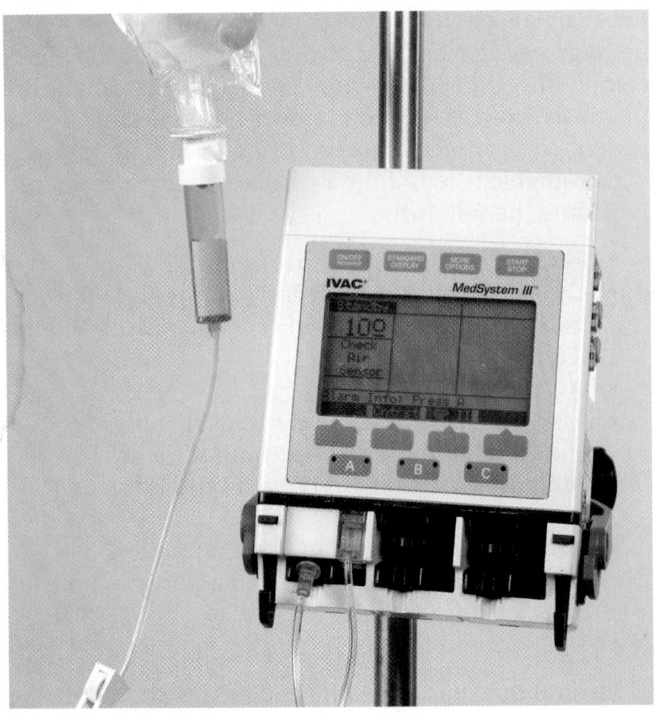

Figure 57-3 Triple-chamber pump.

accommodate the many pieces of equipment that may accompany the patient, such as an intraaortic balloon pump (Figure 57-4). Hospitals have elaborate pieces of equipment such as ventilators, IV pumps, and multiparameter physiologic monitors made specifically for the hospital setting. Critical care ground units must have comparable equipment designed for the confined space of an ambulance.

HISTORY OF AEROMEDICAL SERVICES

[OBJECTIVE 5]

The use of aircraft to transport the sick and injured dates back to World War I, when the French successfully evacuated patients from the battlefield (McNab, 1992). During that time, the United States also converted aircraft to be used as air ambulances. However, these planes were large, old, and costly to maintain. When the planes began to break down, the U.S. military decided not to invest in maintaining the aircraft. The military wanted to use smaller, less-costly aircraft for transporting patients.

Igor Sikorsky, a Russian immigrant, invented the first and perhaps most well-known helicopters for the U.S. military. In 1942 the U.S. Army Corps took delivery of the prototype that would be produced in quantity for the

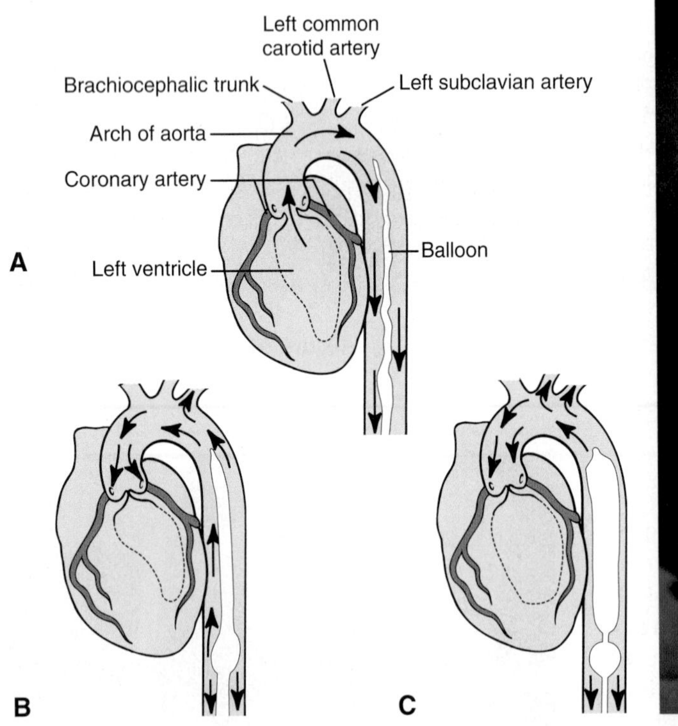

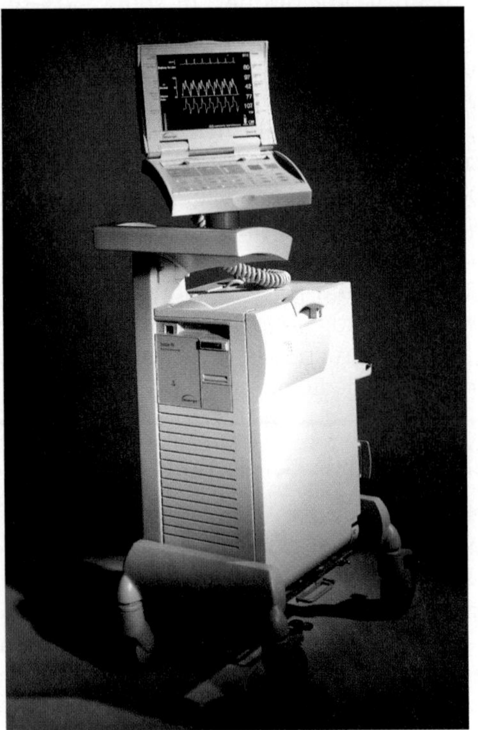

Figure 57-4 Intraaortic balloon pump. **A,** During systole the balloon is deflated, which facilitates ejection of the blood into the periphery where systemic arterial resistance vessels are perfused. **B,** In early diastole, the balloon begins to inflate. **C,** In late diastole, the balloon is totally inflated, which augments aortic pressure and increases the coronary perfusion pressure, with the end result of increased coronary and cerebral blood flow. **D,** Intraaortic balloon pump machine.

U.S. armed forces (Sikorsky, 2006). In 1944 the first patient rescue by helicopter took place in the jungles of Burma (Holleran, 2003). This event marks the beginning of the military use of helicopters for patient transportation. The use of helicopters evolved throughout the Korean and Vietnam military conflicts. During this time medical personnel were placed in the battlefield and on the helicopters to provide immediate triage and treatment of the sick and injured (Carter, 1986).

In the late 1960s civilian air transports began. The Scottish Air Ambulance System had begun transporting patients from the islands to the mainland. The first hospital-based helicopter program started in 1972 at St. Anthony's Hospital in Denver, Colo. During the 1980s hospital-based programs opened at a rapid rate. Today the Association of Air Medical Services (AAMS) estimates that approximately 350,000 rotor-wing flights take place in the United States every year (AAMS, 2006). An estimated additional 100,000 fixed-wing flights occur in the United States annually (AAMS, 2006). The aeromedical industry has grown significantly over the past 40 years to become part of the provision of EMS.

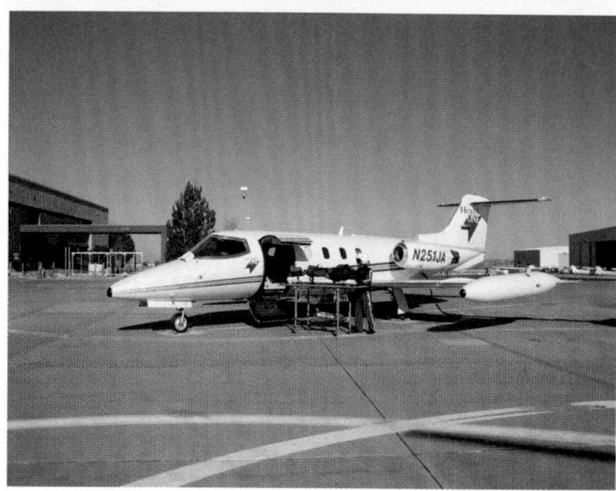

Figure 57-5 Air medical fixed-wing aircraft.

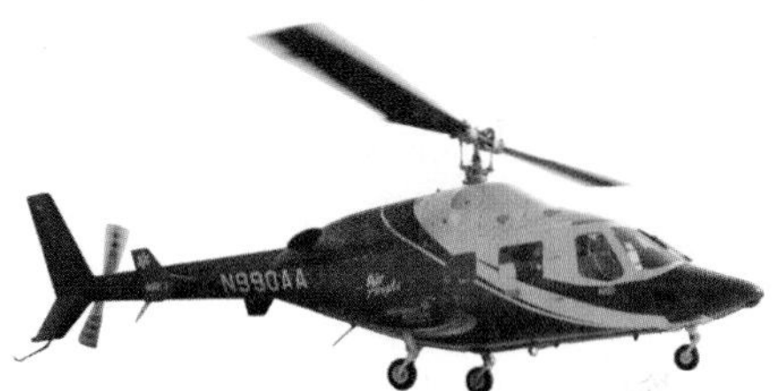

Figure 57-6 Air medical helicopter.

FIXED-WING VERSUS ROTOR-WING AIRCRAFT

[OBJECTIVE 5]

Most people tend to think of helicopters, or rotor-wing aircraft, when considering aeromedical services. However, fixed-wing aircraft play a part in the transport of the sick and injured as well. Both types of aircraft provide important services.

Fixed-Wing Aircraft

Fixed-wing aircraft were the first air medical transport vehicles and have been used as such for almost 90 years (Figure 57-5). Fixed-wing transports differ from rotor-wing transports in a variety of ways. Typically this type of transport involves moving a patient from facility to facility. These aircraft are able to travel farther, fly higher, and fly faster. The type of patient involved in these transports varies. For instance, they may include a stable patient involved in an accident, a patient who has a medical condition and wants to be moved closer to family, or even a critical heart patient who needs a transplant. For the most part, the care rendered in a fixed-wing aircraft is similar to the care rendered in a rotor-wing aircraft.

Rotor-Wing Aircraft

Rotor-wing aircraft, or helicopters, are better known for scene-to-facility transport, although they are used for facility-to-facility transport as well (Figure 57-6). Helicopters fly lower, have a shorter travel radius, and fly slower than fixed-wing aircraft. They can also land in a much smaller space than that required for fixed-wing aircraft, which makes them useful in prehospital care. Helicopters often are activated for trauma patients, especially if extrication is required before the patient can be transported. Medical, burn, and cardiac patients are also flown by helicopter, depending on the circumstances. Much of the care rendered is similar to the care that can be provided in a fixed-wing aircraft. More patients may receive acute procedures, such as intubation, chest tube insertion, and blood transfusion, during helicopter transport, however. As a paramedic, you will find that medical helicopters can be a valuable resource in the field.

FLIGHT CREW CRITERIA

[OBJECTIVE 6]

The typical air medical flight crew consists of a pilot and a combination of a registered nurse, paramedic, respiratory therapist, or physician. The crew's composition is defined by the flight service and local, regional, or state requirements for staffing. The specific training required for each level of licensure, particularly the paramedic, may be defined by state guidelines. Many flight services require their registered nurse and paramedic staff to have special flight certifications.

Nurses

Flight nursing can be traced back to the 1930s, when Laureate M. Schimmoler formed the Emergency Flight Corps in 1933 (Holleran, 2003). The first class of flight nurses graduated from a specialized course of medical training at Bowman Field in Louisville, Ky. (Holleran, 2003). Since then, flight nursing has evolved into a certified specialty. Flight nurses are usually **certified flight registered nurses (CFRN)** and also have met a variety of other educational requirements. Often they must be certified as an emergency medical technician or paramedic. Flight nurses also are expected to have a clinical background in emergency or critical care nursing along with certifications such as ACLS or PALS. Other requirements may exist depending on the location and employer.

Paramedics

The use of paramedics in air medical services dates to the 1970s, when the Maryland State Police implemented the first statewide EMS helicopter service. The requirements for flight paramedics have evolved to include a comprehensive set of expectations. Typically paramedics are expected to have 3 to 5 years of clinical experience before attempting to enter the practice of flight medicine. The specific requirements vary by agency and locality, region, and state.

In an effort to differentiate the critical care paramedic from the flight paramedic, the **National Flight Paramedics Association (NFPA)** has developed the **Certified Flight Paramedic (FP-C)** Exam. The requirements and examination were developed with the premise that most flight paramedics generally function as critical care providers. The NFPA has developed a position regarding the training considered necessary to pass the examination and perform the duties of an FP-C. This position also includes recommendations for continuing education and patient contact hours (Box 57-1) (NFPA, 2000). If a paramedic decides to become an FP-C, the expectations are set very high and demonstrate high-level commitment to the flight medicine profession.

Other Members of the Flight Team

Other potential crew members of an air medical flight team are respiratory therapists and physicians. Respiratory therapists typically work in the hospital setting, but their educational background is conducive to cross-training for critical care transports. Respiratory therapists receive training in gas laws, biology, chemistry, and pharmacology, and they perform a number of clinical procedures. Physicians have a training background that differs from other air medical team members. They have usually attended 4 years of premedical school, 4 years of medical school, and 3 to 5 years of residency. Physicians are often part of flight teams during their residencies to meet procedural requirements and receive exposure to the prehospital environment. Regardless of the composition of the flight team, it consists of highly trained individuals who work together to provide the best care possible in the air to patients.

TRANSPORT PHYSIOLOGY

[OBJECTIVE 7]

The transport of patients by the rotor- or fixed-wing route requires further consideration than for ground transport. Some important factors to consider include the gas laws and the possible effects on patients and the transport team. Flight crews undergo several stressors that should be considered before moving a patient. These factors must be taken into account because of the potential impact on patient care and the well-being of the crew.

Gas Laws

To provide optimal care in the flight environment, you must understand altitude physiology. Atmospheric air is a mixture of gases subject to established laws that govern temperature, pressure, volume, and density. The variables can be defined as follows (Holleran, 2003):

- *Temperature,* when expressed in degrees kelvin (K), indicates the level of energy of a gas sample and is referred to as *absolute temperature.* This is converted from centigrade (Celsius [°C]) or Fahrenheit (°F). When altitude increases, temperature decreases, which affects the rate of molecular movement (energy levels) of gases such as oxygen and nitrogen. *Kelvin* describes the energy level of molecules; absolute temperature expressed in 1 K is the same incremental increase as 1°C on the Celsius scale, which is the common unit of measure for temperature in medical care. The administration of oxygen at higher altitudes is more difficult because of the low energy level of the molecule.
- *Pressure,* defined as absolute or total exerted pressure, is conventionally expressed in atmospheres (torr) or as a given column of mercury in millimeters (mm Hg) or of water balancing the pressure in centimeters (cm H_2O). Pressure is typically considered force per unit area of surface: 1 torr = 1 mm Hg; 1 atm = 760 torr = 760 mm Hg. This concept is important when considering the altitude at which the patient will be flown, the use of pressurized or nonpressurized aircraft, and the delivery of medical gases.
- *Volume* is expressed in cubic units, such as cubic meters (m^3) or cubic centimeters (cc), or in liters (L).
- *Density* is the relative mass of a gas or number of molecules (n) or ions expressed in gram molecules (the molecular weight of the substance in grams).

Gas laws govern the body's physiologic response to barometric pressure changes by these four variables, which become particularly important on ascent and descent.

BOX 57-1 Minimal Recommendations for FP-Cs

The NFPA believes that the FP-C should remain current in the following certifications:

- Basic Cardiac Life Support
- Advanced Cardiac Life Support
- Prehospital Trauma Life Support or Advanced Trauma Life Support (audit)
- Pediatric Advanced Life Support
- Neonatal Resuscitation Program

The NFPA believes that the initial didactic education for the FP-C should include content that has a *minimum* of the following hours in each area:

- History, philosophy, and indications for air medical transport: 1 hour
- Industry associations and standards including the standards of the Commission on the Accreditation of Medical Transport Systems: 1 hour
- Air medical outcome research, trauma systems, and trauma scoring: 1 hour
- Kinematics of trauma and injury patterns: 1 hour
- Aircraft: fundamentals, safety, and survival: 3 hours
- Flight physiology: 1 hour
- Stress management: 1 hour
- Advanced airway management techniques: 2 hours
- Radiographic interpretation: 1 hour
- Management of medical neurologic emergencies: 1 hour
- Management of the critical cardiac patient, including pacemakers and invasive hemodynamic monitoring: 8 hours
- Intraaortic balloon pump theory and transport considerations: 8 hours
- 12-lead electrocardiographic interpretation: 8 hours
- Management of acute respiratory patients, including acid-base balance, arterial blood gas interpretation, capnography, and ventilator management: 6 hours
- Management of septic shock: 1 hour
- Management of toxic exposures: 1 hour
- Management of aortic emergencies: 1 hour
- Management of hypertensive emergencies: 1 hour
- Management of obstetric emergencies: 3 hours
- Management and delivery of the term or preterm newborn: 16 hours
- Neonatal resuscitation program and Pediatric Advanced Life Support and encouraged alternatives (no hourly requirement noted)
- Management of the critical pediatric patient: 5 hours
- Management of adult thoracic and abdominal trauma: 2 hours
- Management of the burn patient: 1 hour
- Management of pediatric trauma: 1 hour
- Management of environmental emergencies: 1 hour
- Trauma in pregnancy considerations: 1 hour

As appropriate, the listed education should include information regarding radiographic findings, pertinent laboratory and bedside testing, and pharmacologic interventions.

The NFPA believes that the FP-C should have initial and annual training in the indications, contraindications, and desired effects and adverse effects of the following skills. Furthermore, the NFPA believes that to ensure competency, the FP-C should have the opportunity to perform the following skills in a laboratory setting:

- Rapid sequence intubation
- Pericardiocentesis
- Escharotomy
- Central venous access through subclavian, internal jugular, or femoral approach
- Chest tube thoracotomy
- Surgical cricothyrotomy

The NFPA believes that the FP-C should be given clinical exposure to critical care suitable to fill a *minimum* of the following number of hours in each area:

- Labor and delivery: 8 hours
- Neonatal intensive care: 8 hours
- Pediatric intensive care: 16 hours
- Adult cardiac care (to include postoperative cardiothoracic surgery patients): 16 hours
- Adult intensive care (to include medical and surgical patients): 16 hours

The NFPA believes that the FP-C should maintain a *minimum* of 24 hours per year of continuing education in areas pertaining to critical care transport and care.

The NFPA believes that the FP-C should maintain a *minimum* of 8 hours per year of patient contact in the following patient population areas (may be met through actual patient contact time during transport or through clinical time spent in the appropriate intensive care or specialty unit):

- Labor and delivery
- Neonatal intensive care
- Pediatric intensive care
- Adult cardiac care
- Adult intensive care
- Emergency and trauma care

The listed curriculum and minimum hours of content should not be considered end points for the FP-C. The NFPA recognizes that individual learning styles and variances in transport program cultures and practices may require additional content to meet the needs of the individual FP-C provider.

Reprinted from NFPA. (2001). The role of the certified flight paramedic (CFP) as a critical care provider and the required education. *Prehosp Emerg Care*, *5*(3), 290-292.

FP-C, Certified flight paramedic; *NFPA*, National Flight Paramedics Association.

The typical gas laws applied to flight physiology are Boyle's law, Dalton's law, Charles' law, Gay-Lussac's law, Henry's law, and Graham's law.

Boyle's law: As long as the temperature is constant, the volume of gas is inversely proportional to its pressure (at moderate temperatures). As pressure increases, volume decreases. Gas expansion within a confined space can cause pain in the teeth and ears and barotrauma to the gastrointestinal tract (Nordian, 2006).

Dalton's law (law of partial pressures): The total partial pressure of the gas mixture is equal to the sum of partial pressures. Think about the atmosphere and all the gases it contains. These gases exert their own partial pressures within the atmosphere. As altitude increases, the partial pressure of these gases decreases. In flight, as the partial pressure of oxygen decreases, it is more difficult for oxygen to transfer from air to blood (Holleran, 2003).

Charles' law: The volume of a fixed mass of gas held at a constant pressure varies directly with absolute temperature. As temperature increases, then so does the volume. Oxygen cylinders in different ambient temperatures can have variations in pressure readings. The mass of the oxygen would remain the same, but the indicated pressure would change with the change in temperature (Holleran, 2003).

Gay-Lussac's law: This law is sometimes combined with Charles' law because it addresses the relation between pressure and temperature. This law states that as the temperature decreases, the pressure decreases. In an oxygen cylinder, as the ambient temperature decreases, so would the pressure reading for the tank (Holleran, 2003).

Henry's law: This law deals with the solubility of gases in liquids. At equilibrium, the amount of gas dissolved in a liquid is proportional to the gas pressure. This law is associated with decompression sickness. If ascension occurs too rapidly, nitrogen bubbles can form in the blood, causing one form of the illness (Holleran, 2003).

Graham's law: Gases move from a higher pressure or concentration to an area of lower pressure or concentration. For example, carbon dioxide is 19 times more diffusible than oxygen, so the uptake of carbon dioxide would occur 19 times faster than the oxygen. This has an impact on simple diffusion or gas exchange at the cellular level (Holleran, 2003).

These laws are important for the flight paramedic to consider when transporting patients, whether on a fixed- or rotor-wing aircraft. Many patients will have an illness or injury that requires the delivery of oxygen, IV fluids, or medications. The paramedic's understanding of the gas laws will help determine the appropriate actions based on flight and patient conditions.

Stress of Transport

The following stressors may be caused by air transport (Holleran, 2003):

- Decreased partial pressure of oxygen
- Barometric pressure changes
- Thermal changes
- Decreased humidity
- Noise
- Vibration
- Fatigue

Decreased Partial Pressure of Oxygen

Patients can have a variety of physical responses when exposed to a decreased partial pressure of oxygen. The flight paramedic must understand such responses to evaluate the changes in patient condition and respond appropriately. The details of this topic are beyond the scope of this text; therefore only a brief overview is presented. First the terms *hypoxia, hypoxemia,* and *hypercapnia* must be understood to be aware of the effects of a decreased partial pressure of oxygen.

Hypoxia is the general term that describes a state in which the tissues have a lack of oxygen. Essentially, the oxygen supply to the tissues is inadequate to meet the body's demand. A variety of conditions can affect the ability of the blood to carry oxygen to the tissues. Some include blood loss from trauma, altitude, alcohol, and heavy smoking.

Hypoxemia refers to the decrease in the arterial blood oxygen tension. A normal PaO_2 in a patient may not mean that he or she is adequately oxygenated, and a low PaO_2 may not indicate tissue hypoxia. The medical history of the patient must be understood to evaluate these findings appropriately in flight.

Hypercapnia refers to an increased amount of carbon dioxide in the blood.

Understanding the three causes of hypoxia, along with the signs, symptoms, and treatment, is most important. The three chief causes of hypoxia are high altitude, hypoventilation, and pathologic conditions of the lungs (Holleran, 2003). Regardless of the cause of the hypoxia, a care provider can observe signs and symptoms that the patient may experience. The flight crew should determine the type of hypoxia they believe the patient to be exhibiting and treat the patient accordingly. Oxygen is the primary treatment for hypoxia (Box 57-2). If the patient is being treated in flight, oxygen may need to be administered under pressure. In flight, one of the more common causes of hypoxia is the malfunction of equipment. As a result, ensure the equipment is checked and properly maintained. Finally, the descent of the aircraft to a lower altitude can help compensate for an equipment malfunction. However, the prevention of hypoxia during flight is the best treatment. If the patient requires transport by aircraft, he or she already is compromised. Therefore any stress related to the transport increases the

BOX 57-2 Treatment for Hypoxia or Hyperventilation

1. Administer 100% oxygen.
2. Begin positive-pressure ventilation, which is the same as supplemental oxygen under pressure.
3. Regulate breathing and watch for hyperventilation.
4. Check equipment.
5. Descend.

If the patient hyperventilates in flight, you may have to assist the conscious patient in controlling his or her ventilatory efforts.

risk of hypoxia. The best deterrent of hypoxia involves continuous monitoring and accurate anticipation of the patient's oxygen requirements during transport (Holleran, 2003).

Barometric Pressure Changes

The ascent and descent of an aircraft can have a variety of effects on a patient being transported. Patients being transported by helicopter are particularly susceptible because the aircraft is not pressurized. The altitude changes of the aircraft create trapped or partially trapped gases in body cavities, especially the gastrointestinal tract, lungs, sinuses, and ears.

Other medical conditions the patient may have that could be affected by barometric changes should be considered. For example, patients being transported who have a recent history of upper respiratory infection are at higher risk of developing **sinus block,** or **barosinusitis.** Sinus block is a condition of acute or chronic inflammation of one or more of the paranasal sinuses (Holleran, 2003). The inflammation produced is typically a negative pressure difference between the air in the sinus cavity and that of the surrounding atmosphere. If this occurs, the patient may report pain in the area of the affected sinus that varies from mild fullness to excruciating. Immediate treatment for this condition is for the aircraft to reascend until the pressure equalizes within the sinuses and atmosphere. Administration of vasoconstrictors to reduce swelling and a gradual descent also may alleviate the problem.

Flight crews also must take into account concerns with the gastrointestinal tract before patient transport. A patient who has had recent abdominal surgery or has a colostomy could be affected by transport. The ascent and descent can cause the gases in the abdominal cavity to expand or contract, causing potential complications during flight. A patient who has had recent abdominal surgery should have a nasogastric tube in place that is vented to ambient air or low intermittent suction. Patients with colostomies should have the bag emptied and adequately vented before transport to prevent rupture of the bag.

Thermal Changes

Patients who are ill or have been injured already have a harder time maintaining an adequate body temperature. An increase in altitude results in a decrease in ambient air temperature, affecting the ability of these patients to stay warm or cool. The vibration of the aircraft can also pose a risk to body temperature regulation. Depending on the environment, where and how high the aircraft is traveling can also have an affect the patient. Fixed-wing aircraft tend to have better climate control than do rotor-wing aircraft. However, the patient should be monitored for body temperature changes throughout the transport. Medications that have been given, such as sedatives and analgesics, can also affect body temperature. If the patient develops hypothermia or hyperthermia, he or she has an even greater energy requirement than before. The increased energy requirements also may change the patient's oxygenation and absorption of administered medications. Ensure that the appropriate equipment to maintain adequate body temperature is available. Many rotor-wing aircraft carry a first-aid thermal blanket, sometimes referred to as a **space blanket** (Holleran, 2003). This blanket resembles a large piece of aluminum foil. It is designed to help reflect body heat and assist the patient in maintaining body temperature.

Decreased Humidity

Humidity is the concentration of water vapor in the air. As air cools, it loses its ability to hold moisture. Therefore, as altitude increases, humidity decreases (Holleran, 2003). In flight, the aircraft draws in air that is quite dry, depending on altitude. The primary sources of moisture in the air at this point are the crewmembers, the patient, and the air-handling system. The relevance of understanding this concept is that the patient may be put at risk for fluid loss. During long flights, he or she may be at risk for dehydration. The administration of nonhumidified oxygen also can increase the risk of fluid loss. The flight crew members must remain adequately hydrated along with the patient, particularly during flights of longer duration.

Noise

The definition of *noise* is subjective. The paramedic who enjoys listening to hard rock while responding to a call with the lights and sirens on may have a different idea of what constitutes noise than the patient who requires transport. Aircraft obviously produce different types of sound than ambulances, none of which are quiet. Be sure to consider the effect that the noise has on the crew members and patient.

Noise affects three primary aspects of the flight environment. It affects the crew members' ability to communicate, which can affect the patient. In addition, noise can alter the ability of the patient and flight crew to hear. Lastly, noise can lead to varying levels of fatigue. All these factors can impair your ability to assess and treat any changes in patient status. The crew must primarily rely on visual cues and monitoring the equipment to assess the patient. The hearing of the crew and patient also should be protected. The use of helmets or earplugs can lessen the potential damage. Note that if earplugs are placed in a patient's ears for transport, they should be removed before descent. When the aircraft descends, the pressure change can pull the earplugs toward the tympanic membrane (Holleran, 2003). The noise fatigue of the flight crew can be combated by ensuring adequate rest between longer flights, monitoring the length of shifts, and not working excessive hours.

Vibration

The motion of an object in relation to a reference point, which is usually the object at rest, is considered a vibration (Holleran, 2003). The relative effect that vibration has on the human body is evaluated in terms of frequency, intensity, direction, and duration of exposure (Holleran, 2003). Whether you are transporting the patient by ground in an ambulance or by flight in fixed- or rotor-wing aircraft, two sources of vibration exist. The first source is from within the vehicle itself, typically from the engine. The second source comes from the environment through which the vehicle travels. By ground, the terrain affects vibration. In the air, the turbulence of the atmosphere further affects vibration. Rotor-wing aircraft are typically affected by an increase in airspeed and with loading.

Fixed-wing aircraft have vibrations coming from the power source that tend to be of higher frequencies than that of helicopters. The main source of vibration in fixed-wing craft is the atmospheric turbulence through which the aircraft flies.

Several problems are caused by the vibration of aircraft. The most common concerns are the transference of mechanical energy to the patient's body and equipment interference. When the human body is in direct contact with a source of vibration, a transfer of mechanical energy occurs. Some of the energy gets degraded into heat within tissues, which have dampening properties. Muscle activity may increase in the body in response to vibration. This increase helps maintain posture and reduce the amplification in body structures. In response to vibration in aircraft, increases in metabolic rate and the redistribution of blood from peripheral vasoconstriction have been noted. This increased metabolic rate can cause an increase in respirations to assist in the elimination of carbon dioxide (CO_2). Visual disturbances and problems with speech and fine muscle coordination can be noted with vibration in aircraft (Holleran, 2003). The best way to decrease the effect is to reduce exposure to the vibration. The equipment in the aircraft, such as blood pressure cuffs and cardiac monitors, can have interference from the vibration as well. The best approach is to ensure that the equipment is secured appropriately and in a manner that would limit the vibrations.

Fatigue

Fatigue is the end product of all the exposures that can occur while a person is in an aircraft. For the flight crew, fatigue is a stressor related to their duties. Patients being flown in medical aircraft already have a variety of stressors on their bodies from their illness or injuries; therefore fatigue is likely to occur. The flight crew must prevent their own fatigue and the fatigue of patients who are flown in their aircraft.

Case Scenario—continued

The patient's skin is pale, cool, and dry. He is unresponsive with a Glasgow Coma Scale (GCS) score of 8. He has shallow, unlabored breathing with periods of apnea. You notice a spidered windshield on the car, an angulated left lower extremity, and various cuts and abrasions to the face and head. Vital signs are pulse, 120 beats/min; blood pressure, 100/58 mm Hg; and respirations, 10 breaths/min.

Questions

4. *Is this patient high priority? Why or why not?*
5. *What safety factors should be considered for air transport?*
6. *How critical is this patient?*
7. *What additional treatment should be initiated?*
8. *What is the ongoing assessment of this patient?*
9. *What destination is most appropriate for this patient?*

CRITERIA FOR PATIENT TRANSPORT

[OBJECTIVE 7]

Several considerations should be taken into account when determining whether to use aircraft to transport an ill or injured patient. Fixed-wing aircraft are typically used for longer distance transport. Although distance criteria may vary by flight service, fixed-wing aircraft are generally used for transports of 100 miles or greater. Additionally the severity of illness and injury of the patients involved can vary widely when using fixed-wing aircraft. The use of rotor-wing aircraft should be considered when

BOX 57-3 Specialty Transport Teams

- High-risk obstetrical (HROB)
- High-risk neonate
- Intraaortic balloon pump
- Stroke

a shorter distance of transport is required and the patient is of a high acuity. The patient criteria examined in this chapter primarily focus on the activation of medical helicopters.

Helicopters can be used for facility-to-facility transport and prehospital scene-to-hospital transport. Many flight services have programs for interfacility transports that can be activated with a phone call. At that time, the necessity of such a flight can be screened. In addition to standard flight services, most flight programs provide specialty transport services. Examples of these can be found in Box 57-3. Paramedics who activate helicopters from the field should be familiar with their local protocols for doing so. However, field paramedics must be aware of some general considerations when determining if a patient meets the criteria for helicopter transport, as well as the advantages and disadvantages of such a decision (Box 57-4).

Medical Patients

Depending on the proximity to the hospital, many patients who are ill enough to be transported by rotor-wing aircraft will be moving from hospital to hospital. Parts of the country have hospitals spread out rather far apart, so helicopters may be used to transport from the scene to the hospital. Patients who are medically unstable or critically ill can be considered for helicopter transport, especially when definitive care by ground transport will be prolonged.

Although the following list does not include all conditions possible, following are some specific medical conditions that warrant helicopter transport (AAMS, 2005):

- Dissecting or bleeding aortic aneurysm
- Intracranial bleeding
- Acute ischemic stroke
- Epiglottitis
- Severe hypothermia or hyperthermia
- Cardiac intervention
- Septic shock
- Status asthmaticus
- Status epilepticus
- Severe poisoning
- Cardiogenic shock
- Any condition in which the patient is unstable and may benefit from hastened transport

BOX 57-4 Advantages and Disadvantages of Air-Medical Transport

Advantages

- Rapid transportation
- Access to remote areas
- Access to specialty units such as neonatal intensive care units and burn centers
- Access to personnel with specialized skills
- Access to specialized equipment and supplies

Disadvantages

- Weather and environmental restrictions to flight
- Limitations on patient weight
- Limitations on number of patients that can be transported
- Altitude limitations
- Airspeed limitations
- High cost
- Difficulties delivering patient care because of limited access and cabin size
- Limitations of the amounts of equipment and supplies that can be carried

Trauma Patients

The most likely patients to be transported by helicopter from the scene to the hospital are trauma patients. Three criteria are typically used to determine helicopter activation: physiologic criteria, anatomic criteria, and mechanism of injury. The criteria listed below are likely considerations but are not necessarily all-inclusive (Vanderbilt LifeFlight, 2008). Physiologic criteria include the following:

- Airway compromise (actual or potential)
- GCS score less than 13
- Signs and symptoms of shock (systolic blood pressure less than 90 mm Hg)

Anatomic criteria include the following:

- Penetrating trauma to the torso
- Amputation proximal to the wrist or ankle
- Limb paralysis
- Suspected spinal cord injury with neurologic deficit
- Burns greater than 15% total body surface area, especially with airway involvement

Mechanism of injury criteria include the following:

- High-speed motor vehicle crash
- Prolonged extrication (typically more than 20 minutes)
- Fatality in same vehicle
- Ejection from a vehicle
- Intrusion into the passenger compartment of more than 12 inches

- Mechanism that includes a physiologic and/or anatomic finding

One absolute contraindication to the activation of a medical helicopter is a patient who is in cardiac arrest. Ground paramedics must be familiar with their local, regional, or statewide air transport activation protocols for exclusion criteria because differences may exist. Other usual contraindications include the following:

- Terminally ill patients with a do not resuscitate order
- Active untreated communicable disease that could put the crew at risk
- Patients who are of sound mind and refuse transport
- Stable patients

Other considerations to weigh when considering ground transport versus air transport include the following:

- Weather conditions in the area of the scene (including wind speed and visibility)
- Availability of a landing zone
- Extrication of the patient, including ground transport time (if the extrication and ground transport time exceed the arrival and air crew treatment time, ground transport may be a wise choice)

A variety of patients may meet aircraft transport criteria. Summoning a helicopter to the scene of an incident is common in the EMS community. Field paramedics should be familiar with their local or regional protocols regarding the activation of medical helicopters to help ensure that the appropriate patients are being transported by this method.

PATIENT PREPARATION

[OBJECTIVE 8]

The mode of transport and the reason for which the patient is being transported have a bearing on what preparation is required before transport. Fixed-wing transportation has subtly different requirements than rotor-wing transportation. As previously described, when a patient is being flown by fixed-wing aircraft it is usually for greater distances and the patient must be delivered to and transported from an airport by ground ambulance. Most of the time rotor-wing transports do not require the use of a ground ambulance to get the patient to the aircraft. Patient preparation largely depends on whether the patient is being transported from a scene to a hospital or from a hospital to another hospital.

Minor variations also exist in what necessary interventions must be completed for medical and trauma patients before moving them. The most important consideration is the safety of the patient and flight crew given the need for transport.

Hospital to Hospital

A patient being transported from hospital to hospital may travel by fixed-wing aircraft or helicopter. The patient may be in an inpatient unit or the emergency department (ED). On arrival at the transferring facility, the flight paramedic should expect that the patient will have his or her airway secured, a minimum of one IV line, and cardiac monitoring in place. Medications being administered may require evaluation. All transfer paperwork, including copies of radiologic testing, should be near completion. Much of the preparedness of the patient depends on the resources that the transferring facility has in place to provide for the patient initially. As the flight paramedic, you may be required to assist with intubation, establish further IV access, or administer medications to prepare the patient for transport. The flight crew is required to prepare the patient for transport on the basis of his or her current condition, mode of transport, weather conditions, and agency expectations. You should expect variable preparatory efforts based on the reason for transport and the transferring facility.

Scene to Hospital

A majority of the time the transport of a patient from a prehospital scene occurs by ground ambulance. Depending on the county, region, or state, different criteria exist for the rotor-wing transport of certain patient groups on the basis of their illness or injury. Transports from a scene to the hospital by fixed-wing aircraft are unlikely because of the landing requirements of the aircraft. As a flight paramedic arriving at the scene of a critically ill or injured patient, you may need to do a fair amount of patient preparation or very little. The preparation of the patient may be as simple as positioning him or her on the transport litter or preparing your equipment. On the other hand, it may be as complex as waiting for the patient to be extricated from a vehicle and using all your paramedic skills. The amount of patient preparation from scene to hospital is related to the EMS service for which you are responding. Advanced life support services may have much of the patient preparation complete before your arrival. This, of course, depends on the situation they faced while treating the patient. Basic life support services may have the immediate life-threatening conditions assessed and may have provided intervention to the level of their ability. However, you may need to establish IV lines and perform intubation and other advanced measures that they are unable to do. What is most helpful in transport from the scene to the hospital is to be aware of your service area and what the provider capabilities are that you would respond to assist. This will allow you, as the flight paramedic, to establish what may be required of you before arrival. Then you will be able to provide swift care for patient transport. As has been established, the preparedness of the patient on your arrival depends on the capabilities of the agencies that respond in your service area.

Case Scenario CONCLUSION

You and your flight crew initiate oxygenate and ventilate the patient's lungs with 100% oxygen by bag-mask device (SpO_2 = 98%). You prepare your intubation equipment, establish two large-bore IVs, and administer normal saline (a total of 1000 mL administered before arrival at the ED). You provide in-line cervical and spinal stabilization on a long backboard with cervical immobilization devices and a rigid cervical collar. Before departure from the scene, you successfully intubate the patient using rapid-sequence induction. On arrival at the ED, the trauma team awaits the patient. His vital signs remains unchanged, but his skin color has improved. The patient is diagnosed with a subarachnoid hemorrhage, left femur fracture, and tibia and fibula fracture and is admitted to the hospital for further evaluation and treatment.

Looking Back

10. *Given the patient's final disposition, was your treatment appropriate? Why or why not?*
11. *What are the advantages and disadvantages of air transport in a patient such as this?*

LANDING SITE PREPARATION

The following information is provided to assist ground EMS crews to prepare a safe landing site for a rotor-wing aircraft. (Fixed-wing aircraft have requirements typically met only by landing at an airport.) Flight paramedics and crews should actively take part in the education of providers in their service area on the important elements of establishing a safe landing site for the arrival of the aircraft. These elements, which are summarized in Box 57-5, include size, location, obstructions, surface conditions, night operations, communications, and general safety.

Size

A landing zone (LZ) should be at least 100 by 100 feet, day or night. If multiple helicopters are called, then the site must increase in size to accommodate them (Figure 57-7).

Location

The LZ should be located at least 100 to 200 feet downwind of the patient care area. This should help prevent loose gravel and debris from blowing into the area. If the LZ is on one side of a two-way roadway, both lanes of traffic should be stopped. Remember that the rotor wash can create a significant downdraft, causing debris to blow into traffic and the patient care area.

Obstructions

The area should be clear of power lines, trees, poles, buildings, stumps, rocks, or anything that could be thrown up into the rotor system of the aircraft. If possible, the LZ should be set up at least 200 feet from bystanders, livestock, or any other motor vehicles (Air Evac Services, 2006). These factors are essential when determining an appropriate site because safety is the most important consideration.

BOX 57-5 Landing Zone and Scene Operations

Landing Zone

- Ensure the landing zone is a minimum of 100 × 100 ft.
- Identify and mark any obstructions in the immediate area.
- Identify the landing zone by GPS coordinates or a major nearby intersection.
- Inform the flight crew of the landing surface and slope.
- Mark the corners of the landing zone with cones or other easily visible objects in the daytime. Place a fifth marker on the upwind side of the landing zone. Make sure markers are secured or heavy enough that they will not blow away.
- For night operations, mark the corners of the landing zone with ground strobes, secured flares, or vehicles with their lights on. Place a fifth lighted marker on the upwind side of the landing zone.

Scene Operations

- Keep spectators at least 200 feet away.
- Assure personal equipment is secured (e.g., no hats).
- Do not approach the helicopter until you are signaled by one of the crew members.
- Always approach from the front of the helicopter, never from the tail.
- Never bend over when approaching the helicopter. The rotors are 10 feet above the ground, and you are more likely to trip and fall if you are looking down.
- Do not hold anything above your head.
- Do not wear a hat.

GPS, Global positioning system.

Surface Conditions

The surface of the LZ should be as level as possible and should not exceed 5 degrees. Concrete is the best choice of surface if it is available. Blacktop or asphalt, sod or grass, and dirt or brush may be used in that order based on what is available where the aircraft is landing. If the

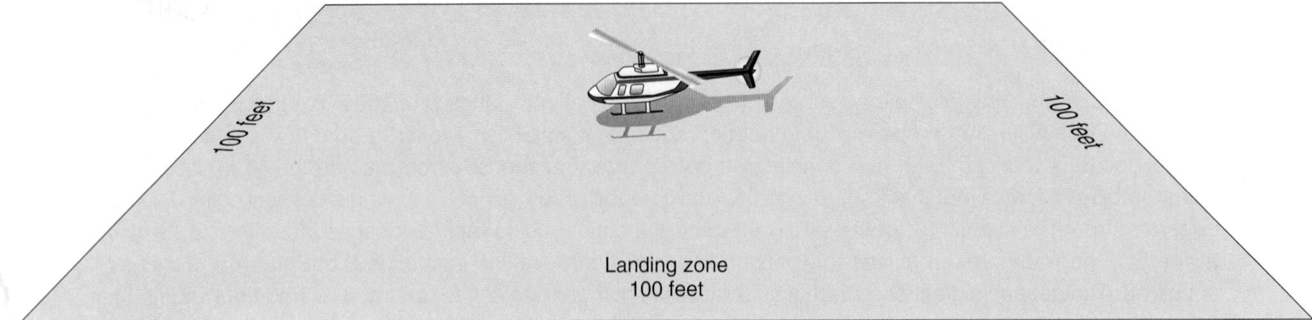

Figure 57-7 Minimum LZ dimensions.

LZ is a dirt surface, ask the fire department to moisten the landing zone with a light water fog. If this is not possible, be aware that the downdraft will limit visibility and possibly kick up small stones and sticks.

Night Operations

When establishing an LZ at night, it should be marked with five lights or secured flares. One flare should be at each corner of the LZ and on the upwind side, indicating wind direction. If it is impossible to mark the LZ in this manner before the arrival of the helicopter, convey this to the pilot and describe how the LZ is marked so that he or she can locate it and determine whether the aircraft can land safely.

Communication

Communication with the pilot of the aircraft is essential to ensure the safety of the flight crew, patient(s), and scene providers. Designate one person to establish radio communications with the pilot to relay the location of the LZ, any obstacles noted, and the type of surface on which the aircraft will land. If possible, provide any known patient information to be conveyed to the flight crew. Notify the pilot immediately if the situation on the ground changes and anything seems unsafe. The pilot can then make an appropriate landing decision. Always provide locations of objects, the LZ, and other factors in relation to the aircraft, in which the nose of the aircraft is the 12 o'clock position and standard clock markings are used for direction. Describing items relative to your location is of no benefit, as the pilot may not be aware of your position.

General Safety

When approaching a helicopter, always do so from the front and only at the signal of the pilot (Figure 57-8). Do not walk around the rear of the helicopter by the tail rotor, and never rush to the aircraft. If the aircraft had to land on a sloped surface, approach from the downhill side, never the uphill side. Take off baseball caps or hats that can be dislodged by the downdraft of the rotor before approaching the aircraft to prevent complications with the aircraft.

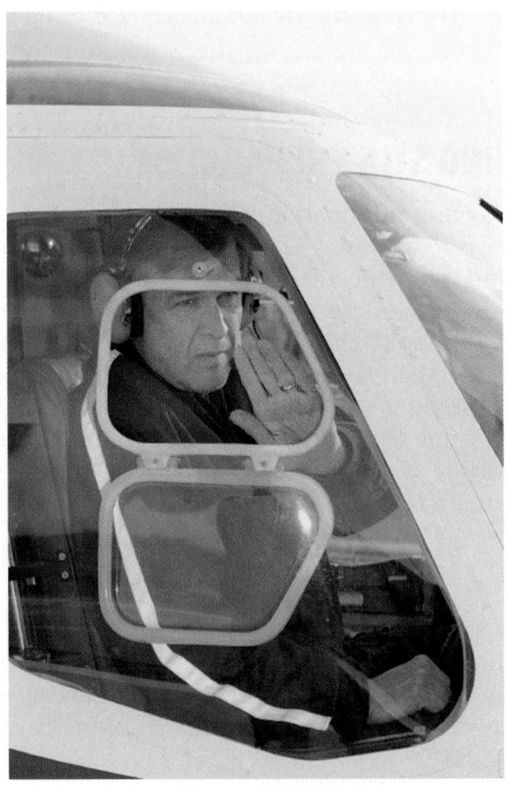

Figure 57-8 Approach a helicopter from the front. Make eye contact with the pilot and wait for him or her to signal that it is okay to approach the aircraft.

You must be familiar with safety procedures when working with flight services. The establishment of an LZ typically rests on the crew that activated the helicopter for service. They should have a clear understanding of the expectation of what the flight services in a responder's area require or what is outlined in local protocols regarding the establishment of a safe LZ. Safety is always the primary concern for the patient, flight crew, bystanders, and road crews when operating in this environment.

The role of the flight paramedic has evolved in recent years. Anyone wishing to become involved with flight medicine must be aware of what is expected in terms of education and skill maintenance. Many considerations should be taken into account, such as the effects of flight physiology on the patients, the effects of flying on the individual and crew, the types of patients that meet the criteria for air transport, and the essential care that is provided. Finally, the flight paramedic must be aware of the capabilities of the responders in his or her service area. He or she can help provide appropriate safety education to ensure that all members of the response team, including the patient, are kept free from harm during an operation. The flight paramedic can be a challenging yet rewarding role in the prehospital care environment.

Case Scenario SUMMARY

1. *What is your general impression of this patient?* Several factors in the initial assessment suggest that this patient is a high priority. First, unresponsiveness often is a sign of brain injury and is your first sign that this patient is a high priority. The second sign is pale skin color. This often is a sign of poor perfusion and the first clue that the patient is in shock. The rapid, thready carotid pulse also confirms the diagnosis of hypovolemic shock.
2. *What additional assessment will be important in the evaluation of this patient?* The primary survey suggested that the patient is in shock and has altered mental status. Further evaluation of mental status, vital signs, and secondary assessment will be important. Complete airway and ventilation evaluation and control to ensure adequacy. Obtain further patient medical history, including current medications and past medical history.
3. *What intervention should you initiate at this time?* The initial impression suggests that this patient is in shock and has a potential head injury. Administration of high-flow oxygen by bag-mask device and IV fluids is the most important treatment at this time.
4. *Is this patient high priority? Why or why not?* Unresponsiveness, the presence of tachycardia with associated signs of shock, prolonged extrication, and an extended transport time confirm that the patient requires emergent treatment and transport.
5. *What safety factors should be considered for air transport?* Weather conditions as well as safe landing site preparation, including location, surface area, size of LZ, obstacles or obstructions, and communications. Also consider general safety when approaching the aircraft.
6. *How critical is this patient?* This patient is significantly critical and requires a skilled air medical crew to provide stabilization, treatment, and transport to the most appropriate trauma facility.
7. *What additional treatment should be initiated?* Administer high-flow oxygen and be prepared for emergent intubation. Administer and maintain IV fluids throughout flight. Provide an early prehospital radio report to the receiving trauma center to provide adequate hospital resources to manage this critically injured patient. Apply a cervical collar and place the patient on a long backboard for spinal immobilization. Apply an extremity traction device for stabilization of extremity trauma.
8. *What is the ongoing assessment of this patient?* Frequently reassess the primary survey, including monitoring vitals signs and neurologic status.
9. *What destination is most appropriate for this patient?* This patient is extremely unstable and should be rapidly transported to a designated trauma center. This patient has potential airway, hemodynamic, and neurologic complications. Carefully prepare the patient for transport. The receiving trauma center should have been notified before departure from the scene. Treatment should not delay transport unless a critical intervention is warranted.
10. *Given the patient's final disposition, was your treatment appropriate? Why or why not?* Yes. Rapid airway control, administration of oxygen, ventilation, and obtaining vascular access to administer fluids for resuscitation and provide medications to facilitate rapid-sequence intubation are important to this case. For patients who are in shock and have head injuries, both airway management and IV fluid administration are appropriate. Spinal immobilization and splinting of the lower extremity also was appropriate.
11. *What are the advantages and disadvantages of air transport in a patient such as this?* The advantages of air transport include trained advanced healthcare professionals who provide the highest quality of patient care possible. Major advantages are the rapid transport of air transport. Specific trauma guidelines support activation of rotary air transport, which includes rapid transport because of airway compromise, GCS score less than 13, and signs and symptoms of shock. Various anatomic criteria and mechanism of injury also support the use of rotary air transport. Disadvantages of air transport include weather conditions, availability of an LZ, and extrication time (if extrication and ground transport time do not exceed arrival of air crew, ground transport may be more beneficial).

Chapter Summary

- The training and availability of the critical care paramedic has allowed agencies to provide critical care grounds units.
- Critical care ground transport may be appropriate for the critical care patient who requires transport to another medical facility.
- Critical care ground transports are conducted by a multidisciplinary team of healthcare professionals.
- The patient compartment of a critical care ground unit should be equipped with all standard equipment found on a mobile intensive care unit.
- The beginning of aeromedical services dates back to the 1940s and continues to present day, with approximately 350,000 rotor-wing and 100,000 fixed-wing transports annually.
- Fixed-wing and rotor-wing aircraft are used to transport ill or injured people to appropriate medical care.
- Fixed-wing aircraft have been used for almost 90 years for medical transport. These transports are typically from facility to facility.
- Rotor-wing aircraft, or helicopters, although sometimes used for facility-to-facility transport, are better known for scene-to-facility transport.
- Flight crew criteria apply to nurses, paramedics, and other members of the flight team.
- Transport physiology includes multiple factors that should be considered before and during the transport of the patient.
- Gas laws govern the body's physiologic response to variables of temperature, pressure, volume, and the relative mass of a gas.
- Boyle's law presumes that if the temperature is constant, the volume of gas is inversely proportional to its pressure.
- Dalton's law, the law of partial pressure, states that "the total partial pressure of the gas mixture is equal to the sum of partial pressures."
- Charles' law expresses that the volume of a fixed mass of gas held at a constant pressure varies directly with absolute temperature.
- Gay-Lussac's law is sometimes combined with Charles' law because it deals with the relation between pressure and temperature.
- Henry's law is associated with decompression sickness.
- Graham's law describes how gases move from a higher pressure or concentration to an area of lower pressure or concentration.
- Seven stressors have been identified that may be caused by air transport.
- The treatment for hypoxia or hyperventilation includes administering 100% oxygen, initiating positive-pressure ventilation, regulating breathing and watching for hyperventilation, checking equipment, and descending.
- Barometric pressure changes can cause several effects during ascent and descent.
- Patients who are already ill or injured can have difficulty maintaining their body temperature. Changes in ambient air temperature during transport can affect the patient.
- Humidity is the concentration of water vapor in the air; changes can require the provider to modify patient care.
- Noise affects the ability of the flight crew to communicate, alters the hearing of the patient, and can promote varying levels of fatigue.
- Vibration is defined as the motion of an object in relation to a reference point, which is usually the object at rest.
- Fatigue is the end product of all the exposures that can occur while a person is in an aircraft.
- The criteria for patient transport are the conditions required for the use of an aircraft for transport.
- Medical patients who are critically ill may require transport by fixed- or rotor-wing aircraft based on defined criteria.
- Trauma patients who have been injured may meet the established criteria for transport by rotor- or fixed-wing aircraft.
- Other considerations, such as weather conditions, may prevent the use of aircraft for transporting patients.
- Patient preparation includes actions to be taken before placing the patient in the aircraft.
- Hospital-to-hospital transport is typically done by fixed-wing aircraft but depends on a variety of factors.
- Scene-to-hospital transport is typically done by rotor-wing aircraft and more commonly involves trauma patients.
- The landing site preparation includes the following factors: size, location, obstructions, surface conditions, night operations, communication, and general safety.

REFERENCES

Air Evac Services, Inc. (2006). Retrieved March 6, 2006, from http://www.airevac.com.

American College of Emergency Physicians. (2005). Retrieved February 20, 2008, from http://www.acep.org.

Association of Air Medical Services. (2006). Retrieved November 1, 2006, from http://www.aams.org.

Association of Air Medical Services. (2005). *Appropriate use of critical care ground transport services. Position paper of the Association of Air Medical Services,* Alexandria, VA. Retrieved February 20, 2008, from http://www.aams.org.

Carter, G. (1986). The evolution of air transport systems: A pictorial review. *Journal of Emergency Medicine, 6,* 499-504.

Department of Health and Human Services. (2007). *Ambulance fee schedule, ground ambulance services, revision to the specialty care transport (SCT) definition.* Retrieved May 28, 2007, from http://www.cms.hhs.gov.

Holleran, R. S. (2003). *Air & surface patient transport principles and practice* (3rd ed.). St. Louis: Mosby.

McNab, A. (1992). Air medical transport: "Hot air" and a French lesson. *Journal of Air Medical Transportation, 11,* 15-16.

Gryniuk, J. (2001). The role of the certified paramedic (FP-C) as a critical care provider and the required education. National Flight Paramedics Association position statement. *Prehospital Emergency Care, 5*(3), 290-292. Retrieved February 20, 2008, from http://www.flightparamedic.org.

Nordian Aviation Training Systems. (2006). *Human performance and limitations: Flight physiology.* Retrieved October 1, 2006, from http://www.nordian.net.

Sikorsky, I. I. (2006). *Our history.* Retrieved March 6, 2006, from http://www.sikorsky.com.

St. Anthony Hospitals. (2005). *Flight for Life Colorado.* Retrieved March 6, 2006, from http://www.stanthonyhosp.org.

Vanderbilt LifeFlight. (2008). Retrieved February 20, 2008, from http://www.mc.vanderbilt.edu.

SUGGESTED RESOURCES

Air Medical Journal: http://journals.elsevierhealth.com/periodicals/ymam

Air Medical Physician Association: http://www.ampa.org

Air & Surface Transport Nurses Association: http://www.astna.org

Association of Air Medical Services: http://www.aams.org.

Hankins, D., & Thomson, D. (1998). National Association of EMS Physicians Position Paper. *Special resuscitation issues encountered during air medical transport, Prehospital Emergency Carem 2*(4), 326-332. Retrieved February 20, 2008, from http://www.naemsp.org.

International Association of Flight Paramedics: http://www.flightparamedic.org.

Memorial Hospital & Health System. *Preparing the landing zone (LZ).* http://www.qualityoflife.org.

National EMS Pilots Association: http://www.nemspa.org

Thomson, D., & Thomas, S. (2003). National Association of EMSP Physicians Position Paper. Guidelines for air medical dispatch, *Prehospital Emergency Care, 7*(2), 265-271. Retrieved February 20, 2008, from http://www.naemsp.org.

Chapter Quiz

1. True or False: The standard of care for critical care ground transport is defined in a national standard curriculum.

2. True or False: Critical care ground transport is defined by the Department of Health and Human Services strictly as interfacility transportation of a critically ill or injured person.

3. True or False: Critical care ground transport units must be equipped with specialty equipment in addition to the equipment required for an ACLS ambulance.

4. True or False: Igor Sikorsky is considered the inventor of the first helicopters used by the United States military.

5. The first use of a helicopter for the rescue of a patient took place in __________.

a. 1941
b. 1944
c. 1943
d. 1945

6. True or False: Henry's law is associated with decompression sickness.

7. List three elements that cause stress of transport.

____

____

____

8. Which of the following conditions is not likely to meet the criteria for air transport?

a. Cardiogenic shock
b. Dissecting and bleeding aortic aneurysm
c. Intracranial bleeding
d. Isolated extremity fracture without neurovascular compromise

9. True or False: Airway compromise is considered *physiologic criteria* for the activation of a medical helicopter.

10. True or False: Prolonged extrication may meet the *anatomic criteria* for the activation of a medical helicopter.

11. True or False: Limb paralysis may meet the *anatomic criteria* for the activation of a medical helicopter.

Chapter Quiz—continued

12. The best surface for an LZ is ________.
- **a.** asphalt
- **b.** concrete
- **c.** dirt
- **d.** grass

13. The typical size of an LZ is ________.
- **a.** 60 feet by 100 feet.
- **b.** 70 feet by 70 feet
- **c.** 100 feet by 100 feet
- **d.** 110 feet by 100 feet

Terminology

Boyle's law Gas law that demonstrates that as pressure increases, volume decreases; explains the pain that can occur in flight in the teeth, ears, and barotrauma in the gastrointestinal tract.

Certified Flight Paramedic (FP-C) A certification obtained by paramedics on successful completion of the Flight Paramedic Exam.

Certified Flight Registered Nurse (CFRN) A nurse who has completed education, training, and certification beyond a registered nurse, with a focus on air medical transport of potentially critically ill or injured patients.

Charles' law Law stating that oxygen cylinders can have variations in pressure readings in different ambient temperatures.

Dalton's law (law of partial pressure) Law relating to the partial pressure of oxygen during transport; defines that it is more difficult for oxygen to transfer from air to blood at lower pressures.

Fixed-wing aircraft Airplanes used for longer distance medical flights; they can travel higher and faster than rotor-wing aircraft.

Gay-Lussac's law A gas law sometimes combined with Charles' law that deals with the relation between pressure and temperature; in an oxygen cylinder, as the ambient temperature decreases, so does the pressure reading.

Graham's law Law stating that gases move from a higher pressure or concentration to an area of lower pressure or concentration; takes into consideration the effect of simple diffusion at a cellular level.

Henry's law Law associated with decompression sickness that deals with the solubility of gases in liquids at equilibrium.

Hypercapnia An increased amount of carbon dioxide in the blood; may be a result of hypoventilation.

Hypoxemia A decrease in the arterial blood oxygen tension; a normal PaO_2 may not indicate adequate oxygenation, and a low PaO_2 may not indicate tissue hypoxia; medical history of the patient is the determinant.

Hypoxia General term that describes a state in which oxygen is lacking in the tissues.

National Flight Paramedics Association (NFPA) Association established in 1984 to differentiate the critical care paramedic from the flight paramedic; has developed a position statement recommending the training considered necessary to perform the duties of an FP-C.

Rotor-wing aircraft Helicopters that can be used for hospital-to-hospital and scene-to-hospital transports; usually travel a shorter distance and are used in the prehospital setting for certain types of transport.

Sinus block (barosinusitis) A condition of acute or chronic inflammation of one or more of the paranasal sinuses; produced by a negative pressure difference between the air in the sinuses and the surrounding atmospheric air.

Space blanket A blanket resembling aluminum foil used to help the patient maintain body temperature.

DIVISION **10**

OPERATIONS

CHAPTER 58

EMS Deployment and System Status Management

Objectives

After completing this chapter, you will be able to:

1. Define *system status management.*
2. Describe how resource planning and deployment methods affect response times.
3. Outline two primary ambulance deployment strategies.
4. Compare the advantages and disadvantages of different deployment strategies.
5. Define *unit hour utilization.*
6. Explain how system coverage costs and customer satisfaction can be balanced.

CHAPTER OUTLINE

Case Scenario

You are an EMS supervisor for Timbuck Township EMS and live in the city of Crabtree. Last night the city of Crabtree received notice from its contract ambulance service provider that it intends to cease operations in the city as of midnight the following Sunday. That provider has served the city with five 24-hour ambulance units operating from a single facility on the northeast edge of town; its ambulances were dispatched by the city's 9-1-1 center. The average week involves approximately 300 dispatches that result in roughly 200 transports per week.

The city council, in emergency session, has voted to form a city-operated EMS agency. Your next-door neighbor, the city manager for Crabtree, has asked you to serve as the city's interim EMS director and to help him prepare for the transition to this city-operated service. You believe this will be a great professional opportunity for you and that the city manager will be a great person to work for. He has told you that he wants excellent response performance, a modern approach to deployment, and a positive workplace environment. In addition, to the extent that you believe appropriate, you can use the paramedics from the departing service to start the operation. The city will initially fund the same number of unit hours from the city-operated service as it did from its contract provider, pending your evaluation of future needs and the development of a 5-year plan.

Questions

1. *What sources of data would you rely on to start evaluating your options?*
2. *What type of deployment model is currently in use? What are its strengths and weaknesses?*
3. *What additional information would you want to gather?*
4. *What is the unit hour utilization for transport for this service? For responses? For time deployed for coverage?*

[OBJECTIVES 1, 2, 3, 4]

One of the key principles of an EMS system is to ensure access and appropriate response for those in need of emergency services and medical transportation. Planning and effectively managing ambulance placement and movement deployment and redeployment are key factors in meeting service response time goals at a reasonable cost.

Airlines schedule planes and flight crews to ensure adequate capacity on busy routes, on-time arrivals, and the safety of both passengers and employees. Although different airlines use different methods, each airline has a well-defined deployment strategy. They all have advantages, disadvantages, and costs associated with them that can be quantified. The result is that American Airlines uses a different strategy than Southwest does, but both are respected airlines.

EMS agencies operate in a similar manner. EMS must arrive safely, strive to have good on-time performance, and deliver quality service at a defined cost. Like the airlines, failure to perform often has significant implications. In extreme situations it can have potentially catastrophic affects on those served.

Webster's dictionary defines *deployment* as a way to extend units, place units in battle formation or appropriate positions, and spread out, use, or arrange units strategically. EMS systems have been involved in strategic vehicle and crew deployment for more than 25 years using a variety of deployment methods.

EMS **deployment** and **system status management (SSM)** can be defined as the art and science of matching the production capacity of an ambulance system to the changing patterns of demand placed on that system. They involve strategies and tactics used to manage the resources available to anticipate and prepare for the next call. Paramedics must understand how deployment planning and SSM can be used to achieve the system goal of improving access and response.

Consider the following scenario. An elderly couple is sitting down at the kitchen table having breakfast. Their daughter had come by over the weekend with the newest grandchild, and they reminisce about the visit. As Mr. Johnson gets up to refill his coffee, he suddenly clutches his chest and falls to the floor unconscious.

Because it is morning rush hour, resources are strained. How does this affect the EMS system's response time? The answer is, that depends.

Everyone wants a quick response, clinically competent personnel, and caring service for their loved ones. Community leaders also want to know that EMS is provided at a reasonable cost. In large measure, the manner in which an EMS system plans to meet the demand for service and the way it deploys ambulance resources has a significant impact on response times and potentially on the patient's ultimate outcome in a critical case.

This hypothetical example can be used to compare three different types of deployment and how each would answer the call to aid Mr. Johnson. Community A uses a **fixed-station deployment** strategy. The station is at a busy highway where accidents frequently occur during the evening rush hour, but ambulances are not staged into position as calls occur (Figure 58-1). Community B uses a mixture of stations and posting locations determined by computer modeling of previous requests for service. This community uses a **combination deployment** approach to deploy its ambulances by using a mix of geographic coverage and demand posts to serve the community, given the number of ambulances available at any one time (Figure 58-2). Community C does not base its ambulances at fixed stations but considers its ambulances **fully deployed** by assigning units to a street corner post, similar to small patrol zones established for police units. All other factors are identical (Figure 58-3).

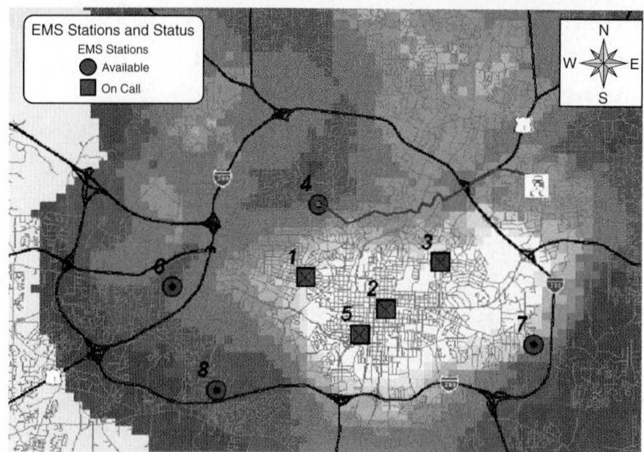

Figure 58-1 Eight fixed stations, no demand posts, four units remaining available.

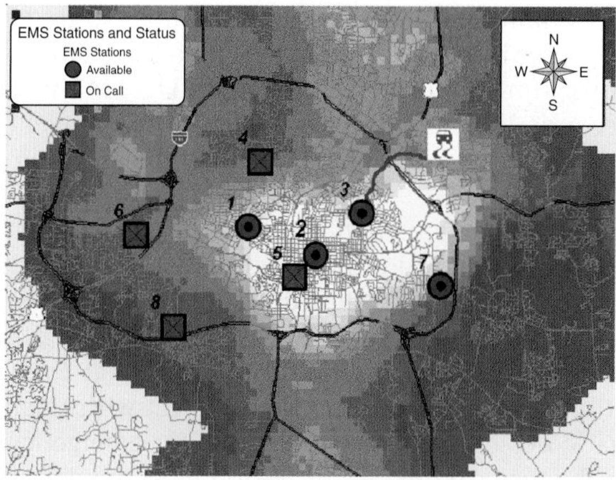

Figure 58-2 Eight fixed stations with high-demand posts, four units remaining available.

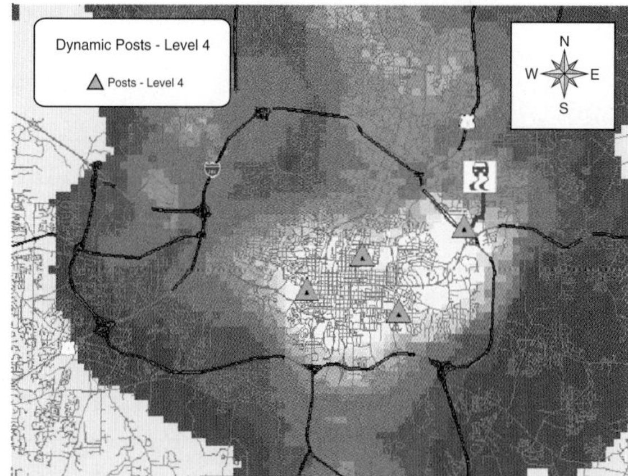

Figure 58-3 Eight demand posts, four units remaining available.

In Community A, because of multiple calls already in progress, the four closest stations' units are on calls. The nearest ambulance is 14 miles away. Its response time to the incident is 19 minutes and 8 seconds, including call processing, chute time, and travel time. Sample system response time includes 1 minute for call processing, 1 minute to leave the station (sometimes referred to as *reflex, turnout,* or **chute time**) and a travel time of 17 minutes and 8 seconds, assuming an average speed of 49 mph.

In Community B, the historic demand has shown a high likelihood of calls in Mr. Johnson's vicinity at this time of day. Two other calls were received before Mr. Johnson's call, so the coverage plan had changed before the hypothetical call was received; the next closest ambulance was moved up to the station where high call volume historically occurs. Now 7.5 miles from the incident, response time is reduced to 11 minutes, 11 seconds. This is based on the same call processing time and speed.

In Community C the scenario is similar to that in B, but the unit is sent to a street corner, not the station. The response time in the incident is reduced to 9 minutes and 11 seconds, including the call processing and travel time. The chute time is eliminated because the crew is already in the vehicle.

Traditionally, ambulance services have constructed stations at different locations within their service areas, with each fixed station staffed 24 hours a day to handle calls. Staffing levels remain constant, with the same amount of ambulances and staff available at the same locations at the same times. The problem with this form of static deployment is that demand for emergency services fluctuates dramatically according to the day of the week, the time of day, and the area of the city. As a result, at times the system is underused, and at times it is overwhelmed by an increase in responses.

In contrast, **flexible deployment,** or SSM, uses computer-aided dispatch records and geographic information systems to ensure that the correct number of ambulances are in the right location when they are needed. By accurately predicting when and where ambulances will be needed, the service is able to minimize response times while maximizing efficiency and distributing workload within the system. In addition to historic information, routing and a wide variety of other factors that can affect response times can be instantly considered and used to maintain optimal coverage as service requests ebb and flow throughout the day.

Different locations of demand within a community are referred to as **geospatial demands.** The measurement of demand by hour of the day is referred to as **temporal demand.** Geospatial demand is illustrated in Figures 58-1, 58-2, and 58-3 by the intensity of the color. In this example, more-rural or less-dense areas of call demand are represented by darker colors. Lighter colors indicate increased demand. Figure 58-4 illustrates this system's ambulances on duty and average number of calls per hour.

There is no single "right" way to deploy ambulances. Many factors must be considered. As a paramedic, you must understand the ethical dimensions of the Hippocratic Oath, which can be paraphrased as "do no harm." Regarding EMS deployment, the goal is to "do the most good." This requires careful balancing of 9-1-1 requests (service demand) with scheduled hours of coverage (service supply), and budgets. How this balance can be achieved and how the organizational culture can be developed must be understood to ensure that employee and employer expectations are well matched (Figure 58-5).

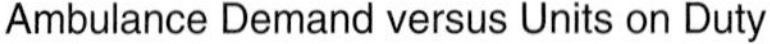

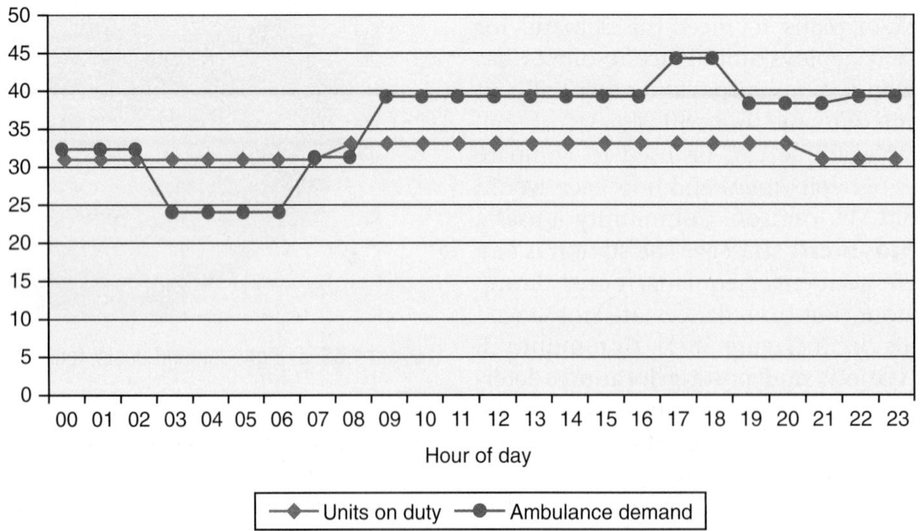

Figure 58-4 Hour of day: lower demand, midnight to 7 AM; higher demand, daytime, peaking at 5 PM.

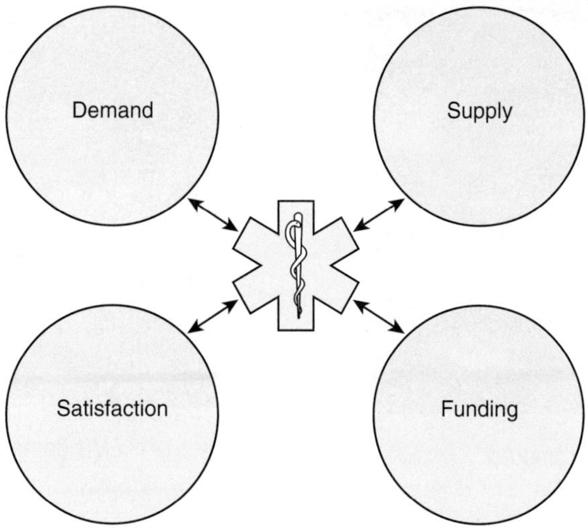

Figure 58-5 Balancing deployment factors.

Case Scenario—continued

After meeting with the employees of the former provider, you learn the following:

- They believe that running five ambulances out of the same location contributes to long response times throughout the city.
- They get along well with the city's firefighters, who provide co-response on medical calls at the emergency medical responder level.
- They enjoy sleeping through the night on most nights but report that at least once per week they have to wait for mutual aid from surrounding communities during the busiest hours of the day.
- They have heard about "street corner posting" and become visibly angry when the subject is raised.

Questions

5. *What geospatial and temporal concerns have you identified in this discussion?*
6. *What tools would you use to analyze and validate those concerns?*
7. *What options could be explored to better meet the needs of the citizens for prompt EMS while addressing the employees' concerns about street corner posting?*

HISTORY OF DEPLOYMENT

Modern deployment strategies originated in studies conducted in the late 1950s by police departments in such cities as New York, Chicago, and Los Angeles. Determining when and where crimes historically occurred helped departments predict future incidents.

Economist and EMS system pioneer Jack Stout first expressed the concept of EMS deployment 25 years ago, originating the idea of SSM (Stout, 1983).

EMS agencies in Tulsa, Okla., and Kansas City, Mo., analyzed historic ambulance calls to create rudimentary demand maps and plans. These plans were loaded on an Apple IIe computer (Figure 58-6). Considered high technology at the time, the Apple IIe had less memory than today's cell phones, and the initial SSM software offered little more than an automated chalkboard. The software prompted dispatchers to move ambulances to certain geographic locations based on historic predictions of where calls would likely occur during certain hours of the day and days of the week.

Instead of all units being assigned 24 hours per day, more units were scheduled during peak demand periods and fewer units when demand was lowest, between 2 and 6 AM. Systems began using a mix of 24-, 12-, 10-, 8-, and even 6-hour shifts, sometimes referred to as *power shifts*. The initial results were dramatic. The same number of budgeted personnel hours was used to improve response times.

Unfortunately, even though demand for service could be predicted, routinely relocating ambulances to cover those high-demand areas proved more challenging. EMS managers decided performance could be improved by predetermining stand-by post locations. A post location could be a fire station, a street corner that offered easy access to a downtown area, or the parking lot of a suburban convenience store that positioned crews equidistant to multiple districts. The key to selecting each post location was the geographic response advantage it offered the EMS system during peak call-volume periods when resources quickly deplete.

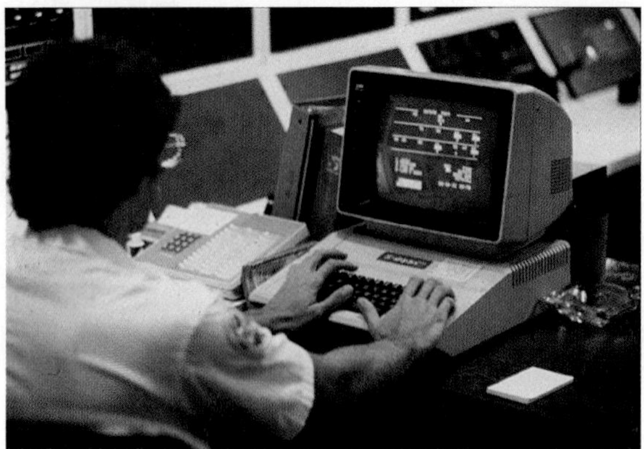

Figure 58-6 Early SSM computer.

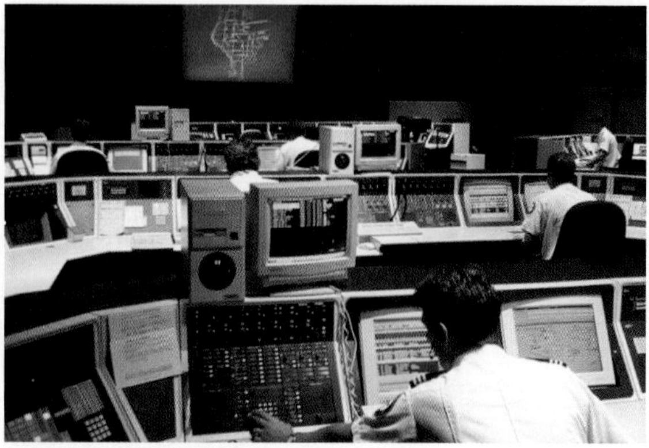

Figure 58-7 EMS Communications Center, Pinellas County, Florida.

The computer generated a unique deployment plan for each of the week's 168 hours. The deployment strategy changed each time a single unit went on an assignment. This necessitated the development of nearly 2400 different posting plans, which were created on the primitive computer. It prompted dispatchers to move units according to each specific plan.

An old myth states that if a little medicine is good, then a lot is better. This is a myth in SSM, too. In many systems the number of post-to-post moves dramatically increased, particularly at night when fewer calls came in and a limited number of ambulances were available. Staff on 24-hour shifts did not get adequate rest but still wanted traditional 24-on, 48-off shift patterns. Aggressive domino-style movements suggested by the computer quickly proved counterproductive. In the middle of the night some crews were moved around faster than a ketchup bottle at a picnic.

The initial SSM euphoria from service improvements and lower costs passed as EMS organizations also recognized the negative side effects. Taken to the extreme, aggressive deployment on long shifts became detrimental. Over time, SSM became derisively known as *street corner deployment,* and EMS personnel angrily resisted vehicle relocations required by the data-driven, systematic deployment approach.

Most individuals entering the EMS profession have a solid work ethic. They expect to work all hours for which they are paid. Compare these different opinions: "I work hard when we get a call, and I should not have to drive all over the area when we are not on an assignment. I work multiple jobs, and when we are not on a call, I should be able to sleep." A more realistic view is "Although I'd rather have downtime in a station, I understand that part of my job is providing coverage, and if I can reduce the response time by being mobile, then that's what I need to do." EMS deployment increased the number of hours each shift that employees were engaged in work-related activity.

In addition to the natural desire to head for the lounge chair between calls, implementing effective deployment planning and management has been hampered by other factors. Chiefs and directors, who often were former EMS workers, were not that knowledgeable about SSM and, until recently, technology to accomplish geographic and temporal (time) analysis of call demand data was expensive. In addition, 9-1-1 and communications personnel, who are critical to the success of managing the system status plan, often worked in another department that was not held accountable for the EMS system's response time performance. Figure 58-7 illustrates a modern EMS communications center that deploys units to match supply (ambulances) with demand (requests).

BASIC PRINCIPLES AND PRACTICES OF DEPLOYMENT

As with many aspects of medicine, topics that seem complex can be better understood if they are broken into their component parts. Effective deployment has three components. These include workload management planning, modern deployment strategies, and dispatch factors (Figure 58-8).

A **workload management** focus means planning resources and support services around demand. Extensive **temporal modeling** (predicting the times when calls occur) helps EMS managers design shifts to meet call volume demand. Other factors that affect workload management include recruiting personnel who expect to work in an event-driven demand system, educating and communicating with existing staff members about deployment strategies, and creatively designing shift patterns and peak-load staffing considerations. Improving fleet management, performing inventory checks, and restocking to reduce nonproductive unit hours also help manage the workload. Well-designed ambulances, access to facilities, and meal breaks also must be considered as part of managing workloads.

Modern deployment considers workload and how available resources can achieve a balance among coverage, response times, and crew satisfaction. Multiple factors must be considered when developing a deployment plan. These include the following:

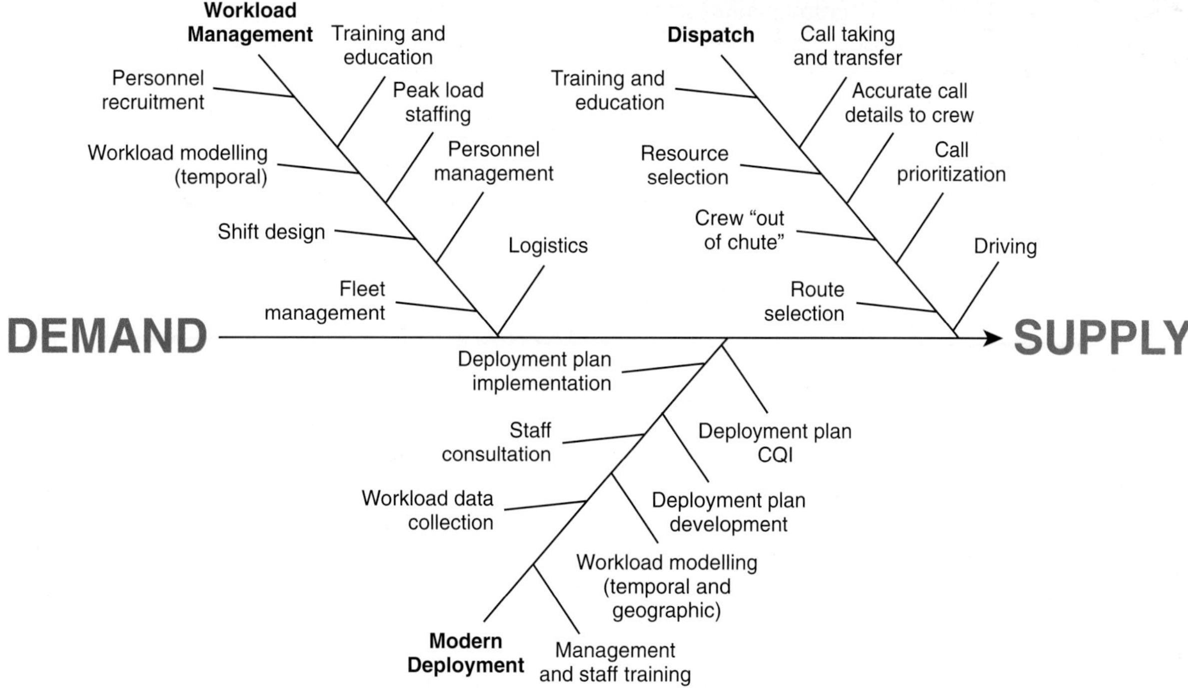

Figure 58-8 Workload management, modern deployment, and dispatch factors. *CQI*, Continuous quality improvement.

- Required response times
- Level-of-care requirements
- Population density
- Geographic density
- Call demand patterns
- Call acuity (severity)
- Road systems
- Location of healthcare facilities

Hard work is required for an EMS system to become truly efficient. Best-practice systems collect and model data before creating a deployment plan. Involving both dispatch and field personnel in plan development and revision stages helps ensure successful implementation. A rational deployment plan will not work if it is not followed. As with other aspects of EMS, the deployment plan must be linked to a service's continuous quality improvement process.

Dispatch factors affecting crew deployment include training and education of communications personnel, rapid call-taking and call prioritization (selecting the most appropriate resource(s) to respond), managing out-of-chute times (getting crews on the road quickly), and providing crews with route selection assistance. Effective communication services are the integration point for planning, deploying, and dynamically redeploying resources.

When all three components are in place, a collaborative effort is still required to achieve success. To achieve efficient and effective resource deployment requires having experienced field and dispatch personnel help design shifts and post locations, developing sophisticated logistics and resupply processes, improving fleet management services, and implementing other strategies to reduce wasted unit hours (a single staffed hour of ambulance coverage), all of which are critical to the success of SSM.

Hundreds of little things can rob systems of needed coverage. These include the hours crews spend out of service dealing with faulty equipment, an inability to start a shift (or put a crew on the road) because the off-going crew is on a late call, and the time crews spend checking ambulances and getting needed supplies. These all negatively affect coverage and, consequently, response times.

Reducing chute times—the time required to get a unit rolling to a call—is critical because it directly affects each call's response time. More difficult, but equally important, is shortening **hospital off-load times**—the time necessary for a crew to become available once they arrive at a hospital. In the past 2 years a number of cities reported increased patient drop-off times caused by emergency department overcrowding and reduced bed capacity. These two factors decrease the efficiency of delivery of EMS because crews cannot quickly transfer their patient to a hospital stretcher or bed and become available for their next assignment.

Reducing hospital off-load times has the net coverage effect of adding ambulances that are staffed on a 24-hour basis to the system and reducing everyone's workload.

Each coverage thief decreases a system's performance. When managed effectively, deployment improvements can be accomplished without the employees shouldering all the responsibility. In a properly designed deployment system, crews no longer have to change post locations every 30 minutes or spend an entire shift in an ambulance.

UNDERSTANDING UNIT HOUR UTILIZATION

[OBJECTIVE 5]

Unit hour utilization (UhU), as a measure of ambulance service productivity and staff workload, has sparked debate for more than two decades. A variety of factors outlined below must be considered to construct a valid comparison that can be used for benchmarking value.

UhU is an indicator of productivity and is defined as a fully equipped and staffed vehicle available or on assignment for the hour. Initially, UhU was used to benchmark systems by considering only the UhU associated with transports (UhU-T). Transports were associated with revenue, productivity, and profitability. But by itself UhU-T is not a true indicator of actual workload.

Calls canceled en route, patients gone on arrival, and patient assessments that did not require transport were not reflected in the UhU-T. To address these factors a complementary ratio was developed, and systems also began measuring UhU for responses (UhU-R) to benchmark the workload associated with nontransport incidents. Some systems also began to include post moves in their measurement or the UhU for the total time deployed for coverage (UhU-TD) to better understand the true workload of field personnel.

Measuring Unit Hour Utilization

The basic UhU-T ratio is determined by dividing the number of transports by the system's net unit hours available for coverage (e.g., UhU = Transports ÷ Available UH). Unit hours lost to the system because of vehicle failures, out-of-service training or meetings, long-distance transfers, and so forth must be factored to determine the net unit hours available to reflect workload accurately.

Assume that the system has 2650 tranports per week and that planned unit hours are 8050. The resulting UhU-T is 0.33. However, the system squanders 1057 unit hours by not paying attention to the amount of time ambulances are unavailable for coverage. The picture changes when lost unit hours are subtracted. A total of 2650 transports are still available, but with only 6993 available hours the UhU-T increases to 0.38. The same mathematical equation can be used to determine UhU-T and UhU-TD.

Time on Task

Time on task also must be considered to benchmark UhU accurately. *Time on task* is defined as the average time a unit is committed to manage an incident (e.g., from dispatch until time the unit is available for another assignment). When the UhU concept was first developed most systems required approximately 60 minutes to manage a transport. The time on task must be factored into the equation when developing UhU ratios. For example, in a rural system in which the average transport takes 90 minutes, using an unadjusted unit hour distorts the productivity picture.

Another common factor that distorts time on task and productivity measures is hospital off-load delays. These delays can be from paperwork, care transfer issues, or staff playing "hide and seek" with dispatch. *Off-load delay is the most common reason for increased time on task throughout North America.* This productivity leakage increases the cost of maintaining response times in some suburban systems between 5% and 10%. In others, response times increase and patients pay the price.

Schedules

Another factor to consider in building a valid comparison is the length of shifts used and the schedule pattern. Typically shorter shifts can tolerate higher UhU measures than can 24-hour shifts. High UhUs coupled with long shifts and little opportunity for rest can be a potential risk factor for employee fatigue, mistakes in patient care, and employee dissatisfaction. Some services use power units during peak demand periods to contribute extremely high productivity, preserve coverage, and maintain a lower overall UhU for the remaining units in the system.

A wide variety of productivity measures, including transports, responses, deployment, and time on task, must be used to determine accurately the appropriate workload for each system. The goal is to balance and optimize multiple variables fully, including caller demand, geographic coverage needs, clinical implications, employee schedules and satisfaction, and fiscal realities. No single right answer or simplified formula can be uniformly applied.

Why Is Unit Hour Utilization Important?

Accurately benchmarking your system can demonstrate value. When buying a home or car, the goal is to get the most value you can by paying a fair price—without overpaying. In some cases a home's fair market value or the Blue Book price for a similarly equipped automobile can be used to establish if the investment is reasonable. For an effective comparison, you must know what specific features were used in the equation. Similarly, accurately measuring UhU, response times, and other productivity factors compared with costs help EMS and community leaders determine whether systems provide communities optimal value.

FUNDING

"It's public safety. Communities should pay whatever it costs without complaint, right?" A variation of this thought is commonly expressed in society. In an ideal world that would be true. In that system, every paramedic would work only 2 hours per week and be paid at least $100,000. Unfortunately, no one knows where that ideal community is located. And, although you might want to work there, you would not want to pay the tax bill.

Providing EMS at an appropriate level of responsiveness and quality requires a significant investment. Because EMS is a public safety and service industry, the majority of costs—between 55% and 80%—are allocated to personnel (Williams, 2005). (The wide variation is linked to the provider type and to whether the service is urban or rural.)

The most expensive aspect of EMS is ensuring that resources are adequate to achieve the target response times. In fact, achieving target response times and the deployment method used to achieve those response times are the primary determinants of cost. Assume the community's response time goal is to place a transport capable ambulance on the scene in less than 9 minutes 90% of the time (90% reliability). If one deployment strategy to accomplish the goal requires eight units to achieve response times and another strategy requires only six units, community leaders take notice. Elected officials are constantly trying to balance the requests for funding from multiple departments. Over a decade, the savings between the two deployment strategies can be significant.

If the community goal is to receive the most value it can obtain by paying a fair price, without overpaying, elected officials must consider alternative deployment approaches. In essence they want to be assured that the EMS funds spent reflect good value for the dollars invested. Even in the wealthiest communities, simply increasing the number of stations and personnel available for response is not the best answer, particularly if they are not properly deployed.

For many communities, changing current workload management, dispatch processes, and deployment strategies is the only cost-effective way to achieve response times that meet goals such as arrival on scene in less than 9 minutes 90% of the time (90% reliability).

ISSUES THAT AFFECT SUCCESS AND SATISFACTION

[OBJECTIVE 6]

When developing an EMS deployment plan, a number of fundamental issues play a role in its success. You must define and measure response times and the processes that make up a response time, UhU, the level of control of field resources, and other human factors.

Response-time calculations, measurement intervals, and benchmarks have been debated for years. Figure 58-9 describes more than key intervals and Table 58-1 outlines recommended benchmarks against which a system can be measured on a fractile (specific time to time) basis. **Fractile response time** measurement involves taking all applicable response times and stacking them in ascending length. The total number of calls generating response times within the preset benchmark are then calculated as a percentage of the total number of calls.

UhU is the measurement of a system's productivity. Calculate UhU for a given period by dividing the number of transports handled by the number of unit hours produced. When adapted or interpreted, comparisons become skewed and less meaningful. Therefore such measures as response utilization, total time deployed, and total workload ratios are additional ways to benchmark and analyze productivity. Vehicle and station amenities also affect crew attitudes about staying in their vehicle longer than usual. For example, some services provide compact disc players, televisions, and small coolers in vehicles. Stations must be clean and comfortable and should be designed for easy egress to reduce chute times. These factors are important in achieving a balance of efficiency, effectiveness, and staff satisfaction.

Resource control is another significant factor. Few, if any, systems can consistently achieve urban response times of less than 8 minutes with 90% fractile reliability without functional control of their field resources. Consolidated dispatch centers that simply process orders (calls) for EMS fail to manage the dynamic deployment and redeployment process adequately. One large North American city developed a sophisticated EMS deployment plan several years ago but found that its communications center followed the plan only 40% of the time. This finding presented them with an internal deficiency that needed to be improved quickly.

Human factors also play a major role in deployment. A major reason that deployment initiatives fail is because of unrealistic expectations on the part of both management and field staff. If either group thinks a new deployment strategy will solve all the system's problems, they are wrong. Commitment, knowledge, available technology, and people also must be considered:

- *Commitment* to develop and properly execute a program can vary. When an organization fails to stay the course, the situation becomes frustrating for all concerned.
- *Lack of baseline knowledge* also can be a factor. EMS organizations sometimes egotistically think, "This can't be that hard." It is. Deployment planning is a statistical process that requires scientific and artistic (leadership) skills.
- *Lack of technology* can prove limiting. The right equipment and software to capture, sort, and interpret large volumes of data are necessary to make good choices.

TABLE 58-1 Benchmarks for Response Times

Time (T)	Description of Time Interval to Measure	Recommended Fractile Benchmark to Measure
T0 to T1	Length of time from 9-1-1 call receipt at PSAP to transfer to an EMS answering point	<30 sec (90% reliability)
T1 to T2	Length of time the phone rang before being answered	<5 sec (90% reliability)
T2 to T3	Elapsed time between picking up the call and verifying the incident location and type by using a recognized process	<25 sec (90% reliability)
T3 to T4	Elapsed time between verification of the incident location and transfer of the call details to the dispatcher's screen or queue	<5 sec (90% reliability)
T4 to T4.1	Elapsed time from location verification and conclusion of dispatch or call taker disconnect (may occur any time between T4 and T7)	Benchmark by call type for quality improvement outliers (e.g., incidents beyond the established norm)
T4.1 to T5	Elapsed time between the call appearing in the queue (to be dispatched computer screen) and dispatching it to a crew	<25 sec (90% reliability)
T5 to T6	Elapsed time between the crew receiving the call and going en route to the call (wheels turning)	<45 sec (90% reliability)
T6 to T7	Elapsed time between the crew going en route and arriving at the incident scene (stopped in front of requested location or designated staging point)	Actual travel time (in an 8:59/90% total response time, this single component would be 434 seconds)
T7 to T7.1	Elapsed time between the crew's arrival at location and arrival at the patient	Benchmark for quality improvement purposes: critical, high-rise, and inaccessible patients
T7.1 to T8	Elapsed time between the crew's arrival at the scene and departure for the destination	<15 min, 90% reliability (protocol dependent)
T8 to T9	Elapsed time between crew departure from the scene and arrival at the destination	Actual travel time
T9 to T10	Elapsed time between the crew's arrival at the destination and their availability for further work	<15 min (90% reliability); call acuity (severity) may require additional benchmarks
T10 to T11	Elapsed time between crew availability and crew departure from destination	Measure to establish internal benchmark
T11 to T12	Elapsed time between crew departure and arrival at designated post or location	Measure to establish internal benchmark

PSAP, Public safety answering post.
When determining the fractile response time for an incident, the elapsed time between T2 and T7 of the first-arriving transport-capable ambulance is typically computed. Measuring and separately reporting the same interval for first responders also is appropriate.

Case Scenario CONCLUSION

In the limited time available, you are able to reach agreement with the city fire chief to co-locate your EMS units at the city's five geographically distributed fire stations. You have reallocated some unit hours so that up to seven ambulances are on duty at the busy times of the day but only three units are on duty from the hours of 1 to 6 AM. Your response performance (T0 to T7) has improved, but not as much as you thought it would. Several employees have resigned because they did not want to work the schedules that came with the unit hour reallocation.

Looking Back

8. *Given this outcome, did you make good decisions? What other information might you have wanted in your possession before you made your decisions?*

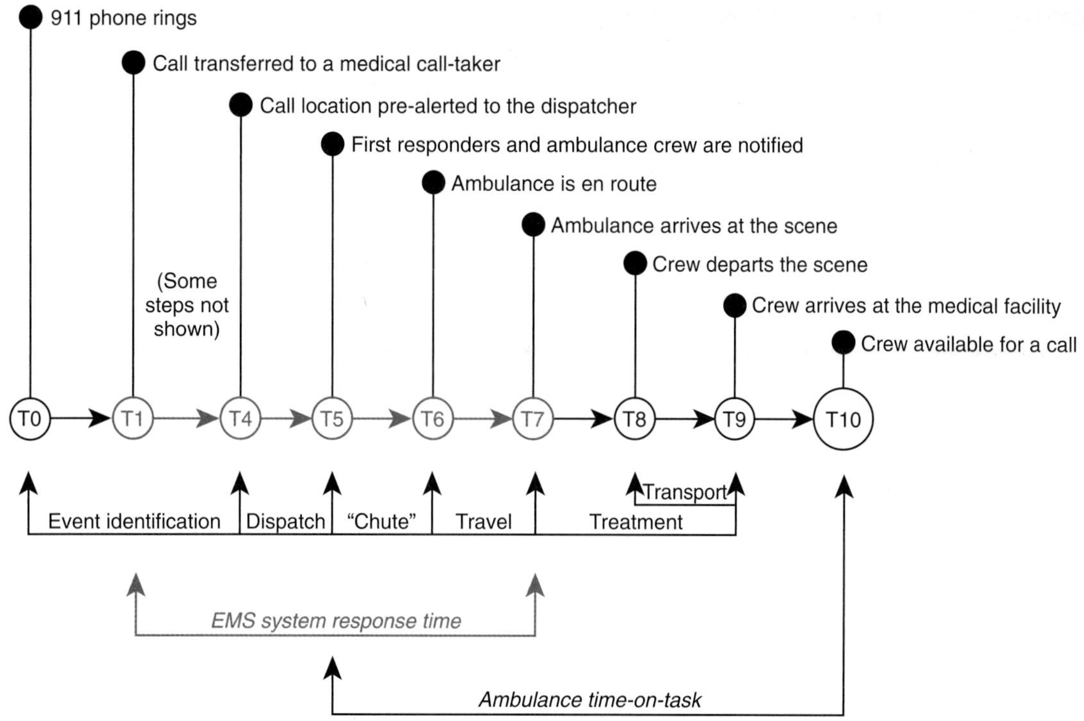

Figure 58-9 Key response time intervals to be measured.

- *Lack of qualified people is a failure point.* Deployment strategies, no matter how aggressive, cannot compensate for a shortage of qualified personnel who care about doing the best possible job for patients.

Understanding deployment and SSM is a fundamental tool to improve EMS system access and response time. It is part of every paramedic's job. Regarding deployment, one size (approach) does not fit all. Progressive public safety and EMS systems recognize that a successful plan can thoughtfully balance community and employee needs.

Case Scenario SUMMARY

1. *What sources of data would you rely on to start evaluating your options?* When beginning to evaluate a service, operational data are of primary importance, particularly when you have not yet been asked to deal with the financial concerns of the organization. Call data from the 9-1-1 center's computer-aided dispatch system, together with data from the service's patient care reporting system, will allow you to perform statistical and geospatial analyses. You will need the ability to use (or find someone to help you use) statistical analysis software such as Microsoft Excel and geographic information systems software such as ArcGIS or MapPoint.
2. *What type of deployment model is currently in use? What are its strengths and weaknesses?* This service is using a fixed-point, static deployment model that accounts for neither the geospatial or temporal needs of the city. It is perhaps the worst-performing model that can be designed in terms of service delivery. Its principal strengths are that it is easy, cheap, and convenient to manage, and it may provide a pleasant social environment for the working personnel.
3. *What additional information would you want to gather?*
   - Number of mutual aid calls and when they occur
   - Hospital turnaround time
   - Performance data for the fire department co-responders
   - Impressions of the quality of the service from the citizens, healthcare providers, and public safety officials in the community

Continued

Case Scenario SUMMARY—continued

4. *What is the unit hour utilization for transport for this service? For responses? For time deployed for coverage?* UhU-T is 0.238 (200/840), and UhU-D is 0.357 (300/840). The UhU cannot be calculated from the information available. Information about move-ups is required to use this measure.
5. *What geospatial and temporal concerns have you identified in this discussion?* Ambulances are not staffed with any regard for demand for service. Too many ambulances are on duty at night and too few during the day. The ambulances are not located with any regard for the location of demand. At least four of these units could be better located to improve response performance across the city.
6. *What tools would you use to analyze and validate those concerns?* A statistical analysis tool such as Microsoft Excel could be used to generate a demand curve showing how many calls can, on the average, be expected in each hour of each day. Geographic information systems software could be used to perform a density analysis for calls during certain parts of the day. This would identify hot spots where EMS units should be located for optimal coverage.
7. *What options could be explored to better meet the needs of the citizens for prompt EMS while addressing the employees' concerns about street corner posting?* De-clustering the EMS units to provide better coverage is an essential concern for this new service. Existing public facilities and healthcare facilities may be simple starting points that can be quickly accessed and provide temporary or longer term solutions, particularly given the good relationship between EMS and fire department staff. Reallocation of unit hours, from the slow middle of the night period to the busy part of the day when mutual aid is required, might make sense and does not require additional funding because the city manager has agreed to continue to fund 840 unit hours per week.
8. *Given this outcome, did you make good decisions? What other information might you have wanted in your possession before you made your decisions?* Given the pressures of time, this was an excellent short-term solution that also may prove effective in the longer term. The city is better served than before, and resource availability has been better matched with demand for service. Given more time, more employee involvement might have been sought. Some level of employee turnover should be expected any time a major organizational change occurs, but efforts should be made to minimize that through communication and involvement. The issue of chute time was not addressed during the transition and may be contributing to the less-than-expected improvement in response performance. The issue of hospital turnaround time also was not addressed, but if hospital turnaround is slow or the local hospitals are diverting patients to hospitals outside the community, these factors may limit the availability of ambulances to respond to emergency calls. This scenario presents a new EMS manager with an opportunity to apply progressive, innovative, yet relatively simple modern ambulance deployment techniques to a very old-school approach to service. Effectively managing the deployment of resources in an EMS system is a hallmark of an excellent EMS organization.

Chapter Summary

- Deployment methods can significantly affect clinical, operational, and financial aspects of an EMS system.
- Key deployment strategies include (1) fixed-station deployment, (2) a mix of geographic and demand deployment when the system is busy, and (3) fully deployed systems that frequently use street corner posts.
- Response times, hours of coverage required to achieve response time, employee satisfaction, and cost are each considered advantages and disadvantages associated with different deployment strategies.
- Flexible deployment, or SSM, is the art and science of matching the production capacity of an ambulance system to the changing patterns of demand placed on that system.
- UhU is an indicator of ambulance service productivity and staff work load.
- A variety of factors must be considered when determining the best deployment strategy for a particular community. These include anticipated call demand, supply or availability of units, funding, and employee satisfaction.

REFERENCES

Stout, J. (1983). System status management. *Journal of Emergency Medical Services, 8*(5), 22-32.

Williams, D. (2005). 2005 JEMS salary and workplace survey. *Journal of Emergency Medical Services, 30*(10), 36-38, 40, 42.

SUGGESTED RESOURCES

American Ambulance Association: http://www.the-AAA.org

Fitch, J. (2004). *Prehospital care administration: Issues, cases, and readings* (2nd ed.). San Diego: Jems/KGB Media.

Fitch, J. (2005). EMS in crisis: Meeting the challenge. *IQ Reports—International City/County Management Association, 37,* 5.

Fitch, J. (2005). Response times: myths, measurement & management. *Journal of Emergency Medical Services, 30*(9), 47-56.

Fitch & Associates, LLC: http://www.fitchassoc.com

International Association of Fire Chiefs: http://www.iafc.org

Kuehl, A. (2002). *Prehospital systems and medical oversight* (3rd ed.). Dubuque, IA: Kendall/Hunt.

National Academies of Emergency Dispatch: http://www.emergencydispatch.org

Chapter Quiz

1. Define SSM.

2. What are two different strategies for ambulance deployment?

3. What is UhU?

4. How does SSM affect response times?

5. How can system costs and employee satisfaction be balanced?

6. What three factors should be considered in developing a deployment plan?

7. What accounts for the majority of the cost of operating an ambulance system?

8. What is the most common reason for increased time on task?

9. What is temporal demand?

10. How is UhU-T measured?

Terminology

Chute time The time required to get a unit en route to a call from dispatch.

Combination deployment Using a mix of geographic coverage and demand posts to best serve the community given the number of ambulances available at any one time.

Deployment Matching production capacity of an ambulance system to the changing patterns of call demand.

Dispatch factors Training and education of communications personnel, rapid call taking, call prioritization (selecting the most appropriate resources to respond), managing out-of-chute times (getting crews on the road quickly), and providing crews with route selection assistance.

Fixed-station deployment Deployment method of using only geographically based stations.

Flexible deployment See System status management.

Fractile response time Method used to determine the time at which 90% of all requests for service receive a response; considered a more definitive measure of performance than averages.

Fully deployed Assigning ambulances to a street corner post.

Geospatial demand analysis Understanding the different locations of demand within a community.

Terminology—continued

Hospital off-load time The time necessary for a crew to become available once it arrives at a hospital.

Modern deployment Deployment that considers workload and how available resources can achieve a balance among coverage, response times, and crew satisfaction.

Response time The time from when the call is received until the paramedics arrive at the scene.

System status management (SSM) The dynamic process of staffing, stationing, and moving ambulances based on projected call volumes; also called *flexible deployment.*

Temporal demand Measurement of call demand by hour of the day.

Temporal modeling Predicting the times when calls occur.

Time on task The average time a unit is committed to manage an incident.

Unit hour utilization (UhU) A measure of ambulance service productivity and staff workload.

Workload management Planning resources and support services around demand.

CHAPTER 59

Crime Scene Awareness

Objectives

After completing this chapter, you will be able to:

1. Explain how EMS providers often are mistaken for the police.
2. Describe warning signs of potentially violent situations.
3. Explain specific techniques for risk reduction when approaching highway encounters, violent street incidents, residences, and dark houses.
4. Explain emergency evasive techniques for potentially violent situations, including threats of physical violence, firearms encounters, and edged-weapon encounters.
5. Explain EMS considerations for the following types of violent or potentially violent situations:
   - Gangs and gang violence
   - Clandestine drug labs
   - Interpersonal violence
6. Explain the following techniques: field contact and cover procedures during assessment and care, evasive tactics, and concealment techniques.
7. Describe police evidence considerations and techniques to assist in evidence preservation.

CHAPTER OUTLINE

Case Scenario

Police at a private residence call you for a 65-year-old woman found unresponsive. On arrival, you see that the police have blocked off the area and they are searching for a perpetrator. While you are grabbing your equipment, the officer in charge informs you that a suspect entered the residence and attacked a woman. He states they believe the woman is dead but they need your confirmation. The officer leads you to the side entry door, asking for your cooperation in minimizing your effect on the crime scene.

Questions

1. *Is the scene safe?*
2. *What equipment would you bring?*
3. *How could you minimize disrupting the crime scene?*
4. *Should crime scene preservation or patient care take priority?*

Violence can occur anywhere and in any form. Whether you work as a paramedic in the inner city, the suburbs, or a rural town, you can be affected by violence. EMS exposure to violence includes street violence, terrorists, interpersonal violence, and unruly mobs. Violence that arises from street gangs, terrorist groups, domestic disputes, and drug users against EMS crews is increasing (Jacobsen, 1997; U.S. Department of Transportation, 1998). EMS crews must be educated in hazard awareness and avoidance because they may arrive at the scene before (or with) law enforcement. As part of hazard awareness, the EMS provider should attempt to identify and respond to dangers before they become threatening. Any emergency response has the potential to be dangerous for EMS crews. Personal safety must be the first priority.

PARAMEDIC*Pearl*

When you are at a crime scene and law enforcement personnel are present, guns are now guaranteed to be on scene. If police need to use them, or in the unlikely event one is taken away from an officer, a significant danger exists for everyone, including EMS.

RESPONDING TO THE SCENE

[OBJECTIVES 1, 2]

Personal safety begins as soon as you are dispatched to a call. Emergency medical dispatchers attempt to keep callers on line to obtain as much information as possible. The dispatching center may have the following information that should alert you to possible dangers:

- Locations of unsafe scenes
- Large crowds
- People under the influence of alcohol or drugs
- On-scene violence
- Weapons

Crew members or other emergency responders monitoring the call who have had previous experience with a particular area or address also can offer additional valuable information.

Your assessment for dangerous situations should begin several blocks from the scene as you look for evidence of possible danger. The paramedic should ensure that warning devices are used, or not used, as appropriate. Warning devices can attract large crowds to an already tenuous situation; additionally when responding to a dangerous scene the paramedic will likely be required to stage until the scene is secured. Responding with lights and sirens to a staging area increases the risk of being involved in a collision with little benefit. Responding in a "silent" emergency mode—using visual warnings only—is not acceptable, as most states require the use of visual and audible warning devices in an emergency response. An alternative to this is to respond to the emergency to a certain point and then turn off all warning devices. When possible danger is suspected or reported by the dispatcher, stage the ambulance and do not approach the scene until it is secured by law enforcement personnel. Ensure your staging area is far enough from the scene that bystanders will not converge upon the ambulance stating "the patient is down there." This can set up a situation where not responding can agitate the bystanders, creating a dangerous situation, yet responding to an unsecured scene is also not acceptable. This is a no-win situation in which the paramedic can become injured, taken hostage, or even killed if they enter the unsafe scene or stay at the staging area with agitated bystanders. Work with law enforcement to determine when to approach the scene. Remember: even when law enforcement is on scene, violence still can occur. Do not let the presence of law enforcement provide a false sense of security. Also keep in mind that people may mistake you for law enforcement because of uniform colors, use of badges, and vehicles with flashing lights and sirens. These people also may show aggression toward you as an authority figure.

Observing Danger on Arrival

Remember that the potential for danger exists even if dispatch has not alerted you of this possibility. The purpose of performing a scene size-up is to search for any potential hazards. These include nonviolent hazards such as downed power lines, dangerous pets, unstable vehicles, or hazardous materials. Your knowledge of past violence in the area or whether the area is known for gangs or drugs is a valuable tool in the scene size-up. When you are in the neighborhood, begin to make observations of the scene you are approaching. Examples of things to look for include the following:

- Crowds in front of the residence
- People running from the residence
- Signs of altercation, such as people fighting or yelling
- Vehicles speeding away from the residence
- Darkened residence
- Unusual silence

PARAMEDIC*Pearl*

As an EMS professional, you spend a lot of time in your jurisdiction and should notice and remember many of the things that occur around you. To maintain focus on situational awareness, consider the memory aid PPTT:

***P**eople*
***P**laces*
***T**hings they do*
***T**imes they do them*

Do not exit your vehicle until you have ruled out all immediate hazards. Some safety strategies to use to minimize your exposure to violence include the following (Figures 59-1 to 59-3):

- Carry a portable radio.
- Do not leave your crew without a way to communicate.
- Use an unconventional path instead of the sidewalk leading to the front of the door.

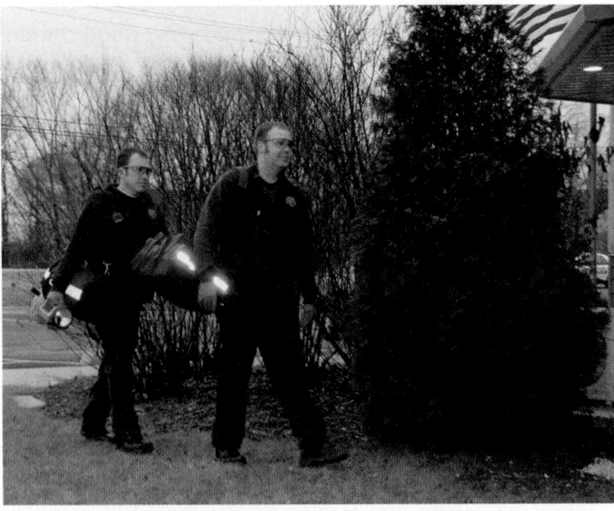

Figure 59-1 Approach unstable scenes single file and use an unconventional path.

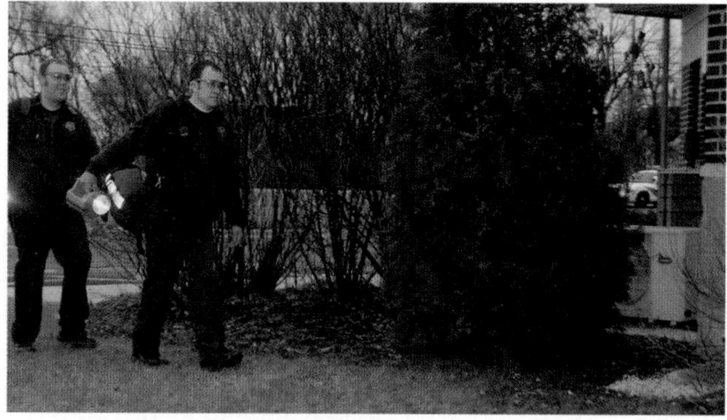

Figure 59-2 Assailants who are armed usually aim at the light. Hold a flashlight to the side of your body, not in front of it.

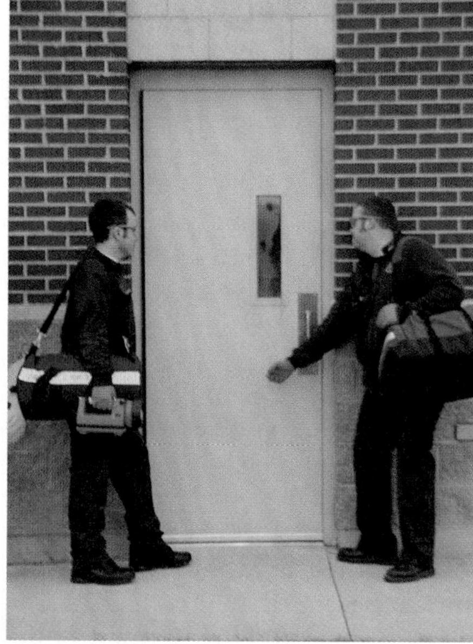

Figure 59-3 When knocking at a door, stand to the side. Never stand directly in front of a door or window.

- Stand to the side of the door when knocking.
- Do not backlight yourself.
- Listen for sounds indicating danger before you announce your presence.

Danger during Patient Care or Transport

The EMS crew must remain alert throughout a call. You may find while caring for the patient that additional combative people arrive on scene, and bystanders or the patient may over time become agitated. These people may begin to threaten the EMS crew. Your safety must come first even if you have begun treatment. If you find yourself in this situation, you have the following two options:

- Leave the scene with the patient as efficiently as possible.
- Retreat to safety without the patient.

Retreating for your or your crew's protection is not considered abandonment; be sure to document and keep accurate records of these incidents.

The EMS crew must always have an escape plan. When entering a building, look for other potential exits if you need to retreat. A failure to have an escape plan can put you at risk of becoming a victim of violence.

POTENTIALLY DANGEROUS SCENES

[OBJECTIVES 3, 4, 5]

Your ability to survive a dangerous scene depends on recognition of potential threats and an ability to provide rescuer and patient safety. Following are some potentially dangerous scenes you may encounter:

- Highway encounters
- Violent street incidents
- Interpersonal violence
- Drug-related crimes

Highway Encounters

Never consider an emergency response to a traffic incident routine. Besides the risks associated with traffic flow, emergency vehicle positioning, and extrication, you must be aware of the potential for violence. The highway encounter can include the risk of violence from fleeing felons, intoxicated or drugged persons, or persons in possession of weapons. Potential warning signs of danger on the highway include the following:

- Persons with an altered mental state
- Arguing or fighting among passengers
- Differences among stories told by occupants
- Grabbing or hiding items inside the vehicle
- Lack of activity where activity is expected
- Open or unlatched trunks (a potential hiding spot for people and weapons)
- Physical signs of alcohol or drug abuse (e.g., liquor bottles, beer cans, syringes)

For a safe approach of a vehicle at a roadside emergency, use the following steps:

- Park your apparatus (engine or ambulance) between you (and your crew) and oncoming traffic.
- Use a one-person approach to the vehicle. The driver should remain in the ambulance, which is elevated and provides greater visibility. It also allows the partner to notify dispatch of the situation, location, license plate number, and state registration of suspicious vehicles. Consider getting in the habit of calling in the plate number as you approach the vehicle—every time, day or night. By doing so on "routine" calls, you are less likely to forget to do so in an unusual or unsafe situation.
- Discuss a plan with your partner for retreat and escape before exiting the ambulance.

- At night use ambulance headlights to illuminate the other interior of the other vehicle and surrounding area. However, do not walk between the ambulance and other vehicle, which will cause you to be backlit and therefore an easy target.
- Consider that parking on the side of the road with your headlights on may blind oncoming drivers so that it is difficult for them to see the medical crews on scene.
- Approach the vehicle from the passenger side, which provides protection from traffic and usually is the opposite approach the driver would expect from law enforcement personnel.
- Use the A, B, and C door posts for cover.
- Observe the front seat from behind the B post and move forward only after ensuring safety.
- If you observe warning signs of danger, retreat to safety and request law enforcement assistance.

Violent Street Incidents

While working on the streets you will encounter many different types of violence. These incidents can range from random acts of violence against individuals to organized acts of terrorism. You must be prepared to respond to some of the following violent street incidents.

Murder, Assault, and Robbery

The crimes of murder, assault, and robbery often occur in the United States. Many of these crimes involve dangerous weapons. In addition, violence may be directed toward EMS personnel from perpetrators at the scene or who return to the scene or from injured or distraught patients.

PARAMEDIC*Pearl*

Individuals may follow an ambulance to the hospital or show up there later after an incident. This creates potential safety hazards for hospital staff and those seeking care from unrelated incidents. This situation should be considered possible in all violent crime situations, not just gang-related incidents. Hospital security, police, and other EMS units should be made aware of the potential danger.

Dangerous Bystanders and Crowds

Awareness of crowd dynamics is crucial for EMS personnel to maintain a safe environment. A crowd can quickly become large and violent. This violence can be directed toward anyone or anything. The following are warning signs of impending danger when a crowd is present:

- Shouting or increasing loud voices
- Pushing or shoving
- Development of hostilities toward anyone on scene
- Rapid increase in crowd size
- Inability of law enforcement officials to control bystanders

EMS personnel should constantly monitor the crowd. Do not antagonize anyone in the crowd; treat people with respect. If possible, remove the patient from the scene as you retreat, which eliminates the need to return later.

Street Gangs

Groups of people who band together and engage in socially disruptive or criminal behavior are considered gangs. Street gangs can be found throughout the country. Some have branched out into smaller towns to escape surveillance and expand their illegal activities.

Gangs operate on the premise of intimidation and extortion. Most are heavily involved in drug trafficking, which finances their activities. Some of the commonly observed gang characteristics include the following:

- *Appearance*. Members of a gang wear unique clothing specific to their group. The clothing is often a particular color and is referred to as the gang's color. Examples of styles common among gang members are shaved heads, tattoos, jewelry, bandanas, oversized t-shirts or jeans, and baseball caps worn backwards. Tattoos or other body markings are of the gang's logo or motto and in their colors. Gang experts recommend that you explain and ask for permission before cutting the colors in front of other gang members. Gangs have a strong system of values based on respect. By explaining and asking for permission they perceive that you respect them. This can possibly prevent repercussions toward EMS personnel.
- *Graffiti*. Gangs have territories defined as *turfs*. Members mark their territories with graffiti. Often the graffiti is used to show their logo, warn away other gangs, brag about crimes, insult other gangs, or even taunt police.
- *Hand signals and language*. Gangs have established their own method of communication. They create their own codes and meanings for words. Hand signs are used to provide quick identification among gang members, warn about approaching law enforcement, or show disrespect to other gangs.

EMS personnel who enter gang territory must be aware of the increased potential for violence. Gangs may attempt to prevent you from transporting one of their members to a hospital beyond the reach of the gang. If your safety is at stake, do not force the issue.

Interpersonal Violence

Violence that occurs between persons in a relationship is considered interpersonal violence. Victims of interpersonal violence may be male or female, and the violence can be physical, emotional, sexual, verbal, or economic. It may be directed against spouses, partners, children, or older relatives who live in the residence. Indicators of interpersonal violence include the following:

- Apparent fear of a household member
- Different or conflicting accounts by parties at the scene
- One party preventing another from speaking
- A patient who is reluctant to speak
- Injuries that do not match the reported mechanism of injury
- Unusual or unsanitary living conditions or personal hygiene

When responding to a scene of interpersonal violence, EMS personnel should be aware that acts of violence may be directed toward them by the perpetrator. Take all safety precautions; once the scene is considered safe, treat the patient's injuries and notify medical direction along with any other authorities consistent with protocol. Remember to not be judgmental about the situation. Document as soon as possible (during and after the call) and always be factual.

Drug-Related Crimes

Violence as a result of the sale of drugs kills many people each year. You must be aware that drug dealers will protect their operations with booby traps, automatic weapons, and dogs trained to attack. Violence toward EMS personnel can erupt by unknowingly walking onto the scene of a drug deal or uncovering an illicit drug operation.

Signs of Drug Involvement

Some signs that can alert you to the involvement of drugs at a call include the following:

- Prior history of drugs in the neighborhood of the call
- Clinical evidence that the patient has used drugs of some kind
- Drug-related comments by bystanders
- Drug paraphernalia at the scene, such as vials, syringes, and needles

If any of these signs occur, you must assume the use or presence of drugs at the scene. Some patients who use drugs will be seeking help and will not harm you. If the patient is not involved, others at the scene may pose a danger. You must carefully evaluate each situation.

PARAMEDIC*Pearl*

Remember PPTT in these situations. Another resource is the computer-aided dispatch premise history. Seasoned dispatchers are in the habit of checking the history often and reporting the information to street units. Also, most systems have a feature that allows automatic pop-up caution notes for premises. Communication during incidents is important, but also be sure to feed back the information from the field to dispatch so they can add notes.

Clandestine Drug Laboratories

Laboratories are set up by drug dealers to manufacture or convert controlled substances with the intent to sell them for profit. A common substance manufactured in these drug laboratories is methamphetamine (also called *crank, speed,* or *crystal*). A clandestine drug laboratory needs privacy, utilities, and equipment (e.g., glassware, chemical containers, heating mantels, match heads and match striker plates, burners). Often these laboratories are discovered by neighbors who report suspicious odors, deliveries, or activities.

Clandestine laboratories can turn into hazardous material operations because they contain toxic fumes and volatile chemicals. People found on scene can contribute to the dangerous situation by fighting or shooting at EMS personnel. Drug dealers are also known to set booby traps for police or EMS personnel. Take the following actions when you come across a clandestine drug laboratory:

- Leave the area immediately.
- Do not touch anything.
- Do not stop any chemical reactions already in progress.
- Do not smoke or bring any source of flame near the laboratory.
- Notify law enforcement.
- Initiate the incident command system and hazardous materials procedures.
- Consider evacuation of the area.

Case Scenario—continued

You and your partner follow the officer into the kitchen. You observe chairs turned over, dented paint cans, and a significant amount of blood splattered on the floor and walls. The officer leads you through the kitchen and into the living room, pointing to the stairs. You look to your right and find the victim lying halfway up the stairs, unresponsive. As you approach her, you notice the carpet is soaked in blood. You find the victim is not breathing and has no pulse. Her skin temperature is warm and color is cyanotic.

Questions

5. *What is your general impression of this patient?*
6. *What examples of evidence can be found at this crime scene?*
7. *Should you move the victim? Why or why not?*

TACTICAL SAFETY AND TACTICAL PATIENT CARE

[OBJECTIVES 4, 5, 6]

The best tactical response to violence for EMS personnel is observation and avoidance. When the dispatcher advises you of danger in advance, stage your ambulance outside the danger area until advised that the scene is secured by law enforcement. Despite your best attempts, you may still find yourself in situations with a potential for danger. Always have a plan in place regarding how to handle potentially violent situations. Below are some actions you can take to protect yourself while attempting to provide patient care.

PARAMEDIC*Pearl*

Remember that when police have the scene secured, their weapons are still a potential hazard.

Safety Tactics

Your response to dangerous situations will cause extreme stress. Your response to the danger will be based on how you practiced preparing for it. You must practice your response to danger on a frequent basis. Many training programs specialize in teaching tactical considerations for safety and patient care.

PARAMEDIC*Pearl*

Consider leaving a piece of equipment outside the door or turn on the scene lights on only the side to which you went, to mark your position. If you need to call for help, responders will be better able to know which way you went (by the lights) and through which door you entered (stair chair or other equipment left outside or propping door).

Retreat

The best strategy is to **retreat** when you observe indicators of violence. The decision to retreat is a decisive action and must be immediate. When you choose to retreat it should be done in a calm, safe manner and include cover. When you retreat, the risks you are retreating from are now located behind you and you must be alert for other associated dangers. A safe distance should accomplish the following:

- Protect the crew from any potential danger
- Keep the crew out of immediate line of sight
- Provide cover
- Allow reaction if danger reappears

When you have retreated to a safe area, notify the other responding units and agencies. Follow your department's standard operating procedures and interagency agreements. Thorough documentation is essential to reducing charges of abandonment or liability if injuries or deaths occur. Document your observations of danger and your specific responses. Be sure to include the following information in your documentation:

- Actions taken while on scene
- Reasons you retreated
- Accurate times that retreat and return to scene occurred
- Personnel and agencies contacted

Retreating for appropriate circumstances is not considered abandonment. Once the scene is determined safe by law enforcement, you can respond from staging again.

PARAMEDIC*Pearl*

When necessary, consult audiotapes and computer-aided dispatch information for times when completing prehospital care reports to ensure accuracy.

Cover and Concealment

Two strategies you can use when faced with danger are cover and concealment. **Cover** hides your body and offers ballistic protection. Examples of cover include large trees, telephone poles, and a vehicle engine block. **Concealment** also hides the body but offers no ballistic protection. Examples of concealment include hiding behind bushes, wallboards, and vehicle doors. Applying the following general rules allows you to apply cover and concealment properly:

- Remain constantly aware of the surroundings.
- Place as much of your body as possible behind adequate cover.
- Constantly look for ways to improve protection and location.
- Be aware of reflective clothing that may draw attention or serve as a target.

Distraction and Evasion

Distraction and evasion can be used as a self-defense measure during retreat. Some distraction and **evasive tactics** to avoid dangerous situations include the following:

- Wedging a stretcher in a doorway to block aggressor
- Throwing equipment to trip or slow an aggressor
- Using an unconventional path while retreating
- Anticipating the moves of the aggressor and taking counter moves

You must be in good health to ensure you will have the strength to outrun or defend yourself against an attacker. Regular exercise and proper nutrition play an important part in your overall health. Take advantage of any self-defense training that is offered. Because policies pertaining to the application of force to restrain a patient vary widely, you must know your local protocols related to the application of force.

Contact and Cover

The concept of contact and cover is used to handle threats of physical violence, firearms, and edged-weapon encounters. EMS providers have preassigned roles in which one provider initiates and provides direct patient care (contact) while the second provider serves as the safe cover for the contact provider (cover). The roles of each provider are outlined in Box 59-1.

Warning Signals and Communication

Communication is a vital part of EMS and is an invaluable safety tool. All EMS personnel must develop methods of alerting other providers to danger without alerting the aggressor. You should devise prearranged verbal and nonverbal clues and regularly practice them. Dispatch should be included in the danger signal process. Choose signals that will sound harmless to the attacker but will alert the dispatcher to have additional appropriate personnel respond. For example, consider using first names on the radio instead of unit numbers in these situations. If dispatch calls and asks if you are OK, you can respond, "Yes Cheryl, we're fine." Doing so alerts everyone, not just dispatch, that a situation has developed, and the aggressors may not notice it. Developing this form of communication can be life saving for you, the crew, and the patient.

Tactical Patient Care

Tactical training and protections offered to EMS have increased over time because of continued involvement in dangerous situations. The duties and roles of EMS and law enforcement agencies at crime scenes, riots, and terrorist events must be clarified in advance through interagency planning and agreements. **Tactical patient care** includes the use of body armor by EMS crews and specially trained tactical EMS personnel.

Body Armor

An increasing number of EMS agencies are supplying body armor to their personnel. Body armor is also known as a *bullet-resistant vest*. Body armor is soft and is made from a series of fibers woven tightly together to form a vest. It offers protection from handgun bullets, most knives, and blunt trauma. Body armor does not protect against high-velocity bullets (e.g., rifles) or thin or dual-edged weapons (e.g., ice pick), and protection is reduced when wet. Remember the following:

- Body armor does not work if it is not worn.
- Never do anything you would not do without body armor.
- Body armor does not cover all your body. You can still be critically injured or killed.
- You may still sustain severe cavitation injury.

BOX 59-1 Contact and Cover

Contact Provider

- Initiates and provides direct patient care
- Performs patient assessment
- Handles most interpersonal scene contact

Cover Provider

- Observes the scene for danger while the contact provider cares for the patient
- Generally avoids patient care duties that would prevent observation of the scene
- In small crews, may perform limited functions such as handling equipment

Tactical EMS

Tactical EMS refers to the provision of care inside the scene perimeter or hot zone. It requires special training, authorization, body armor, and compact functional equipment. This type of care may require risks not taken in the standard EMS situation. Tactical patient care differs from routine EMS calls in the following ways:

- A priority of extraction of the patient from the hot zone
- Frequent care of trauma patients
- Modified care to meet tactical considerations
- Treatment and transport interventions coordinated with the incident commander
- Patients moved to tactically cold zones for complete assessment, care, and transport
- Metal clipboards, chemical agents, or other tools used as defensive weapons

Local protocols, standing orders, and medical direction must be developed and implemented before the deployment of a tactical EMS team. A tactical EMS team may be composed of EMTs, paramedics, and physicians who operate as part of a tactical law enforcement team. Some teams use persons cross-trained in law enforcement and tactical EMS. Tactical EMS certifications are offered by some organizations. The training required of tactical EMS personnel involves strenuous physical activity under extreme conditions. Tactical EMS personnel may be trained in the following:

- Raids on clandestine drug labs
- EMS in barricade situations
- Wounding by weapons or booby traps
- Special gear for tactical operations
- Use of chlorobenzylidenemalononitrile (tear gas), oleoresin capsicum (pepper spray), or other gas
- Blank-firing weapons
- Helicopter operations
- Pyrotechnics
- Operating under extreme conditions (e.g., extreme hot or cold weather, extended operations, darkness, psychological stress)
- Firefighting and hazardous materials operations

Case Scenario CONCLUSION

The cardiac monitor shows asystole in three leads. You run an ECG strip to document your findings. Further assessment finds that the patient has several puncture wounds along the right side of her neck where the carotid artery is located. You contact medical direction and receive permission not to resuscitate. Custody of the victim is turned over to the medical examiner's office. The police take pictures of the soles of your shoes, as well as those of your partner. You complete the patient care report and then head back to the station to complete the rest of your shift. The next day the medical examiner's report states that the patient had more than 50 stab wounds along her carotid artery from scissors, and the cause of death was exsanguination.

Looking Back

8. *Should the victim have been resuscitated? Why or why not?*
9. *Are your observations and documentation important?*

EMS AT CRIME SCENES

[OBJECTIVE 7]

A **crime scene** can be defined as a location where any part of a criminal act has occurred and where evidence relating to a crime may be found. At a crime scene you should provide high-quality patient care while preserving evidence. Do not jeopardize patient care to preserve evidence, but do not perform patient care with disregard of the criminal investigation that will follow.

EMS and Police Operations

At times, emergencies require the response of both EMS and law enforcement. Remember that both are there for a reason. EMS is on scene to treat patients and the police are on scene to protect the public and solve a crime. Sometimes tension will result between EMS and law enforcement. You must be aware of the nature and significance of evidence at the scene and, if possible, keep it intact. Police should be aware that the first priority of EMS is to save the life of the victim. EMS and law enforcement must communicate to find common ground. Developing a good rapport on every call is important in situations such as this. If police understand when you say the situation is life threatening, they will work with you if they know you will work with them when the situation is not.

Preserving Evidence

When on the scene of a crime, be aware that anything you touch, walk on, pick up, cut, wipe off, or move could be evidence. If you must touch something, remember it and tell law enforcement. An awareness of evidence affects the way you treat patients. Carefully observe the patient and disturb as little evidence as possible. If you must remove clothing, do not cut through gunshot or knife wounds. Cut along seams if possible. Place any cut garments in a brown paper bag, not a plastic bag. A plastic bag may destroy evidence.

Types of Evidence

The main categories of evidence include the following: prints, blood and body fluids, particulate evidence, and on-scene observations.

Prints. Prints include fingerprints and footprints. No two people have identical fingerprints, which are composed of the distinctive ridge characteristics left behind on a surface with oils and moisture from the skin. Try not to disturb any fingerprint evidence and do not leave behind your own fingerprints. You can preserve fingerprints by minimizing what you touch at the crime scene. Wearing disposable gloves as a part of standard precautions prevents you from leaving any fingerprints. Footprints have value for law enforcement because patterns may be matched to the footwear used by an alleged perpetrator.

Blood and Body Fluids. Much information about a crime can be gleaned from blood and body fluids. DNA is routinely used to match blood samples or other body fluids to the DNA of a suspect. Matching is highly accurate; only a one in several-million chance exists that the DNA could be from someone else. ABO blood typing of samples found at the scene, on the victim, or on the perpetrator also can narrow the field of suspects. Blood splattered at the scene provides additional clues for law enforcement. It can indicate the type of weapon used, the position of the attacker in relation to the victim, and the direction or force used in the attack. Blood evidence can be preserved in the following ways:

- Avoid mixing samples of blood.
- Avoid tracking blood on your shoes.
- Place bloody clothing in a brown paper bag.
- Do not throw clothes stained with blood or other body fluids in a single pile or in a puddle of blood.
- Do not clean up or smudge blood splatters left at a scene. Do remove your trash (e.g., IV supplies, bandage and dressing wrappers, gloves) if approved by police.

- If you leave behind blood from a venipuncture or accidental needle stick, notify police.

Particulate Evidence. *Particulate evidence* is defined as microscopic or trace evidence that cannot readily be seen by the human eye. Examples of particulate evidence are hairs and fibers from carpets and clothing. Minimal handling of a victim's clothes by EMS personnel may help preserve this type of evidence.

On-Scene Observations. Your observations can serve as evidence and become part of the law enforcement record. Be sure to record the following information:

- Patient (victim) position and injuries
- Conditions at the scene, including the absence or presence of lights, open or closed curtains, or signs of forced entry
- Statements of persons at the scene
- Statements by the patient or victim
- Dying declarations
- Suspicious persons at, or fleeing from, the scene
- Presence and/or location of weapons

Documentation

Only record the facts about the scene of a crime. You must record them accurately because they will be used in court. Record any remarks made by the patient or bystanders in quotation marks. Avoid opinions and keep the documentation objective. Be aware of protocols, local laws, and ethical considerations in reporting crimes such as child abuse, elder abuse, rape, interpersonal violence, and other violent crimes. In many cases threats of violence are crimes. They must be taken seriously and followed up. Follow local policies and regulations regarding the issue of confidentiality.

Case Scenario SUMMARY

1. *Is the scene safe?* Yes, the scene is safe even though the perpetrator has not been caught. The police have secured the area. Always maintain a level of awareness that the scene may become dangerous or pose a threat to you.
2. *What equipment would you bring?* At a minimum you should bring airway equipment, a defibrillator/cardiac monitor, medications, and a backboard.
3. *How could you minimize disrupting the crime scene?* You can minimize disrupting the crime scene by working with police and only allowing the minimal number of personnel needed to enter the scene. Walk single file, use one path in and out of the residence, and touch as little as possible.
4. *Should crime scene preservation or patient care take priority?* Patient care is the priority, but always attempt to minimize the amount of disruption to a crime scene.
5. *What is your general impression of this patient?* The patient is clinically dead.
6. *What examples of evidence can be found at this crime scene?* The appearance of the room with chairs knocked over, dented paint cans in the kitchen, and splattered blood can be considered possible evidence at this crime scene. In addition, fingerprints, footprints, or other body fluids may be present.
7. *Should you move the victim? Why or why not?* Movement of the victim depends on whether you will attempt resuscitation. If you attempt resuscitation, you must move the victim to allow full resuscitation efforts. You should work with police to remove the victim carefully from the crime scene, disrupting as little as possible. If you do not attempt resuscitation, do not move the victim to help preserve the crime scene.
8. *Should the victim have been resuscitated? Why or why not?* The decision on whether to resuscitate is a decision based on local protocols and medical direction. Based on the information given, successful resuscitation is highly unlikely.
9. *Are your observations and documentation important?* Yes, your observations and documentation are very important. Your observations can help keep you from getting hurt if any danger is still at the scene. Documentation is extremely important because the prehospital care report can be used as evidence. Note observations objectively; avoid opinions not relevant to medical care.

Chapter Summary

- Your first priority at any crime scene is your own safety.
- Scene safety starts by identifying and responding to dangers before they threaten (***p***eople, ***p***laces, ***t***imes, ***t***hings). If the scene is known for violence, stage the ambulance at a safe distance until it is secured by law enforcement.
- EMS personnel must look for warning signs of violence during a response to a residence and retreat from the scene if danger is evident.
- Responding to highway encounters may present danger from violence as well as traffic and extrication.
- Monitor for warning signs of danger in violent street incidents and retreat as necessary.

Chapter Summary—continued

- EMS personnel often resemble law enforcement officers, so always be extremely cautious about personal safety when working in gang areas.
- Clandestine drug laboratories can produce explosive and toxic gases. Additional risks include booby traps that can maim or kill.
- When responding to scenes of interpersonal violence, be aware that acts of violence may be directed toward you.
- Safety tactics include retreat, cover and concealment, distraction and evasion, contact and cover, and warning signals and communication.
- Patient care in the hot zone requires special training, authorization, body armor, and equipment.
- Your observations at a crime scene are important and should be carefully documented. Evidence protection can be performed while caring for the patient by not unnecessarily disturbing the scene or destroying evidence.

REFERENCES

Jacobsen, B. (1997). Street smarts. *Emergency, 29*(11), 12.

National Highway Traffic Safety Administration. (1998). *EMT-Paramedic national standard curriculum,* Washington, DC: U.S. Department of Transportation.

SUGGESTED RESOURCES

EMSNetwork: http://www.emsnetwork.org
EMSResponder: http://www.emsresponder.com
EMSvillage.com: http://www.emsvillage.com
Journal of Emergency Medical Services: http://www.jems.com
Merginet: http://www.merginet.com
U.S. Immigration and Customs Enforcement: http://www.ice.gov

Chapter Quiz

1. The difference between cover and concealment relates to the degree to which you _____.
  a. can rapidly exit if needed
  b. are protected from bullets
  c. can be seen by others
  d. can be identified by law enforcement

2. The best material in which to collect potential evidence is _____.
  a. a plastic bag
  b. a brown paper bag
  c. any airtight container
  d. a glass container

3. When should assessment of the potential for violence at the scene begin?
  a. If the patient threatens the crew
  b. On arrival to the scene
  c. When the patient is encountered
  d. En route to the call

4. Which represents the safest approach to a single vehicle stopped on the highway?
  a. Approach from the passenger side of the vehicle
  b. Simultaneous approach by both crew members
  c. Ambulance lights turned off to eliminate glare
  d. Walking between the ambulance and the other vehicle

5. What types of physical evidence may be found on scene?

____

____

6. You are providing care to an injured fan at a large soccer match when irate fans begin to hurl bottles at you and your partner. Which tactic is indicated to increase your safety?

____

7. What strategies can you use to increase safety as you approach a darkened residence?

____

8. True or False: Body armor does not protect against high-velocity bullets.

9. Record only the ______ at the scene of a crime, and record them accurately.

10. What are the signs of impending danger in the setting of a crowd?

____

Terminology

Concealment To hide or put out of site; provides no ballistic protection.

Cover A type of concealment that hides the body and offers ballistic protection.

Crime scene A location where any part of a criminal act has occurred or where evidence relating to a crime may be found.

Distraction A self-defense measure that creates diversion in a person's attention.

Evasive tactic A self-defense measure in which the moves and actions of an aggressor are anticipated and unconventional pathways are used during retreat for personal safety.

Retreat Leaving the scene when danger is observed or when violence or indicators of violence are displayed; requires immediate and decisive action.

Tactical EMS EMS personnel specially trained and equipped to provide prehospital emergency care in tactical environments.

Tactical patient care Patient care activities that occur inside the scene perimeter or hot zone.

CHAPTER 60

Dispatch Activities

Objectives

After completing this chapter, you will be able to:

1. Explain how the communications center fits into the overall EMS system.
2. List the standard functions of the emergency medical dispatch center.
3. Explain the difference between a primary 9-1-1 center and a secondary 9-1-1 center.
4. Describe the common challenges of address verification.
5. List the five elements of an effective emergency medical dispatch program.
6. Explain the role of states in an emergency medical dispatch program.
7. Explain the basics of a continuing education program.
8. Describe the differences among protocols, guidelines, and telephone aid.
9. Describe the conditions, benefits, public expectations, and legal implications of prearrival instructions.
10. Describe how best practices are achieved in an emergency medical dispatch center.
11. Explain the basics of call triage and prioritization.
12. Identify patient conditions that would trigger a high-priority, intermediate-priority, and low-priority response.
13. Identify the primary objectives of a response assignment plan.
14. Identify the common response types in a response assignment plan.
15. Explain how a response assignment plan is consistently applied.
16. Identify the four goals of a quality improvement program.
17. Identify the importance of a physician medical director.
18. Explain the need for case evaluation and feedback.
19. Explain the role of the quality improvement unit.
20. Describe the factors in choosing a random sample for case audits.
21. Identify the key clinical performance indicators and the significance of each.
22. Define the call processing time.
23. Identify some common controllable and uncontrollable factors that determine call processing time.
24. Identify the need for differentiated call processing times.
25. Identify the different components of call processing.
26. Describe the process of unit selection and incident tracking.
27. Identify the process of nonemergency call taking.
28. Describe a performance-based EMS response system.
29. Explain a demand-based unit deployment process.
30. Describe the primary technology components of a state-of-the-art communications center.
31. Explain how dispatch agencies can get useful information for public health authorities on a contagious disease outbreak.

Chapter Outline

Case Scenario

You and your partner are assigned a special detail to visit a local school for its career day. You are to display the ambulance and answer questions the students may have as well as stimulate interest in a career in emergency medical services. The grade levels range from fifth grade to eighth grade.

You park the ambulance in the designated area and proceed to the auditorium to set up a special booth where students will meet you and your partner. As the career day event begins, you are approached by several students asking what being a paramedic is like. Occasionally you take interested students to the ambulance for a quick tour. The day has gone well, but after lunch you are approached by an eighth-grade girl who asks you about what happens when you call 9-1-1. She has several questions that seem to be based on something that recently happened. She asks, "Who answers the 9-1-1 call? Where is the call answered?"

Questions

1. *How do you respond to the girl's initial questions about calling 9-1-1?*
2. *If the girl hints about a recent event, what information would you need to be able to answer her questions?*

[OBJECTIVE 1]

The communications center is the central nervous system of EMS (Figure 60-1). It serves as the first point of contact for callers and patients in the continuum of patient care and controls the call triage, response, and even the initial treatment for most cases the system handles. The EMS dispatcher is a highly trained professional. He or she must determine the correct response location, complete the prearrival patient assessment, and provide prearrival instructions and treatment—often for many minutes before the arrival of EMS crews at the scene. He or she must assign and alert responding crews, track the progress of every case, and manage the system's mobile resources. EMS dispatchers are experts in remote patient care and provide cardiopulmonary resuscitation (CPR), choking, emergency childbirth, and bleeding control instructions over the phone as well as routine safety and patient care activities.

To accomplish this multitude of tasks, the emergency medical dispatcher relies on specialized training and skills as well as state-of-the-art technology that provides "virtually there" functionality and control. Enhanced 9-1-1, computer-aided dispatch (CAD) with links to mobile data devices, electronic geographic information systems and street indexes, digital paging systems, computerized patient triage and prearrival instruction protocols, **global positioning systems (GPS),** and automated system status management with system demand and response-time modeling are only a few of the high-tech tools commonly used in the modern EMS communications center.

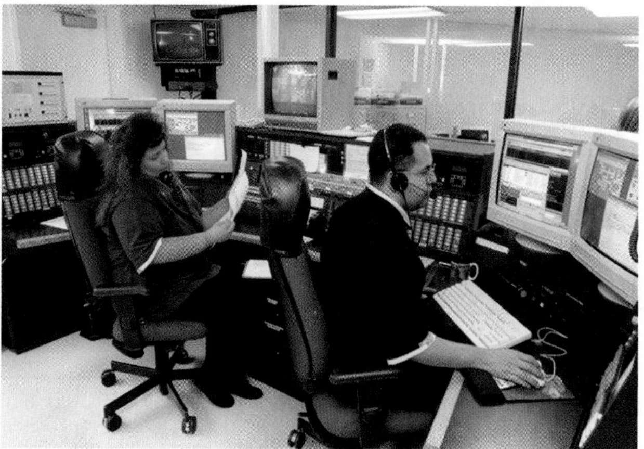

Figure 60-1 9-1-1 Emergency medical dispatch center.

ROLES AND RESPONSIBILITIES OF AN EMERGENCY MEDICAL DISPATCH CENTER

[OBJECTIVES 2, 3]

The standard functions of the **emergency medical dispatch (EMD)** center include the following:

- 9-1-1 and emergency call receiving
- Incident address verification
- Patient assessment and call triage
- Identification of scene hazards
- Responder case assignment and unit alerting
- Prearrival instructions
- Incident communication and coordination
- Response time measurement
- Unit status tracking
- Critical staff notifications
- Posting and deploying available units
- Scheduling interfacility and nonemergency transports

The dispatch model used is often dependent upon the EMS system model used. For example, in EMS systems that are part of a city or county government, generally a single 9-1-1 center performs the above functions for all emergency response agencies (e.g., EMS, police, fire) within that governmental structure. In other cases, such as when a governmental body contracts EMS to a private agency, these roles may be handled by more than one emergency communications center. For example, a citywide or countywide 9-1-1 center may receive all public safety calls—police and fire emergencies as well as EMS calls—and transfer its EMS callers to a secondary center that processes and manages only EMS-related incidents.

Once the EMS center receives the transferred caller from the primary 9-1-1 center, it is responsible for completing the above functions. State and local laws and regulations often dictate specific terms of the 9-1-1 transfer process (e.g., in the state of California, a 9-1-1 call cannot be transferred more than once). Any communications center that receives 9-1-1 calls is known as a *public safety answering point (PSAP)*. Not all EMS communications centers are PSAPs. Some centers receive calls from 10-digit phone numbers only. In those cases, the 9-1-1 center may notify the EMS communications center when an EMS response is needed, and the EMS center handles the unit selection and alerting as well as all incident tracking and status changes for the ambulance assigned to the case.

Address Verification in the EMD Center

[OBJECTIVE 4]

Because there can be no response to an EMS incident without an accurate address or location, correctly determining this information is a critical first step that can make the difference between patients and victims getting care at the right time or being subjected to unnecessary response delays that may prove disastrous. Because victims and patients can be found virtually anywhere within a given geographic region—inside a six-story apartment complex, trapped in a vehicle on a lonely stretch of highway, or stuck on the side of a cliff—the dispatcher must rely on several technical tools as well as knowledge and skill to identify the incident address or location correctly. For many calls, 9-1-1 systems provide the emergency call taker with **automated number identification (ANI)** and **automated location identification (ALI).** A type of detailed caller ID system, the ANI/ALI information, when available, is generally the most reliable tool for verifying the incident location. Extending ANI/ALI service to mobile telephones has created a unique challenge for 9-1-1 centers around the globe. Phase II of this technology uses the cell phone's GPS to send a signal to the dispatch center with latitude and longitude coordinates. Location resolutions can vary from 30 to 3000 meters. Mobile location technology (sometimes known as *phase II 9-1-1 service*) is still being installed in many 9-1-1 centers. Internet phone service (or **voice over Internet protocol**)—expected to be widespread in coming years—will be the next technologic challenge for ANI/ALI systems. Discussions are currently underway between 9-1-1 officials and Internet phone service providers to facilitate building ANI/ALI-compatible programs for this emerging technology.

Case Scenario—continued

The girl tells you about an instance in which her father had chest pain and she had to call 9-1-1. She asks, "How come they ask so many questions? Why can't they just get the address and send you?"

Questions

3. *What are the initial steps in answering a call to 9-1-1?*
4. *Why does the dispatcher need to verify the address?*
5. *How would you answer the girl's question about the number of questions asked by the emergency medical dispatcher?*

EMD STANDARDS AND TRAINING

[OBJECTIVE 5]

The National Institutes of Health (NIH) has published a detailed document that covers the practice of EMD. This document, *Emergency Medical Dispatching: Rapid Identification and Treatment of Acute Myocardial Infarction,* describes the practice this way: "Effective emergency medical dispatching has the goal of sending the right EMS resources to the right person, at the right time, in the right way, and providing the right instructions for the care of the patient until help arrives" (NIH, 1994).

This goal ideally can be accomplished through the trained dispatcher's careful use of a protocol that contains the following elements:

- Systematized caller interrogation questions that are chief complaint specific
- Systematized prearrival instructions
- Protocols that determine vehicle response mode and configuration based on the dispatcher's evaluation of the injury or illness severity
- Referenced information for dispatcher use

The NIH recommends the following five elements as key to an effective EMD program (NIH, 1994):

1. Use of medical dispatch protocols
2. Provision of **dispatch life support** (prearrival instructions)
3. Dispatcher training
4. Dispatcher certification
5. Quality control and improvement processes

State Regulations

[OBJECTIVE 6]

To date, 20 states have passed legislation regulating EMD training, certification, oversight, and practice standards, and numerous other states are planning similar laws. States normally require dispatchers to complete an approved certification course for those persons operating in an EMD center. For example, the legal code in Indiana that regulates EMD centers says, in part, "An individual may not furnish, operate, conduct, maintain, or advertise services as an emergency medical dispatcher unless the individual is certified by the [Indiana] commission as an emergency medical dispatcher" (State of Indiana, 2005). States also may require oversight by a physician medical director, case evaluation for quality assurance, and approved continuing education programs.

Continuing Education

[OBJECTIVE 7]

Trained and certified dispatchers, like their paramedic and EMT counterparts, must receive regular continuing education to maintain and enhance their skills. Most standard-setting bodies require a minimum of 12 hours per year of approved continuing education. A state or local EMS authority should approve continuing EMD education. Topics covered may include protocol review of specific elements, such as chief complaint selection, prearrival instruction delivery, compliance issues and concerns, and audio case review. Continuing education hours also can be approved for ambulance ridealongs, observation time spent in a hospital emergency department, disaster preparedness training, and similar courses.

PROTOCOLS AS A STANDARD OF CARE

[OBJECTIVE 8]

A **protocol** is a predictable, reproducible process for addressing a medical problem with specific, sequenced actions and a definable, measurable result. A significant difference exists between EMD call-taking protocols and less-structured, more subjective processes, often referred to as **guidelines.** Call-taking protocols, properly applied and followed, accomplish several important objectives, including accurate and orderly information gathering, proper call **triage** and prioritization, and delivery of scripted, carefully designed prearrival instruction sequences.

Protocols also differ substantially from ad-libbed instructions, sometimes referred to as **telephone aid.** Telephone aid has been most often used in centers where dispatchers have had previous training as paramedics, EMTs, or CPR providers. It strictly relies on the dispatcher's experience and prior knowledge of a particular situation or medical condition. According to the NIH, telephone aid "often provides only the illusion of correct help by telephone without predictably ensuring consistent and accurate instructions to all callers. Telephone aid, therefore, is usually considered an inappropriate and unreliable form of dispatcher-provided medical care" (NIH, 1994).

PROVISION OF PREARRIVAL INSTRUCTIONS AS A STANDARD OF CARE

[OBJECTIVE 9]

Prearrival instructions have become a public expectation for situations of sudden cardiac arrest and choking and even certain cases of emergency childbirth. Tens of thousands of dispatchers in North America have received training and protocols on instructing untrained layperson callers in delivering such care. And in many cases in which victims are without oxygen, effective prearrival instructions are perhaps the best hope for patient survival. In their book *Principles of Emergency Medical Dispatch,* Clawson and Dernocouer discuss the impact of early intervention through prearrival instructions:

> The [dispatcher] is the sole authority over an emergency scene until the first responding crew can make initial assessments and establish scene control. An excellent average response time once wheels are rolling to the address would range from five to ten minutes. Then, additional time (average one and a half minutes) ticks by while crews leave the emergency vehicle and make actual patient contact. Thus the best to-the-patient time often exceeds eight minutes during which the patient may not be receiving any care.
>
> A properly trained EMD can effectively eliminate this time gap for many situations. Willing bystanders can provide first aid via telephone instruction. In fact, callers increasingly expect to be coached this way. If oxygenated blood can be pumped to a clinically dead brain within one minute because of the combined efforts of [a dispatcher] and the people at the scene, that is obviously better than waiting seven—and sometimes 10 or more—minutes for trained people to arrive at the patients side. This concept, trademarked as the Zero-Minute Response, is changing the complexion of emergency care (Clawson & Dernocouer, 2004).

One concern that has surfaced regarding the provision of prearrival instructions is that this practice may increase legal risk or liability for the 9-1-1 center and its managing body, whether a private entity or a local, state, or national government organization. This concern is a fear that has largely been dispelled by the body of legal evidence and opinion. In fact, many state laws and statutes now require the provision of prearrival instructions by trained and certified dispatchers for situations in which

BOX 60-1 EMD Medicolegal Danger Zones

- Failure to verify address and callback number
- "No sending" (no response or appropriate follow-up referral)
- Dispatch "diagnosis"
- Significantly delayed responses
- More than one call for help
- No protocols to follow
- Failure to follow protocol exactly
- Requesting permission to give prearrival instructions
- Asking to talk with the patient (distrusting the caller)
- Attitude problems or argumentative interrogation
- Preconceived notions of caller's motives and situation
- Problems at shift changes
- First party "gone on arrival" situations

those instructions are warranted and the EMD protocol directs their use. Therefore the legal liability is greater when necessary prearrival instructions are not given. Potential EMD medicolegal risks have been called *dispatch danger zones* (Box 60-1). Dispatch danger zones are discussed in detail during EMD training programs.

BEST PRACTICES AND BENCHMARKING

[OBJECTIVE 10]

Accreditation through an established, widely accepted, formal program is a proven method for attaining significantly improved service quality in an EMD communications center. For example, the National Academies of Emergency Dispatch (NAED) has created an internationally recognized, performance-based accreditation process that has given agencies the standards and incentives to implement protocols, policies, and procedures consistent with industry best practices. Accredited sites are required to achieve and maintain protocol compliance percentages at or above 90% to 95% in six key performance areas (NAED, 2004). Oversight processes include a steering and dispatch review committee and implementation of dispatch prioritization procedures and response assignment plans that provide for differentiation of responses based on specific incident types. Another advantage to accreditation is that it provides **benchmarking** opportunities for centers involved in such a process. They can compare their operating policies, procedures, protocols, and performance to one another and, in so doing, improve their own results.

CALL TRIAGE PROCESSES: PATIENT ASSESSMENT AND CASE PRIORITIZATION

[OBJECTIVE 11]

Triage, or classifying patients on the basis of severity of illness or injury, is a familiar practice in emergency medicine. Because the dispatch patient assessment is done remotely—often with a caller who is not the patient and generally not medically trained—the dispatcher must rely on a specific set of skills, procedures, and protocols to obtain correct information and make accurate dispatch decisions.

Once the correct location is determined, the dispatcher's patient assessment begins by getting basic case information, starting with a description of the problem. For cases in which a single patient is involved, the dispatcher must determine the age, level of consciousness, and breathing status of the patient.

After this initial assessment, the dispatcher asks a series of complaint-specific questions that lead to an assigned prioritization level and specific call typing. A thorough caller interrogation process requires completing a protocol that determines the presence of high-priority conditions: those that require a maximum response from the EMS system. For example, any patient who is not breathing or who is unconscious with signs of severe circulation or oxygenation problems is assigned the highest priority level. Lower-priority signs and symptoms are assigned a corresponding prioritization level that fits the urgency of the case and need for specific EMS resources. The EMD assessment process ends when all high-priority conditions have been either identified or excluded and other relevant conditions have been recorded.

RESPONSE PRIORITIZATION AND RESOURCE ASSIGNMENT PLANS

[OBJECTIVES 12, 13, 14, 15]

Below are several common examples of specific dispatch call types with a corresponding dispatch priority:

- Sudden cardiac arrest: Priority 1
- Chest pain with cardiac history: Priority 2
- Traffic accident with injury: Priority 3
- Unknown problem: Priority 4
- Diabetic patient with high blood sugar: Priority 5
- Minor trauma with injured ankle: Priority 6

Assigning the correct responders to an EMS case, in the correct **response mode,** is a critical function of the dispatch center. A properly triaged case is followed by an equally appropriate resource assignment using a predefined response scheme. Local EMS authorities, including a physician medical director, should develop this comprehensive resource assignment plan.

Any such plan should be constructed with two primary objectives: first, it must match the EMS resource used to the patient's clinical need; second, it must adequately limit the use of lights and siren responses to only the most critical cases. Excessive use of lights and sirens carries special risks that can put the driving public and responders in harm's way. Hence a well-constructed resources assignment plan is an effective risk management tool for the EMS agency.

Table 60-1 gives an example of a typical **response assignment plan.**

TABLE 60-1 Typical Response Assignment Plan		
Priority	Personnel and Equipment	Mode
1	Engine/ALS ambulance/ QRU/PD	Red
2	Engine/ALS ambulance	Red
3	Engine/ALS ambulance	Closest unit red/second unit yellow
4	ALS ambulance	Red
5	ALS ambulance	Yellow
6	BLS ambulance	Yellow

Engine, Closest fire engine first responder (usually basic life support–trained personnel); *ALS,* advanced life support; *QRU,* ALS quick response unit (single paramedic, no transport capability); *PD,* defibrillator-equipped police unit; *red,* lights and siren response; *yellow,* no lights and siren response; *BLS,* basic life support.

Modern-day CAD systems are capable of storing response tables that contain the response priority and predetermined response assignment for each individual call type. This information can be automatically displayed to the dispatcher at a workstation monitor for every incident dispatched. In this way, consistency of response is ensured for each case and each incident of a specific type. An EMD oversight committee that includes the physician system medical director should review response assignment plans annually, at a minimum (NAED, 2004).

QUALITY IMPROVEMENT

[OBJECTIVE 16]

The NIH lists the following four goals for EMD quality control and improvement programs:

1. Dispatchers understand policy, protocol, and practice.
2. Dispatchers comply with policy, protocol, and practice.
3. Compliance deficiencies are corrected.
4. Policies, protocol, and practices are updated regularly (NIH, 1994).

Physician Oversight

[OBJECTIVE 17]

An EMD quality improvement program should be directed by a qualified physician medical director responsible for monitoring EMD performance, ensuring compliance to protocols, and providing direction in the medical supervision and ongoing education of dispatchers (Figure 60-2). The physician medical director is generally

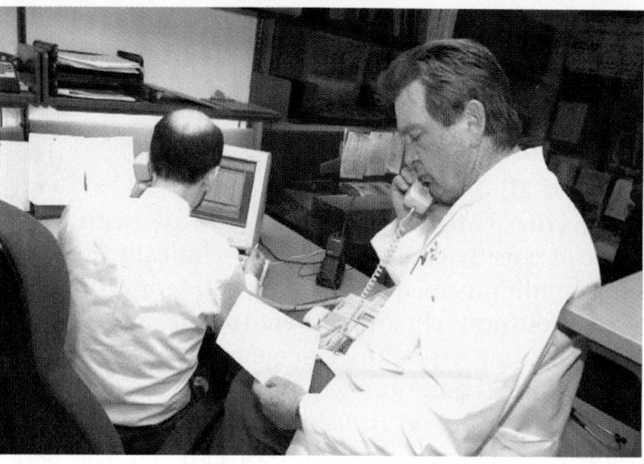

Figure 60-2 Medical director.

employed by the local EMS provider agency and also may have government-mandated authority to adopt EMD protocols and approve and update EMS responses to specific incident types.

Performance Monitoring and Feedback

[OBJECTIVES 18, 19]

Consistent case evaluation coupled with timely, objective feedback is the most effective way to improve dispatcher performance.

A number of professional standard setting organizations, including the NAED, the National Association of Emergency Medical Physicians, the NIH, and the American Society for Testing and Materials have requirements or position statements covering this practice.

For a case evaluation process to succeed, there must be an official **quality improvement unit (QIU)** formally tasked with the case evaluation function. The individuals who comprise this group should be trained and certified quality specialists who have the knowledge and skills to measure dispatcher performance against established standards accurately and consistently. This group selects audio records and evaluates cases for EMD compliance to protocol. The evaluator also provides case narrative to assist the individual dispatcher in performance improvement. Individual dispatchers receive the case evaluations as official performance feedback.

The information provided by the QIU also is entered into a master database and used to manage and improve overall system performance. Hence the information produced by the QIU must be consistent and unquestionably accurate.

Random Case Selection

[OBJECTIVE 20]

Effective case evaluation begins by choosing a random sample of cases for a comprehensive audit by QIU personnel. Typically this means capturing the audio record of incoming 9-1-1 calls. The NIH recommends auditing 7%

to 10% of each dispatcher's cases. The NAED has a sliding scale that uses total EMS call volume to determine the number of monthly audits required (NAED, 2005).

Key Clinical Performance Indicators

[OBJECTIVE 21]

An effective EMD protocol will identify—with a high degree of sensitivity and specificity—clinically life-threatening conditions such as cardiac arrest, agonal breathing, unconsciousness, choking, severe trauma, acute myocardial infarction, respiratory emergencies, and severe hemorrhage. These conditions require immediate intervention by the EMD using prearrival instruction protocols.

One straightforward measure of EMD clinical performance is how often dispatchers correctly identify these life-threatening conditions. This is determined by case evaluation audits and comparison of EMD coding to ambulance crew findings on arrival at the scene.

A related but more specific key indicator of EMD system clinical effectiveness is correct identification of cardiac arrest patients. A published study evaluated the ability of one EMD system, the Medical Priority Dispatch System (MPDS), to identify cardiac arrest victims (Heward et al., 2004). The study demonstrated that use of the MPDS resulted in a 200% rise in the number of patients accurately identified as having a cardiac arrest. The relation between factors identified suggests that complying with protocol is an important factor in the accurate recognition of patient conditions (Heward et al., 2004).

EMD **clinical performance indicators** should include the following:

- Correct chief complaint identification
- Compliance to basic case information protocols
- Correct final call typing
- Compliance to interrogation protocol for all cardiac arrest cases
- Compliance with prearrival instruction protocol for all cardiac arrest cases
- Compliance with prearrival instruction protocol for all near arrests and cases of respiratory failure

Case Scenario CONCLUSION

The girl tells you about a time she and her friends called 9-1-1 to see what would happen. 9-1-1 answered the call and the girl hung up. She was surprised and a little scared when the 9-1-1 dispatcher called her back.

You and your partner answer the girl's questions and continue with your career day assignment. You have sparked the student's interest in EMS as well as 9-1-1 dispatching.

Questions

6. *Why would the 9-1-1 dispatcher call back?*
7. *How would the 9-1-1 dispatcher know where to call?*
8. *What happens if the dispatcher called back and no one answered the phone?*
9. *Does this happen when using a cell phone?*

CALL PROCESSING TIME

[OBJECTIVES 22, 23, 24, 25]

The **call processing time** is the elapsed time from the moment an emergency call is received at the 9-1-1 center until the closest available responder crew(s) has been notified with all incident information necessary to respond.

The latest state-of-the-art interfaces between phone equipment and computerized dispatch systems are capable of capturing the exact time the phone is answered and how much time elapses to answer the call. They also can record elapsed time from call pickup to address verification in the CAD system and time to first unit alerted.

Not all EMS cases can be processed in seconds. It often takes well over 1 minute to obtain accurate location information from the caller, particularly when callers are not at a fixed location (where no numeric address exists), such as a hiker in a park, a boater on a lake, or a driver on a highway.

The widespread use of wireless phones has lengthened the time required for a call taker to obtain and record a correct address or location. Mobile phone callers are not always stationary, and ANI technology is much less reliable for wireless phones. Factors that affect call processing time that are difficult to control include the following:

- Language barriers
- Level of activity in the system
- Nature of the call
- Caller's state of mind and knowledge of the incident type and location

Factors that affect call processing time that EMS communications centers can control include the following:

- Emergency call center staffing
- Type of telephone and call-processing technology used in the communications center
- Availability and reliability of a geographic information database
- Proper use of dispatch protocols

Just as response time expectations for public safety responders vary on the basis of the priority assigned to a particular incident type, so should expectations for 9-1-1 staff consistent with case urgency. A sound EMD protocol identifies the most time-critical cases early in the call-taking process and prompts the call taker to initiate immediate notification of the closest available responders. For example, all other factors being equal, a confirmed case of sudden cardiac arrest should have a faster call processing time than an injured ankle case.

Finally, call processing time in an emergency communications center is only a fraction of the total response time to the victim, patient, or caller. Driving time to the incident location, average turnout time (sometimes referred to as *chute time*) for responding crews, and even the time necessary for responders to get from the curbside to the victim's side exceed the total call processing time in many emergency responses. Call processing times therefore must be evaluated in their proper context—as a percentage of total response time.

In general, EMS communications centers can ensure reasonable and efficient call processing times by implementing state-of-the-art technology, providing adequate training, and enforcing compliance to specific established policies, protocols, and procedures.

Components of EMD call processing are shown in Table 60-2.

TABLE 60-2 Components of EMD Call Processing

Task or Event	Time in Task (Seconds)	Typical Elapsed Time (Seconds)
Call received at EMD center	0	0
Call answered by dispatcher	5-10	7
Address (and phone number) verification	15-75	37
Dispatcher evaluation of patient(s) and scene conditions	45-60	90
Case queued for dispatch	10-30	110
Unit selected and EMS crew notified	5-20	120

Times in table are only estimates of average times. Actual processing times vary from center to center and on a case-by-case basis.

UNIT SELECTION AND INCIDENT TRACKING

[OBJECTIVE 26]

In addition to call-taking responsibilities, most EMS communications centers also handle unit alerting, incident tracking, and electronic communication with responding and transporting paramedic crews. Unit selection is done when an incident address has been verified and the call taker has recorded either a preliminary or final incident type code. The EMS dispatcher selects and alerts the closest available ambulance (and sometimes the **first responder unit**) to the call. Initial information given at dispatch includes an address—with specific information on apartment or building number when necessary and any special access instructions—the call type, and any information about safety hazards given to the EMD call taker. A dispatcher tracks the times units are responding, arriving on scene, transporting to the hospital, arriving at the hospital, available at the hospital, returning to post, and at post. Because the dispatcher's unit selection for each incoming case is based on the posted location of all the available units, the dispatcher must maintain current status and location of all units in the system.

Nonemergency Care in the Communications Center

[OBJECTIVE 27]

For many centers a large portion of the workload is managing nonemergency ambulance transportation between medical facilities. This function requires several specialized dispatcher skills and tasks. Although nonemergency transportation does not require a detailed patient assessment or emergency prearrival instructions, it does necessitate careful documentation and knowledge of medical facilities and their particular needs. Call center software specifically designed for nonemergency transports is typically used to record patient pickup information, relevant medical histories, and any special equipment needs.

UNIT DEPLOYMENT PRACTICES

[OBJECTIVES 28, 29]

A number of private EMS services operate as **performance-based response systems.** In such a system the municipality or local government sets specific response time requirements for emergency and nonemergency calls. For example, an EMS provider agency may be required to respond to emergency calls in less than 9 minutes 90% of the time and nonemergency calls in less than 15 minutes 90% of the time on a monthly basis. Under such a contract, the EMS provider agency provides monthly response time reports subject to audit by the local governmental authority. To maintain a performance-based contract in an efficient manner, EMS managers must develop unit deployment plans that match EMS responder resources to call demand. Typically historic data are used to look at patterns of demand by geographic area, time of day, and day of week. The unit deployment plan dictates the number of units staffed at any given time and posting locations of those units.

The communications center is responsible for executing the unit deployment plan. In a dynamic deployment model (known as *system status management*) ambulances are moved, or posted, to positions in areas with a high probability of calls occurring (see Chapter 58). Once an ambulance is assigned to a call in a high call load area, another available ambulance may be moved into the area to backfill. In this way the fastest response can be provided to the greatest number of patients. Some deployment plans may balance their coverage between high-demand areas and geographically isolated areas. For example, a large urban area may have a bedroom community (one isolated from the rest of the city) that generates relatively few ambulance runs; but because the ambulance response time from other, busier areas of the area is great, an ambulance may be posted in the center of that community on a regular basis to reduce response times for the occasional calls that occur there.

TECHNOLOGY

[OBJECTIVE 30]

New technology has brought about sweeping change to EMS communications centers. Only a few decades ago dispatching was a difficult and inexact science. Today, by contrast, sophisticated computer technology, satellite systems, ultra-high radio frequencies, and speedy digital devices all play a major role in the operation of the modern communications center. In addition to ANI/ALI telephone technology, some common state-of-the-art technologic components of a communications center include the following:

- CAD systems
- **800-MHz,** two-way radio systems
- DVD audio recording systems
- Mobile data devices (mobile data terminals and mobile data computers)
- Digital paging
- GPS vehicle tracking
- Real-time unit deployment and demand displays

The CAD system is the main dispatch computer in an up-to-date, automated communications center. It contains the primary hardware and software to enter cases; store incident records; master streets files, unit deployment plans, and response grids; as well as control many interface devices that communicate with other connected hardware, software programs, telephone equipment, and remote terminals. All cases are processed and tracked in the CAD system. CAD screens display active calls, unit status and locations, staffing information, and other real-time information used by the dispatcher. CAD systems process so much information they often are referred to as "the dispatcher's second brain."

Radio systems of 800 MHz operate on ultra-high-frequency radio signals that allow for multiple talk groups. Each talk group is a separate voice communication link that gives dispatchers and EMS responders more flexibility than standard very-high-frequency radio systems. When properly controlled, 800-MHz technology simplifies two-way voice communications among dispatchers, responders, hospitals, and other personnel in the network.

Virtually every telephone conversation and radio transmission in a dispatch center is recorded. The clunky reel-to-reel magnetic tape machines of early dispatch centers have been replaced, mostly with DVD recording devices that can store hundreds, sometimes thousands, of hours of audio records on a single disk. These records are often retrieved and reviewed to check the accuracy of CAD incident entries and for legal evidence in criminal cases involving 9-1-1 calls. The dispatcher often is the first to gather evidence of a crime scene based on information obtained from the caller, sounds in the background, and the time of various calls.

Mobile data devices are stand-alone computers or semismart terminals connected to the main CAD system and placed in remote locations, such as ambulances, fire and police vehicles, and crew stations (Figure 60-3). Mobile data devices, also known as **mobile data terminals** or **mobile data computers,** typically provide responding crews with updated incident information for active calls as well as past incident information. With a keyboard or mouse, crews also can make status changes for their units, including placing themselves responding to a call, on the scene of a call, transporting to the hospital, or available for another call. Additionally, if the vehicle is equipped with GPS or an automated vehicle locator (AVL) system, the mobile terminal can provide real-time maps and directions to the scene.

Digital paging systems are a fast, reliable method of alerting crews to respond to a call. EMS crews often are

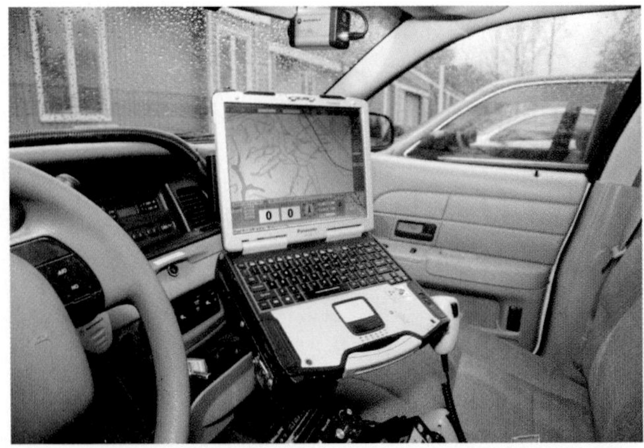

Figure 60-3 Mobile data device and terminal.

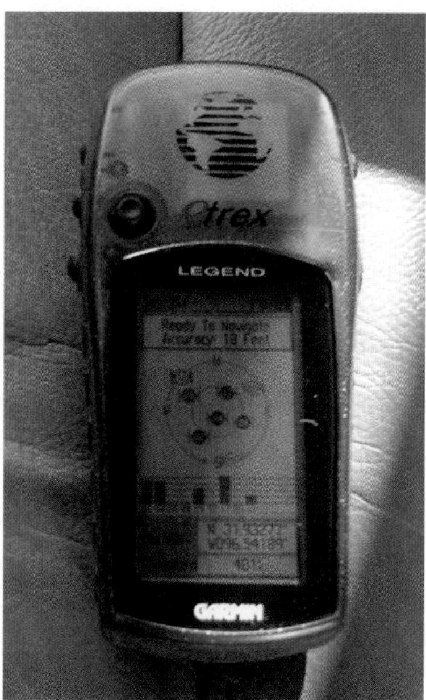

Figure 60-4 Handheld GPS device.

not in their stations or vehicles and therefore cannot always be reached by phone or two-way radio. Compact pagers can be carried by crew members and toned-out with short text messages to provide basic run information. Most digital paging systems are connected to the dispatch CAD and can be activated with a few keystrokes by a dispatcher.

Many modern dispatch centers are equipped with vehicle tracking software that runs by GPS (Figure 60-4). Ambulances and first responder units are frequently polled by the system to measure their location, speed, and proximity to the location of an active or pending call. Some CAD systems have the ability to recommend the closest unit to respond to any given location by using GPS readings and mapping coordinates. In most situations lost or stolen vehicles equipped with GPS devices can be readily located.

Real-time deployment and demand displays are a relatively new technology that allows dispatchers to view a dynamic electronic map of the region, with ambulance locations and estimated response time coverage areas for each available unit. The display also overlays color-coded shading for regions with high call volumes. They allow dispatchers to see immediately the available system coverage and predicted system demand for any given time of day.

NEW HORIZONS IN EMD: BIOSURVEILLANCE, PUBLIC HEALTH, AND EARLY WARNING SYSTEMS

[OBJECTIVE 31]

The millions of callers in North America who annually call EMS communications centers for help sometimes report symptoms consistent with contagious, potentially pandemic diseases such as tuberculosis or sudden acute respiratory syndrome. They represent an important group from which to draw valuable public health information. Research done on biosurveillance concludes that a pressing need exists for better methods and practices of collecting and interpreting disease information among populations. The use of data from 9-1-1 calls is attractive to public health officials because the data come from a centralized, standardized database in near real time (Patterson & Scott, 2003).

Rapidly evolving technology provides new tools to meet the need for a faster, more reliable early warning system. Standardization, speed, sensitivity, specificity, and ethical considerations are all important factors in developing early warning surveillance systems in an emergency communications center. First-generation models of integrated surveillance software systems are already installed in a number of 9-1-1 centers in the United States, covering more than 12 million citizens. Such software is used to poll 9-1-1 data in real time, searching for recorded symptoms that may be associated with a specific contagious disease. These data are then compared with historic records to see if any significant anomalies occur, and the system automatically triggers an alert when they do. These integrated systems are designed so that an agency may turn on the enhanced features on the basis of need, such as an elevated national alert status or a local, regional, or statewide threat. When posted on a secure Web site, these data can be reported to and monitored by public safety agencies in an effort to discover trends that may signify an actual threat.

Case Scenario SUMMARY

1. *How do you respond to the girl's initial questions about calling 9-1-1?* Depending on how the 9-1-1 dispatch system is set up, the initial call can answered by a countywide 9-1-1 dispatching center or a local law enforcement agency or sent to a PSAP. If the call is medical in nature, the caller can be immediately connected to a dispatcher.
2. *If the girl hints about a recent event, what information would you need to be able to answer her questions?* If the girl seems distressed about an event or has some questions about a specific event, encourage her to give more specifics, such as the nature of the call, where the emergency took place, time of day, and any other relevant information. This information will help pinpoint the

Continued

Case Scenario SUMMARY—continued

actual questions that the girl has and enable you to provide the answers she is seeking.

3. *What are the initial steps in answering a call to 9-1-1?* A number of processes are involved when someone places a call to a 9-1-1 center. These processes include answering the call, verifying the address, performing patient assessment and call triage, assigning emergency vehicles to the call, giving prearrival instructions, and monitoring the response from beginning to end.
4. *Why does the dispatcher need to verify the address?* Verifying the address is important because EMS does not want to respond to the wrong place. In an emergency, the caller might be upset and give the wrong street name or number. For example, the caller could confuse northeast with northwest and responding personnel might go to the wrong place. If that happens, the crew may not arrive in time.
5. *How would you answer the girl's question about the number of questions asked by the emergency medical dispatcher?* Additional information needed by the dispatcher can help save a person's life. For example, if someone is having a heart attack, the dispatcher can give the caller information and instructions to care for the patient while waiting for help to arrive.
6. *Why would the 9-1-1 dispatcher call back?* When someone calls 9-1-1, dispatchers assume the caller needs help. Sometimes a caller has to hang up before speaking with the 9-1-1 dispatcher because of a medical emergency or a crime taking place in which the caller is unable to speak. If a person calls 9-1-1 and hangs up, the 9-1-1 dispatcher will call back to make sure help is needed.
7. *How would the 9-1-1 dispatcher know where to call?* 9-1-1 dispatchers know where to call because a computer system provides that information. ANI/ALI information tells the dispatcher the number the caller is calling from and where that number is located.
8. *What happens if the dispatcher called back and no one answered the phone?* If a person calls 9-1-1 and hangs up and the dispatcher calls and gets no answer, a police officer is dispatched to the location of the call. Again, the dispatcher knows where the call came from and therefore knows where to send the police officer.
9. *Does this happen when using a cell phone?* Not all areas have the capability to identify the location of a cell phone when it is used to call 9-1-1. Technology is becoming available to provide the location of a cell phone through a GPS. Remaining on the line is important when using a cell phone to call 9-1-1.

Chapter Summary

- EMD communications centers have rapidly evolved into complex operations with sophisticated technology, requiring staffing by highly skilled emergency medical dispatchers.
- The communications center is the starting point for EMS care in a community, serving as a critical link between patients in need and EMS responders, including paramedic crews.
- Dispatchers are now widely accepted as full EMS professionals with specific training, certification, quality improvement, and continuing education requirements.
- Federal, state, and local governments, as well as numerous professional organizations, have produced both binding and nonbinding standards that define the roles of the dispatcher and the EMS communications center.
- Included in those roles are the use of patient assessment protocols, call typing, response prioritization, and the provision of prearrival instructions.
- New technologies that provide automation of previously manual processes, reliable and rapid geographic information, and better communication links with responders and other public safety agencies have replaced less-efficient systems and made the dispatch center the focal point of all information moving through the EMS system.

REFERENCES

Clawson, J. J., & Dernocouer, K. (2004). *Principles of emergency medical dispatch (3rd ed.).* Salt Lake City: Priority Press.

Heward, A., Damiani, M., & Hartley-Sharpe, C. (2004). Does the use of the advanced medical priority dispatch system affect cardiac arrest detection? *Emergency Medicine Journal, 21,* 115-118.

National Academies of Emergency Dispatch. (2004). *Twenty points of accreditation.* Retrieved March 3, 2008, from http://www.emergencydispatch.org.

National Academies of Emergency Dispatch. (2005). *Random case review calculator.* Retrieved March 3, 2008, from http://www.emergencydispatch.org.

National Institutes of Health. (1994). *Emergency medical dispatching: Rapid identification and treatment of acute myocardial infarction.* Washington, DC: National Institutes of Health.

Patterson, B., & Scott, G. (2003). Using academy dispatch protocols as an early warning system. *The Journal of Emergency Dispatch, 5*(4).

State of Indiana. (2005). *Emergency medical dispatch regulations.* Indiana State Code; IC 16-31-3.5-3.

SUGGESTED RESOURCES

Colwell, C. B., Pons, P., Blanchet, J. H., & Mangino, C. (1999). Claims against a paramedic ambulance service: A ten-year experience. *Journal of Emergency Medicine, 17*(6), 999-1002.

National Academy of Emergency Medical Dispatch. (2001). *Model EMD rules and regulations.* Salt Lake City, UT: National Academy of Emergency Medical Dispatch.

National Highway Traffic Safety Administration. (1996). *Emergency medical dispatch: National standard curriculum.* Washington, DC: U.S. Department of Transportation.

National Association of Emergency Medical Service Physicians. (1989). Emergency medical dispatching [position paper]. *Prehospital and Disaster Medicine, 4*(2), 163-166.

Stratton, S. J. (1992). Triage by emergency medical dispatchers. *Prehospital and Disaster Medicine, 7*(3), 263-269.

Chapter Quiz

1. Name four of the standard functions of an EMD center.

   ____
   ____
   ____
   ____

2. What does the acronym ANI/ALI mean?

   ____

3. True or False: The standard continuing education requirement for a certified emergency medical dispatcher is 6 hours per year.

4. True or False: Delivering prearrival instructions can create a significant legal liability for the EMD center.

5. How does telephone aid differ from a structured set of prearrival instructions?

   ____
   ____

6. What is the critical first step in EMD call taking?

   ____

7. Name two of the five elements of an effective EMD program according to the NIH.

   ____
   ____

8. True or False: A patient with chest pain and cardiac history is given a higher priority response than a diabetic patient with high blood sugar.

9. What is the most effective way to improve dispatcher performance?

   ____

10. What term is given to the main dispatch computer in a state-of-the-art communications center?

    ____

Terminology

800 MHz A type of radio signal in the ultra-high-frequency range that allows splitting a frequency into individual talk groups used as communication links with other system users.

Accreditation Recognition given to an EMD center by an independent auditing agency for achieving a consistently high level of performance based on industry best practice standards.

Automatic location identification (ALI) Telephone technology used to identify the location of a caller immediately.

Automatic number identification (ANI) Telephone technology that provides immediate identification of the caller's 10-digit telephone number.

Benchmarking Comparison of operating policies, procedures, protocols, and performance with those of other agencies in an effort to improve results.

Call processing time The elapsed time from the moment a call is received by the communications center to the time the responding unit is alerted.

Clinical performance indicator A definable, measurable, skilled task completed by the dispatcher

Terminology—continued

that has a significant impact on the delivery of patient care.

Computer-aided dispatch (CAD) The main dispatch computer in an EMD center; used to complete numerous call-taking, dispatching, monitoring, and electronic communication tasks.

Dispatch life support The provision of clinically approved, scripted instructions by telephone by a trained and certified emergency medical dispatcher.

Emergency medical dispatching (EMD) The science and skills associated with the tasks of an emergency medical dispatcher.

First responder unit The closest trained persons and vehicle assigned to respond to a call; often the closest available fire department vehicle.

Global positioning system (GPS) A satellite-based geographic locating system often placed on an ambulance to track its exact location.

Guidelines For emergency medical dispatchers, an unstructured, subjective, unscripted method of telephone assessment and treatment; a less-effective process than protocols.

Mobile data computer A device used in an ambulance or first responder vehicle to retrieve and send call information that has its own memory storage and processing capability.

Mobile data terminal A device used like a mobile data computer but without its own memory storage and processing capability.

Performance-based response system A contractual agreement between the EMS provider and the government authority to provide ambulance response to a particular municipality or region with time requirements for each response and total responses on a monthly basis.

Prearrival instructions Clinically approved instructions provided by telephone by a trained and certified EMD.

Protocol A predictable, reproducible process for addressing a medical problem with specific, sequenced actions and a definable, measurable result.

Quality improvement unit (QIU) Trained and certified quality specialists who have the knowledge and skills to measure dispatcher performance against established standards accurately and consistently.

Quick response unit A type of responder with paramedic-level skills but no transport capability.

Response assignment plan An approved, consistent plan for responding to each call type.

Response mode A type of response, either with or without lights and sirens use.

Telephone aid Ad-libbed instructions most often used in EMD centers by dispatchers who have had previous training as paramedics, EMTs, or cardiopulmonary resuscitation providers; strictly relies on the dispatcher's experience and prior knowledge of a particular situation or medical condition and is considered an ineffective form of telephone treatment.

Triage Classifying patients based on the severity of illness or injury.

Very high frequency A type of radio signal used to make two-way radio contact between the communications center and the responders. Now considered old technology compared with more contemporary 800 MHz radio systems.

Voice over Internet protocol Telephone technology that gives Internet users the ability to make voice telephone calls.

CHAPTER 61

Emergency Vehicle Operations

Objectives

After completing this chapter, you will be able to:

1. Identify current local and state standards that influence ambulance design, equipment requirements, and staffing of ambulances.
2. Identify and discuss the benefits and drawbacks of the three types of ambulances.
3. Identify local and state standards for ambulance marking.
4. Discuss the importance of regular vehicle cleaning and maintenance.
5. Identify the potential liability for the paramedic as it pertains to vehicle maintenance and operation.
6. Discuss the importance of completing a daily emergency vehicle equipment and supply checklist.
7. Discuss the factors to be considered when determining ambulance stationing within a community.
8. Discuss the importance of district familiarization and route planning.
9. List factors that contribute to safe vehicle operations.
10. Describe the considerations that should be given to the following:
    - Using escorts
    - Working in adverse environmental conditions
    - Using lights and siren
    - Proceeding through intersections
    - Parking at an emergency scene
11. Discuss the concept of due regard for the safety of all others while operating an emergency vehicle.
12. Differentiate proper from improper body mechanics for lifting and moving patients in emergency and nonemergency situations.
13. Describe the advantages and disadvantages of air medical transport and identify conditions and situations in which air medical transport should be considered.

Chapter Outline

Case Scenario

At 2:05 PM on a spring afternoon your crew responds to a call for a car and motorcycle collision on a two-lane road approximately 5 miles outside of town. Because today is a workday, traffic is usually moderate to heavy along that stretch of road. Just after beginning your response, the dispatcher notifies you that police on scene state the motorcycle rider's condition is critical. You are approximately 5 minutes away from the scene. Your route of travel is mostly four-lane surface streets. However, the last 1.5 miles are on the two-lane road. The weather is clear with mostly sunny skies and the roads are dry.

Once on the two-lane road, you note that the road has a narrow but useable shoulder on your right side. The left side of the road is lined with a guard rail aimed at preventing motor vehicles from sliding down a rather steep embankment. At this point, traffic is light and no vehicles are oncoming.

Questions

1. *What are the hazards that may interfere with your prompt response to the scene?*
2. *What information about the road might be beneficial in determining your best response?*
3. *What scene hazards are you contemplating during your response?*

All the cardiology learned, the drug doses memorized, and the tools you use are useless if you cannot bring them safely, quickly, and in good working order to the scene and to the patient. Operating and maintaining an emergency vehicle is an important responsibility. The paramedic is responsible for ensuring that all needed and required equipment is on the vehicle and in good working order. The operational status of the vehicle must be evaluated and mechanical problems addressed. You must be familiar with the location of equipment and supplies in the vehicle. You also must make certain that the vehicle is clean and safe. En route to a call, you must drive with the safety of the public in mind. When arriving on the scene, the vehicle must be positioned in a place where the safety of those on the scene will not be jeopardized. Although this chapter reviews emergency vehicle operations, emergency medical services and vehicles are different. Ensure you are familiar with your vehicle, agency, and local governmental requirements for its operation.

AMBULANCES

[OBJECTIVE 1]

From horse-drawn carts, trucks with camper shells, and Cadillac station wagons, ambulance design has come a long way. Three types of ambulances are currently in use and are regulated by the federal government. These guidelines are outlined in the document *Federal Specifications for Ambulances, KKK-A-1822E,* which is prepared by the General Services Administration (National Highway Traffic Safety Administration, 1995). In addition to federal standards, each state and local government may impose specific requirements regarding the design of ambulances for their area of governance. It would be impossible to address all the state and local variations in this text; therefore the paramedic must be familiar with these requirements for the area in which he or she works.

Types

[OBJECTIVES 2, 3]

Type I ambulances are a regular truck cab and frame with a modular ambulance box mounted on the back. These ambulances commonly have a pass-through window from the cab to the ambulance box so that the driver can communicate with the medic in the back. One of the benefits of a type I ambulance is that the truck chassis and the ambulance can be purchased and replaced individually. For example, if the ambulance is involved in a crash and the truck is damaged but the ambulance box is not, the ambulance box can be placed on a new truck chassis, so a new ambulance does not have to be purchased. Another benefit is that plenty of space is available to work in the back. One drawback is that communication between the driver and the medic in the back is limited and the driver has a limited ability to see what is happening in the back (Figure 61-1).

Type II ambulances are vans. Vans are narrower and have less space to work in the back. The benefits are that they offer better gas mileage than type I and type III ambulances and they are relatively inexpensive to purchase, making them more affordable to purchase and operate. Type II ambulances also have an open passageway from the driver's compartment to the patient compartment, allowing the driver to see clearly into the back and better communication between the crew (Figure 61-2). A drawback of this type of ambulance is that not a lot of space is available to work in the back. If more than one EMS professional is needed in the back, working space becomes tight.

Type III ambulances are a combination of type I and type II ambulances. They are on a van chassis with a modified modular back (Figure 61-3). The patient care compartment is large, similar to a type I, with ample room to provide patient care. An open passageway runs

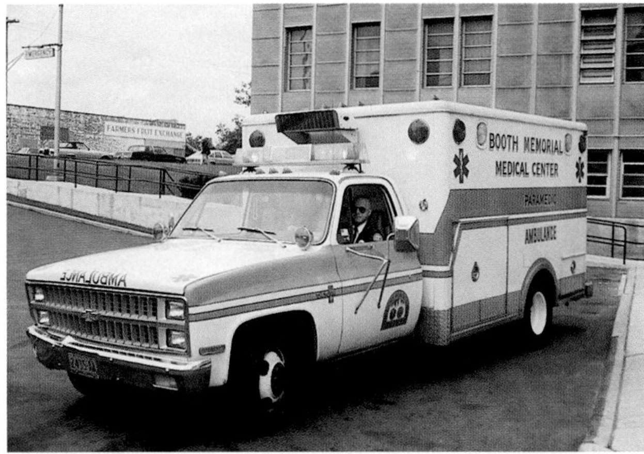

Figure 61-1 Type I ambulance.

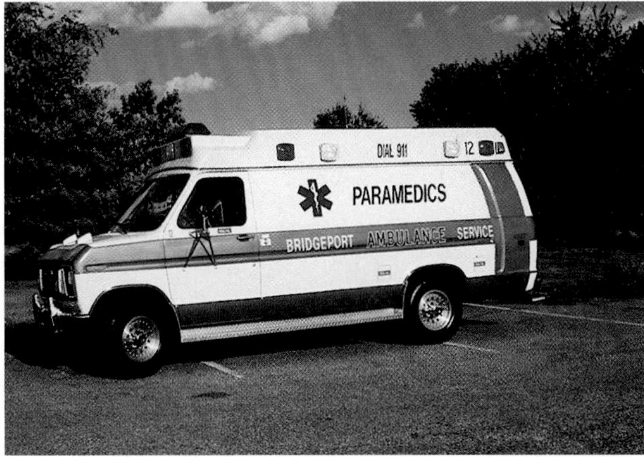

Figure 61-2 Type II ambulance.

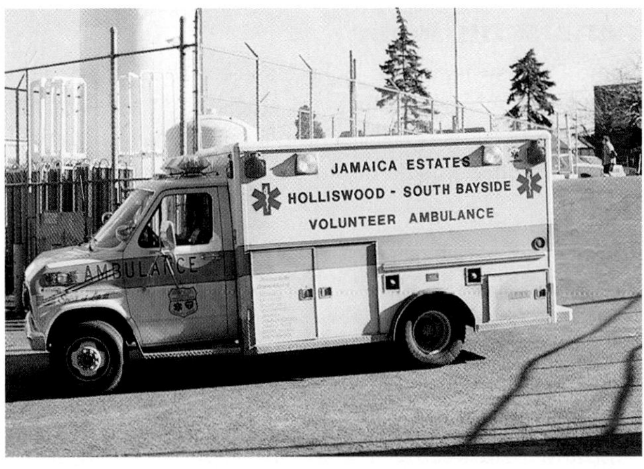

Figure 61-3 Type III ambulance.

from the driver's compartment to the patient care compartment, allowing easy communication. The drawbacks are that type III ambulances tend to be more expensive than type I and type II ambulances and they tend to be heavier and thus use more fuel than a type II.

When the KKK-A-1822E standards were rewritten in June 2002 (replacing KKK-A-1822D) the type I and type III categories were expanded to include "additional duty" classes, or type I-AD and type III-AD (General Services Administration, 2002). These categories pertain to what were formally referred to as *medium duty ambulances*. These ambulances are mounted on large chassis such as a freightliner. This allows for a larger ambulance box, the ability to carry heavier equipment, and the ability to store more equipment on the ambulance, including rescue equipment. Many EMS services have also found that these vehicles last longer and have lower operating costs.

BOX 61-1 Factors That Influence Type of Ambulance Selection

- Agency's call volume
- Size of the service area
- City driving versus rural driving
- Average number of EMS professionals expected to be caring for the patient in the back
- Agency budget

The ambulance type selected by an EMS service is determined by considering a variety of factors (Box 61-1). Whatever type of vehicle is selected, the ambulance must meet KKK-A-1822E guidelines to be allowed to display the Star of Life.

CLEANING AND MAINTENANCE

[OBJECTIVES 4, 5]

Daily emergency vehicle maintenance and cleaning are commonly the responsibility of the paramedic. At the beginning of each shift, check the vehicle and perform any needed routine maintenance. Tasks such as checking the oil, transmission fluid level, and tire pressure and radiator fluid levels can be performed quickly and easily. Add fluid and air if necessary. Always ensure the ambulance has enough gasoline.

Emergency lights are necessary when responding and transporting emergent patients. All the emergency lights must be in working order. If a light is out, replace it with a working light.

Medical equipment should be tested every shift. Cardiac monitors, suction devices, and all other equipment must be charged as appropriate and in good working order. All battery-operated equipment such as laryngoscopes, pulse oximeters, and glucometers must be checked. Medical equipment that is not working must be replaced. Ensure there is adequate oxygen in both the main and portable tanks. Also ensure that the gurney is clean and in proper working order.

If you notice any malfunction or failure of any mechanical or electrical component of the vehicle, take the vehicle out of service to have it repaired or replaced by a qualified technician. A vehicle that is not in good working order is a danger to you, the patient, and the public.

PARAMEDIC*Pearl*

If a paramedic knows of a malfunction and does not address it, he or she may be held legally liable for any injuy incurred because of the malfunction. For example, at the beginning of the shift the paramedic recognizes that the gurney is not locking correctly. The paramedic does not have the issue corrected and chooses to leave the problem for the next day's crew. During the paramedic's shift, a patient is loaded onto the gurney. The gurney slips from the upright position and slams to the ground, causing the patient back pain. The paramedic could be held liable for this injury.

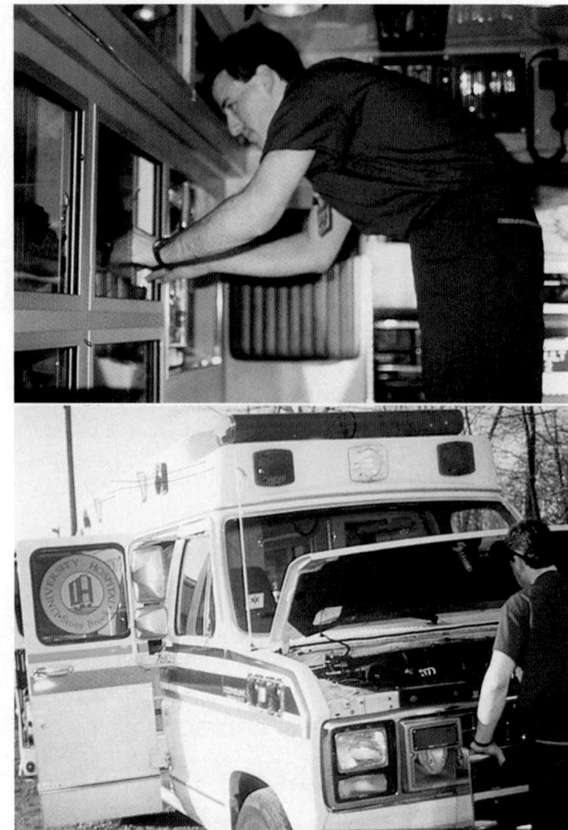

Figure 61-4 An emergency transport vehicle must be cleaned to reduce the risk of infection.

Although an ambulance is not a **sterile** environment, it needs to be a **medically clean** environment. Because invasive procedures are sometimes performed in the ambulance, you must ensure that these procedures can be carried out with minimal risk of contamination (Figure 61-4). Because patients with different illnesses are transported in the ambulance, they may contaminate the vehicle with the virus or bacteria causing their illness. After the patient is out of the ambulance, bacteria and viruses can linger, posing a contamination risk for other patients and EMS professionals.

PARAMEDIC*Pearl*

A dirty ambulance increases the risk of infection.

The back of the ambulance should be cleaned at the beginning of the shift and after every call. Cleaning should consist of mopping the ambulance, wiping down equipment as necessary, and cleaning the seats and walls. Spray disinfectants are easy to use and ensure a safe working patient care area.

INVENTORY

[OBJECTIVE 6]

During a shift you have the potential to care for and transport many patients with a variety of injuries and illnesses. You must be prepared for anything, which includes having all the necessary equipment and supplies. Most EMS agencies have minimal stocking levels for the emergency vehicles in their system. An example of an ambulance inventory sheet is shown in Table 61-1. At the beginning of each shift, check all equipment and supplies to ensure the vehicle is stocked appropriately. All cabinets as well as the **jump kit** must be checked.

Check the drug box to verify it is stocked and that the drugs within it have not been damaged. In many areas, exposure to temperature extremes is a concern for the drugs. In addition to daily inventory, all the drugs on the vehicle should have their expiration dates checked at least once a month and replaced as necessary. The Schedule II drugs should be checked to ensure they are sealed and secure. These drugs must be signed for with every shift change.

PARAMEDIC*Pearl*

Some EMS systems use locked, sealed, and tamper-proof drug boxes. A hospital pharmacy stocks and then signs and dates the box. As a result, the paramedic can only check the date on the outside of the paramedic drug box.

EMERGENCY VEHICLE STATIONING

[OBJECTIVE 7]

Society expects a quick response from an EMS vehicle. To ensure EMS vehicles arrive on scene as quickly as possible, they must be stationed or positioned appropriately. Ambulance stationing is a dynamic process that should be regularly reevaluated. Two of the more common positioning or stationing models are discussed here. In both models, factors such as population, roads and access, and businesses must be evaluated.

Fixed Positioning

Fixed positioning is used by most volunteer and fire-based systems or ambulance services that work 24- or 48-hour shifts. In a fixed positioning model, the EMS

TABLE 61-1 Ambulance Equipment Checklist

Item	Description	Quantity
Burn sheet	Sterile	2
Cold pack	Chemical	4
Surgical clothing	Goggle, gown, mask, hat, eyewear	4 each
Bandages, gauze	Two sizes	10 each
Bandages, triangular		10
HEPA respirator		4
Obstetrics kit	Disposable	1
Obstetrics pad	Sterile	6
Swaddler	Infant, commercially prepared	1
Incontinence pads	Disposable	4
Dressings and tape	Multitrauma, 4 × 4, occlusive	4 each
Tissue	Facial	1 box
Restraint	Vest, extremity	1 pair
Scissors, bandage		1 pair
Multiple-casualty incident kit	Sealed	1
Vest-type immobilization device		1
Oxygen tank	Full E cylinder Regulator on tank On-board oxygen tank	2 1 1
Linen	Towel, sheet, blanket, pillowcase Pillow	4 each 2
Oral and nasal airways	Adult, pediatric	4 each
Nasal cannulae	Adult, pediatric	4 each
Nonrebreather masks	Adult, pediatric	4 each
Bag-mask unit	Adult with $ETCO_2$ detector Pediatric with $ETCO_2$ detector Neonatal	1 1 1
Masks for bag-mask device	Sizes: premature, infant, child, adult	4 (1 of each)
Bed pan	Regular Fracture	1 1
Emesis basin	Small, large	2 each
Blood pressure cuff, stethoscope		1 each
Urinal	Plastic	1
Sharps container	Mounted forward end squad bench	1
Spine board	Adult, pediatric	1 each
Traction splint	Adult, pediatric	1 each
Rigid splints	4 ft × 3 in, 3 ft × 3 in, 15 in × 3 in	2 each
Head immobilizer	Adult, pediatric	1
Padded board splint	Small, medium, large	6 (2 of each)
Scoop stretcher	With three sets of straps	1
Strap	6-ft long	5
Cervical spine immobilization collars	Tall, regular, short, no-neck, pediatric, baby no-neck	12 (2 of each)
Immobilizer	Pediatric	1

HEPA, High-efficiency particulate air; *$ETCO_2$*, end-tidal carbon dioxide.

Continued

TABLE 61-1 Ambulance Equipment Checklist—continued

Item	Description	Quantity
Flashlight	Large	1
Jumper cable	Heavy-duty	1
Flare, road	Emergency, 30-min	12
Screwdriver	Large, straight blade	1
Transport folder	Passenger side	6
Portable suction	Various Suction tubing, suction catheters: 5F to 18F and rigid	1 1 each
Stair chair	Folding	1

system must evaluate its service area to determine geographic centers. For example, if a system has one EMS vehicle, it looks at its response area and determines a central point from which the vehicle can respond. The vehicle is stationed at this point 24 hours a day. Larger systems have multiple stations, all covered 24 hours a day. Station call volumes vary based on time and day. For example, during the week when most people leave a residential neighborhood to go to work, the station in the residential area is slow. On the weekends, the call volume at that station predictably increases because more people are at home. This method of positioning has the potential for a fair amount of downtime or time when the vehicle and crew are not running calls.

System Status Management

System status management (SSM) is a more dynamic method of positioning ambulances. This system is used by many larger cities with high call volumes and whose EMS system is primarily focused on medical response. With this version of positioning, the response area is evaluated geographically and based on the numbers of calls in each area. The calls are monitored and tracked on the basis of location and time of the call. After a large amount of data has been collected, staffing is based on predicting calls. For example, if every weekday evening during rush hour two to five motor vehicle crashes (MVCs) occur in a busy commuting area, then EMS vehicles should be stationed in this area during the week at rush hour. If no or few MVCs occur in the same area on the weekend, then that area does not need to be covered during the weekend. Vehicle staffing varies according to time of day and predicted call volume for that time. This system continually evaluates vehicle efficiency with a formula to determine **unit hour utilization (UhU).** This formula calculates how many calls a vehicle will run in 1 hour. If a vehicle ran one call every hour, its UhU would be 1. Most services using system status management strive for a UhU of at least 0.4 to 0.5, in which all vehicles in service run one call every 2 hours. This version of EMS vehicle positioning tends to be more cost effective than fixed positioning.

Several systems use fixed positioning systems and supplement their response area with extra ambulances during busy times. These extra ambulances move throughout the response area according to call volume, similar to an SSM approach. Staffing an extra ambulance for 8 or 10 hours is cheaper than building an additional station and staffing it for 24 hours.

Remember that no system can predict without error the exact location, time, and number of all calls. Nor can they predict multiple-casualty incidents. All systems must establish mutual aid and backup agreements with neighboring agencies and EMS systems. These backup agreements help ensure an ambulance response if the primary agency is busy or overwhelmed. Factors that are taken into consideration when deploying an ambulance fleet are listed in Box 61-2.

DISTRICT FAMILIARIZATION

[OBJECTIVE 8]

No matter the type of EMS system or type of emergency vehicle positioning used, EMS professionals must know their **response area** or district. They must be familiar with the roads—which go through and which may stop at a dead end. They must know the best way to get on and off a highway as well as the location of mile markers on the highway. They also should be familiar with local businesses and neighborhoods.

The response area can change according to traffic patterns and weather. Knowing which roads may become congested during rush hour is important, as is knowing which roads are maintained first during inclement weather (e.g., snowfall).

Road maintenance and construction can change a response area as well. The EMS crew should obtain regular updates regarding where road crews are working and how traffic will be diverted. If an EMS crew comes across road

BOX 61-2 Factors in Ambulance Deployment

- Location of facilities to house ambulances
- Location of hospitals
- Anticipated volume of calls
- Local geographic and traffic considerations

work, they should inform the dispatch center so that other emergency vehicles can be notified.

Knowing the response area is important. Also important is having a complete and accurate set of maps to guide you to the scene.

PARAMEDIC*Pearl*

Become familiar with your response area or district. Drive around the district at different times of the day to familiarize yourself with the roads, businesses addresses, and traffic patterns.

ROUTE PLANNING

[OBJECTIVE 8]

When an EMS crew is dispatched to a call, the most direct route should be taken. As the driver heads in the general direction of the call, the passenger can navigate with maps. All the criteria previously discussed, such as traffic patterns, construction, and weather, should be taken into account when planning a response route. If the crew becomes lost responding to a call, resulting in a delayed response, the crew could be found guilty of negligence and held liable for a negative patient outcome. If an EMS crew becomes lost or disoriented, many dispatch centers have maps and may help with an appropriate response route. Newer technology available in some dispatch centers and on some emergency vehicles maps response routes. Typically these computer-generated routes do not take into account variables such as traffic and weather. Ultimately an appropriate, timely response is the responsibility of the EMS crew.

PARAMEDIC*Pearl*

Many emergency vehicles are equipped with a mobile data device, also known as a *mobile data terminal* or *mobile data computer.* In addition to providing responding crews with updated incident information for active calls, this device can provide map navigation and road condition information.

SAFE VEHICLE OPERATION

Responding

[OBJECTIVES 5, 9, 10, 11]

The tones go off; the lights come on in the station and the pager on your belt gives an address at which a patient is requesting emergency medical care. No delay should occur getting to the emergency vehicle. Backing the vehicle into its parking space lets you drive straight out when you receive a call.

Before moving the vehicle, the driver and passenger should have a good idea where they are heading and the best route to take. They should determine the mode of response as well; not all calls require the use of lights and sirens. Sirens should be used only when responding to a medical emergency. The *U.S. Department of Transportation Emergency Vehicles Operators Guide* defines a true emergency as a situation with a high probability of death or serious injury to an individual or significant property loss and in which action by an emergency vehicle operator may reduce the seriousness of the situation (National Highway Traffic Safety Administration, 1995).

Notify dispatch as soon as you respond. Dispatch may have additional information such as updated patient data or a change in address.

The driver should drive with **due regard** for others on the road. Due regard is remembering that lights and sirens only *request* the right of way. The driver of the emergency vehicle is responsible for ensuring that other drivers and pedestrians see and hear the lights and sirens and yield the right of way. If you hit another vehicle while responding to a call, you can be found liable even if your lights and sirens were running. The paramedic driver is responsible for watching for others on the road. The medic riding as the front seat passenger should also watch to ensure all vehicles yield the right of way.

The emergency vehicle can exceed the speed limit when responding to a call. Laws vary regarding the degree to which an emergency vehicle can exceed the speed limit. In addition, ambulances are generally allowed to pass through a stop sign or red traffic signal after ensuring it is safe to do so, disregard restrictions on turning and direction of travel, and stop or park the ambulance in areas that would be prohibited for nonemergency vehicles. Paramedics must be familiar with their local laws. All laws, however, require you to drive with due regard, and in most states the use of all warning devices is required to exercise these privileges.

PARAMEDIC*Pearl*

Although laws may vary, in most states ambulances are not permitted to pass a school bus that is displaying its red flashing lights. In this situation the paramedic must stop, leave the emergency lights on, turn off the siren, and wait until the bus driver motions you to pass.

Change the siren sound when approaching intersections. Between intersections, use a long wail sound. When approaching an intersection, change the sound to a shorter, faster yelp or, in some states, the Hi-Lo siren sound. This warns other motorists of your arrival at the intersection. Be sure to slow down when approaching an intersection. When traveling though an intersection with a green light, the driver of the emergency vehicle should slow down and enter the intersection with one foot covering the brake in case a sudden stop is needed. The driver is responsible for ensuring that all other vehicles have stopped. At red lights and stop signs, stop the emergency vehicle to ensure that all other vehicles have yielded. Only after all other vehicles have stopped should the emergency vehicle proceed though the intersection. It must be appreciated that intersections are the most dangerous situations, as traffic is crossing in differet directions, and intersections are the location of most ambulance collisions. A list of other common collisions involving ambulances can be found in Box 61-3.

Pass on the left side toward the center of the road as much as possible. Passing on the right may catch drivers off guard because they are used to seeing emergency vehicles in the center of the road.

Remember you are driving a heavy vehicle and stopping distances are longer than for a regular vehicle. When approaching vehicles from behind, the driver of an emergency vehicle must be prepared to stop, leaving the vehicle in front enough room to react and move out of the way. When following another vehicle, a good idea to use is the 4-second rule. Watch as the vehicle in front of you passes an object on the side of the road, such as a telephone pole. Then count "one thousand one, one thousand two, one thousand three, one thousand four." As you finish counting, your front bumper should be passing the same object. If you reach that object sooner, you should slow down.

PARAMEDIC*Pearl*

An average type III ambulance weighs just over 10,000 lb. At a speed of 45 mph, at least 200 feet is required to stop a vehicle of this size. That is two thirds the length of a football field.

When responding with a convoy of multiple emergency vehicles or with a police escort, extra caution is required at intersections. Drivers commonly see one emergency vehicle pass and assume they are clear but end up pulling directly in front of the next emergency vehicle. Allow adequate distance between emergency vehicles to avoid intersection confusion and an embarrassing, injurious, and costly emergency vehicle collision.

When multiple emergency vehicles are responding from different directions, such as in a tiered response system (Box 61-4), the vehicles should communicate with each other as they get closer to the scene. Multiple emergency vehicles from different directions can converge on an intersection at the same time, once again resulting in an emergency vehicle collision.

BOX 61-3 Common Types of Ambulance Collisions

- Other drivers "timing" lights
- Emergency vehicles following each other
- Multiple emergency vehicles converging on same location
- Motorists going around stopped traffic
- Vision of pedestrians in crosswalk obstructed by other vehicles

PARAMEDIC*Pearl*

Many EMS services are using cameras mounted on the dashboard in their emergency vehicles. Activated by a collision or abrupt maneuvering of the vehicle, the camera will record 10 seconds before and 10 seconds after the event. If the crew sees crash occur in front of them, a switch can activate the recorder to provide valuable information on what exactly happened.

On Scene

Once an emergency vehicle is on the scene, notify the dispatch center. Park the vehicle to allow easy access to the patient as well as safety for the EMS crew. Do not let the ambulance be blocked by structures or other vehicles. Park to allow easy egress from the scene.

Several factors must be considered in regard to the placement of an ambulance at the scene of an MVC; however, the priority is the safety of the crew. In a situation where there is no evidence of fire, leaking liquids, or fumes the following general guidelines should be followed: If the ambulance is the first unit on scene, it should be parked 50 feet behind the collision to provide protection for the crew. If a police or fire apparatus arrive on scene first, it should be parked behind the scene, and the ambulance should be parked 100 feet in front of the scene. If there is any evidence of fire, leaking liquids, or fumes the ambulance should be parked a minimum of

BOX 61-4 Tiered Response System

A tiered response system is an EMS system that operates units with several different levels of patient care and transport capability. Typically a tiered system includes a larger number of units with basic life support (BLS) capability than with advanced life support (ALS) capability. When a request for service is received, the dispatcher uses a protocol to determine which types of units to send. Frequently, both a BLS unit and an ALS unit will respond to the same call. If the patient needs care by a paramedic, the ALS unit will transport the patient. If the patient requires only basic care, the BLS unit will transport the patient, and the ALS unit will return to service.

100 feet from the scene regardless of the presence of another apparatus. If the involvement of hazardous materials in the collision is suspected, the ambulance should be parked uphill and upwind of the scene at the distance recommended in the *DOT Emergency Response Guidebook*.

In the cases of crime scenes, hazardous materials, or multiple-causality incidents, a staging zone is usually identified. Arriving emergency vehicles should wait in the staging area until called to the scene. More information on crime scenes, incident command, hazardous materials, and multiple-casualty incidents is discussed in Chapters 59, 62, 64, and 67, respectively.

On the scene of traffic accidents, fire apparatuses are usually positioned to protect the scene. The apparatus should be visible to other drivers. The vehicle's spotlights also can offer light to the scene. Leave emergency lights on while on the scene of an MVC. The EMS crew must work on scene with caution, always watching for passing traffic.

Lifting, Moving, and Loading

[OBJECTIVE 12]

Lifting and moving patients is a common action required by paramedics. Helping patients up from a sitting position in a chair, lifting patients off the floor, and carrying patients down flights of stairs are some examples of the different situations in which you must lift patients. Back injuries caused by lifting and moving patients are one of the most common injuries in EMS professionals. You must make every effort possible to avoid such injury.

You must work to stay in good physical shape. A training program should consist of a combination of aerobic, strength, and flexibility training (Figure 61-5). Staying in good physical shape will help to reduce injury. The well-being of the paramedic is discussed in more detail in Chapter 1.

You must also be aware of your personal limitations. When faced with a situation you know is beyond your physical capabilities, call for assistance. You can injure yourself attempting to lift beyond your own physical abilities. In addition, the patient and other people lifting with you can also be hurt.

You must know how your equipment operates. Several different versions of **gurneys,** or stretchers, are used in EMS. All have similar functions but may load differently or may raise and lower differently. Not knowing how to operate the gurney properly can result in injury to all involved. The same is true for other lifting devices such as **stair chairs.**

Two-person dead-lift stretchers are rarely used any more because of the high incidence of back injury associated with their use. With this type of stretcher, paramedics lower the stretcher to the ground and then lift the stretcher from the sides to the level of the back of the ambulance. They then slide the stretcher into the floor locks.

One and a half–person stretchers are more common. With this type of stretcher, a set of wheels is under the head of the stretcher. These wheels are rolled into the back of the ambulance. The foot end of the stretcher is then lifted and the wheels are released. A second paramedic lifts the wheels up, and the stretcher is rolled into the ambulance. One-person stretchers are similar to the one and a half–person version. With the one-person version, the stretcher is simply pushed into the ambulance. As the wheels meet the ambulance, they fold under the stretcher. Because this can jolt the patient, use caution when pushing the gurney into the ambulance.

Newer stretchers have motors that raise and lower the bed. This adds weight to the stretcher but alleviates much of the lifting done by paramedics. **Bariatric ambulances** are ambulances designed for transporting morbidly obese patients (Figure 61-6). These ambulances have winches that can pull the gurney up a ramp for easy loading.

Regardless of the stretcher being used, always use good lifting posture (see Chapter 1). Keep your back straight and lift with the legs. Bending over or twisting while lifting increases the risk of back injury. Do not begin the

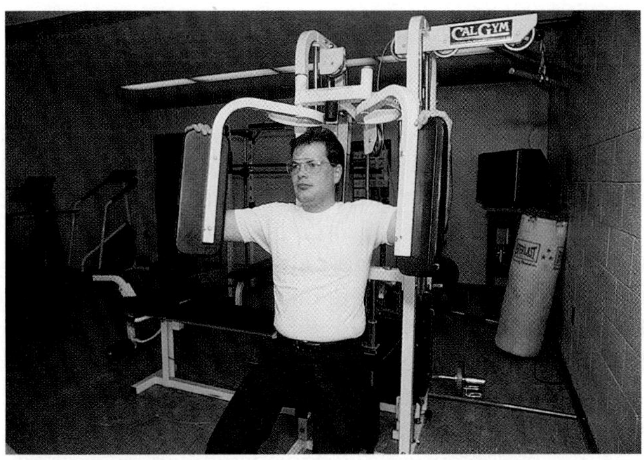

Figure 61-5 Staying in good physical shape will help reduce the risk of injury to the paramedic.

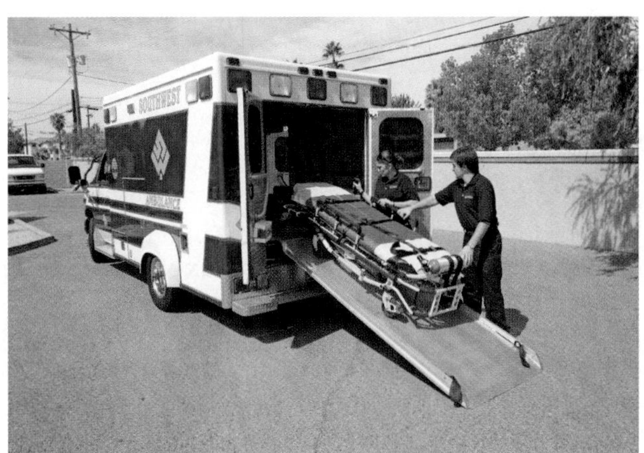

Figure 61-6 A bariatric ambulance is specially designed and equipped for transporting morbidly obese patients.

lift until all persons lifting are ready. The person at the head should initiate the lift with a three count. When lifting patients on the stretcher, the persons lifting should not release the stretcher until they are positive the wheels have locked. Wheels not being locked can result in the stretcher falling to the ground, injuring the patient.

Transporting

Once the patient has been loaded and the ambulance is heading for the hospital, notify dispatch. The EMS driver must remember another EMS professional is in the back of the ambulance attempting to provide medical care. The ride to the hospital should be as smooth as possible using the most direct route. If the driver sees a need to stop or turn suddenly, the EMS personnel in the back should be notified in advance of the maneuver. The driver must make every effort to avoid the risk of sudden stops or turns. The driver also must monitor the patient compartment to determine the type of treatment being given. For example, if the paramedic is about to use a defibrillator, a turn or stop may cause injury to the paramedic.

When attending the patient on the way to the hospital, wear a safety restraint. Several different versions of nets and harnesses are available but work with varying degrees of effectiveness. Use the seat belts on the bench and captain's chair whenever possible. The laws pertaining to ambulances generally do not provide exemption from laws that require the use of restraints. Additionally the patient should be secured to the stretcher using all straps, including shoulder straps if they are available. All loose equipment should be secured to avoid injury in the event of a sudden stop, turn, or collision.

Once at the hospital, notify dispatch. Make every attempt to provide a good patient hand-off to receiving facility staff, clean and restock the ambulance, and get back in service as quickly as possible.

PARAMEDIC*Pearl*

What a person does commonly speaks louder than what he or she says. When driving an emergency vehicle, remember that you are in a large billboard representing your company, fire service, or ambulance district.

General Driving

Paramedics must drive with due regard at all times. The driver is obligated to ensure other drivers see the vehicle. Paramedics are EMS professionals, and that should be reflected in their driving, both emergent and nonemergent.

All paramedics responsible for driving an ambulance should take an emergency vehicle operating course. In 1995 the National Highway Traffic Safety Administration approved an emergency vehicle operating course for ambulance operations.

Case Scenario—continued

The speed limit on the road is set at 30 mph. Your speedometer reads 45 mph. You continue on the two-lane road and, approximately one-quarter mile ahead, you notice brake lights and stopped traffic. You estimate you are approximately 1 mile from the actual scene. You slow as you approach the stopped traffic. Your emergency lights and siren are still operating.

Questions

4. *What laws pertain to exceeding the speed limit when responding to an emergency call?*
5. *If traffic cannot move, what options do you have to continue your response?*
6. *What is your legal obligation to other drivers on this emergency response?*

AIR MEDICAL TRANSPORT

[OBJECTIVE 13]

Transporting patients by air is an option available to paramedics in many EMS systems. **Fixed-winged** aircraft (airplanes) and **rotor-wing** aircraft (helicopters) are the transport options. Transporting from the scene of a call most commonly is done by helicopter. The first hospital-based helicopter transport service was established in October 1972 at St. Anthony's Hospital in Denver, Colo. By 1986 a total of 140 hospital-based helicopter transport services were in operation throughout the United States. Most helicopters can provide service within a 130-mile radius from the base facility. Airplanes are used for long distance interfacility transports. Transport ranges for airplanes commonly are limited to a 500-mile radius. Staffing for medical aircraft varies widely from service to service. Most are staffed with at least one registered nurse. The Emergency Nurses Association and the Air and Surface Transport Nurses Association report that approximately 30% of medical helicopters in the United States are staffed with at least one paramedic (Emergency Nurses Association, 2001).

Many factors must be considered when making a decision to call a helicopter to the scene. You must first consider transport time. Many patients may require a

specialty center such as a level I trauma center, tertiary pediatric center, or burn center. Air transport may be of benefit in this situation, but several factors should be considered. Helicopters obviously can fly faster than an ambulance can drive, but other times must be considered as well. How long before the helicopter arrives and lands on the scene? Once on the scene, how close to the scene can the aircraft land? Will the patient need to be shuttled to the aircraft? Finally, how long is the flight to an appropriate facility? In many cases, even if you are 30 minutes by ground to an appropriate facility, if scene times can be kept short an emergent response to the hospital may be faster than calling, waiting, loading, and then transporting by helicopter.

In some EMS systems, helicopters can bring a higher level of care to the scene than the paramedic on scene can provide. For instance, the flight teams in some states carry fibrinolytic drugs. These drugs can be brought to the bedside of a patient having a heart attack when time is of the essence.

If a helicopter would be a benefit to the patient, then logistic concerns must be considered. An extra EMS or fire crew is usually required to be on the scene to land the helicopter. Extra police may be required to control traffic. A **landing zone** must be established. A landing zone must be at least 100 feet by 100 feet and free of power lines and phone lines. It should be a flat area away from hills and free of debris. Many scenes in mountainous regions or in larger cities are not suited for landing a helicopter.

Weather is another factor to consider when using air transport. Different aircraft have different criteria for flying in inclement weather. Some general conditions that would preclude air medical transport of a patient would be low clouds causing decreased visibility, excessive precipitation such as rain or snow, and extreme wind. Temperature also plays a role in flight. Typically the cooler the air, the easier it is for a helicopter to lift. Conversely, the hotter the air, the more difficult it is for a helicopter to lift.

Once the helicopter has landed, the EMS crew on the scene must be familiar with how to approach the aircraft. The EMS crew should have eye contact with the pilot. Depending on the aircraft and the situation, the pilot may stop the rotors before loading and unloading the patient. Other times the EMS crew may need to do a **hot load,** which means loading the patient with the rotors still turning. The pilot will signal the crew when approach is safe. Always approach the front of the helicopter, keeping your head low. Avoid the rear of the craft to prevent injury from the tail rotor. If the terrain is not completely flat, approach the helicopter from the downhill side. Use caution in windy situations because the wind can cause the rotors to dip and cause injury.

Case Scenario CONCLUSION

As you approach the stopped traffic, you note no oncoming traffic, probably because of the collision ahead. You opt to use the oncoming traffic lane to reach the scene even though the road bends to the right and your vision is somewhat obscured. As you round the bend, you are approximately one half mile away from the scene and can see some of the police vehicles. You also notice an intersection on your right approximately 250 feet ahead. At the intersection, a dump truck wants to turn left. The driver, waved onto the road by a stopped motorist, begins his slow left turn directly into your path.

You apply hard pressure to your brakes. No room is available on the right because of the stopped cars, and the left side of the road is on the edge of a drop-off. As your speed drops, your vehicle starts to skid and you lose control of it. As the skid continues, the rear of the ambulance strikes the front fender of the dump truck. Fortunately no one is injured; however, a second ambulance must be dispatched to the motorcycle crash. Because of the delay, the driver of the motorcycle dies from his injuries.

Looking Back

7. *What are your options at this point?*
8. *Is the dump truck driver failing to yield the right of way?*
9. *What should you have done differently during the last stages of this emergency response?*

PARAMEDIC LIABILITY

[OBJECTIVE 5]

Paramedics can be held liable for decisions made or actions taken while operating an ambulance that result in harm to a patient or society. Many areas of liability are discussed in this chapter. Actions that may seem minor, such as not checking the ambulance before the beginning of the shift, open the door for legal action against you. If the drug box was incomplete and was not recognized and corrected at the beginning the shift and during the shift a patient required the missing medication, you could be found negligent.

Responding to a call, driving without due regard for others on the road, and causing an accident or being involved in an accident can have dire consequences for you. Paramedics have been stripped of their licenses, lost the ability to practice prehospital medicine, and even been incarcerated because of their misjudgments while operating an emergency vehicle. Several questions have been raised in the EMS community about the benefits versus liabilities of responding emergently to calls.

Paramedics must value all aspects of emergency vehicle operation just as much as reading ECG strips or reviewing drug doses. Operating an emergency vehicle is a large part of the paramedic's job. Failure to uphold the responsibilities of that job may result in poor outcomes for the paramedic, patient, and society.

Case Scenario SUMMARY

1. *What are the hazards that may interfere with your prompt response to the scene?* Hazards include stopped cars that may decide to turn around and head the other direction. Another hazard is the guard rail on the left side of the road designed to prevent rolling down a drop-off. The narrow shoulder on the right side of the road is hazardous if used for a main route of response. Stopped cars may pull to the right, directly in your path, requiring an emergency stop.
2. *What information about the road might be beneficial in determining your best response?* You need to know the topology of the road such as turn, bends, intersections, and speed limits. Being aware of these features can help in your overall emergency response.
3. *What scene hazards are you contemplating during your response?* Scene hazards usually involve spilled fuel, fire or potential for fire, downed electrical wires, trapped victims, and other problems that interfere with reaching the patient.
4. *What laws pertain to exceeding the speed limit when responding to an emergency call?* Most states allow emergency vehicles responding to a bona fide emergency to exceed the speed limit as long as the emergency vehicle does not endanger the lives and property of others. Some states set a specific limit on the speed of an emergency vehicle, such as 15 mph over the limit.
5. *If traffic cannot move, what options do you have to continue your response?* Depending on the situation, one or more options may be available. Allowing the motorists in front of you to pull to the side of the road may take longer than desired but may be the safest option. Using the shoulder on the right side may be an option but could pose a problem if a motorist opts to move to the shoulder in an effort to yield the right of way. You could also use the oncoming lane of traffic. This option should be a last resort because it is fraught with danger. When using an oncoming traffic lane, do not travel more than 10 to 15 mph.
6. *What is your legal obligation to other drivers on this emergency response?* As the driver of an emergency vehicle, you have the obligation to operate the ambulance with due regard for the safety and property of others. Do not exceed the speed limit or ignore driving laws if such actions would put the lives and property of other drivers at risk. Operating an emergency vehicle without due regard can mean the liability for injury or property damage is yours.
7. *What are your options at this point?* You may not have many options if the dump truck is turning into your path. If you were traveling at a slow rate of speed, coming to a complete stop is a lot easier. You must allow time for the dump truck driver to recognize and react to your presence. A low speed permits this.
8. *Is the dump truck driver failing to yield the right of way?* Remember that emergency lights do not go around corners or curves in the road. Also remember that the siren may not be heard in a closed vehicle when using the radio and air conditioning. Similarly, the noise of a dump truck's engine can easily hide the sound of an approaching siren. The dump truck driver, moving on what he believed to be a safe situation, was not failing to yield the right of way.
9. *What should you have done differently during the last stages of this emergency response?* As previously mentioned, if you choose to use oncoming traffic lanes to pass stopped cars, do so at a very low rate of speed. This allows you to make changes in your course or come to a complete stop to avoid hitting another vehicle.

Chapter Summary

- The importance of safe and proper operation of the ambulance and its equipment cannot be overstressed. It can mean the difference between arriving safely and timely versus not arriving at all.
- The timely and appropriate care of the patients served by paramedics depends on the emergency vehicle being in good operating condition, well stocked, and clean.
- Paramedics must remember that they are liable for the condition of their emergency vehicle and the way it is operated.

REFERENCES

Emergency Nurses Association. (2001). *Staffing of critical care air medical transport services.* Des Plaines, IL: Emergency Nurses Association.

General Services Administration (2002). *Federal Specification for the Star of Life Ambulance. KKK-A-1822D.* Retrieved Date August 4, 2008, from http://www.gsa.gov.

National Highway Traffic Safety Administration. (1995). *Federal specifications for ambulances, KKK-1822E.* Washington, DC: U.S. Department of Transportation.

National Highway Traffic Safety Administration. (1995). *Emergency vehicle operators course.* Washington, DC: U.S. Department of Transportation.

SUGGESTED RESOURCE

U.S. Department of Health, Education, and Welfare. (1999). *Essentials and guidelines for the education and training of the emergency medical technician-paramedic.* Washington, DC: U.S. Government Printing Office.

Chapter Quiz

1. Which of the following ambulance types is typically the most affordable to purchase and operate?
   a. Type I
   b. Type II
   c. Type III
   d. They are all similar

2. When responding to a call, when should lights and sirens be used?
   a. In a life-threatening emergency
   b. On all 9-1-1 calls
   c. When the ambulance is out of position
   d. When traffic is heavy

3. Stopping distances in an ambulance are longer than in a car. How much space should be left between the ambulance and the vehicle it is following?
   a. 1 second
   b. 2 seconds
   c. 3 seconds
   d. 4 seconds

4. What is the recommended size for a helicopter landing zone?
   a. 10 feet × 10 feet
   b. 100 feet × 100 feet
   c. 200 feet × 200 feet
   d. The largest space available

5. While responding to a call with light and sirens, the ambulance approaches an intersection with a red light. What actions should be taken by the paramedic driving?
   a. Come to a complete stop, check for other vehicles, then proceed
   b. Come to a complete stop, wait for a green light.
   c. Continue through the red light with no need to slow down
   d. Slow down, check for other vehicles, then proceed

6. True or False: A bariatric ambulance is designed to transport morbidly obese patients.

7. At the beginning of the shift, you notice that the right rear emergency flasher is out. What should you do?
   a. Do not use the flashers today
   b. Have the light replaced
   c. Not worry because the other emergency lights will be enough
   d. Request only nonemergent calls for the shift

8. A two-person crew is called to transport a patient who weighs 500 lb. How should the crew proceed?
   a. Attempt to carry the patient
   b. Call for a lift assist
   c. Fabricate a slide device from backboards
   d. Leave the patient

9. True or False: Responding with other emergency vehicles can increase the risk of being involved in a collision at intersections.

10. When should the transport vehicle be cleaned?
   a. At the beginning of each shift, after each call, at the end of each shift
   b. Only after each call
   c. Only at the beginning of each shift
   d. Only at the end of each shift

Terminology

Bariatric ambulance Ambulance designed to transport morbidly obese patients.

Due regard Principle used when driving an emergency vehicle of ensuring that all other vehicles and citizens in the area see and grant the emergency vehicle the right of way.

Fixed positioning Establishing a single location in a central point to station an emergency vehicle, such as a fire station.

Fixed-winged aircraft An airplane.

Gurney Stretcher or cot used to transport patients.

Hot load Loading a patient into a helicopter while the rotors are spinning.

Jump kit A hard-sided or soft-sided bag used by paramedics to carry supplies and medications to the patient's side.

Landing zone An area used to land a helicopter that is 100 × 100 feet and free of overhead wires.

Medically clean Disinfected.

Response area The geographic area assigned to an emergency vehicle for responding to the sick and injured.

Rotor-wing aircraft A helicopter.

Specialty center A hospital that has met criteria to offer special care as a burn center, level I trauma center, stroke center, or pediatric center.

Stair chair A collapsible, portable chair with handles on the front and back used to carry patients in sitting position down stairs.

Sterile Free of any living organism.

System status management (SSM) Dynamic process of staffing, stationing, and moving ambulances according to projected call volumes.

Type I ambulance Regular truck cab and frame with a modular ambulance box mounted on the back.

Type II ambulance Van-style ambulance.

Type III ambulance A van chassis with a modified modular back.

Unit hour utilization (UhU) Mathematic calculation used to determine the effectiveness of an ambulance; one call per hour = 1 UhU.

CHAPTER 62

EMS Operations Command and Control

Objectives

After completing this chapter, you will be able to:

1. Explain the need for the incident management system or incident command system in managing EMS incidents.
2. Compare command procedures used at small-, medium-, and large-scale medical incidents.
3. Define the term *multiple-casualty incident.*
4. Explain the local or regional threshold for establishing command and implementation of the incident management system, including threshold multiple-casualty incident declaration.
5. Define the term *disaster management.*
6. Describe the functional components of the incident management system in terms of command, finance, logistics, operations, and planning.
7. Describe the role of the paramedic and EMS system in planning for multiple-casualty incidents and disasters.
8. Describe the role of table-top exercises and small and large drills in preparation for multiple-casualty incidents.
9. List the physical and psychological signs of critical incident stress.
10. Describe the role of critical incident stress management sessions in multiple-casualty incidents.
11. Describe the role of command.
12. Compare singular and unified command and describe when each is most applicable.
13. Describe the methods and rationale for identifying specific functions and leaders for these functions in the incident command system.
14. Describe the role of command posts and emergency operations centers in multiple-casualty incidents and disaster management.
15. Describe the need and procedures for transfer of command.
16. Describe essential elements of scene size-up when arriving at a potential multiple-casualty incident.
17. Describe modifications of telecommunications procedures during a multiple-casualty incident.
18. List and describe the functions of the following groups and leaders in an incident command system as they pertain to EMS incidents:
    - Safety
    - Logistics
    - Rehabilitation
    - Staging
    - Treatment
    - Triage
    - Transportation
    - Extrication or rescue
    - Disposition of deceased (morgue)
    - Communications
19. Describe the role of the physician at multiple-casualty incidents.
20. Describe the need for and techniques used in tracking patients during multiple-casualty incidents.
21. Describe techniques used to allocate patients to hospitals and track them.
22. List and describe the essential equipment to provide logistical support to multiple-casualty incident operations, including airway, respiratory, and hemorrhage control; burn management; and patient immobilization.
23. Define and describe the principles of triage.
24. Given a list of 20 patients with various multiple injuries, determine the appropriate triage priority with 90% accuracy.
25. Define *primary triage* and *secondary triage.*
26. Describe when primary and secondary triage techniques should be implemented.
27. Describe the START method of initial triage.
28. Given color-coded tags and numeric priorities, assign the following terms to each: immediate, delayed, hold, and deceased.

Chapter Outline

Case Scenario

You are called to an accident on an expressway that involves a fuel tanker and multiple cars. Because of fire, the overpass has collapsed on the highway. You are called to the scene and are instructed to wait at triage for further instructions. Dispatch provides information that multiple cars are trapped under the collapse. The incident commander has announced that he has established command.

Questions

1. *What are the differences among a multiple-patient incident, a multiple-casualty incident, and a disaster?*
2. *What is the National Incident Management System?*
3. *What are the basic elements of the National Incident Management System?*

[OBJECTIVES 1 TO 10]

EMS Command and Control formalizes a crucial process that ensures optimal patient care and positions the right people in the right place doing the right tasks. EMS Command and Control principles are used daily, and over the course of a career paramedics will use this system in response to both minor incidents and disasters. The system is designed to accommodate small, everyday incidents (e.g., a routine motor vehicle crash) or once-in-a-lifetime, large-scale events (e.g., the Oklahoma City bombing) while the incident commander manages resources and allows the system to expand and contract. Incident command is not limited to supervisors or managers. Anyone in the system can be "in charge" while the incident is in its early stages. As the situation escalates and supervisors arrive, the incident command function may be, and often is, transferred to a person of higher training. When the principles are applied properly with a building blocks approach and without regard for jurisdictional or geographic boundaries, the EMS professional can be prepared to deal with an incident of any scale.

This chapter explains the responsibilities toward achieving that goal. In addition, you will learn how to integrate triage, treatment, and transportation elements into the incident command system effectively.

The **span of control** within the incident command system is the amount of resources that one person can effectively manage. This may be as few as three or as many as seven, but five is optimal. Resources are a group of equally trained personnel performing common tasks within the framework of a set of standard operating guidelines.

The routine, everyday incident is easily managed with few resources; there is not much harm in calling a vehicle collision a car crash. However, a big difference exists between a car crash and an incident involving 10, 20, or 100 patients. The EMS community must have a clear understanding of the magnitude of the incident.

In many systems common definitions are used to describe certain events according to the number of ill or injured patients. For example, a **multiple-patient incident** involves two to 25 persons. A **multiple-casualty incident** involves 26 to 99 persons, and a **disaster** describes incidents that involve 100 or more patients. The role of the incident commander remains constant, but the command staff is different at each of these incident types.

Many systems are in place to provide guidance and structure to the personnel who respond to incidents. The successful systems identify the supervisor and the workers and provide a template of responsibility for each member. Two of the more popular systems are the incident command system (ICS) and the National Incident Management System (NIMS). Although the terminology varies between systems, ICS and NIMS are both flexible and can be adapted to a host of incidents ranging from a bus accident to a hurricane. NIMS provides a standardized strategy to approach incident management and response and is the template for the National Response Framework. All local, state, tribal, and federal governments were required to be trained in NIMS and its use by the end of 2007. This levels the playing field and ensures that all responders have an identical foundation for coordinated incident response to manage a host of situations from an all-hazards perspective. Additionally, NIMS provides a common language and terminology to address different incident types and identify the resources needed to manage each type of incident (Federal Emergency Management Agency, 2004).

Different communities are prone to different large-scale events. California is at risk for earthquakes and devastating wildfires, Oklahoma is in the heart of tornado alley, and Florida is susceptible to massive hurricanes. Regardless of location, each community should have a disaster management plan in place with a goal to mitigate, prepare for, respond to, and recover from major incidents and disasters (Box 62-1). This plan should include local and regional EMS systems and personnel. The incident commander and command staff should have a familiarity with the local disaster management plan and be able to put that plan into action when needed.

BOX 62-1 Phases of the Emergency Response

Mitigation is preventing or limiting the impact of emergencies. Examples of mitigation activities include zoning ordinances, building codes, and safety inspections.

Preparedness consists of activities occurring before an emergency that are intended to ensure an efficient, effective response. Preparedness includes development of evacuation and emergency response plans, training, exercises, and stockpiling of essential equipment and supplies.

Response consists of activities following an incident that are intended to save lives and property and stabilize the situation that is producing the emergency.

Recovery involves restoring the responding agencies and the community to normal. Activities taken during the recovery phase can also be used to mitigate the impact of future incidents.

BOX 62-2 Common Problems at Large-Scale Incidents

- Failure to adequately provide widespread notification of the event
- Lack of rapid initial stabilization of all patients
- Failure to move, collect, and organize patients rapidly at a treatment area
- Failure to provide proper triage
- Overly time-consuming care employed
- Premature transportation of patients
- Improper use of personnel in field
- Lack of proper distribution of patients to medical facilities
- Lack of recognizable EMS command in the field
- Lack of proper pre-planning and lack of adequate training of all personnel

Critical components to any ICS include a uniform, consistent set of rules, and a common language. A standardized approach may be to divide the incident into geographic or functional locations (or sectors) and designate sector officers with titles based on their location or function, such as "Command to Medic 1, you will be East Sector," or "Command to Medic 1, you will be Treatment Sector." Early sectorization of an incident prepares the incident commander by not placing too many resources into one area or function and prevents members from "freelancing" or acting on their own authority. Sectorization allows the span of control (and the sanity of the incident commander) to be maintained. In many systems, Sector officers are identified by easily distinguishable helmets, vests, or bibs. This clearly identifies who is in charge of that particular area and minimizes confusion.

Major functional areas of any ICS should include the following:

- Command
- Finance
- Logistics
- Operations
- Planning
- Safety

The most important component to any ICS is communications. The EMS professional should be trained to understand the rules of engagement and know what to say, when to say it, and how it should be said. This allows all other participants to have a clear understanding of what it happening and how it affects the big picture. A proven tool is found in the **standard operating procedures (SOPs),** which become the playbook of the organization. SOPs offer a clear, concise description of the incident command process. Each EMS agency should have its own set of SOPs, and every member should be trained in their application. Technology, systems, and treatment methods are constantly evolving; therefore SOPs should be reviewed and updated frequently.

Because large-scale events occur infrequently, most agencies and their personnel do not use their multiple-patient, multiple-casualty, or disaster skills with any regularity. In an effort to maintain the readiness required, ongoing training must take place. This often comes in the form of tabletop discussions or mock practical drills. Both of these practices help maintain the knowledge and skills necessary to prepare for small- and large-scale incidents. Each drill should begin with an overview of the desired result and end with a post-incident review to discuss positive and negative experiences as well as offer a chance to incorporate new or different strategies into the SOPs. Post-incident reviews of drills and real events also create lessons learned that will benefit others for many years. Many problems can present themselves during a large-scale incident without proper preparation before the event, or preplanning. Common problems are listed in Box 62-2.

Planning to provide for the physical and mental health of prehospital responders is as critical as planning for the incident itself. An often overlooked and mismanaged aspect of a multiple-casualty incident—and specifically during post-incident review—is to address adequate critical incident stress management. Large-scale incidents can have a profound impact on responders regardless of how many years of experience they may have. The effects on rescuers may be physical (e.g., difficulty sleeping, eating, or focusing; weight gain/loss) or psychological (e.g., difficulty coping, personality changes). The response may be different for different people. What may affect some may not affect others in the same manner—if at all. Some form of critical incident stress management should be considered at each incident, especially after a large-scale, high-profile incident.

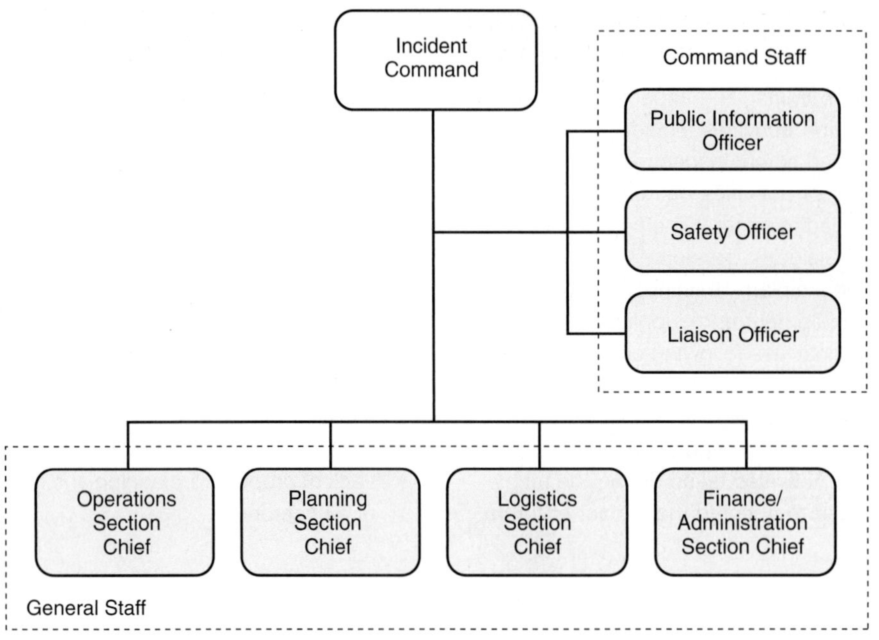

Figure 62-1 Incident command system: command staff and general staff.

BASIC ELEMENTS OF THE INCIDENT COMMAND SYSTEM

Nearly every ICS contains several basic components. NIMS breaks the major components into several parts, which are easily remembered by the mnemonic CFLOPS:

Command
Finance
Logistics
Operations
Planning
Safety

All of these elements are in place during every event, but some may be less obvious during smaller incidents and not have a specifically assigned person. Figure 62-1 shows the relationship among these components.

Command

[OBJECTIVES 11, 12, 13]

The **incident commander (IC)** is the boss, or the person ultimately responsible for managing the event. Regardless of the size of the incident, someone *must* be in charge. The IC is responsible for or delegates the creation of an action plan and manages the event at the highest level by establishing strategic objectives (e.g., treat and transport all patients, put the fire out) and tactical priorities (e.g., treat the most severely injured first, find and control the fire). The IC should call for additional resources and expand the command structure (e.g., get more ambulances/paramedics, sound the second alarm) as dictated by the event and release units as they are no longer needed.

Case Scenario—continued

On arriving at the staging area, you notice many people from various organizations. Police, fire, EMS, the military, construction companies, the Federal Emergency Management Association, Disaster Medical Assistance Team, the Red Cross, and the media are all present. An individual is making announcements on the public address system and providing assignments. He makes an announcement that this incident will use a unified command.

Questions

4. *Define singular command and unified command.*
5. *Who will manage large equipment from the construction companies?*
6. *Which of these groups will report to the operations commander?*

Within every incident management system should be two basic types of control: singular and unified. A **singular command** system is used in most events because it works well when only one agency responds, such as a rescue and ambulance service or fire department. A **unified command** system is used for large-scale, long-duration events and often involves many diverse agencies such as police, fire, and rescue and ambulance services. The benefit to a unified command system is that it allows the right agency to lead at the appropriate time.

Finance

Although seldom used, the finance component should not be overlooked and should be considered early as events escalate. The **finance officer** is responsible for providing accurate accounting and monitoring of all costs associated with the incident. This is an essential position in large-scale, long-term events because personnel, equipment, and supply costs often may be recovered.

Logistics

The logistics support function is responsible for the procurement, stockpiling, and distribution of equipment and supplies. This is used mainly during long-duration, large-scale events. Items the logistics function is responsible for include the following:

- Supplies and equipment
- Facilities
- Food
- Communications support
- Medical support for workers

Operations

Operations is where the hands-on work occurs in most EMS events. Through incident action planning, **operations** carries out the tactical objectives as directed by the incident commander. Divisions that fall under operations include branches, divisions and groups, and resources. These are shown in Figure 62-2 and described in Box 62-3. Most, if not all, EMS activities take place under the supervision and direction of operations, including the following:

- Carries out tactical objectives
- Directs front-end activities
- Participates in planning
- Modifies the action plan
- Accounts for personnel

Planning

Planning is typically a staff function and is used during large-scale or long-duration incidents. The **planning officer** supports the operation by providing the IC with

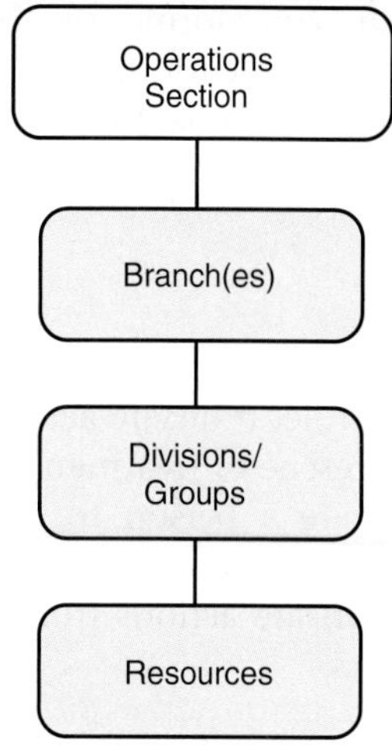

Figure 62-2 Major operational elements of operations sector.

BOX 62-3 Operational Divisions

Branches may be functional, geographic, or both, depending on the circumstances of the incident. In general, Branches are established when the number of Divisions or Groups exceeds the recommended span of control. Branches are identified by the use of Roman numerals or by functional area.

Divisions and/or Groups are established when the number of resources exceeds the manageable span of control of Incident Command and the Operations Sector Chief. Divisions are established to divide an incident into physical and/or geographic areas of operation. Groups are established to divide the incident into functional areas of operation. For certain types of incidents, for example, Incident Command may assign evacuation or mass care responsibilities to a functional group in the operations Sector. There also may be additional levels of supervision below the Division or Group level.

Resources may be organized and managed in three different ways, depending on the requirements of the incident:

- Single Resources are individual personnel or equipment and any associated operators.
- Task Forces are any combination of resources assembled in support of a specific mission or operational need. All resource elements within a Task Force must have common communications and a designated leader.
- Strike Teams are a set number of resources of the same kind and type that have an established minimum number of personnel. All resource elements within a Strike Team must have common communications and a designated leader.

The use of Task Forces and Strike Teams is encouraged when appropriate to optimize the use of resources, reduce the span of control over a large number of single resources, and reduce the complexity of incident management coordination and communications.

From FEMA (2007). *National incident management system* (pp. 53-54). Washington, DC: U.S. Department of Homeland Security.

past, present, and future information about the incident. Planning also is responsible for maintaining resource and situation status reports and having them available to the IC and other members of the command team.

Safety

Regardless of the size or magnitude of an incident, safety plays an important role. If unsafe acts are permitted, the rescuers may need rescue or treatment themselves. Many EMS systems dedicate a person to the role of **safety officer.** The sole function and responsibility of this position is to prevent unsafe actions from occurring during emergency incidents.

Additional Components

If the incident increases in size, additional components can be added to the command structure as needed. For example, a public information officer (PIO) may be identified to interact with the media based on the direction of the incident commander. A liaison officer may be identified to coordinate activities of those agencies outside the command structure. This may include utility companies or public relief agencies such as the Salvation Army or Red Cross. Figure 62-3 demonstrates the flexibility of the command system and how it may be expanded as the incident requires.

ROLE OF THE INCIDENT COMMANDER

[OBJECTIVES 13 TO 18]

The assumption of command is the first step in bringing an out-of-control situation (e.g., a major medical incident) back into control. Command is a role, not a person. The IC should select a location that affords a quiet, safe workspace (e.g., inside a vehicle) and provides visibility of the incident and the workers. As the incident escalates, the command structure becomes more pronounced. During these times, the command team should consider moving to a stationary post such as a command van (Figure 62-4). The largest of incidents require additional emergency managers and support staff. The most suitable location for this to occur is the **emergency operations center.**

Regardless of the size of the incident, the IC stays in that position until he or she passes it to a higher-ranking or more qualified person or the event is under control and command is terminated. The incident command process should be established early in the incident. Although no concrete rules exist on when command should be established, good practice suggests establishing it more often than not. This creates a higher degree of comfort with the system for both supervisors and workers. The IC is afforded practice in working with tactical worksheets and knowing which sectors to assign depending on the complexity of the event. This prepares the EMS

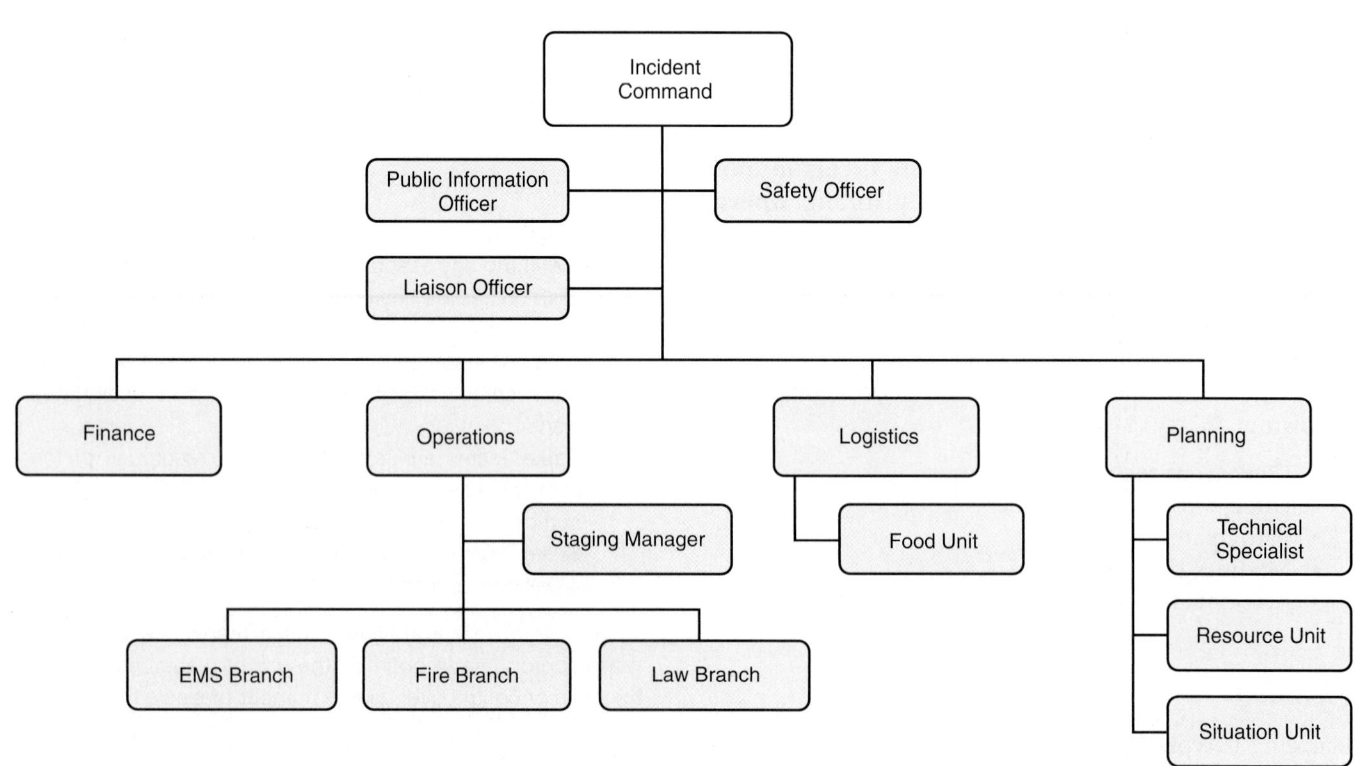

Figure 62-3 Incident command structure.

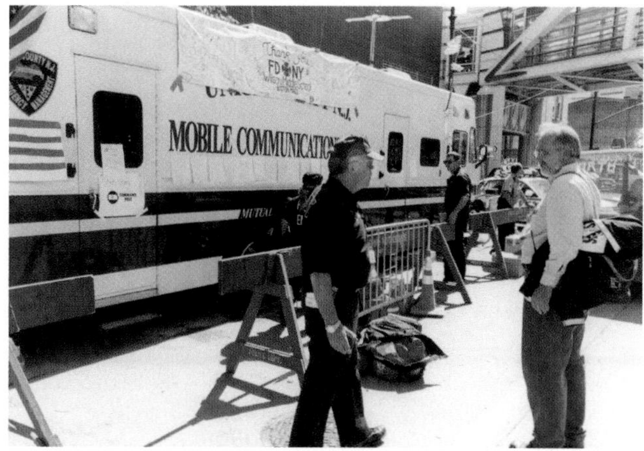

Figure 62-4 As an incident escalates, the command team should consider moving to a stationary post such as a command van.

professional for situations when a formalized command system is needed.

On arrival, the first unit should immediately size up the scene through the windshield and relay this information to others who are responding. This size-up should include the following:

- What do you have?
- What are you doing (or going to do) about it?
- What do you need?
- Where should additional responding apparatuses stage?
- Announce that you are the incident commander and the location of the command post. For example, "Medic 1 is on scene of a large tour bus . . ."

After the initial size-up, conduct a more detailed assessment of the scene. This should include the number and severity of patients as well as any special considerations such as entrapment or extrication needs. Additionally, the type of incident and incident priorities should be determined if possible. These are described in Boxes 62-4 and 62-5, respectively.

If the situation cannot be effectively managed with the resources dispatched or assigned, request additional help sooner rather than later. In many jurisdictions this may require the use of mutual aid from neighboring communities. Each agency and the appropriate communications centers should have SOPs that address mutual aid responses. If they are not needed, they can be cancelled. Updated information should be transmitted as time permits.

The IC should realize that excessive or unnecessary radio transmissions could have an adverse impact on the ability of the sector officers to manage their areas. It additionally creates a distraction for the workers within the sectors to perform effective triage, treatment, and transportation. Good communication is a skill; a difference exists between "nice to know" and "need to know" information. In dynamic, rapidly changing events, the IC may assign an aide to assist him or her in managing communications. This is especially useful if mutual aid agencies operate on different radio channels.

Assigning sectors (or divisions) early into a mass casualty event allows the IC to divide the overwhelming scene into manageable pieces. The IC places responsibility and accountability of achieving tactical objectives with the sector officer.

BOX 62-4 Types of Incidents

Closed Incident

Also referred to as a *stable incident,* this type of incident is one that is not expanding and is unlikely to generate additional patients, hazards, or damages. An example would be a motor vehicle collision.

Open Incident

Also referred to as an *unstable incident,* this type of incident is in the process of expanding or likely to expand. There is the potential for the generation of additional patients, hazards, and damages. An example would be a continuing natural disaster.

BOX 62-5 Incident Priorities

Life Safety

The first priority at any scene is the safety of emergency responders and the public.

Incident Stability

Once the safety of all persons involved has been assured, the focus can shift to stabilizing the incident. This phase can be the most varied, and the ease or difficulty in stabilizing an incident depends on if the incident is open or closed.

Property Conservation

The last priority in an incident is the conservation of property. Once life safety has been established and the incident has been stabilized, the incident commander should make attempts to minimize damage to the property surrounding the incident.

Triage

The triage officer is responsible for conducting a thorough assessment of the scene, identifying all injured or ill patients, and categorizing them by severity. These finding are reported back to the incident commander in the form of a triage report, and the patients are taken to a central location for treatment. In some jurisdictions during long-duration events, physicians may be used to aid EMTs and paramedics in making complex triage decisions.

Case Scenario CONCLUSION

Your first assignment is the triage of patients using the START triage system. You arrive at the first patient and notice that he is walking comfortably and tells you that he is okay. He does not appear in distress.

Looking Back

7. *What is the definition of triage?*
8. *What is the START triage system?*
9. *What is the most appropriate triage color for your first patient?*

Extrication and Rescue

[OBJECTIVE 19]

In many incidents extrication and rescue is needed before patients can be transferred to the treatment sector. Generally, extrication is first performed for those patients identified by the triage sector as the most critically injured. The extrication officer is responsible for coordinating extrication and rescue and determines the types of equipment and resources needed, as well as the need for specialized equipment and personnel such as a confined space rescue team or a structural collapse team. The extrication officer will work closely with personnel from the triage sector and treatment sector to determine if triage and treatment can begin while patients are entrapped or must wait until the patient is safely extricated.

Treatment

[OBJECTIVES 20, 21]

The treatment officer is responsible for coordinating the treatment of all injured and ill patients and ensuring each patient is delivered to the transport area. During most large-scale incidents the patients outnumber the paramedics. As a result, the treatment officer initially may be an EMT. In some cases a physician may be assigned to assist. Physicians may be used in the treatment area in certain situations.

As a general rule, the treatment area should be away from the incident scene. The treatment officer should maintain constant communication with the triage and transportation officers to maintain a constant flow of patients. A division of the treatment sector may include a field morgue for the deceased. Individuals involved in this division should work closely with the medical examiner, coroner, law enforcement, and other individuals to coordinate the movement of the deceased to the field morgue. When possible the field morgue should be geographically separated from the treatment area, and deceased individuals should be left where they are found until coordinated plans for their removal are made.

Transportation

The movement of patients to medical facilities is the responsibility of the transportation officer. During a large-scale incident, patients may be transported by air or ground ambulances. Coordination of these resources and connecting the right patients with the right hospitals are vital functions. The transportation officer must select a site that has adequate space and facilitates easy entrance and exit (easy in, easy out) of ambulances from the incident scene. Additionally the transportation officer is responsible for tracking the destination of patients. For this purpose a transportation log must be maintained and each patient be assigned a unique identifier. The log should include the patient identifier, destination, transporting unit, and transport priority.

Staging

In an effort to prevent bottlenecks and congestion at the incident scene, a staging area should be identified and a staging officer assigned to manage it. The staging area provides a \location for all later-arriving units to park—away from the incident scene—and be called into action as needed by the incident commander. A staging guideline should be included in the SOPs. The staging officer should track the arrival and departure of units in the staging area.

Rehabilitation

A rehabilitation (rehab) area is a key component to maintaining the health and safety of EMS professionals. The rehab area is a place where workers are provided hydration, nourishment, and medical monitoring. In addition, the rehab area offers protection from the elements. It is removed from public view whenever possible.

Safety

[OBJECTIVE 22]

A **safety officer** is a valuable resource to the incident commander. The safety officer should be empowered to

How to Use the NYS-EMS Triage Tag

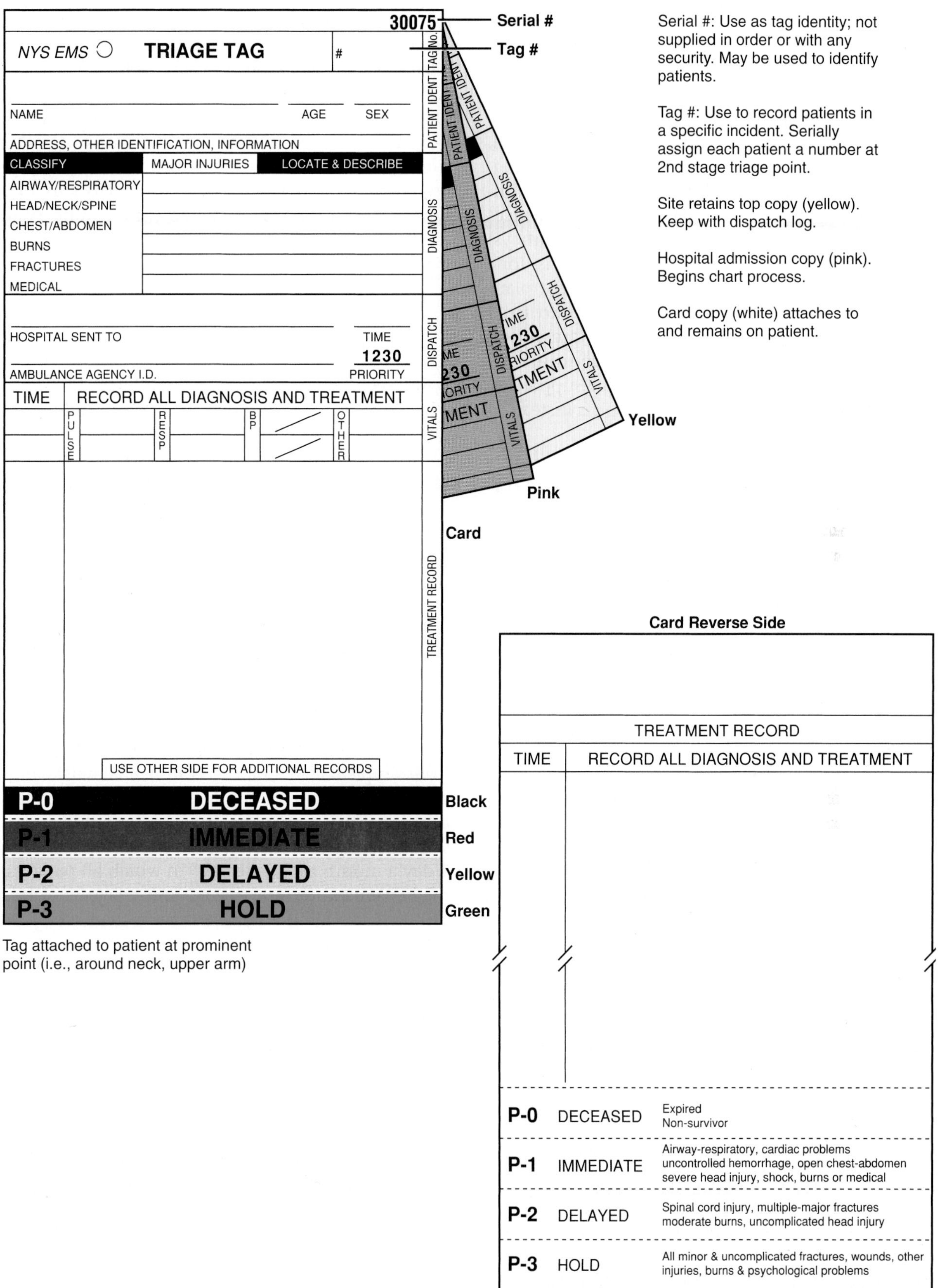
30075 — Serial #

NYS EMS TRIAGE TAG # — Tag #

PATIENT IDENT TAG No.

NAME AGE SEX

ADDRESS, OTHER IDENTIFICATION, INFORMATION

CLASSIFY	MAJOR INJURIES LOCATE & DESCRIBE
AIRWAY/RESPIRATORY	
HEAD/NECK/SPINE	
CHEST/ABDOMEN	
BURNS	
FRACTURES	
MEDICAL	

DIAGNOSIS

HOSPITAL SENT TO — TIME 1230

AMBULANCE AGENCY I.D. — PRIORITY

DISPATCH

TIME	RECORD ALL DIAGNOSIS AND TREATMENT
	PULSE / RESP / BP / OTHER

VITALS

TREATMENT RECORD

USE OTHER SIDE FOR ADDITIONAL RECORDS

P-0	DECEASED	Black
P-1	IMMEDIATE	Red
P-2	DELAYED	Yellow
P-3	HOLD	Green

Yellow

Pink

Card

Tag attached to patient at prominent point (i.e., around neck, upper arm)

Serial #: Use as tag identity; not supplied in order or with any security. May be used to identify patients.

Tag #: Use to record patients in a specific incident. Serially assign each patient a number at 2nd stage triage point.

Site retains top copy (yellow). Keep with dispatch log.

Hospital admission copy (pink). Begins chart process.

Card copy (white) attaches to and remains on patient.

Card Reverse Side

TREATMENT RECORD

TIME	RECORD ALL DIAGNOSIS AND TREATMENT

P-0	DECEASED	Expired Non-survivor
P-1	IMMEDIATE	Airway-respiratory, cardiac problems uncontrolled hemorrhage, open chest-abdomen severe head injury, shock, burns or medical
P-2	DELAYED	Spinal cord injury, multiple-major fractures moderate burns, uncomplicated head injury
P-3	HOLD	All minor & uncomplicated fractures, wounds, other injuries, burns & psychological problems

Figure 62-5 START color-coding system.

institute safety practices and stop unsafe acts from taking place during EMS events.

Logistics

The **logistics officer** is responsible for providing required equipment, materials, and supplies to the scene of an incident. Items that should be prepurchased and, in some cases, predeployed include airway, breathing, circulation, and bandaging and burn supplies. Additionally, disposable, single-use backboards and other devices used to transport patients (e.g., cots, litters, gurneys) should be considered. The majority of this work is done before the event as part of disaster or preincident planning. The value of predeployment of supplies to fixed locations (e.g., medical supply caches, warehouses) cannot be overemphasized. During the large-scale incident, the logistics officer focuses efforts on supporting the event by using those predeployed supplies instead of having to procure them.

PRINCIPLES AND TECHNIQUES OF TRIAGE

[OBJECTIVES 23 TO 28]

Triage is the sorting of patients into categories according to the severity of their injury or illness to prioritize who receives treatment in which order. Triage methods used at the major incident scene should be simple, quick, and require minimal equipment or tools. Most triage programs in use by EMS systems throughout the United States use some sort of method to identify patient condition at a glance.

During a large-scale incident, the first personnel to arrive should conduct a **primary triage** to separate the most critically injured from the other patients. After this is completed, a **secondary triage** is performed to identify the most critical (of those remaining) and the order of treatment.

Over the past several years, a triage method called *START* (***s***imple ***t***riage ***a***nd ***r***apid ***t***reatment) has gained wide acceptance by EMS professionals across the nation. START was developed by the Hoag Memorial Hospital in Newport Beach, Calif., to triage patients quickly during a major medical event. START quickly differentiates critically ill victims from the less severely injured.

Following a specific process, an EMS professional quickly assesses airway, respiration, pulse, and mental status (RPM) to categorize patients into one of four categories: immediate, delayed, minor, or dead/dying. Using START, a triage team of two EMS professionals should be able to triage an average of one patient every 30 seconds. The only treatment rendered by the triage team is to open a patient's airway by head tilt/chin lift or placing an oral airway or by applying direct pressure to stop obvious bleeding.

START has been adopted by many jurisdictions throughout the United States and has been successfully used during many large-scale events. START uses the following internationally accepted color-coding system to identify patients (Figure 62-5):

- Immediate: Red
- Delayed: Yellow
- Minor: Green
- Dead or dying: Black

Immediate patients have an altered RPM. Patients who have intact RPM but are unable to follow instructions to move to a treatment area are delayed, which is the most common category. Patients with significant mechanism of injury but an intact RPM are placed into the delayed category. Minor (not to be confused with pediatric) patients are the "walking wounded"—those who are able to leave the area on the instruction of EMS personnel. The dead or dying are those who cannot breathe after the airway is opened or are mortally wounded.

As patients are triaged, their priority should be identified with some type of colored marking or "tag" so that personnel from the extrication and or treatment sector can quickly identify which patients should be treated first. There are many variations of triage tags available, from simple flagging tape to commercial wrist bands. The paramedic should be familiar with the type of tag used by his or her service in order to be familiar with the system when it is needed. Many EMS services designate 1 day a month as "triage day" in which all patients paramedics encounter are triaged and triage tags are used. This ensures familiarity with the system when a large-scale event occurs. Regardless of the method used, the tag should meet the following criteria:

- Be easy to use
- Rapidly identify priority
- Allow for easy tracking
- Allow for some documentation
- Prevent patients from re-triaging themselves

Case Scenario SUMMARY

1. *What are the differences among a multiple-patient incident, a multiple-casualty incident, and a disaster?* A multiple-patient incident involves two to 25 persons. A multiple-casualty incident involves 26 to 99 persons, and a disaster describes incidents that involve 100 or more patients. In this scenario determining the type of incident is impossible from this dispatch information.
2. *What is the national incident management system?* NIMS provides a standardized strategy to approach incident management and response. All local, state,

tribal, and federal governments were required to be trained in NIMS and its use by the end of 2007. This levels the playing field and ensures that all responders have an identical foundation for coordinated incident response to manage a host of situations from an all-hazards perspective. Additionally, NIMS provides a common language and terminology to address different incident types and identify the resources needed to manage them.

3. *What are the basic elements of NIMS?* Command, finance, logistics, operations, planning, and safety.
4. *Define singular command and unified command.* A singular command system is used in most of events because it works well when only one agency responds, such as a rescue and ambulance service or fire department. A unified command system is used for large-scale, long-duration events and often involves many diverse agencies such as police, fire, and rescue and ambulance services. The benefit to a unified command system is that it allows the right agency to lead at the appropriate time.
5. *Who will manage large equipment from the construction companies?* The logistics officer is typically responsible for supplies, equipment, facilities, food, communications support, and medical support for workers. EMS providers do not typically report to logistics unless the incident is very large and a separate location is designated for medical support for workers. In any large-scale event, focus your attention on directions, your assignment, and your reporting location.
6. *Which of these groups will report to the operations commander?* The operations officer is responsible for the Federal Emergency Management Association, EMS, fire, police, and the Disaster Medical Assistance Team. In general, operations carries out tactical objectives, directs front-end activities, participates in planning, modifies the action plan, and accounts for personnel.
7. *What is the definition of triage?* Triage is the sorting of patients into categories according to the severity of their injury or illness to prioritize who receives treatment in which order. Triage methods used at the major incident scene should be simple, quick, and require minimal equipment or tools. Most triage programs in use by EMS systems throughout the United States use some sort of method to identify patient condition at a glance. Many think triage is simple. However, in mass casualty incidents or disasters it can be a daunting task. Triage should be practiced during training and planning sessions.
8. *What is the START triage system?* START stands for ***s**imple **t**riage **a**nd **r**apid **t**reatment. This method quickly distinguishes critically ill victims from the less severely injured. Following a specific process, an EMS professional quickly assesses RPM to categorize a patient into one of four categories: immediate, delayed, minor, or dead or dying. The only treatment rendered by the team is to open a patient's airway by head tilt/neck lift or by placing an oral airway or applying direct pressure or elevating the extremities to stop obvious bleeding. The purpose is to identify people who are the most critical and need medical attention first.
9. *What is the most appropriate triage color for your first patient?* The patient in this scenario should receive a green tag. All patients found in the area should be tagged, which will avoid triaging people twice.

Chapter Summary

- Basic elements of the ICS include command, finance, logistics, operations, planning, and safety.
- The incident commander's role includes triage, treatment, transportation, staging, rehabilitation, safety, and logistics.
- Critical components to any ICS include a uniform, consistent set of rules, and a common language.
- The most important component to any ICS is communications.
- The incident commander is responsible for or delegates the creation an action plan and manages the event at the highest level by establishing strategic objectives and tactical priorities.
- The finance officer is responsible for providing accurate accounting and monitoring of all costs associated with the incident.
- The planning officer supports the operation by providing the incident commander with past, present, and future information about the incident.
- The incident commander places responsibility and accountability of achieving tactical objectives with the sector officer.
- The logistics officer is responsible for providing required equipment, material, and supplies to the scene of an incident.
- The triage officer is responsible for conducting a thorough assessment of the scene, identifying all injured and ill patients, and categorizing them by severity.
- The treatment officer is responsible for coordinating the treatment of all injured and ill patients and ensuring each patient is delivered to the transport area.

Chapter Summary—continued

- The movement of patients to medical facilities is the responsibility of the transportation officer.
- In an effort to prevent bottlenecks and congestion at the incident scene, a staging area and a staging officer should be identified. The staging officer should track the arrival and departure of units in the staging area.
- A rehabilitation area is a place where workers are provided hydration, nourishment, and medical monitoring.
- The safety officer institutes safety practices and stops unsafe acts from taking place during EMS events.
- Principles and techniques of triage are applied in two stages in large-scale incidents.

REFERENCE

Federal Emergency Management Agency. (2004). *National Incident Management System (NIMS), an introduction.* Retrieved April 11, 2007, from http://training.fema.gov.

SUGGESTED RESOURCES

FEMA National Incident Management System
FEMA 500 C Street SW
Washington, DC 20472
Phone: 800-621-FEMA
Website: http://www.fema.gov

Department of Homeland Security
National Response Plan
Washington, DC 20528
Operator: (202) 282-8000
Comment line: (202) 282-8495
Website: http://www.dhs.gov

Chapter Quiz

1. What is the optimal number of resources the incident commander can effectively manage within the span of control?

2. What is the difference between a multiple-patient incident and a multiple-casualty incident?

3. What does CFLOPS stand for? Give a one-sentence summary of its use within the ICS.

4. What are the two types of command within the ICS?

5. During the largest of incidents, what is the most suitable location for incident commanders and support staff?

6. What are the components of the first unit's size-up of an emergency scene?

7. Discuss the importance of good communications.

8. What is the method of triage, developed in California, that has gained wide acceptance in the last several years?

9. How are patients categorized by START triage?

10. What is the role of the safety officer during an emergency incident?

Terminology

Disaster An incident involving 100 or more persons.

Emergency operations center A gathering point for strategic policymakers during an emergency incident.

Finance officer The person responsible for providing a cost analysis of an incident.

Incident commander The person responsible for the overall management of an emergency scene.

Logistics officer The person responsible for assembling supplies used during an incident.

Multiple-casualty incident An incident involving 26 to 99 persons.

Multiple-patient incident An incident involving two to 25 persons.

Operations Carries out the tactical objectives of the incident commander.

Planning Supplies past, present, and future information about the incident.

Primary triage The initial sorting of patients to determine which are most injured and in need of immediate care.

Safety officer The person responsible for ensuring that no unsafe acts occur during the emergency incident.

Secondary triage Conducted after the primary search; determines the order of treatment and transport of the remaining patients.

Singular command Command type involving one agency.

Span of control The amount of resources that one person can effectively manage.

Standard operating procedures (SOPs) An organized set of guidelines distributed across the organization.

Unified command Command type involving multiple agencies.

CHAPTER
63

Vehicle Rescue and Rescue Awareness Operations

Objectives *After completing this chapter, you will be able to:*

1. Define the term *rescue.*
2. Explain the medical and mechanical aspects of rescue situations.
3. Explain the role of the paramedic in delivering care at the rescue site and continuing through the rescue process to definitive care.
4. Describe the three levels of skills for responders to a technical rescue incident and how they differ.
5. Describe in order the priorities for safety in any rescue.
6. Describe the phases of a rescue operation.
7. List the three capabilities that situational awareness gives the emergency responder.
8. List and describe the types of personal protective equipment needed to operate safely in the rescue environment, including head protection, eye protection, hand protection, personal flotation devices, thermal protection and layering systems, high-visibility clothing, and specialized footwear.
9. Integrate the principles of rescue awareness and operations to rescue patients from highway incidents.
10. Have a working knowledge of various technologic improvements found on vehicles today that can affect emergency medical, safety, and extrication and rescue operations at motor vehicle incidents.
11. Explain supplemental restraint and airbag systems as well as methods to neutralize them.
12. Describe the necessary practices and procedures to resolve concerns presented by a hybrid gasoline and electric vehicle involved in a fire, crash, or extrication incident.
13. List and describe the major categories of safety hazards related to EMS personnel working at vehicle crash, fire, and rescue incidents.
14. Describe the electrical hazards (above and below ground) commonly found at highway incidents.
15. List the four phases of rescue for dealing with entrapment and extrication at a crash scene and describe the individual extrication tasks that comprise each phase of the process.
16. Explain typical door anatomy and methods to access stuck doors.
17. Develop specific skills in emergency stabilization of vehicles and access procedures and an awareness of specific extrication strategies.
18. Explain assessment procedures and modifications necessary when caring for entrapped patients.
19. Explain the differences in risk between moving water and flat water rescue.
20. Given a picture of moving water, identify and explain the features and hazards associated with hydraulics, strainers, and dams and hydroelectric sites.
21. Explain the effects of immersion hypothermia on the ability to survive sudden immersion and self-rescue.
22. Explain the phenomenon of the cold protective response in cold water drowning situations.
23. Given a list of rescue scenarios, identify the victim survivability profile and differentiate rescue versus body recovery situations.
24. Explain specific methods for assessment and spinal stabilization.
25. Explain why water entry techniques are methods of last resort.
26. Explain the rescue techniques associated with "talk, reach, throw, row."
27. Explain the self-rescue position if unexpectedly immersed in moving water.
28. Given a series of pictures, identify which would be considered confined spaces and potentially oxygen deficient.
29. Identify the hazards associated with confined spaces and risks posed to potential rescuers, including oxygen deficiency, chemical or toxic exposure or explosion, engulfment, machinery entrapment, and electricity.
30. Identify the poisonous gases commonly found in confined spaces, including hydrogen sulfide, carbon dioxide, carbon monoxide, low and high oxygen concentrations, methane, ammonia, and nitrogen dioxide.
31. Identify components necessary to ensure site safety before confined space rescue attempts.
32. Explain the hazard of cave-in during trench rescue operations.
33. Define *low angle, high angle, belay, rappel,* and *scrambling.*
34. Explain the different types of rescue litters and the advantages and disadvantages associated with each.
35. Describe the procedure for basket litter packaging for low-angle evacuations.
36. Develop proficiency in patient packaging and evacuation techniques that pertain to hazardous or rescue environments.
37. Explain the procedures for low-angle litter evacuation, including anchoring, litter and rope attachment, and lowering and raising procedures.
38. Explain nontechnical high-angle rescue procedures with an aerial apparatus.

Chapter Outline

Case Scenario

You and your partner are dispatched to a construction site for a "construction accident." As you drive through the gate, you initially see only a small group of workers looking down at something. Some of the workers motion you to come to the area. As you get closer, you see that the men are looking down into a trench. You get out of your vehicle and walk to the edge. You see that a portion of the approximately 10-foot-wide trench has collapsed. At approximately 11 feet down is a worker in soil up to his groin. He appears unresponsive, but breathing. His construction helmet was knocked off in the collapse. Also in the trench are two workers with shovels trying to uncover the victim. You notice that in the soil along the edge of the trench are cracks running parallel to the trench. The weather is warm, the first warm temperatures after a long cold spell. You and your partner are trained at the "awareness" level of technical rescue skill.

Questions

1. *What is your initial size-up of the scene?*
2. *What are your priorities?*
3. *What should your first actions be?*

Paramedics often are called for patient care at the scene of technical rescues. A rescue might be relatively simple, such as a rescue involving a motor vehicle accident. In contrast, it could be more complex, such as one involving a trench collapse or a confined space accident. The latter rescue may involve many responders and take a long time to complete. This chapter introduces you to the types of rescue you may encounter as a paramedic as well as the roles and responsibilities of paramedics in rescue.

ROLE OF THE PARAMEDIC IN RESCUE OPERATIONS

[OBJECTIVE 1]

The definition of **rescue** is the act of delivery from danger or entrapment. The sequence of rescue activities includes locating endangered persons at an emergency incident, removing those persons from danger, treating the injured, and transporting the injured to an appropriate healthcare facility.

Rescue: A Patient-Driven Event

Rescue is a patient-driven event. Without a patient, rescue is not needed. Most rescue situations usually require patient care. Additionally, each rescue situation requires understanding of the hazards to rescuers and patients. These situations also require knowledge of the specialized needs of the patient and the skills needed for the particular rescue.

Throughout the rescue operation, you must continue to relate to the patient both physically and through communication to reassure and carefully explain what is happening regarding to the progress of the rescue. You also must show your awareness of the patient in the physical sense. This means making the patient as comfortable as possible and making sure that all elements of the operation show concern for the patient. Just as in a routine EMS call, medical personnel in a rescue must monitor the patient and provide care throughout the rescue operation.

Medical and Technical Skills of Rescue

[OBJECTIVES 2, 3]

Most rescues involve medical skills along with mechanical skills, commonly known as *technical skills*. Depending on the particular rescue, a combination of medical and mechanical skills must be applied in the correct amount and at the appropriate time. Medical care and rescue are sometimes referred to as two different actions. However, this artificial separation does not reflect real-life conditions in which medical care and rescue functions need to be performed at the same time. The rescue patient usually needs both rescue and urgent medical care. The patient's medical condition may be critical, and medical care cannot be delayed until the rescue is completed and the patient transported.

On occasion some rescuers may become so engrossed in the technical challenges of rescue that they lose sight of the reason why they are there—the patient. Rescuers and medical providers must together evaluate the rescue techniques for their effects on the patient's medical outcome. On occasion you may have to decide which has priority: a rescue technique or a medical procedure. For example, should intravenous (IV) lines be established before the patient is moved? Is the environment too hazardous to begin medical care?

The roles of the paramedic include awareness of the situation of the rescue, an understanding of the hazards involved for the paramedic and the patient, and knowledge of the rescue skills needed to take part in the physical rescue.

Managing rescue and providing medical care at the same time requires careful preparation and realistic training. In addition, some rescue environments are hazardous both to the patient and rescuers. Consequently, you must tend to your safety and survival while helping with the patient's safety and survival. In some cases the rescued patient is a good distance from the ambulance or helicopter, so you often must improvise medical equipment and be able to tend to the patient over an extended period.

Rescue often involves an individual who also needs urgent medical care. Following are important basic points regarding the rescue process:

- Patients must be accessed and assessed for treatment needs. As with other EMS calls, rescue patients first must be assessed for the nature of their injuries and medical conditions before treatment is begun.
- Assessment and treatment must begin at the accident site, except in cases in which the patient and rescuers are in immediate danger.
- The patient must be released from entrapment.
- Medical care must continue throughout the incident.

As first responders to many rescue incidents, paramedics need to do the following:

- Understand hazards associated with various environments
- Know when gaining access or attempting rescue would be safe or unsafe
- Have skills to carry out a rescue when safe and necessary
- Understand the rescue process and when certain techniques are indicated or contraindicated

Each skill or technique requires specialized training to perform and to avoid injury to the rescuer and further injury to the patient. A rescue that requires specialized knowledge and skills often is called a *technical rescue* (Box 63-1).

BOX 63-1 What Is Technical Rescue?

Technical rescue is the application of special knowledge, skills, and equipment to resolve unique or complex rescue situations safely. Technical rescue disciplines include rope rescue, swift water rescue, dive rescue, confined space rescue, snow and ice rescue, cave rescue, and trench or excavation rescue, among others. In the United States, technical rescues often have multiple jurisdictions operating together to carry out the rescue and often use the ICS to manage the incident and resources at the scene.

ICS, Incident command system.

BOX 63-2 Who Decides Who Is Qualified?

According to NFPA 1670 (2004 edition), the "authority having jurisdiction" shall establish levels of operational capability needed to conduct operations at technical rescue incidents. These capabilities are based on a community hazard analysis, risk assessment, training level of personnel, and availability of internal and external resources.

From National Fire Protection Association. (2004). *NFPA standard on operations and training for technical search and rescue incidents.* Quincy, MA: National Fire Protection Association.

SKILL LEVELS FOR RESCUERS

[OBJECTIVE 4]

Three levels of skills for responders to a technical rescue incident are recognized: *awareness, operations,* and *technician.* Local disagreement may exist regarding how these skill levels are defined. However, the National Fire Protection Association (NFPA) standard 1670, *Standard on Operations and Training for Technical Rescue Incidents* (NFPA, 2004), provides standardized definitions. Similar skill levels are outlined by the Safety and Health Administration and Environmental Protection Agency for hazardous materials response (see Chapter 64). This chapter focuses on the awareness and operations levels (Box 63-2).

The NFPA standard does not detail specifics of the training and qualifications from responders at each level but leaves that to the **authority having jurisdiction (AHJ).** The AHJ is the local agency that has legal authority for the type of rescue and the location where it occurs.

Awareness

According to the NFPA, the awareness level represents "the minimum capability of a responder who, in the course of his or her regular job duties, could be called upon to respond to, or could be the first on the scene of, a technical rescue incident. This level can involve search, rescue, and recovery operations. Members of a team at this level generally are not considered rescuers" (NFPA,

2004). This level of provider usually remains safe in the cold zone, and the rescuers bring the patient to them.

Operations

The operations level represents "the capability of hazard recognition, equipment use, and techniques necessary to safely and effectively support and participate in a technical rescue incident. This level can involve search, rescue, and recovery operations, but usually operations are carried out under the supervision of technician-level personnel" (NFPA, 2004). When properly trained and equipped, this level of provider may participate in the rescue in a support manner.

Technician

The technician level represents "the capability of hazard recognition, equipment use, and techniques necessary to safely and effectively coordinate, perform, and supervise a technical rescue incident. This level can involve search, rescue, and recovery operations" (NFPA, 2004).

The 1670 standard states that minimal training for all members of EMS should include the awareness level, leaving training for the higher levels to interested rescuers (NFPA, 2004). The technician level of provider may have planning and direction responsibility.

As a possible responder to a technical rescue, you must know under whose authority you are working and what skill level of response you are qualified to provide. You should plan for technical rescue calls with the appropriate training and equipment.

All responders to technical rescue incidents should be trained at least to the awareness level. This means that everyone involved in the rescue, not just those at the technician level, are aware of safety issues, understand the resource needs, can assist the responders at operations and technical levels, and can assist in managing the scene. Paramedics at this level often are called on to provide medical support to the other rescue personnel who may be more directly involved in the rescue.

SAFETY IN RESCUE OPERATIONS

EMS responders tend to be action-oriented people, so when they arrive at the scene of a rescue and see a person in distress, they believe they must do something. Unfortunately numerous responder injuries and deaths have occurred because the potential rescuer did not step back and evaluate the dangers before rushing in to rescue. The hard decision for a responder is to sometimes simply stand and watch while the site is cleared of dangers or more qualified personnel arrive. The first responders at any scene should perform a risk analysis to determine the risk versus benefit of gaining immediate access to a patient or awaiting the arrival of trained, competent technical rescue personnel.

Priorities for Safety in Rescue

[OBJECTIVE 5]

The most critical concern in any rescue is safety. Numerous kinds of hazards are found at rescue sites. Common hazards include hazardous materials, electrical hazards, fire, unstable structures, and traffic. The priorities for safety in any rescue are as follows:

1. Personal safety
2. Safety for the rescue team
3. Safety of bystanders and other uninvolved persons
4. Safety of the rescue patient

The reasons for this priority include the following:

- By being alert to your own safety, you avoid injury or death, which would add another person to be rescued and reduce the number of capable rescuers.
- With rescue team members involved in a joint effort for safety, they avoid injuries to the team members, which would complicate the rescue (risk versus benefit).
- Bystanders and others not directly needed for the rescue unnecessarily complicate the rescue and endanger themselves, so they must be moved from the rescue area.
- The last concern is that of the patient or the person who is entrapped and/or injured. The first three priorities must be achieved before the rescue of the patient so that no one is further injured, complicating the rescue.

PHASES OF A RESCUE OPERATION

[OBJECTIVE 6]

Arrival and Scene Size-Up

When EMS personnel are the first at the rescue site, they must first size up the scene for any risks to rescuers and report them to incoming responders. Size-up begins as soon as a unit is dispatched, continues during response, and continues after arrival on scene.

During response, the responders must obtain as much specific information as possible. Dispatch should provide the basic information, including nature of the incident, known patient condition, and location. As with other EMS calls, you may find on the scene that the circumstances are completely different from the information first provided in dispatch. Mistakes may exist in location or patient condition, so be alert to updates and corrections.

Rescue environments pose risks to responders. In some cases the risks are not obvious to those without training. Rescuers must know the potential risks they face as well as the risks to the patient.

Command and Scene Assessment

Every rescue requires coherent coordination and management. If you are first at the scene, establish an incident command system (see Chapter 62). The incident command system allows the command structure to be stepped up if the incident becomes larger and more complicated. You must establish the immediate priorities, particularly the safety needs for incoming responders and the patient.

Number of Patients and Triage

If the rescue is a multiple-casualty incident, begin triage. If the rescue is for one person, then assess the patient's medical needs and establish priorities if it is safe to do so.

Search and Rescue versus Body Recovery

If the location of the victim is unknown, then you must begin a search. Depending on the nature of the incident, the search may be as simple as establishing the specific area of an industrial plant in which the patient is located, or searching a collapsed building or backcountry.

If the victim is dead, the urgency diminishes. You must not risk injury or death for a body recovery.

Risk versus Benefit Analysis

One important step is a risk versus benefit analysis. This means determining whether the potential rescue strategy is worth the potential dangers. For example, does the patient's condition warrant the risk of a helicopter rescue?

Additional Resources

With information from the previous steps, you must decide if additional resources are needed. One way that rescues commonly go wrong is when initial responders miscalculate the needed resources because they "don't want to bother other people." This attitude can lead to serious consequences, including delays in rescue and threats to the life of the patient or the potential rescuers.

Command and Control

Management of the incident begins at the initial response by using the incident command system (ICS). Because of the modular nature of ICS, management of the incident can be maintained as the incident escalates.

Among the first steps is establishing the immediate priorities, especially the safety of responders, other emergency workers, and other persons. This includes establishment of safe zones and exclusion of all persons not immediately involved in the emergency. These zones should be made visible to all. This often is done with scene control tape or barricades.

An incident action plan should include overall incident objectives, strategies, and tactics to deploy. The plan should evolve and be updated through ongoing size-up of the incident and its needs.

Time to Access and Evacuate

One common pitfall in technical rescue is making an overly optimistic prediction of how long the operation will take. This may come from inexperienced technical rescue personnel or pressure on rescue personnel from the incident commander to "get it done." Continuous status and progress reports should be provided to the incident commander from the tactical-level rescue personnel.

Hazard Control

In the hazard control phase of the rescue, the first arriving personnel identify the hazards and make the scene as safe as possible. The units first on scene also must identify the hazards for the units being dispatched or en route. This may involve shoring up partially collapsed buildings or removing debris from the top of a cliff.

Situational Awareness

[OBJECTIVE 7]

Most accidents that happen during rescue operations are caused by human error, not equipment failure. Rescuers commit errors during emergency operations because of stress, poor communication, and the responsibility for too many tasks.

Military pilots often are faced with similar problems, which can lead to crashes. To reduce the number of crashes, the military developed the concept of **situational awareness** (Box 63-3). This concept has now been adopted throughout aviation and increasingly in other dynamic, complex situations requiring human control.

Situational awareness is being aware of everything occurring in the surrounding environment and the relative importance of all these elements. Because your environment is constantly evolving, you also must be aware of any changes and the relevance of these changes.

Situational awareness is essential for safe operations and effective decision making. This is true for all EMS calls, not only those involving rescue operations.

One important function on the incident command staff is that of the safety officer. As stated by the Occupational Safety and Health Administration (OSHA) (2004),

> The safety officer's role is to develop and recommend measures to the [incident commander] for ensuring personnel health and safety and to assess and/or anticipate hazardous and unsafe situations. The safety officer also develops the site safety plan, reviews the incident action plan for safety implications, and provides timely, complete, specific, and accurate assessment of hazards and required controls. This safety plan has a component to provide medical care to other rescuers that are part of the rescue operation.

One reason for placing the safety function with the incident commander staff instead of operations, for example, is so that the safety officer has an overall view of the rescue and is not drawn into the specific functioning of another portion of the rescue.

Gaining Access to the Patient

Access refers to the safest and most expedient way to reach the patient. You must determine the best method to gain access to the patient, deploy personnel to the patient, and stabilize the physical location of the patient.

BOX 63-3 Maintaining Situational Awareness in Emergencies

Situational awareness refers to the emergency responder's ability to do the following:

- Maintain an accurate perception of the external environment.
- Identify the source and nature of problems.
- Detect a situation requiring action.

Factors That Diminish Situational Awareness

- Insufficient communication
- Fatigue and stress
- Task overload
- Task underload and boredom
- Group mindset
- A philosophy of "press on, regardless"
- Degraded operating conditions
- Rapidly changing and unplanned operational conditions

Ways to Prevent Loss of Situational Awareness

- Actively question and evaluate the progress of the mission.
- Analyze one's own individual situation.
- Update and revise one's image of the mission.
- Use assertive behavior when necessary.
  - Make suggestions.
  - Provide relevant information without being asked.
  - Ask questions as necessary.
  - Confront ambiguities.
  - State one's opinion on decisions and procedures.
  - Refuse unreasonable requests.

Remember: It Is OK to Say No!

Modified from the U.S. Navy Situational Awareness Training Program. Prepared by Ken Phillips, Grand Canyon National Park Search and Rescue.

In some types of rescue, such as confined space rescue, access to the patient may be the most difficult phase of the rescue. Access also means freeing the patient from entrapment or hazardous situations.

Stabilization

Stabilization involves medical stabilization and monitoring of the patient. It also might involve physically stabilizing the patient in a litter so that the transport of the litter does not add to the injuries. This is often called *patient packaging.* The stabilization phase of the rescued patient continues during transport. In some rescue environments, such as in a vertical rescue, this phase may be challenging.

Medical Treatment

You should provide medical treatment appropriate to the rescue situation. Patient treatment must begin at the site and continue from first contact with the patient until definitive medical care. On reaching the patient, perform a rapid initial assessment to identify and manage life-threatening issues. If possible, initiate critical stabilization, such as airway management and oxygenation, spinal stabilization, and IV fluid therapy. In a longer evacuation, this could involve temperature control, nutrition, and elimination.

In addition to the medical needs of the patient, you must deal with the technical challenges of extrication. You, as a paramedic, may not be directly involved in the physical aspects of the rescue. However, you have primary responsibility for patient care, so you must be aware of any hazards to the patient during rescue. Unless hazards (e.g., rock fall, rising floodwaters) or overwhelming medical needs are present, you must evaluate and treat urgent conditions before the patient is moved.

Disentanglement

Disentanglement is releasing the patient from physical entrapment. It may mean, for example, clearing a pathway through wreckage to reach the patient. The disentanglement techniques must be driven by the patient's needs and take into account both rescuer and patient safety. Disentanglement could involve the use of specialized equipment and techniques.

Patient Packaging

Patient **packaging** is preparing the patient for transport by physically securing him or her to prevent additional injury. It involves stabilizing the patient in a litter or other transport device. This stabilizing includes making the patient as comfortable as possible, protecting the patient from environmental factors, and protecting any medical equipment that must accompany the patient.

Patients should be packaged to ensure their medical needs are addressed and to make them physically secure to prevent additional injury. Depending on the nature of the rescue, patient packaging could involve the use of specialized equipment and techniques.

Transportation and Evacuation

The transport of the patient may be as quick and simple as placing the patient in an ambulance or helicopter. In contrast, it could involve hours of lengthy transport from a backcountry area. The nature of the patient transportation, such as in a litter, must be planned before the patient is secured.

During some types of transportation advanced medical procedures, such as intubation or insertion of IV lines, may be difficult to perform. You must decide whether to perform these procedures before or after transportation. In addition, the patient should be packaged so that you can monitor airway, pulse, and other medical conditions.

The route of evacuation may not be the same one the rescuers used to access the patient, and as such the rescuers must continually evaluate the best route by which to deliver the patient to the transporting unit.

RESCUER PERSONAL PROTECTIVE EQUIPMENT

[OBJECTIVE 8]

Personal protective equipment (PPE) includes clothing and equipment used by a responder that protect the wearer from injury and death. A variety of rescue environments is always possible; note that the same PPE is not appropriate in all situations. The PPE must be appropriate for the type of situation encountered. EMS personnel potentially involved in rescue operations should have access to PPE described below.

Personal Protection from Blood-Borne Pathogens

See Chapter 31 for a full description of PPE that is appropriate in a setting at risk for blood-borne pathogens.

Helmets

Head protection is one type of PPE that often is forgotten in EMS, with devastating consequences. Currently no standard exists for head protection specific to ground EMS responders, but NFPA's *Standard on Protective Ensemble for USAR Operations* includes guidelines for helmets used in urban search and rescue (USAR). This guideline is part of the NFPA recommendations. A compact firefighter's helmet that meets NFPA standards is adequate for most vehicle and structural applications.

Helmets for High-Angle Rescue

Helmets to be used in high-angle rescue protect the wearer from injury and can reduce the severity of injury from falls by the wearer as well as falling objects found in many rescue situations. Avoid fire helmets with extended brims because they can obstruct vision. High-angle helmets should have a secure chin strap to prevent the helmet from falling off the head when the wearer falls or is hit by falling objects.

Helmets for Water Rescue

Water rescue helmets should be compact but have a wraparound design to protect the skull, temple, and base of neck. These helmets should have ports that drain water and a lining that does not absorb water. The chin strap should have a quick-release buckle.

Eye Protection

The rescuer's eyes must be protected from a variety of hazards, including falling and flying debris, dust and metal particles, smoke and noxious gases, chemicals, and blood-borne pathogens. Ordinary prescription glasses and the face shield on most fire helmets do not provide adequate protection. The best eye protection in most rescue environments would be American National Standards Institute (ANSI) approved safety glasses or goggles with side shields (ANSI Z87.1). Some wraparound styles of goggles fit comfortably over prescription glasses.

Hearing Protection

You often will be subjected to high-noise environments in extrication situations. As a result, you should have earplugs or earmuffs with you. In some environments auscultation may require specially adapted stethoscopes. Patient communication also may require special systems.

Hand Protection

Finding the right hand protection for all rescue situations is a challenge. Gloves need to protect the hands from cuts and punctures yet allow dexterity and protection from blood-borne pathogens. Medical examination gloves may need to be worn under outer protective gauntlets.

To cover all situations, you should have three types of gloves: examination gloves for patient care; work gloves for situations that pose higher physical hazards, such as extrication (NFPA 1999 indicates cut-resistant leather); and cleaning gloves for handling and cleaning contaminated EMS equipment for barrier protection.

Foot Protection

Foot protection depends on the expected rescue environment. Backcountry rescues that may require hiking require different footwear from water rescue or vehicle rescue. All footwear should have ankle support to limit range of motion and reduce the chances for ankle injury. The footwear should be cut and puncture resistant and provide toe safety and barrier protection.

Standards for footwear include NFPA 1999 EMS standards (footwear) and ANSI Z41, 1991 American National Standard for Personal Protective Footwear.

Clothing

Clothing for rescuers must provide a variety of services:

- Protection from blood and body fluids.
- Resistance to chemicals commonly found at accident scenes, including battery acid, gasoline, hydraulic fluid, aqueous film–forming foam, and swimming pool chlorine solution.
- Resistance to wind chill. Clothing must block the wind, keeping the wearer warmer and more protected from the elements. Clothing should remain windproof after repeated use and laundering.

- Resistance to rain (may be required in certain circumstances to allow for sweat to "breathe" away from clothing to maintain inner insulation value in cold environments).
- High visibility.
- Resistance to tearing and cutting.
- The ability to wick sweat away from the skin. This is especially important in extended and backcountry operations.

Fire and Flight Operations

Polybenzimidazole flame-retardant cotton and Nomex (DuPont, Wilmington, Del.) are designed to provide limited flash protection as jumpsuits and coveralls. This clothing does not provide complete protection from punctures or cuts. The thermal protection provided by this type of clothing may increase heat stress.

Highway Operations

For safe operations, you should be particularly concerned with being visible, especially on roads. Clothing should include reflective trim on all outerwear. High-visibility yellow clothing or safety vests should be used during highway operations.

Cold Weather

Most EMS personnel are accustomed to working in relatively warm areas, such as heated ambulances and hospitals, so their work uniforms tend to be rather light. Outside the ambulance, however, EMS personnel are as susceptible to cold injury as anyone else, and you must take the time to dress appropriately for outside exposure.

Hypothermia can quickly mean less dexterity in limbs and confused decision making. Less-obvious hazards include helicopter downdrafts and airplane prop wash, which can create intense wind chill dangers.

The cold weather ensemble should include cold weather gloves, because handling of litters and other equipment can contribute to frostbite. Moreover, you should wear a hat because up to 40% of body warmth can be lost through the head. Insulated boots or other warm footwear are also recommended.

For EMS personnel working for extended periods in the cold, the basic principle is to maintain warmth when needed but also allow the body to lose warmth before becoming overheated. Responders in the cold can wear an insulating layer with a windproof and water-resistant shell over that to protect the insulating layer from precipitation. The shell should have a means of venting in case of overheating, such as zippers in the front and at the armpits.

Underwear made from artificial fibers such as polyester pile is commonly used by people in the outdoors. But responders in an environment with the danger of flashover, such as in a helicopter, should be cautious of wearing this type of fabric next to the skin because it can melt when subjected to high heat.

Personal Flotation Devices

A personal flotation device (PFD) is a necessity for anyone responding to a water rescue and working on and around water. The PFD must meet Coast Guard standards for flotation. The type III PFD is preferred for most rescue work. The PFD should have an attached whistle, strobe light, and safe cutting knife.

Never wear turnout gear, turnout boots, or wildland or structure fire helmets when working in the water or within 10 feet of water. Each of these items makes swimming in moving water more hazardous.

Dehydration can occur even in cold weather, so rescuers should have access to water. In addition, they should have high-energy snacks. A rehabilitation unit should be established under the ICS with designated EMS personnel assigned to monitor the environment and provide screening and health monitoring for all responders as well as treatment of any responder illness or injury. NFPA standard 1984 as well as the U.S. Fire Administration have guidelines to address this level of responder support. Additional EMS resources may be required to facilitate and support long-term technical rescue operations in this area.

Fatal Incident Example 1

On August 17, 2000, a 37-year-old male career firefighter drowned while attempting to rescue a civilian stranded in flood waters. The fire department was notified of several cars that were stranded because of heavy amounts of rain and subsequent flooding. A crew was dispatched to the scene at approximately 1700 hours to assist motorists stranded by the flood waters. After the crew determined that no civilians were in the cars, they waited until the police arrived to take over scene control. While two firefighters (Firefighter #1 and the victim) were waiting for the police to arrive, they were verbally summoned by a civilian bystander to help a female civilian stranded in the water. The civilian was observed holding onto a pole in a pool of water that appeared to be approximately 3 feet deep. Because of the flooding conditions, it was not obvious to the firefighters that she was standing at the top edge of a culvert approximately 10 feet deep. Both firefighters responded to the location of the female civilian and attempted a rescue. Firefighter #1 was the first to enter the water, and he was quickly pulled under by the undertow. The victim entered the water to aid Firefighter #1 to safety, then reentered the water to retrieve the civilian. While doing so, the victim was pulled under the water, into the culvert, and through a large-diameter pipe. For several hours, Firefighter #1 and other crews made numerous attempts to rescue and recover the victim. At approximately 2245 hours, the victim was found several blocks from the original location of the attempted rescue. He was pronounced dead at the scene.

From National Institute for Occupational Safety and Health (2002). *Death in the line of duty.* Retrieved March 3, 2008, from http://www.cdc.gov.

VEHICLE CRASH RESCUE AND EXTRICATION

[OBJECTIVE 9]

A vehicle crash scene can present some unique and challenging problems. As always, safety is the primary concern. You must concentrate on providing patient care under what can be extremely difficult and challenging conditions and locations as well as continually assess the safety of the work environment and whether the responders present and the patient(s) receive additional injuries during the rescue process.

The following information is not intended as an extrication training program. It is written with the EMS responder in mind—the person at the scene who accepts responsibility for the care, treatment and, most importantly, the safety of all EMS providers and the patient(s). This rescue and extrication segment explains some of the most common safety and responder hazards found at crash scenes, including undeployed airbag systems, leaking gasoline and vehicle fluids, unstable vehicles, sharp metal, broken glass, and hazards involving the vehicle's battery or electrical system. The phrase *new technology* is used to describe new features, designs, components, or systems on modern vehicles. Each new technology item can affect the safety of all responders, whether the call is for a vehicle fire, a person injured at a crash scene, or extensive extrication work.

An overview of vehicle rescue and extrication from the paramedic point of view is presented as well. Known as the phases of rescue, these four basic steps for dealing with the most common crash scenarios are described. When fire and rescue personnel work in a coordinated effort with EMS crews to free a trapped occupant, they become part of an efficient and safe responder team.

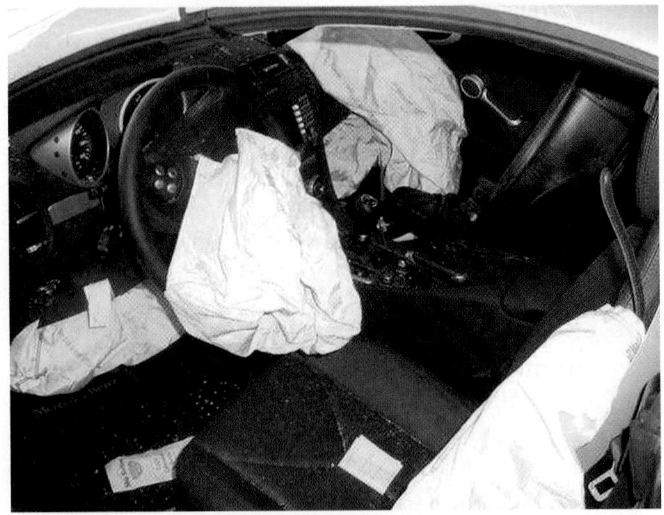

Figure 63-1 Several supplemental restraint system airbags deployed inside this Mercedes automobile. Visible are frontal airbags, the dual knee bags, and one of the two seat-mounted side-impact airbags.

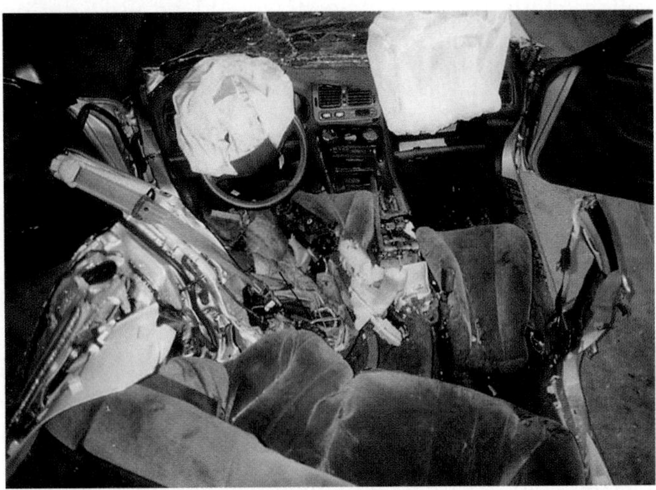

Figure 63-2 This view of the Mitsubishi Galant sedan shows the extent of impact on the driver's side. The red cables on the center console are connected to the airbag control module, which short circuited, causing the frontal airbags to deploy.

Airbags

[OBJECTIVES 10, 11]

Airbags, also known as *supplemental restraint systems,* are one of the most common new technology items confronting responders at crash scenes. Frontal airbag systems are designed to supplement the protection of the front seat occupants during head-on and near head-on crashes (Figure 63-1). **Side-impact airbags** can be located inside any or all vehicle doors, front and rear outboard seatbacks, as well as along all or a portion of the roof line. Side-impact airbags provide a cushion of protection between the occupants and the object crashing into the vehicle. Many side airbag systems use a stored gas pressurized vessel to inflate the airbag during the crash. These cylinder-like containers can contain upwards of 4000 psi of pressure. If accidentally cut during an extrication, they have the potential to fail violently (Figure 63-2). Special airbags known as **knee bags** also can be located low on either side of the front instrument panel. These are designed to deploy during a frontal collision. They make contact with the front occupants' knees and lower legs, helping hold them back in their seat. To address driver foot injuries, a new carpet airbag design deploys beneath the carpet of the driver's pedal area to protect the feet and ankles.

Airbags do save lives and reduce the chance of injury. In fact, occupants walk away from crashes today that would not have been survivable in years past. Responders arrive to find everyone already out of their mutilated vehicles, usually with no injuries or only minor complaints. Occupants today who are restrained by a properly worn seat belt system and are also protected by airbags have the greatest chance of survival in a motor vehicle crash.

Undeployed Airbag Hazard

Airbags present a challenge to fire, EMS, rescue, and law enforcement responders. The possibility of having undeployed airbags within the immediate patient care area is a reality now at almost every crash scene. Accidental deployment of an airbag during extrication has already happened and can happen again. This can even occur after vehicle electrical systems have been disabled.

Fatal Incident Example 2

The Dayton Airbag Incident

On Monday morning, August 21, 1995, at 5:49 AM in Dayton, Ohio, firefighters received a call reporting people trapped in a motor vehicle accident on Hoover near McGee. The four-member crew of Rescue One responded in their rig to meet Engine 17, Truck 13, and Medic 4 at the scene. For firefighters Jim Kohler and Tom Trimbach responding with Rescue One, little did they know that in a few moments they would be making history and that the next fire department vehicle they would ride in would be an ambulance.

In what has become the most widely known vehicle extrication incidents of modern day, the two firefighters were injured when the dual airbags deployed on the 1994 Mitsubishi Galant automobile on which they were working. Both firefighter Trimbach and Kohler were struck by the airbags, with Trimbach thrown through the air by the inflation force of the passenger front airbag.

This was the first documented incident of airbag deployment caused by the actions of fire and rescue personnel. Lessons learned from this response reinforced the need for fire and rescue personnel to shut down the electrical system of any vehicle on which they perform extrication operations at a crash scene.

From Moore R. (1997). *The Dayton airbag incident*, from http://www.firehouse.com.

Emergency Procedures for Airbag-Equipped Vehicles

For emergency responders the question is no longer, "Does this vehicle have airbags?" The question now is "Where are the loaded airbags?" A **loaded airbag** is one that has not deployed during the initial crash. By design, a vehicle with front- and side-impact airbags would likely not have all bags deploy in the initial crash. Fortunately for emergency responders, although more than 180 different makes and models of vehicles are sold today, enough similarities exist between airbag systems that standard operating procedures can be developed to cope with most situations that may be encountered.

Vehicle Crash Procedures

Responders often arrive at the scene of a vehicle crash and find one or more deployed airbags along with one or more undeployed airbags in the same vehicle (Figure 63-3). Bags that have not deployed present obvious safety concerns for both you and the patient. Some vehicles have an airbag system that can either automatically shut off the passenger front airbag or allow the occupant to deactivate this airbag manually (Figure 63-4). With the advent of **dual-stage airbags,** even a deployed airbag can be dangerous to work around during patient care activities. A dual-stage airbag has two inflation charges inside. Potentially only one of the two charges may deploy during the initial crash. That deployment causes the bag to inflate. The safety concern for responders,

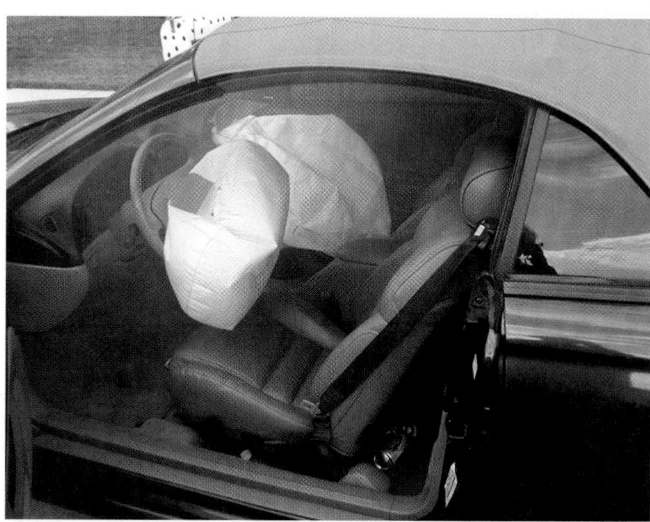

Figure 63-3 Airbags that use a chemical reaction to generate the nitrogen gas to inflate the airbags also yield a dust as the bags deploy. This atmosphere inside a closed vehicle after airbag deployment can cause slight respiratory irritation and breathing difficulties for patients susceptible to respiratory problems.

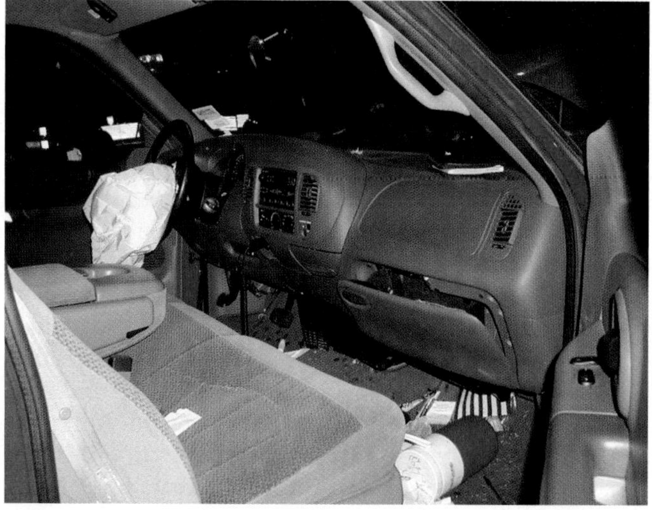

Figure 63-4 The driver of this pickup truck used the ignition key and manually deactivated the passenger front airbag. During this head-on collision, that bag remained loaded. EMS personnel inside the vehicle must use caution in this area.

however, is that the second charge of the dual-stage airbag may remain untriggered. During extrication or patient care activities, this charge could inadvertently fire off, causing a second deployment of the already-deployed airbag.

You should consider several specific safety actions when working in and around an airbag-equipped vehicle at a crash scene. The most effective activity to minimize the chance of any airbag deploying while a responder is inside performing patient care or while extrication is taking place is to shut down the vehicle's electrical system. Your airbag safety activities should include the following:

- Electrical system shutdown
- Scanning for airbags
- Determining the status of every airbag (deployed or undeployed)
- Maintaining a 10 × 18 × 5-inch inflation zone (explained below)

Once access is gained to the passenger compartment of the damaged vehicle, the inside rescuer should determine the need for the operation of any electrically powered features of the vehicle and activate features as deemed appropriate. Unlock all doors with the electric door lock switch. Lower door window glass with the electrically powered window switch. Move electrically powered seats as necessary. Unlock and release the inside trunk, hatchback, or tailgate latch. To ensure that the vehicle engine is not running even though the vehicle has crashed, move the gear selector to the park position and turn the ignition switch off if possible. Remove the key from the ignition and place it on the dashboard above the steering column.

Outside personnel should determine the location of the battery, being aware that the battery may not be under the hood within the engine compartment. In addition, the potential exists for the vehicle to have multiple batteries in different locations. To assist fellow responders in shutting down the electrical system of the vehicle, the inside rescuer should operate the inside hood release mechanism. If the hood is jammed, those assigned to shut down the power should forcibly open the hood if the battery is located there. If the battery is not located in the engine compartment, rescuers must determine the alternate location and gain access to the battery. Potential alternate battery locations include inside the front wheel well, under the front or rear seat, and inside the trunk.

Once the battery has been located and outside rescuers are prepared to shut down the electrical system, the inside rescuer must be told to coordinate the timing of the electrical system shutdown. He or she should cut or disconnect the **negative battery cable** first, being careful not to touch any metal part of the chassis with the cable or the hand tool, thus minimizing the risk of creating a spark. The negative or ground cable typically is black and completes the positive and negative electrical circuit of the vehicle's 12-volt electrical system.

If the rescuer cuts the negative battery cable, the same cable should be cut a second time to remove a minimum 2-inch section (Figure 63-5). If the rescuer choses to disconnect the cable at the battery terminal, he or she should fold the loose cable end back on itself. The rescuer should securely wrap it with insulating tape to protect the bare cable clamps from reestablishing a ground.

During any battery disconnection, an arc can be created. Even with the ignition key in the off position and the engine shut down, a slight current is always drawn on the battery. In addition, because the battery is discharging, it is generating some flammable hydrogen gas around the battery area. This can pose an additional safety concern for fire and rescue personnel.

Next, to accomplish total electrical system shutdown, the rescuer should cut or disconnect the **positive battery cable(s).** If he or she cuts the cable, he or she should cut the hot cable a second time to remove a minimum 2-inch section. If the rescuer choses to disconnect the cable at the battery terminal, he or she should fold the loose cable end back on itself. The rescuer should look for any evidence that power from the battery is still running any part of the electrical system of the vehicle. He or she should check for still-operating headlights, parking lights, dome light, or dash instrument panel lights to ensure that power shutdown has been accomplished. In a severe crash, the rescuer must also make certain the battery case has not been penetrated by metal parts, which could reestablish the electrical circuit. If the electrical system remains energized after this action, the rescuer should determine the location of additional batteries and repeat shutdown tactics for the second battery. Some supplemental restraint systems may still discharge after as long as 20 minutes because of a capacitor in the circuit.

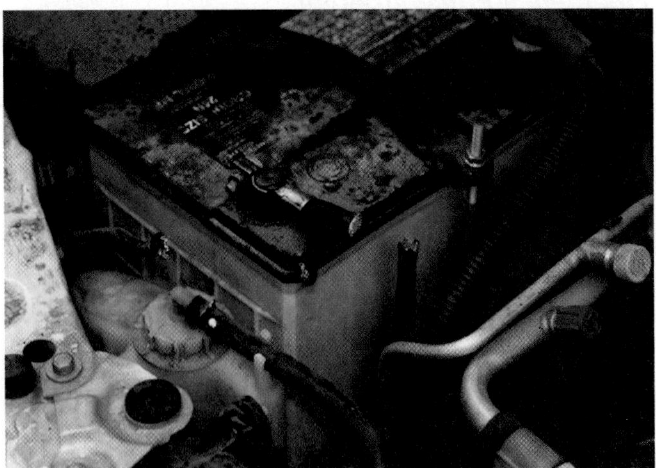

Figure 63-5 If a rescuer cuts the negative battery cable, he or she must cut the same cable a second time to remove a minimum 2-inch section. This creates a gap, making it less likely that the battery cables will reestablish an electrical circuit.

Determining Airbag Locations

With the introduction of the 2002 Mercedes sedan, as many as 12 airbags can now exist inside a single vehicle. If a vehicle could have an airbag in every possible location, responders would encounter as many as 16 different bags. If they all deployed at once, the occupants would feel as though they were in a bag of marshmallows during the crash. *Scanning* refers to the process of looking around the interior of the vehicle in an attempt to determine the location of both deployed and undeployed airbags. Scanning, similar to a patient assessment, is brief but efficient, systematic, and complete and establishes the degree of risk from airbag systems for both the rescue personnel and the patient.

Airbag Identification

Before you can scan the vehicle's interior for the presence of airbags, you first must know what you are looking for. Auto manufacturers offer various shapes, sizes, colors, and styles of visual identification labels indicating that an airbag is present (Figure 63-6). Unfortunately, no standardization exists regarding the type or location of these **airbag identification** labels. The process of airbag scanning focuses your attention on the airbag systems in the vehicle. If loaded airbags are located, you must ensure that everyone at the scene avoids placing any medical or rescue equipment, any portion of his or her body, or the patient within the airbag's inflation zone.

The generally accepted guideline for emergency responder safety when working near undeployed airbags is to remember that the inflation zones are $10 \times 18 \times 5$ inches. This safety reminder emphasizes that driver airbags typically deploy to a depth of 10 inches from the steering wheel hub assembly (Figure 63-7). The second number refers to the 18-inch depth that a typical passenger front airbag deploys outward at its full inflation. This 18-inch distance is measured rearward from the instrument panel. The thickest portion of a side-impact airbag is 5 inches, whether it is the tubular BMW unit, a drop-down, curtain-style airbag, or an airbag that deploys from the seat or door panel (Figure 63-8). Knee airbag systems deploy rearward at knee level approximately 5 inches. The curtain-style, roof-mounted side-impact airbags, although only 5 inches in thickness, deploy downward to cover much larger areas along both driver and rear passenger windows. Roof-mounted airbags reach from the roof rail down to the bottom of the window opening and can extend from the front of the front windshield to the rear of the rear door window. Depending on design, this provides coverage from the front A pillar to the rear C or D pillar of the vehicle.

Police, fire, and medical personnel as well as patients must remain clear of these invisible 10-, 18-, and 5-inch inflation zones at all times. In addition to anticipating the deployment depth, rescuers must visualize the size,

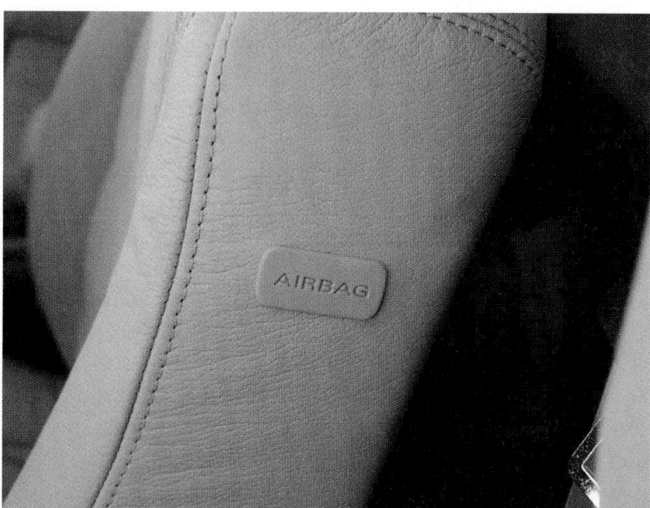

Figure 63-6 This airbag identification for a seat-mounted airbag is a plastic button sewn to the upholstery of the seat itself. Airbag identifications do not indicate the actual location of the airbag but rather that an airbag is present somewhere within this vicinity of the vehicle.

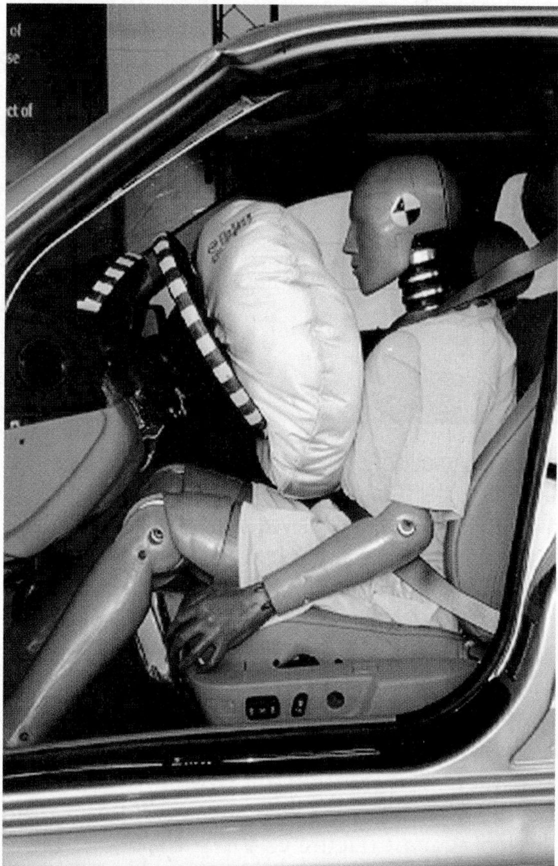

Figure 63-7 The generally accepted guideline for emergency responder safety when working near undeployed airbags is to remember the inflation zones $10 \times 18 \times 5$ inches. The driver's frontal airbag typically deploys to a depth of 10 inches from the steering wheel center hub.

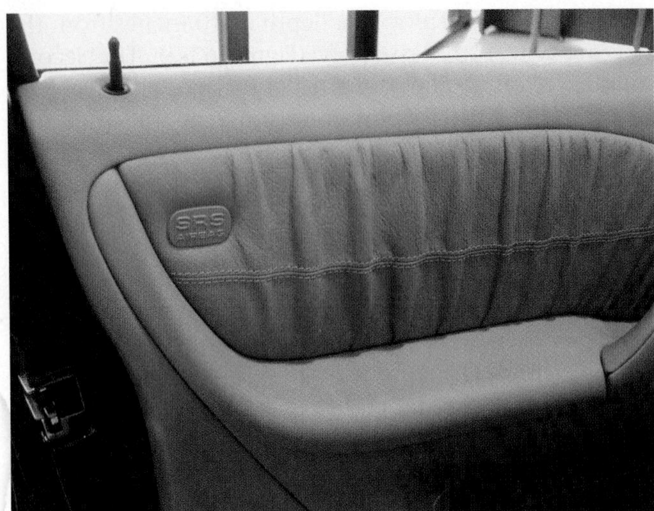

Figure 63-8 The airbag identification and the seam that will tear open as the side-impact airbag deploys are visible on the door of this Mercedes sedan. All door-mounted airbags are positioned above the armrest and toward the latch end of the door.

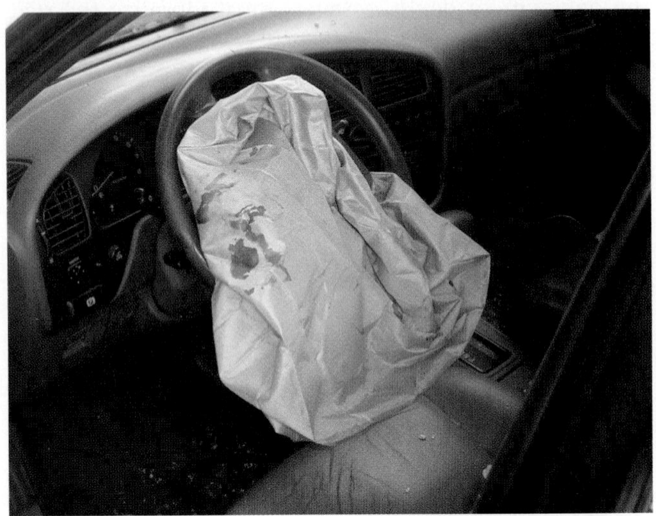

Figure 63-9 An out-of-position driver was seated too close to this steering wheel before the head-on crash. When the driver's frontal airbag deployed, he received significant facial injuries, including a facial fracture.

shape, and area that a deploying airbag will occupy. If the patient displays facial injuries inconsistent with the crash scenario, he or she may have been physically positioned within an airbag's inflation zone. Because the patient was out of position and within the 10 × 18 × 5-inch zone, he or she may have received injures from the airbag deployment (Figure 63-9).

Do not place yourself, the patient, or any piece of his or her rescue or medical equipment within this inflation zone. Loaded airbags must be thought of as being active at all times. Under extremely rare circumstances, loaded airbags can deploy while rescue and EMS personnel work inside and around the vehicle.

If an airbag were to deploy at an extrication scene, one fact is known: no possible chance exists for anyone within the zone of a deploying airbag to react quickly enough to avoid being struck, injured, and potentially killed.

Extrication with Undeployed Airbags Present

In crash situations involving any vehicle with side-impact airbags, loaded airbags are always present somewhere inside the vehicle. Law enforcement, medical personnel, and fire and rescue personnel must anticipate encountering undeployed frontal or side-impact airbags at any crash scene. For a vehicle equipped with undeployed airbags, several procedures are recommended to ensure maximal safety for personnel and patients while completing the necessary tasks in a most efficient manner. The following four potential hazards should be avoided when working around undeployed airbags:

- Unintentionally powering the electrical firing circuit, causing airbag deployment
- Causing the propellant to react by mechanical force, exposure to heat, spark, or static electricity
- Puncturing or cutting into the high-pressure cylinder of a stored gas airbag system
- Placing oneself, the patient, or equipment within the 10 × 18 × 5-inch inflation zone

Shutting down the vehicle's electrical system addresses the concern of accidentally shorting out the airbag electrical circuit. Even with the electrical system disabled, the risk is always present that an undeployed airbag will accidentally fire off from stray static electric charges. Because of this hazard, you must never trust an airbag. Always believe that the airbag can and will deploy at the worst possible time. Respect its inflation zone and keep the patient and all equipment clear of the deployment area.

The concern about accidentally cutting into the stored gas inflator units for a side impact airbag can be alleviated if rescue teams strip before they cut. This means that the headliner trim and any molding or trim panels on any roof line or roof support member must be peeled away or removed before any cutting task being initiated. Stripping the trim exposes any undeployed airbags and, most importantly, shows rescue personnel where a stored gas inflator module may be located. Once located, rescue teams can safely cut above or below the inflator during a roof removal operation. Rescue personnel can still accomplish all required tasks necessary to access, treat, and extricate occupants of a vehicle even though undeployed airbags are present. A few additional practices and procedures must be in place during the process.

Gasoline and Electric Hybrid Vehicles

[OBJECTIVE 12]

Hybrid vehicles are one of the newer challenges that confront EMS personnel at vehicle crash scenes. **Gasoline and electric hybrid vehicles** are specially designed, low-emission vehicles that combine a smaller than normal internal combustion gasoline engine with a special electric motor to power the vehicle. From a safety standpoint, responders are most concerned with the high-voltage rechargeable battery contained inside the hybrid vehicle. Voltages can be up to 500 volts DC, enough to kill on contact. The electric motor is energized by a newly designed high-voltage battery pack. The gasoline engine and the electric motor work either separately or together to provide power to the drive wheels of the vehicle.

Hybrid vehicles contain two electrical systems: the standard 12-volt system and a high-voltage system. Each hybrid therefore also has two separate batteries: a 12-volt unit and a high-voltage battery for the electric motor (Figure 63-10). All components of a hybrid vehicle that can contain potentially hazardous high voltage, up to 500 volts DC current, are color coded with a high-visibility orange color. All high-voltage cables, wires, and electrical connectors prominently display this safety color. You must avoid touching, moving, or cutting any electrical system component on a hybrid vehicle that is orange (Figure 63-11).

The normal 12-volt battery in each vehicle is similar to that found in a conventional vehicle. To power the electric motor, hybrids use a high-voltage nickel metal hydride battery. It is typically located toward the rear of the vehicle (Figure 63-12). The rear trunk and the area directly behind the rear seat are common mounting locations. The high-voltage battery can weigh as much as 110 pounds and is secured inside a steel case. High-voltage batteries are considered dry cell batteries and are not classified as a hazardous material by the U.S. government.

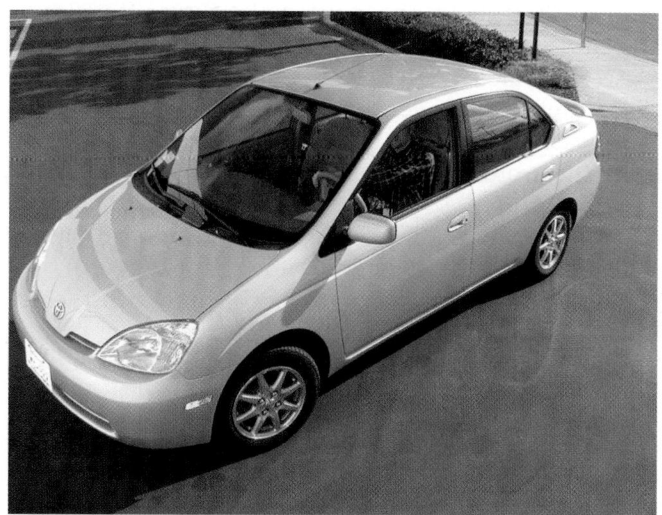

Figure 63-10 Toyota introduced their first gasoline hybrid vehicle in 2001, the Toyota Prius. It carries a special 274-volt electric battery inside the trunk area along with a standard 12-volt battery.

Crash Procedures

General crash procedures have been developed for hybrid vehicles. Although each make and model of hybrid vehicle is different because of manufacturer design and construction, the overall goals remain the same. These procedures represent the new concept of hybrid vehicle "lock out, tag out" protocols that maximize safety and minimize risks to personnel and patients at hybrid vehicle incidents.

Recommended vehicle crash procedures applicable to hybrid vehicles include the following:

- Identifying the hybrid vehicle
- Stabilizing the vehicle

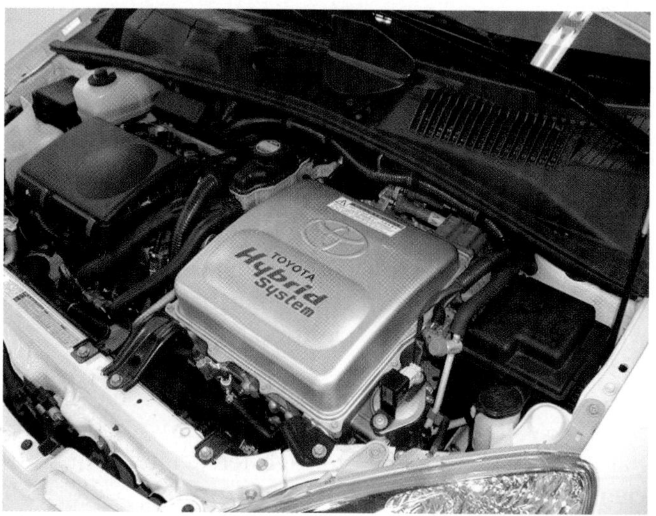

Figure 63-11 Responders must avoid touching, cutting, or in any way working with anything on a hybrid vehicle that is bright orange in color. Orange indicates the item is part of the high-voltage hybrid electric system.

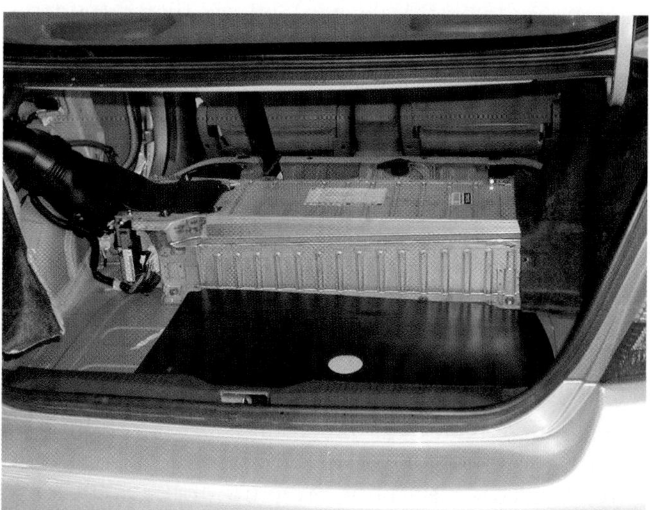

Figure 63-12 With the trunk of a Toyota Prius open and the carpeting removed, the 274-volt battery is visible.

- Gaining access to the passenger compartment
- Shifting the gear selector lever to park
- Turning the ignition off and placing the key on the dashboard
- Verifying that the dash light indicating an energized hybrid system goes out
- Shutting down the vehicle's 12-volt electrical system at the battery

Emergency Procedures at a Fire Incident

A fire involving a hybrid vehicle can be handled by following normal vehicle firefighting procedures. In a typical vehicle fire incident the engine compartment area, interior of the vehicle, or vehicle trunk area is burning. By following generally accepted fire suppression guidelines, crews attack the fire with an adequate water flow rate, working from a safe position of approach. A breathing apparatus is worn throughout the duration of the fire incident. The wheels of the vehicle are chocked as soon as safely possible to prevent forward or rearward movement.

Some possible fire situations involving a hybrid can present unique concerns. One example is any fire in which a direct flame is impinging on the high-voltage battery pack. A fire that has originated within the battery pack itself or an electrical fire that begins somewhere within the high-voltage electrical system also requires special precautions.

Radiant heat could cause the plastic modules inside the high-voltage battery to melt just as any plastic material would when exposed to high temperatures. If sufficiently heated, the plastic module casings could melt down, exposing the inner components of the high-voltage battery.

The fire service has already experienced lead acid batteries melting down during fully involved engine compartment fires. Unlike the meltdown of a 12-volt battery, however, responders who encounter a melted nickel metal hydride battery may want to notify the nearest appropriate hybrid dealership and ask that their designated battery recovery specialists be notified to deal with the damaged battery properly after the fact.

When a fully involved hybrid vehicle fire is encountered, large amounts of water are generally the extinguishing agent of choice. Water eliminates the radiant heat and begins cooling the metal battery box and the plastic battery cell modules inside the high-voltage battery pack. Fire suppression crews will not be shocked or electrocuted during direct attack on a hybrid vehicle fire even if flames impinge on the battery pack.

Emergency Procedures at a Crash Incident

What differentiates the procedures for a conventional vehicle crash from one involving a hybrid vehicle begins with vehicle identification. **Size-up** of the scene must include efforts to view the rear area of each crashed vehicle. This is the most common area that denotes a vehicle as being a hybrid, typically by the word itself in chrome trim along their rearmost edge of the trunk lid or hatchback.

Vehicle stabilization is important at any vehicle crash. In the case of a hybrid vehicle, particularly one found in a condition responders refer to as *sleep mode,* stabilization efforts must immediately prevent any forward or rearward movement. Wheels must be quickly blocked or chocked to remove the possibility that the energized vehicle may suddenly wake up and lurch forward.

After hybrid vehicle stabilization is accomplished, the passenger compartment must be accessed. As with any vehicle, scan the vehicle interior for airbags, remaining especially aware of the side-impact airbags that may be present within the seatbacks or roof line areas.

If a door opens normally, particularly the driver's door, open it. If all doors are jammed, gain access to the interior by taking out the window glass. Once inside, you can move the transmission lever into the park position.

With the vehicle stabilized to prevent movement and the gear selector properly set, responders can now initiate a special hybrid vehicle **lock out, tag out** process. This refers to the systematic process of ensuring that all sources of power and energy are turned off and/or shut down. Because medical personnel typically work in the interior of the vehicle to treat the patient, this next step can be an important function easily completed without compromising patient care.

Once the selector lever has been moved, the inside rescuer must attempt to turn the ignition off. Once the vehicle is turned off, he or she must remove the key completely from the ignition. The rescuer must check that a green or amber light on the instrument panel goes out. This signifies that the high-voltage electrical system of the hybrid has been effectively shut off. This simple action turns off the engine and the high-voltage electric motor, which prevents electric current from flowing into the cables from either the motor or the high-voltage battery. Shutting off the ignition also turns off power to the airbags and the seat belt pretensioners.

Selected models of hybrid vehicles have no ignition key. Instead, responders may find a large button on the dashboard to the right of the steering column. Labeled with the word *POWER,* this button turns the vehicle power on and off just as a standard ignition key does. To turn the hybrid off, the responder can depress the button and check that the green indicator light goes out.

The responder must now work to shut down the 12-volt electrical system on the hybrid just as is done on any conventional vehicle. He or she can begin by locating the 12-volt battery. The battery may be located inside the driver's rear wheel well area, within the trunk area, or under the hood.

If the responder's agency has a battery shutdown policy that requires responders to disconnect cables, he or she should locate the negative battery terminal and disconnect this ground cable. The responder should do the same for the positive cable. If the agency's battery shutdown policy is to cut cables, the responder should double cut the negative cable first, followed by double cuts to the positive one. With either technique, both 12-volt battery cables must be disconnected or cut to ensure rescuer safety at vehicle rescue or car fire operations. The responder should not cut any portion of the high-voltage orange wiring harness. Moreover, he or she should not touch any bare or exposed wires of this high-voltage system.

With the ignition key turned off and removed and the 12-volt battery disconnected, it is safe to work on the hybrid vehicle for medical and rescue evolutions. High-voltage electricity still exists but is isolated to the battery pack in the trunk or rear of the vehicle.

EMS Responder Safety at Vehicle Crash Scenes

[OBJECTIVE 13]

Any situation or set of circumstances with the potential to do harm is a hazard. All vehicle crash scene hazards fall in one of three general categories: environmental hazards, scene hazards, and hazards presented by the vehicle itself.

Environmental hazards are related to the weather and time of day and include extremes of heat, cold, wetness, dryness, and darkness that increase risks to crews and patients.

Incident scene hazards directly relate to the specific incident scene and include control of crowds, traffic, the danger of downed electrical wires, the presence of hazardous materials, and the location of the emergency. A vehicle precariously perched on the edge of a bridge railing or one that has crashed into a structure, causing a partial building collapse, are examples of scene hazards requiring special safety activities early in the incident.

The final category is extremely important and includes the hazards that most often confront emergency service personnel. **Vehicle hazards,** those directly related to the vehicle itself, include undeployed airbags; fuel system concerns; electrical system and battery electricity; stability of the vehicle; sharp glass and metal; leaking fluids, hot antifreeze, engine oil, or transmission oil; and antifreeze spills (Figure 63-13). Even contents inside the vehicle's trunk or cargo area are typical vehicle hazards that can be encountered.

Each emergency vehicle driver and crew member must be held responsible for the safe and efficient operation of that vehicle. For the safety of the responding personnel, the operator should be required to check and confirm that all personnel riding in the vehicle are fully dressed in appropriate protective clothing and are seated and belted before the vehicle begins its response. Crew members must remain seated and belted throughout the entire response to the incident. The senior person on the EMS unit is ultimately held responsible for the overall safe operation of the vehicle while responding to and returning from an incident.

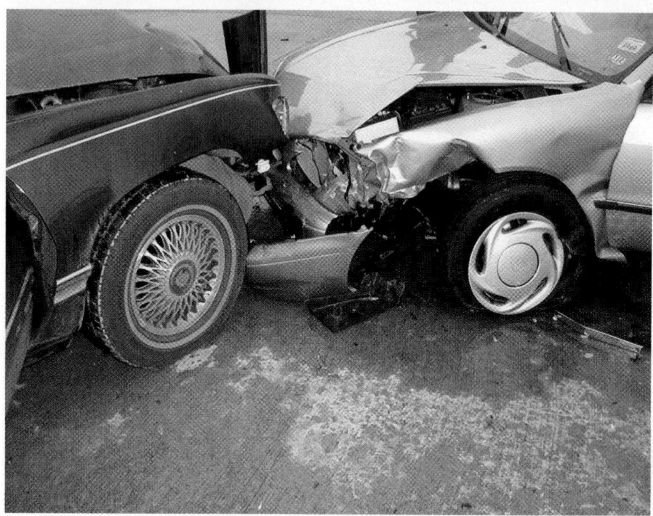

Figure 63-13 Fluids leaking from these vehicles include antifreeze and engine oil. Gasoline, diesel, and transmission fluid are other liquids that may be encountered leaking from a crashed vehicle at an incident. Responders should know how each possible fluid looks, feels, and smells.

Safety While Working in or near Moving Traffic

Emergency service personnel working in or near moving traffic are killed every year. **Struck-by** situations in which responders are working in or near moving traffic and are struck, injured, or killed by vehicles passing the incident scene are a significant safety risk. Prompt traffic control reduces traffic problems at the scene of a highway emergency and prevents secondary collisions. Although crowd and traffic control is considered a basic police agency function, lack of control of traffic seriously affects the safety of all concerned. Traffic control must be an integral part of hazard control activities and is necessary even when personnel are limited in number. Personnel on the emergency scene must learn to use their vehicles as initial traffic control devices. This concept is referred to as *safe parking* and involves using the responder vehicle to block oncoming traffic.

Blocking is the most critical initial action that can be taken to minimize these unfortunate struck-by occurrences. A block position places the emergency vehicle at an angle to the approaching traffic, across several lanes if necessary. This position begins to shield the work area and protects the crash scene from some of the approaching traffic (Figure 63-14). Under normal circumstances, the initial emergency vehicle to arrive at the crash scene should block on the **upstream,** or approaching traffic side, of the damaged vehicles and the crash scene. A **right block** or **left block** means that as the responding vehicle arrives on scene, it turns at a right or left angle. In this block position, the emergency vehicle's lights warn approaching traffic of the presence of the incident as vehicles approach. Most importantly, the vehicle acts as a physical barrier between the crash scene work area and approaching traffic. Ideally, a large vehicle such as a

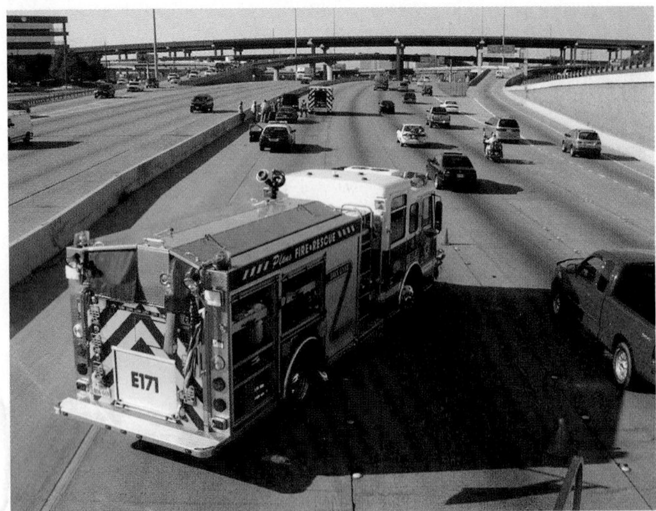

Figure 63-14 Engine 171 blocks to the right upstream of the crash scene. This creates a protected work area for the ambulance, police car, and all responding personnel.

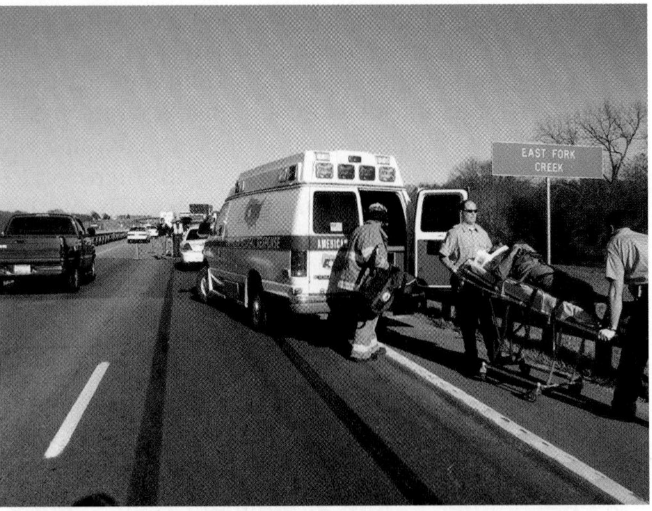

Figure 63-15 Once within the protected area created by a blocking fire apparatus, this ambulance parked in a slight block to the left position. This maneuver places the patient loading zone even farther from the moving traffic.

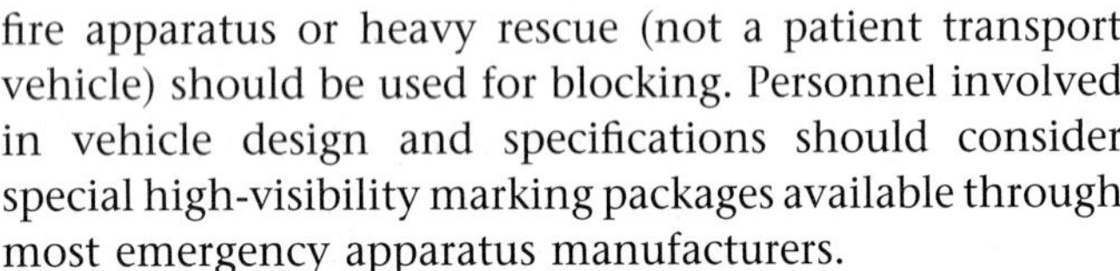

fire apparatus or heavy rescue (not a patient transport vehicle) should be used for blocking. Personnel involved in vehicle design and specifications should consider special high-visibility marking packages available through most emergency apparatus manufacturers.

When an ambulance first arrives at a crash scene, it must be parked in a safe position. The ambulance must block at least the lane that the damaged vehicle is positioned in plus one additional lane. This concept is called **obstructed lane + 1** blocking. This initial block, which can be as far as 100 feet upstream of the actual damaged vehicles and the crash scene, begins to provide a protected area around the damaged vehicles. EMS personnel can conduct initial patient care activities with this initial block. Their vehicle, however, is severely exposed to approaching traffic. The next arriving emergency vehicle, whether it is a police squad car or a fire department engine company, must also block farther upstream of the initial blocking ambulance. That action warns approaching traffic even earlier and offers some degree of safety for the initial ambulance.

If the fire department is already on scene when the ambulance arrives, safe parking is much easier and the scene is significantly safer for all responders. The driver of the ambulance pulls past the blocking fire department vehicle, drives past the crash scene, and parks in a protected position on the departure side, or downstream side, of the incident. The ambulance must stop at a slight blocking angle that also places the rear patient loading area as far away as possible from any moving traffic (Figure 63-15). With this safe parking of the ambulance, patient loading is safer and, when loaded, the ambulance is able to depart from the scene.

In addition to protective positioning with emergency vehicles, personnel themselves should don high-visibility reflective apparel. These garments can be vest or jacket style and should be rated as an ANSI class II or class III. This verifies that the vest or jacket is of a lime-green and bright-orange color combination, with a reflective trim to improve visibility of personnel. Fire service PPE does not typically meet this standard, and when it becomes worn over time it loses much of its intended reflectivity. An ANSI-compliant garment such as a class II or III vest as a minimum should be worn instead of or in addition to normal structural PPE.

Establishing the Hot Zone

The area of highest risk for EMS personnel at a crash scene is closest to the crashed vehicles and typically where the patients are located. This primary danger zone is commonly referred to as the **hot zone,** a familiar term used by hazardous materials teams. When no fuel, fire, or spill hazards are present at a crash scene, the hot zone extends approximately 50 feet in all directions from the wreckage. The emergency vehicle initiating the first upstream block maintains this 50-foot hot zone spacing if possible. If one or more vehicles involved in the crash are burning, the hot zone distance increases to approximately 100 feet. The hot zone should be expanded whenever doubts exist about the safety and stability of a scene.

A recommended hot zone clear area of 2000 feet in all directions should be initially maintained if a hazardous material is or may be involved in the incident. This includes the presence of any pressurized storage cylinders or toxic, reactive, or explosive materials. This minimal distance may increase to 3000 feet or more in all directions depending on the nature of the incident. In hazardous materials situations such as these, emergency vehicles and personnel are best positioned uphill and upwind of the scene.

If the crashed vehicle is leaking gasoline, the fumes typically travel downhill and downwind to low-lying areas such as sewer drains, curbs, ditches, and gullies. Because these low-lying areas must be evacuated and must have all sources of potential ignition near them isolated, these areas become extended hot zones. Low-lying areas downhill or downwind from a leaking fuel situation should be avoided when positioning emergency vehicles or patients. Safe parking at a crash scene involving a utility company power pole requires vehicles and crews to avoid any area under overhanging transmission lines and near power transformers, which could short out. The hot zone should extend one intact pole beyond both affected poles when wires are down at a crash. Command personnel must quickly ascertain the stability of overhead wires, the damaged pole, adjacent power poles, and adjoining spans of transmission wires.

In all situations that are unclear regarding how much space to put between the damaged vehicles and the ambulance, a rule of excess should prevail. If in doubt, you should stay back for safety's sake. Moving the ambulance forward is far easier and safer than rapidly backing it up or abandoning it entirely if an unanticipated, life-threatening situation develops.

Traffic should be kept moving by being detoured or rerouted if possible. Immediate traffic merging into an open lane or quickly established detours that move approaching traffic around and away from the crash scene are recommended. If traffic is detoured and kept far enough away from the crash area, congestion at the incident scene can be minimized. What should be avoided is the complete stopping of traffic, especially for any extended period. If traffic is completely stopped on a typical high-volume interstate highway or expressway, the traffic jam can extend 1 mile for each minute that traffic is not moving. After 5 minutes of total shutdown, the possibility of getting additional emergency service units into or out of the immediate crash scene area becomes extremely difficult and time consuming. A detour around the area minimizes traffic congestion and maximizes scene protection. Although rescuers may need to initiate traffic management, remember that this is a primary function of law enforcement and/or the local Department of Transportation agency. Some areas of the country have specialized fire or police units within their emergency services that augment or support this strategic area.

Need for Standby Protection

The fire hazards on a vehicle, its quantity of fuel, undeployed airbags, and the many potential sources of ignition at a crash scene mandate that a fire department engine company be dispatched to any crash serious enough to result in personal injury to the occupants. If an ambulance is needed at the scene, EMS responders on scene also need the safety and security provided by having a standby fire department engine company on location. Simply having a large engine park in a two-lane upstream block position improves the safety of all at the scene.

Vehicle Fluid Leaks and Spills

Leaks and spills of vehicle fluids can be a minor inconvenience or present a serious safety problem. Leaks can be hot antifreeze from the radiator, oil from the engine, fluid from the transmission, acid from the battery, or fuel from the fuel system. The leak can be a small spill or can cover a large area of the crash scene. An important safety procedure for at least one EMS responder at the vehicle incident scene is to conduct a hazard survey of the scene and the damaged vehicles. Among other things, the responder wants to find out if liquid leaks or spills beneath the vehicle are a hazard.

Once a leak or spill is observed, the next step is to identify the nature of the liquid. Antifreeze and leaking motor oil cause the roadway surface to become slippery, but they are not considered a fire hazard. If the liquid comes from the fuel system, it most likely is gasoline. A diesel fuel spill or a leak of any of the alternate fuels such as propane, butane, or natural gas also is a possibility. If a leak hazard or potential leak can be confirmed, the fire department engine crew that was simultaneously dispatched should be notified when they arrive on scene.

Until the fire department arrives, positioning a multipurpose, dry chemical fire extinguisher nearby is a quick way to establish a basic level of standby fire suppression at a crash scene. The extinguisher may be the first line of defense while a protective hose line is being stretched and readied for service by the fire department.

Vehicles on Fire

A vehicle fire is a serious safety threat. A burning vehicle can be considered a time bomb with a fuse that has been burning long before the arrival of emergency personnel. Initial actions at a vehicle fire must therefore be directed at snuffing out this fuse. Vehicle fire hazards include the possibility of large amounts of fuel on vehicles equipped with large-capacity gasoline or diesel tanks. A large sport utility vehicle can carry as much as 44 gallons of gasoline. Some larger commercial vehicles, especially those with auxiliary fuel tanks, may have as much as 150 gallons or more of fuel on board. Some fuel tanks are made of plastic; these tanks are more susceptible to melting and rupturing when exposed to high heat. Older pickup trucks may have an extra fuel tank in the cab behind the seat.

Alternative fuels such as liquefied petroleum gas, butane, and natural gas present unique safety concerns during a fire situation. Travel trailers, motor homes, and catering vehicles, for example, also may contain liquefied petroleum gas fuel storage. Magnesium can be found in vehicle wheels, engine blocks, and other automotive accessories. Magnesium ignites at approximately 1200°F and burns a brilliant white color, generating temperatures in excess of 4000°F. If a burning vehicle or potential burning vehicle can be confirmed, the fire department engine crew that was simultaneously dispatched should be notified so they can attack the fire and render the scene safe when they arrive on scene.

Wires Down at the Crash Scene

[OBJECTIVE 14]

At an incident with utility lines down, consider the danger zone as any area in which persons and vehicles could make contact with wires that are or may be energized or the current extending outward from the energized wires. Electricity can leave an energized wire and travel invisibly through the ground. When this happens at a crash scene, the ground becomes energized with what is referred to as *ground gradient.* The current traveling through the ground can electrocute a person without the individual ever touching the actual downed wire. Downed wires also are dangerous because determining if a downed wire is energized or not is difficult. If it is arcing and sparking, it obviously is energized. Energized wires can appear motionless and dead, yet they can have fatal amounts of current running through them. A once-dead wire can be reenergized and become lethal in less than 1 second.

Electricity is transmitted through transmission and distribution wires. These wires, which are higher up on the power pole, routinely carry up to 19,900 volts of current in residential neighborhoods, with greater currents moving through major distribution lines. Amperage is the measure of flow of current through an object—the wire in the case of power lines. This amperage is the killing factor in electrical shock. The voltage is only important in that it determines how much amperage or current flows through a given body of resistance.

As little as $\frac{1}{10}$ amp of current flowing through the human body can be fatal; some authorities set this figure as low as $\frac{1}{20}$ amp. A person making contact with a downed 19,900-volt line at a crash could have a current of 19 amp flowing through his or her body to the ground. This is 190 times the amperage needed to be fatal. Wires containing common household 120-volt or 220-volt service also have sufficient amperage to be fatal to human beings.

In electrocution cases, the current flows through the path of least resistance as it reaches the ground. In an electrocution case, the parts of the body through which the current flows as it grounds itself can be severely damaged. If a person is standing in water, which reduces the resistance to the ground and allows more current to pass, the resistance to the ground when contact is made with a 19,900-volt line can increase to 130 amp or more. The potential effects of electrical current on the body are shown in Box 63-4.

Whether electrocution has occurred cannot be determined by simply looking at the patient. The patient may show no visible signs of electrocution if, for example, he or she had stepped into energized water. If energized wires may be down or a power pole has been damaged, personnel initially should not get close to the scene. As a general rule, a hot zone extending one intact pole beyond the damaged lines should be established. All crew members should remain in their emergency vehicles until the area is determined to be safe. All other responding personnel should be notified immediately of the situation. Personnel should proceed as though all power wires as well as the guy wires that support the power pole are energized. Because of modern power transmission line technology, circuit breakers can automatically reenergize a downed line multiple times as the power company's system attempts to reset itself. What was once a dead line can become reenergized multiple times as the circuitry attempts to restore power to the system.

If you can confirm that power poles at the crash scene are damaged or that power lines are down, you must notify the responding fire department and ensure that the local utility company is notified and requested to respond to the scene. Establish a hot zone to control scene safety, treating all wires as energized. No responder should touch an involved vehicle until it is determined that the vehicle and the ground around it are not energized and will not become energized. Personnel must maintain adequate clearance around all sides of the electrical danger zone. Traffic and crowd control measures must be enforced. Communication among all emergency service personnel must make everyone fully aware of the danger and the exact location of the danger zone.

BOX 63-4 Potential Effects of Electrical Current on the Body

- 1 mA causes no sensation and is not felt.
- 2 to 8 mA causes sensation of shock but is not painful. The individual can release contact at will.
- 8 to 15 mA causes painful shock. The individual can let go at will.
- 15 to 20 mA causes painful shock. Control of adjacent muscles is lost.
- 20 to 70 mA causes painful shock. Severe muscular contractions with extremely difficult breathing occur.
- 100 to 200 mA causes painful shock and ventricular fibrillation of the heart.
- 200 mA or more causes severe burns and muscle contractions so severe that chest muscular reaction clamps the heart and stops it for the duration of the shock.

PARAMEDIC*Pearl*

Always consider any downed wire as energized until secured by the local electric utility.

If safe to do so, approach victims or damaged vehicles by "duck walk"—moving forward by slowly sliding the feet side by side. This waddling movement may allow you to detect electrical current flowing through the ground.

As the distance closes between you and a charged wire, you may feel a tingling sensation in the feet, as though your toes have gone to sleep. This tells you that the ground on which you are standing is energized. Going any closer would be dangerous, placing you at risk of injury. The invisible ground gradient force field runs outward in all directions from the electrical source. If these force fields were visible, they would resemble waves created by the splash of a rock thrown into a pond. The closer you get to the electrical source, the greater the amount of current that flows through the ground. The ground gradient current will enter the body through one leg and discharge through the other.

Current may be transmitted through objects other than the ground. Take special precautions when you suspect that steel supporting wires, steel highway guide rails, metal fences, telephone lines, or even cable television transmission wires are in contact with a downed transmission wire. The wire can readily energize everything it comes in contact with, extending the electrical strike zone great distances. The Niagara Mohawk Power Company, headquartered in Syracuse, N.Y., conducts a training school specifically designed for emergency service personnel. The program's instructors relate the story of a telephone repairman electrocuted 15 miles from the scene of a car crash. His death occurred when broken power lines at the crash site made contact with telephone lines on a nearby utility company pole. The current energized the innocent-looking phone lines that transmitted the fatal electrical current to the lineman working on the lines in the next community.

At any incident with wires down, resist the temptation to move the wire, particularly when the wire is not moving, arcing, or showing any signs of being energized. Remember, do not touch or move any downed wire, even if it appears dead. Never trust downed wires. They can be quick and silent killers.

When occupants are inside an electrically energized vehicle, take quick action to ensure their safety. Establish and maintain immediate visual and verbal contact with the occupants, even if those inside do not acknowledge the communication or are unconscious. The use of a bullhorn or public address system on the emergency vehicle may be necessary. Convince these victims to stay inside the vehicle if possible. Their best chance of not being electrocuted lies in waiting for the electricity to be shut off. Despite popular misconception, there is no safe way to jump clear.

PARAMEDIC*Pearl*

For those entrapped in a vehicle to feel secure, they must always be able to see a concerned rescuer paying attention to them. If they look around and see no one, they may feel abandoned, panic, and attempt to get out of their predicament on their own.

Because of the higher carbon content in the rubber used today for vehicle tires, a steel-belted radial tire can spontaneously burst into flames from high amperage flowing through it. This presents an immediate danger for those inside the vehicle. Engine company personnel may be instructed to discharge water from a high-volume fog stream onto the tire fire in an effort to control the flames and prevent extension into the vehicle.

As emphasized, electrical hazards are not to be taken lightly. Take the utmost care to ensure safe operations at an emergency scene.

PARAMEDIC*Pearl*

As a general rule, you should never move a downed electrical wire. The preferred action is to secure the scene, communicate with any stranded occupants of the vehicle, and await the arrival of professional utility company personnel.

Four Phases of Rescue

[OBJECTIVE 15]

Real-world experiences demonstrate that a typical vehicle crash does exist. It is probably on a dry, level road surface and more than likely at an intersection. The vehicles involved have either experienced a head-on collision, a side collision, or a rear-end crash. A vehicle may have rolled over. On EMS arrival, the vehicle may still be resting on its side or roof, or it may have rolled completely and be back on its wheels.

The most common patient encountered at a crash is the driver of the vehicle. Vehicle occupant capacities range from a lone individual in the vehicle to full-size sedans, which seat six; a minivan, which can carry eight; an extended van, which has a 15-passenger capacity; to a bus, which can carry 84 to 100 occupants.

If you analyze all the activities that take place at a typical motor vehicle crash with entrapment, approximately 36 to 40 tasks you may be called on to accomplish become apparent. To understand better what happens at an extrication scene and promote improved training for vehicle rescue, all these tasks can be organized into four categories. These groupings are known as the four **phases of rescue.** Each phase includes related activities that may have to be done for the patient to be extricated from a crashed vehicle. Since its creation by Chief Ron Moore in the mid-1990s, the phases of rescue have become an unofficial national extrication training drill used by fire and rescue organizations across the United States (Moore, 2003). For the purposes of this chapter, the "phases" concept is used to explain the overall process of vehicle extrication at a typical crash scene. The example vehicle is a sedan with two front-seat occupants that has undergone a head-on collision. It now rests on its four wheels on a level surface. The driver is trapped by the steering wheel, steering column, and instrument panel assembly. The unbelted front-seat passenger slid forward on the seat and is now trapped between the floorboard and the dash and firewall structure on the passenger's side of the car.

Phase 1

Phase 1 activities are those that responding crew members are initially involved in on arrival. These activities are the first actions done at the scene, and they set the stage for the challenges that will be faced while working to free the trapped occupants. Phase 1 activities include the following:

- Arrival and safe parking at the crash scene
- Scene size-up, assessment, and 360-degree walk around
- Command establishment
- Scene and vehicle stabilization
- Airbag scanning
- Battery access and electrical system shutdown
- Hazard control (fluid leak or spill) assessment
- Initial patient access opening (removal of window glass)
- Initial interior access and patient contact
- Patient protection and safety
- Determination of contents of trunk

For a medical care provider, phase 1 means remembering to approach the scene and the damaged vehicles carefully while assessing the scene for safety-related hazards. Once the scene is safe and the vehicle stabilized, access must be gained to the interior of the vehicle. Rescuers prefer to use a door that opens normally if possibly. If no door readily opens, the rescuer must break out side or rear window glass to climb in the vehicle. This allows the medics to contact the patient(s) and begin an initial assessment of condition. Emergency medical care continues to the extent possible within the confined space of the damaged vehicle. The inside medic also can readily scan for airbags, both deployed and undeployed, and can ensure the ignition key is turned off and put the vehicle in "park." In reality, initial rescue activities are more involved than this, but from an EMS point of view think scene safety, vehicle stabilization, patient access, and initial medical care.

Phase 2

[OBJECTIVE 16]

Phase 2 is the disentanglement phase. It involves all the tasks necessary to open doors and the sidewall of the vehicle on one or both sides. The goal of phase 2 is total sidewall removal on one side of the vehicle. When finished, phase 2 tasks give EMS providers maximal room for patient care and sufficient space for efficient patient packaging and removal (Figure 63-16). Phase 2 tasks include the following:

- Verifying vehicle stabilization
- Verifying patient protection and safety
- Removing side window glass
- Cutting or removing seat belts
- Removing interior trim panel materials (B pillar)
- Removing the sidewall, including:
  - Front door
  - Rear door
  - B pillar
- Covering exposed metal

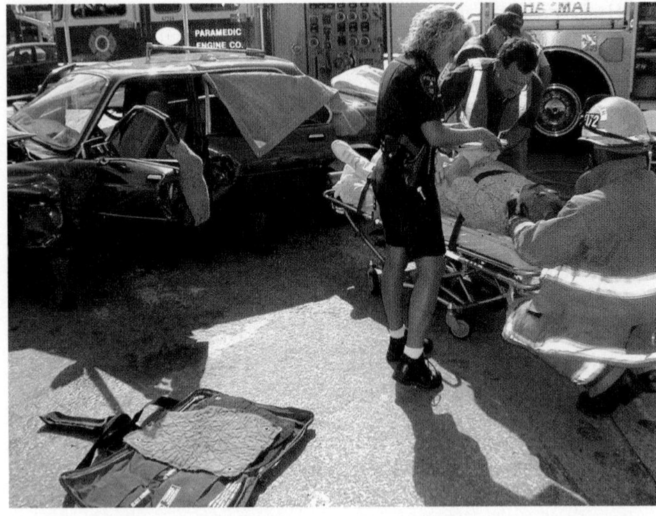

Figure 63-16 A rescuer must do what is necessary to make sufficient space to extricate the patient—in this case forcing the door open at the latch was sufficient for the patient to be taken out of the car on a long board.

Think of the phrase "buy one, get one free." In regard to doors, if opening one jammed door is good, opening the entire side of the vehicle is generally even better. With a two-door automobile, opening one door and the sidewall of the vehicle provides a safe and efficient operating room on that side of the vehicle. With a two-door vehicle, the opening or removal of the front door is accompanied by sidewall removal along that same side back seat area in what is referred to as a *three-door evolution*. With total sidewall removal on a four-door automobile, both doors are opened and the center post is moved or removed to open up that side of the vehicle from the front door hinge area to the rear door latch (Figure 63-17). Phase 2 also requires that interior trim panels be removed on any roof pillar to be cut, in this case, the **B pillar.** The B pillar is the roof support member at the latch end of the front door. The rear is also hinged to it. Stripping plastic trim with a tool such as a screwdriver or small pry bar exposes the inner structure. Rescuers are then able to see the pillar's thin or thick areas, any airbag stored gas inflator units, pyrotechnic seat belt pretensioner devices, thick door latch pins, or seat belt spools and reinforced metal areas. Stripping the interior trim also can reveal the location of the roof-mounted airbag inflator modules. If the roof must be removed, it is done in phase 3. Stripping the trim in phase 2, however, ensures that the hazard areas are exposed.

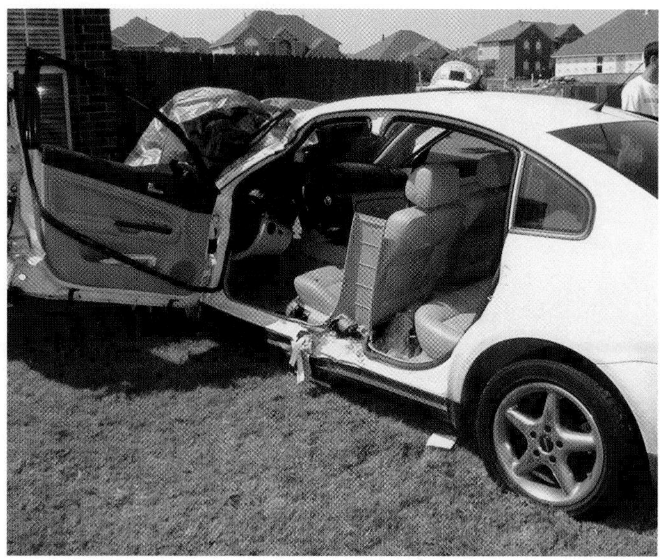

Figure 63-17 An off-duty female police officer received serious injuries in this broadside collision that forced her vehicle through a yard and into a house. Rescue crews performed a total sidewall removal, which included both doors and the B pillar, to extricate her.

PARAMEDIC*Pearl*

Pillars, or posts that support the roof of a vehicle, are referred to in alphabetical terms. The pillar at the windshield is referred to as the *A pillar* (or *post*), the next pillar toward the rear is the B pillar, and so on.

Phase 3

[OBJECTIVE 17]

Phase 3 activities remove the roof (Figure 63-18). Total roof removal is the single most effective vehicle rescue task that provides the greatest degree of patient access for all occupants of a vehicle on its wheels. Total roof removal is especially effective for vehicles with thin roof pillars or roofs with power sunroofs. Total removal is preferred in situations in which roof-mounted heating and cooling units are encountered, such as in the newer model sport utility vehicles. Total roof removal is recommended when working on a new vehicle that has an airbag system mounted along its roof line. Exposing roof pillars and removing the entire roof minimally disturbs the roof airbag system.

Phase 3 activities can be accomplished quickly and efficiently with even the simplest tools. All tasks related to total roof removal are accomplished during phase 3 activities and *must* include the following:

- Verifying vehicle stabilization
- Verifying patient protection and safety
- Removing side and rear glass
- Cutting or removing windshield glass
- Cutting or removing seat belts
- Removing interior trim panel materials at roof pillars

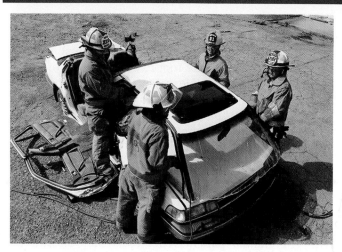

Figure 63-18 During phase 3, crews conduct a partial or total roof removal evolution. The windshield was only cut along the dashboard so that it moves away with the roof. Note the total sidewall removal along the passenger's side.

- Severing roof pillars
- Removing roof to debris area
- Covering exposed metal

PARAMEDIC*Pearl*

The side and rear glass of vehicles are made of tempered glass. Therefore they are easily broken by applying a high force on a small surface area. When broken they shatter into many small pieces. The windshield is made of laminated safety glass that remains intact when broken. To remove the windshield it must be "cut out."

Rather than delaying roof removal, a well-trained rescue officer orders roof removal early in the rescue incident. Roof work may be initiated even before all the doors have been opened. With partial roof removal, the roof section above the trapped patient is flipped rearward. Complete cuts of several roof posts and some effective cuts of side roof channel in the rain gutter area are all that is necessary to accomplish partial roof section removal. The other possibility is total roof removal, which involves completely cutting all roof posts and removing the entire roof structure. This gives the vehicle a convertible-like appearance.

Whether to complete partial or total roof removal is a tactical decision made by EMS and rescue personnel at the emergency scene. The design of the vehicle's rear posts is probably the most significant factor to consider in determining which roof opening to use. Vehicles with large rear C posts are better handled by flipping the roof rearward. Vehicles with thin roof posts are best accessed by total roof removal. Medical personnel must add their input to the roof removal decision as they consider the patient's medical condition and physical positioning within the passenger compartment. With a car containing two adult trauma patients, as in the example scenario, no other single rescue job can compare with the effectiveness of total roof removal. With any trauma patient with suspected head, neck, or spinal injuries inside an automobile, the roof removal process of phase 3 allows the best possible patient immobilization and packaging efforts to be completed.

With the roof of the vehicle partially moved or removed, the serious trauma patient whose life is ticking away may now be rapidly extricated from the interior of the vehicle directly onto a long board. However, completely immobilize the patient who is relatively stable before removal. The concept of rapid patient extrication is now possible because of the massive opening that roof removal afforded the medical crew members working with the trauma patient. The doors may all still be jammed, but the trauma patient may be well on his or her way to the medical facility because of the early and aggressive roof removal.

For phase 3, crews must cut or remove the laminated windshield glass as part of roof removal. In an effort to increase efficiency and decrease the overall rescue time, crews should consider cutting the glass low along the dash from A pillar to A pillar. With this technique, the windshield remains attached to the roof as both are lifted off the vehicle. If the windshield remains attached to the roof, crews should lift the roof and move forward. This takes the broken windshield glass away from the patient area rather than dragging the glass over the heads of patients.

Phase 4

[OBJECTIVE 18]

Phase 4 requires movement of the dashboard, instrument panel, and firewall structure of the vehicle away from the front seat passengers. Phase 4 activities include the following:

- Verifying vehicle stabilization
- Verifying patient protection and safety
- Cutting or bending the steering wheel ring
- Cutting the A pillar and/or rocker channel
- Rolling or jacking the dashboard
- Covering exposed metal

In this final rescue phase, strategic cuts are made in the firewall structure, and pushing, spreading, or even pulling equipment is used to move the dashboard, firewall, steering wheel and column, and pedals away from front seat occupants simultaneously. Rescue teams typically refer to this as **rolling the dash.** An alternate method that in many cases may be quicker and just as effective as rolling the dash is referred to as **jacking the dash.** In this process rescue crews use spreading or lifting equipment at a 90-degree angle to the side of the firewall and dashboard and vertically spread or lift all the front structure of the vehicle up and away from the occupants (Figure 63-19).

Some of these standardized activities are basic, whereas others involve complex and technical rescue work. The preplanned standard operating procedures that comprise the phases of rescue are primarily designed for the common scenario of a passenger automobile or automobiles involved in a head-on, side, or rear-end collision in which the vehicles remain on their wheels. Rescue and medical personnel can adapt the four rescue phases to other types of vehicles. The suggested four-phase rescue guidelines presented address the true concept of vehicle rescue today. Handling an incident with people trapped can be likened to eating a banana. The delicate core of the banana represents the patient trapped within his or her vehicle. The banana peel represents the tangled and twisted wreckage of the automobile. The person who wants to eat a banana, like the emergency service teams who want to free the trapped patient, must peel the various sections of the banana skin away one strip at a time until the fruit is exposed and ready to be eaten. At a typical vehicle rescue incident, rescuers "peel the banana" as they open or remove the roof, lay the doors and sidewalls out, and move the dashboard and firewall structure of the vehicle to release the patient from entrapment.

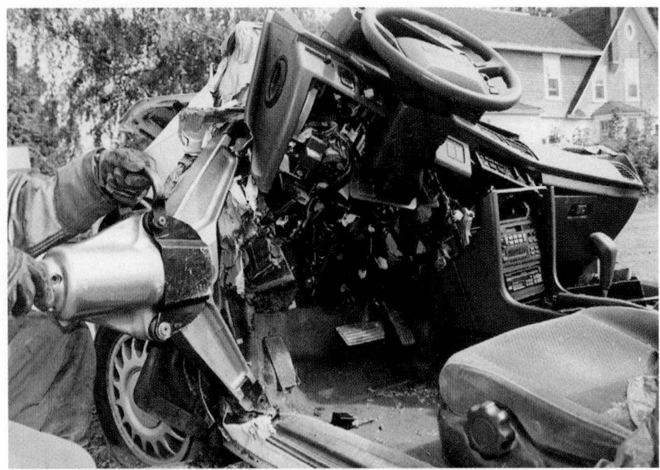

Figure 63-19 Jacking the dash involves making cuts into the front pillar and A pillar and lifting the dash, instrument panel, steering wheel and column, and even the pedals off a trapped driver or front seat passenger.

SURFACE WATER RESCUE

[OBJECTIVE 19]

Surface water presents hazards for many people, including EMS responders. Most drownings happen to people who never intended to even get wet. The number of drownings of well-intentioned potential rescuers are numerous. People are drawn to moving water for recreation, but many underestimate its power. Unaware rescuers also underestimate the power of water and fail to understand the hazards involved.

Moving Water and Common Hazards

[OBJECTIVE 20]

Moving water (rivers, creeks, and streams) is especially dangerous to individuals and rescuers. Moving water creates different kinds of forces, depending on depth, velocity, and obstructions to flow. Obstructions such as small ledges, dams, and low-water bridges can trap potential rescuers. When entering moving water, responders are at risk for drowning regardless of their ability to swim.

The forces in moving water are often hidden and deceptive. Water rescue is a dangerous activity that should never be attempted by rescuers without special training and equipment. A part of this training includes how to read moving water and its hidden dangers.

Drowning Machines

One of the most dangerous types of water hazards is commonly referred to as a *drowning machine,* or **hydraulic** (Figure 63-20). Hydraulics are caused by water moving over a uniform obstruction to flow and are commonly found on lo-head dams (i.e., dams with a low height). They are a common hazard and are present on many rivers and streams. They are particularly hazardous because they do not appear to be dangerous and often cannot be seen from upstream by boaters and swimmers. They have been the cause of death by drowning of many victims and rescuers.

Hydraulics form when water flows over an obstruction, causing water to flow back upstream. This recirculation effect can easily trap objects and people, resulting in drowning even for individuals wearing PFDs. Persons trapped in a hydraulic become fatigued and hypothermic, which can lead to drowning. Patients trapped in the recirculation also may suffer trauma from hitting structures of the dam and being struck by debris caught in the backwash.

Strainers

Strainers are another type of water hazard that result in rescue calls. Like hydraulics, strainers tend to be hazardous to rescuers. Strainers are formed by an object or structure in the current that allows water to flow but strains out large objects, such as boats and people. A number of objects create strainers, including trees, fences, grates, dam intakes, and broken structures. Strainers also can be formed in the stream by natural features such as boulders and natural ledges. People are pulled into the strainer and cannot escape because the current holds them against the strainer. Rescue often is difficult because of the force of water holding the victim against the strainer. This is a hazardous rescue and responders must be careful not to be sucked into the strainer.

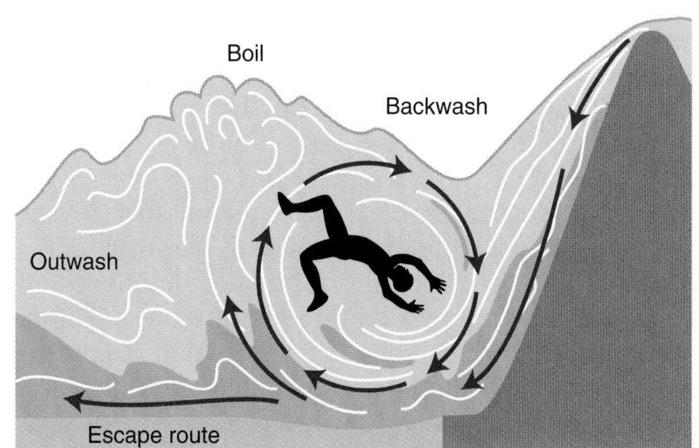

Figure 63-20 "Drowning machines," or hydraulics, are formed by water moving over a uniform obstruction to flow.

Foot or Extremity Pin

The force of the water's current can be hard to read, and individuals and rescuers can quickly become trapped by a variety of mechanisms. One of these dangerous mechanisms is the foot or extremity pin. This occurs when a person is wading in the water and gets a foot or other extremity caught between rocks or under another structure. The current then forces the body forward and into the stream. The pin becomes even more severe and the person succumbs to fatigue or cold, eventually loses strength, goes under the surface and drowns. Rescuers or bystanders may attempt to hold the victim up out of the water but they, too, lose strength and become hypothermic. Usually the only way to rescue the patient is to pull the entrapped body portion out the same way it went in, usually on the upstream side.

The potential for foot or extremity pin is one reason that rescuers should never wade in streams that are more than mid-tibia deep.

Dams and Hydroelectric Intakes

Other water rescue situations that are hazards for rescuers involve dams and hydroelectric and irrigation intakes (also known as *head gates*). Both the upstream and downstream sides of a dam are potentially dangerous. On the upstream side, individuals can get sucked into the intake or spillway. The upstream side of a dam also is often invisible from water level. On the downstream side, the bottom of a spillway can create hydraulics. The height of the dam is no indicator of the degree of hazard. In addition, dam spillways often open automatically and without warning.

Flat Water (Slow-Moving or Still Water)

Most people who drown never planned on being in the water. Many lives would be saved if individuals routinely wore and properly used PFDs when on or around water. Having the PFD available but unworn is useless.

Many accidents on land result from alcohol use, which alters mental ability and reason. This also is true on water where accidents often result in fatalities (Box 63-5).

Water Temperature and Drowning

[OBJECTIVE 21]

Immersion in cold water can rapidly lead to hypothermia, which can lead to drowning. Any water temperature

BOX 63-5 Alcohol Use in Drownings

Alcohol use is involved in approximately 25% to 50% of adolescent and adult deaths associated with water recreation. Boating carries risks for injury. In 2004, the U.S. Coast Guard received reports for 4904 boating accidents; 3663 participants were reported injured and 676 killed in boating accidents. Among those who drowned, 90% were not wearing life jackets (United States Coast Guard, 2005).

From United States Coast Guard. (2005). *Boating statistics—2004, Comdpub P16754.18.* Washington, DC: United States Coast Guard.

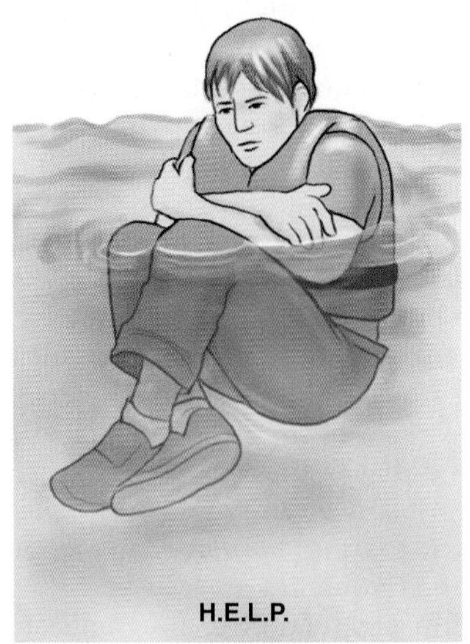

Figure 63-21 A person wearing a life jacket can increase survival time with the ***h****eat* ***e****scape* ***l****essening* ***p****osition* (HELP).

less than 98°F will cause hypothermia. The human body cannot maintain its heat in water less than 92°F. Colder water causes a faster rate of heat loss. Water causes heat loss 25 times faster than air. Moving water can cause even greater heat loss.

Hypothermia victims rapidly lose the ability for self-rescue. They are often unable to follow directions, and grabbing anything that might save them becomes difficult. A 15- to 20-minute immersion in water at 35°F is likely to be fatal.

Water temperature varies widely with seasons and runoff. Even on warm days, water temperature can be very low. PFDs lessen heat loss and energy required for flotation.

Cold Protective Response

[OBJECTIVE 22]

Cold protective response is the mechanism by which individuals can survive extended periods of submersion. It has been called a "metabolic icebox" because the response slows the deterioration of body parts such as the brain. This mechanism increases the chance of a cold water drowning victim's survival. One child has been resuscitated after submersion of 66 minutes with full or partial neurologic recovery. However, the cold protective response depends on how long the victim's head was above water during the cooling process.

Protective Physiologic Response. In some individuals cold water stimulation of the temperature receptors in the skin triggers the mammalian diving reflex. The younger the patient, the stronger the reflex. It triggers the shunting of blood to the brain and heart from the skin, gastrointestinal tract, and extremities. The victim's heart rate slows in response to the increased volume of blood in the body's core. These actions help the body conserve oxygen and may help the victim survive.

Survivability

[OBJECTIVE 23]

The factors influencing whether a victim survives include age (the younger the victim, the more active the mechanism), length of time the victim is submerged, presence of trauma, the contaminants inhaled from the water, posture in the water, and physical condition.

A number of individuals, particularly children, have been successfully resuscitated after being submerged for 30 minutes. Most individuals recovered in cold water near-drowning cases display signs of death, including cyanosis, no detectable breathing or pulse, and dilated pupils.

Unless physical signs of death are present, such as decapitation, putrefaction, or rigor mortis, the hypothermic victim should be considered salvageable. Until rewarming confirms death, *a patient is never cold and dead—only warm and dead.* The patient must be rewarmed and an assessment made before death can be confirmed. Before such an event, EMS personnel should consult available healthcare facilities regarding their capabilities to resuscitate an immersion hypothermia victim, which requires specialized equipment and specifically trained physician and nursing personnel as well as a standing protocol to receive and manage such patients.

Cold Water Survival

A person who accidentally falls into cold water should use some basic tactics to help survive long enough for help to arrive. To delay loss of body heat, the individual should not remove clothing, except for heavy items such as an overcoat.

A person wearing a life jacket can increase survival time with the ***h****eat* ***e****scape* ***l****essening* ***p****osition* (HELP) (Figure 63-21). In this position the knees are flexed and drawn toward the chest, with the arms pressed firmly against the sides of the chest. This position delays heat loss by protecting the most vulnerable areas: the head, the sides of the chest, and the groin.

Groups of three or more people can use the huddle position, which is based on the same principle as the HELP position. In the huddle position, the sides of the chest, the groin, and the lower body are pressed together.

If swimmers must stay in deep water without a life jacket for a long period, they should remain as still as possible, conserving energy and, if possible, staying in a tucked position. As the body's core temperature drops, making rational decisions will become increasingly more difficult.

Moving Water Rescue Training

In-Water Spinal Stabilization

[OBJECTIVE 24]

Spinal stabilization in water requires special training. Only rescuers who have training in water rescue should attempt rescue that includes in-water immobilization.

Head Splint Technique. Following are the steps of the head splint technique, which is used when the rescuer's PFD prohibits other techniques:

1. Approach the victim from the side.
2. Move the victim's arms over his or her head.
3. Hold the victim's head in place by using the victim's arms as a splint.
4. If victim is face down, perform steps 1 to 3, then rotate the victim toward the rescuer to the face-up position.
5. Ensure an open airway.
6. Maintain this position until a cervical collar is applied.

Cervical Collar Application. A cervical collar is then applied as follows:

1. The second rescuer determines collar size.
2. The second rescuer holds an open collar under the victim's neck.
3. The primary rescuer maintains immobilization and patent airway.
4. The second rescuer brings the collar up to the back of the victim's neck; the primary rescuer allows the second rescuer to bring the collar around the victim's neck and throat while the second rescuer maintains airway.
5. The second rescuer secures the fastener on the collar while the primary rescuer maintains airway.
6. The second rescuer secures the victim's hands at his or her waist.

Back Boards and Victim Extrication. Apply a back board and extricate the victim as follows:

1. Submerge the board under the victim at his or her waist.
2. Never lift the victim to the board; allow the board to float up to the victim (if the board does not float, lift it gently to the victim).
3. Secure the victim with straps, cravats, or other devices.
4. Move the victim to the extrication point at the shore or boat.
5. Always extricate the victim head first so that body weight will not compress possible spinal trauma.
6. Avoid extrication of the victim through the surf because the board could capsize.
7. Maintain airway management during extrication.

Overview of Water Rescue Techniques

[OBJECTIVE 25]

Basic Principles of Water Rescue

Following are the basic principles of water rescue:

- Never underestimate the power of moving water. The force of moving water combined with underwater hazards create a deadly mix.
- Do not enter moving water without highly specialized training and equipment.
- As in other rescues, the priorities at the scene are always self-rescue first, rescue and security of fellow rescuers second, and the victim last.
- All rescuers must wear a PFD even if using shore-based rescue techniques.

Swimming to perform rescues is hazardous to both the rescuer and the victim. Trained and equipped personnel should attempt these rescues only if other efforts fail.

Basic Water Rescue Model

[OBJECTIVE 26]

The following basic rescue model can be summarized as talk, reach, throw, row and, only as a last resort, go:

- *Talk.* Attempt to establish voice contact. If the victim is capable of self-rescue, provide encouragement and directions.
- *Reach.* From the shore, use a pike pole or other item to reach to the victim and pull him or her to shore. If using this technique the rescuer must keep his or her feet spread and body angled perpendicular to the water and keep weight as low as possible and balanced backward to avoid being pulled in.
- *Throw.* From the shore, throw a rope or throw bag to the victim and pull him or her to shore. To use a throw bag effectively, a rescuer needs instruction and practice in its use. This technique of rescue also has the danger of the rescuer being pulled in; use the stance described above.
- *Row.* If one is available, use a boat (row) to reach the victim. Practice and experience in handling a boat are necessary. Technique will depend on the type of boat. The pilot should not be the rescuer, and a minimum of two people should be on board. Always have a backup plan and have the resources present or en route to accomplish this plan immediately.

Rescue Safety Equipment

- Properly fitting PFD (U.S. Coast Guard approved)
- Helmet for head protection
- Knife for entanglement protection
- Whistle for location if in trouble
- Thermal protection

Victim Safety Equipment

- Flotation for victim
- Immobilization equipment
- Extrication equipment
- Thermal protection equipment
- Resuscitation equipment
- Transportation equipment

Self-Rescue

[OBJECTIVE 27]

If you accidentally find yourself in dangerous water, use the following self-rescue techniques if you have fallen into flat or moving water:

- Cover your mouth and nose during entry.
- Protect your head and keep your face out of the water.
- If you are in flat water, assume the HELP position.
- If you are in moving water, do not attempt to stand up.
- Float on your back with feet downstream and head pointed toward the nearest shore at a 45-degree angle.

HAZARDOUS ATMOSPHERES

Fatal Incident Example 3

At approximately 1000 hours, two sewer workers (27 and 28 years of age) entered a 50-foot-deep underground pumping station. Neither worker was wearing personal protective clothing or PPE. The two workers proceeded to remove the bolts of an inspection plate from a check valve. The plate blew off, allowing raw sewage to flood the chamber, overwhelming one of the workers. The second worker exited the pumping station and radioed the police department requesting assistance. He again entered the station and also was overcome. Two police officers responded to the call at approximately 10:09 AM, and one officer entered the pumping station. Later the sewage systems field manager arrived on the scene and followed the first officer into the pumping station. None of the rescuers returned to the top of the ladder. A construction worker passing by the site stopped and entered the station in a rescue attempt. After descending approximately 10 feet into the shaft, he called for help. The second police officer assisted the construction worker out of the shaft. None of the responding men was wearing a respirator.

Fire department personnel arrived at the accident site at approximately 10:11 AM. One firefighter, wearing self-contained breathing apparatus (SCBA), entered the shaft but could not locate the four men. By this time, sewage had completely flooded the underground room. The fireman exited the pumping station. A second volunteer fireman (6 feet, 8 inches tall, 240 lb) entered the shaft wearing an SCBA and a lifeline. As he began his descent, he apparently slipped from the ladder and became wedged in the shaft approximately 20 feet down. (His body was folded with his head and feet facing upward.) Not being able to breathe, he removed the face mask and lost consciousness. After a 30-minute effort, rescuers at the site extricated the fireman, who lived. No further rescue attempts were made until professional divers entered the station and removed the bodies. Autopsy results revealed a considerable amount of sewage in the lungs of the sewer workers and only a trace of sewage in the lungs of the field manager and the police officer.

Modified from National Institute for Occupational Safety and Health. (2005). FACE 85-31: *Three sanitation workers and one policeman die in an underground pumping station in Kentucky.* Retrieved February 28, 2007, from http://www.cdc.gov.

Oxygen-Deficient Environments and Confined Spaces

[OBJECTIVE 28]

Confined spaces and other hazardous environments may be the most dangerous situation to which a responder can be called. The National Institute for Occupational Safety and Health (NIOSH) estimates that 60% of the fatalities associated with confined spaces involve people attempting to rescue someone else (NIOSH, 1994).

Because of the high rate of fatalities, OSHA has created regulations regarding confined spaces. In some places, OSHA regulation 29 CFR1910.146, Permit-Required Confined Spaces, may not apply to certain responders. But all responders, whether required to or not, should use the OSHA regulations as guidelines for the safety of all involved. NFPA Standard 1670 also provides guidelines for confined space response.

According to OSHA, a **confined space** meets the following requirements:

- Is large enough and configured so that an employee can bodily enter and perform assigned work
- Has limited or restricted means for entry or exit (e.g., tanks, vessels, silos, storage bins, hoppers, vaults, and pits are spaces that may have limited means of entry)
- Is not designed for continuous employee occupancy

Some examples you may encounter are listed in Box 63-6.

Permit-Required Confined Space

A **permit-required confined space** (permit space) refers to a confined space that has one or more of the following characteristics:

1. Contains or has a potential to contain a hazardous atmosphere
2. Contains a material with the potential for engulfing an entrant

BOX 63-6 Examples of Confined Spaces

- Septic tanks
- Silos and grain bins
- Utility vaults
- Boilers
- Pits
- Sewers
- Tunnels
- Sewage digester
- Reaction vessel
- Ship ballast tanks
- Wells and cisterns
- Storage tanks

3. Has an internal configuration such that an entrant could be trapped or asphyxiated by inwardly converging walls or a floor that slopes downward and tapers to a smaller cross-section
4. Contains any other recognized serious safety or health hazard

OSHA uses the term *permit space* to describe spaces that meet the definition of confined space and pose health or safety hazards.

Confined Space Hazards

Hazardous Atmospheres

[OBJECTIVE 29]

Atmospheric problems are most often the danger in confined space situations. They account for approximately 60% of fatalities in confined spaces. In confined spaces, toxic gases present a condition known as immediately dangerous to life or health, both in the form of inhalation dangers as well as flame and explosion dangers.

One reason rescuers are sometimes unaware of the danger is that oxygen-deficient atmospheres often are not a visible problem, so rescuers assume the atmosphere is safe. Many of these gases, which displace the oxygen, are colorless, odorless, and tasteless but are deadly. Another problem is that increased oxygen levels can cause atmosphere-monitoring meters to give false readings.

Atmosphere oxygen levels are considered dangerous when the percentage of oxygen falls below 19.5% or rises above 23.5%. Slight changes in oxygen levels can cause behavioral changes in an individual, resulting in confusion and inability to help oneself. Before entering a space, the oxygen levels must be tested by qualified personnel.

Poisonous Gases

[OBJECTIVE 30]

Poisonous gases commonly found in confined spaces include the following:

- Hydrogen sulfide
- Carbon dioxide
- Carbon monoxide
- Low/high oxygen concentrations
- Methane
- Ammonia
- Nitrogen dioxide

Fire and Explosion

Toxic gas also can cause fire and explosion. The minimal concentration of fuel in the air that will ignite is measured in terms of *lower explosive limit.* Below this point, too much oxygen and not enough fuel are present to burn (the mixture is too lean). *Upper explosive limit* refers to the concentration of fuel in the air above which the vapors cannot be ignited. Above this point, too much fuel and not enough oxygen are present to burn (the mixture is too rich).

Engulfment

Another hazard is engulfment, which occurs when loose products such as grain or coal become unstable and cover a person, resulting in suffocation. In addition, some products, such as flour and coal, present the danger of dust explosion. A dust explosion occurs when a combustible material is dispersed in the air, forming a flammable cloud. With ignition, flame propagates through the cloud, resulting in explosion.

Machinery Entrapment

Confined spaces often have augers, screws, blades, gears, conveyer belts, and other moving parts that can entrap and injure a person.

Electricity

High levels of electricity are used in industrial processes, in running large motors, and in moving products from one area to another. Stored energy, such as large battery units, presents another danger.

Structural Hazards

Confined spaces may contain structural hazards that can impede or endanger rescuers. Many spaces have cross-beams, piping, and trays that can entangle rescue systems. Some spaces are not symmetrical but have structures shaped like an L, T, or X.

Fall Hazards

Most confined space configurations are below ground or elevated. These spaces must be accessed by steep ladders, which can become slippery and have small footing surfaces.

Emergencies in Confined Spaces

OSHA requires what is known as a *permit process* before a rescuer can enter a confined space. This is a step-by-step list of actions that must be done before confined space

Confined Space Entry Permit			
Location and description of confined space: Reason for entry: Permit issued to: Supervisor's name: Attendant's name: Permit issuer's name:			
% oxygen:	% lower explosive limit:	ppm CO:	H2S:
Requirements:			
Emergency rescuer	yes	no	
Continuous gas monitor	yes	no	
Barrier for ground openings	yes	no	
Warning signs	yes	no	
Safety harness with life line	yes	no	
Tripod/hoist/pulley	yes	no	
Access (ladders/other)	yes	no	
Eye protection	yes	no	
Respiratory protection	yes	no	
Continuous ventilation	yes	no	
Body protection	yes	no	
Hand protection	yes	no	
Foot protection	yes	no	
Weather protection	yes	no	
Ground fault circuit	yes	no	
Interrupters	yes	no	
Lockout of hazardous energy	yes	no	

Figure 63-22 Confined space entry permit.

entry. Only trained and qualified persons can take the steps to secure a confined space entry permit (Figure 63-22).

Steps for Safe Entry into a Confined Space

[OBJECTIVE 31]

Specific criteria must be met before EMS can enter a confined space.

Environmental monitoring of the site must occur before entry. Before anyone enters the space, any threats to human life in the space must be known. In addition, the internal atmosphere must be tested with a calibrated direct-reading instrument for oxygen content, flammable gases and vapors, and potential toxic air contaminants, in that order.

Atmospheric monitoring must occur continuously or at frequent intervals to determine the following:

- Oxygen concentration
- Hydrogen sulfide level
- Explosive limits
- Flammable atmosphere
- Toxic air contaminants

A "lock out, tag out" process must occur for all power. The term *power* here includes hydraulic or compressed gas–powered devices, not just electrically powered. Lock out is the placing of a locking device on an energy-isolating device, ensuring that the energy-isolating device and the equipment being controlled cannot be operated until the device is removed. Tag out is the placing of a tagging device on an energy-isolating device that indicates the energy-isolating device and the equipment being controlled may not be operated until the device is removed.

After the power source has been locked and tagged, all flow into the site must be stopped. Hydraulic lines must be secured to prevent even minor leakage. All stored energy must be dissipated, and the area must be ventilated.

At this point, no EMS rescuers are allowed to make entry until a rescue team has made the area safe. Access to confined spaces often is limited, making access and extraction difficult.

The use of a self-contained breathing apparatus (SCBA) in a confined space is a dangerous practice. All SCBAs have a limited air supply, which means that if the air runs out while the wearer is in a confined space the wearer is in danger of dying. Because of small entryways and obstructions, a person may have to remove that SCBA to fit through some areas. In most cases a supplied air apparatus is preferred. Supplied air is a system of air hoses that run from an air supply usually outside the space to the user inside the space.

Finally, a rescuer lowering and retrieval system must be in place. A way to retrieve a person in the space who becomes incapacitated must exist. Each authorized entrant must wear a chest or full body harness with a retrieval line attached at the center of the entrant's back near shoulder level, above the entrant's head, or at another point that presents a profile small enough for the successful removal of the entrant.

First Actions for Arriving EMS Personnel

When EMS personnel arrive on the scene of a rescue emergency, they should immediately perform the following actions:

1. Establish a safe perimeter.
2. Restrict any additional entry to the space.
3. Assist in attempting remote retrieval.
4. Determine from the permit or entry supervisor the type of work being done when the accident happened.
5. Determine from the entry supervisor the number of workers inside.
6. Ensure the area for workers to don PPE is safe. The space must be cleared of any threats or access by outside persons. Entrants must have the PPE to protect against any threats that remain in the space.
7. Ensure retrieval devices are in place.
8. Ensure a standby person is at each entry in case problems develop. The standby person should be equipped with rescue equipment, including a safety line attached to the worker in case the worker needs to be retrieved.

EMS personnel should evaluate the following elements:

- Confirm that a confined space emergency is what it appears to be.
- Determine if any patients are present and the number.
- Establish whether the emergency is a rescue or a recovery.

Roles and Responsibilities of the First Responder

Begin ICS early. Request adequate resources, especially trained confined space personnel and equipment. Know their availability and location before such an incident occurs.

Hazards

You must identify any hazards present, the extent to which they are present, and any special considerations relating to the hazards. You also must consider whether any type of contamination is present or possible (hazardous materials). If contamination is present, you must determine the type, extent, and problems the contamination may create, such as where contaminants are going if they are moving.

Access to confined spaces often is limited, making access to the victim and extraction difficult. Confined spaces typically involve constricted spaces and tight entrances. This means that conventional litters cannot be maneuvered through many confined spaces. You may need a flexible litter or ridged litter with a small profile. You must practice using this type of litter before a real emergency.

RESCUE FROM TRENCHES AND CAVE-INS

[OBJECTIVE 32]

Excavating is one of the most hazardous activities in the construction industry. Likewise, response to trench collapse is one of the most dangerous calls for EMS personnel.

A look at the simple physics of trenching shows why an excavation collapse is so dangerous. The average weight of one cubic foot of soil is approximately 100 pounds. Only 2 feet of soil pressing on the trunk of a person can weight 700 to 1000 pounds. Obviously this quickly leads to impaired breathing and asphyxia along with other medical problems.

A person buried for longer periods may develop crush syndrome, requiring careful monitoring, particularly when his or her body is completely uncovered. Deep soils are often cooler than the air, so the patient also may develop hypothermia.

Causes of Trench Cave-In and Collapse

OSHA regulations require that when workers are in an excavation deeper than 5 feet the trench walls must be supported by a system made with posts, beams, shores, or planking and hydraulic jacks or a trench box (a preassembled structure, usually of metal, that can be moved where needed). However, contractors, in an attempt to save time and/or money, may miss this critical safety step.

A number of mechanisms cause trench collapse, but the most common are the following (Figure 63-23):

- The lip of one or both sides of the trench caves in.
- A wall shears away and falls in.
- A spoil pile is too close to edge, causing collapse.

Factors contributing to collapse include the following:

- Previously disturbed soil
- Intersecting trenches
- Ground vibrations from trucks or machinery
- Dirt (spoil) pile too close to edge of trench
- Water seepage

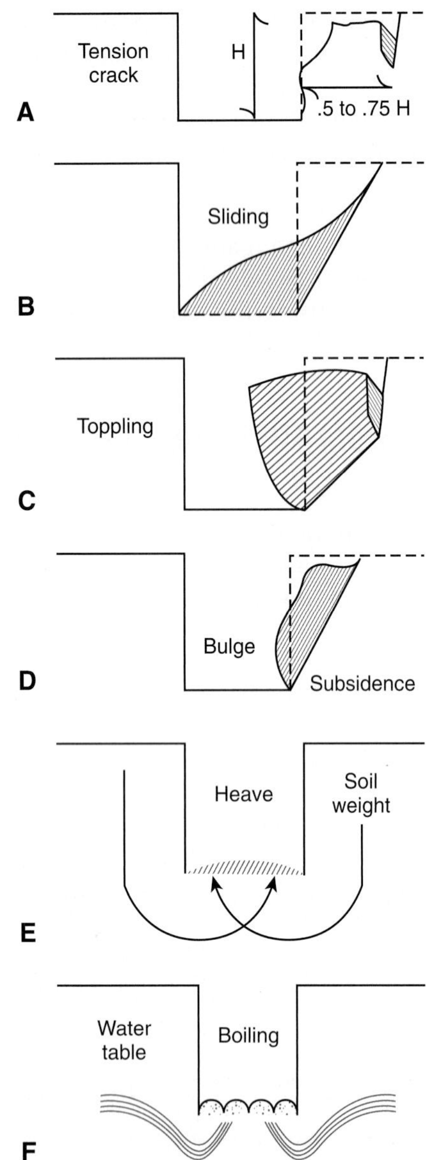

Figure 63-23 A number of mechanisms cause trench collapse. **A,** Tension cracks. **B,** Sliding. **C,** Toppling. **D,** Subsidence and bulging. **E,** Heaving or squeezing. **F,** Boiling.

Initial Response

Anyone responding to a trench collapse must realize that if a collapse has already occurred, a secondary collapse is likely. This will endanger responders who enter the trench or get too close to the edge. As with a confined space incident, the first steps on arriving at the scene of a trench collapse are to secure the scene, initiate command, and secure a perimeter. Only qualified personnel directly involved in the rescue are allowed inside the perimeter. All vehicles should be staged at a designated staging area, and initially arriving units should shut down where possible to minimize vibration to the ground that could precipitate a secondary collapse.

BOX 63-7 OSHA Definition of Competent Person for Trenching

Competent Person. The designated competent person should have and be able to demonstrate the following:

- Training, experience, and knowledge of soil analysis, use of protective systems; and requirements of 29 CFR Part 1926 Subpart P.
- Ability to detect conditions that could result in cave-ins, failures in protective systems, hazardous atmospheres, and other hazards including those associated with confined spaces.
- Authority to take prompt corrective measures to eliminate existing and predictable hazards and to stop work when required.

Modified from Occupational Safety and Health Administration. *Competent person.* Retrieved October 30, 2008, from http://www.osha.gov.

If a qualified trench rescue team is not already on scene, first responders should call for one. Prevent anyone, including workers and emergency personnel, from entering the trench until it has been made safe with appropriate shoring (Box 63-7).

Medical Considerations in Trench Rescue

One major medical issue in trench collapse is crush injury. This means that a cave-in victim must be continuously monitored and treated during the rescue operation, which could take hours. All medical resources and transportation must be ready when the patient is freed.

Another medical concern in trench collapse is hypothermia because soil tends to be below the normal human body temperature. It is usually impossible to get protective clothing around the patient, so you may want to consider warm air inhalation systems. If IV access can be obtained, consider providing warmed IV solutions. In addition, monitor both intake and output (if possible) to assess both hydration and renal function. If blood sampling is accessible, obtain serial samples and take to a local facility so that blood electrolyte levels can be monitored. This may be a consideration in determining crush syndrome and other physiologic affects of long-term entrapment. Core rewarming in such a rescue is sometimes best accomplished by using exterior warming. Ventilation fans with heated air are usually found with trench collapse teams and, if unavailable, can be obtained either from a local excavation contractor or from a contractor supply. EMS and rescue agencies should maintain a resource listing, and the logistics section of an ICS should be able to coordinate specialized resources such as this. For long-term collapse rescue, an urban search and rescue trained physician team should be considered and deployed as available.

Case Scenario—continued

Fire department rescue units have arrived at the scene and begun shoring operations. Command announces that the area around the victim has been stabilized but shoring is not complete, so no one is allowed in the trench yet. Plywood has been placed along the edges of the trench, so you can come to the edge of the trench. The patient has regained consciousness.

The rescue team has stabilized the trench so that EMS personnel can approach the patient. However, the patient remains covered to his groin by damp, clay-type soil. The soil is cool to the touch and the air is cooler at the bottom of the trench than at the surface. The rescuers are using an air knife to loosen the soil and a vacuum hose to remove it from the trench. Command reports that the patient may be completely exposed in 1.5 hours. This means he will have been partially covered by soil for a total of 3.5 hours. The patient is alert and oriented and reports that he feels cold and has no feeling in his legs. Signs of shock are present. You observe that he is shivering.

Questions

4. *Was there anything you could do for the patient before the trench was stabilized?*
5. *What sort of physical protection must be provided for the patient now that the trench is stabilized?*
6. *What can be done for environmental factors (chill)?*
7. *What medical care should be considered?*
8. *How should you prepare for when the patient is completely released from entrapment?*
9. *What destination and level of medical transportation are most appropriate for this patient?*

HAZARDOUS TERRAIN

Fatal Incident Example 4

This incident involved response for an injured individual who had fallen 180 feet down a steep slope. When the medical evacuation helicopter landed, the flight paramedic left the aircraft to attend to the patient. Using skills he had learned in high school Reserve Officers' Training Corps, he rappelled down the cliff to the patient. He attended to the patient and assisted in packaging him in a litter. Using a mechanical ascending system provided by other responders, he began ascending a rope to return to the aircraft. Night was approaching, so the rescuers asked the helicopter crew to help by taking off and providing "night sun" to assist in their hauling and raising operations. The responders began hauling the litter, but two litter attendants on the basket overloaded its capabilities. The noise and downdraft from the helicopter negated all communication and put the scene into what one investigator later termed "a whirlwind of confusion and noncommunication."

When the paramedic had ascended to a wide ledge approximately 15 to 20 feet from the top, he was asked to surrender his ascending system so it could be used by another responder to get up the cliff. The paramedic then was handed a white line and told to hand-over-hand the rest of the way up.

Meanwhile, the litter had gotten snagged on a rocky outcrop. Adding to the confusion, one of the litter attendants panicked, unhooked himself from the litter package, and stepped off in a pocket on the rock face. The downdraft had turned the location into an on-scene tornado.

Using the line he had been handed, the paramedic pulled on it so he could scramble to the top. Suddenly the line broke and the paramedic fell backward 160 feet to his death.

Investigation revealed that the broken "rope" was not designed for life support, but rather was a piece of boiler plate gasket made of 100% asbestos, with no strength to speak of. It had been taken from a rescuer's truck and placed in service by one of the EMS persons.

Rescue in hazardous terrain can be challenging and dangerous. This kind of rescue activity requires specialized training along with management coordination and continuous situational awareness.

Types of Hazardous Terrain

The site of a rescue in a hazardous area may contain elements of more than one type of terrain.

Steep Slope or Low-Angle Terrain

A steep slope, or **low-angle terrain,** is an environment in flat or mildly sloping areas. In low-angle operations, rescuers primarily support themselves with their feet on the terrain surface. They are not usually supported by a rope system; however, they may use one or more ropes as a safety or for evacuating a litter with a patient.

In most low-angle environments rescuers can navigate without having to use their hands to balance themselves. In some areas footing may be difficult, so a rope may be used for stability. In a low-angle environment, carrying a litter may be difficult, even with several people, so a rope may be used for stability during evacuation. If a rescuer were to make an error in most low-angle environments, the consequences would likely be no more serious than a fall and tumble. Rescue in low-angle terrain also is known as *slope evacuation* or *scree evacuation.*

Rescue in the Low-Angle Environment

Low-angle rescues often occur in locations easily reached by walking or scrambling (i.e., a way of moving in hazardous terrain that is between walking and climbing). Scrambling may involve using the hands for balance and occasionally using rope for added safety in some of the more hazardous areas.

Rescuers in the low-angle environment need appropriate footwear because slopes often are grassy or have loose rock. In addition, they should wear a helmet. In many cases, a rope hand line, running from top to bottom, can assist rescuers in keeping their balance and can speed up operations.

High-Angle or Vertical Terrain

High-angle, or **vertical terrain,** is an environment such as a cliff or building side where hands must be used for balance when ascending (Figure 63-24). High angle is an environment in which the load is predominantly supported by the rope rescue system.

If a rescuer makes a mistake in high-angle terrain, it could lead to serious injuries or death. In a high-angle environment, litter movement completely depends on rope systems. Some of the environments in which a high-angle rescue might be used include the following:

- Cliffs
- Buildings
- Industrial sites, either outside a structure or inside a vessel
- Construction sites such as tower cranes
- Other structures such as stacks, silos, or towers
- Vertical caves

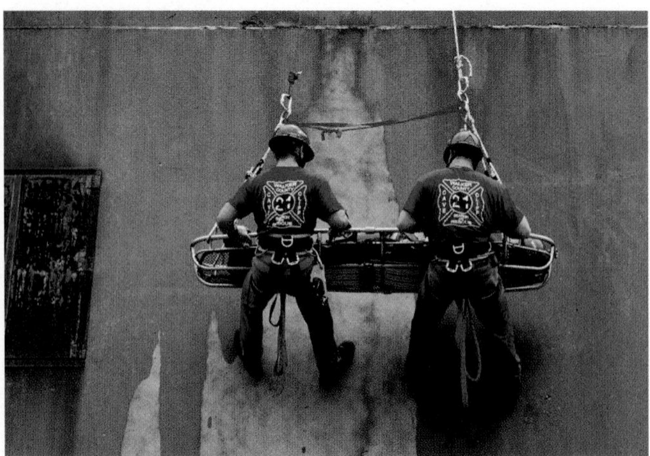

Figure 63-24 High-angle terrain. Rescue in high-angle terrain requires the use of rope systems.

Flat Terrain with Obstructions

Some rescue areas may be mostly flat but with isolated areas with obstructions such as rocks, loose soil or rock, and creeks.

Patient Access in Hazardous Terrain

[OBJECTIVE 33]

Potential rescuers must have specialized training and equipment to operate safely and efficiently in the high-angle environment. Among the personal skills needed in high-angle rescue are belaying, rappelling, and ascending.

Belaying

Belay is a safety technique used to safeguard personnel exposed to the risk of falling. A belay uses an unload rope (belay rope) attached to the person or persons being belayed. The rope used should be a dynamic rope, meaning it will absorb some energy of a fall in stretch. These are specially designed and maintained ropes called lifelines.

The belayer is the person responsible for operation of the belay. The belayer may use a belay device, a braking mechanism through which a secondary line, also called the *belay line,* is rigged. Being a belayer is a serious commitment, meaning the well-being, perhaps even the life, of the person at the end of the rope is in the hands of the belayer.

Rappelling

Rappelling is controlled descent on a rope by using the friction of the rope through a descender (also known as a *rappel device*). Rescuers rappel to get from the top to the bottom of a vertical face. Rappelling is used in combination with other essential vertical skills for performing a rescue. Rappelling is a potentially hazardous activity and requires training by a qualified instructor. Rappelling and raising of persons are also done on a lifeline but one that has no stretch, called *static rope.* This rope must not be interchanged with the belay rope.

High-Angle Litter Evacuation

High-angle lowering, also sometimes called *vertical lowering,* refers to the controlled lowering of a rescue patient with a rope. If the patient's injuries are severe enough, the lowering is done with the patient secured in a litter.

In some cases in which the subject is uninjured or only slightly injured, he or she may be lowered without the litter, either alone or with a rescuer.

By its nature, the high-angle environment is hazardous both for rescuer and patient. To perform rescues safely in a high-angle environment, responders must have training from a qualified source and use equipment specific to the high-angle environment.

Patient Packaging

[OBJECTIVE 34]

Rescue usually means dealing with an injured or sick person. Transporting the injured or sick person from the rescue environment to an ambulance or helicopter usually requires a litter. Knowing how to package the patient in the litter and how to move the litter containing the patient are essential skills of rescue.

Basket Litters

The basket litter is the standard stretcher for hazardous terrain rescue. It sometimes is called a *Stokes litter* or *Stokes basket.* Basket litters for rescue are constructed of a rigid frame and strong materials that help protect the patient and resist damage when used in the rescue environment. Basket litters may be constructed of a wire frame and covered either with a metal or plastic mesh.

Most basket litters have handholds along each side and at either end so that several rescuers can carry the litter. These and other connection points can be used to attach a rope rescue system to the litter.

Metal Basket Litters. The metal basket litter has been the litter most commonly used by rescuers and is generally the stronger type. Many military surplus litters are available to rescuers, but rescuers should avoid a metal litter unless they know its history. Some metal litters have hidden rust or faulty welds that could fail in rescue conditions.

If possible, rescuers should avoid the military style litters with a leg divider and chicken wire mesh. The leg divider keeps this type of litter from accepting a conventional spine board and requires additional padding for the patient's groin area. The wire mesh often has sharp ends, which can puncture skin and medical equipment.

Plastic Basket Litters. Most plastic litters weigh less than most metal litters (Figure 63-25). The advantages of a plastic litter include the fact that they slide more easily over rough ground or snow. Because of their solid bottoms, they usually provide better patient protection under the patient. Their disadvantages include the fact that they are not as resistant to damage as the stronger metal litters and they can collect water and snow, creating more challenges in patient packaging.

Flexible Litters

Unlike a basket litter, a flexible litter does not have an inherent rigid structure but wraps closely around the patient. Because of their flexibility, these litters often are easier to work with in confined spaces.

One flexible litter is the Sked (Skedco, Inc., Tualatin, Ore.). When it is conformed around the patient like a cocoon, the litter becomes more rigid (Figure 63-26). The Sked can be rolled into a compact shape that is stored or transported in its own backpack, which is 9 inches (22.9 cm) in diameter and 36 inches (91.4 cm) long. This means that one person can backpack the litter to remote locations.

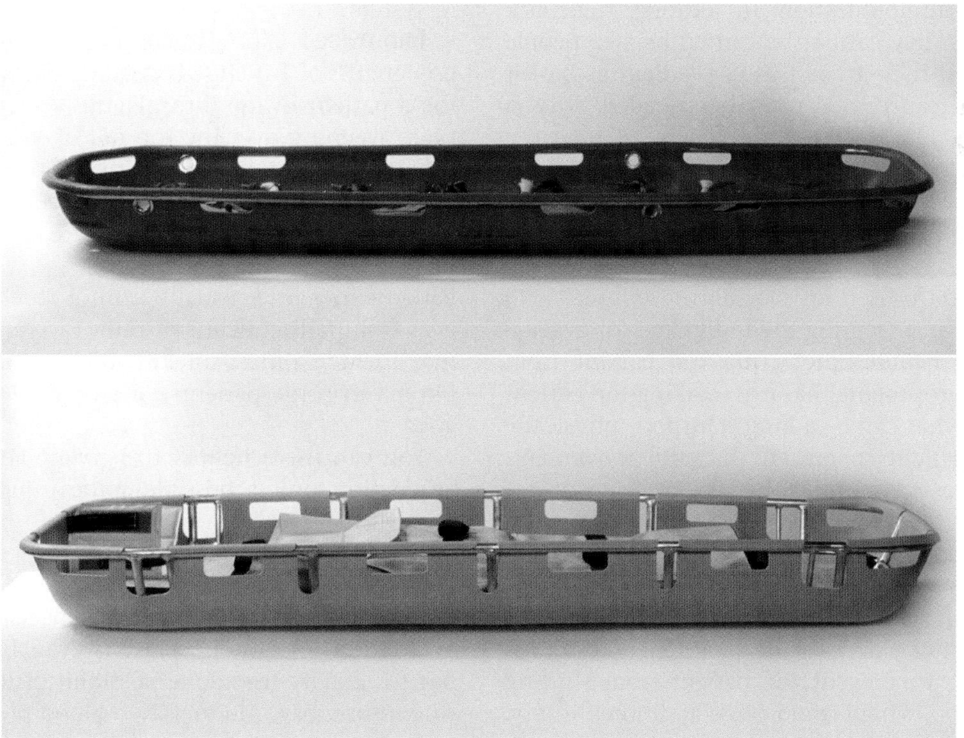

Figure 63-25 Plastic basket litters slide easily over rough or frozen ground and may offer more protection to the patient. They may retain water and snow if not properly drained and can be blown about in high winds and helicopter downdraft.

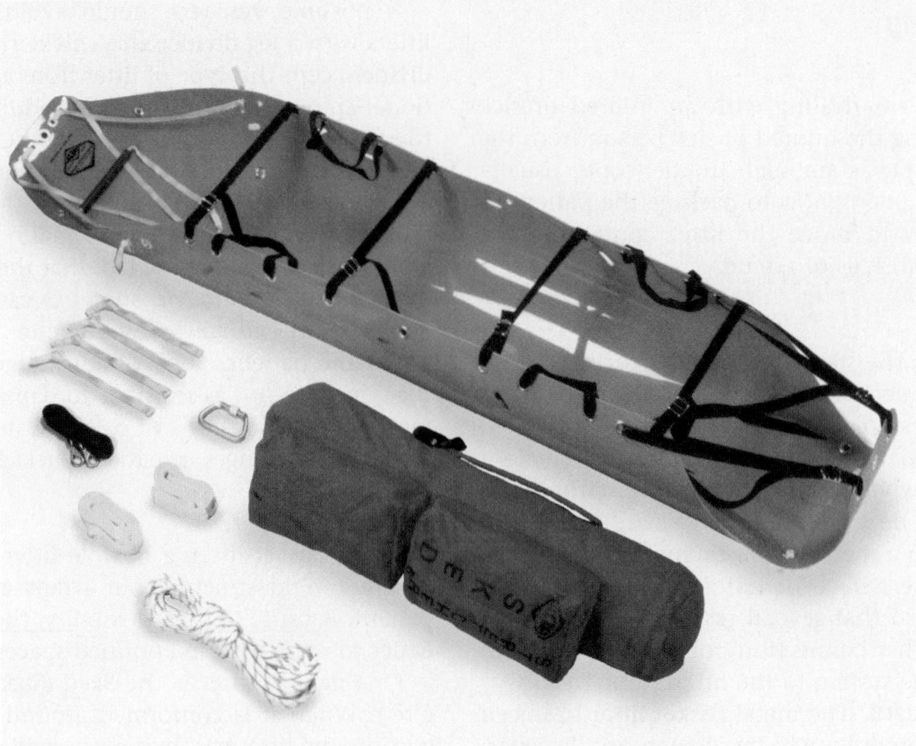

Figure 63-26 Flexible litters do not have an inherent shape but are wrapped closely around the patient. Flexible litters often are easier to work through confined spaces. Shown here is the Sked basic rescue system.

Disadvantages of flexible litters include the need for additional spine immobilization. In addition, their lack of rigidity means they cannot be carried by two people at either end, and they are not as convenient as basket litters for litter teams to carry when loaded with a patient.

Packaging and Securing the Patient in the Litter

[OBJECTIVE 35]

Packaging is the term used for placing the injured or ill person in a litter and securing the individual for evacuation. Packaging includes protecting the patient from physical and environmental hazards, making the patient comfortable for what can be a long transport, physically stabilizing the patient to prevent harmful movement, and allowing access to monitor the patient.

Litter Patient Restraint

[OBJECTIVE 36]

During rescue in hazardous terrain, rescuers may need to tilt and turn the litter. Consequently, a system of restraints must be in place to prevent the patient from shifting around in the litter, which could cause additional injury. Most basket litters are not equipped with adequate restraints. All require additional strapping or lacing for rough terrain evacuation and extraction, so the choice is usually a manufactured patient restraint system, which can save time in packaging, or an improvised patient tie-in system.

Improvised Litter Patient Tie-In. Rescuers commonly use lengths of 1-inch (24 mm) tubular webbing for securing a patient in the litter (Figure 63-27). Avoid running tie-in webbing over the top rail of the litter, where it is subject to abrasion and cutting. Also, tie-in webbing on the top rail could conflict with rescue rigging.

Protecting the Patient

Patients in a litter usually cannot shield their faces and eyes from falling debris or rain. Face and eye protection may include a litter shield (which can produce claustrophobia in some patients), a face shield or, at the least, goggles.

You can use a helmet to prevent head injury during evacuation unless possible spine injury considerations prevent its use.

Fluids

Managing fluids (IV or oral) takes special care during litter evacuation. Usually no place is available to hang an IV bag for gravity feed. One possibility is the use of a pressure infuser bag. Alternately, a blood pressure cuff can be used, but it requires monitoring to make certain it has the right pressure to keep fluids running. If IV fluids are pressurized, extra care must be taken to prevent air embolism. As an alternative, a J loop or saline lock may be

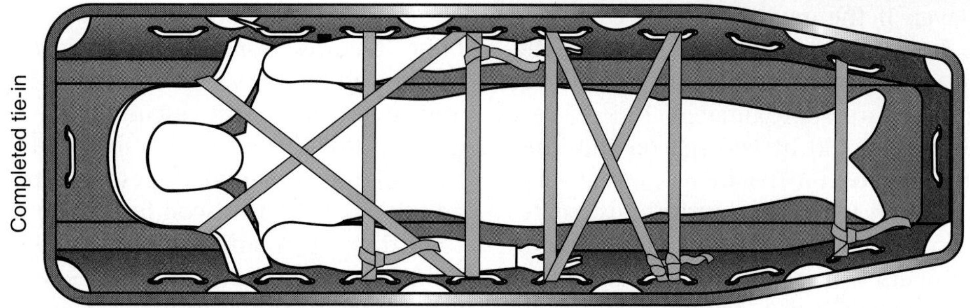

Figure 63-27 Rescuers commonly use 1-inch wide webbing to create an improvised litter patient tie-in, although many different improvisations are possible.

appropriate with fluid boluses instead of continuous infusion.

Of special concern is the freezing of fluids in cold weather. IV lines are particularly susceptible to freezing, but whole bags may end up frozen, making them useless. Special devices can keep IV bags from freezing in cold weather. When these are not available, some responders keep the bags inside their clothing. EMS responders also should be conscious of the possible temperature of the fluids because they would not want to administer cold fluids into a patient already at risk from a cold environment. General hypothermia also should be considered when deciding if fluid therapy is indicated. In a cold environment, the process itself may expose the patient to unnecessary cooling, and the presence of hypothermia may significantly compromise peripheral venous access.

Accessibility

As rescuers are packaging the patient, they must do so with consideration for monitoring the patient during the evacuation. The patient should be packaged for easy access for checking blood pressure and perfusion and performing airway management.

Airway Management

All patients in any circumstance should be packaged with concern for airway management. Patients should be packaged such that they can be rolled in case of vomiting or other airway threats. Suction should be placed at the head of the litter so that it can be quickly accessed. An option is packaging the patient in a lateral recumbent position. This is difficult to do with conventional strapping techniques, but it can be done with a vacuum mattress.

Padding

During a rescue evacuation, the patient may be in the litter for long periods, so rescuers should make every effort to make the patient comfortable and prevent additional injury. To prevent additional pain and possible tissue damage in areas of tissue pressure, rescuers must pad areas of tissue pressure.

Patient Restraint for Other Terrain

The patient packaging for low-angle and flat, rough terrain is the same as for high-angle terrain. The goal in all types of restraint in rough terrain is to prevent the patient from sliding around in the litter.

Packaging the Patient with Possible Spinal Injuries

A full spine board is not always required in most rigid basket litters. Effective stabilization can be accomplished by using half-length spinal immobilization devices such as a Kendrick extrication device (Ferno, Wilmington, Ohio) or the Oregon spine splint (Skedco).

Most spine boards are flat and hard, and immobilization of patients on rigid spine boards can be painful for the patient even for a short period. Immobilization on rigid spine boards for longer periods can result in tissue interface pressure, or pressure points. Over time, sufficient pressure at these points can result in pressure necrosis, or bedsores. The vacuum mattress is preferable for immobilization during long evacuations.

Vacuum Mattress. Vacuum mattresses are air-tight splint devices filled with polystyrene beads that interlock when air is sucked out of the mattress. Vacuum mattresses provide the same degree of immobilization as spine boards but conform to the patient's body. Because they contour to the body's curves, they are less likely to cause pain and tissue damage from pressure points.

Vacuum mattresses have the same overall weight as full spine boards and have other advantages than immobilization. For example, they also help insulate a patient in a litter from the cold. The disadvantages of vacuum mattresses include potential for puncture (although they can be repaired in the field) and restricted access to some areas of the patient, particularly the posterior aspects.

Protecting from Environmental Concerns

A patient in a litter is particularly susceptible to cold, both from his or her injuries and from the inability to move around and warm himself or herself. Protect the patient from wind, cold, and rain with a waterproof and windproof outer layer. If the environment is cold, line the bottom with a foam pad or blankets to provide extra insulation. One means of providing this waterproof layer is to use a large plastic tarp approximately 15 × 15 feet (4.5 × 4.5 m). The tarp should be laid out on the litter before the patient is placed in it (Figure 63-28).

In providing insulation for patient warmth, use material that provides access to all sides of the patient. Sleeping bags should have zippers or hook-and-loop closures that open all around the patient's torso. Commercially made hypothermia bags used in hospital transport work well, as do disaster pouches that are sealed and air tight.

Protecting the Patient in the Litter

Litter Underside. Protecting the underside of the patient is of particular concern in a wire basket litter. This litter is uncomfortable to be in and offers little protection on the bottom from protruding objects such as twigs, branches, and stones. To protect the bottom and make it more comfortable, material such as a closed-cell foam pad and/or blankets can be used to line it. Be sure to pad hollow spaces along the body, such as behind the knees and the small of the back.

Packaging for Long Bone Fractures

All suspected fractures must be protected by using rigid splints and protective bandages. Basket stretchers with hard shells provide the best protection for suspected long bone fractures. Some femur traction splints commonly used in urban ambulance transport have too much bulk and length to use in rescue litters. When applied to a patient, they often extend above the litter top rail and beyond the foot end of rescue litters. This can cause additional patient discomfort, expose the affected limb to further injury, and complicate rescue rigging and handling. More compact and portable femur traction devices are available. Some examples are the Sager emergency traction splint (Sager, Redding, Calif.) and the Kendrick extrication device.

Patient Movement

If the terrain is flat enough, a nontechnical/nonrope evacuation or carry out is usually faster because rope systems are time consuming to set up. A number of techniques can make a carry out easier on the litter bearers.

Litter Slings. Rescuers often must carry a litter with a patient from the rescue site to a vehicle or helicopter. Carrying a litter with one hand on the litter rail can be extremely tiring. A litter sling can help relieve the load by spreading it to the shoulder (Figure 63-29). Depending on the size of the litter bearer, a litter sling can be made with a 14- to 18-foot (4.5 to 6 m) length of tubular webbing. With a ring bend (water) knot, you can create a continuous loop in the webbing. Then attach the loop to the litter

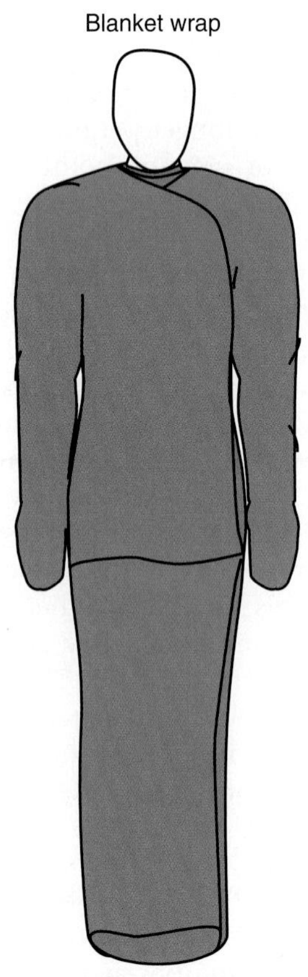

Figure 63-28 Packaging patients in a litter includes protecting them from environmental concerns.

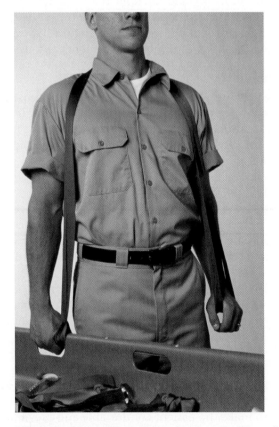

Figure 63-29 Carrying a litter with one hand on the litter rail can be extremely tiring. Litter slings can relieve the load by spreading it to the shoulder.

rail with a large carabiner or by cinching it on the rail. Then run the line over the carrier's shoulder and grasp the other end of the web with the hand away from the litter.

Even with litter slings, carrying a litter with an adult patient can be an exhausting process. This usually requires six litter bearers at one time. If possible, additional bearers should be available to relieve other bearers for carries longer than half a mile. This relief is often accomplished by a process of rotation, with the two relief bearers approaching the rear of the litter to take up the position of the two rear bearers. The bearers then move forward on the litter until the two front bearers move off the litter and go on ahead. In this position, they serve as scouts, looking for obstacles and alerting the other bearers to hazards. At the next rotation, the two scouts move to the rear, and the process continues. Frequent timed switches will be less exhausting and move the litter faster than waiting for rescuers to ask for relief.

Litter Wheels. The litter wheel is a device that can help save rescuers' energy and expedite the evacuation. The litter is attached to a wheel with either a clamping device or straps. When using the wheel, rescuers walk beside or at the ends of the litter (or in both places), holding and balancing the litter because the wheel supports most of the weight.

If a wheeled litter is to be used on a flat, smooth surface to transport a patient who requires only a minimum of care, only two litter tenders may be needed, one at each end. However, handling a wheeled litter in more rugged terrain usually requires a minimum of four rescuers, two on each side. More difficult terrain may require additional attendants.

Rescuers should practice using the wheel before a rescue. Such practice can help rescuers understand aspects of wheeled litter handling, including how to find the center of gravity for proper balance.

Case Scenario CONCLUSION

Rescuers are in the process of removing that last of the soil from around the patient's feet. They have positioned an aerial unit above the patient with a rope attached. The plan is to place a full body harness on the patient and lift him from the trench. The patient is lifted from the trench and placed in an ambulance, which takes him a short distance to the helicopter. Shortly after extrication, his vital signs begin to deteriorate and he loses consciousness. He is taken to the trauma center and his vital signs are stabilized. He is then admitted to the intensive care unit.

Looking back

10. *What was your most important medical consideration for the patient?*
11. *What was the level of transport urgency for this patient?*

Low-Angle and High-Angle Evacuation

[OBJECTIVE 37]

Anchors are the means of securing the ropes and other elements of the high-angle system. The place where an anchor is connected is the **anchor point.** Anchor points take a number of forms. They can be manmade, such as with structural beams, or natural anchors, such as trees or rocks. Or they may be **artificial anchors** that people have placed in rock walls. Without suitable and secure anchors, the remainder of the high-angle system (ropes, hardware, and other gear) is in danger of failure, no matter how well they are established. Always use multiple anchors; do not depend on a single anchor. The greater the load and consequences of failure, the more complex anchors may need to become.

Rope Lowering Systems

The objective of a lowering system in rope rescue is the controlled lowering of what is called the *rescue load.* The rescue load could be a patient or a patient in a litter with the litter attendant.

Braking Systems

Braking devices are devices through which the rope is run for a controlled lowering of the rescue load. One commonly used braking device is the **brake bar rack** (Figure 63-30). By changing the number of bars on the brake bar rack, a rescuer can adapt to changing rescue load. It can be used in steep-slope evacuation as well as high-angle evacuation. In terrain that varies between steep and gentle, the brake bar rack can easily vary friction. Figure 63-31 shows a typical lowering of a litter in a high-angle environment.

Hauling

Not all litter evacuations go down slope. Many must go up slope. Hauling techniques use many of the same principles as lowering. However, hauling systems may involve slightly more complex rope work and additional personnel.

The type of hauling system is usually expressed in mechanical advantage. Mechanical advantage is the advantage created by a machine that enables people to

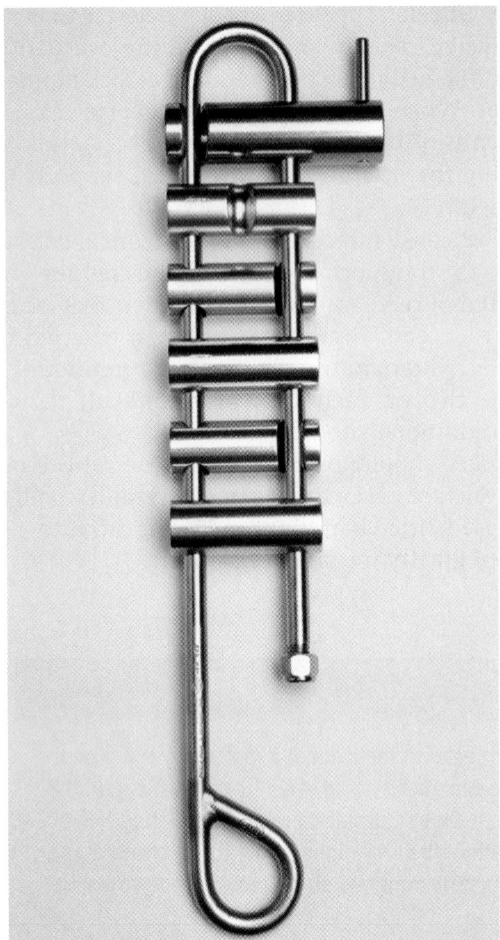

Figure 63-30 A brake bar rack is a descending device that offers a large amount of control and the ability to greatly vary the amount of friction.

BOX 63-8 Harness Suspension Pathology

Everyone potentially involved in high-angle rescue should be aware of harness suspension pathology, a potentially fatal condition that can occur when a person hangs motionless in a seat harness for a long period. The condition results when the individual's position in the harness, along with harness strap compression, reduces venous blood flow from the extremities (particularly the legs) to the right side of the heart, with subsequent reduction in cardiac output. This can result in unconsciousness and possibly death in minutes. Most at risk are individuals who are unconscious, hypothermic, dehydrated, or fatigued. Anyone who appears to be in danger of harness suspension pathology should be brought down and unclipped from the harness as quickly and safely as possible. Reports have been made of victims of harness suspension pathology dying suddenly after being brought down and released from the harness; affected individuals therefore must be carefully handled and closely monitored.

One potential medical consequence of harness suspension pathology is crush syndrome, which can lead to renal failure and other life-threatening conditions. Medical responders should consider the potential for crush syndrome in their treatment, closely monitor vital signs, and have the patient examined by a physician.

Rescuers who must hang in a harness for long periods can reduce the potential for harness suspension pathology by repositioning and moving about in the harness to facilitate blood flow. Individuals involved in high-angle rescue should consult their medical control officer regarding treatment of the condition and conduct their own research into this condition.

do work while using less force. Mechanical advantage is expressed as a ratio. For example, if the load is 100 pounds and rescuers can raise it with 50 pounds of force, the mechanical advantage would be 2:1.

Mechanical Advantage Hauling System. One of the simplest hauling systems to be used in low-angle evacuation is the 1:1 hauling system. In essence, the 1:1 ratio means that the force needed to haul the load (litter, subject, and attendants) is approximately the same as the weight of the load. Rescuers must take into consideration one important fact: hauling systems create enormous forces on the rope rescue system. Unnoticed problems can quickly result in catastrophic system failure.

Hauling Low-Angle Evacuation Figure 63-32 illustrates a 2:1 hauling system for low-angle evacuation. In theory, the force needed by the haul team to move the litter system is only half the force needed in the 1:1 hauling system. But with the 2:1 hauling system, the haul team will have to travel twice as far.

The 2:1 hauling system is created by anchoring a rope at the top, running it back down to the litter through a pulley attached to the litter yoke, and then running the rope back to the top through a primary direction change on a separate anchor and near the first anchor. The haul team may be able to pull uphill on the rope, but Figure 63-33 shows them going off to the side to make travel a little easier. This sideways pull is made possible by running the rope over a directional pulley anchored near the anchor point of the top end of the rope.

Belay

Both lowering and hauling usually need a belay, but in very-low-angle environments the litter may need only a braking system or a belay.

Training and Equipment

The failure of rope rescue systems can be catastrophic, possibly resulting in severe injury and death. All rope rescues require appropriate training and equipment (Box 63-8).

Use of an Aerial Apparatus

Tower Ladder or Bucket Trucks

[OBJECTIVE 38]

In areas where they can be positioned, tower ladder or bucket trucks can help expedite vertical evacuation.

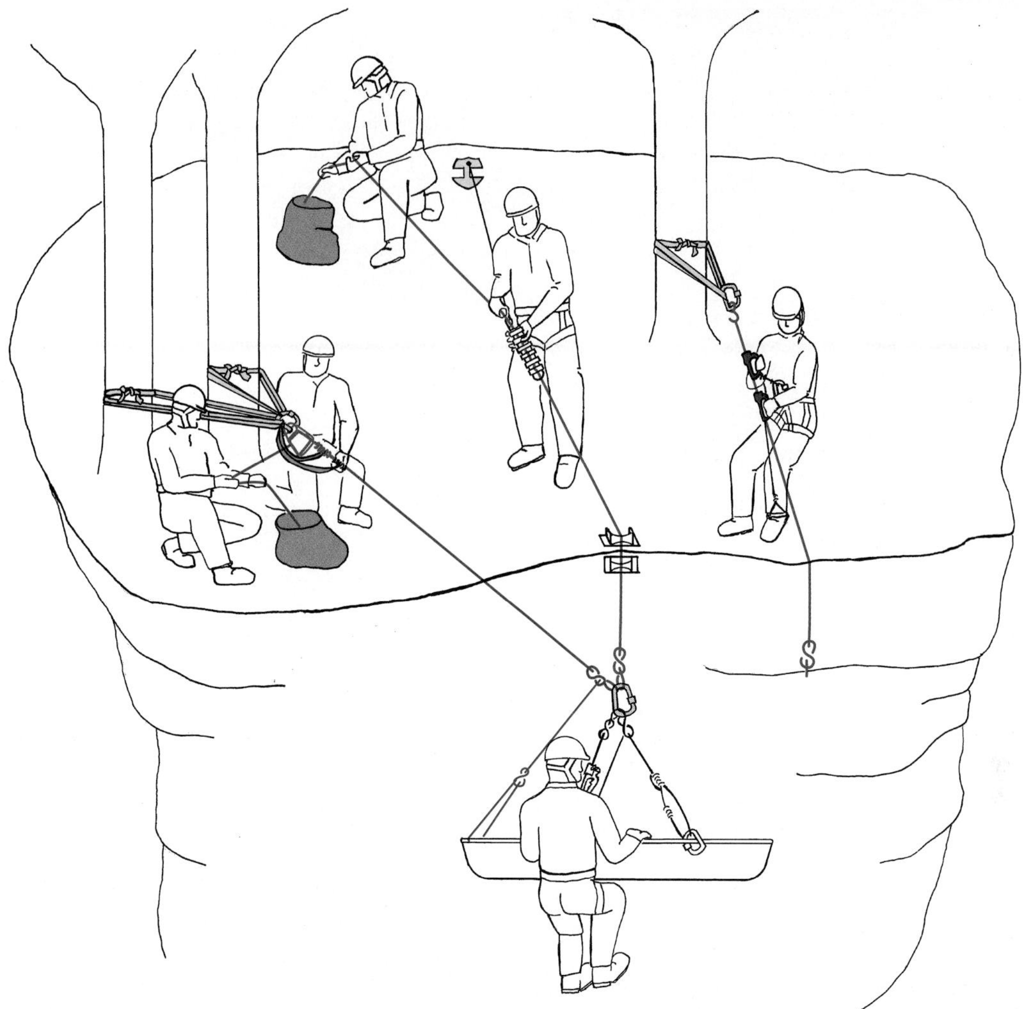

Figure 63-31 High-angle lowering is the controlled lowering of the litter in a high-angle environment.

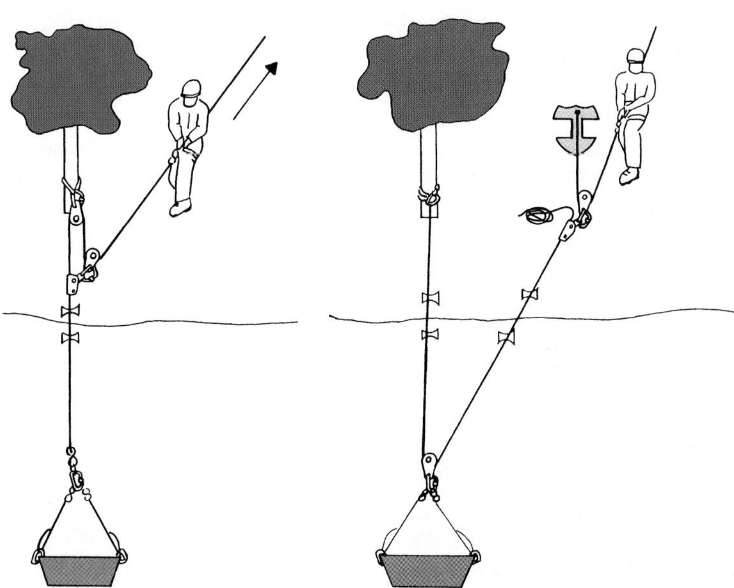

Figure 63-32 A 2:1 hauling system enables the rescue load to be raised with less force.

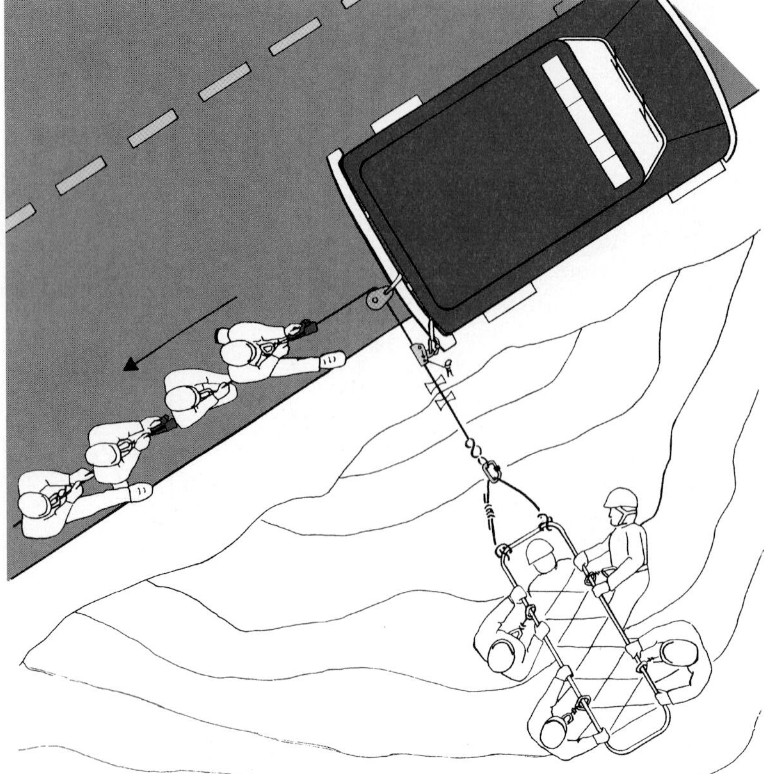

Figure 63-33 By using a directional pulley, the haul team can pull to the side instead of uphill.

Personnel in the bucket with the litter patient and the litter must be belayed during movement to the bucket. Aerial ladders can be used for evacuation, but the litter must be belayed as it is moved down the ladder, and a litter tender should accompany the foot end of the litter to help guide it up or down.

In rescue situations in which a patient must be moved only a short distance, such as one story, roof ladders could be an option. The ladder must be securely anchored, and rescuers should use a safety rope controlled from the top.

Use of Helicopters in Hazardous Terrain Rescue

Fatal Incident Example 5

A 28-year-old male fire department paramedic died after falling approximately 50 to 75 feet from a helicopter during an attempt to retrieve medical equipment in a state park. The victim worked in the air operations division of the county fire department. The victim was using a tether strap harness and carabiners to secure himself to the helicopter. This was a routine operation procedure for personnel in the air operations division. The restraining system failed, causing the victim to fall. On recovery, no emergency medical kits were found on board to begin first aid.

Helicopters have both life-saving and life-destroying potential. The EMS responder must have the knowledge of helicopter potential, which includes their dangers.

Most EMS responders will eventually be familiar with the medical evacuation helicopters that transport seriously injured patients from the field to the hospital. Most medical evacuation helicopters do not have the capability to perform rescue tasks. To perform rescues, a helicopter must have an extra margin of power and greater maneuverability. In addition, the pilot must have the training and experience needed to perform helicopter rescues.

When calling a helicopter for rescue, the pilot must be given the precise location (geographic coordinates if possible); weather information, including visibility and winds; hazards, including utility lines and towers; and, if working in mountainous terrain, the altitude.

Many military helicopters have the power and range to conduct a mission, and many have hoist capability. However, the pilot also must possess the training and experience (Box 63-9).

Because of hazards involved and the complexity of helicopter rescue operations, responders must be acquainted with helicopter operations. If possible, EMS responders should train with helicopter units before a real rescue operation. In addition to training, this experience provides the opportunity for the pilot and other crew members to know the EMS responder and trust him or her.

BOX 63-9 Twelve Standard Aviation Questions That Could Save Your Life

1. Is this flight necessary?
2. Who is in charge?
3. Have all hazards been identified and have you made them known?
4. Should you stop the operation or flight because of:
   - Inadequate and unclear communications
   - Hazardous weather
   - Turbulence
   - Insufficient or untrained personnel
   - Conflicting priorities
   - Deceased rescue subject
5. Is there a better way to do it?
6. Are you driven by an overwhelming sense of urgency?
7. Can you justify your actions?
8. Are other aircraft in the area?
9. Do you have an escape route?
10. Are any rules being broken?
11. Are communications getting tense?
12. Are you deviating from the assigned operation or flight?

Remember: When in Doubt—Don't!

Courtesy Ken Phillips, National Park Service Aviation.

Ground Safety

Safety on the ground during a helicopter rescue includes the following guidelines:

- Keep well clear of helicopter rotors.
- Always get the approval of a flight crew member before approaching a starting or operating helicopter. Only approach and depart as directed, in a slightly crouched position and in full view of a crew member.
- Keep seat belt and shoulder harness fastened until instructed by the pilot to unbuckle.
- Wear eye protection when working around helicopters.
- Aircraft must be loaded by qualified personnel only.
- Do not smoke within 100 feet of an aircraft.
- Do not throw objects to or from an aircraft.

Air Safety

Safety in the air during a helicopter rescue includes the following guidelines:

- Do not smoke.
- Keep clear of controls.
- Hold loose objects securely while in flight.
- Stay alert for hazards, particularly towers, transmission lines, and other aircraft. Inform the pilot of their presence.
- Avoid unnecessary talk with the flight crew.
- Keep seat belt and shoulder harness fastened until instructed by the pilot to unbuckle.
- Perform movement within or in or out of the aircraft only at the direction of the pilot or other designated flight crew member.
- Remain in visual contact with the pilot at all times.

Helicopter Maneuvers

A helicopter one-skid landing is the placing of one skid of the helicopter on the ground while the other remains above the ground; it is typically performed in steep terrain. When the skid is in contact with the ground, the center of gravity can shift laterally, so this maneuver requires a great deal of pilot skill and experience.

In a **hover,** a helicopter remains fairly stationary over a given point, moving neither vertically nor horizontally. A skilled pilot and adequate power are required to perform a hover, which requires low wind conditions and relatively flat terrain.

A hover is most stable when the helicopter is said to be operating in **ground effect,** at an altitude at which the positive influence of ground effect is attained (usually equal to one half the rotor diameter above the surface). In this condition the helicopter is operating on a cushion of air created by its prop wash.

A hover out of ground effect is hovering at a high enough altitude that the added benefit of ground effect is not obtained. This is much more difficult in terms of pilot skill and engine power and is not as stable as operating in ground effect.

Short Haul

A **short haul** is the transport of one person or more externally suspended below a helicopter. It also involves the use of a helicopter and an externally attached line to insert or extract personnel in areas that preclude a normal landing.

Sling Load

A sling load is an external load supported by a sling, net, bag, or some combination of these that is attached with a long line to the helicopter by means of a cargo hook.

Hoist Rescue

A hoist rescue involves insertion or extraction of personnel on a lightweight cable with an electric or hydraulic hoist anchored to a helicopter. Patients must be protected from prop wash, and all loose items around helicopter operations must be secured.

Case Scenario SUMMARY

1. *What is your initial size-up of the scene?* This is a hazardous and unstable situation involving an apparent trench collapse with entrapment. The patient has a potential cervical spine injury and possible head injury. Secondary collapse often occurs after an initial trench collapse. The cracks in the ground indicate this strong possibility.
2. *What are your priorities?* The safety of you and your partner is first. Do not go into the trench. Use appropriate PPE (helmet and appropriate footwear). The safety of bystanders is next. Those in the trench must exit and those at the edge must move away to a safety zone. The safety of the patient is last. Any source of vibration, such as heavy equipment, must be stopped. Incoming vehicles must not approach the trench.
3. *What should your first actions be?* Back up. Get people away from the edge. If properly qualified and equipment trench rescue personnel are not en route, they must be immediately requested. Describe to them the situation and the hazards involved. Initiate ICS. Set up for cervical spine stabilization and potential head injury and crush syndrome care.
4. *Was there anything you could do for the patient before the trench was stabilized?* Reassure the patient. Explain the steps being taken for his rescue.
5. *What sort of physical protection must be provided for the patient now that the trench is stabilized?* Protect his airway from soil and dust. Place a helmet to protect his head. Provide eye protection and hearing protection if needed. Once you have made physical contact with the patient, someone should stay with him as much as possible to reassure and explain the steps being taken to rescue him.
6. *What can be done for environmental factors (chill)?* Provide clothing or a space blanket wrap for the exposed part of his body. Provide warm IV fluids. Warmed oxygen can be administered by wrapping the oxygen tubing around hot packs.
7. *What medical care should be considered?* Considering the circumstances, crush syndrome is a distinct possibility. Furthermore, having his helmet knocked off and becoming unresponsive, then reawakening, shows strong potential for traumatic brain injury. Follow local protocols for crush syndrome and traumatic brain injury management and contact medical direction.
8. *How should you prepare for when the patient is completely released from entrapment?* Time aggressive medical care with rescue personnel actions. This should include establishing IV access with large-bore catheters and preparing to give fluid boluses (even if the vital signs are currently stable) according to orders from medical direction. Once the patient is released from the entrapment, patients can quickly become hypotensive and go into cardiac arrest as a result of the release of toxins generated by the lack of blood supply to the extremity.
9. *What destination and level of medical transportation are most appropriate for this patient?* This patient needs transport to a trauma center, with advance notice of possible spinal complications, crush syndrome, and traumatic brain injury. Depending on the distance to a trauma center, aeromedical transport may be necessary if ground transport is extended.
10. *What was your most important medical consideration for the patient?* The existence of prolonged immobilization and compression of large muscle mass (the legs) indicate the strong potential for crush syndrome. A patient who appears alert and oriented with stable vital signs may, upon release, suddenly go into arrest and die despite rapid transport to a trauma center. Responders must make a thorough assessment of the patient before extrication, provide appropriate treatment, and be ready with aggressive treatment once the patient is released from entrapment. You should maintain communication with a physician familiar with the pathologic process involved with crush syndrome.
11. *What was the level of transport urgency for this patient?* This patient requires rapid transport to a trauma center. If ground transport time to a trauma center is extensive, the patient should be transported by air. In some jurisdictions a physician may be called to the scene to evaluate the patient during extended extrication times. During transport, support circulation and treat aggressively for shock. Maintain body heat. Follow local protocols for crush syndrome. Maintain contact with medical direction.

Chapter Summary

- Rescue is a patient-driven event, so you must continue to relate to the patient throughout the rescue both physically and emotionally.
- A rescue must combine both technical and medical skills. Everyone involved in a rescue must be aware of the rescue's effect on the patient. You must be aware of the situation of the rescue and the hazards for both paramedic and patient.
- Rescue often involves a patient needing medical care. This means careful preparation and realistic training.

At a rescue, you must understand the hazards, know when it is safe or unsafe to access the patient, and have the necessary skills.

- The three levels of skills for responders to a technical rescue incident are awareness, operations, and technician.
- The priorities for safety in any rescue are personal safety, rescue team safety, safety of bystanders, and patient safety, in that order.
- The phases of a rescue operation are arrive and size up the scene, establish command and conduct scene assessment, determine the number of patients and triage if necessary, determine if the situation is search and rescue or body recovery, conduct a risk versus benefit analysis, request additional resources, establish ICS as command/control mechanism, and estimate time to access and evacuate.
- Phase 1 activities are those that responding crew members would initially be involved in on arrival: scene safety, vehicle stabilization, patient access, and initial medical care.
- Phase 2 is a disentanglement phase to remove the sidewall on one side of the vehicle, giving EMS providers maximal room for patient care and sufficient space to package and remove the patient.
- Phase 3 activities remove the vehicle roof.
- Phase 4 requires movement of the dashboard, instrument panel, and firewall structure of the vehicle away from the front seat passengers.
- You must maintain situational awareness throughout the rescue by being aware of everything happening in the environment.
- Patient packaging prepares the patient for transport and involves physically stabilizing the patient to prevent additional injury.
- PPE includes clothing and equipment to protect the wearer from injury and death and may include helmets, hearing protection, hand protection, foot protection, and protective clothing.
- A downed electrical wire should never be moved by responders. The preferred action is to secure the scene, communicate with any stranded occupants of the vehicle, and await the arrival of professional utility company personnel.
- Airbags that have not deployed present responders with obvious safety concerns for both the responders and their patient.
- Recommended vehicle crash procedures applicable to hybrid vehicles include hybrid vehicle identification, vehicle stabilization, access to passenger compartment, shift gear selector lever, turning ignition off and placing key on dash, checking that dash light indicating an energized hybrid vehicle system goes out, and shutting down hybrid vehicle's 12-volt electrical system at the battery.
- Because of the forces it creates, moving water is dangerous to individuals and rescuers. Hydraulics and strainers create particularly dangerous hazards.
- Water causes heat loss 25 times faster than air, and water temperature lower than 98°F will cause hypothermia.
- Cold protective response can result in individuals surviving extended periods of submersion. A patient is never cold and dead—only warm and dead.
- Individuals who accidentally fall into cold water should use basic tactics to survive, including such techniques as HELP and huddle.
- Spinal immobilization in water requires special training, and only trained water rescue responders should attempt rescue, including in-water immobilization.
- The basic principles of water rescue include the following: never underestimate the power of moving water, do not enter water without specialized training and equipment, and always wear a PFD. The basic rescue model for untrained rescuers is talk, reach, throw, and row. For their own safety, rescuers need a PFD, a helmet, knife, and thermal protection. For victim safety, they need flotation along with equipment for immobilization, extrication, and thermal protection.
- Confined spaces are particularly dangerous for rescuers. OSHA has defined confined space (permit space). Among the hazards in confined spaces are atmospheric dangers, fire and explosion, engulfment, electricity, structural hazards, and fall hazards. OSHA requires a permit process before a rescuer can enter a confined space.
- Among the first actions for EMS personnel at a confined space emergency are to establish a safe perimeter, prevent additional entry to the space, assist in remote retrieval, and determine from the permit or entry supervisor the type of work being done at the time of the accident.
- Trench collapse is one of the most dangerous calls for EMS personnel. The first steps are to secure the scene, initiate command, and secure a perimeter.
- Rescue in hazardous terrain can be challenging and dangerous and requires specialized training for the individual and team.
- A rescue often involves transporting the patient in a litter. Rescuers must know which litters are appropriate, how to package and secure and protect the patient, and how to arrange medical equipment for use during transport.
- Among the skills needed in low-angle or high-angle evacuation are knowledge of placing anchors, rope lowering systems, braking systems, and hauling systems.
- In working with helicopters, rescuers must understand helicopter limitations, ground safety, and air safety. Among the helicopter rescue techniques are one-skid landing, hovering, short haul, and sling load.

REFERENCES

Moore, R. E. (2003). *Vehicle rescue & extrication* (2nd ed.). St. Louis: Mosby.

National Fire Protection Association. (2004). *NFPA standard on operations and training for technical search and rescue incidents.* Quincy, MA: National Fire Protection Association.

National Institute for Occupational Safety and Health. (1994). *Worker deaths in confined spaces: summary of NIOSH surveillance and investigative findings, publication no. 94-103.* Washington, DC. Retrieved August 9, 2008, from http://www.cdc.gov.

National Institute for Occupational Safety and Health. (2002). *Death in the line of duty: A fire fighter drowns after attempting to rescue a civilian stranded in flood water—Colorado.* Retrieved March 3, 2008, from http://www.cdc.gov.

National Institute for Occupational Safety and Health. (2005). FACE 85-31: *Three sanitation workers and one policeman die in an underground pumping station in Kentucky.* Retrieved February 28, 2007, from http://www.cdc.gov.

Occupational Safety & Health Administration. (2004). *What is an incident command system?* Retrieved February 28, 2007, from http://www.osha.gov.

United States Coast Guard. (2005). *Boating statistics—2004, Comdpub P16754.18.* Washington, DC: United States Coast Guard.

United States Department of Health and Human Services, Centers for Disease Control and Prevention: *Water-Related Injuries: Fact Sheet.* Retrieved March 20, 2008, from http://www.cdc.gov.

SUGGESTED RESOURCES

Phillips, K. (Editor). (2005). *Basic technical rescue (10th ed.).* Grand Canyon National Park: U.S. National Park Service.

Ray, S. (2002). *Swiftwater rescue: A manual for the rescue professional (3rd ed).* Asheville, NC: CFS Press.

Roop, M, Vines, T, & Wright, R. (1998). *Confined space and structural rope rescue.* St. Louis: Mosby.

Vines, T., & Hudson, S: *High angle rescue techniques (3rd ed.).* St. Louis: Mosby.

Chapter Quiz

1. Rescue is a __________-driven event.

2. Name the three levels of skills for responders at a technical rescue incident.

____

____

____

3. Name the four priorities for safety in any rescue.

____

____

____

____

4. Who identifies on-scene hazards for the arriving units?

____

5. Name five types of PPE.

____

____

____

____

____

6. What type of PFD is preferred for most rescue work?

____

7. Airbags also are known as ____________.

a. deployable cushions
b. inflatable bags
c. supplemental crash systems
d. supplemental restraint systems

8. Many side-impact airbag systems use a stored gas pressurized container system to inflate the airbag during the crash. These cylinder-like containers can contain pressurized gas at _______.

a. 1000 psi
b. 2000 psi
c. 3000 psi
d. 4000 psi

9. A vehicle's battery may not be under the hood within the engine compartment. List three potential alternate battery locations.

____

____

____

10. When shutting down a vehicle's electrical system, battery cables may need to be cut. If the rescuer cuts the negative battery cable, he or she should ____________.

a. cut into the battery casing to drain the battery fluid
b. cut it after first cutting the positive battery cable
c. cut the red cable, then the positive cable
d. cut the same cable a second time to remove a minimum 2-inch section

11. The vehicle rescue term that refers to the process of looking around the interior of the vehicle in an attempt to determine the location of both deployed and undeployed airbags is called __________.

a. airbag identification
b. assessment
c. inflation zone
d. scanning

12. The airbag inflation zone distances for front driver, front passenger, and side-impact airbags are ____________.
   a. 5, 10, and 20 inches
   b. 10, 5, and 18 inches
   c. 10, 18, and 5 inches
   d. 18, 10, and 5 inches

13. The concern about accidentally cutting into a stored gas inflator unit for an undeployed side-impact roof airbag can be alleviated if rescue teams ____________.
   a. locate the airbag identification and cut above or below the marker
   b. strip away the roof pillar trim before cutting a roof pillar
   c. use a power rescue system cutter to sever the inflator module
   d. use a saw to cut the inflator

14. True or False: Hybrid gasoline and electric vehicles contain two electrical systems: the standard 12-volt system and a high-voltage system.

15. At a hybrid vehicle crash incident, once the gear selector lever has been moved to the park position, the inside rescuer must attempt to ____________.
   a. open the jammed door and get out
   b. open the hood
   c. remove the roof of the vehicle
   d. turn the ignition off

16. All vehicle crash scene hazards fall into one of three general categories: environmental hazards, scene hazards, and _________.
   a. hazards presented by leaking fuel
   b. hazards presented by patient blood and body fluids
   c. hazards presented by the vehicle itself
   d. hazards presented by weather

17. Personnel arriving at a crash scene must learn to use their vehicles as initial traffic control devices. Placing the emergency vehicle at an angle to approaching traffic is referred to as ____________.
   a. blocking
   b. fending off
   c. safe parking
   d. upstream positioning

18. The area of highest risk for EMS personnel at a crash scene is closest to the crashed vehicles and typically where the patients are located. This primary danger zone is commonly referred to as the ____________.
   a. cool zone
   b. crash zone
   c. hot zone
   d. warm zone

19. True or False: Electricity can leave an energized wire and travel invisibly through the ground. When this happens at a crash scene, the ground becomes energized with what is referred to as ground gradient.

20. True or False: Real-world experiences demonstrate that a typical vehicle crash does exist. It probably will be on a dry, level road surface and more than likely at an intersection.

21. To better understand what happens at an extrication scene and promote improved training for vehicle rescue, all tasks that take place can be organized into four categories known collectively as the ____________.
   a. phases of rescue
   b. plan of rescue
   c. stages of rescue
   d. steps of rescue

22. List three types of hazards presented by moving water.

____

____

____

23. List the basic principles of water rescue.

____

____

24. The basic water rescue model is _____, ______, ______, and ______.

25. What is the most common danger in confined space situations?

____

26. Describe what takes place in lock out, tag out.

____

____

27. Name the two common medical issues in trench collapse.

____

____

28. Name three personal skills needed in high-angle rescue.

____

____

____

29. What negative consequence for the patient can result from immobilization on a rigid spine board for a long period?

____

____

30. __________ are the means of securing the ropes and other elements in the high-angle system.

31. Name six ground safety concerns for EMS personnel working around helicopters.

____________________ ____________________

____________________ ____________________

____________________ ____________________

Terminology

Airbag identification The various shapes, sizes, colors, and styles of visual identification labels indicating that an airbag is present.

Airbags Inflatable nylon bags designed to supplement the protection of occupants during crashes; one of the most common new technology items confronting responders at crash scenes; also known as *supplemental restraint systems.*

Anchor point A single secure connection for an anchor.

Anchors The means of securing the ropes and other elements of the high-angle system.

Artificial anchors The use of specially designed hardware to create anchors where good natural anchors do not exist.

Authority having jurisdiction The local agency having legal authority for the type of rescue and the location at which it occurs.

Belay A safety technique used to safeguard personnel exposed to the risk of falling; the **belayer** is the person responsible for operation of the belay.

Blocking A position that places the emergency vehicle at an angle to the approaching traffic, across several lanes of traffic if necessary; this position begins to shield the work area and protects the crash scene from some of the approaching traffic.

B pillar The structural roof support member on a vehicle located at the rear edge of the front door; also referred to as the *B post.*

Brake bar rack A descending device consisting of a U-shaped metal bar to which several metal bars are attached that create friction on the rope. Some racks are limited to use in personal rappelling, whereas others also may be used for lowering rescue loads.

Cold protective response The mechanism associated with cold water in which individuals can survive extended periods of submersion.

Confined space By OSHA definition, a space large enough and configured so that an employee can enter and perform assigned work but has limited or restricted means for entry or exit (e.g., tanks, vessels, silos, storage bins, hoppers, vaults, and pits are spaces that may have limited means of entry); not designed for continuous employee occupancy.

Dual-stage airbags An airbag with two inflation charges inside; only one of the two charges may deploy during the initial crash, causing the bag to inflate; the second charge of the dual-stage airbag may remain.

Environmental hazards Hazards related to the weather and time of day, including extremes of heat, cold, wetness, dryness, and darkness, that increase risks to crews and patients.

Gasoline and electric hybrid vehicle Vehicle designed to produce low emissions by combining a smaller than normal internal combustion gasoline engine with a special electric motor to power the vehicle.

Ground effect The cushion of air that is created by downdraft when a helicopter is in a low hover. Ground effect benefits the helicopter flight because it increases lift capacity, meaning less power is required for the helicopter to hover. When the helicopter has ground effect, it is said to be in ground effect. If a helicopter does not have ground effect, it is said to be operating out of ground effect.

High angle An environment in which the load is predominantly supported by the rope rescue system.

High-angle terrain (vertical terrain) A steep environment such as a cliff or building side where hands must be used for balance when ascending.

Hot zone The primary danger zone around a crash scene that typically extends approximately 50 feet in all directions from the wreckage.

Hover The condition in which a helicopter remains fairly stationary over a given point, moving neither vertically nor horizontally.

Hydraulic A water hazard caused when water moves over a uniform obstruction to flow.

Incident scene hazards Hazards directly related to the specific incident scene, including control of crowds, traffic, the danger of downed electrical wires, the presence of hazardous materials, and the location of an emergency.

Jacking the dash Making cuts into the front pillar and A pillar and lifting the dash, instrument panel, steering wheel and column, and even the pedals off a trapped driver or front seat passenger.

Knee bags Airbags mounted low on the instrument panel designed to deploy against the driver's and front seat passenger's knees in a frontal collision.

Loaded airbag An airbag that has not deployed during the initial crash.

Lock out, tag out An industrial workplace safety term describing actions taken to shut off power to a device, appliance, machine, or vehicle and to ensure that power remains off until work is completed.

Low-angle terrain An environment in flat or mildly sloping areas in which rescuers primarily support themselves with their feet on the terrain surface.

Negative battery cable An electrical power cable that allows the vehicle's electrical system to be grounded or neutral as an electrical circuit.

Obstructed lane + 1 Blocking with an emergency vehicle to stop the flow of traffic in the lane in which the damaged vehicle is positioned plus one additional lane or the shoulder of the roadway.

Packaging Placing the injured or ill patient in a litter and securing him or her for evacuation.

Permit-required confined space A confined space with one or more of the following characteristics: (1) contains or has a potential to contain a hazardous atmosphere; (2) contains a material with the potential for engulfing an entrant; (3) has an internal configuration such that an entrant could be trapped or asphyxiated by inwardly converging walls or by a floor that slopes downward and tapers to a smaller cross-section; or (4) contains any other recognized serious safety or health hazard.

Phases of rescue The training and organizational concept that groups all the activities that take place at a typical vehicle crash with entrapment into four categories, with each known as a phase of rescue.

Positive battery cable Also known as the *hot cable,* this electrical power cable allows the vehicle's electrical system to carry the current or electrical energy from the battery to the electrically powered appliances throughout the vehicle.

Rescue The act of delivery from danger or entrapment.

Right block or left block Terms describing a responding vehicle arriving on scene and turning at a right or left angle. In this block position, the emergency vehicle acts as a physical barrier between the crash scene work area and approaching traffic.

Rolling the dash Rescue tasks involving strategic cuts to the firewall structure followed by pushing, spreading, or even pulling equipment to move the dash, firewall, steering wheel and column, and pedals away from front seat occupants.

Short haul The transport of one or more people externally suspended below a helicopter.

Side-impact airbags Deployable airbags located inside any or all vehicle doors, front and rear outboard seatbacks, as well as along all or a portion of the roof line.

Situational awareness The state of being aware of everything occurring in the surrounding environment and the relative importance of all these events.

Size-up The art of assessing conditions that exist or can potentially exist at an incident scene.

Strainer A water hazard formed by an object or structure in the current that allows water to flow but that strains out large objects, such as boats and people.

Struck-by A situation in which a responder, working in or near moving traffic, is struck, injured, or killed by traffic passing the incident scene.

Upstream A term describing the approaching traffic side of the damaged vehicles and the crash scene.

Vehicle hazards Hazards directly related to the vehicle itself, including undeployed airbags; fuel system concerns; electrical system and battery electricity; stability of the vehicle; sharp glass and metal; leaking hot antifreeze; and engine oil, transmission oil, or antifreeze spills. Even the contents inside a vehicle's trunk or cargo area are typical vehicle hazards that can be encountered.

Vehicle stabilization Immediate action taken to prevent any unwanted movement of a crash-damaged vehicle.

CHAPTER 64

Response to Hazardous Materials Incidents

Objectives

After completing this chapter, you will be able to:

1. Identify training regulations regarding EMS and hazardous materials response and contact agencies that may provide additional information.
2. Identify commonly used recognition and identification clues.
3. Identify the international and Department of Transportation hazard classes.
4. Use physical properties to assess the movement of hazardous material.
5. Use chemical properties to determine a chemical's hazard potential.
6. Identify the properties used to determine a chemical's toxicity.
7. Identify written and verbal resources that can be accessed to obtain chemical information.
8. Determine the safest way to approach a hazardous materials incident.
9. Identify the exclusion (hot), contamination reduction (warm), and support (cold) zones at a hazardous materials or weapon of mass destruction incident and describe the EMS actions performed in each zone.
10. Identify the types of personal protective equipment that should be used by EMS responders at a hazardous materials incident.
11. List the four Environmental Protection Agency designated levels of protection and discuss the use and limitations of each.
12. Identify the procedures necessary for proper responder monitoring and rehabilitation at a hazardous materials incident.
13. Describe responder decontamination procedures.
14. Discuss the need for patient decontamination and explain how it is carried out.
15. Describe how effective mass casualty decontamination may be carried out.
16. Identify the proper treatment for commonly encountered hazardous materials.
17. Discuss the need for early scene-to-hospital communication.
18. Identify ways to reduce secondary exposure risk during patient transportation.
19. Identify the procedures that must take place at the end of the incident.

Chapter Outline

Case Scenario

It is 5:10 PM on a fall afternoon and your crew responds to a call at a metal shop where someone has lost consciousness. On arrival, the only person on the scene other than the patient is the shop manager, who claims to have found the patient while closing up for the evening. The manager states that he does not know why his employee suddenly fell ill. The manager leads you through the shop and shows you where the patient is located.

The shop is a metal working plant specializing in electroplating chrome on bumpers of older model cars and applying chrome on various metals for distribution to other companies.

Your initial impression reveals a well-nourished man who appears to be in his mid-30s. His clothing is soiled from work, but the patient appears to be in reasonably good health. No obvious signs of trauma are present; however, your partner detects a slight scent of bitter almond.

Questions

1. *What is your initial impression of the patient?*
2. *Does any particular hazard suggest prompt evacuation?*
3. *What other information is needed to complete your assessment?*

Although what constitutes a hazardous material has been defined many ways, the most basic defintion is probably the best. A **hazardous material** is a solid, liquid, or gas substance that, when released from a container, is capable of harming people, the environment, and property. Hazardous materials may be found nearly everywhere, including industrial locations, swimming pools, hospitals, agricultural areas, and homes. Hazardous materials are transported by rail, boat, truck and, in limited quantities, air.

Incidents involving hazardous materials may occur during transportation or at any location where hazardous materials are stored or used. They may occur in residential areas with commonly used household cleaning chemicals or pesticides. Incidents involving illegal drug laboratories are becoming increasingly commonplace, and terrorist activities involving chemicals are now a frightening reality. Incidents may involve a single patient or multiple casualties or, in the event of a disaster, a large segment of the community.

EMS RESPONDERS

When a hazardous materials incident occurs, EMS responders may come in contact with patients exposed to or contaminated by hazardous materials. EMS personnel also may be dispatched to a situation in which the presence of hazardous materials has not yet been recognized. They must understand what hazardous materials are and what potential harm they present.

The adequate management of patients exposed to hazardous materials may require changes in your normal response practices. Different toxic materials may affect the way the body responds to trauma and medical conditions, necessitating triage protocol changes. Standard treatment protocols may need to be modified to provide effective patient management. Patients may be contaminated. Decontamination protocols must be developed to limit injury to contaminated patients and reduce the likelihood of secondary contamination to emergency responders and hospital personnel.

Hazardous materials may cause harm in multiple ways. They may be flammable, corrosive, toxic, radioactive, reactive, or any combination of these. Exposed patients may exhibit various problems. Besides the chemical threat, many other hazards may be present at the scene of a hazardous materials incident. Chemical releases usually occur because the container has been damaged. The physical cause of the incident may have resulted in trauma to individuals. The response process itself generates some physical risks and psychological stress.

Another hazard to responders in protective equipment at hazardous materials incidents is heat stress. When responders wear chemical protective equipment, they may be at high risk for heat-induced injuries.

TRAINING REQUIREMENTS

[OBJECTIVE 1]

Occupational Safety and Health Administration and the Environmental Protection Agency

Response to hazardous materials or weapon of mass destruction incidents is inherently dangerous, and EMS personnel must be trained to respond safely and effectively. The **Occupational Safety and Health Administration (OSHA)** and the Environmental Protection Agency (EPA) have established mandatory safety procedures for personnel who deal with problems involving hazardous materials. OSHA's **Hazardous Waste Operations and Emergency Response (HAZWOPER)** standard (CFR 1910.120) provides for the safety of personnel who work on hazardous waste cleanup sites or hazardous waste treatment storage and disposal sites or who respond to hazardous materials emergencies. The EPA also has a parallel HAZWOPER standard (40 CFR 311) that extends coverage to governmental employees and volunteers who would not normally be covered under OSHA standards.

Under the HAZWOPER standard, training for emergency responders is broken down into the following five levels. The requirements for these levels are outlined in CFR 1910.120(q)(6).

1. **Awareness.** Responders who may come upon a hazardous materials incident are trained to recognize hazardous materials, isolate the area, and call for appropriate assistance. Although this the awareness level has no set training hour requirement, OSHA has defined specific objectives that must be met in this training. In general these courses are 8 hours in length. The paramedic must realize that the awareness level is designed for the recognition of hazardous materials incidents. Responders trained to this level may not be initially dispatched to a scene that is known to involve hazardous materials (OSHA, 2003). Awareness level providers must wait until higher trained technicians have made the scene safe before approaching the scene. The objectives for this level of training, as defined by OSHA, are:
   - An understanding of what hazardous substances are, and the risks associated with them in an incident
   - An understanding of the potential outcomes associated with an emergency created when hazardous substances are present
   - The ability to recognize the presence of hazardous substances in an emergency
   - The ability to identify the hazardous substances, if possible
   - An understanding of the role of the first responder awareness individual in the employer's emergency response plan, including site security and control and the U.S. Department of Transportation's *North American Emergency Response Guidebook*
   - The ability to realize the need for additional resources and make appropriate notifications to the communication center
2. **Operations.** Personnel who respond to protect nearby people, property, and the environment from the effects of a hazardous materials incident are trained to operate in a defensive manner and not make direct, intentional contact with the hazardous substance. The operations level has a minimum 8-hour training requirement. However, because of the combination of cognitive and practical training required to meet the objectives established for this level of training, most courses are a minimum of 40 hours in length. Because of the limitations imposed on responders trained at the awareness level, many EMS agencies provide this level of training for paramedics. Paramedics must be trained to the operations level if they might treat patients who have been only partially decontaminated or not decontaminated at all (OSHA, 1995). The objectives for this level of training, as defined by OSHA, are:
   - Knowledge of the basic hazard and risk assessment techniques
   - Knowledge of how to select and use proper personal protective equipment provided to the first responder operational level
   - An understanding of basic hazardous materials terms
   - Knowledge of how to perform basic control, containment, and/or confinement operations within the capabilities of the resources and personal protective equipment available in their unit
   - Knowledge of how to implement basic decontamination procedures
   - An understanding of the relevant standard operating procedures and termination procedures
3. **Technician.** Responders who are usually members of a hazardous materials team make direct, intentional contact with a spilled material to lessen the problem. The technician level has a minimum 24-hour training requirement. Because of the amount of training needed to meet the objectives established for this level of training, most courses are a minimum of 80 hours in length. OSHA-defined objectives for the technician level are:
   - Knowledge of how to implement the employer's emergency response plan
   - Knowledge of the classification, identification, and verification of known and unknown materials by using field survey instruments and equipment
   - Ability to function within an assigned role in the Incident Command System
   - Knowledge of how to select and use proper specialized chemical personal protective equipment provided to the hazardous materials technician
   - Understanding of hazard and risk assessment techniques
   - Ability to perform advanced control, containment, and/or confinement operations within the capabilities of the resources and personal protective equipment available in the unit
   - Understanding of and ability to implement decontamination procedures
   - Understanding of termination procedures
   - Understanding of basic chemical and toxicologic terminology and behavior
4. **Specialist.** Senior hazardous materials responders who respond in support of technicians have a

specialized, focused knowledge about an aspect of the response. They also act as liaisons to state and federal response agencies. The specialist level has a minimum 24-hour training requirement equal to the technician level as well as competency in additional objectives. As a result, the length of specialist level training can vary greatly. The following are additional objectives:

- Knowledge of how to implement the local emergency response plan
- Understanding of classification, identification, and verification of known and unknown materials by using advanced survey instruments and equipment
- Knowledge of the state emergency response plan
- Ability to select and use proper specialized chemical personal protective equipment provided to the hazardous materials specialist
- Understanding of in-depth hazard and risk techniques
- Ability to perform specialized control, containment, and/or confinement operations within the capabilities of the resources and personal protective equipment available
- Ability to determine and implement decontamination procedures
- Ability to develop a site safety and control plan
- Understanding of chemical, radiologic, and toxicologic terminology and behavior

5. **Incident command.** An incident commander is a responder who is trained to take control of the incident and direct the response operation. The incident command level has a minimum 24-hour training requirement that is equal to the operations level as well as competency in the following areas:
   - Knowledge of and ability to implement the employer's incident command system
   - Knowledge of how to implement the employer's emergency response plan
   - Knowledge and understanding of the hazards and risks associated with employees working in chemical protective clothing
   - Knowledge of how to implement the local emergency response plan
   - Knowledge of the state emergency response plan and the Federal Regional Response Team
   - Knowledge and understanding of the importance of decontamination procedures

Under the HAZWOPER standard, EMS responders must be trained to the awareness level at a minimum. Some states require that EMS personnel be trained to the operations level because they respond to protect life and safety at a hazardous materials emergency. In some areas EMS agencies have decided to take an active role in hazardous materials response and have trained selected responders to the technician or specialist level. Although most of the HAZWOPER curriculum is designed for fire and hazardous materials team response and may not be appropriate for the EMS responder, a program can be designed that combines specific medical and hazardous materials information.

National Fire Protection Association

In addition to OSHA and EPA regulations, the **National Fire Protection Association (NFPA)** has developed voluntary training competencies for personnel who respond to hazardous materials incidents. Of special interest to EMS responders is NFPA 473. This standard is designed for EMS personnel who respond to hazardous materials incidents.

NFPA 473 designates two levels of training, level 1 and level 2. EMS personnel at EMS/hazardous materials (HM) level 1 would be expected to perform patient care activities in the **cold zone** at a hazardous materials incident. This zone should be free of contamination. Response activities in this area represent a minimal risk. EMS personnel at the EMS/HM level 2 could operate in personal protective equipment and perform patient care activities during decontamination procedures in the **warm zone** (the area where personnel and equipment decontamination takes place) at hazardous materials incidents. Personnel in this zone have a greater chance of being exposed to the hazardous material and are at higher risk than personnel in the cold zone.

HAZARDOUS MATERIALS RECOGNITION

[OBJECTIVE 2]

The presence of hazardous materials may not always be apparent at the scene of an incident. EMS personnel may be dispatched to a situation at which the presence of hazardous materials has not yet been recognized.

Certain indicators may suggest the presence of hazardous materials at an emergency scene. The types of reported injuries may be an indication of hazardous materials involvement. The presence of multiple patients with similar symptoms, such as difficulty breathing, seizures, nausea, disorientation, eye irritation, blisters, or rashes, is a common example.

Dead animals, birds, fish, and insects may be an indication of chemical release. Areas that look different in appearance, such as dead vegetation, lawns that are discolored or withered, or low-lying clouds or foggy conditions not explained by normal surroundings are signs of possible chemical presence. Numerous surfaces exhibiting oily droplets or film or numerous water surfaces that have an oily film may be present. Responders may sense unexplained odors or symptoms of irritation. Obviously by the time responders can determine if some of these indicators are present, they will be in close proximity to the release and probably exposed. The sooner responders realize that hazardous materials are present and take appropriate precautions, the safer they will be. Personnel must always be aware of their surroundings and be on the lookout for the presence of hazardous materials.

An understanding of how chemicals are transported, stored, and handled assists responders recognizing and identifying hazardous materials at an incident scene. The recognition and identification of hazardous materials involvement at an emergency scene is the most important element of the response. Safe operating procedures, protective equipment needs, response techniques, and patient care all depend on this step.

Transportation of Hazardous Materials

Hazardous materials transportation is governed by the U.S. Department of Transportation (DOT) regulation known as the Hazardous Materials Transportation Act (HMTA) under Chapter 49 of the Code of Federal Regulations. This standard regulates the types of containers used, the markings of those containers, the mode of transportation used, and the types of documentation needed.

Transportation Containers

Containers are used to transport hazardous and nonhazardous materials. They include bulk and nonbulk containers. Nonbulk containers are smaller, individual packages (Figure 64-1). Bags and sacks are mainly used for solid materials. Bottles are used for solids and liquids. Boxes are used for outside packaging for other nonbulk packages. Drums may be used for solids and liquids. Fiber drums and open-top drums are commonly used to contain solids. Tight, or closed-head, drums with bung openings are commonly used to transport liquids. Drums can be made from plastic (commonly used for corrosives) or steel (commonly used for solvents and fuels). **Carboys** are glass or plastic bottles that may be encased in outer packaging. These are commonly used to transport corrosive products.

Cylinders are nonbulk containers that normally contain liquefied gases, nonliquified gases, or mixtures under pressure. Cylinders also may contain liquids or solids. Typical cylinder types include aerosol containers, uninsulated cylinders, and **cryogenic** (products cooled to less than –90°C [–130°F]) cylinders. Service pressures can range from a few **pounds per square inch (psi)** to several thousand psi.

Bulk containers are larger containers and tanks used to transport large quantities of hazardous materials. Large bulk bags are used for transporting solids such as pesticides and fertilizers. Portable tanks, often called *intermodal tank containers,* are enclosed in a metal supporting frame (Figure 64-2). These tanks are bulk containers that can be transported by highway, rail, or water. Intermodal tank containers may be of the following types: nonpressure, pressure, refrigerated tank container, or high-pressure tube module.

Portable bins are portable tanks used to transport bulk solids. Ton cylinders are pressure tanks approximately 3 feet by 8 feet that transport liquefied gases such as chlorine, sulfur dioxide, and phosgene (Figure 64-3).

Protective packaging for **radioactive** materials includes boxes, overpacks, and casks. Shipping boxes are used for low-level shipments. Overpacks may be cylindrical or boxlike. Casks are rigid metal packages that range in size up to 10 feet in diameter and 50 feet in length.

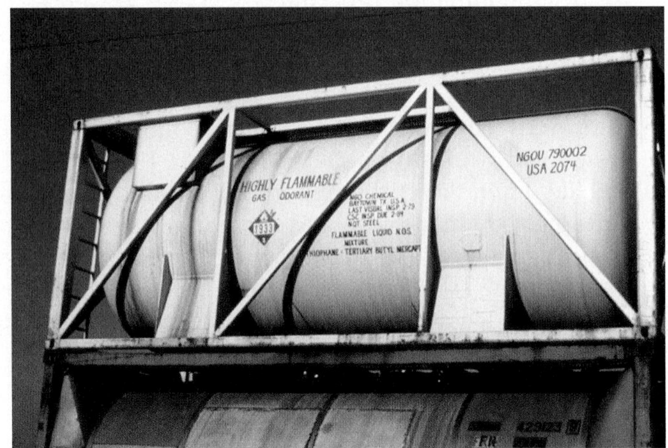

Figure 64-2 Intermodal container.

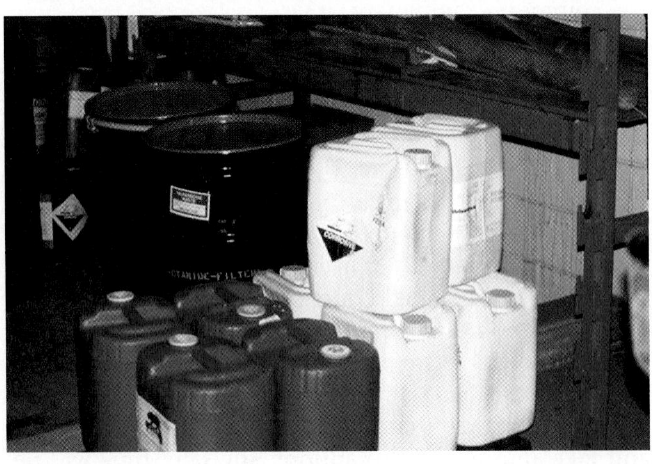

Figure 64-1 Various types of nonbulk containers.

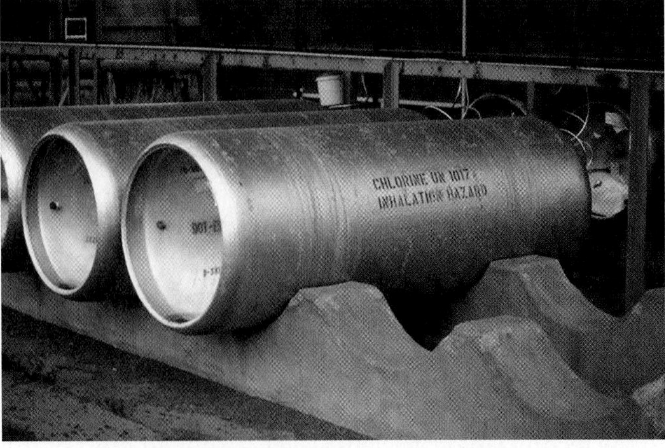

Figure 64-3 Ton cylinders of chlorine.

Cargo tanks transport bulk liquefied or compressed gases, liquids, solids, or molten materials. They may be nonpressurized, pressurized, or of specialized design. Nonpressurized cars transport liquids. The design of the tank is indicative of the types of products they transport. Tank trailers designated as motor carrier (MC) 306/DOT 406 are commonly seen on the highway (Figure 64-4). These trailers have an elliptical-shaped cross section with flat ends and are commonly constructed of aluminum. They are usually compartmentalized and hold up to 9000 gallons of a product that is lighter than water, such as hydrocarbon products (e.g., gasoline or diesel fuel).

MC 307/DOT 407 tank trailers have a circular-type cross section and flat ends and are general-purpose chemical carriers (Figure 64-5). MC 311 and 312/DOT 412 tank trailers have a smaller, rounded cross section with visible supporting rings and flat ends (Figure 64-6). Occasionally the supporting rings are concealed by an outside jacket. These trucks commonly carry 5000 to 6000 gallons of a product that is heavier than water, such as corrosive products.

Pressurized tank trailers transport liquefied and compressed gases. MC 331 tank trailers have rounded cross sections and rounded ends and carry liquefied gas such as liquefied petroleum gas or anhydrous ammonia (Figure 64-7).

Specialized cargo tanks include cryogenic carriers, tube trailers, and hopper trailers. MC 338 trailers are heavily insulated, cylindrical tanks with a characteristic wagon-like structure on the rear end. These trailers are used to transport cryogenic products (Figure 64-8). Cryogenic products (e.g., liquid oxygen and nitrogen) are stored and transported in an extremely cold state. **Tube trailers** are trailers carrying multiple cylinders of pressurized gases (Figure 64-9). Pneumatic hopper trailers have V-shaped compartments with bottom openings. They are commonly used to transport dry solids (Figure 64-10).

Trucks and semi-trailers include flatbed and box designs. Flatbed trailers can carry intermodal containers, ton cylinders, or nonbulk containers. Box semi-trailers may carry any type of nonbulk container.

Rail freight cars can be nonpressure type; pressure type; specialized types, such as hopper and gondola cars; flatcars; and boxcars. Nonpressure cars transport liquid products (Figure 64-11). Even though these containers are classified as nonpressure, they may hold vapor

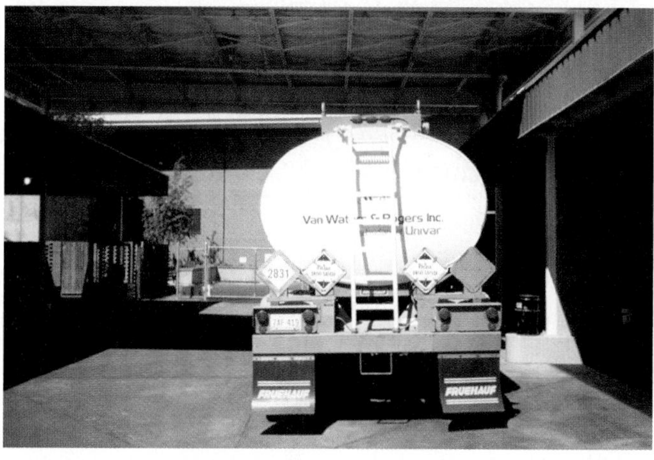

Figure 64-4 MC 306 tank trailer.

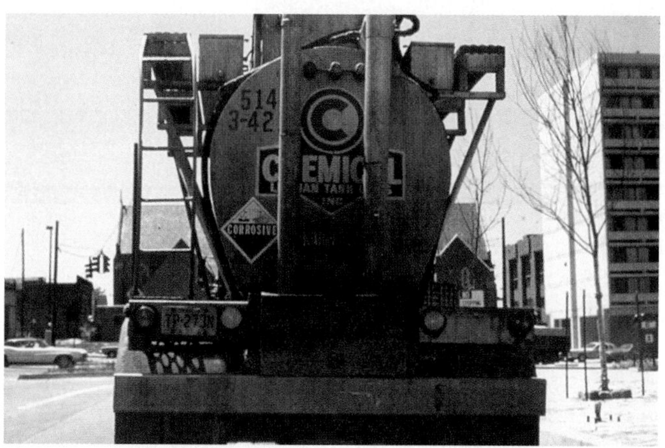

Figure 64-6 MC 311 tank trailer.

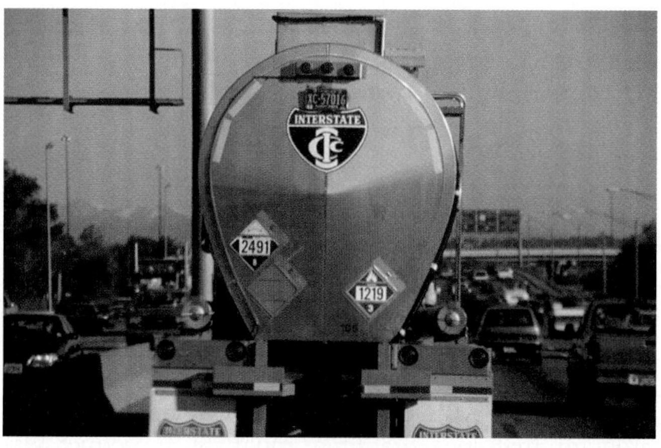

Figure 64-5 MC 307 tank trailer.

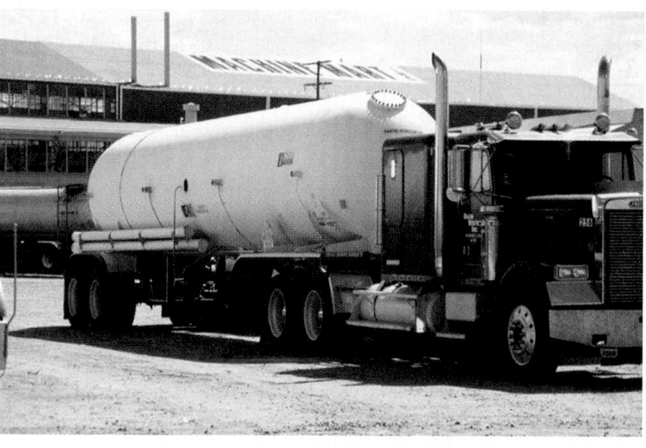

Figure 64-7 MC 331 tank trailer.

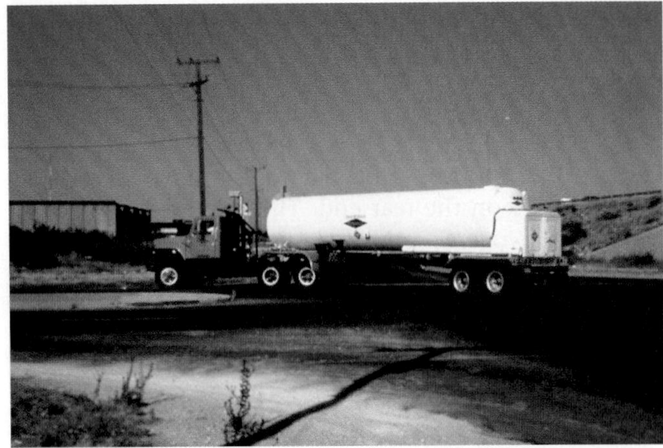

Figure 64-8 MC 338 tank trailer.

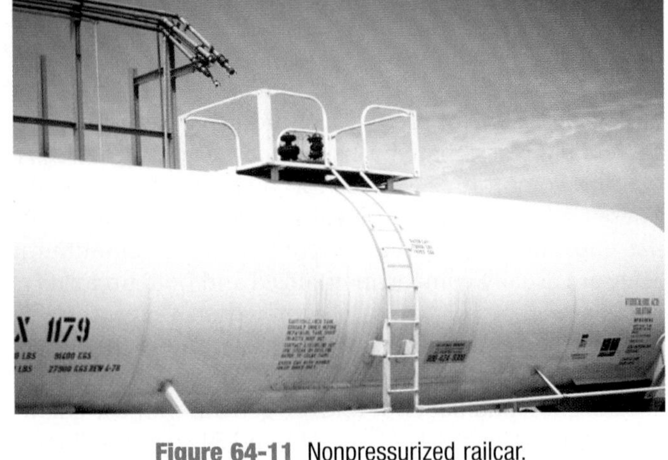

Figure 64-11 Nonpressurized railcar.

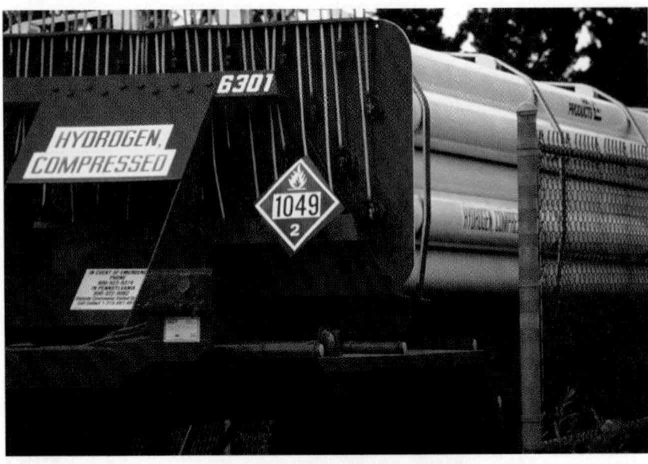

Figure 64-9 Tube trailer.

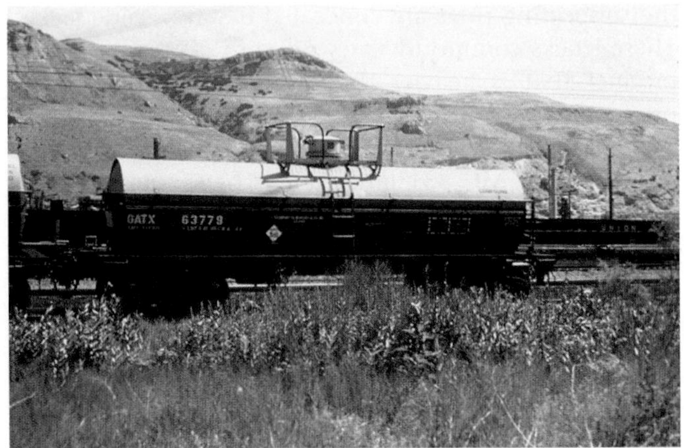

Figure 64-12 Pressurized railcar.

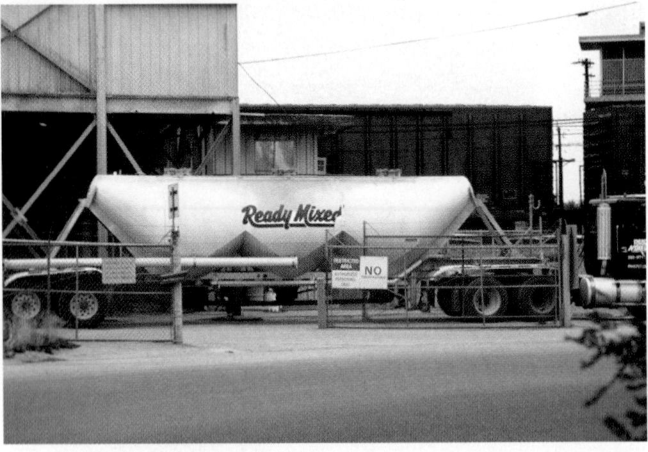

Figure 64-10 Pneumatic hopper trailer.

pressure up to 100 psi. They may be insulated or thermally protected. Most nonpressure cars can be identified by visible fittings on the top of the car and unloading valves on the bottom of the car.

Pressurized tank cars transport liquefied gases (Figure 64-12). Some of these cars are thermally protected. These tanks are typically identified by the presence of a single protective housing (dome) on the top of the car that contains all the valves and fittings.

Specialized tank cars include cryogenic and high-pressure (tube) cars. Cryogenic cars transport extremely cold liquids. These are heavily insulated tanks within a tank and are usually identified by the lack of fittings on the top of the car.

Hopper cars transport bulk solids. They have two or more sloping sided bays on the bottom. They may be open top, closed top, or pneumatically unloaded. Flatcars are commonly used to transport intermodal containers and van trailers. Boxcars are enclosed rail freight cars with doors. They are used to transport nonbulk containers.

Pipelines also are transport containers. Pipelines should be marked with the product, owner, and emergency telephone number (Figure 64-13). The emergency telephone number connects the caller with a control room, where an operator monitors pipeline operations and can begin shutdown procedures in case of an emergency. Many pipeline systems are monitored through a computerized program that logs the time and date a product was injected into the pipeline and its estimated delivery date

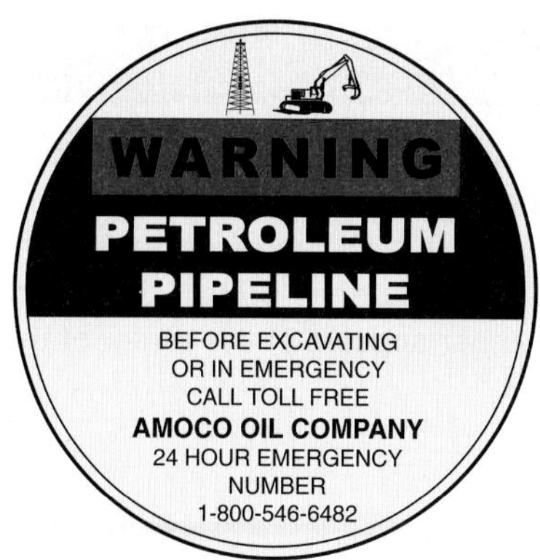

Figure 64-13 Pipeline identification sign.

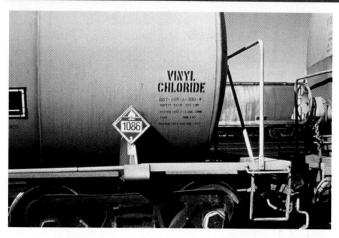

Figure 64-14 Placard and four-digit ID number.

and time. Although most pipelines are dedicated to a single product, some pipelines can carry different materials at different times.

Transportation Identification Systems

[OBJECTIVE 3]

Hazard Classes. Under DOT 49 CFR, containers carrying hazardous materials must be identified. To assist with identification of hazardous materials, the DOT organizes hazardous materials according to the international hazard classes. This classification system is composed of nine classes of hazardous materials. Many of these classes are further divided into categories that represent various degrees or types of hazards. An understanding of these classifications and the types of hazards that they represent allows responders to anticipate the potential harm if the hazardous materials are released from their container. To assist responders in remembering the different hazard classes and placards, they are listed in the *North American Emergency Response Guidebook*. The nine classes of hazardous materials are shown in Table 64-1.

The DOT has adopted a placarding and labeling system to assist emergency responders in identifying the possible hazards involved in an incident involving hazardous materials. **Placards** are diamond-shaped signs placed on the sides and ends of bulk transport containers that carry hazardous materials. They relay information by four means: color background, a symbol on the top, the international hazard class number on the bottom, and the hazard class wording or a four-digit identification number, known as the identification (ID) number, in the center. DOT and international labels are smaller versions of the placards. They are used on individual, nonbulk containers (see Table 64-1).

Certain hazardous materials, regardless of the quantity, must always be placarded when transported. These materials include most explosive products, poisonous gases, water-reactive flammable solids, and most radioactive substances. Other products do not have to be identified by a placard unless more than 1001 lb gross weight is carried. Under certain circumstances, when a mixed load is carried a placard that reads "dangerous" may be used. Many products can fit into multiple hazard classes (e.g., flammable and poison). In most cases the DOT has determined that only one placard (the greatest hazard) is needed on the outside of the bulk container. For example, containers of fuming red nitric acid require three labels: corrosive, oxidizer, and poison, but the truck carrying the containers only requires a corrosive placard. Empty tank trucks must remain placarded until they are cleaned. Empty rail tanks may be placarded as residue. These tanks may contain up to 3% of the tank's capacity.

Four-Digit Identification Numbers. Four-digit ID numbers (also known as *United Nations, North American,* or *product identification numbers*) often can be found on the sides and ends of bulk transport containers. These numbers often are found on the placard or an orange panel located adjacent to the placard (Figure 64-14). They are used to identify the product according to the *North American Emergency Response Guidebook, Emergency Response for Hazardous Materials Exposure,* or other reference. They also may be found in the center of a placard-sized white panel for hazardous substances and wastes not requiring a placard.

Transportation Documentation. Under DOT regulations, shipments of hazardous materials must be accompanied by shipping papers or proper documentation to identify the materials being transported (Figure 64-15). Shipping papers contain the proper shipping name, hazard classification, ID number, number and type of packages, packing group, and correct weight.

Shipping papers identify hazardous materials in the shipment either by listing them first on the manifest, listing them in a contrasting color, or by check marks placed in a hazardous materials identifying column. A notation of *RQ* identifies that chemical as having a reportable quantity listed in EPA regulations. If a specified quantity of an RQ chemical is released, the party responsible for the release must immediately notify the National Response Center in Washington, DC, by calling 800-424-8802.

In truck shipments, papers can be found in the cab. Most often they are in a plastic envelope attached to the

TABLE 64-1 Classes of Hazardous Materials

Class/Division	Notes
Class 1: Explosives Division 1.1: Mass detonation hazard Division 1.2: Mass detonation hazard with fragments Division 1.3: Fire hazard with minor blast or projectile hazard Division 1.4: Explosive substances that present no significant hazard Division 1.5: Very insensitive explosives Division 1.6: Extremely insensitive explosives	Explosive placards and labels are orange and have a symbol showing an exploding ball with fragments on the top and a division number (1.1 to 1.6) on the bottom. The word "explosive" or a four-digit ID number appears in the center of the symbol.
Class 2: Gases Division 2.1: Flammable gases Division 2.2: Nonflammable gases Division 2.3: Poisonous gases	Compressed or liquefied gas placards and labels are red (flammable), green (nonflammable), or white (poison); have a fire symbol, gas cylinder symbol, or a skull and crossbones on the top; and a division number (2.1 to 2.3) on the bottom. These symbols have "flammable gas," "nonflammable gas," or "poison gas" labeling or a four-digit ID number in the center.
Class 3: Flammable or Combustible Liquids Division 3.1: Liquids with flash points <0°F Division 3.2: Liquids with flash points from 0° to 73°F Division 3.3: Liquids with flash points from 73° to 141°F Combustible liquids	Flammable or combustible liquids placards and labels are red, have a flame symbol on the top, and a division number (3.1 to 3.3) on the bottom. They have the wording "flammable liquid" or "combustible liquid" or a four-digit ID number in the center.
Class 4: Flammable Solids Division 4.1: Flammable solids Division 4.2: Spontaneously combustible or pyrophoric solids and liquids Division 4.3: Dangerous when wet	Flammable solid placards and labels are red and white striped (flammable solids), red over white (spontaneously combustible solids and liquids), or blue (dangerous when wet); have a flame symbol on the top; and a division number (4.1 to 4.3) on the bottom. They have the wording "flammable solid," "spontaneously combustible," or "dangerous when wet" or a four-digit ID number in the center.
Class 5: Oxidizing Substances Division 5.1: Oxidizing substances Division 5.2: Organic peroxides	Oxidizing substances placards and labels are yellow, have a symbol showing an "O" with flames on the top, and a division number (5.1 to 5.2) on the bottom. They have the wording "oxidizer" or "organic peroxide" or a four-digit ID number in the center.
Class 6: Poisonous and Infectious Substances Division 6.1: Poisons Division 6.2: Infectious substances	Poison liquid and solid material and infectious material placards and labels are white; have either a skull and crossbones, biomedical symbol, or grain stock with an × through it (depending on material) on the top; and a division number (6.1 to 6.2) on the bottom. These symbols have the wording "poison," "infectious material," "keep away from foodstuffs" or a four-digit ID number in the center.
Class 7: Radioactive Substances	Radioactive materials placards and labels are yellow over white, have the radioactive "propeller" symbol on the top, and the number 7 on the bottom. Labels must identify the radionuclide and the amount of activity in the package. They will have the Roman numerals I, II, or III in the center to identify the level of hazard and type of container and space to write in specific information. The I, II, or III numbering designates the amount of radiation detectable from outside the package. Labels have the wording "radioactive material" or a four-digit ID number in the center.

TABLE 64-1 Classes of Hazardous Materials—continued

Class/Division	Notes
Class 8: Corrosive Materials	Corrosive materials placards and labels are white over black, have a symbol showing a test tube spilling liquid onto a human thumb, and a piece of steel on the top and have the number 8 on the bottom. The word "corrosive" or a four-digit ID number appears in the center.
Class 9: Miscellaneous Hazardous Materials	Miscellaneous hazardous materials placards and labels are black and white striped over white and have the number 9 on the bottom. They have a four-digit ID number in the center.

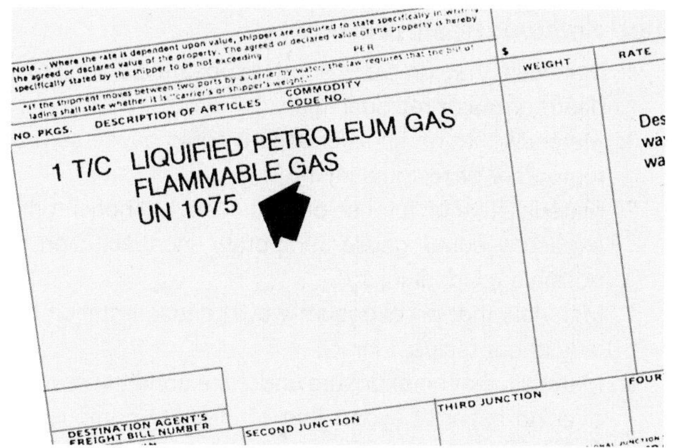

Figure 64-15 Hazardous materials shipping papers.

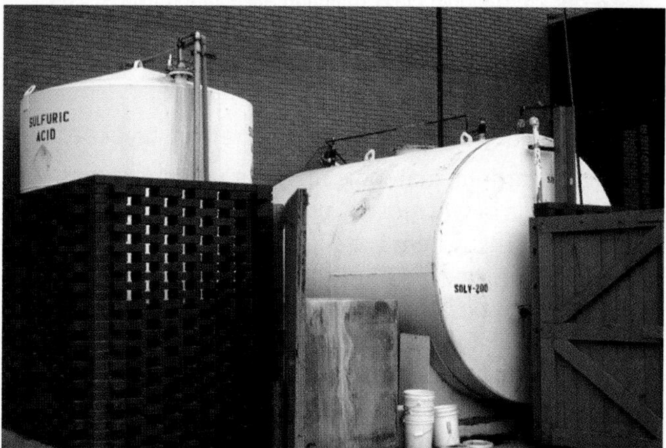

Figure 64-16 Nonpressurized tanks.

inside of the driver's door. On trains they are located in the lead engine. On air shipments, they can be found in the cockpit. On ships, papers are found on the bridge or wheelhouse. Under current DOT regulations, shipping papers must have a 24-hour emergency contact telephone number. Regulations also state that written emergency response information must accompany the shipment.

Storage and Handling of Hazardous Materials

As in transportation, the way that hazardous materials are stored and handled provides information to emergency response personnel. Understanding the types of containers and marking systems in use at fixed facilities can assist in hazard assessment.

Storage Containers

Chemicals are stored at fixed facilities in nonbulk and bulk containers. Bulk storage tanks include both pressure and nonpressure containers. Nonpressure, or atmospheric, storage tanks include above-ground vertical tanks with various types of roof designs, horizontal tanks, and underground storage tanks (Figure 64-16). Low-pressure tanks include spheroid (round) and noded, spheroid tanks. High-pressure tanks include spheres and rounded-end pressure vessels (Figure 64-17).

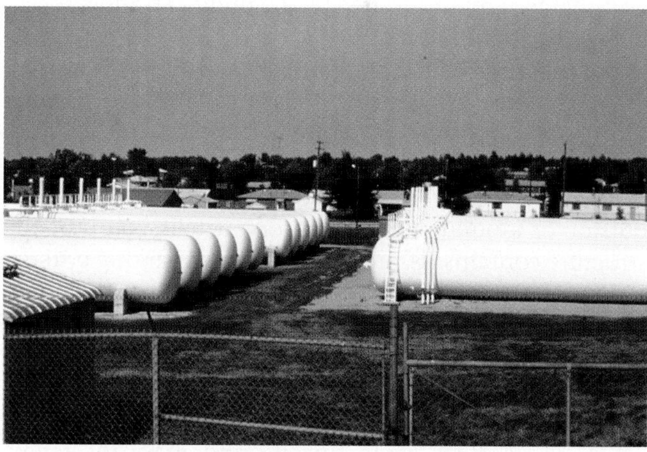

Figure 64-17 Pressurized tanks.

Bulk containers may display marking systems, ID numbers, or the name of the product. Many bulk containers also may be marked with the storage capacity. Some pipelines at facilities may be marked to show the chemical that they transport, but it is not required by federal law.

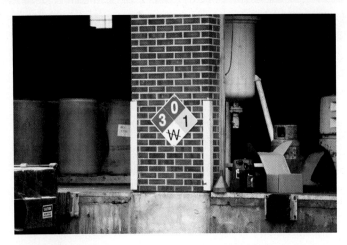

Figure 64-18 National Fire Protection Association (NFPA) 704 system.

Fixed Facility Marking and Labeling Systems

Various hazardous materials marking systems are used at facilities. One of the most popular is the NFPA 704 system (Box 64-1). This system is designed to provide responders with information regarding the material inside the tank, building, or laboratory. It uses a diamond-shaped sign divided into color-coded quadrants (Figure 64-18). The red quadrant on top indicates fire hazard, the blue quadrant on the left indicates health hazard, the yellow quadrant on the right indicates reactivity, and the white quadrant on the bottom is for special information. Numbers in the red, blue, and yellow quadrants indicate the degree of hazard. These numbers range from 0 to 4 and indicate specific levels of hazard. In general, a minimal hazard is indicated by the number 0 and a severe hazard by the number 4.

Special information symbols, such as OXY for an oxidizing product or a W with a slash indicating a product that is dangerous when wet, may be found in the white quadrant. Although this system provides useful information, it does have its limitations. When used on the outside of a building or laboratory, it tells you that the structure contains hazards that meet the marking criteria. It does not specify exactly what the material is, the quantity, or the exact location. When used on a single container, such as a tank, the information is specific. The system is designed under strict criteria and sometimes is not properly interpreted. For example, the health hazard often is based on acute toxicity and may not reflect chronic toxicity. The reactivity hazard is based on the susceptibility of materials to release energy either by themselves or in combination with water. Water reactivity, fire exposure, shock, and pressure were factors considered. This system may not identify reactivity with other chemicals. For example, chlorine is highly reactive with almost everything, but it carries a zero reactivity hazard in the NFPA 704 system.

Labels are often found on hazardous substance containers. The OSHA Hazard Communication Standard (29 CFR 1910.1200), commonly referred to as **HAZCOM,** requires that containers of hazardous substances be labeled so that workers are informed of their respective hazards. Many types of labels are used to accomplish this. Manufacturers usually include a label on their containers that specifies the name of the manufacturer, name of the

BOX 64-1 NFPA 704 System

Red Section: Flammability Hazard

4: Materials that rapidly or completely vaporize at atmospheric pressure and normal ambient temperature or that are readily dispersed in air and that burn readily.
3: Liquids and solids that can be ignited under almost all ambient temperature conditions.
2: Materials that must be moderately heated or exposed to relatively high ambient temperatures before ignition can occur.
1: Materials that must be preheated before ignition can occur.
0: Materials that do not burn.

Blue Section: Health Hazard

4: Materials that on very short exposure could cause death or major residual injury.
3: Materials that on short exposure could cause serious temporary or residual injury.
2: Materials that on intense or continued, but not chronic, exposure could cause temporary incapacitation or possible residual injury.
1: Materials that on exposure would cause irritation but only minor residual injury.
0: Materials that on exposure under fire conditions would offer no hazard beyond that of ordinary combustible material.

Yellow Section: Reactivity Hazard

4: Materials readily capable of detonation or of explosive decomposition or reaction at normal temperatures and pressures.
3: Materials capable of detonation or explosive decomposition or reaction but require a strong initializing source, or that must be heated under confinement before initiation, or that react explosively with water.
2: Materials that readily undergo violent chemical change at elevated temperatures and pressures, or that react violently with water, or that may form explosive mixtures with water.
1: Materials that are stable but can become unstable at elevated temperatures and pressures.
0: Materials that are normally stable, even under fire explosion conditions, and are not reactive with water.

Reprinted from Currance, P. L., & Bronstein, A. C. (1999). *Hazardous materials for EMS*, St. Louis: Mosby–Year Book.
NFPA, National Fire Protection Association.

chemical, major hazards associated with the chemical, and a telephone number to call for additional information. A common method is to supplement the manufacturer's label with Hazardous Materials Identification System or Hazardous Materials Identification Guide labels (Figure 64-19).

These two systems use a label similar to the NFPA 704 system. These labels contain the product name and protective equipment needs and use a system similar to the NFPA system to supply information on the health, flammability, and reactivity hazards of the substance. Another label that responders may encounter is the EPA Hazardous Waste Label (Figure 64-20). This label contains the name of the waste, ID numbers, the name of the generator of the waste, and the accumulation start date (the date when the waste first was placed in the container).

Under EPA regulations, specific information must be available on a label for pesticide containers (Figure 64-21). This information must include the name of the pesticide, a signal word indicating toxicity (e.g., Danger–High, Warning–Moderate, Caution–Low), the EPA registration number, a precautionary statement, hazard statement, and the names of the active ingredients.

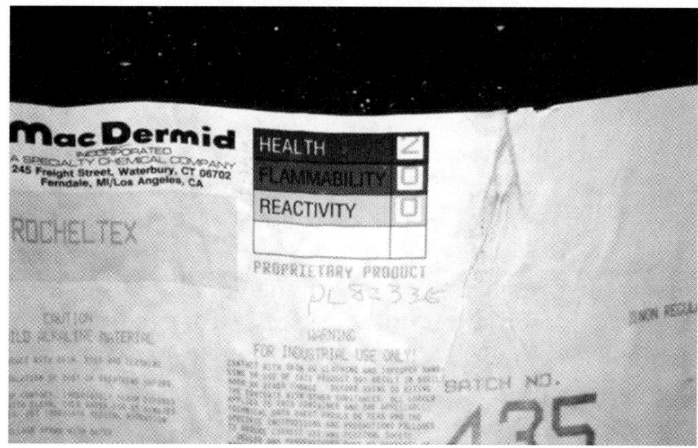

Figure 64-19 Container with Hazard Communication Standard (HAZCOM) and Hazardous Material Identification System (HMIS) labels.

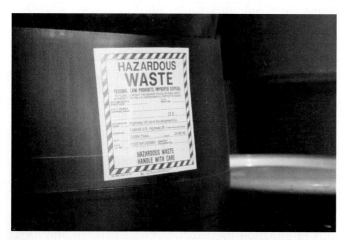

Figure 64-20 Environmental Protection Agency (EPA) hazardous waste label.

Use of Recognition and Identification Clues

An understanding of how chemicals are stored, used, and transported helps EMS responders in recognizing and identifying hazardous materials; however, the concept must be used in an organized manner. The National Fire Academy/National Emergency Training Center manual, *Recognizing and Identifying Hazardous Materials,* outlines the following six clues that may confirm the presence of hazardous materials:

- Occupancy and location
- Container shape
- Markings and colors
- Placards and labels
- Shipping papers and manifests
- Use of senses

These clues are based on increasing risk; that is, as emergency responders approach the scene, they can gather more information but the risk increases. These clues provide limited pieces of information, which then must be used with other sources to provide a clear picture of the situation. In many ways they are like pieces of a jigsaw puzzle. With only one or two pieces, visualizing what the completed puzzle looks like is impossible. The more pieces that are added, the more complete the picture looks. Although these clues provide valuable information, they have their benefits and limitations.

Occupancy and Location

The first and safest clue to hazardous substance involvement is knowledge of the types of materials that may be present in the community. Manufacturing facilities, refineries, laboratories, construction sites, hazardous waste sites, and agricultural areas are examples of locations where hazardous substances are commonly found. Responders should be aware of the hazards in their

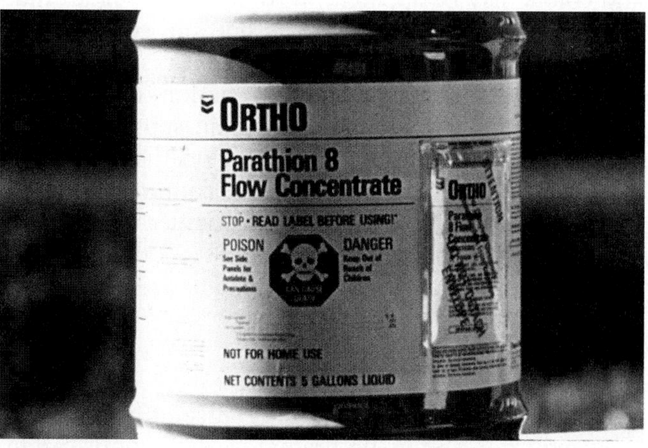

Figure 64-21 Pesticide label.

response area before a problem occurs. Obviously this clue has some major limitations.

Inspections provide information only on the chemicals present on the day and time of the inspection. This may change daily. Chemical reporting requirements usually involve only extremely hazardous substances as defined by the law and then only in certain quantities. In an emergency situation, other chemicals may prove to be extremely dangerous. The accuracy of this clue depends on the adequacy of the inspection or report. Many things can be overlooked or missed. Another concern is the transportation of hazardous materials through the area. Information may be available from area users, transporters, and local police agencies. However, these sources will not be able to track all the chemicals moving through the area.

Containers

Containers are one of the first clues to look for when responding to a hazardous materials incident. The presence of hazardous materials containers at an incident is an indication that chemicals may be involved, and the shape of the containers may help determine the type of hazardous material(s) present. Containers also provide information on the state of matter that may be released. In most cases solids, liquids, and gases are packed in distinctive containers. What the container is made of may provide additional information. For example, plastic drums usually contain a corrosive material. Fixed facility tanks also are an indicator of the type of chemical contained within. Some containers are indicative of certain types of hazardous materials; truck trailers are excellent examples. Tank shape can be an important clue in some cases, whereas in others, such as a boxcar or standard cargo truck, the individual containers that they carry are not visible. Although the container shape may not identify the exact chemical involved, it may provide preliminary information with which to assess the scene. For example, pressurized products usually present a greater hazard during a release than do liquid products.

Markings and Colors

As responders move closer to the scene, certain markings and colors may be apparent, possibly providing an indication of the product located inside the container. At fixed facilities the four-color NFPA 704 system is commonly used. The American Association of Railroads requires that railcars that carry certain substances have the name of the substance stenciled on the side of the car. Colors also may be used to relay information. In addition to these markings, company names, ID numbers, and telephone numbers often are found on containers. The license number of the vehicle can be used to identify the owner and eventually the cargo.

Placards and Labels

Although placards are a valuable source of information, they may not always be present. Legally, only certain hazardous materials must be placarded, no matter what the quantity. Many hazardous materials do not have to be placarded unless a gross weight of more than 1001 lb is carried. A placard with the word "dangerous" can be used on certain mixed loads of hazardous materials. The exact label and placard needed is specified in DOT regulations. Remember that placards and labels may not always be present and the container or vehicle may be improperly labeled or placarded.

Shipping Papers

Shipping papers are usually an extremely accurate source for determining the identity of hazardous cargos. They can clarify what is labeled as dangerous on placards. Shipping papers should accompany all shipments of hazardous substances. Under new DOT regulations, shipping papers must list a 24-hour emergency information telephone number. The problem with shipping papers is their location. In most cases, responders come in close proximity with the hazardous substances when retrieving shipping papers. Responders should never attempt to enter a hazardous materials scene to obtain shipping papers unless they have received proper training and are wearing appropriate protective equipment. Although shipping papers are usually accurate, they may be improperly filled out or missing.

Senses

Senses include any personal physiologic reactions. Visual signs, such as visible vapor clouds, liquids, or solid products; dead or incapacitated people or animals; dead vegetation; or odor and irritation to the skin or eyes can signal the presence of hazardous materials. Because the use of most senses requires that responders be near the incident, relying on senses may result in exposure and therefore is not recommended. The use of sight, preferably aided by binoculars, can provide valuable information from a safe distance. Determine if anyone who was on site at the time of the release noted any unusual sights, sounds, or smells.

Some substances do not have adequate warning properties. Many are colorless, odorless, and tasteless. Many are not detectable until a toxic level has been reached. Some are able to impair the sense of smell, such as hydrogen sulfide. It is detectable at low concentrations but at higher levels causes **olfactory fatigue** (desensitization of the sense of smell). The odor will disappear, leading responders to believe they are in a safe area.

HAZARD ASSESSMENT

Safe and efficient response to a hazardous materials incident mandates a basic knowledge of chemistry and toxicology. The knowledge of where the agent will go and what it is capable of doing is essential. Responders need this information to predict exposure patterns and levels and to anticipate the potential injuries that may occur with specific products.

Chemical Movement

[OBJECTIVE 4]

Probably the most important issue for responders is being able to predict chemical movement. This allows them to stage equipment in a safe area and predict the pattern of exposure.

The state of matter of the chemical has a direct impact on the type of victim exposure. Chemicals can be found in solid, liquid, or gas or vapor form. Vapors present the greatest exposure risk. Liquids and solids present a secondary contamination risk when making contact with contaminated patients. State of matter is determined by assessing the chemical's melting point and boiling point. The **melting point** is the temperature at which a solid changes to a liquid. An example is ice melting to water at 0°C (32°F). The **boiling point** is the temperature at which the vapor pressure of the material being heated equals atmospheric pressure (760 mm Hg). Water boils to steam at 100°C (212°F).

Once the state of matter has been identified, movement of the agent can be predicted by assessing other physical properties. Movement of a liquid contaminant in water can be predicted by looking at the chemical's specific gravity and water solubility. How quickly the chemical will evaporate and present an inhalation hazard can be assessed by looking at the chemical's vapor pressure and sublimation (transforming from solid to vapor) ability.

Specific gravity is the ratio of a liquid's weight compared with an equal volume of water. Water is given a constant value of 1. Materials with a specific gravity of less than 1.0 float on water, and materials with a specific gravity greater than 1.0 sink. Most hydrocarbons, such as gasoline, float on water (Figure 64-22). **Water solubility** is the degree to which a material or its vapors are soluble in water. Materials that are completely soluble in water are called *miscible,* or *polar,* solvents. Alcohols are miscible in water. Insoluble materials are called *immiscible,* or *nonpolar,* solvents.

Volatility is a measure of how quickly a material passes into the vapor or gas state. The greater the volatility, the greater its rate of evaporation. Vapor pressure is a measure of volatility. Examples are gasoline and diesel fuel. Gasoline is more volatile and evaporates faster than diesel fuel. **Vapor pressure** is the pressure exerted by a vapor against the sides of a closed container. It is temperature dependent. As the temperature increases, so does vapor pressure. Vapor pressure is used as an indication of how quickly a liquid evaporates. Water has a vapor pressure of approximately 20 mm Hg at 21°C (70°F) and evaporates slowly at room temperature. If a chemical has a higher vapor pressure, it evaporates faster and presents an increased inhalation hazard.

Of special importance to medical responders are the properties of water solubility and vapor pressure. Inhaled chemicals that are highly water soluble result in upper airway symptoms, and chemicals with lower solubility have a tendency to result in lower airway symptoms. Chemicals with a high vapor pressure evaporate quickly, resulting in an increased inhalation risk. The importance of these properties cannot be underestimated

Boiling point and vapor pressure are closely related. Vapor pressure controls the product's boiling point. This is the reason that liquefied gases, such as chlorine, ammonia, and liquefied petroleum gas, can be kept in a liquid state inside a container even though the temperature is well above its boiling point. Liquefied gases usually have an extremely high expansion ratio. The expansion ratio determines how much vapor results when liquids evaporate. For example, 1 cubic foot of liquid expanding to 100 cubic feet of pure gas has an expansion ratio of 100:1. Liquefied petroleum gas expands 270:1, chlorine expands 450:1, and anhydrous ammonia expands 840:1. Once a liquefied gas is released from its container, it will create an extremely large vapor cloud. When containers of liquids and liquefied gases under pressure are suddenly breached, the product may rapidly boil and expand. If the product is **flammable,** a large fireball may result. This is known as a **boiling liquid expanding vapor explosion** (Figure 64-23).

Physical properties also can be used to predict the movement of gases and vapors. The property of vapor

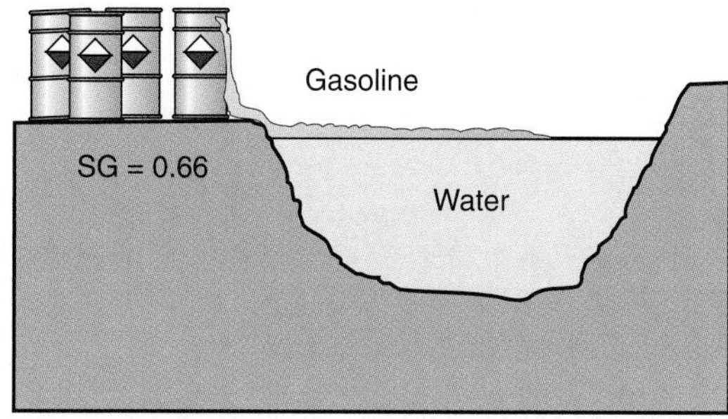

Figure 64-22 Liquid chemicals either float or sink in water depending on their specific gravity (SG).

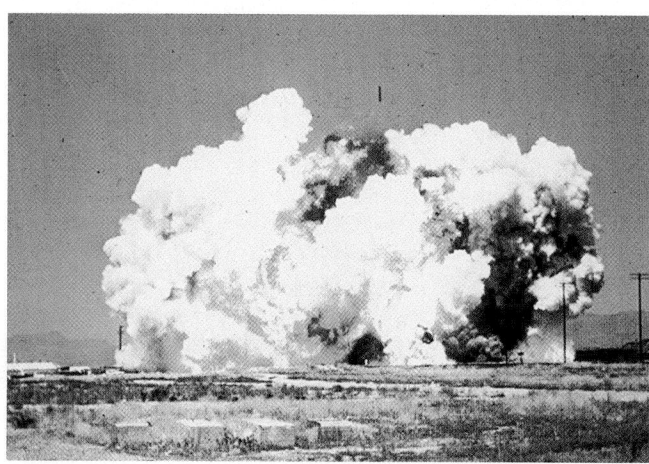

Figure 64-23 Boiling liquid expanding vapor explosion.

density is similar to specific gravity. **Vapor density** is the weight of a volume of pure gas compared with the weight of an equal volume of pure dry air. Air is given a constant value of 1. Materials with a vapor density less than 1.0 are lighter than air and rise when released. Materials with a vapor density greater than 1.0 are heavier than air and sink when released. Most vapors have densities greater than 1.0. Heavier air vapors can flow and settle in low areas, presenting a greater risk of exposure and fire if they reach an ignition source (Figure 64-24). With this information the responder can better predict dispersion patterns and exposure risk.

Hazard Potential

[OBJECTIVE 5]

To prepare for injuries properly, responders must be able to predict the type of damage a chemical can do. Responders should always assess the hazard potential of a chemical by checking its properties. Responders should assess flammability, corrosivity, reactivity, radioactivity, and toxicity.

Flammability

A chemical's flammability can be assessed by knowing its flash point, autoignition temperature, lower flammable limit, and upper flammable limit (Box 64-2).

Corrosivity

Another injury hazard is corrosivity. The DOT defines a **corrosive** product as one that damages human tissue or has a severe corrosion rate on steel. A more in-depth assessment of a corrosive product can be accomplished by determining the chemical's pH. The pH scale is used to define corrosivity and determine if the product is an acid or base (Figure 64-25).

On the pH scale 7 is neutral. **Acids** are materials with a pH value less than 7. Examples include hydrochloric acid and sulfuric acid. **Bases,** or *caustics,* are materials with a pH value greater than 7. Examples include sodium hydroxide and potassium hydroxide. On the pH scale, the lower the number the stronger the acid, and the higher the number the stronger the base. The EPA defines an extremely corrosive product as one with a pH value of 2 or less or 12.5 or greater. Both strong acids and strong alkalis cause extensive tissue damage.

Remember that both sides of the scale are corrosive. Strong alkalis usually result in deeper burns because of their ability to penetrate tissue. When assessing the hazards of a corrosive chemical, also assess vapor pressure. Chemicals with high vapor pressure evaporate, and the corrosive vapors cause inhalation exposure and tissue damage.

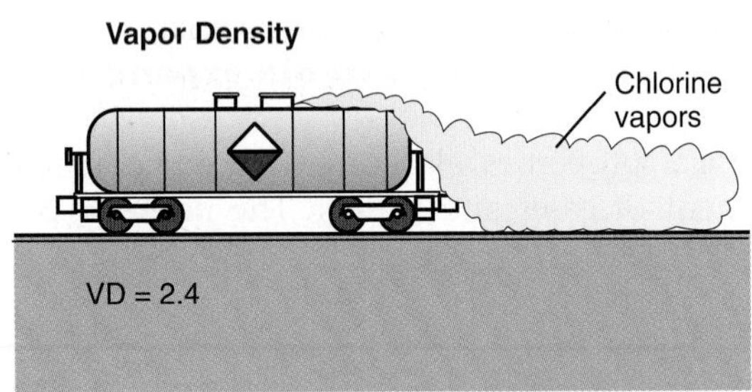

Figure 64-24 Gases and vapors either rise or sink to the ground depending on their vapor pressure. *VD,* Vapor density.

BOX 64-2 Flammability

- **Flashpoint:** The minimal temperature at which a substance evaporates fast enough to form an ignitable mixture with air near the surface of the substance.
- **Autoignition point:** The temperature at which a material ignites and burns without an ignition source.
- **Lower flammable limit** or **lower explosive limit:** The minimum concentration of fuel in the air that will ignite. Below this point too much oxygen and not enough fuel are present to burn (too lean).
- **Upper flammable limit** or **upper explosive limit:** The concentration of fuel in the air above which the vapors cannot be ignited. Above this point too much fuel and not enough oxygen are present to burn (too rich).
- **Flammable range:** The concentration of fuel and air between the lower flammable limit and the upper flammable limit. The mixture of fuel and air in the flammable range supports combustion.

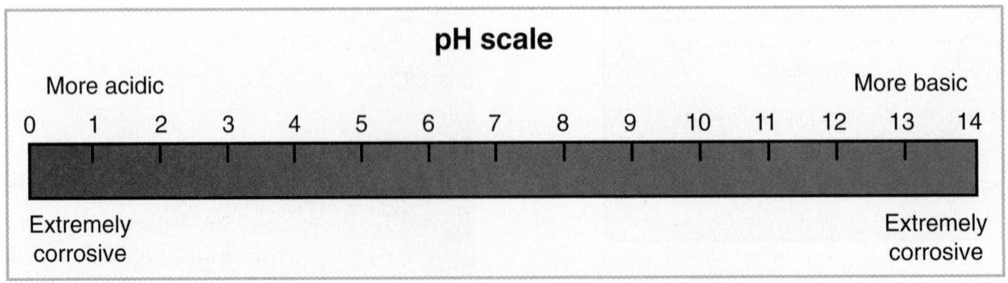

Figure 64-25 Acids have a pH value of less than 7. Bases have a value greater than 7.

PARAMEDIC*Pearl*

Hazardous materials response teams frequently neutralize corrosive chemicals. Although this is an effective way to deal with the released chemical on the ground, corrosive chemicals on skin should *never* be neutralized. Neutralization causes an exothermic (release of heat) reaction that generates a tremendous amount of heat, increasing the amount of tissue damage. Immediate flushing with copious amounts of water is the treatment of choice.

Reactivity

Chemicals also can present a reactivity hazard. Chemicals may interact to produce heat, increased corrosivity, or increased toxicity when mixed with other chemicals. Some chemicals may ignite and burn when exposed to air or water. Chemicals also frequently become more toxic when they decompose under fire or heat conditions (toxic products of combustion). Commonly used terms related to chemical reactivity are shown in Box 64-3.

With the large number of chemicals in use, predicting reactivity can be a major problem. Labeling systems do not always accurately relate reactivity hazards. The yellow section on the NFPA 704 marking indicates reactivity but uses strict criteria. The NFPA reactive criteria include reaction with water and the ability to explode. They may not reflect reactivity when multiple chemicals are mixed.

Radioactivity

Responders also may come in contact with **radioactive substances. Radioactivity** is the spontaneous disintegration of unstable nuclei accompanied by the emission of nuclear radiation. **Ionizing radiation** is in the form of particles or pure energy that produces changes in matter by creating ion pairs.

Following are the most common types of radioactive sources encountered:

- **Alpha particles** are the largest of the radioactive particles, being the same size as the nucleus of the helium atom. They can travel no further than 10 inches and can be stopped by a sheet of paper.
- **Beta particles** are the same size as an electron and can travel approximately 10 feet and be stopped by a piece of aluminum 1 mm thick.
- **Gamma rays** are weightless forms of pure energy that can travel great distances and are stopped by heavy shielding, such as lead.
- **Neutron radiation** is very penetrating and can result in whole-body irradiation. Few natural emitters exist, but neutron radiation can be found in reactors, in research accelerators, and after nuclear detonations.

Half-life is a measure of the rate of decay of a radioactive material. It indicates the time needed for half of a given amount of a radioactive material to change to another nuclear form or element.

Time, distance, and shielding are means of protection against ionizing radioactive materials. The exact periods of time, distance, and thickness of shielding depend on the type and amount of radioactive source present.

For particle radiation such as alpha, beta, and neutrons, respirators, protective clothing, and decontamination procedures must be used to prevent the contamination from entering the body. Responders and patients exposed to electromagnetic radiation sources emitting gamma rays are irradiated. They are not contaminated and pose no risk of secondary contamination. Conversely, exposure to particle radiation sources (alpha and beta particles, neutrons, protons, and positrons) in the form of dust, liquid, or gas results in contamination and presents a secondary contamination risk because of the contamination particles on the person. Radiation experts using special detection equipment can assist with these determinations. In all cases, the shorter the exposure time, the further the distance from the source, and/or the greater the shielding, the lower is the absorbed dose.

BOX 64-3 Commonly Used Terms Related to Chemical Reactivity

- **Water-reactive materials:** Materials that violently decompose and/or burn vigorously when they come in contact with moisture.
- **Air-reactive materials:** Materials that react with atmospheric moisture and rapidly decompose.
- **Pyrophorics:** Substances that form self-ignitable flammable vapors when in contact with air.
- **Oxidation ability:** The ability of a substance to release oxygen readily to stimulate combustion.

Toxicology

[OBJECTIVE 6]

Toxicity is a major concern when dealing with hazardous materials. Just as with other hazards, toxicity can be identified by assessing chemical properties. Guides are available to the agent's level of toxicity.

Dose/Response Relation. Probably the most important concept in toxicology is known as the *dose/response relation.* The toxic effects of a chemical exposure can be estimated according to the level of exposure. One measure of toxicity is known as the *lethal dose system.* This system has been developed from animal research studies to determine fatal exposures with oral, dermal, and inhalation exposures and rates chemicals on the measure of lethal dose (LD50) and lethal concentration (LC50) (Box 64-4). Although this system can be used to compare toxicity of chemicals, it does have limitations. The results are based on animals, not human beings. In addition, the

BOX 64-4 Measures of Toxicity

- **Lethal dose 50% (LD50):** The oral or dermal exposure dose that kills 50% of the exposed animal population in 2 weeks time.
- **Lethal concentration 50% (LC50):** The air concentration of a substance that kills 50% of the exposed animal population. This also is commonly noted as LCt50. This denotes the concentration and the length of exposure time that results in 50% fatality in the exposed animal population.

BOX 64-5 Levels That Identify Potentially Dangerous Exposure

- **Threshold limit value:** The airborne concentrations of a substance; represents conditions under which nearly all workers are believed to be repeatedly exposed day after day without adverse effects.
- **Permissible exposure limit:** Allowable air concentration of a substance in the workplace as established by OSHA. These values are legally enforceable.
- **Immediately dangerous to life or health concentrations (IDHLs):** Maximal environmental air concentration of a substance from which a person could escape within 30 minutes without symptoms of impairment or irreversible health effects.

OSHA, Occupational Safety and Health Administration.

studies are based on lethal effects, not the amount of agent that would cause harm or injury.

Although the LD50/LC50 system uses a lethal end point, dose/response guidelines exist for safe occupational exposures. These levels have been developed by governmental, industrial, and private groups to identify potentially dangerous levels of exposure (Box 64-5).

The immediate danger to health and life (IDHL) level was established by the EPA and the National Institute of Occupational Safety and Health (NIOSH). Immediate evacuation and the use of appropriate-level **personal protective equipment (PPE)** must be emphasized when dealing with IDHL concentrations.

Many private companies establish their own in-house exposure limits. These exposure levels have been developed with the healthy adult subject in mind. The safe level of exposure may vary from agency to agency, so the lowest established level should be used. In addition, these levels do not consider individual differences such as age, individual sensitivity, and preexisting medical conditions. Some people experience adverse effects at or below the established limits. They also are developed for workplace exposures, not home situations, where people spend many more hours.

These limits are usually reported in parts per million (ppm) (parts of gas or vapor per million parts of air) or parts per billion (ppb) (parts of gas or vapor per billion parts of air) for gases and vapors. These are obviously quite small amounts. One ppm can be visualized as one drop of water in a swimming pool. They also may be found in milligrams of a substance per cubic meter of air (mg/m^3) for substances that are respirable as a liquid mist or solid particle mass.

Some chemicals are known or suspected to have the ability to cause cancer. These chemicals are known as carcinogens. NIOSH and OSHA designate potential carcinogenic chemicals with a "Ca" notation.

Duration of Exposure. The duration of the chemical exposure is another important part in assessing the level of toxic threat. The shorter the exposure, the less the absorbed dose and, presumably, the lower the response. Exposures are commonly referred to as *acute* and *chronic*. An **acute exposure** occurs over a short time (less than 24 hours), usually as a result of a spill or release. A **chronic exposure** is exposure to low concentrations over a long period, usually occurring on a daily basis in the workplace.

PARAMEDIC*Pearl*

Take care to avoid confusing exposure with the onset of symptoms. Acute exposures often, but not always, result in the immediate onset of exposure symptoms. Acute exposures also can result in a delayed onset that occurs hours to days later or long-term symptoms that do not show up until years later.

Routes of Exposure. The route of exposure that the agent uses to enter the body is important to consider when evaluating an agent's toxicity potential. Damage may be localized to the exposed area, systemic, or both. **Local damage** is present at the point of chemical contact. **Systemic damage** is remote to the site of exposure or absorption.

Hazardous agents usually attack or enter the body by the following routes: inhalation, ingestion, skin or eye absorption, or injection (subcutaneous, intramuscular, or intravenous).

Inhalation. Inhalation is the quickest and most common route of chemical exposure. The human pulmonary system has an enormous surface area available for absorption. Gas, vapor, and liquid water solubility determine how far into the respiratory tract the substance reaches and the onset of symptoms. Chemicals that are highly water soluble, such as ammonia, react with water in the upper respiratory tract, resulting in upper airway irritation and damage with immediate onset of symptoms such as coughing. Lower water-soluble agents such as phosgene usually penetrate the lower respiratory tract. This usually results in direct lung damage, leading to pulmonary edema, often with a delayed onset.

Another aspect of inhalation toxicity deals with asphyxiants. **Asphyxiants** are chemicals that impair the body's ability to get or use oxygen. **Simple asphyxiants** are inert gases and vapors that displace oxygen in inspired air. Examples include carbon dioxide and nitrogen. **Chemical asphyxiants** prevent the transportation of oxygen to the cells or the use of oxygen at the cellular level. Carbon monoxide is an example of a chemical asphyxiant.

Ingestion. Although ingestion is not the most common way for hazardous chemicals to enter the body, it is certainly a possibility in an intentional release. Food or water supplies may be contaminated by a hazardous materials release. Ingestion may occur when victims or responders fail to decontaminate before smoking, eating, or drinking. Ingestion also may occur when particulate matter is breathed in, impacts in the oropharynx, and is then swallowed.

Skin or Eye Exposure. Unlike the respiratory and gastrointestinal systems, intact skin is usually an effective barrier to many hazardous chemicals and toxic agents. Many chemicals, such as corrosives, can cause skin and eye damage. If the chemical is absorbable across the skin and eye membranes it may cause systemic toxicity. Some chemicals can easily pass through the skin. Certain parts of the body absorb chemicals faster than other areas. For example, the eyes, scalp, and groin absorb chemicals many times faster than the feet or hands. Skin absorption is increased in hot weather and in cases of skin damage.

Injection. How quickly a chemical enters the body when injected depends on the route of injection. From the slowest to the fastest, injections can be by subcutaneous, intramuscular, or intravenous routes. Most hazardous materials exposures by injection or lacerations or puncture wounds are made by contaminated objects. These act in the same manner as subcutaneous or intramuscular injections. Accidental injections also may occur, such as when a piece of metal that has the chemical on it punctures the patient.

Once a chemical is absorbed across a body membrane (such as the lungs, skin, eyes, or gastrointestinal tract), it is distributed throughout the body. It can then be metabolized, stored in organs or adipose (fat) tissue, excreted, and/or cause damage to specific organs. Chemicals are usually metabolized by the liver. The byproducts of this metabolism may be more toxic than the original compound. Chemicals can be stored in organs or fat tissue and released over an extended period. Excretion occurs by the lungs, kidneys, skin, and gastrointestinal system. Specific organs that can be damaged are referred to as *target organs*. Typical target organs include the brain, heart, lungs, liver, and kidneys.

PARAMEDIC*Pearl*

You cannot memorize chemical data on all the chemicals with which EMS responders may come in contact. Likewise, a "see this—do this," or "cookbook" approach to hazardous materials emergency response is too general and does not work. Successful hazardous materials management and treatment of the resultant injuries depend on specific information. Each chemical and situation must be evaluated on its own merits. By researching the physical and chemical properties of the hazardous material, decisions can be made on its exposure potential and ability to cause harm.

HAZARDOUS MATERIALS REFERENCES

[OBJECTIVE 7]

North American Emergency Response Guidebook

The *North American Emergency Response Guidebook* is the reference most familiar to responders (Figure 64-26). It has been available for many years in the United States as the *DOT Emergency Response Guidebook.* In Canada a similar reference was available as the CANUTEC *Dangerous Goods Initial Emergency Response Guide.* In 1996 these two references, as well as information from Mexico, were combined into the *North American Emergency Response Guidebook.* This reference, which is available from the U.S. Government Printing Office or numerous private sources, is a quick-response guide written for first responders to use at a hazardous materials emergency. A chemical can be referenced by placard, chemical name, or a four-digit ID number. Information can be found in guidelines that have been developed for chemicals with similar

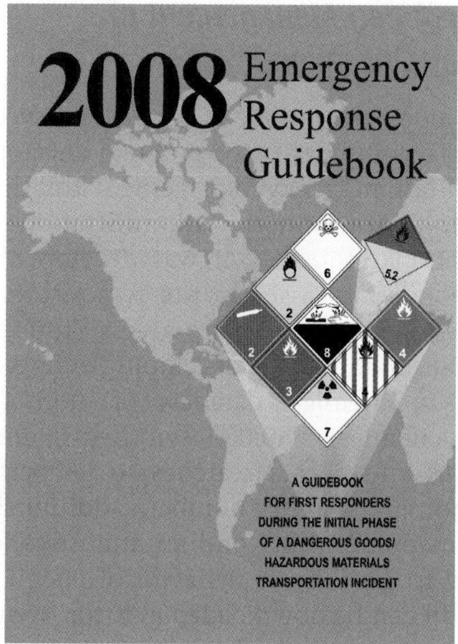

Figure 64-26 2004 *North American Emergency Response Guidebook.*

hazards and management needs. This information includes the following:

- Fire and explosion hazards
- Health hazards
- Public safety information
- Protective clothing needs
- Evacuation concerns
- Fire response
- Spill or leak response
- Basic first aid information
- Protective distances

Material Safety Data Sheets

Under OSHA's Hazard Communication Standard (also known as the *Worker Right to Know*), employers must provide chemical information to their employees by ensuring that containers are labeled and a **Material Safety Data Sheet (MSDS)** is readily available for each chemical with which workers may come in contact. MSDSs are supplied by the chemical manufacturer. This valuable resource usually can be found in industrial settings. Responders may find MSDSs with highly detailed information or quite limited information. The following information is required on the MSDS:

- Chemical name
- Physical data
- Chemical ingredients
- Fire and explosion hazard data
- Health hazard data
- Reactive data
- Spill or leak procedures
- Special protection information
- Special precautions

Computer-Aided Management of Emergency Operations

Computer-aided management of emergency operations (CAMEO) is a computer-based program developed by the EPA's Office of Emergency Management and the National Oceanic and Atmospheric Administration Office of Response and Restoration. It was developed for emergency responders to assist in the response to chemical emergencies and can be used to access, store, and evaluate information critical for developing emergency plans. It contains a chemical database of more than 6000 hazardous chemicals, 80,000 synonyms, and product trade names and allows searches to be performed by name, synonym, and ID number. Additional modules include a mapping utility and an atmospheric distribution model to predict the behavior of chemical vapors. The program can be downloaded at http://www.epa.gov/oem/content/cameo/index.htm. An online version of the program is available at http://cameochemicals.noaa.gov. The base CAMEO program provides a wealth of chemical-specific information in the following six categories:

- Chemical identifiers section
- Hazards section
- Response recommendations
- Physical properties
- Regulatory information
- Alternate chemical names

Telephone References

Telephone references can be extremely valuable to responders who do not have the room to carry multiple written texts or the budget to purchase a laptop and all the necessary software. One drawback of telephone references is the mistakes that can occur when transcribing information. The availability of a fax or cellular fax minimizes this problem.

DOT regulations require that shipping papers for hazardous materials transport contain an emergency contact telephone number accessible 24 hours a day.

Chemical Manufacturers Association

The CHEMTREC and MEDTREC programs are telephone contact resources sponsored by the Chemical Manufacturers Association. These programs are designed to provide emergency responders with immediate response information and make contacts with manufacturers, shippers, and product experts when more detailed information is necessary. Under the MEDTREC program, medical responders can access medical information from the San Francisco Poison Center by calling the CHEMTREC number at 800-424-9300.

Regional Poison Control Center

A valuable resource for EMS responders needing immediate toxicologic information is the regional Poison Control Center. Regional Poison Control Centers are staffed by specially trained medical personnel, including toxicologists. The nationwide phone number to connect to any regional Poison Control Center is 800-222-1222.

SAFE RESPONSE PRACTICES

[OBJECTIVE 8]

Initial Response

The first priority is to protect responders. Response must be to a safe area away from obvious and foreseeable dangers. A safe zone that is upwind, uphill, and upstream from the incident should be established. Because gases and vapors spread the fastest and go the farthest, upwind is the most important factor in selection of a safe zone.

If no other personnel are on site, EMS responders must establish a command post and set up an incident command system (ICS) (see Chapter 62). If an ICS is already established, EMS responders should report to the incident commander or staging area as directed. Rescues from contaminated areas should not be attempted until the chemical has been identified and properly trained responders with appropriate PPE are available.

Remember that bystanders, witnesses, and well-meaning individuals who stopped to assist may be exposed or contaminated. These people must be screened for possible exposure and injuries. If a possibility of contamination exists, decontamination is necessary. Note names and addresses in case future information indicates they were exposed.

Mass evacuations may complicate the response by exposing the evacuating population to the agent or by choking off access to emergency responders. In some cases a better strategy may be protection in place (also called *in-place sheltering*). In all cases, decisions must be approved by the incident commander.

Scene Management

[OBJECTIVE 9]

Site security is necessary to limit scene access to properly trained and equipped response personnel. These types of events are newsworthy and attract a lot of attention. Bystanders and news media personnel may easily end up in the wrong area and become unwilling participants. Protection of the responders also is necessary.

Three zones are typically established: the hot zone, warm zone, and cold zone (Figure 64-27).

Hot Zone

The **hot zone** (also known as the *exclusion zone*) is the area in which contamination currently exists or areas that may be contaminated in a short period (Box 64-6).

Warm Zone

The **warm zone** (also called the **contamination reduction zone**) is the transition area between the contaminated and clean areas. It is designed to reduce the probability that the clean areas will become contaminated or affected by scene hazards (Box 64-7). This is an area of potential contamination and must be adequately controlled.

BOX 64-6 Patient Care Activities in the Hot Zone

- Rapid patient removal with attention to possible spinal injuries.
- If patient is trapped or pinned, medical or trauma stabilization care may be required (medical procedures must be carried out by qualified personnel). Because of the contaminated environment, invasive procedures must be kept to an absolute minimum.
- Airway control.
- Isolation of spontaneously breathing patient's airway with an escape mask, SCBA, filtered bag-mask, or ventilator.
- Rapid removal when extrication procedures are complete.

Activities in this zone require proper preplanning, training, and personal protective equipment (PPE).
SCBA, Self-contained breathing apparatus.

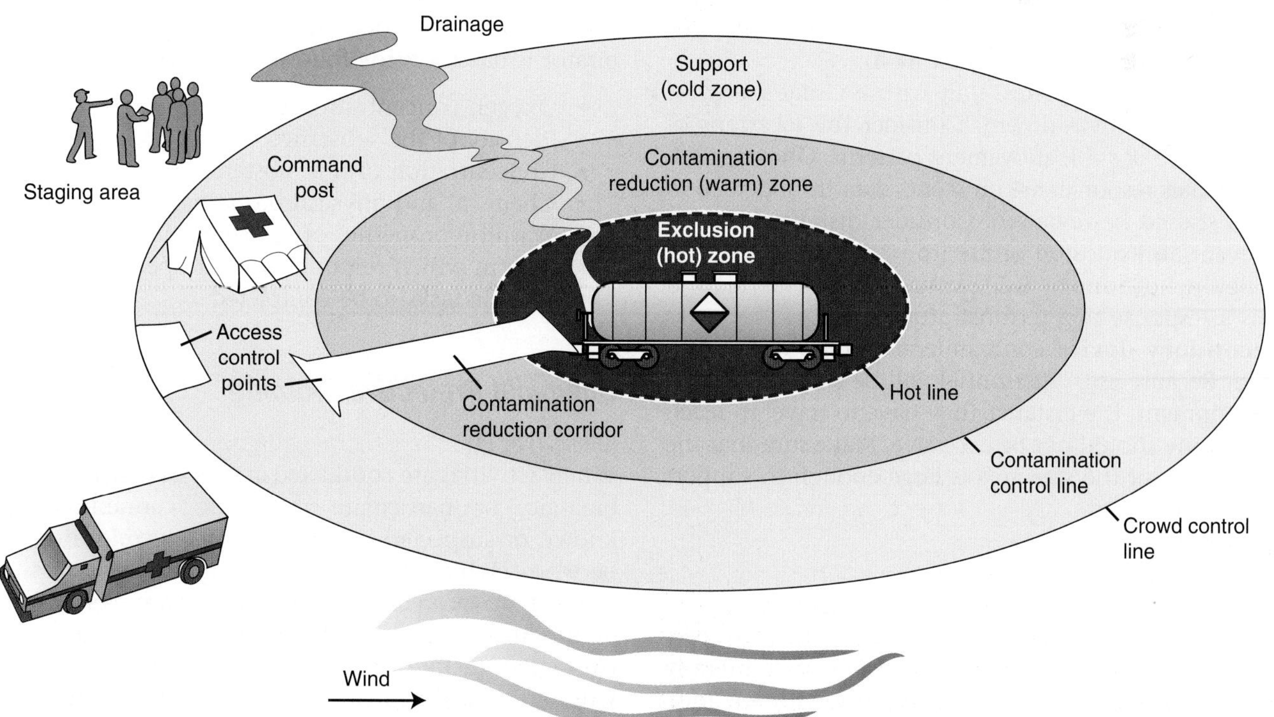

Figure 64-27 Response zones.

BOX 64-7 Patient Care Activities in the Warm Zone

- Medical care during decontamination
- ABC^{2}DE
  - ***A***irway
  - ***B***reathing
  - ***C***irculation (hemorrhage control)
  - ***C***ervical spine stabilization
  - ***D***econtamination
  - ***E***valuate for systemic toxicity
- Oxygen administration
- Limited invasive procedures
- Cardiopulmonary resuscitation as necessary and feasible

Activities in this zone require proper preplanning, training, and personal protective equipment (PPE).

BOX 64-8 Patient Care Activities in the Cold Zone

- Ensure that adequate decontamination has been performed.
- Transfer patient from decontamination personnel to medical caregivers to limit contamination spread.
- Place patient on clean backboard or stretcher.
- Perform basic and advanced life support functions as required.

Activities in this zone require proper preplanning, training, and minimal personal protective equipment (PPE).

Cold Zone

The **cold zone** (also called the *support zone*) is an area under responder control but is located safely away from the emergency. All support and rehabilitation functions are located in the cold zone (Box 64-8).

To establish these zones, start with a visual survey of the immediate environment. Consider the locations of the agent and possible movement patterns. Once hazardous materials resources are on scene, data from detection devices should be reviewed. Consider distances needed to prevent an explosion or fire from affecting personnel outside the hot zone by using your reference manuals. If this is a response to a terrorist attack, the possible areas of **secondary device** concealment should not be overlooked. Because entry personnel will be wearing protective equipment, the distance they have to travel to reach the hot zone should not be excessive. Make sure that the physical area of the safe area is large enough to support site operations.

Safety Plan

Scene operations should be managed by an incident-specific safety plan. The safety plan must be user friendly and should be a guide or checklist for resolving the incident. It also serves to document the response activities and serves as a briefing tool for responders. The safety plan is a dynamic document that should change as scene conditions change. Checklists can be established to assist in the development of the safety plan.

PERSONAL PROTECTIVE EQUIPMENT

[OBJECTIVE 10]

Responders at hazardous materials incidents must be adequately protected from potential exposure and injury. The purpose of PPE is to shield or isolate individuals from the chemical, physical, and biologic hazards that exist when responding to hazardous materials incidents. Exposure to the chemical agent itself is considered primary exposure or primary contamination. PPE concerns must be addressed before any response activity.

PPE decisions must be based on responder involvement. Activities in clean, safe areas, such as management of decontaminated patients, can be safely carried out in PPE commonly used for standard precautions. This equipment includes gloves, mask, eye protection, and a suit to keep liquids from getting on the responder's uniform. This type of PPE is not adequate for use in the contaminated area or during primary decontamination activities. In these areas, chemical protective equipment is needed, including chemical-resistant clothing and gloves specifically compatible with the chemical and either an air-purifying respirator or a self-contained breathing apparatus (SCBA). The use of this equipment requires special training and selection by a knowledgeable, experienced person.

Respiratory Protection

Respiratory protection can be provided by air-purifying respirators, positive-pressure SCBA, or positive-pressure supplied-air respirators. The selection of the proper respirator is based on the following factors:

- Oxygen concentration in the area
- Identity of the substance
- Concentration of the substance
- Chemical and physical properties of the substance
- Warning properties of the substance
- Area in which responders must operate
- Specific tasks to be completed

Chemical Protective Clothing

[OBJECTIVE 11]

When activities are conducted at sites in which chemical, biologic, or particulate radiologic contamination is known or suspected, chemical protective clothing must be worn (Table 64-2). Street clothing or uniforms offer little or no protection from these exposures. The predominant physical and chemical or toxic properties of the agent dictate the type and degree of protection required. The maximal level of protection can only be determined when complete identification of a hazard has been made.

TABLE 64-2 Chemical Protective Clothing

Description	Notes
Vapor protective clothing	Designed to provide the highest level of protection against skin-destructive and skin-absorbable substances Consists of a fully encapsulating, vapor-tight suit Provides highest degree of respiratory protection
Chemical splash protective clothing	Designed to provide protection against liquid splash or particulates Provides very limited protection against vapors

PARAMEDIC*Pearl*

The exact level and type of PPE needed at an incident is dictated by the type of incident and contaminate. Do not attempt to use PPE without proper preplanning, training, medical examinations, and fit testing as required. Selection of equipment by an informed and knowledgeable individual using appropriate reference sources is essential. Initial hands-on training and repeated practice with all PPE is essential for safe and effective use.

The EPA has divided protective clothing and respiratory protection into four categories (levels A through D) according to the degree of protection afforded. Level A protection should be worn when the highest level of respiratory, skin, eye, and mucous membrane protection is needed (Figure 64-28). This level is typically used for protection against skin-toxic or corrosive vapors. It also is needed when gross liquid contact is possible and for extremely hazardous materials. PPE for this level includes a positive-pressure SCBA and a fully encapsulating, vapor-tight, chemical-resistant suit; inner gloves; chemical-resistant outer gloves; and chemical-resistant boots.

Level B protection should be selected when the situation requires the highest level of respiratory protection but a lesser level of skin and eye protection (Figure 64-29). This level is typically used for protection against inadvertent liquid splash or particulates. PPE for this level includes a positive-pressure SCBA and chemical-resistant clothing (overalls and long-sleeved jacket; coveralls; hooded, two-piece, chemical splash suit; disposable, chemical-resistant coveralls; or fully encapsulated, non-vapor-tight suit).

Level C protection should be selected when the type of airborne substance is known, its concentration has been measured, the criteria for using an air-purifying respirator have been met, and skin exposure is unlikely (Figure 64-30). PPE for this level includes a full-face air-purifying respirator or a powered air-purifying respirator and chemical-resistant clothing (one-piece coverall; hooded, two-piece, chemical splash suit; disposable, chemical-resistant overalls).

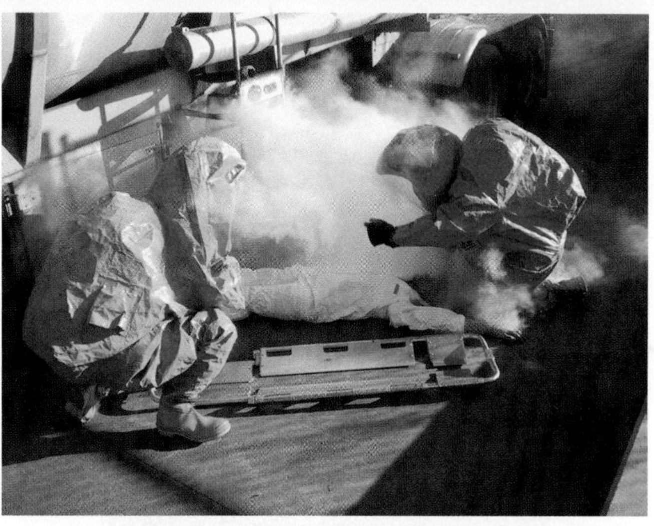

Figure 64-28 During a training exercise, responders using level A personal protection equipment rescue a victim from the hot zone.

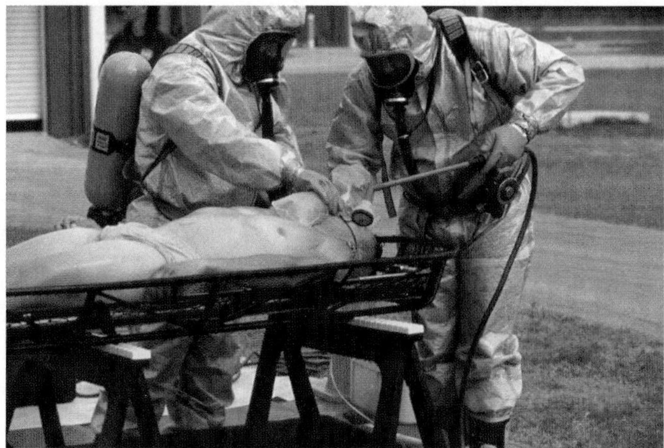

Figure 64-29 EMS responders using level B personal protection equipment provide treatment during patient decontamination.

Level D protection is primarily a work uniform or turnout gear. It should not be worn on any site where respiratory or skin hazards exist (Figure 64-31).

PARAMEDIC*Pearl*

The use of PPE can create significant worker hazards such as heat stress; physical and psychological stress; and impaired vision, mobility, and communication. In general, greater levels of PPE protection can cause the associated risks to increase. For any given situation, equipment and clothing should be selected to provide an adequate level of protection. Gross overprotection, as well as underprotection, can be hazardous and should be avoided.

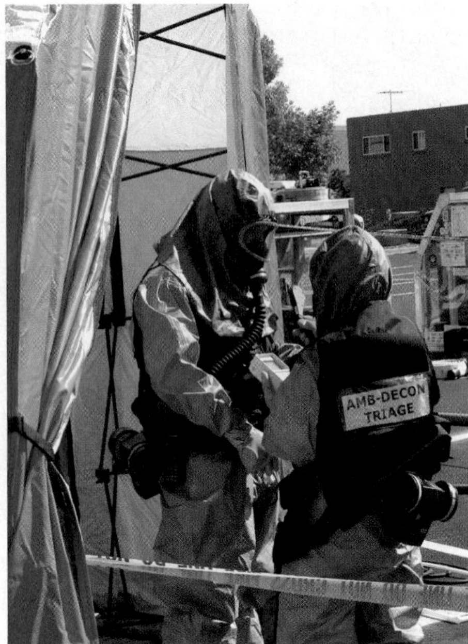

Figure 64-30 EMS responders using level C personal protective equipment (PPE) with a powered air-purifying respirator.

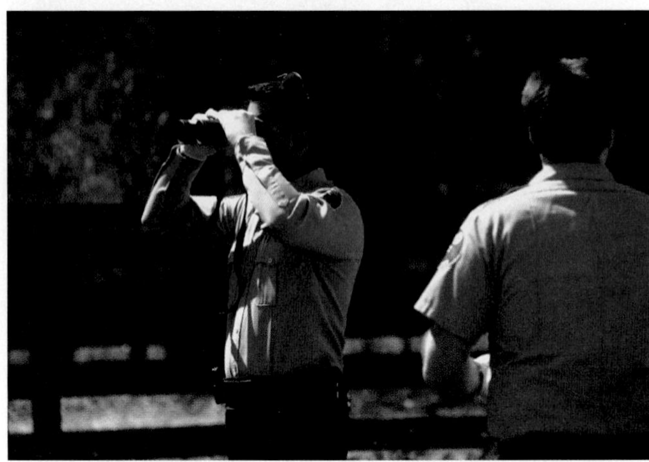

Figure 64-31 EMS responders in level D personal protective equipment (PPE), otherwise known as their work uniforms. Level D offers no chemical protection.

HAZARDOUS MATERIALS TEAM SUPPORT

[OBJECTIVE 12]

In addition to patient care activities for those exposed to a chemical incident, the paramedic will likely be involved in the medical monitoring and rehabilitation of members of the hazardous materials team, as required by OSHA. This is an ongoing process to evaluate the response of personnel who are at risk from exposure to the chemical substance and the effects of heat, cold, stress, and increased physical activity in protective clothing.

BOX 64-9 Reasons to Deny Entry into the Hot Zone

- The body temperature is greater than 99.2°F
- The pulse is greater than 110 beats/min
- The blood pressure is greater than 150/90 mm Hg
- The respiratory rate is greater than 24 breaths/min
- There is a new onset of:
  - Cardiac complaints
  - Respiratory complaints
  - Hypertension
  - Nausea
  - Vomiting
  - Diarrhea

Pre-Entry Examination

Before entry into the hot zone, all personnel required to use level B protection must have a brief health screening conducted to determine baseline levels. This should include an evaluation of the vital signs, temperature, and weight, which can provide early indications of heat stress and dehydration. The skin should be examined for open wounds, rashes, or irritations that may allow entry of a chemical substance. Mental status, gait, and other neurologic functions should be evaluated to determine any change after exiting the hot zone. In addition, a baseline ECG should be obtained. Determine whether the patient has had any signs of recent illness in the last 72 hours, such as fever, diarrhea, cough, nausea, or vomiting, as well as any medications that have been taken. Pay particular attention to the presence of diuretics or other medications that can lead to dehydration and heat stress. If any findings of the preentry physical examination are abnormal, entry to the hot zone should be denied. Findings that would result in the team member being denied entry can be found in Box 64-9. In addition, the team member should ensure adequate hydration by prehydrating with 8 to 16 oz of water or a diluted sports drink to offset the losses that will occur while in chemical protective clothing.

Postentry Examination

If team members demonstrate any changes in gait, speech, or behavior, they should be immediately removed from the hot zone, decontaminated, and evaluated, as should any member with a report of chest pain, dizziness, shortness of breath, weakness, nausea, or headache. Any of these can be indicators of heat stress or exposure to a chemical agent.

After the team member exits the hot zone and is decontaminated (either because of symptoms or a completed assignment), postentry monitoring must take place to determine if the member has been affected by heat stress or chemical exposure. This also is done to determine if the member can be given another

BOX 64-10 Common Postentry Care

- Body temperature greater than 100°F: have the team member rest in cool environment
- Body temperature greater than 102°F: have the team member rest in cool environment and apply cold packs to neck, groin and underarms
- Weight loss less than 3% without signs and symptoms: give 8 oz water for each ½ lb of body weight lost
- Weight loss greater than 3% with signs and symptoms: rehydrate with IV fluids and consider transport

assignment during the incident or immediately after the incident. Note the onset of any signs or symptoms that were not present before entry into the hot zone and monitor vital signs every 5 to 10 minutes until they return to the preentry levels. Determine the team member's weight after exiting the hot zone and perform a thorough neurologic examination. If the team member shows no adverse effects or indicators of chemical exposure at the post-entry evaluation, he or she should remain in the rehabilitation area until rested and rehydrated, with vital signs returned to normal. Increases in temperature and weight loss are commonly found on the postentry examination because of the environment of chemical protective clothing. Treatment specific to these findings is listed in Box 64-10.

Documentation for each team member should include the findings of the preentry and postentry examinations as well as any treatment provided, the response to treatment, and the recommendations of the paramedic to the team member and incident commander regarding the ability of the team member to accept additional assignments.

Heat Stress

One of the greatest risks to hazardous materials team members is heat stress. Wearing chemical protective clothing does not allow heat loss and is similar to being in a sauna. The ambient air temperature is the prime factor in determining the likelihood of developing heat stress; however, heat stress should not be discounted on cool or even cold days. In addition, the surface on which the team member is working also plays a factor. For example, if the incident occurs on pavement a greater amount of radiant heat will be absorbed by the team member than if the incident occurred in a grassy area.

The physical nature of chemical protective clothing does not allow heat loss by radiation. The air within the chemical suit simply heats up and creates a warm pocket of air that surrounds the occupant. Similarly, convective heat loss does not occur because air currents cannot move across the skins surface, and evaporative losses cannot occur because the chemical suit is impermeable. In addition to preventing heat loss, chemical protective clothing adds weight to the team member. This requires greater energy expenditure and an increase in the production of heat by the body.

Other factors that contribute to the development of heat stress include the physical condition of the team member and the degree and duration of activity while in chemical protective clothing. Members who are acclimated to higher temperatures will fare better than those who are not. Body type also plays a role; thin individuals do not generate as much heat as larger individuals and, as a result, temperatures within the chemical suit may be higher for a larger person than a thinner person in the same environment. The duration and activity are important factors as well; the longer the duration or more intense the activity, the higher the body temperature. Heat production increases approximately 13% for each 1°F rise in body temperature. As previously mentioned, this heat cannot be dissipated; therefore the development of heat stress increases exponentially the longer the team member is in protective clothing.

Although heat stress is the primary temperature-related condition associated with chemical incidents, the paramedic also must realize that hypothermia can develop. This can be to the result of prolonged decontamination with cold water or the removal of chemical protective clothing. In this situation the team member is thrust into an environment that is relatively cold compared with the hot environment of the chemical protective clothing. Team members should be monitored for signs of hypothermia while in the rehabilitation area.

PARAMEDIC*Pearl*

A rule of thumb often used by hazardous materials teams with level A protective equipment is to take a rest period after each SCBA bottle is used, approximately every 20 to 30 minutes. A rehabilitation schedule also should be established for decontamination team members and support personnel. During the rehabilitation time, team members should move to a safe area and replenish fluids.

DECONTAMINATION

Decontamination operations should be established before allowing entrance into the hot zone for any reason, including rescue. As victims or personnel exit the hot zone, they must be decontaminated. Contaminated equipment also must be decontaminated as it leaves the hot zone.

A contamination reduction corridor, in which decontamination procedures are carried out, should be established in the warm zone. The decontamination corridor should contain separate areas to decontaminate patients, responders, and heavy equipment as necessary. Selection of a decontamination site should be based on availability;

water supply; ability to contain runoff; and the proximity of drains, sewers, streams, and ponds. Shelters such as schools, firehouses, garages, indoor car washes, and swimming pools may be used after initial rinse at the scene for thorough decontamination. Hospital decontamination can be conducted outside the emergency department with portable equipment. An alternative to outside decontamination is a specially designed room with a separate entrance, contained drains, and separate ventilation system.

The product, life threat, route of exposure, and need for decontamination should be identified. If the exposure is from an unknown material, a worst-case scenario should be considered. Trained, protected responders can manage essential patient treatment at the same time as decontamination. The route of exposure also must be assessed. Products that attack the body only through inhalation present a minimal risk of further exposure once patients are removed from the area.

Responder Decontamination

[OBJECTIVE 13]

All personnel, clothing, and equipment leaving the hot or warm zone must be decontaminated to remove any harmful chemicals or infectious organisms that may have adhered to them (Figure 64-32). Patient care equipment should be changed to clean equipment when the patient is transferred to clean providers in the cold zone. Vehicles and heavy equipment also must be decontaminated before leaving the warm zone.

Dry decontamination is sometimes used in cases in which the contamination is minimal. Dry decontamination involves using disposable clothing and systematically removing these garments in a manner that precludes contact with the contaminant.

Patient Decontamination

[OBJECTIVE 14]

Ambulatory Patient Decontamination

Have ambulatory patients exit the contaminated area. Provide shelter and assist patients if necessary in quickly removing clothing, jewelry, and shoes. Isolate these items in plastic bags. Mark the bags to indicate patient name. Responders who are assisting must use proper PPE. Patients should rinse with copious amounts of water (Figure 64-33). If possible, warm water, 32°C to 35°C (90°F to 95°F), should be used so that extensive washing can be accomplished. A high risk of hypothermia exists if cold water is used. Never use hot water. Use low water pressure and a gentle spray to avoid aggravating any soft tissue injuries. Contact lenses should be removed as soon as possible once the patient's hands are clean. Patients should wash with baby shampoo or a mild liquid soap. They should pay special attention to hair, nail beds, and skin folds. Soft brushes and sponges may be used. Patients should then rinse with copious amounts of water.

Nonambulatory Patient Decontamination

Nonambulatory patients must be removed from the contaminated area. Responders conducting rescue activities or carrying out decontamination procedures should wear proper PPE.

Quickly remove and isolate the patient's clothing, jewelry, and shoes. Then brush off solid or particulate contaminants as completely as possible before washing to reduce the likelihood of a chemical reaction with water. Blot visible liquid contaminants from the body with absorbent material before washing. Use care not to damage skin. Then rinse the patient with copious amounts of warm water (Figure 64-34). Use low water pressure on hose lines to control the spray and avoid

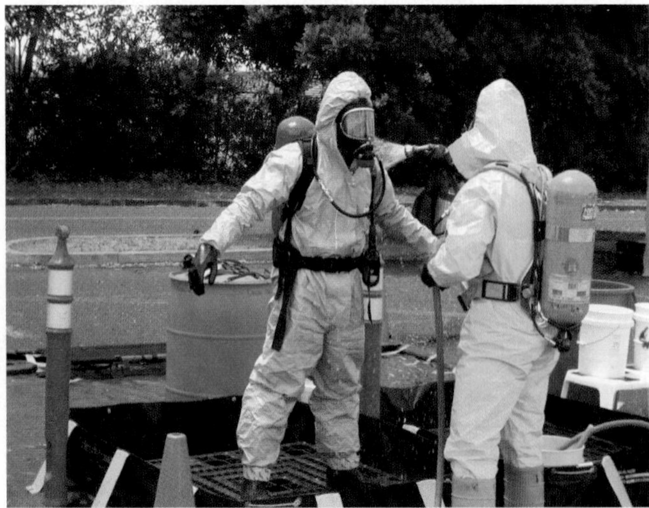

Figure 64-32 Hazardous materials responder going through decontamination.

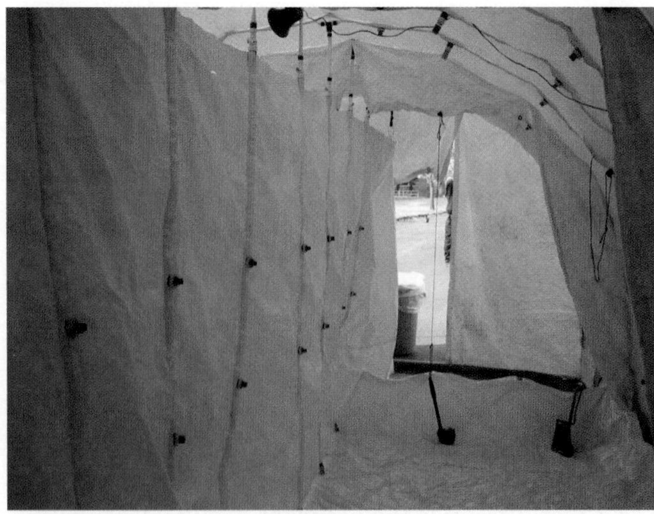

Figure 64-33 Multiple shower nozzles inside a specialized ambulatory patient decontamination tent.

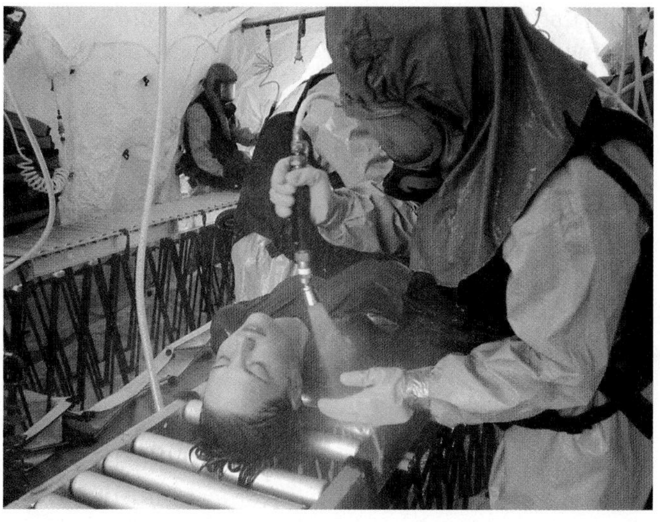

Figure 64-34 Responders performing nonambulatory patient decontamination.

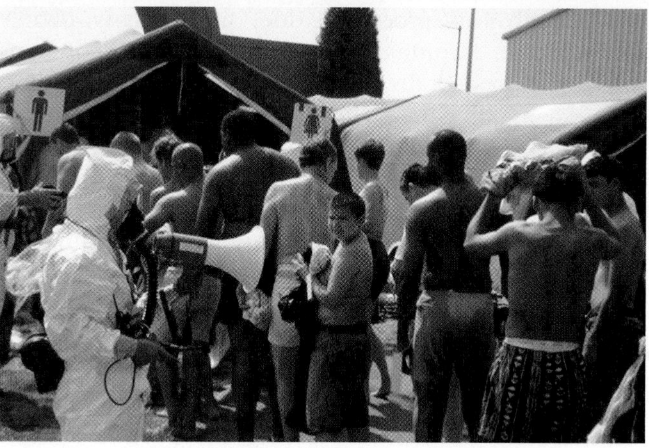

Figure 64-35 Patients waiting to enter the ambulatory patient decontamination tent at a weapons of mass destruction emergency exercise.

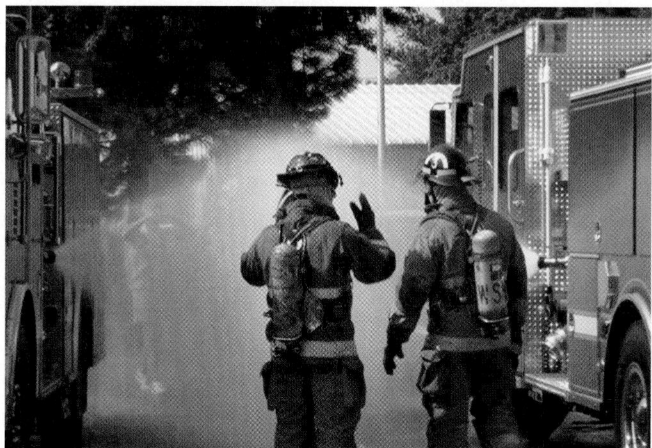

Figure 64-36 Two-engine emergency decontamination system.

aggravating any soft tissue injuries. Avoid overspray and splashing. Use gentle running water from midline to lateral face for eye decontamination. Remove contact lenses as soon as possible. Wash the patient with baby shampoo or a mild liquid soap. Pay special attention to hair, nail beds, and skin folds. Soft brushes and sponges may be used. Be careful not to abrade the skin, and use extra caution over bruised or broken skin areas. Damaged skin areas can enhance the dermal absorption of toxic products.

Decontaminate the head and face first. Brush or blot visible contaminants away from the mouth and nose, and then soap and rinse in the same manner. Isolate the patient's airway with an oxygen mask, bag-mask, or SCBA as soon as possible. Decontaminate areas of skin damage or gross contamination next. Take care not to allow contamination into areas of tissue damage. Gently covering areas of tissue damage with a plastic cover or wrap helps prevent this. Decontaminate the rest of the body as necessary. Finally, rinse the patient with copious amounts of water.

EMS personnel may not be the ones to carry out patient decontamination, but they should be familiar with the process. They may be trained to provide patient care during the process. They also need to evaluate the process to ensure that complete decontamination is taking place.

Mass Casualty Decontamination

[OBJECTIVE 15]

Mass decontamination remains one of the significant bottlenecks in mass casualty incidents or weapons of mass destruction response (Figure 64-35). Some agencies use a procedure known as **emergency decontamination.** This procedure uses fire department apparatus or hoses to decontaminate extremely large numbers of patients in a short period.

An emergency decontamination operation can be established in a number of ways. The simplest way to establish this system uses one fire department engine. One 1.5-inch fire hose is deployed to spray water from one side and a second nozzle is placed on a discharge gate to provide water spray from two directions. A less manpower-intensive system can be rapidly established by parking two fire department engines side by side approximately 20 feet apart (Figure 64-36). This establishes a decontamination corridor and a focal point for victims to move toward. Hose nozzles are placed on the engine's discharge gates so water from each engine sprays to the center of the corridor. Patients are then directed to walk though the water spray. If time allows, ladders can be placed across the top of the engines bridging the tops. Hoses are run over the top of the ladders with nozzles pointing down. This establishes a more conventional overhead shower spray. Tarps can be placed over the ladders to allow male and female separation and some privacy.

Although this procedure does move many people through the decontamination process, some concerns must be addressed. Because cold water is used, hypothermia is a major concern even in temperate weather. If clothes are left on during this type of decontamination operation, contamination could be driven into the skin; therefore patients should disrobe before going through the decontamination process. Many patients are unwilling to disrobe without some form of privacy. Adding to this concern is the probable presence of media at the incident site. This procedure is not effective with nonambulatory patients. Because they must be carried through the water spray, only the front of the patient is cleaned, and patient care during the process is next to impossible. The incident commander should weigh the need for and consequence of using this type of emergency decontamination.

Because of these concerns, many teams use decontamination trailers or special, rapidly deployed tents to provide more effective patient decontamination (Figure 64-37). These systems are easy to set up and provide shelter and privacy during the decontamination process. Water heater and decontamination solution mixer units are available to supply heated decontamination and rinse water through fixed shower nozzles to improve decontamination efficiency and reduce the effects of hypothermia. Air heaters can be used to warm the structures during cold weather. Patient roller systems or carts can be used to increase the efficiency and the throughput of the decontamination process. If these systems are not immediately available at the scene, they can be used for a more thorough decontamination after an initial emergency decontamination.

Decontamination Runoff

Runoff should be contained if possible. Small children's wading pools, commercially manufactured units or tables, draft tanks, or improvised plastic and frame units may be useful during responder decontamination. Patient decontamination should not be delayed to obtain containment pools. If no containers are immediately available, try to channel runoff to a containment area.

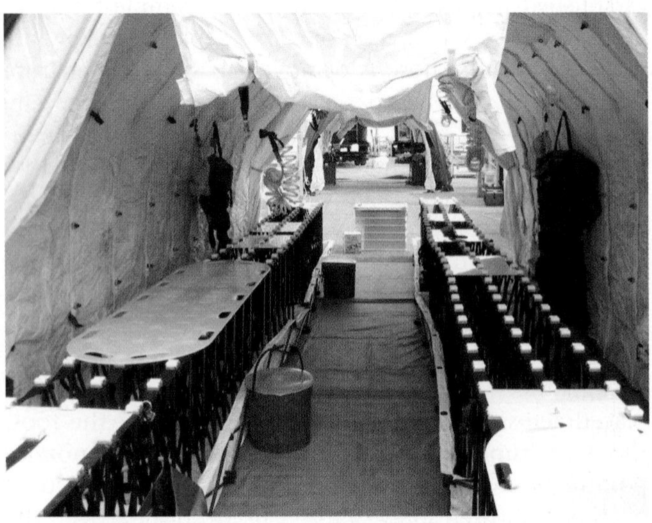

Figure 64-37 Nonambulatory patient decontamination setup with patient roller systems and water heaters.

Local and state water officials should be notified as soon as possible if the runoff cannot be contained. Because of the amount of runoff associated with mass decontamination operations, this may be an extremely difficult task. The EPA has published a position paper stating that patient care comes first. First responders are not held liable for environment regulations if runoff water cannot be contained during a mass casualty decontamination operation. If possible, runoff should be contained, but it should not delay the implementation of decontamination operations. Proper authorities must be notified if the water is allowed to run from the site. In all cases, runoff must not be allowed to run into patient treatment and responder staging areas.

TREATMENT FOR COMMONLY ENCOUNTERED HAZARDOUS MATERIALS

[OBJECTIVE 16]

Corrosives

Any liquid or solid that causes visible destruction of human skin tissue or has a severe corrosion rate on steel or aluminum is a corrosive. As previously mentioned, the EPA defines a corrosive product as having a pH of 2 or less or 12.5 or more. Corrosives include both acids and bases. Some products may cause systemic toxicity. Examples include hydrochloric acid, sulfuric acid, hydrofluoric acid, sodium hydroxide (lye), and caustic potash.

These chemicals can cause damage by inhalation, ingestion, or contact with the skin or eyes. Exposure can result in severe irritation to tissue, which can cause upper airway burns and edema, circulatory collapse, and severe skin burns. Ingestion can cause gastrointestinal perforation, hemorrhage, and peritonitis. Absorption of some products may cause toxic systemic effects (Currance et al., 2005) (Box 64-11).

Pulmonary Irritants

Both chlorine and ammonia act as pulmonary irritants and can cause severe damage to lung tissue. These products also can cause corrosive damage to the eyes or any moist tissue. Chlorine is widely used in the manufacture of chemicals, plastics, and paper. It also is used in water purification and in swimming pools. Chlorine gas is greenish-yellow gas with a characteristic odor. Chlorine reacts with water to form hydrochloric acid.

Anhydrous ammonia is a colorless, water-soluble, alkaline gas. It is used as a fertilizer and as an industrial refrigerant. Ammonia is also used in dyeing, synthetic fibers, and as a neutralizing agent. Ammonia reacts with

BOX 64-11 Treatment of Corrosive Chemical Exposure

- With corrosive chemical exposure, adequate decontamination is essential to limit the patient's tissue damage and the chance of secondary exposure to the caregiver.
- Establish an open airway. Consider orotracheal or nasotracheal intubation for airway control in the patient who is unconscious, has severe pulmonary edema, or is in severe respiratory distress. Early intubation at the first sign of upper airway obstruction may be necessary.
- Ventilate as necessary. Positive-pressure ventilation with a bag-mask device may be beneficial.
- Do not induce vomiting or use emetics.
- Monitor for pulmonary edema and treat if necessary.
- Monitor cardiac rhythm and treat dysrhythmias if necessary.
- Start an intravenous line at 30 mL/hr. For hypotension with signs of hypovolemia, give fluid cautiously. Watch for signs of fluid overload.
- Treat seizures with diazepam (Valium) or lorazepam (Ativan) per local protocol.
- For eye contamination, flush eyes immediately with water. Irrigate each eye continuously with normal saline during transport.
- Cover skin burns with dry, sterile dressings after decontamination.
- Do not attempt to neutralize products because of exothermic reaction.

Reprinted from Currance, P. L., Clements, B., & Bronstein, A. C. (2005). *Emergency care for hazardous materials exposure (3rd ed.).* St. Louis: Mosby.

BOX 64-12 Treatment of Pulmonary Irritant Exposure

- Carry out decontamination if any indications of skin irritation are present.
- Establish an open airway. Consider orotracheal or nasotracheal intubation for airway control in a patient who is unconscious, has severe pulmonary edema, or is in severe respiratory distress. Early intubation at the first sign of upper airway obstruction may be necessary.
- Ventilate as necessary. Positive-pressure ventilation with a bag-mask device may be beneficial.
- Consider the use of a bronchodilator such as albuterol for severe bronchospasm (per local protocol).
- Monitor for pulmonary edema and treat as necessary.
- Monitor cardiac rhythm and treat dysrhythmias as necessary.
- Start an IV and infuse at 30 mL/hr. For hypotension with signs of hypovolemia, administer fluid cautiously. Watch for signs of fluid overload. Consider a vasopressor if the patient is hypotensive with a normal fluid volume, per local protocol.
- For eye contamination, immediately flush eyes with water. Continuously irrigate each eye with normal saline during transport.

Reprinted from Currance, P. L., Clements, B., & Bronstein, A. C. (2005). *Emergency care for hazardous materials exposure (3rd ed.).* St. Louis: Mosby.
IV, Intravenous line.

water to form ammonium hydroxide, a strong alkali. On skin contact, liquefied ammonia may cause frostbite.

These chemicals can cause damage by inhalation, ingestion, or skin and eye contact. Exposure can result in pulmonary edema, hypotension, eye irritation, and chemical skin burns (Currance et al., 2005) (Box 64-12).

Pesticides

Chemicals of the organophosphate and carbamate classes are widely used pesticides. They are found as liquids, dusts, wettable powders, concentrates, and aerosols with a garlic-type odor. The organophosphates are among the most poisonous chemicals and are commonly used for pest control. They are related to the chemical warfare agents soman, sarin, tabun, and VX.

These chemicals can cause damage by inhalation, ingestion, skin and eye contact, and skin absorption. Exposure to organophosphate or carbamate insecticides can result in respiratory failure caused by chemically mediated pulmonary edema and respiratory muscle paralysis. They inhibit acetylcholinesterase, causing overstimulation of the parasympathetic nervous system, striated muscle, sympathetic ganglia, and the central nervous system. This can result in miosis, bradycardia, hypotension, and pulmonary edema (Box 64-13). The following classic set of signs and symptoms known as *SLUDGE-BBM syndrome* may be seen after exposure to these chemicals:

- ***S***alivation
- ***L***acrimation
- ***U***rination
- ***D***efecation
- ***G***astrointestinal distress
- ***E***mesis
- ***B***radycardia
- ***B***ronchoconstriction
- ***M***iosis

Chemical Asphyxiants

Although cyanide and carbon monoxide are chemical asphyxiants, they work in different ways. Cyanide can cause damage by inhalation, ingestion, skin absorption, and skin and eye contact. Cyanide may be found in liquid, solid, or gaseous form. In solid form, it is white, with a faint bitter almond odor (an estimated 20% of the population is genetically unable to detect this odor). It is

BOX 64-13 Treatment of Pesticide (Organophosphate/Carbamate) Exposure

- Adequate decontamination is essential to limit the patient's exposure and the chance of secondary exposure to the caregiver.
- Establish an open airway. Consider orotracheal or nasotracheal intubation for airway control in the patient who is unconscious, has severe pulmonary edema, or is in severe respiratory distress.
- Ventilate as necessary. Positive-pressure ventilation with a bag-mask device may be beneficial.
- Monitor for pulmonary edema and treat as necessary.
- Monitor cardiac rhythm and treat dysrhythmias as necessary.
- Start an IV and infuse at 30 mL/hr. For hypotension with signs of hypovolemia, administer fluid cautiously. Consider vasopressors if the patient is hypotensive with a normal fluid volume, per local protocol. Watch for signs of fluid overload.
- Administer atropine per local protocol. Correct hypoxia before giving atropine.
- **Mydriasis** should not be used to determine the end point of atropine administration; the end point for atropine administration is the drying of pulmonary secretions.
- Administer pralidoxime chloride per local protocol.
- Treat seizures with adequate atropinization and correction of hypoxia. In rare cases, diazepam (Valium) or lorazepam (Ativan) may be necessary per local protocol.
- Succinylcholine, other cholinergic agents, and aminophylline are contraindicated.
- For eye contamination, immediately flush eyes with water. Continuously irrigate each eye with normal saline during transport.

Reprinted from Currance, P. L., Clements, B., & Bronstein, A. C. (2005). *Emergency care for hazardous materials exposure* (3rd ed.). St. Louis: Mosby.
IV, Intravenous line.

BOX 64-14 Treatment of Chemical Asphyxiant Exposure

- Patients exposed to CO usually do not require any decontamination. Because of cyanide's toxicity, patients should undergo decontamination. With liquid or solid cyanide exposure, adequate decontamination is essential.
- Establish an open airway. Consider orotracheal or nasotracheal intubation for airway control in the patient who is unconscious, has severe pulmonary edema, or is in severe respiratory distress.
- Ventilate as necessary. Positive-pressure ventilation with a bag-mask device may be beneficial.
- Do not induce vomiting or use emetics.
- Monitor for pulmonary edema and treat as necessary.
- Monitor cardiac rhythm and treat dysrhythmias as necessary.
- Start an IV and infuse at 30 mL/hr. For hypotension with signs of hypovolemia, give fluid cautiously. Consider vasopressors if the patient is hypotensive with a normal fluid volume, per local protocol. Watch for signs of fluid overload.
- Administer cyanide antidote kit per local protocol for symptomatic patients with cyanide exposure.
- Treat seizures with diazepam (Valium) or lorazepam (Ativan) per local protocol.
- For eye contamination, immediately flush eyes with water. Continuously irrigate each eye with normal saline during transport.
- Pulse oximetry readings may not be accurate in these exposures.
- Hyperbaric oxygen may be required for optimal treatment.

Reprinted from Currance, P. L., Clements, B., & Bronstein, A. C. (2005). *Emergency care for hazardous materials exposure (3rd ed.).* St. Louis: Mosby.
CO, Carbon monoxide; *IV,* intravenous line.

used as a fumigant, in metal treatment, and in the welding and cutting of heat-resistant metals. Cyanide also is used in paper manufacturing, photography, electroplating, blueprinting, and engraving. It is a byproduct liberated during ore extraction and metal purification. Cyanide is a thermal decomposition product of many plastics and other combustible products and is present in most smoke inhalation cases. Cyanide brings cellular respiration to a halt.

Carbon monoxide (CO) is a colorless, tasteless, and odorless gas formed when organic material undergoes incomplete combustion. It is found in exhaust fumes of internal combustion engines and furnace flues. CO also is used in metallurgy, organic synthesis, and the manufacture of metal carbonyls. CO enters the body by inhalation. With CO, the oxygen transport function of hemoglobin in the blood is reduced when it binds with CO, forming carboxyhemoglobin (Box 64-14). Carboxyhemoglobin cannot bind with oxygen. CO causes death by hypoxia (Currance et al., 2005).

Hydrocarbon Solvents

Hydrocarbons are colorless, clear liquids with a faint odor. They are found in solvents, degreasers, wetting agents, agricultural chemicals, laboratory reagents, and antifreezes. They also are used in the application and manufacture of varnishes, lacquers, paints, and detergents.

These chemicals can cause damage by inhalation, ingestion, skin absorption, and skin and eye contact. Exposure may result in skin and eye irritation, dysrhythmias, respiratory failure, pulmonary edema, seizures, and paralysis. Some hydrocarbon solvents also may cause brain and kidney damage (Box 64-15) (Currance et al., 2005).

BOX 64-15 Treatment of Hydrocarbon Solvent Exposure

- Adequate decontamination is essential to limit the patient's tissue damage and eliminate the chance of secondary exposure to the caregiver.
- Establish an open airway. Consider orotracheal or nasotracheal intubation for airway control in the patient who is unconscious, has severe pulmonary edema, or is in severe respiratory distress.
- Ventilate the patient's lungs as necessary. Positive-pressure ventilation with a bag-mask device may be beneficial.
- Consider giving a bronchodilator such as albuterol for severe bronchospasm per local protocol.
- Do not induce vomiting or use emetics.
- Monitor for pulmonary edema and treat as necessary.
- Monitor cardiac rhythm and treat dysrhythmias as necessary.
- Start an IV and infuse at 30 mL/hr. For hypotension with signs of hypovolemia, give fluid cautiously. Watch for signs of fluid overload.
- Treat seizures with diazepam (Valium) or lorazepam (Ativan) per local protocol.
- For eye contamination, immediately flush eyes with water. Continuously irrigate each eye with normal saline during transport.
- Avoid epinephrine and related beta agonists (unless the patient is in cardiac arrest or has reactive airway disease refractory to other treatment) because of the possible irritable condition of the myocardium. Use of these medications may lead to ventricular fibrillation.

Reprinted from Currance, P. L., Clements, B., & Bronstein, A. C. (2005). *Emergency care for hazardous materials exposure* (3rd ed.). St. Louis: Mosby.
IV, Intravenous line.

***Case Scenario*—continued**

After promptly moving the patient outside the building from his initial location, you remove any potentially contaminated clothing. As a precaution, hazardous materials personnel have provided an initial decontamination of the patient. Fortunately, nothing indicates that you and your partner have been exposed to any toxins. A primary assessment of the patient reveals no response to verbal commands but withdrawal from noxious stimuli, a patent airway, extremely rapid but shallow breathing, and a rapid pulse. A head-to-toe assessment reveals no indication of trauma. However, signs of cyanosis are present around the patient's lips and under his fingernails. You administer high-flow oxygen by nonrebreather mask at a rate of 15 L/min. His condition does not improve. Other than the cyanosis around the lips and nails, the patient's skin is normal to flushed in color and dry. Vital signs are pulse, 126 beats/min; respirations, 28 breaths/min; and blood pressure, 122/60 mm Hg. Pupils are sluggish. While you are continuing your assessment, the patient has a clonic seizure.

Questions

4. *Has your first impression changed?*
5. *What conditions are you considering that might cause the cyanosis or apparent hypoxia?*
6. *What additional assessment and treatment options should be considered?*

PATIENT TRANSPORT

[OBJECTIVES 17, 18]

Hospital Communication

Make early contact with the receiving hospital in a hazardous materials emergency (Box 64-16). In large incidents, victims may already have exited the area and may be on their way to the hospital before emergency responders have time to arrive and set up at the scene. Once the news media broadcast the details of the incident, patients who were on the periphery of the incident may think they were exposed and will call local hospitals for advice. Early in the incident, hospital emergency departments will be swamped with potentially contaminated patients and requests for information. Obviously they have a need for information, and they need it as quickly as they can get it. Even if no patients are initially involved in the incident, early communication provides the emergency department with the time needed to carry out research on the chemicals and obtain needed equipment and expertise. All hospitals in the area should be contacted if possible. Your base hospital may be able to make the contacts to the other hospitals.

BOX 64-16 Information to Be Communicated to Receiving Hospitals

- Number of patients and potential additional patients
- Nature of incident
- Agent involved
- Route of exposure
- Duration of exposure
- Associated trauma
- Victim examination findings and vital signs
- Initial signs and symptoms
- Treatment administered
- Current signs and symptoms
- Decontamination carried out?
- Need for further decontamination?
- Estimated time of arrival

Case Scenario CONCLUSION

You assess the patient's oxygen saturation level, and the SpO_2 reads 88 while using a nonrebreather mask. Your partner begins to ventilate the patient's lungs with a bag-mask device as you prepare to intubate. After a few moments of positive-pressure ventilation, the seizure subsides; otherwise the patient's condition remains unchanged. You successfully intubate the trachea and verify tube placement by using an esophageal detector and capnography. You establish intravenous access with D_5W and infuse the solution at a keep-open rate. Per local protocol, you administer the cyanide antidote kit.

Looking Back

7. *What is your final impression of the patient?*
8. *What treatment options are available for this patient?*
9. *Are specific concerns present about toxic exposure during transport or decontaminating the ambulance?*

Reducing Secondary Contamination Risk

Patients with known contamination require decontamination for proper and safe treatment. Unfortunately, determining if the patient is completely decontaminated is difficult in the field. Special precautions should be taken to ensure that the patient and crew are protected during transport. Nonessential equipment should be removed before transport.

Because inhalation is the quickest and most vulnerable route of exposure, adequate ventilation in the transport vehicle is essential. Ambulances should have both intake and exhaust fans operating to ensure maximal ventilation in the patient care compartment. Another suggestion in many protocols is to cover the walls and ceiling of the entire ambulance patient compartment in plastic. Unless time is taken to cut holes for ventilation units and adequately tape down the plastic so no flaps occur, however, ventilation in the patient compartment is radically decreased, resulting in an increase of the secondary inhalation hazard to patients and EMS responders. Plastic may be useful on the stretcher, floor, and bench to reduce contact exposure from patients who are wet with decontamination water.

Another method sometimes recommended is reverse isolation. These procedures include postdecontamination isolation of the patient in specially designed contaminated-patient transportation bags, plastic, sheets, blankets, or zip-front body bags. Although this process reduces the risk of secondary contamination of EMS responders, it may increase the risk of further contamination to the patient. When wrapped, especially in plastic or a body bag, the patient's temperature increases, resulting in sweating, open pores, and dilated peripheral blood vessels. If the patient has not been adequately decontaminated, skin absorption may be increased, which, in turn, increases the patient's chemical exposure risk. Some have argued that if adequate patient decontamination has been carried out, reverse isolation procedures are not needed. Because determining whether the patient has been adequately decontaminated is nearly impossible in the field, a combination of good decontamination and reverse isolation procedures may be useful. Check with your medical control physician and follow his or her recommendations.

Even patients with toxic ingestions and no other exposure may present a secondary contamination hazard. The patient may vomit during transport. The vomitus (as well as burps, hiccups, and flatulence) may contain volatile compounds, leading to an inhalation hazard. Immediately isolate any vomitus in a sealed plastic bag.

EMS personnel may wish to wear respiratory-protective and chemical-protective clothing when transporting patients who may have been contaminated. Chemical-protective equipment, such as respirators and heavy chemical gloves, complicates patient care procedures. If protective equipment is to be used, responders should practice with the equipment before actual use. In all cases, responders should never attempt to wear respirators or protective clothing unless they have received specific training and fit testing, as necessary, on that piece of equipment.

PARAMEDIC*Pearl*

PPE should never be used as a reason or excuse not to decontaminate a patient.

Transporting patients from hazardous materials incidents by air involves risk. The helicopter may travel through an unsafe area, or the rotor wash from the helicopter may affect vapors or fumes at the scene. If decontamination is not complete, the flight crew could experience symptoms of exposure. Because of this, air transportation of patients from a hazardous materials emergency is usually considered to be contraindicated unless rapid transport is absolutely necessary and the patient is *completely* decontaminated or was exposed to a chemical with no risk of **secondary contamination.** Flight services should not be ignored in hazardous materials response planning. They may be the only reasonable way to transport severely injured patients from rural areas or to distant special care centers. Air medical crews may be called to an unrecognized hazardous materials incident and be on scene very quickly. As with all field responders, air medical crews should receive adequate training in hazardous materials recognition and safe response practices.

POST-INCIDENT CONCERNS

[OBJECTIVE 19]

After a hazardous materials incident has ended, numerous items must still be addressed. Procedures must be in place to prevent secondary contamination after the incident is concluded. Residual contamination may still exist on the ambulance and patient care equipment and present a significant hazard. An incident debriefing and post-incident analysis and review should follow every hazardous materials response. The cause of the incident and response procedures should be assessed. Procedures also should be in place to deal with any emotional stress created by the incident.

Case Scenario SUMMARY

1. *What is your initial impression of the patient?* Your initial impression is a patient who may have been exposed to a toxin while working in the metal shop. The most likely toxin is cyanide.
2. *Does any particular hazard suggest prompt evacuation?* The immediate hazard to you, your partner, the shop manager, and any bystanders is exposure to cyanide. You should note any evidence of exposure to all individuals. The cyanide may have been inhaled by the patient before your arrival. Notify the hazardous materials team and promptly evacuate the area. In this situation, if you or any member of the responding crew suspected poisoning by a hazardous material, you should have backed out of the hazardous scene, evacuating everyone as you go but leaving the contaminated patient to be removed by personnel in proper hazardous materials clothing.
3. *What other information is needed to complete your assessment?* Information that may be helpful in determining the nature of the patient's illness and treatment options includes a head-to-toe assessment, vital signs, pulse oximetry, and a SAMPLE history.
4. *Has your first impression changed?* The initial impression may be confirmed by the additional information. The cyanosis around the lips and nails is common with significant hypoxia caused by the cyanide. In addition, a normal to flushed skin from high oxygen levels in the blood may be misleading because the oxygen cannot be used by the cells.
5. *What conditions are you considering that might cause the cyanosis or apparent hypoxia?* In addition to cyanide intoxication, the patient's condition also could be attributed to CO poisoning. The seizure is most likely from cerebral hypoxia.
6. *What additional assessment and treatment options should be considered?* Additional information needed includes blood glucose assessment and pulse oximetry. Blood glucose levels are not critical during this phase of patient assessment and treatment. Beware of falsely elevated oxygen saturation levels. Initial treatment options to be considered include oxygen by endotracheal intubation, intravenous access, and use of a cyanide antidote kit depending on local protocols.
7. *What is your final impression of the patient?* The final impression of this patient is cyanide poisoning.
8. *What treatment options are available for this patient?* Prehospital care includes oxygen, intravenous access, cyanide antidote kit, and monitoring. Hypoxic seizures may recur and the patient should be protected during the clonic seizure.
9. *Are specific concerns present about toxic exposure during transport or decontaminating the ambulance?* In this case, initial decontamination of the patient and crew (if necessary) should be sufficient. Continued or subsequent exposure to cyanide among the crew is highly unlikely as long as the source has been removed. Ventilating the patient's lungs should not result in off-gassing or releasing cyanide by the patient in his exhaled air. Decontaminate the ambulance as you normally would after each patient.

Chapter Summary

- A hazardous materials incident is one of the most challenging emergencies that EMS face. Hazardous materials responses involve out-of-the-norm activities such as the use of PPE and decontamination.
- Responders must be able to recognize the presence of hazardous materials at an incident.
- Responders must be able to use available references and understand the importance of chemical and physical properties when assessing the hazards at an incident involving hazardous materials.
- Proper approach and scene management practices are essential to responder safety at hazardous materials incidents.
- Special training is required before responders may operate at this type of emergency.
- EMS personnel must be able to select and use proper PPE if they will operate in the warm or hot zones of a hazardous materials incident.
- EMS responders should be able to provide the hazardous materials team with medical support and responder rehabilitation at a hazardous materials incident.
- Proper decontamination of both responders and patients is essential to limit harm and the chance of secondary contamination.
- EMS responders should have an understanding of the proper treatment practices for commonly encountered hazardous materials.
- Responders must understand the need for interaction with local hospitals and the need for proper transport procedures when transporting patients from the scene of a hazardous materials incident.
- Post-incident procedures such as debriefing, analysis, and review are vital pieces of a hazardous materials response.

REFERENCES

Currance, P. L., Clements, B., & Bronstein, A. C. (2005). *Emergency care for hazardous materials exposure* (3rd ed.). St. Louis: Mosby.

Occupational Safety and Health Administration. *CFR 1910.120.* Retrieved February 29, 2008, from http://www.osha.gov.

Occupational Safety and Health Administration. *Firefighter training requirements to respond to emergency releases, or potential emergency releases, of hazardous substance.* Retrieved February 29, 2008, from http://www.osha.gov.

Occupational Safety and Health Administration. (1995). *Clarification on who must receive first responder awareness level training.* Retrieved February 29, 2008, from http://www.osha.gov.

SUGGESTED RESOURCES

Briggs, S. M., & Brinsfield, K. H. (Eds.). (2003). *Advanced disaster medical response: Manual for providers.* Boston: Harvard Medical International Trauma & Disaster Institute.

CHEMTREC/American Chemistry Council
1300 Wilson Boulevard, Arlington, VA 22209
Phone: 800-424-9300
Website: http://www.chemtrec.org

Currance, P. L., & Bronstein, A. C. (1999). *Hazardous materials for EMS.* St. Louis: Mosby–Year Book.

Currance, P. L. (2005). *Medical response to weapons of mass destruction.* St. Louis: Mosby.

Hawley, C. (2002). *Hazardous materials incidents.* Albany, NY: Delmar.

Occupational Safety and Health Administration. (1989). *29 CFR 1910.120, Hazardous Waste Operations and Emergency Response, Final Rule, March 6, 1989.* Washington, DC: U.S. Government Printing Office.

Chapter Quiz

1. EMS responders must be trained to a minimum of the ________ level to care for patients during decontamination procedures in the warm zone.

a. awareness
b. operations
c. technician
d. specialist
e. incident command

2. What is the first priority when responding to a hazardous materials emergency?

a. Evaluation of the patient
b. Evaluation of the chemical
c. Notification of the receiving hospital
d. Ensuring response crew safety

3. True or False: The NFPA 704 system is a nationally recognized method of identifying specific chemicals.

4. A simple asphyxiant ________.
  a. displaces oxygen
  b. has no biologic effect on its own
  c. may be an explosion hazard
  d. all the above

5. Which of the following is *not* one of the six hazardous materials recognition clues?
  a. Placards and labels
  b. Container shape
  c. MSDS
  d. Occupancy and location
  e. Markings and colors

6. In what zone should the command post be located?
  a. Warm zone
  b. Cold zone
  c. Transition zone
  d. Hot zone

7. The responder's safest position at a hazardous materials or weapon of mass destruction incident scene is ________.
  a. upwind and uphill
  b. upwind and downhill
  c. crosswind and uphill
  d. downwind and downhill

8. The *most* important reason that control zones are set up at a chemical or radiation incident scene is ________.
  a. to make sure that incoming equipment and apparatus are staged in a safe location
  b. because it is mandated by various federal agencies such as DOT, OSHA, and NFPA
  c. to isolate and minimize risks to the public and emergency response personnel
  d. to control members of the press

9. Which of the following types of PPE are used with level A?
  a. Air-purifying respirator
  b. SCBA and Tyvek suit
  c. Full face mask
  d. SCBA and vapor-tight total encapsulating suit
  e. None of the above

10. The difference between level A and level B PPE is ________.
  a. the degree of respiratory protection
  b. the degree of skin protection
  c. the type of respirator worn
  d. a and b

11. True or False: Overprotection with PPE can be just as dangerous as underprotection.

12. Using the concept of the dose/response relation, which of the following is true?
  a. The chemical structure determines the toxicity.
  b. The vapor pressure determines the toxicity.
  c. The larger the dose, the greater the toxicologic response.
  d. The solubility determines the response.

13. Which of the following statements regarding emergency decontamination operations is *incorrect?*
  a. Patients are usually completely decontaminated.
  b. Large numbers of patients can be quickly decontaminated.
  c. Patients will be wet and cold.
  d. Many patients will object to the procedure.

14. True or False: Patients should be decontaminated before transportation to the hospital.

15. True or False: Responders trained to the competencies required in NFPA 473 level I can operate in the warm zone.

16. The top section of the NFPA 704 symbol is ___________ and represents __________ danger.
  a. yellow; reactivity
  b. red; fire
  c. blue; health
  d. white; special information
  e. none of the above

17. True or False: The nose is a good detection device for assessing hazardous materials exposure.

18. True or False: A gas with a vapor density of 1.87 will sink in air (at the same temperature) and is likely to be found near the ground.

19. The lowest level at which a flammable gas will burn is the ____.
  a. LEL
  b. TLV
  c. UEL
  d. IDHL

20. Which chemical property is an indication of how quickly a chemical will evaporate?
  a. Vapor density
  b. Specific gravity
  c. Vapor pressure
  d. Water solubility

21. A liquid with a specific gravity of 1.27 will ________.
  a. float on water
  b. sink in water

22. Which route of exposure is seen in most hazardous materials exposures?
  a. Dermal
  b. Inhalation
  c. Oral
  d. Intravenous

Chapter Quiz—continued

23. Patient care in the hot zone should include all the following except ________.

a. airway management
b. rapid cervical spine immobilization
c. decontamination
d. rapid removal

24. The purpose of patient decontamination is ________.

a. to reduce the exposure
b. to decrease the risk of secondary exposure
c. to minimize the spread of contamination
d. all the above

Terminology

Acids Materials that have a pH value less than 7 (e.g., hydrochloric acid, sulfuric acid).

Acute exposure An exposure that occurs over a short timeframe (less than 24 hours); usually occurs at a spill or release.

Air-reactive materials Materials that react with atmospheric moisture and rapidly decompose.

Alpha particle A positively charged particle emitted by certain radioactive materials.

Asphyxiants Chemicals that impair the body's ability to either get or use oxygen.

Autoignition point The temperature at which a material ignites and burns without an ignition source.

Bases Materials with a pH value greater than 7 (e.g., sodium hydroxide, potassium hydroxide).

Beta particle A negatively charged particle emitted by certain radioactive materials.

Boiling liquid expanding vapor explosion An explosion that can occur when a vessel containing a pressurized liquid ruptures.

Boiling point The temperature at which the vapor pressure of the material being heated equals atmospheric pressure (760 mm Hg); water boils to steam at 100°C (212°F).

Bulk containers Large containers and tanks used to transport large quantities of hazardous materials.

Carboys Glass or plastic bottles commonly used to transport corrosive products.

Chemical asphyxiants Chemicals that prevent the transportation of oxygen to the cells or the use of oxygen at the cellular level.

Chronic exposure An exposure to low concentrations over a long period.

Cold zone A safe area isolated from the area of contamination; also called the *support zone*. This zone has safe and easy access. It contains the command post and staging areas for personnel, vehicles, and equipment. EMS personnel are stationed in the cold zone.

Contamination The deposition or absorption of chemical, biologic, or radiologic materials onto personnel or other materials.

Contamination reduction zone See *Warm zone*.

Corrosive Any liquid or solid that can destroy human flesh on contact or has a severe corrosion rate on steel.

Cryogenic Pertaining to extremely low temperatures.

Cylinders Nonbulk containers that normally contain liquefied gases, nonliquified gases, or mixtures under pressure; cylinders also may contain liquids or solids.

Decontamination The physical and chemical process of reducing and preventing the spread of contamination from persons and equipment used at a hazardous materials incident; also referred to as *contamination reduction*.

Emergency decontamination The process of decontaminating people exposed to and potentially contaminated with hazardous materials by rapidly removing most of the contamination to reduce exposure and save lives, with secondary regard for completeness of decontamination.

Explosive Any chemical compound, mixture, or device, the primary or common purpose of which is to function by detonation or rapid combustion (i.e., with substantial instantaneous release of gas and heat); found in liquid or solid forms (e.g., dynamite, TNT, black powder, fireworks, ammunition).

Flammable The capacity of a substance to ignite.

Flammable gases Any compressed gas that meets requirements for lower flammability limit, flammability limit range, flame projection, or flame propagation as specified in CFR Title 49, Sec. 173.300(b) (e.g., acetylene, butane, hydrogen, propane).

Flammable range The concentration of fuel and air between the lower flammable limit or lower explosive limit and the upper flammable limit or upper explosive limit; the mixture of fuel and air in the flammable range supports combustion.

Flammable solids A solid material other than an explosive that is liable to cause fires through friction, retained heat from manufacturing or processing, or that can be ignited readily; when ignited, they burn so vigorously and persistently that they create a serious transportation hazard (e.g., phosphorus, lithium, magnesium, titanium, calcium resinate).

Flashpoint The minimum temperature at which a substance evaporates fast enough to form an ignitable mixture with air near the surface of the substance.

Gamma rays A type of electromagnetic radiation that can travel great distances; can be stopped by heavy shielding, such as lead.

Half-life The measure of the rate of decay of a radioactive material; indicates the time needed for half of a given amount of a radioactive material to change to another nuclear form or element.

Hazard Communication Standard (HAZCOM) OSHA standard regarding worker protection when handling chemicals.

Hazardous materials A substance (solid, liquid, or gas) capable of posing an unreasonable risk to health, safety, environment, or property.

Hazardous Waste Operations and Emergency Response (HAZWOPER) OSHA and EPA regulations regarding worker safety when responding to hazardous materials emergencies.

Hot zone The area in which contamination currently exists or areas that may be contaminated in a short period; also called the *exclusion area*. Patients are removed from this area to the warm zone for decontamination. Entrance to the hot zone requires proper PPE.

Immediately dangerous to life or health concentrations (IDHLs) Maximal environmental air concentration of a substance from which a person could escape within 30 minutes without symptoms of impairment or irreversible health effects.

Ionizing radiation Particles or pure energy that produces changes in matter by creating ion pairs.

Lethal concentration 50% (LC50) The air concentration of a substance that kills 50% of the exposed animal population; this denotes the concentration and the length of exposure time that results in 50% fatality in the exposed animal population; also commonly noted as LCt50.

Lethal dose 50% (LD50) The oral or dermal exposure dose that kills 50% of the exposed animal population in 2 weeks.

Local damage Damage present at the point of chemical contact.

Lower flammable limit The minimal concentration of fuel in the air that will ignite; below this point too much oxygen and not enough fuel to burn (too lean) are present; also called the *lower explosive limit*.

Material safety data sheet (MSDS) A document that contains information about the specific identity of a hazardous chemical; information includes exact name and synonyms, health effects, first aid, chemical and physical properties, and emergency telephone numbers.

Melting point The temperature at which a solid changes to a liquid (e.g., ice melting to water at 0°C [32°F]).

Mydriasis Dilation of the pupils.

National Fire Protection Association (NFPA) International voluntary membership organization that promotes improved fire protection and prevention and establishes safeguards against loss of life and property by fire; writes and publishes national voluntary consensus standards.

Neutron radiation Penetrating radiation that can result in whole-body irradiation.

Olfactory fatigue Desensitization of the sense of smell.

Occupational Safety and Health Administration (OSHA) A unit of the U.S. Department of Labor that establishes protective standards, enforces those standards, and reaches out to employers and employees through technical assistance and consultation programs.

Oxidation ability The ability of a substance to readily release oxygen to stimulate combustion.

Permissible exposure limit Allowable air concentration of a substance in the workplace as established by OSHA; these values are legally enforceable.

Personal protective equipment (PPE) Clothing and equipment worn to protect against environmental hazards.

Placards Diamond-shaped signs placed on the sides and ends of bulk transport containers (e.g., truck, tank car, freight container) that carry hazardous materials.

Poisonous Describes gases, liquids, or other substances of such nature that exposure to a very small amount is dangerous to life or is a hazard to health; also known as *toxic* (e.g., cyanide, arsenic, phosgene, aniline, methyl bromide, insecticides, pesticides).

Pounds per square inch (psi) The amount of pressure on an area that is 1 inch square.

Pyrophorics Substances that form self-ignitable flammable vapors when in contact with air.

Radioactive The ability to emit ionizing radioactive energy.

Radioactive substances Any material or combination of materials that spontaneously emit ionizing radiation and have a specific activity greater than 0.002 μCi/g (e.g., plutonium, cobalt, uranium 235, radioactive waste).

Radioactivity The spontaneous disintegration of unstable nuclei accompanied by the emission of nuclear radiation.

Secondary contamination The risk of another person or healthcare provider becoming contaminated with a hazardous material by contact with a contaminated victim.

Secondary device An explosive, chemical, or biologic device hidden at the scene of an emergency and set

Terminology—continued

to detonate or release its agent after emergency response personnel are on scene.

Simple asphyxiants Inert gases and vapors that displace oxygen in inspired air (e.g., carbon dioxide, nitrogen).

Specific gravity The ratio of a liquid's weight compared with an equal volume of water (which has a constant value of 1); materials with a specific gravity of less than 1.0 float on water, and materials with a specific gravity greater than 1.0 sink.

Systemic damage Damage remote to the site of exposure or absorption.

Threshold limit value The airborne concentrations of a substance; represents conditions under which nearly all workers are believed to be repeatedly exposed day after day without adverse effects.

Tube trailers Trailers that carry multiple cylinders of pressurized gases.

Upper flammable limit The concentration of fuel in the air above which the vapors cannot be ignited; above this point too much fuel and not enough oxygen are present to burn (too rich); also called the *upper explosive limit.*

Vapor density The weight of a volume of pure gas compared with the weight of an equal volume of pure dry air (which has a constant value of 1); materials with a vapor density less than 1.0 are lighter than air and rise when released; materials with a vapor density greater than 1.0 are heavier than air and sink when released.

Vapor pressure The pressure exerted by a vapor against the sides of a closed container; a measure of volatility.

Volatility A measure of how quickly a material passes into the vapor or gas state; the greater the volatility, the greater its rate of evaporation.

Warm zone Area surrounding the hot zone that functions as a safety buffer area, decontamination area, and as an access and egress point to and from the hot zone; also called the *contamination reduction zone.*

Water-reactive materials Materials that violently decompose and/or burn vigorously when they come in contact with moisture.

Water solubility The degree to which a material or its vapors are soluble in water.

CHAPTER 65

Tactical EMS

Objectives

After completing this chapter, you will be able to:

1. List the types of missions to which civilian special weapons and tactics teams respond.
2. Define *tactical EMS.*
3. List at least five duties of a tactical EMS medic.
4. Describe the three sides of the tactical EMS triangle.
5. Recognize the difference between cover and concealment.
6. Define *tactical casualty care.*
7. List the three most common causes of preventable death on the battlefield.
8. List the priorities of tactical casualty care.
9. Match the tactical casualty care stages of care to the incident command system hot, warm, and cold zones and describe the appropriate care in each stage.
10. Identify the appropriate training for the tactical EMS medic.
11. Formulate an inventory of tactical EMS equipment, including tactical medical equipment, prioritized into four distinct lines.
12. Discuss the advantages and disadvantages of arming the tactical EMS medic.

Chapter Outline

Case Scenario

You are a senior paramedic and your crew receives a call to stand by at a strip mall shopping center where a man has reportedly barricaded himself in his dry cleaning shop. You arrive on the scene and find the special weapons and tactics (SWAT) police team standing in front of the shop's front door. The SWAT leader is talking with a middle-aged man who is brandishing what appears to be a large knife. He is swinging the knife about wildly and periodically yelling obscenities at the officers. You watch the process intently from across the street in the outer perimeter. After several prolonged minutes of attempted negotiations, SWAT moves forward and rushes the armed man. They proceed with a prompt takedown and, fortunately, no one is injured. After the call has ended, you are talking with one of the SWAT medics who assessed the man before incarceration. He is also a paramedic with your agency and tells you that SWAT is expanding the tactical EMS team. The SWAT medic asks if you would be interested in joining the tactical EMS team. You indicate an interest but need to know more.

Questions

1. *What is the purpose of a tactical EMS team?*
2. *What are the types of duties or responsibilities of a tactical EMS medic?*
3. *What is required to become a tactical EMS medic?*
4. *What type of training does a tactical EMS medic undertake?*

This chapter introduces an established and growing specialty within prehospital care and local and federal law enforcement most commonly referred to as **Tactical Emergency Medical Support (TEMS).** By its name, TEMS may seem to limit the providers of such care to emergencies only, and the term tactical medicine may be more correct and all encompassing; however, for the purposes of this text, TEMS is the nomenclature used.

Maximum proficiency in field advanced life support in a busy paramedic unit is required before applying to a tactical team as a TEMS medic. Experienced paramedics will find that this chapter can help clarify whether your motivation and ability are sufficient to render the appropriate medical aid safely and effectively on the inner perimeter of SWAT missions.

This chapter examines certain general tactical concepts. However, no specific tactics, techniques, and procedures or standard operating procedures are disclosed. These are proprietary and are dictated by the individual law enforcement agencies that use TEMS medics. General medical procedures and capabilities are identified in the chapter. However, as with any medical capability, the TEMS scope of practice is always dictated by the local, state, or federal medical directors in the jurisdictions in which the TEMS medics practice.

INTRODUCTION TO SPECIAL WEAPONS AND TACTICS TEAMS

[OBJECTIVE 1]

TEMS medics serve on local, state, or federal tactical or special operations teams. These teams are most commonly referred to as **special weapons and tactics (SWAT)** teams (Box 65-1). Although several acronyms are generic to law enforcement special operations, SWAT remains the most widely used (Carmona, 2003a). SWAT sounds aggressive and hostile, as though the main purpose of such a team is to wipe out an enemy, like exterminating an insect. Indeed, decisive, aggressive actions are necessary in many SWAT missions; yet the main goals are providing protection and safety for the community, hostages, officers, and suspects. SWAT officers or agents are precision shooters; however, they frequently do not have to use lethal force to carry out the various extreme missions they are assigned. In fact, their self-control and sound judgment in the face of a potentially deadly situation usually results in success. Most tactical incidents are resolved by establishing control, containment, coordination, and communication.

SWAT teams carefully consider each contingency and take all reasonable safety precautions before an action plan is carried out. At the point at which suspects must be taken down, it happens swiftly and often without major injuries. Even when resistance is encountered, many less-than-lethal weapons and tactics often can be employed. Considering American, Canadian, and British SWAT units as functioning rescue teams is appropriate. Sometimes hostages are rescued, and sometimes suspects must be rescued from themselves. In addition, various agencies use SWAT teams to serve warrants on people who are known to be heavily armed and dangerous. These missions involve the arrests of suspected felons. SWAT teams are activated in many other types of missions as well.

Following are examples of SWAT missions:

1. Barricaded suspects
2. Hostage situations
3. Felony warrants
4. Tactical search and rescues
5. Officers and casualties down in the line of fire
6. Dignitary and political protection
7. Mobile field force (riot control) (Figure 65-1)
8. Extraordinary deployments (mass casualty shootings with one or more active shooters)
9. Weapons of mass destruction or terrorism

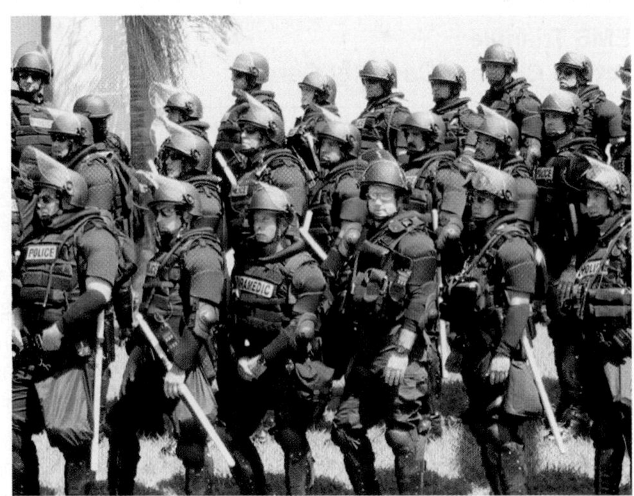

Figure 65-1 Mobile field force (riot control) is one type of SWAT mission.

BOX 65-1 Examples of Three Different Models of TEMS Teams

Sworn Law Enforcement "Organic" TEMS Medic Model

The organic model typically produces the most tactically sound TEMS medics, provided they are sworn officers or agents already assigned to a tactical team. This model has no issue with the TEMS medics being armed on the inner perimeter because they are law enforcement officers and/or agents first and paramedics second. The challenge with this model is with the TEMS medics developing and sustaining paramedic skills, which take numerous patient contacts to develop and are perishable without continual ALS training and regular patient contacts.

One team that has overcome the medical proficiency challenge is the Los Angeles County Sheriff Department's Emergency Services Detail (ESD). This is a specialized unit attached to the Special Enforcement Bureau Special Weapons Team

TEMS, Tactical emergency medical support; *ALS*, Advanced life support; *SWAT*, special weapons and tactics.

BOX 65-1 Examples of Three Different Models of TEMS Teams—continued

(their name for SWAT). Established in 1966, ESD is staffed by 20 full-time deputy sheriffs. In addition to their general law enforcement duties, they also are licensed paramedics with the added duties of mountain and remote area search and rescue, swift water rescue, helicopter search and rescue, helicopter medical evacuations, underwater search and recovery, offshore homeland security, ocean rescue, investigation of self-contained breathing apparatus deaths, and special weapons team tactics, including tactical medical support on all special weapons team activations. The ESD is one of the few full-time law enforcement TEMS teams in which the team members are able to maintain their medical skills. This is because they respond to more than 1000 calls for service each year. These calls include 200 tactical EMS deployments and hundreds of 9-1-1 helicopter responses in the mountains and other remote areas around Los Angeles County.

Fire Service TEMS Medic Model

The fire service TEMS medic model produces medics who are physically fit enough for SWAT duties. In addition, as long as they come from active fire service or paramedic programs that focus on EMS, the medics are usually experienced enough to be proficient clinicians. The issues that sometimes arise in this model are political. For example, the medics are employed by one agency (fire service) but fall under the chain of command of another agency (law enforcement) during SWAT missions.

One team that has overcome such political issues and has maintained excellent rapport with tactical agencies is the San Diego Fire Department Special Tactics and Rescue (STAR) Team. The STAR Team has 12 firefighter/paramedics with TEMS qualifications spread across three shifts who respond in pairs while on duty or off duty to San Diego Police Department SWAT missions. Each STAR Team TEMS medic runs several hundred regular EMS calls per year, rotating between fire/paramedic engines and ambulances. A medic/rescue ambulance is exclusively outfitted and set aside for the team. It is staged in a central fire station and is automatically dispatched with the STAR Team on more than 70 calls per year. STAR Team members must graduate from the San Diego Police Department SWAT Academy as well as several other law enforcement and TEMS courses. The team provides medical support on the inner perimeter of all San Diego SWAT missions and training. The STAR Team is also part of the Weapons of Mass Destruction Metropolitan Medical Strike Team and the San Diego Police Department Mobile Field Force. The STAR Team also responds to U.S. Coast Guard deep-water missions (onboard either Coast Guard helicopters or boats) when critical patients are reported off the coast of San Diego. Over the years the STAR Team has been used by federal agencies such as the U.S. Secret Service; the Federal Bureau of Investigation; and Alcohol, Tobacco, and Firearms tactical teams.

The STAR Team was established in 1982 after the delayed resuscitation attempts of two slain San Diego police officers. The original STAR Team paramedics worked for a private company that held the City of San Diego paramedic contract at the time. In July 1997, when the San Diego Fire Department won the city paramedic contract, all STAR Team members made the transition to firefighter/paramedic selection, training, and duty without any break in tactical support.

Hospital-Based, or Third Service, TEMS Model

The hospital-based model generally yields the most proficient paramedics because they are exclusively focused on EMS and have daily contact with the patients and hospitals in their area. The challenge is that sometimes the physical strength and stamina of the personnel are not at a level required for SWAT duty. In addition, their jobs are often in jeopardy because of ongoing paramedic contract negotiations between public and private entities.

One paramedic third service that has established a consistent and expanding TEMS team is the Tactical Response Unit (TRU) in York, Penn.

Medic 97 TRU functions as part of York Hospital Medic 97 paramedic response team. York Hospital is part of the Wellspan Health Organization based in York, Penn. Medic 97 is a paramedic response service that provides ALS to area basic life support ambulance companies. Their providers respond in squad trucks, which carry ALS equipment to the sick and injured of York County. They respond to more than 6000 calls per year and continue to grow with the population. Medic 97 TRU responds to approximately 100 tactical responses per year.

TRU was formed in 1991 after a hostage situation tragedy in which the paramedics were staged blocks away and not close enough to save lives after shots were fired. Eight York Hospital paramedics with more than 5 years of street experience were selected, trained by the Counter Narcotics and Terrorism Operational and Medical Support program and their local tactical team, and began responding to tactical calls by the York City Police Department Quick Response Team. Five years of paramedic street experience continues as one of the minimum requirements for TRU.

In 1994, the TRU began responding with the Pennsylvania State Police Special Emergency Response Team East. The TRU continues to grow and currently covers the entire eastern half of Pennsylvania.

The TRU is an unarmed entity. Commonwealth EMS law prohibits EMS providers from carrying offensive weapons. They function inside the inner perimeter with an assigned cover trooper or officer.

INTRODUCTION TO TACTICAL EMS TEAMS

[OBJECTIVES 2, 3]

Well-developed SWAT teams plan for every contingency. If they are prospectively planning to deploy tear gas, detonate explosive diversionary devices, or make dynamic entries, an emergency medical contingency also must be considered. However, regardless of how well a situation is planned for and rehearsed, injuries do occur. If a suspect is determined to end life in a violent way, sudden critical injuries are sometimes unavoidable. The best way to plan for the medical contingency is to incorporate TEMS medics into the team during the training, planning, and execution of tactical missions. In fact, this has become the standard of care.

The National Tactical Officers Association, TEMS Section, defines TEMS (or more appropriately, tactical medicine) as "the comprehensive out-of-hospital medical support for law enforcement's tactical teams during training and special operations" (National Tactical Officers Association, 2006). The best type of medical support is advanced life support (ALS) medical support. Furthermore, the best providers of ALS during tactical missions are experienced paramedics who are comfortable immediately assessing and providing rapid, appropriate field treatments in hostile environments. Emergency physicians, physician assistants, and registered nurses may have the right medical skills in a controlled hospital setting, but they lack the kind of field experience required for TEMS medics. That is, they lack the experience unless they also do regular field EMS work, such as on an active medical helicopter program, or they are part of an even smaller subset of active reserve law enforcement. A small, unique group of these kinds of practitioners serve alongside paramedic TEMS providers on a few teams. However, more important than having a physician as a teammate on missions is having a physician as an involved medical director for the team's scope of practice (Carmona, 2003b).

When critical injuries occur during a SWAT mission, the first medical priority is to immediately assess any SWAT officer injured, regardless of the potential injuries to any suspect (Figure 65-2). This is called SWAT assessment triage (Meoli, 2000). This practice is practical and legally defendable. The first priority is personal safety. Therefore the SWAT officer is assumed to be less of a threat to medical personnel than a suspect. In addition, SWAT officers are well known as being mission intensive. Consequently, they may not even be aware of their own physical condition when involved in a critical mission. In fact, officers can be shot in vital areas of the body and compensate up to their last moment of consciousness. In other words, they may be unaware that they have sustained a critical injury. Once a complete assessment is performed on all patients and no tactical concerns exist, treatment triage continues along conventional guidelines. Although minor injuries occur somewhat frequently, critical wounds to SWAT officers are thankfully rare.

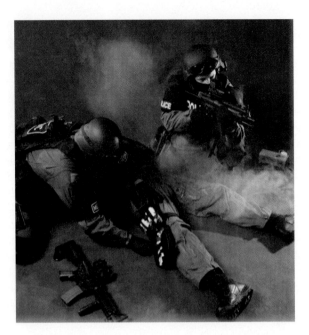

Figure 65-2 When critical injuries occur during a SWAT mission, the first medical priority is to immediately assess any SWAT officer injured.

The typical critically injured patients encountered at SWAT missions are, in fact, suspects. Moreover, their injuries are almost always a direct result of their own suicidal actions (Rathbun, 2003). They are usually the only patients on scene. Furthermore, it is morally and legally essential that TEMS medics use every skill in their scope of practice to save the lives of properly secured suspects regardless of their actions before being injured. The SWAT commander relies on the dedication of TEMS medics in this area specifically because all contingencies must be covered, including limiting liability. In addition to wanting the best care for their tactical teams, law enforcement agencies realize that incorporating TEMS medics into their missions mitigates liability, whereas not doing so causes them to assume all liability if critical injuries occur.

The main function of the TEMS medic is to be able to assess and treat critical patients immediately in the most austere environments. However, the injuries the TEMS medic most often encounters are minor injuries or medical complaints from extended missions or training evolutions. As a result, TEMS medics should have a good handle on minor wound care, sports injuries, allergies, and the common cold. Paramedics cannot prescribe or recommend medications not within their EMS scope. However, most medical directors allow their TEMS medics to carry appropriate over-the-counter medications for their teammates to be available on request during extended missions or training sessions. These would include non–blood-thinning analgesics (acetaminophen),

BOX 65-2 Types of TEMS Duties

- Casualty care on the inner perimeter of tactical missions and during high-risk training
- Medical intelligence and threat assessment before missions
- General assessment and health maintenance of team members during extended training or missions
- Remote assessment of casualties in the line of fire
- Medical assessment and clearing of suspects before incarceration
- Medical training of tactical operators
- Physical readiness qualification at the tactical operator level (many tactical teams also require TEMS medics to qualify on weapons at the operator level)

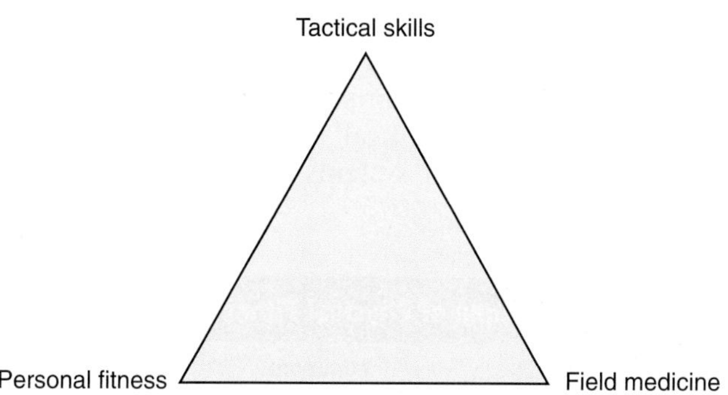

Figure 65-3 TEMS triangle.

nonsedative decongestants (pseudoephedrine), antitussives, and antacids.

Types of TEMS duties are shown in Box 65-2.

TEMS TRIANGLE

[OBJECTIVE 4]

The fire service uses a fire triangle (now a tetrahedron). Wilderness rescue uses the survival triangle. The TEMS triangle represents the three main areas of focus (tactical skills, personal fitness, and field medicine) to be a safe, effective TEMS medic (Meoli, 2001) (Figure 65-3).

Tactical Skills

[OBJECTIVE 5]

A TEMS medic has valuable portable assets unique to law enforcement. However, the medic must be sure that these assets are self-contained. Moreover, he or she must be sure they are, in fact, assets and not liabilities that slow the team at critical points. One way to ensure this is by developing a sound base of tactical knowledge, skill, and mastery of tactical equipment.

TEMS personnel must first acquire a working knowledge of the difference between cover and concealment. Moreover, they must know how these actions apply to the different scenarios they encounter. After working in EMS for several years and approaching potentially dangerous scenes, this knowledge should already be somewhat intuitive. Following is a quick review.

The U.S. Army defines cover as "protection from enemy fire" and concealment as "protection from enemy observation" (U.S. Army, 2005).

Natural concealment involves hiding behind trees, bushes, tall grass, or shadows. Facilitated concealment involves wearing camouflage, hiding underneath windowsills, and taking other similar actions. TEMS medic uniforms should be nonreflective and similar to or exactly like the uniforms of their respective SWAT officers, but with something unique that identifies the medic to other officers or agents (Vayer, 2003). All the medic's gear should be soundproof. To check this, the medic must don all his or her gear, jump up and down, and jog for a few paces. If excess sounds are present, he or she should relocate and quiet the gear. This helps concealment, but no action can protect the medic from stray bullets.

Hard cover, or complete protection from enemy fire, even in the civilian SWAT setting must take into account that the enemy (perpetrator or suspect) could have the ability to shoot with high-velocity rifle rounds. Therefore the only true cover would be level 4 armor, which can stop rifle rounds. Most body armor is level 3A, which can stop only handgun rounds. The medic would need to slide in level 4 plates to protect from rifle rounds, and then only his or her chest and back would be fully protected (some of the latest plates protect shoulders and legs but generally are considered too cumbersome for most operators to wear). Most armored vehicles are designed to withstand rifle rounds but some are not. Many SWAT teams carry level 4 protective shields that can be advanced into the scene.

Therefore the TEMS medic must find places along the way where he or she has cover, concealment, or both and know the difference. For example, as the medic approaches a residence, he or she can find cover and concealment behind the engine block of a vehicle. Once the medic has made it to the door alongside the structure, he or she can find concealment by keeping a quiet, low profile around and under windows, but only relative cover positions. Handgun rounds can easily penetrate drywall or plaster. The medic can find some relative cover at the corners of buildings or near doorjambs where several studs line up within the outer wall. However, the medic must realize that high-velocity rounds from rifles and some handguns will be merely slowed down by two-by-fours.

The TEMS medic also must possess a working knowledge of how to operate in and around tear gas, weapons, and other noise-producing equipment. Whether a TEMS medic should carry a weapon is examined later in the chapter.

Certain topics related to the procedures for tactical entries, enemy fire, and tactical retreat are not appropriate for this text. For these, the TEMS medic must learn the specific tactics, techniques, and procedures of his or her particular team and gain their trust that he or she can follow directions and maintain operational security.

Personal Fitness

One component of overall personal fitness is physical fitness. On SWAT missions, a TEMS medic may be staged in many pounds of armor and equipment for hours and then suddenly have to negotiate walls and other obstacles while accessing and extricating a patient.

TEMS personnel should meet or exceed the same physical standards of the SWAT team. A typical annual physical fitness test is provided in Table 65-1.

The other component of personal fitness is psychological fitness. TEMS medics must have a similar mindset as the law enforcement officers and agents on the teams on which they serve. Many SWAT teams require their TEMS medics to pass the same psychological examination as employees of their law enforcement agency. However, psychological fitness is broader than testing. As EMS professionals, you see many people who are grossly injured, dismembered, or killed. When an adult who is a perfect stranger becomes a critical casualty, you typically do not carry the emotional burden around with you. However, three kinds of critical casualties usually result in EMS worker stress: uniformed public safety personnel, children, and people you know. Furthermore, if you have young children, then seeing dead children is the worst, and the worst of these is when the child is murdered—especially when the perpetrator is the child's parent or guardian. A TEMS medic who runs enough SWAT missions will likely see any or all of these scenarios.

Some situational stressors are unique for the TEMS medic. For example, the medic may be delayed in treating an innocent hostage who eventually ends up dead because knowing whether he or she was alive or injured was impossible while the perpetrator refused to talk to negotiators during a long standoff. When the final showdown occurs, the medic is then only able to save the life of the perpetrator. The medic responds in a professional manner on scene by triaging the obviously dead hostage(s) and not disturbing the crime scene. Intellectually, the medic knows he or she did the right thing by performing life-saving skills on the perpetrator and facilitating a stat transport to the closest trauma hospital. The morbid jokes shared with teammates, in private, may help the situation. However, the medic still carries around the internal stress of knowing that the innocent died, the perpetrator lived, and the medic was the primary caregiver.

All the previous scenarios highlight the importance of knowing the difference between a normal EMS call and one that can lead to posttraumatic stress. Some mainstream stress reduction therapies (e.g., exercise, massage) can help make the EMS provider more effective at his or her job—whether he or she experiences horrifying calls or not. However, if a traumatic call occurs, knowing in advance the kind of critical incident stress debriefing or confidential support systems available in the area is helpful.

TABLE 65-1 Example of Physical Fitness Test Results

Fitness Test	Minimum Points: 40*	Maximum Points: 100
440 Run	90 seconds	55 seconds
Push-ups (in 1 min)	40	60
Sit-ups (in 1 min)	40	60
Pull-ups	6	15
SWAT obstacle course	4 minutes	2.5 minutes

*You must exceed the minimums in several events to get the required minimum combined score of 300 points.

The Importance of Critical Incident Stress Debriefing: The Last Missions of Two TEMS Medics

This vignette is about two tactical medics who responded to two horrific SWAT missions early in the history of their TEMS team. Their experience on these calls and the kind of support that was not available at that time were factors in the career decisions that both paramedics ultimately made. The following was written with their permission.

Mark and Dan had plenty of life experiences before becoming paramedics and later helped establish their system's first TEMS team. They both served in the U.S. military during the late 1960s, and Dan saw action in Vietnam. In the 1970s they worked together as ocean lifeguards. They became paramedics and ran more than 2000 9-1-1 calls (many of them together as partners) before establishing their TEMS team. Mark and Dan were both married with growing families around the same time that the following calls took place.

First SWAT Mission: Extraordinary Deployment—Active Shooter with Mass Casualties

On July 18, 1984, James Huberty walked into a McDonalds in a southern suburb of San Diego and shot everyone he encountered. Before he had finished, he had killed 23 people.

On arrival, Mark and Dan were placed with the entry team on the inner perimeter. Several minutes passed before the green light was given to enter the structure. During the wait, gunshots could be heard echoing from the structure as the gunman walked around and systematically fired additional rounds into victims who still had signs of life.

Once Huberty presented himself in the front window of the McDonald's, two things happened simultaneously. A SWAT sniper took his shot through glass, while the entry team (including Mark and Dan) approached the building. Huberty was firing three different weapon systems that day and had reloaded dozens of times, so no one could tell whether only one gunman or many were in the building. In addition, at the time of entry whether the sniper had neutralized his target was unknown because he had to take his shot through glass.

Once inside, only a few seconds of room clearing was necessary to determine that Huberty was dead. All around him was a bloodbath of motionless people, many of them clinging to each other in what appeared to be piles of families. When Mark and Dan saw that the scene was safe, they called in a flood of EMS resources and began the grim task of triaging patients. Most of the patients were already dead, and they were mostly children.

After the last living patient was transported by ambulance or helicopter, Mark and Dan went back in service as a regular paramedic crew in the city. Critical incident stress debriefing had not been developed at this time, but a police psychologist organized a crisis debriefing. EMS personnel and officers were taken off line and invited to attend. After the debriefing, all the EMTs and paramedics involved were allowed to go home. That is, all except for Mark and Dan. In fact, Mark and Dan were never taken off line at all, presumably because it was assumed that they were "too tough to care." They spent a few minutes at the debriefing just as it was starting and then began running back-to-back calls in the southern districts of San Diego and continued this until their 24-hour shift ended the following morning.

During all the media hype, Mark and Dan had very little to say when asked about their experience.

Second SWAT Mission: Barricaded Suspect with Hostage Executions

Less than 2 weeks after the McDonalds massacre, another multiple homicide on a smaller, more intimate scale, transpired in San Diego. This one received no media attention. Again, Mark and Dan happened to be on duty and were called to the scene for their TEMS skills.

The incident involved a father who took his three children hostage. He abused them at gunpoint and then shot each one to death. He subsequently turned the gun on himself.

Once again, Mark and Dan were on the entry team. On entry and immediate clearing of all rooms, they began their duty of carefully assessing each victim and found each of them dead and the children grossly mutilated.

In a two-week span of time, Mark and Dan saw more dead children than most soldiers see in war. The victims they found were not in a foreign country, but right in their hometown. Mark and Dan were not detached observers of these massacres. They were the primary caregivers assigned to attempt to save the lives of dozens of innocent children who were slaughtered.

None of their managers had any training in critical incident stress debriefing at the time. Consequently, Mark and Dan received no support for their ordeal, were not offered any time off, and were not even asked how they were doing.

A few days after the last mission, Dan resigned his paramedic position without fanfare and started an emergency training business. A short time after that, Mark also left the field to pursue a career in multimedia. They both continued to teach EMS topics, kept their families intact, and successfully raised their children.

Field Medicine

[OBJECTIVE 6]

Proficient field medicine is the portable asset for which the TEMS medic is needed. Everything else is simply a means of transporting that asset. A TEMS medic should be at the pinnacle of his or her local scope of practice. The TEMS medic should take part in every form of relevant continuing education possible. Before applying to become a tactical medic, the paramedic should be confident with his or her assessment and treatment skills and have made thousands of patient contacts. The paramedic should be an integral part of the system served with a sound working knowledge of local hospitals, trauma facilities, and other medical resources. He or she should also have a sound working knowledge of the local incident command system in case he or she responds to a multiple casualty incident. If the paramedic is in an area that does not run many calls, then he or she should augment patient contacts by accumulating additional experience. Some potential activities to consider include working in emergency departments, in medical military reserve units that deploy to combat zones, and on paramedic ridealongs in adjacent busy systems.

The most important part of field medicine is the emergency medical component, specifically tactical casualty care, which is fully examined in the next section. Furthermore, the most important skill a medic possesses, especially in a high-stress emergency setting, is assessment. This skill is the gateway to all other skills and the one that prioritizes which skill, if any, comes next. Proficiency in patient assessment, as with other skills, can only be gained by contact with many hundreds of patients. As with others it is a perishable skill and can only be maintained by regular patient contact.

One expectation of the TEMS medic is that he or she will be able to perform a trauma assessment in less than 5 seconds. In those 5 seconds, a determination must be made whether the team has time to continue with the mission or must expend operator resources to extricate the casualty immediately. TEMS medics also are expected to be able to perform a remote assessment with binoculars (or more sophisticated visualization equipment) on casualties who are down in the line of fire (Figure 65-4). Then the medic must give the SWAT team leader information to help determine whether sending out a rescue team at that moment is worth the risk. That key piece of information is the medic's best assessment regarding whether the casualty is salvageable or not. He or she is expected to give the assessment with confidence, sometimes with something as simple as a thumbs up or down. Although the medic needs training to make this kind of assessment, actual experience working on literally thousands of patients and seeing many critically sick or injured patients is essential. This is one of the reasons why most TEMS teams require their medics to have a minimum of 2 years or more in busy EMS systems before applying.

In addition, the TEMS medic is expected to handle common minor medical complaints from officers on extended missions or training exercises. The medic should have a working knowledge of fundamental sports injury care, such as RICE (***r***est, ***i***ce, ***c***ompression, and ***e***levation). If the medic is dealing with a potential strain, sprain, or fracture and the officer does not want to be taken off-line, the medic must be clear about the fact that the proper place for a definitive diagnosis and treatment is a medical facility that can perform radiographs. Most TEMS providers carry a small cache of over-the-counter medications for team members who know what to ask for while on extended operations. Thus these medics must have a sound knowledge of the proper dosage and precautions of any medication they carry. Moreover, their own medical director must be involved with any practice of providing over-the-counter medications.

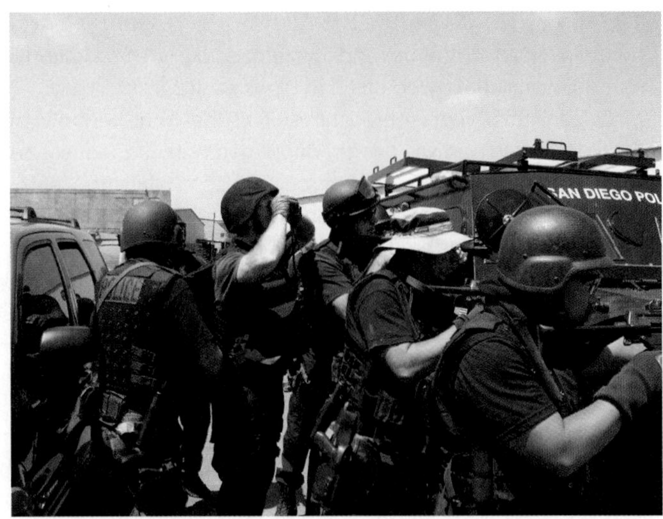

Figure 65-4 TEMS medics are expected to be able to perform a remote assessment with binoculars or more sophisticated visualization equipment.

Case Scenario—continued

You and your team (TEMS and SWAT) are called to the scene of a robbery attempt at a fast food restaurant. The robbery was aborted when a customer called 9-1-1 from a cell phone to report the incident. The robber fired a handgun from inside the restaurant at the first responding police officer on the scene, who received a superficial wound on his right arm. The perpetrator has taken several hostages. He threatens to kill them unless his demands for money and safe transportation are met. As the perpetrator is talking with police negotiators, he repeatedly fires his weapon toward you and other responders. During one barrage of fire, a responding police officer is wounded in the leg, fracturing bone and causing arterial hemorrhage, requiring immediate care. Triage and transport areas are created on the other side of a building adjacent to the restaurant.

Questions

4. *What areas are considered the hot zone, warm zone, and cold zone?*
5. *You and a SWAT officer get closer to the downed officer while crouching below the windows of the squad cars. Is this technique known as cover or concealment?*
6. *If a decision were made to care for the fallen officer, what care would you provide?*

TACTICAL COMBAT CASUALTY CARE

Tactical Combat Casualty Care (TCCC) is military nomenclature usually simplified to tactical casualty care for civilian TEMS, but the principles are the same.

Before 1996, a tenet of battlefield medicine held that 90% of all soldiers killed in action die on the battlefield before reaching a field treatment facility (Vayer, 2003). TCCC encompasses all appropriate field care rendered to casualties of war from the point of injury until they are out of the combat zone and delivered to the closest appropriate treatment facility.

In 1996 the guidelines for TCCC were first issued to military special operations (Army Special Forces and Rangers, Navy SEALs, U.S. Air Force Pararescuemen) medics by U.S. Special Operations Command (Butler & Hagman, 1996). Since then, conventional U.S. Army, Navy, Marine Corps, and Coast Guard forces have embraced TCCC principles and have civilian tactical teams. Consider how civilian trauma systems were roughly patterned after military battlefield medicine pioneered during the Korean and Vietnam Wars. Similarly, TCCC, which represents the field care portion of battlefield medicine, directly applies to the care given to casualties incurred during civilian tactical law enforcement operations (Giduck, 2008).

Causes of Preventable Battlefield Death

[OBJECTIVE 7]

TCCC principles center around managing the top three causes of preventable death on the battlefield. **Preventable death** in this case refers to death that could have been avoided if the casualty were given the right care at the right time. A comprehensive study of preventable deaths in Vietnam and Mogadishu, Somalia (Butler, 1996), concluded that the most common causes of preventable battlefield death are the following:

1. Exsanguination from extremity wounds (60%)
2. Tension pneumothorax (33%)
3. Airway obstruction (6%)
4. All other (1%)

Therefore all tactical operators should train to perform self-aid and buddy aid and carry tactical tourniquets and dressings. All medics, however, should be trained and carry tactical medical equipment to perform higher levels of hemostasis, chest decompression, and airway control (Cain, 2008).

Tactical Combat Casualty Care Priorities

[OBJECTIVE 8]

To fully understand when treating a casualty is important, you must know the following TCCC priorities:

1. *Fire superiority.* Shoot all lethal perpetrators or have enough weapons pointed downrange so that perpetrators cannot position themselves to shoot without being immediately hit by cover fire.
2. *Prevent further casualties.* Get the casualty and all uncovered personnel out of the line of fire.
3. *Triage.* Decide which casualties to treat and which life-threatening conditions to treat first.
4. *Treat according to TCCC guidelines.* On the battlefield and the inner perimeter of SWAT missions, "tactics drive medicine."

Notice that treating a casualty is the last priority.

Stages of Care

[OBJECTIVE 9]

TCCC doctrine states three distinct stages of care that dictate the kind of casualty care that should or should not be rendered at each stage. The stages are roughly comparable to the civilian incident command system hot zone, warm zone, and cold zone model. Understanding that nothing is absolute, the bottom line is that "tactics drive medicine."

Stage 1: Care Under Fire (Hot Zone)

In this phase, the casualty is exposed to effective or potentially effective enemy fire. All efforts are directed at getting the casualty and the team out of the line of fire or eliminating the threat. Assuming the team has established fire superiority, the only appropriate treatment would be to stop uncontrolled extremity hemorrhage. This should be accomplished with a tourniquet that can be applied in less than 15 seconds. If fire superiority cannot be reasonably assured, the casualty should simply be immediately extracted without medical aid (Figure 65-5). If that is not possible at the point of injury, the extraction may be delayed until the threat is eliminated.

Stage 2: Tactical Field Care (Warm Zone)

In this phase, the casualty is still on the inner perimeter of a live mission but is in a position of cover and concealment, not exposed to enemy fire. Some appropriate actions at this stage include applying effective tactical dressings, chest sealing and/or decompression, and advanced airway control. These should be accomplished without setting anything down or giving away the position. Starting intravenous (IV) lines and splinting may be appropriate if no immediate pathway to a medical evacuation platform is clear. However, as in any trauma system, starting IVs on scene should not delay transport to a trauma center once a form of transport is available and accessible.

Stage 3: Medical and Casualty Evacuation (Cold Zone)

In this phase the casualty and the medic are now out of the inner perimeter and heading to the trauma center (in military areas of operation, this may not mean out of

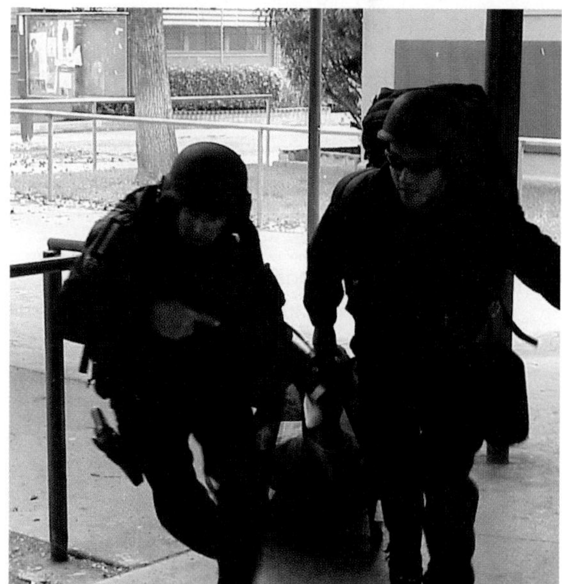

Figure 65-5 Care under fire. If fire superiority cannot be reasonably assured, the casualty should be immediately extricated without medical aid. If that is not possible at the point of injury, the extrication may be delayed until the threat is eliminated.

harm's way). Whether the medical evacuation platform is a helicopter, ambulance, or armored victim rescue vehicle, it should be staged with additional medical gear. It also should be staffed with an ALS-level medic who can fully stabilize the victim en route. In civilian tactical missions, the casualty is sometimes handed off to a paramedic ambulance or helicopter in the outer perimeter. If a TEMS medic does go with the patient and the mission is still hot, at least one TEMS medic should remain on scene until everything is secure.

The most exhaustive live tissue studies for tactical medical procedures and efficacious products are performed at the U.S. Army Institute of Surgical Research (ISR) at Fort Sam Houston, Texas. Sadly, the wars in Iraq and Afghanistan have provided numerous after action reports (AARs) that validate these studies. The well-respected Committee on Tactical Combat Casualty Care analyzes all such data on a quarterly basis. You can stay abreast of the latest information by visiting the ISR seb site.

TRAINING

[OBJECTIVE 10]

TEMS medics who are not already law enforcement officers should attend at least a reserve level peace officer course. These courses are taught in a matter of days or weeks at community colleges that usually run full police academies. One example of such a course is California's Penal Code 832. This course covers the basic principles of the powers of arrest, search and seizure, and the application of lethal force. A basic handgun qualification occurs at the end of the course.

Many SWAT teams will run a mini-academy for new TEMS members. Typically these teams eventually send all their TEMS medics through their own full SWAT academy at the officer level. In addition, TEMS medics should attend the monthly or periodic training of the team they support. That way they are on hand for training emergencies and can also rotate into training evolutions, especially full mission simulations.

Advanced trauma life support, a course designed for in-hospital trauma staff, provides certification on the kinds of individual advanced medical skills required of TEMS medics. However, it is set up for a hospital setting in which the priorities are completely different from those of TCCC. Prehospital trauma life support (PHTLS) has now developed a military version that addresses TCCC and is incorporated into the Special Operations Combat Medical (SOCM) Skills Course at Fort Bragg, NC. Although you must be selected as a special operations combat medic to attend the SOCM course, other military and tactical courses certify PHTLS-Military and the text is available to the public.

Box 65-3 lists some available medical courses for TEMS medics.

BOX 65-3 A Selection of Medical Courses for TEMS Medics

Each of these courses is professionally run and mindful of operational security. Therefore you must be already chosen for a tactical team and be officially sponsored by a tactical law enforcement agency to be admitted.

- Tactical Operator Care (TOC) Course, Medical College of Georgia: http://www.mcg.edu/ems/com/Tactical/TOCCourse.pdf.
- Basic and Advanced Tactics and Medicine, International School of Tactical Medicine: http://www.tacticalmedicine.com
- Tactical Emergency Medical Operator, The Tactical Element: http://www.tacticalelement.com
- TEMS Basic Course and TEMS Advanced Course, National Tactical Officers Association: http://www.ntoa.org/tems
- Operational EMS, Deployment Medicine International: http://www.deploymentmedicine.com

Case Scenario CONCLUSION

After a 1-hour standoff with repeated threats to kill hostages, the perpetrator makes a mistake and positions himself in the restaurant doorway. A SWAT sniper fires at the suspect. Within seconds, you are summoned into the restaurant to assess the perpetrator. The suspect has sustained a single entrance wound on his forehead just above the right eye. He has no pulse and is not breathing. You can hear screams and moans from the hostages within the restaurant. The suspect is triaged out as you continue with your SWAT team. You and the other TEMS and SWAT team members reach the hostages and find a few with minor cuts and bruises and a few others deeper in the restaurant who have been pistol whipped in the head and have altered mental states. The scene is quickly cleared as safe by SWAT and you activate your local mass casualty plan.

Questions

7. *The TEMS medic knows when treating a casualty is important. What are the four TCCC priorities?*
8. *What are the four lines of tactical medical equipment accessible to TEMS medics?*

Examples of Civilian TEMS Medical Cases

Following are summary case studies of actual SWAT missions that occurred in the United States. Specific names, dates, addresses, tactics, techniques, and procedures have been omitted because they are not relevant to the TEMS aspects of these incidents. If such details are needed, contact the Tactical EMS Chairperson of the National Tactical Officers Association at http://www.ntoa.org. Given the legitimacy of your agency and need for such details, they may be provided.

Type of SWAT Mission: Felony Warrant

TEMS Casualties: One Officer Shot during Dynamic Entry and One Suspect Shot in Counter Fire

TEMS after Action Report

The SWAT team was tasked with serving simultaneous warrants for the arrest of several violent street gang members. One of the locations was in a government housing project known for its significantly violent gang presence. The team had determined that a dynamic entry was the best tactical method. On initial entry, the team cleared the living room and was confronted with closed doors, which led to a bedroom and bathroom area. On opening the door, the first officer through was fired on and struck by a suspect who had concealed himself by sitting on the floor in a recessed alcove just to the right of the entry area. The officer returned fire, striking the suspect. The remainder of the entry element removed the injured officer from the threat zone and immediately locked down the small bedroom and bath while the remainder of the team held the rest of the residence. The team leader then called for immediate TEMS support.

Two paramedic TEMS providers responded from their posting inside the inner tactical perimeter. They first evaluated the officer who had been struck twice in the chest by handgun rounds. The officer denied any injury and a rapid trauma assessment confirmed no obvious penetration or gross bruising of the affected areas beneath the level 3A vest. In addition, no signs or symptoms indicating any injury were present.

Next, a rapid trauma assessment was conducted on the suspect who had been secured by the entry team. He had suffered at least two 9-mm gunshot wounds: one to the upper abdomen and one to the pelvic area. The suspect met major trauma criteria. The paramedics applied an occlusive dressing to the upper abdomen and facilitated a rapid extrication to a predetermined safe rally point. TEMS paramedics continued treatment during the rapid transfer of care to a local ALS/EMS transport unit. The suspect was loaded and transported with law enforcement in attendance. The TEMS team then immediately returned to the scene of the shooting until the location was completely secure. They then made themselves available to augment other TEMS elements participating in continuing tactical warrant service operations within the housing project until all locations had been completely secured.

Conclusions

- A potentially chaotic situation was mitigated by proper medical mission planning and rehearsal.
- SWAT Assessment Triage was appropriately provided to the officer.
- TEMS intervention and transport was appropriately provided to the suspect, saving his life.

Type of SWAT Mission: Barricaded Suspect and Gun Battle

TEMS Casualties: One Suspect Down with Critical Injuries

TEMS after Action Report

An intoxicated suspect had battered his wife. She escaped and called 9-1-1 from a neighbor's apartment. The suspect fired a 0.22 caliber semiautomatic pistol at the first responding officers from his upstairs apartment. SWAT set a perimeter and attempted to call him out. The suspect refused to talk to negotiators, occasionally discharging his weapon inside the apartment. He later indicated that he was about to kill himself. Tear gas was deployed into the apartment and a SWAT element made a dynamic entry, trailed by a second SWAT element with two TEMS paramedics. The suspect fired at the entry team officers from behind a bathroom door. Entry team officers returned fire through the door, hitting him twice in the chest and four times in his extremities with 9-mm rounds.

The casualty was handcuffed on his side with two entry wounds noted on his right chest, one on his right shoulder, one in the upper arm, and one in the right thigh. Four exit wounds were evident on various parts of his back and posterior extremities as well as a 4-inch linear incision on the inner aspect of his right bicep with blood continuing to flow. Approximately 500 mL of blood was on the bathroom floor. The patient responded to painful stimulus by moaning. He was pale, cool, and drenched in sweat with a rapid carotid pulse, no peripheral pulse or blood pressure, respirations more than 30 breaths/min, and equal lung sounds.

Hemorrhage was controlled by applying a pressure dressing and bandage to the suspect's arm wound before completing assessment. A nasal airway was inserted. The casualty was immobilized on a scoop stretcher with flex-cuffs and rapidly extricated down stairs to a staged ambulance. The total time from crisis entry to casualty transport was less than 8 minutes.

Treatment en route involved high-flow oxygen mask, large-bore external jugular IV wide open (no extremity veins visible or palpable), flushed face with water to decontaminate tear gas, and warming measures. The patient arrived at the trauma center with a blood pressure greater than 90 mm Hg systolic, still tachycardic, dry skin, and rapidly speaking a non-English language.

Follow-up revealed that none of the 9 mm rounds destroyed any vital organs or vessels. The patient incurred a simple

SWAT, Special weapons and tactics; *TEMS,* tactical emergecy medical support.

Continued

Examples of Civilian TEMS Medical Cases—continued

pneumothorax without complication. He initially presented in a profound state of shock because of external bleeding from his severed brachial artery. This turned out to be a self-inflicted wound he had incurred by smashing out a window a few minutes before the team's entry. TEMS medics treated this man in a gas-charged apartment, with gas masks on their faces, and were aware only of the relatively small pool of blood in the bathroom. Later, remaining SWAT officers found several larger pools of blood in various rooms where he had walked about squirting his blood onto walls and furniture and apparently trying to write with it on several walls. This man's life was saved by the crisis entry of SWAT officers and the immediate medical intervention to stop the hemorrhage.

Type of SWAT Mission: Felony Warrant Service

TEMS Casualty: SWAT Officer Down

TEMS after Action Report

A city SWAT team was called to serve a warrant for a narcotics team who had information that the gang suspects, whom they wanted for dealing crack cocaine, were heavily armed. Also, the house out of which the suspects were operating was fortified with steel bars on every door and window and required special breaching capabilities. In fact, two metal doors needed to be breached—an exterior door and another at the end of an interior hallway.

All squads deployed to their designated locations just after dawn. One officer, who was assigned to breach the interior door, was in the process of igniting a gas cutting torch when the exterior door was breached. Because of an unexpected variation in the construction of the breaching equipment that was used, the heavy metal door became a flying missile, which struck the torch officer in the back of the head and sent him head first into a wall and on top of another officer. Another entry team officer immediately grabbed the cutting torch and continued the dynamic entry while TEMS medics were called to treat the officer who was in plain view of the front windows of the house, making it a potential care under fire scenario. Within 10 seconds two TEMS medics were tending to the first injured officer.

Casualty 1: The officer was lying prone across a pile of rubble. He was unconscious and unresponsive, with stertorous breathing and long periods of apnea. He had a strong radial pulse and was flaccid from the neck down.

Casualty 2: The officer who was hit by the first officer later developed neck pain but did not notice it during the assessment and treatment of the first officer.

On-Scene Treatment

Casualty 1: Because of the mechanism of injury, the TEMS medics decided to override the normal protocol and immobilize the casualty before extrication. With two SWAT officers holding cover fire positions, another officer was assigned to hold neutral stabilization of the casualty's head. A nasal pharyngeal airway was placed, which aided spontaneous breathing. An extrication collar was placed and a scoop stretcher placed inverted across the casualty's backside. When everything was in place, the officer was rolled as a unit (holding in-line spinal stabilization), quickly secured to the stretcher, and extricated to the staged ambulance. One TEMS medic rode to the trauma center with the casualty with an officer driving while the other remained on scene until the scene was secured. The total time from injury to transport was less than 4 minutes.

Casualty 2: After the mission was secured, the other officer noticed he had acute neck pain. On assessment he was immobilized and transported.

Treatment en route for casualty 1 was as follows. Because he was head injured, the officer was clenching down and not able to be intubated, and no rapid-sequence intubation protocols existed at the time. He was kept immobile and 100% oxygen was delivered by nonrebreather mask, assisting with positive-pressure ventilation when necessary. Two large-bore IVs were placed in each arm. Verbal reassurance remained constant during the transportation to the trauma center regardless of whether the officer could verbally respond.

Officer 1 had incurred injuries to his skull, neck, and left shoulder. He remained in a coma for 7 days while family and friends kept a constant positive vigil. Once he regained consciousness, he immediately engaged in an aggressive physical therapy program. He turned down the opportunity to retire on disability, returned to full duty within 6 months, and eventually returned to full SWAT duty.

Conclusion: The decision to override the normal procedure of immediately dragging the casualty out of the line of fire and taking the extra minutes to immobilize him saved him neurologic deficit and possibly his life.

Type of SWAT Incident: Felony Warrant, Gun Battle, and Structure Fire with Exposures

TEMS Casualties: Two Suspects Burned to Death in Structure Fire

TEMS after Action Report

Multiple simultaneous warrants were served at three different locations on heavily armed members of a gang who were wanted for multiple high-profile robberies and at least one murder. Four TEMS medics were assigned to the operation at two target locations. Two target locations went without incident but a third did not, which was the residence of the gang leader who reportedly claimed he would never be taken alive.

As soon as SWAT deployed teams, the suspect and his girlfriend opened fire with automatic weapons, pinning down two officers. Officer rescues were immediately performed with no injuries. The suspects stopped firing and released two hostages who were relatives of the suspects. As soon as the hostages were safe, the gang leader and his girlfriend began spraying rounds in all directions. SWAT officers responded in kind and sent in tear gas canisters. More than 400 rounds were estimated to have been exchanged in the gun battle.

A fire started inside the structure, which eventually ventilated itself through a side window. Fire crews were standing by on both ends of the residential block but could not come any closer than five houses in any direction because of the danger of high-velocity submachine gun rounds. Radiant heat started to blister paint on the walls of the house next door, and the danger of losing exposed structures throughout the neighborhood became evident. The decision was made to form two tactical teams on either side of the structure and advance 2.5-inch-diameter hose lines from the engines, with firefighters standing hundreds of feet back. One team consisted of three SWAT officers. The other consisted of two TEMS medics. Both were flanked by SWAT shooters.

By the time the two teams reached the front driveway and accessed water, the structure was fully involved, with fire burning through the roof of the garage and extending into bedrooms. Firefighters were confronted with a solid wall of flame more than 30 feet high. The two houses on both sides were showing signs of spalling (i.e., they were generating smoke and paint started to blister off the walls facing the burning structure).

Once the hose lines were charged, the first streams were directed at the exposed houses next door to the fully involved structure. Next the water streams were directed at the main seat of the fire in the garage and then into the bedrooms. The main part of the fire was put out in less than 10 minutes. When both suspects were determined to be dead, regular fire crews extinguished the smoldering remains.

The main structure was already burned beyond repair, so water damage was not a consideration. Hence the SWAT and TEMS teams were given 2.5-inch hose lines, which are as large as can be used and still controlled by hand. The nozzles on the hoses were set at 250 gal/min, which puts out more than 1 ton of water each minute. This provided the ability to stand back far enough to not get burned but left plenty of power to protect exposures and drown the main part of the fire. This intervention saved many houses in the neighborhood. (In addition to houses exposed on each side, a hill in the backyard was filled with overgrown brush and lead up to a school.)

This call highlights the need for tactical team members to have a basic skill level in handling firefighting hand lines and, at a minimum, be able to perform "surround and drown" fire suppression.

Type of SWAT Incident: Barricaded Suspect with Hostage

TEMS Casualties: Hostage Dead, Perpetrator Sustains Multiple Trauma from Suicide Attempt

TEMS after Action Report

A suspect visited his girlfriend while she was at work cleaning a suburban house. An altercation ensued, which ended with the suspect shooting his girlfriend in the head with a 9-mm semiautomatic handgun. Police officers were called and they activated SWAT.

While establishing the perimeter, SWAT officers found a gun in the backyard wrapped in a bloody T-shirt. The suspect seemed to have escaped because of the evidence outside the house and the fact that absolutely no sounds were heard in the house after many attempts by negotiators to call the suspect out. TEMS medics accompanied the entry team to the back door. A dog was sent in and immediately went upstairs and found the suspect, who was hiding in a closet.

Casualty 1: Woman in her late 20s, lying on her side at the base of a stairwell, with her head in a 2-L pool of coagulated blood. She was mottled with full rigor mortis. Shell casings were on the stairs.

Casualty 2: Man in mid-30s, sitting, handcuffed from behind, and trembling. The patient spoke only Spanish. He had a full-thickness incision across each wrist, which he said he did with a knife that was later found in the backyard. Minimal bleeding was present from both wounds, which seemed to be caused by him pulling on his handcuffs. A 2-inch bloody depression was found in his hair on his right occipital skull, which he said he was not aware of. An iron was found in the living room; a corner of it was bloodstained and seemed to match the pattern mark on his head. A reasonable assumption was that he was hit with the iron, but he never admitted that fact. The patient's only subjective complaint was pain in his neck. He had a completely normal set of vital signs and good sensation and movement in all extremities. He was covered in dried blood from head to toe, some of which was from his girlfriend, whom he apparently embraced after shooting.

Treatment of the woman involved crime scene preservation only. Treatment of the perpetrator included placing an extrication collar, removing his handcuffs, and bandaging his wounds. He was immobilized supine and flex-cuffed to a scoop stretcher. He was extricated down the stairs, being careful to avoid stepping on any casings or spots of blood.

Treatment en route included 100% oxygen by nonrebreather mask, large-bore IV in each arm, and transportation to a trauma center. Serial vital signs, including electrocardiogram and SPO_2, all remained stable.

To everyone's amazement, investigation later discovered that the perpetrator had put his 9-mm automatic in his mouth and pulled the trigger more than 2 hours before SWAT entry. No soot was found around his mouth, and no teeth were fractured. A small hole was discovered in the back of his throat 40 minutes after his neck radiograph at the trauma center. The bullet fragmented on his cribriform plate, and the computed tomography scan revealed a bullet fragment in his brain and two in his cervical spine, which explained his neck pain. This man sustained a point-blank gunshot wound to the head from a 9-mm round and remained hemodynamically stable and neurologically intact for hours.

From a technical standpoint, the TEMS team was glad they had taken all trauma precautions.

EQUIPMENT

[OBJECTIVE 11]

The personal protective equipment for TEMS medics should include body armor, helmet, and gas mask. Furthermore, it should be equal to whatever the SWAT operators are wearing. The TEMS medic also should have the same level (or higher) of hazardous material chemical protection equipment, up to level C with an air-purifying respirator and a small cache of decontamination equipment to set up for a hasty decontamination in case the entry team is hit with chemical agents.

Based on TCCC concepts, four lines of tactical medical equipment should be accessible to TEMS medics and SWAT operators, staged with the following minimums.

Operator Level, Quick Draw

The first line of medical equipment is composed of one tactical tourniquet and one tactical battle dressing. Every SWAT officer, agent, and medic should carry these items in an easy-to-access place. Tactical dressings are essentially bulky dressings already attached to bandages with rigged cinching and fastening devices (Figure 65-6). They should be vacuum packed, lightweight, and easily deployed. Tactical tourniquets are similarly set up, with the constricting band woven into a sheath and the windless attached and rigged (Figure 65-7). Because the tourniquet is mainly used for the rare exsanguinating hemorrhage in the care under fire scenario, it must be placed on the operator's or medic's tactical gear in a place that can be quickly drawn, like a weapons magazine, and applied with one hand in less than 20 seconds on an arm and less than 30 seconds on a leg. Everyone on the team should stage his or her first-line gear in the same place. If possible, the casualty should perform self-aid with his or her own first-line gear. If not, the closest teammate (who is not covering a field of fire) will perform buddy aid with the casualty's first-line gear.

Medic Level, Quick Draw

The second level of gear includes the following:

- One additional tourniquet (see Figure 65-7)
- One additional tactical battle dressing (see Figure 65-6)
- Two shrink-wrapped gauze (S-Rolled Gauze; North American Rescue, Greer, S.C.)
- Hemostatic dressing or granules (Combat Gauze [Z-Medica Corporation, Wallingford, Conn.] or WoundStat [TraumaCare, Bethesda, MD.])
- Two chest seals (with or without relief valves)
- Two chest decompression needles (3.25 inches, 14 g)
- Nasal and oral airways
- Supraglotic airway (Combitube or King)
- Cricothyroidotomy kit
- Trauma shears

Second-line medical equipment should be staged in pockets of tactical vests or body armor (Figure 65-8), which ensures that all equipment can be drawn with one hand without looking and without putting anything down. The medic can quickly begin treating the top three causes of preventable battlefield death in a tactical field care setting. He or she also will be able to move the casualty immediately if the situation changes without leaving anything behind.

Third-line medical equipment is carried in a tactical backpack (Box 65-4). Three main scenarios occur in which the medic would access medical supplies from the backpack. The first is a tactical field care scenario with one or more critical casualties. In this situation the medic is still in the inner perimeter but in a secure place of cover, remaining there for a minimum of 5 minutes because of tactical considerations or because he or she is awaiting the arrival of a transport platform. Therefore the medic has time to do more definitive care until the patient is relatively stabilized and the tactical team has cleared a safe pathway to the outer perimeter. The second scenario is when all suspects are in custody and the entire scene is secure. At this point the medic does not have the pressure of tactical considerations but, as with any EMS call, should not spend time starting IVs, for example, if a clear pathway to a safe transport platform exists. In the third

BOX 65-4 Third Line: Medic Level, Backpack Contents

- Additional trauma dressings for mass casualty
- Bandages: four each of roller gauze, Ace, and triangular
- Water gel burn dressings
- Bag-mask device
- Endotracheal intubation kit
- Two bags of 1000 mL normal saline with IV start kits attached
- One bag 500-mL hetastarch (Hespan) or other colloid/isotonic
- Chest tube kit
- Minor wound cleaning and closure kit
- Epinephrine/diphenhydramine autoinjectors
- Mark 1 antidote kits (atropine/pralidoxime autoinjectors)
- Morphine, naloxone, nitroglycerin, aspirin, albuterol
- Over-the-counter medications (antacids, non-antihistamine decongestants, acetaminophen, etc.)
- Extrication collar
- Two formable/SAM splints (SAM Medical Products, Tigard, Ore.)
- Blood pressure cuff and stethoscope
- Ear, nose, and throat kit with tactical otoscope
- Examination gloves and other standard precautions supplies
- Sound suppression ear plugs (enough for several teammates during training)
- Two flex cuff–type restraints

IV, Intravenous.

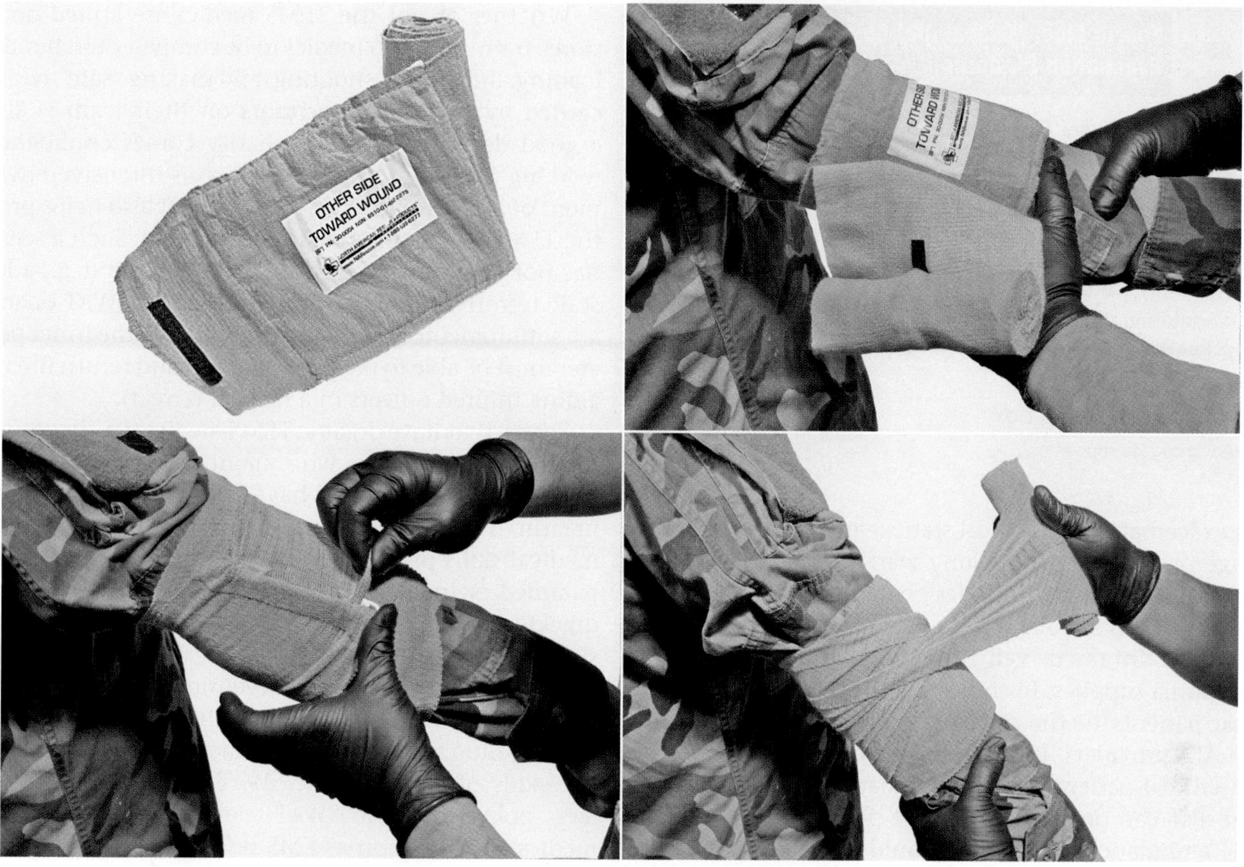

Figure 65-6 Tactical dressings are essentially bulky dressings already attached to bandages, some with rigged cinching and fastening devices. They should be vacuum packed, lightweight, and easily deployed.

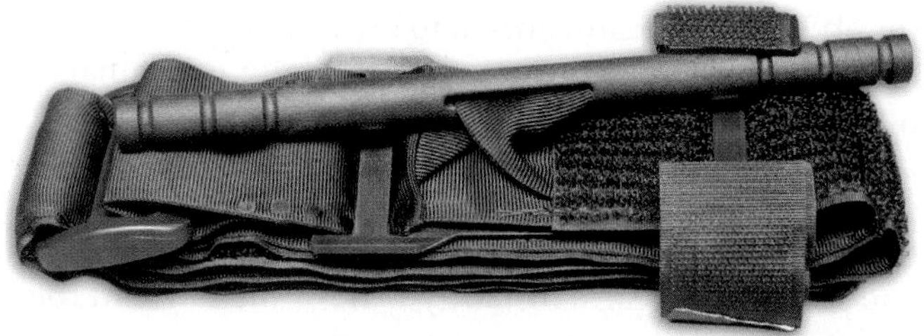

Figure 65-7 Tactical tourniquets are similarly set up with the constricting band woven into a sheath and the windless attached and rigged.

scenario, the medic's backpack should also double as a coverage bag for extended missions or training. In these cases the medic can take it off his or her back and stage it in places where it is available for minor medical problems or injuries for the team.

Ideally the transport platform, considered the fourth line, should be a fully stocked paramedic rig already staged on scene (Box 65-5). The medic can then adequately treat major trauma as well as any critical medical emergency en route to the hospital. Cardiac medical problems are rare in SWAT operators. However, this is not the case for hostages, suspects, and incidental subjects present at the incident. People with preexisting medical problems may have their respiratory or cardiac condi-

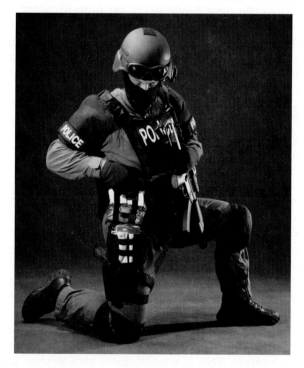

Figure 65-8 Second-line medical equipment should be staged in pockets of tactical vests or body armor.

BOX 65-5 Fourth Line: Medical and Casualty Evacuation Platform

- All the previously listed third-line equipment (see Box 65-4)
- Oxygen cylinders and delivery supplies
- Full spinal immobilization equipment
- Blankets and warming supplies
- Total body water gel burn blanket
- Decontamination equipment
- 12-Lead electrocardiograph/SPO_2 monitor with defibrillation and pacing
- Complete ALS drug box

ALS, Advanced life support.

tions exacerbated to a critical status when they are taken hostage or drawn into a felony warrant scenario. If the TEMS team does not have a designated paramedic rig, an alternative is to retrofit a law enforcement vehicle (e.g., armored victim rescue vehicle, van, sport utility vehicle) with trauma supplies. In this mode the medic can extract critical patients to the outer perimeter and hand them off to ALS providers. If the scene is secure and the medic has a critical patient and no ambulance is on scene, he or she also can opt not to pass the patient off to a paramedic ambulance. The medic would then continue ALS care in the back of the law enforcement vehicle all the way to the appropriate treatment center. This type of scenario must be preplanned by the TEMS medics with a designated, competent driver who knows the quickest routes to the right hospitals, or no time is gained and time is potentially lost.

A list of outfitters that provide tactical medical equipment for TEMS is available in the Suggested Resources section at the end of this chapter.

ARMED MEDICS

[OBJECTIVE 12]

Probably the most controversial issue within tactical EMS is whether to arm the bulk of TEMS providers who are not sworn law enforcement officers (Carmona, 2003b; Vayer, 2003). No right or wrong answer exists regarding whether arming medics on the inner perimeter of SWAT missions is appropriate. The issue is not moral; it is a safety and legal issue with advantages and disadvantages. Ultimately the decision is made by the individual law enforcement agencies that oversee the SWAT operators and the agencies that provide the TEMS medics. Below are some general guidelines.

If TEMS medics are not armed going into SWAT missions, they must be accompanied at all times by armed SWAT officers. This is usually not a problem on large teams. Large teams have numerous perimeter shooters, snipers, and an entry team (where medics should not be placed) that goes in before an arrest team (which is an appropriate place for the TEMS medics).

Whether or not the TEMS medics are armed on missions, training TEMS medics to be competent in handling, loading, unloading, shooting, and making "safe" weapons carried by the SWAT operators on their team is always a good decision. With familiarity comes confidence in working in and around the weapons-intensive environment of SWAT training and missions. It also helps prepare the TEMS medic for an extreme scenario. Such a scenario has not yet occurred in the Western world (e.g., a large-scale terrorist ambush in which multiple SWAT operators are simultaneously shot and everyone on the inner perimeter must be able to pick up a weapon and return fire while aiding injured officers in a tactical retreat).

Teams that have organic TEMS medics (i.e., law enforcement SWAT operators who maintain EMT or paramedic certifications) obviously have no issue with carrying a firearm. The main issue with this setup is maintaining medical skills proficiency. Even if they were experienced paramedics in a prior career, skill decay occurs rather quickly in EMS when a paramedic is not treating a consistent number of patients each year. It is only partially a matter of maintaining intervention skills and mostly a matter of developing and maintaining assessment skills. A small number of law enforcement teams can maintain the skills of their organic SWAT paramedics. These are large police or sheriff SWAT teams in which their TEMS medics also function as EMS rescue medics and perform numerous rescues and medical transports.

If the TEMS medic who is not a sworn law enforcement officer is armed, then he or she must be trained and qualify to the operator level on whatever firearm is carried. The most important initial and ongoing training issue is the ability to determine when to use deadly force. In some areas attaining a reserve peace officer status is optimal but not always a requirement. The TEMS medic should not carry a rifle unless the TEMS medic is supporting a very small SWAT team with not enough operators to cover all fields of fire. The TEMS medic should be able to holster and secure the firearm instantly so he or she can shift roles and focus on patient assessment and care.

Extraordinary Deployment

Active Shooter and Mass Casualty

Because of the current climate of the United States and other free countries, the topic of extraordinary deployments unfortunately requires special attention.

Tactical operators are mission-driven individuals who are highly motivated to engage and kill active shooters who may threaten their community. TEMS medics are similarly motivated to take calculated risks to intervene immediately if a tactical operator or citizen sustains life-threatening injuries while engaging such dangerous criminals. However, the extraordinary deployment scenario is the type of callout to which no law enforcement or EMS personnel wants to respond. This is because, by definition, many of the victims cannot be saved by the time the tactical team arrives because the active shooter planned and carried out numerous murders before the tactical callout was even dispatched. Examples of these situations include the following:

- April 16, 2007—Virginia Tech massacre, Blacksburg, Va.; 33 killed, 28 wounded
- March 21, 2005—Red Lake High School massacre, Red Lake, Minn.; 10 killed, 13 wounded
- April 26, 2002—Guttenberg High School massacre, Erfurt, Germany; 17 killed, unknown number wounded
- November 2, 1999—Xerox massacre, Honolulu, Ha.; seven killed, unknown number wounded
- April 20, 1999—Columbine massacre, Littleton, Colo.; 15 killed, 18 wounded
- October 16, 1991—Luby's Diner massacre, Killeen, Tex.; 24 killed, 20 wounded
- December 6, 1989—University of Montreal Massacre, Quebec, Canada; 15 killed, 14 wounded
- July 18, 1984—McDonald's massacre, San Diego, Calif.; 22 killed, 19 wounded
- January 29, 1979—Cleveland Elementary School massacre, San Diego, Calif.; three killed, nine wounded
- August 1, 1966—University of Texas tower massacre, Austin, Tex.; 13 killed, 31 wounded

Some of these shooting sprees were handled by experienced, well-trained law enforcement agencies that secured the scene in a matter of minutes. Some were not. As previously stated, discussing specific tactics, techniques, and procedures is not appropriate for this text. Well-developed SWAT teams, however, do train to engage and kill active shooters immediately and now train the regular patrol officers in their respective agencies to take decisive actions even before the SWAT team arrives. Either way, TEMS medics must be trained, equipped, and know their roles in these scenarios. At a minimum, proper preparation includes the following:

1. A reliable communications system that ensures interoperability with all agencies
2. Prepackaged mass casualty medical supplies that can be backpacked into a scene
3. Active shooter immediate action drills based on the respective SWAT team tactics, techniques, and procedures
4. Mass casualty drills based on the regional EMS incident command system

The rest of this section presents best practice recommendations based on two types of active shooter scenarios (Figure 65-9): (1) active shooter(s) who are alive and still shooting and (2) active shooter(s) who are dead or in custody.

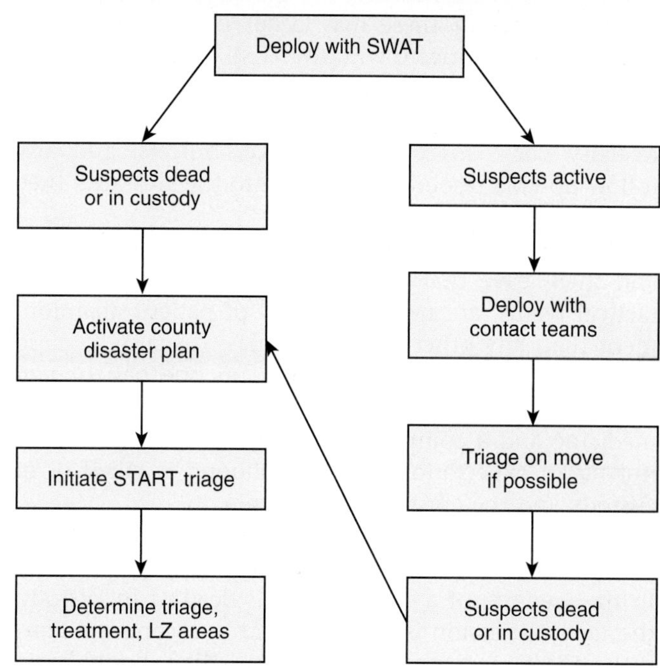

Figure 65-9 Active shooter scenario algorithm. *LZ,* Landing zone.

Shooter Alive and Still Shooting

In the scenario of a shooter who is still firing a weapon, the TEMS medics are assigned to either tactical contact teams or rescues teams. In either case, the primary mission of the TEMS medics remains the same as any other tactical mission—to support the team by being immediately available to treat any tactical officer who becomes a casualty. This means that one or more TEMS medics advances with the team into the hot zone and does not become bogged down in the triage and treatment of civilian mass casualties.

In large facilities such as schools, the tactical team likely will encounter civilian casualties congregating in areas of cover and concealment on their way to the suspect. The TEMS medic is expected to at least give a size-up to responding EMS resources while advancing with the team. Follow-up law enforcement officers should secure enclosed areas with large numbers of casualties, whether they are SWAT trained or not. Once secured, these areas would be synonymous with warm zone incident command settings.

If the tactical decision is to wait briefly in an area where casualties are located, then the TEMS medic should immediately perform the following:

1. Initiate simple triage
2. Initiate primary care based on TCCC guidelines
3. Give a brief size-up to EMS responders in the cold zone based on the regional incident command system

Ideally, additional medical resources would be advanced into warm zones and take over casualty care from the TEMS medic before he or she advances with the tactical team. Another option is to perform appropriate TCCC and move casualties and other civilians into the cold zone, as directed and covered by law enforcement officers along the way. However, because of tactical considerations, neither of these may occur before the tactical element moves forward with the TEMS medic to stop the shooter.

Well-equipped TEMS teams can leave behind mass casualty packs for casualties, cover officers, and any follow-up EMS resources brought into the area after they move forward (Figure 65-10).

Note that TEMS medics who initiate care on a casualty and then leave that casualty, at the direction of their tactical teams, are no more guilty of patient abandonment than any other medic in a mass casualty scenario who performs a triage assessment on one patient and moves on to other patients. Tactics must always drive medicine and a complete triage of all casualties should not be an expectation until the shooter is killed or in custody and the entire scene is secure.

Shooter Dead or in Custody

In the scenario of a shooter who is dead or in custody, the tactical mission is complete and the scene is secure. If the TEMS medics are first on scene, they should begin simple triage and rapid transport according to the National Incident Management System protocols in their regional EMS system.

The key to preparing for any extraordinary deployment is planning and rehearsing with all agencies that will be dispatched to such incidents. The key to interoperability when the unthinkable happens is a reliable communications system among all agencies. A good resource for networking best practices between tactical teams is the National Tactical Officers Association.

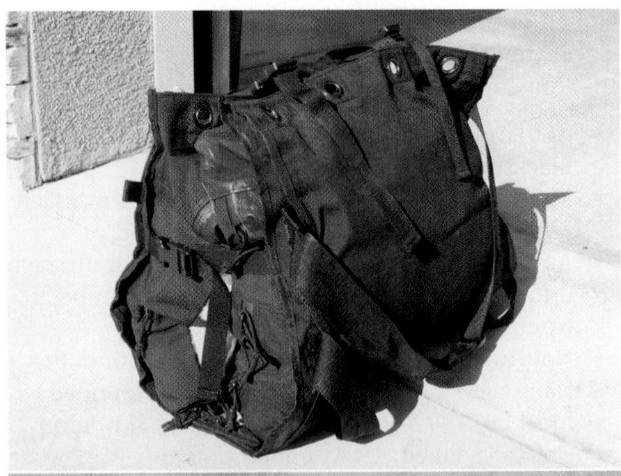

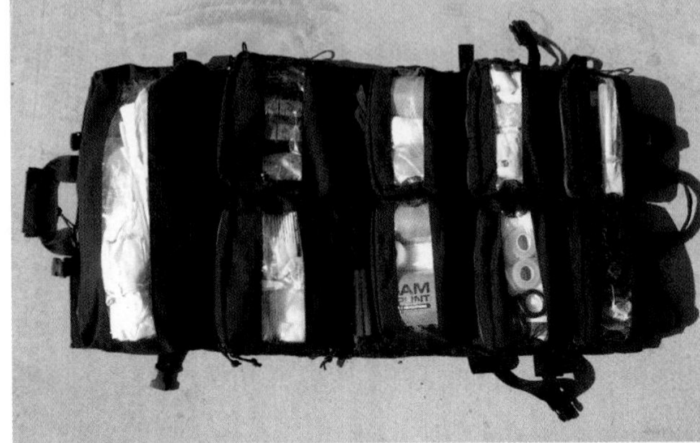

Figure 65-10 Mass casualty bag.

Case Scenario SUMMARY

1. *What is the purpose of a TEMS team?* According to its definition, the primary purpose of a TEMS team is to provide prehospital medical support for law enforcement tactical teams while the teams are in training or on a special operation.
2. *What are the types of duties or responsibilities of a TEMS medic?* The types of duties or responsibilities of a TEMS medic include (1) casualty care on the inner perimeter of an operation, (2) medical intelligence and threat assessment, (3) assessment and health maintenance of team members on prolonged training or missions, (4) remote assessment of casualties, (5) medical clearance of suspects, (6) medical training of tactical operators, and (7) physical readiness qualification at the operator level.
3. *What is required to become a TEMS medic?* Requirements for a TEMS medic include extensive direct patient contact experience as a field ALS practitioner (paramedic) and successful completion of the local SWAT physical abilities test.
4. *What type of training does a TEMS medic undertake?* Training for the TEMS medic may include law enforcement training, PTLS, and tactical medical training from a variety of resources.
5. *What areas are considered the hot zone, warm zone, and cold zone?* The hot zone is the zone under fire, which has a substantial risk of being exposed to effective enemy fire. The warm zone, while still within the inner perimeter, is in a position of cover and concealment. The cold zone is the medical evacuation or transportation zone outside the perimeter of all containment police officers.
6. *You and a SWAT officer get closer to the downed officer while crouching below the windows of the squad cars. Is this technique known as cover or concealment?* The officer crouching below the windows of a squad car is using concealment. Cover is completely out of the line of fire where no weapon can penetrate the cover mechanism. Armor-piercing bullets may go through the squad car and strike the officer. The only position of hard cover

on unarmored vehicles would be the opposite side of the engine block and, even then, stray rounds could skip under the vehicle and hit your lower extremities.

7. *If a decision were made to care for the fallen officer, what care would you provide?* Care provided to the fallen officer would be line-of-fire care and consist of quick drawing and applying a tourniquet to control bleeding followed by immediate extraction from the area.

8. *The TEMS medic knows when treating a casualty is appropriate. What are the four TCCC priorities?* The four TCCC priorities include (1) fire superiority, (2) prevention of further casualties, (3) triage, and (4) treatment according to TCCC guidelines.

9. *What are the four lines of tactical medical equipment accessible to TEMS medics?* The four lines are (1) operator level, quick draw, consisting of a tourniquet and battle dressing; (2) medic level, quick draw, consisting of equipment to control bleeding, airway equipment, and equipment to seal and/or decompress a chest; (3) medical equipment carried in a backpack, including burn dressings, IV access, intubation equipment, and medications; and (4) medical evacuation platform consisting of third-line equipment plus oxygen cylinders, 12-lead electrocardiogram, and pulse oximeter, along with all other paramedic rig gear.

Chapter Summary

- Civilian special operations teams, most commonly referred to as *SWAT teams,* respond to unusually hazardous threats. These threats are beyond the capabilities of normal law enforcement. They include snipers, barricaded armed suspects, hostage situations, felony warrants on well-armed suspects, weapons of mass destruction, and other extraordinary deployments.
- TEMS, or more appropriately, tactical medicine, is defined as "the comprehensive out-of-hospital medical support for law enforcement's tactical teams during training and special operations."
- Although TEMS medics provide tactical casualty care on the inner perimeter of SWAT missions, their duties are usually much broader. They include medical threat assessments before missions, remote assessment of downed casualties during missions, health maintenance of team members, and assessment before incarceration of suspects.
- TEMS providers should be experienced paramedics who maintain numerous patient contacts each year and are well rounded in all parts of the TEMS triangle, including tactical skills, medical skills, and personal fitness.
- TEMS medics should wear proper personal protective equipment. In addition, they should have a working knowledge of cover, which is protection from enemy fire, and concealment, which is defined as protection from enemy observation.
- TCCC represents the field care portion of battlefield medicine. It directly applies to the care given to casualties incurred on the inner perimeter of civilian SWAT operations.
- The most common causes of preventable death on the battlefield are (1) exsanguination from external bleeding (60%), (2) tension pneumothorax (33%), (3) airway compromise (6%), and (4) all other (1%).
- The priorities of TCCC are (1) fire superiority (suppress the threat), (2) prevent further casualties (get out of the line of fire), (3) triage, and (4) treat the life threats.
- TCCC under fire is comparable to the incident command system hot zone. All efforts are made to get the casualty out of the line of fire, and the only appropriate care rendered should be stopping exsanguinating bleeding with a quick-draw tourniquet.
- TCCC tactical field care is comparable to the incident command system warm zone. Casualties are protected until a clear route to medical transport is secured, and emergency care is rendered in a tactical manner without putting anything down or giving away the position.
- TCCC medical and casualty evacuation is comparable to the incident command system cold zone. Casualties are en route to a hospital or await transport in the outer perimeter.
- TEMS medics should participate in all appropriate and authorized tactical law enforcement and medical training. Most importantly, they should train with the tactical team they serve and provide self-aid and buddy aid training to their tactical operators in case of mass casualty catastrophes.
- TEMS medics should stage their equipment so that all care under fire and tactical field care equipment can be quickly drawn with one hand without looking and without setting anything down.
- No right or wrong answer exists regarding whether TEMS medics should be armed. It is a matter of the needs and policies of the tactical team they serve.

REFERENCES

Butler, F., & Hagman, J. (1996). Tactical combat casualty care in special operations. *Military Medicine, 161*(suppl 1), 1-19.

Cain, J. S. (2008). From the battlefield to our streets. *Journal of EMS*, October (Suppl.), 16–19.

Carmona, R. H. (2003a). History and evolution of tactical emergency medical support and its impact on public safety. *Topics in Emergency Medicine, 25*(4), 278.

Carmona, R. H. (2003b). Controversies in tactical emergency medical support. *Topics in Emergency Medicine, 25*(4), 342-346.

Giduck, J. (2008). Terror in American Schools. *Journal of EMS*, October (Suppl.), 9–10.

Meoli, M. R. (2000). *San Diego TEMS, California Association of Tactical Officers News, 7.*

Meoli, M. R. (2001). *San Diego TEMS, California Association of Tactical Officers News, 11.*

National Tactical Officers Association. (2008). *Tactical emergency medical support.* Retrieved November 6, 2008, from http://www.ntoa.org.

Rathbun, D. (2003). The clinical practice of tactical medicine and care under fire. *Topics in Emergency Medicine,* 25(4), 309-310.

United States Army. (2005). *Combat skills of the soldier,* USA Field Manual FM 3-21.75, Chapter 1. Retrieved March 14, 2007, from http://www.globalsecurity.org.

Vayer, J. S. (2003). Developing a tactical emergency medical support program. *Topics in Emergency Medicine Journal,* 25(4), 283, 289, 292.

SUGGESTED RESOURCES

Battlelab Tactical Nylon: http://www.diamondbacktactical.com

Blackhawk International: http://www.blackhawk.com

Butler, F. K. (2001). Tactical medicine training for SEAL mission commanders. *Military Medicine* 166(7):625-631.

Butler, F., & Hagman, J. (1996). Tactical combat casualty care in special operations. *Military Medicine* Aug;161 Suppl:3-16.

Heck, J. (2003). The role of preventative medicine in TEMS. *Topics in Emergency Medicine, 25*(4), 299-305.

Hughey, J. M. (2001). Operational medicine 2001: Health care in military settings (NAVMEDPUB 5139), Washington, DC: United States Navy Bureau of Medicine and Surgery.

Llewellyn, C. H. (2003). Antecedents of tactical emergency medical support. *Topics in Emergency Medicine, 25*(4), 274-276.

London Bridge Trading Company: http://www.londonbridgetrading.com

Meoli, M. R. (Winter 2000/Spring 2001). San Diego TEMS, *California Tactical Officers Association News.*

National Association of Emergency Medical Technicians. (2007). *PHTLS: Prehospital trauma life support Military version,* (6th ed.). St. Louis: Mosby.

National Tactical Officers Association: http://www.ntoa.org/tems

North American Rescue Products: http://www.narescue.com

Special Operations Medical Association: http://www.somonline.org

Yevich, S., Whitlock, W., Broadhurst, R., & Thompson, G. D. (Eds.) (2001). *Special Operations Forces medical handbook* (2nd ed.). Fort Gordon, GA: Center for Total Access.

Rathbun, D. (2003). The clinical practice of tactical medicine and care under fire. *Topics in Emergency Medicine, 25*(4), 306-315.

United States Army. *Camouflage, concealment and decoys,* U.S. Army Field Manual FM 3-58.1.

United States Army. (2003). *Combat lifesaver handbook 2003,* U.S. Army Interschool Subcourse IS0824.

United States Army. *First aid for soldiers,* U.S. Army Field Manual FM 21-11.

United States Army. *Medical evacuation in a theater of operations,* U.S. Army Field Manual FM 8-10-6.

United States Army Institute of Surgical Research: http://www.usaisr.amedd.army.mil.

Vayer, J. S. (2003). Developing a tactical emergency medical support program. *Topics in Emergency Medicine, 25*(4), 282-298.

Chapter Quiz

1. What are the three main areas of proficiency in the TEMS triangle on which a TEMS provider must focus to be an asset and not a liability on SWAT missions?
   a. Field medicine, firearms qualification, and personal fitness
   b. Field medicine, firearms qualification, and personal integrity
   c. Field medicine, tactical skills, and personal integrity
   d. Field medicine, tactical skills, and personal fitness

2. Keeping a low profile beneath the windowsill of a single-family house with a suspect inside is an example of using ________.
   a. cover
   b. concealment
   c. cover and concealment
   d. neither cover nor concealment

3. How important is physical fitness for a TEMS medic?
   a. Somewhat important; a TEMS medic should be somewhat fit.
   b. Not important; the SWAT officers on the team will help a TEMS medic with any physical limitations.
   c. Critically important; a TEMS medic must qualify to the same physical and psychological standards of the SWAT team.
   d. Important; however, if a person is fit enough to perform regular paramedic duties, he or she will have no problem performing at a SWAT level.

4. What is the most important medical skill for the TEMS medic?
   a. Endotracheal intubation in confined space situations
   b. Starting IV lines in the dark
   c. Assessment; a TEMS medic should have years of experience with thousands of field patients
   d. Basic life support skills, such as controlling exsanguinating hemorrhage

5. Before 1996, what percentage of American war casualties who were killed in action died on the battlefield before reaching a field medical hospital?
   a. 90%
   b. 80%
   c. 60%
   d. 40%

6. What accounts for the highest percentage of preventable deaths on the battlefield?
   a. Head injuries
   b. Airway compromise
   c. Tension pneumothorax
   d. Exsanguination from external hemorrhage

7. What is the first priority of TCCC?
   a. Tactical triage
   b. Open airway
   c. Fire superiority
   d. Extricate casualty from the line of fire

8. In a care under fire scenario, what are the only appropriate treatment modalities?
   a. Insert a nasal airway, control exsanguinating hemorrhage with trauma dressings, immobilize the cervical spine, place a chest seal on a sucking chest wound, extricate from the line of fire
   b. Insert a nasal airway, control exsanguinating hemorrhage with trauma dressings, extricate from the line of fire
   c. Control exsanguinating hemorrhage from an external bleed with a tourniquet, extricate from the line of fire
   d. No treatment modalities are ever appropriate in a care under fire scenario. The only appropriate move is to extricate from the line of fire.

9. In a tactical field care scenario, TEMS medics should be able to quickly draw supplies from tactical pockets without looking and without putting anything down. What are the minimum supplies they should be able to draw?
   a. Tourniquets and tactical battle dressings
   b. Tourniquets, tactical battle dressings, airways, chest seals, 3.25-inch 14g needles, trauma sheers
   c. Tourniquets, tactical battle dressings, airways, chest seals, 3.25-inch 14g needles, trauma sheers, IV bags and start kits
   d. Tourniquets, tactical battle dressings, airways, chest seals, 3.25-inch 14g needles, trauma sheers, IV bags and start kits, splinting equipment

10. Who decides whether TEMS medics who are not sworn law enforcement officers or agents should be armed on SWAT missions?
   a. The TEMS medics and their families
   b. The law enforcement agency and the agency that employs the medics
   c. The medical director in the county or state where the medics practice
   d. No one; it is immoral for medics to be armed

Terminology

Autoinjector A self-contained, compact injection system containing a single dose of an antidote or medication.

Critical incident stress debriefing Allows personnel affected by job stress as a result of a crisis or emergency situation to work through their experiences with their peers and/or mental health professionals.

Casualty Any person who is lost to the organization by having been declared dead, whereabouts unknown, missing, ill, or injured.

Killed in action A casualty category applicable to a hostile casualty, other than the victim of a terrorist activity, who is killed outright or who dies as a result of wounds or other injuries before reaching a medical treatment facility.

Tourniquet A device used to control bleeding that cannot be stopped with direct pressure and elevation.

Mark1 antidote kit Self-injected nerve agent antidote kit consisting of atropine and pralidoxime chloride.

Formable splint A splint made from a flexible material, usually with a thin metal core, that can be formed around an injury to provide stability and support.

Preventable death Death that could have been avoided if the casualty were given the right care at the right time.

Special Weapons and Tactics (SWAT) The division of a law enforcement agency equipped to handle especially dangerous, violent situations.

Tactical Combat Casualty Care (TCCC) A set of guidelines for use in providing trauma care in combat situations.

Tactical Emergency Medical Support (TEMS) Offers medical support to law enforcement tactical operations.

TEMS triangle The diagram that represents the three main areas of focus (tactical skills, personal fitness, and field medicine) to be a safe, effective TEMS medic.

US Special Operations Command Leads, plans, synchronizes, and, as directed, executes global operations against terrorist networks; also trains, organizes, equips, and deploys combat-ready special operations forces to combatant commands.

DIVISION 11

DISASTER AND DOMESTIC PREPAREDNESS ISSUES

CHAPTER 66

Disaster Response and Domestic Preparedness

Objectives *After completing this chapter, you will be able to:*

1. Explain the importance of disaster response preplanning and preparedness.
2. Describe the purpose of the National Response Plan.
3. Describe the federal medical resources available from the National Disaster Medical System.
4. Discuss the need for and the use of an incident command system.
5. Describe the role of EMS in the incident command system.
6. Identify the different types of natural disasters and the emergency medical needs associated with each.
7. Identify chemical weapons of mass destruction agents first responders should be concerned about.
8. Identify the five classes of chemical warfare agents and give examples from each class.
9. Identify the epidemiologic clues that may indicate an act of bioterrorism is occurring.
10. List the biologic agents considered the most critical threats.
11. Identify particular concerns that exist with large-scale radiologic events.
12. Explain why explosive and incendiary devices are used most often by terrorists.
13. Describe blast injuries and the human response.

Chapter Outline

Case Scenario

A bomb deploys at an airport during holiday travel. It destroys three jets and part of a terminal. You are a paramedic in a nearby community and are called to assist in this disaster. You are told that hazardous materials teams, disaster medical assistance teams, the Federal Emergency Management Agency, and the National Response Plan have been deployed. They are currently setting up the incident command system. You are to report to staging at the airport until further notice.

Questions

1. *Define the National Response Plan.*
2. *What is a disaster medical assistance team?*
3. *What is an incident command system?*
4. *What is the Federal Emergency Management Agency?*

Disaster response presents numerous challenges for emergency personnel. The safety of responders may be in jeopardy. The number of victims may be much greater than the number of available responders. Equipment may be in short supply. Fortunately, disaster and mass casualty incidents are uncommon. Unfortunately, that presents a problem. Because of the limited number of mass casualty incidents, responders do not get much practice experiencing these events.

Disasters can be natural or manmade. Natural disasters include earthquakes, floods, hurricanes, and tornadoes. Manmade disasters include structural collapses, hazardous materials incidents, and terrorist attacks. Responder safety needs and response procedures vary with each type of disaster.

This chapter discusses disaster response preparation and safe response practices, such as the use of the incident command system. Types of common injuries and

BOX 66-1 Natural and Manmade Disasters

Natural
- Earthquakes
- Floods
- Hurricanes
- Tornadoes
- Avalanches
- Typhoons
- Cyclones
- Droughts
- Tsunamis
- Storm surges
- Eruptions
- Landslides

Manmade or Technologic
- Structural collapse
- Hazardous materials incidents
- Nuclear incidents
- Terrorist attacks
- Airplane crashes
- Shipwrecks

treatment are presented. Special emphasis is placed on incidents involving weapons of mass destruction (WMD). Recognition methods for terrorist attacks are discussed. Descriptions of chemical, biologic, radiologic, nuclear, and explosive agents are presented. Examples of natural and manmade disasters are shown in Box 66-1.

DISASTER RESPONSE PREPAREDNESS

Local and State Response

[OBJECTIVE 1]

Preplanning is a vital part of safe and effective response to these types of incidents. Many aspects of disaster response should be determined far in advance of an actual emergency. Response to these types of incidents is a team effort, and many agencies are likely to become involved. Local response will likely involve EMS, fire, and police responders. Additional responders from the state level may include electrical and water utility workers, state office of emergency management, and possibly National Guard troops. In a hazardous materials incident or release of WMD, other local resources such as highway department personnel, local or state health department representatives, the county hazardous materials team, and private hazardous materials cleanup contractors all may be present. The capabilities of all primary response agencies (e.g., police, fire, hazardous materials) must be assessed and developed into a response plan. The roles of other agencies, such as the local health department and utility company, also must be ascertained and included in a response plan.

Preplanning also includes the development of operating procedures. All responders should be trained beforehand to the level of action they would be expected to take during a response. Specific training needs should be guided by area hazards. The Hazardous Waste Operations and Emergency Response (HAZWOPER) standard required training and National Fire Protection standard 473 discussed in Chapter 64 are focused on hazardous materials emergency response. They are the backbone of a safe and efficient WMD response training program. Some programs are more specific to WMD response. The National Domestic Preparedness Consortium, which is part of the Department of Homeland Security Office of Grants and Training, has presented training to scores of emergency responders across the country. It offers specific training for various levels of fire and hazardous materials response, emergency medical response, and hospital providers. Other programs such as the Noble Training Center in Alabama and programs from Texas A&M University, Louisiana State University, and many others are helping EMS quickly come up to speed in this crucial area. Because of the rapidly changing face of this problem, more quality training programs and texts are becoming available.

Response procedures should be developed to guide safe scene operations. Checklists can be a valuable addition to standard operating procedures. Patient decontamination, treatment, medication, and destination protocols must be developed by your local medical advisor.

Disaster response requires large amounts of medical equipment. The type of equipment needed depends on the type of disaster. A hazard vulnerability analysis should be conducted to determine the type of incidents that may occur in the area, and appropriate caches of supplies should be established. Hazardous materials and WMD incidents require special supplies, including personal protective equipment, mass decontamination supplies, and antidotes.

In many cases local hospitals may be overwhelmed when a disaster occurs. In the last 2 years, most states have started to establish plans for **surge capacity** hospitals to handle the increased number of patients. These may be composed of equipment caches to set up hospitals in existing facilities such as convention centers and sports facilities, portable tent hospitals, or elaborate trailer units.

One of the most important tools to help ensure efficiency and the safety of personnel in an emergency is an emergency response plan. This plan should be developed, rehearsed, modified as necessary, and rehearsed again. It should establish the response agency's actions when faced with a disaster situation. Emergency response organizations may use the local emergency response plan or the state emergency response plan as a model to avoid duplication. If the local or state plan is used, it must be modified to be specific to the emergency response organization.

Federal Response

National Response Plan

[OBJECTIVE 2]

The federal response to disasters is managed by the National Response Plan (NRP). The NRP describes the structure and processes that comprise a national approach to domestic incident management. It is designed to join the efforts and resources of federal, state, local, tribal, private sector, and nongovernmental organizations. The NRP includes planning assumptions, roles and responsibilities, concept of operations, incident management actions, and plan maintenance. It represents a concerted national effort to accomplish the following:

- Prevent terrorist attacks within the United States
- Reduce America's vulnerability to terrorism, major disasters, and other emergencies
- Minimize the damage from attacks, major disasters, and other emergencies
- Facilitate recovery from domestic incidents that occur

The NRP applies a functional approach that groups the capabilities of federal departments and agencies as well as the American Red Cross into emergency service functions (ESFs). ESFs provide the planning, support, resources, program implementation, and emergency services that are most likely to be needed during major incidents. The federal response to these incidents is typically provided through the full or partial activation of the ESF structure as necessary. The ESFs (Box 66-2) serve as the coordination mechanism to provide assistance to state, local, and tribal governments.

National Disaster Medical System

[OBJECTIVE 3]

Of special interest to medical providers is ESF 8, Public Health and Medical Services. This ESF is coordinated by the Department of Health and Human Services. Personnel for this task come from this agency and the **National Disaster Medical System.** The National Disaster Medical System response includes field units, coordination of patient transportation, and provision of hospital beds. The field component is composed of many volunteer teams of medical professionals.

Disaster medical assistance teams (DMATs) are field-deployable teams that include physicians, nurses, emergency medical technicians, and other medical and nonmedical support personnel (Figure 66-1). Specialty DMATs concentrate on areas such as burns, pediatrics, and mental health concerns.

National medical response teams for WMD are quick-response specialty teams trained and equipped to provide mass casualty decontamination and patient care after the release of a chemical, biologic, or radiologic agent. **International medical surgical response teams** are specialty surgical teams that can respond both in the United States and internationally. **Disaster mortuary operations teams** are composed of forensic and mortuary professionals trained to deal with human remains after disaster situations. **National Veterinary Response Teams (NVRTs)** are designed to provide animal care and assistance during disasters.

The Federal Emergency Management Agency (FEMA) also has field teams known as *urban search and rescue teams,* which specialize in the location, rescue, and initial medical stabilization of victims trapped in confined spaces resulting from structural collapse and other incidents. They are considered multiple-hazard teams that may respond to a variety of disasters, including earthquakes, hurricanes, tornadoes, floods, terrorist attacks, and hazardous materials releases.

Many groups and organizations respond to disasters. The coordination of these resources at the emergency scene is vital and is managed by a program called the *National Incident Management System* (NIMS).

BOX 66-2 ESFs

- ESF 1: Transportation
- ESF 2: Communications
- ESF 3: Public works and engineering
- ESF 4: Firefighting
- ESF 5: Emergency management
- ESF 6: Mass care, housing, and human services
- ESF 7: Resource support
- ESF 8: Public health and medical services
- ESF 9: Urban search and rescue
- ESF 10: Oil and hazardous materials response
- ESF 11: Agriculture and natural resources
- ESF 12: Energy
- ESF 13: Public safety and security
- ESF 14: Long-term community recovery and mitigation
- ESF 15: External affairs

ESF, Emergency service function.

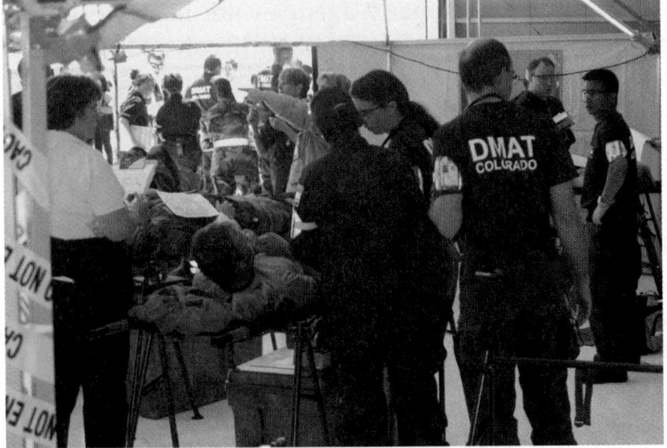

Figure 66-1 Colorado disaster medical assistance team (DMAT) working with military resources.

INCIDENT MANAGEMENT SYSTEM

National Incident Management System

NIMS is a recently created program that provides a set of protocols, concepts, terminology, and organizational processes to enable effective, efficient, and safe incident management. The system provides a consistent, nationwide approach for federal, state, and local governments and the private sector to prepare for, respond to, and recover from incidents, regardless of cause, size, or complexity. NIMS includes the following core set of concepts, principles, and terminology:

- The incident command system
- Multiple-agency coordination systems
- Training
- Identification and management of resources (including systems for classifying types of resources)
- Collection, tracking, and reporting of incident information

This system combines preincident planning, such as preparation, training, resource identification, and incident management activities, as well as postincident activities, such as information collection and reporting. The incident management activities are handled under the incident command system.

Incident Command System

[OBJECTIVE 4]

The **incident command system (ICS)** is designed to focus the actions of all responders on safely and efficiently mitigating an incident. ICS originated in the 1970s to manage California wildfires. Since then it has been adopted nationwide as an all-hazard and all-incident system. This means that it is designed for use in all types of incidents, regardless of type or size. The use of ICS principles in small, routine incidents serves as practice to ensure that the system works when it is needed on large incidents.

The use of an ICS at a hazardous materials incident is mandated by the Occupational Safety and Health Administration regulation and the HAZWOPER standard. An Environmental Protection Agency parallel standard extends HAZWOPER coverage to volunteers and government workers not covered by Occupational Safety and Health Administration rules.

The usefulness of the ICS has been recognized by hospital systems. A version of the ICS system was adapted for hospital facilities and is called the **Hospital Incident Command System.** The basic structure of the ICS is the foundation of the new NIMS.

Incident Command System Structure

ICS is a management tool consisting of procedures for organizing personnel, facilities, equipment, and communications at the scene of an emergency. It is organized in a modular format. It should be a top-down organizational structure that can be used for any incident. Modules are typically organized according to function, with five primary functional areas or sections. These five functional areas include command, operations, planning, logistics, and finance and administration. Each functional area is recognized in any implementation of the ICS; however, each area does not require independent staffing. In a small incident one person may be responsible for several functions. As the incident expands, so does the ICS, with an individual in charge of each area.

Command. The command function involves directing, ordering, and/or controlling resources. The senior person at the scene is usually considered the **incident commander (IC)** (Figure 66-2). As previously mentioned, an ICS is a top-down structure. An IC is always present; the remaining sections are added as needed. The first arriving responder assumes the role of the IC. As personnel who are more qualified arrive on the scene, the person assuming the role of IC may change, but the responsibilities remain the same. The IC has the primary authority for the overall control of the emergency event. All response operations are conducted under the control of this person. The IC position is sometimes held by more than one person representing more than one agency. This concept is known as *unified command.* The IC may appoint staff positions to assist in the command function. These include the safety officer, public information officer, and the liaison officer (Box 66-3).

Operations Section. The Operations Section is responsible for managing all tactical operations at the incident. This section is coordinated by the operations section chief, who reports to the IC. Depending on the incident, fire control, police operations, public works, and EMS and hazardous materials team activities may all report to the operations section chief. Depending on the incident, the operations section may be divided into branches,

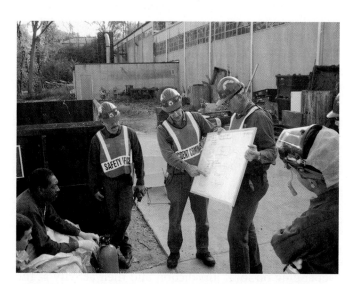

Figure 66-2 Incident commander briefing emergency response team.

BOX 66-3 Staff Positions to Assist in Command Function

Safety Officer

The safety officer is responsible for all safety concerns at the incident. The safety officer must have the ability to stop or modify any unsafe acts, then immediately report those changes to the IC. The safety officer reports to the IC.

Public Information Officer

The public information officer is responsible for developing and presenting information to the news media. The news media can be of major assistance in getting information to the public. The media can alert the public and provide them with information on exposure effects. Real-time medical information provided by qualified experts through the media can help the public differentiate real from somatic symptoms of the incident.

Liaison Officer

The liaison officer is a member of the command staff responsible for coordinating with representatives from cooperating and assisting agencies. He or she must have immediate access to the IC. This position becomes extremely important at large, multiple-agency incidents.

IC, Incident commander.

BOX 66-4 Possible Divisions of Operations Section

Branch

The organizational level with functional, geographic, or jurisdictional responsibility for major parts of the incident operations. The branch level is organizationally between section and division or group in the operations section and between section and units in the logistics section. Branches are identified by the use of Roman numerals, function, or jurisdictional name.

Division

The organizational level with responsibility for operations within a defined geographic area. The division level is organization between the strike team and the branch.

Group

Groups are established to divide the incident into functional areas of operation. Groups are located between branches (when activated) and resources in the operations section.

Unit

The organizational element with functional responsibility for a specific incident planning, logistics, or finance and administration activity.

Task Force

A group of resources with common communications and a leader that may be preestablished and sent to an incident or formed at an incident.

Strike Team

Specified combinations of the same kind and type of resources with common communications and a leader.

Single Resource

An individual piece of equipment and its personnel complement or an established crew or team of individuals with an identified work supervisor that can be used on an incident.

divisions, groups, units, task forces, strike teams, and single resources (Box 66-4).

Planning and Intelligence. Responsibilities of the planning and intelligence section include collecting and evaluating information about the response. The planning and intelligence section also is responsible for developing a suggested action plan for approval by the IC. This section is coordinated by the planning and intelligence section chief, who reports to the IC. At smaller incidents the planning function often is combined with the operations function.

Logistics. The logistics section is responsible for locating, organizing, and providing facilities, services, and materials needed for mitigation of the incident. This section is coordinated by the logistics section chief, who reports to the IC.

Finance or Administration. The finance, or administration, section is responsible for tracking all incident costs and evaluating the financial considerations of the incident. This section also may be responsible for securing resources that are unavailable to the logistics section chief. This section is coordinated by the administrative section chief, who reports to the IC.

Role of EMS

[OBJECTIVE 5]

Depending on local jurisdiction and their activity at the scene, EMS providers may fall into many of these functional areas. For example, the EMS providers managing injuries that occurred at the incident will most likely be assigned to a medical sector or group under the operations section (Figure 66-3). The senior EMS provider on the scene may be assigned to be the medical sector supervisor or leader. EMS providers supporting the responders at an incident may be assigned to the logistics section. EMS providers also may be assigned to the planning section to assist in identifying patient needs.

The IC must be informed of all activities that deviate from the established plan. Final approval of any actions must come from the IC. Medical responders *must* determine their actions under the local ICS in preplanning before an incident takes place.

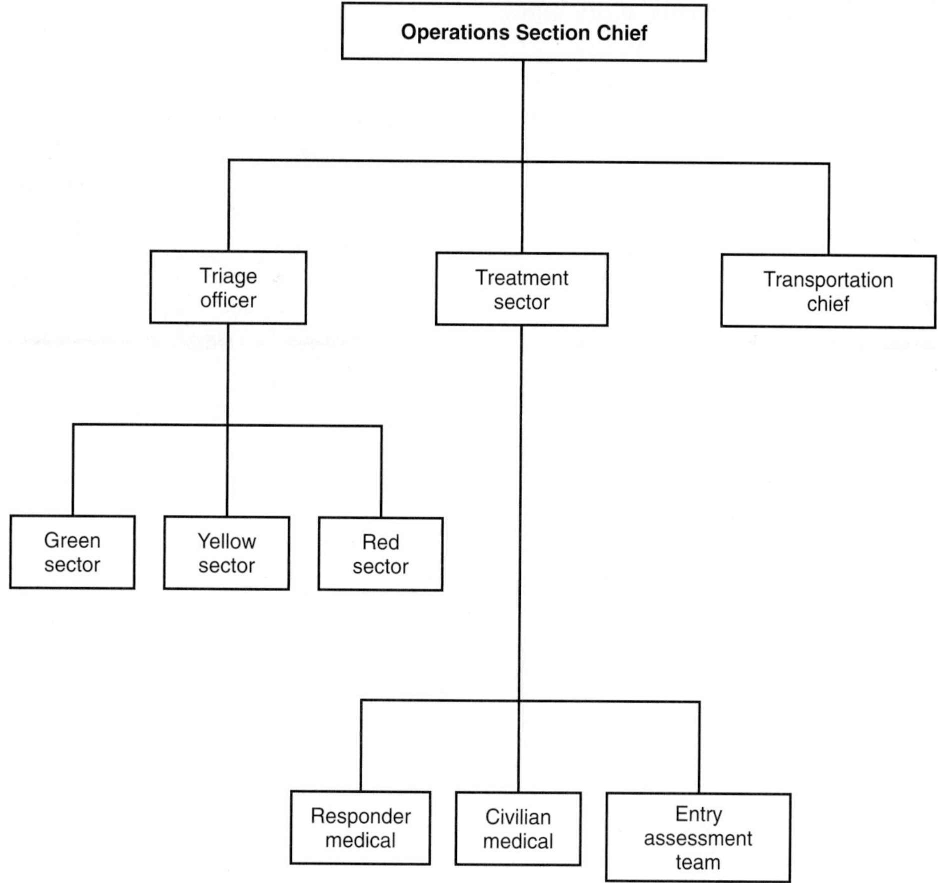

Figure 66-3 Example of medical sector in the incident command system (ICS).

Concepts

Certain concepts are essential to the successful implementation of an ICS. These concepts allow the ICS to function no matter which agencies are involved in the response.

Common Terminology. Common terminology is essential to the effectiveness of the system. The "10 codes" used in the past only cause confusion with agencies that do not use them. Communications must be done in plain English, both on the scene and on the radio, to reduce the possibility of confusion between agencies.

Command Post Operations. The establishment of a command post is an important benchmark. The **command post** is the location from which incident operations are directed. At small incidents, this may be the car of a senior officer. At larger incidents a specially designed mobile command post, command tent, or even a nearby structure may be used. Only one incident command post is set up at an incident. The command post is usually marked with a green flag or light. In large or complex incidents, an emergency operations center may be established to support the IC.

Unified Command. The unified command concept is used when a number of agencies have an overall responsibility to the incident. Senior representatives from each involved agency compose the unified command group. The unified command group makes the decisions for the goals, objectives, and priorities for the response to the incident. With the concept of unified command, a leader managing it is still required. The agency with the current incident focus usually takes the lead of the unified command group.

Consolidated Response Plan. A plan is necessary when responding to any type of emergency. Each responding agency and the local, county, and state government all have response plans. The coordination of these plans must be handled as a preplanning concern. These plans can help identify who will be responsible for each aspect of the incident. They also can help obtain resources during the emergency.

Span of Control. An ICS also helps organize response activities and ensure that safety procedures are followed at the scene. It suggests a range of control, defined as the number of subordinates one supervisor can effectively manage, to ensure that the safety of every responder is maximized. The guidelines describe a desirable range of three to seven persons reporting to a supervisor, with an optimal number of five.

Integrated Communications. Communication has always been a major problem at a large incident. Many different agencies respond with different radio systems. Advances in the communications field have resulted in the development of mixing units. Mixing units allow radios with different frequencies to communicate with each other. If they are not available, the "old-fashioned" concept of sharing radios or placing a person from each unit with a radio in the command post can be used.

Staging Areas. For EMS responders, an important concept of the ICS is the staging area. A staging area is a resource marshaling area to which units report while awaiting specific assignments and direction (Figure 66-4). Only resources immediately needed at the scene of the emergency should be on the site. Different personnel and resources are needed at different times and in different locations. Staging areas are under the control of a staging area manager, who must be in direct contact with the operations section chief.

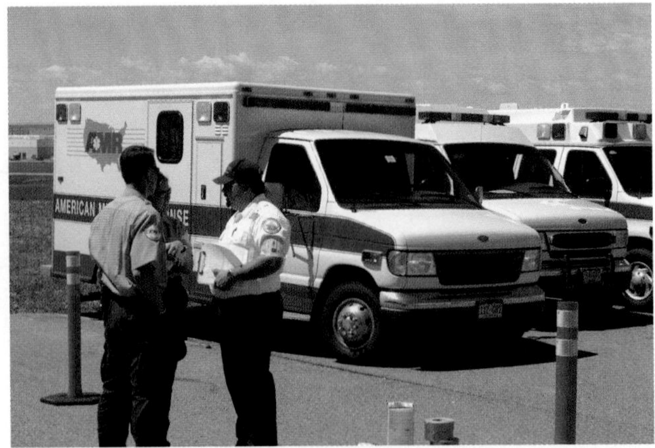

Figure 66-4 EMS unit receiving assignment at the staging area.

Case Scenario—continued

You arrive at the staging area, which is approximately 1 mile away from the airport. Also arriving are police units, FEMA members, DMAT teams, the Red Cross, construction equipment, and the media.

Questions

5. *Where should the police, FEMA, and DMAT report in the ICS?*
6. *Who is in charge of the construction equipment location and the Red Cross?*
7. *Who is in charge of the media?*

NATURAL DISASTERS

[OBJECTIVE 6]

Sudden-onset natural disasters such as earthquakes, hurricanes, tornadoes, floods, and volcanoes can strike with little or no warning and leave their impact over a short period (Ryan et al., 2002). The amount of damage left in their wake can be enormous. The number of injured and dead can be devastating, as witnessed in the 2004 South Asia tsunami, where hundreds of thousands were killed or remain missing.

Many of these events render the local emergency response system ineffective. Response may involve the establishment of field hospitals to augment or replace the damaged medical system. Patients may need to be evacuated to other cities to receive medical care. In most of these incidents the injuries will be familiar, but the settings in which care is provided may be different. Medical personnel may find themselves working in austere environments. Resources, transport, access, and the entire social and economic infrastructure may be damaged or destroyed. These conditions impose severe constraints on the immediate care of injured patients.

Triage procedures, the prioritizing of patients based on severity of injury, is mandatory. Triage is covered in Chapter 62.

Earthquakes

Most injuries resulting from earthquakes come from structural collapse. Suffocation from the building rubble and asphyxia from the large clouds of dust generated account for a substantial number of deaths. Immediate injuries include crush injuries to the head, chest, and extremities; external or internal hemorrhage; chest compression; and burns from resulting fires. Many patients may survive for a time in the collapsed structure. This has been termed the *fade away time*. Extensive information on survival times in different types of structures does not exist. Most authorities agree that victims who are not removed within 12 hours have a low probability of survival. Delayed deaths can be caused by conditions such as dehydration, hypothermia, hyperthermia, crush syndrome, and postoperative sepsis. Past earthquakes have shown that injuries seen 7 days after the earthquake are commonly minor orthopedic and soft tissue injuries sustained in recovery work, psychological trauma, respiratory infections, diarrhea, and chronic diseases aggravated by the incident (Ryan et al., 2002).

Hurricanes and Tornadoes

Hurricanes can cause massive disruption of the existing medical system, as seen in Florida in the 2004 hurricane season and during hurricanes Katrina and Rita in 2005.

Damage to hospitals, relocation of hospital and long-term care patients, traumatic injuries from building collapse, and flying debris can be expected. However, the greatest number of deaths and severe injuries result from flooding caused by extensive rainfall, landslides, and sea surge (Ryan et al., 2002). Hurricane and storm path prediction can allow time for evacuations and the establishment of surge capacity care centers.

Tornadoes can result in damage similar to hurricanes but on a much smaller scale, causing potentially severe damage locally rather than regionally. Traumatic injuries are common. Tornadoes have little or no warning time, so patients injured in collapsed structures are common.

In both cases existing hospital resources may be damaged by the storms. Patients with minor injuries sustained in recovery operations and chronic diseases aggravated by the incident may need supportive care until hospital resources have recovered.

Floods

Drowning is obviously the primary cause of deaths in floods, but trauma from impact with floating debris and hypothermia from cold exposure can be expected. In these types of disasters the number of patients with severe injuries is usually minimal. Minor injuries are much more common. Secondary illness and/or infection from contaminated water is possible. As in the other types of natural disasters, support of damaged medical resources is needed.

RESPONSE: HAZARDOUS MATERIALS INCIDENTS VERSUS WEAPONS OF MASS DESTRUCTION

The threat of a terrorist attack with a WMD on U.S. soil is a relatively new concept. However, EMS has been responding to incidents involving hazardous materials for many years. These two responses have many things in common. Specific training, safe response tactics, personal protective equipment, decontamination procedures, and patient treatment needs are all similar. In some cases even the chemicals can be the same. The same chlorine and anhydrous ammonia used in industry can easily be used as a chemical weapon (Figure 66-5).

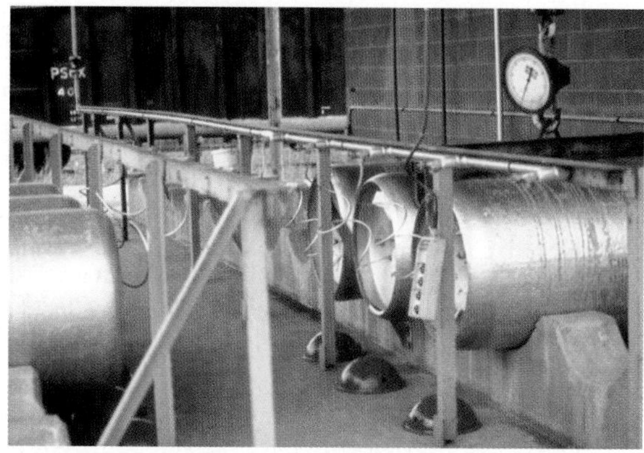

Figure 66-5 Chlorine at an industrial facility. Some of the same chemicals used in industry also can be used as a weapon.

Case Scenario CONCLUSION

The IC provides direction to all his key officers and commanders. An announcement is made that a unified command will be used, and they will follow the consolidated response plan. The command post will be a mobile van with a large green flag near staging.

Questions

8. *What is a unified command?*
9. *What is a command post?*
10. *What is a consolidated response plan?*

WEAPONS OF MASS DESTRUCTION

[OBJECTIVES 7, 8]

Chemical Agents

Blood Agents

Blood agents are chemicals absorbed into the body through the action of breathing, skin absorption, or ingestion. Once in the body and bloodstream they cause lethal damage at the cellular level by inhibiting the cellular use of oxygen. The blood agents include the two cyanides: **hydrogen cyanide (AC)** and **cyanogen chloride (CK).** The two-letter code listed in parentheses after the chemical name is the North Atlantic Treaty Organization designation for that chemical. This designation often is used in military chemical references manuals.

At room temperature, hydrogen cyanide is a colorless liquid that is predominately absorbed through inhalation, but gaseous, liquid, and crystallized cyanide can also be absorbed through the skin. Hydrogen cyanide is highly volatile, meaning that it evaporates very quickly. Along with being volatile, hydrogen cyanide also is considered nonpersistent. Chemical warfare agents have been divided by the military into nonpersistent and persistent categories. Persistent agents stay active in the environment as liquids for more than 24 hours. Hydrogen cyanide has a faint odor similar to bitter almonds that is not detectable by all people. Cyanogen chloride, like hydrogen cyanide, is a colorless, highly volatile liquid that is soluble in water and nonpersistent. Both of these bind to the iron ion in cytochrome a3, interfering with the transfer of electrons to oxygen. This blocks the process of electron transport, shutting down the cell's ability to make adenosine triphosphate (ATP).

The symptoms of cyanide exposure vary depending on several factors, including the total dose of the poison, the route of poisoning, and the exposure time. In the initial stages of cyanide poisoning several things occur. An individual becomes restless and has an increased respiratory rate. Other early symptoms are similar to hypoxia and include giddiness, headaches, heart palpitations, and respiratory difficulty. Patient oxygen saturation levels may be normal or near normal because of the cell's inability to use oxygen. As time progresses, vomiting, convulsions, respiratory failure, and coma typically occur. In cases of high concentrations, an increase in respiration occurs within seconds of exposure, followed by 20 to 30 seconds of convulsions and, within 1 minute, the patient would rapidly deteriorate into cardiac arrest.

Persons who do not immediately die after exposure to hydrogen cyanide must be treated rapidly. The patient must first be removed to a fresh air environment by responders wearing the appropriate levels of personal protective equipment. If the agent was released as a liquid, decontamination is vital. Airway and circulatory system management is vital in the early stages of treatment. One antidote for cyanide exposure is the Taylor Cyanide Antidote Package (Taylor Pharmaceuticals, San Clemente, Calif.), formerly known as the Lilly or Pasadena Cyanide Antidote Kit (Figure 66-6). The kit contains three separate medications: amyl nitrite, sodium nitrite, and sodium thiosulfate. Amyl nitrite reacts with hemoglobin to form approximately 5% methemoglobin. Amyl nitrite is included in aspirols that are broken and held in front of the patient's nose. In case of respiratory arrest, the aspirol can be placed inside a bag-mask and the patient's lungs ventilated (remove after 15 seconds, ventilate for 15 seconds, and repeat) until sodium nitrite can be administered.

Sodium nitrite reacts with hemoglobin to form approximately 20% to 30% methemoglobin. Methemoglobin attracts cyanide ions from tissue and binds with them to become cyanmethemoglobin. The sodium nitrite is in liquid form that should be administered by intravenous (IV) push over a 5-minute period.

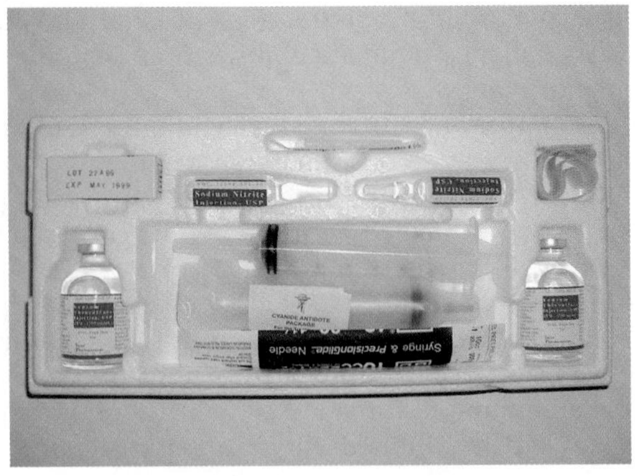

Figure 66-6 Cyanide antidote kit.

The final medication in the cyanide antidote kit is sodium thiosulfate, which converts cyanmethemoglobin to thiocyanate, which is excreted by the kidneys. It also is found in liquid form that should be administered by IV push over a 5-minute period. Both sodium nitrite and amyl nitrite in excessive doses can induce a dangerous methemoglobinemia and can be fatal, especially in children. Unlike hemoglobin, methemoglobin does not carry oxygen. Sodium nitrite also can cause hypotension. Correct administration of the cyanide antidote kit is complex, especially when treating children. Detailed instructions are on a label found inside the kit. Remember that when treating a cyanide exposure, the antidotes themselves are poisonous and can damage the body, so you must be sure you are dealing with a cyanide exposure. Antidote therapy should be in addition to ventilation, oxygen therapy, and rapid transport. Because of the hazards associated with the Cyanide Antidote Kit, a new cyanide antidote called the Cyanokit (EMD Serono, Inc., Rockland, Mass.) has recently been approved by the Food and Drug Administration. The Cyanokit includes the drug hydroxocobalamin, IV tubing, and saline for reconstituting the drug product. In France the kit has been used for more than a decade, more typically to treat cyanide poisoning resulting from smoke inhalation. In the presence of cyanide, hydroxocobalamin takes up the cyanide and becomes a form of vitamin B_{12}, which is then easily excreted from the body.

In general, a patient who has had inhalation exposure and survives long enough to reach medical care needs little treatment.

Pulmonary Agents

Pulmonary agents are the chemicals first responders should fear the most. These chemicals are easy to obtain and usually do not require any manufacturing process to turn them into a weapon. These agents (also referred to as **choking agents** or *pulmonary irritants*) primarily attack the lungs and lung tissue after inhalation and are characterized by pronounced irritation of the upper and lower respiratory tract.

Phosgene. Phosgene is a chemical widely used today in the manufacturing of dyes, coal tar, pesticides, and pharmaceuticals. It was used in World War I until mustard gas was introduced on the battlefield. The Bhopal, India, disaster of 1984 at the Union Carbide plant involved an industrial accident that caused the release of 50,000 lb of methyl isocyanate. This incident resulted in the immediate death of more than 3000 people and more than 10,000 deaths since the accident occurred. This chemical is composed of phosgene and methylamine. Phosgene has the following properties:

- It is a colorless gas with an odor of newly mown hay.
- It is a highly volatile, nonpersistent agent.
- It is heavier than air and remains in low-lying places for long periods.
- It is a gas at temperatures greater than 47°F.
- It is easy to produce but is unstable in storage and therefore must be kept refrigerated.

Directly after an individual is exposed, symptoms include coughing, choking, feeling of pressure on the chest, nausea, vomiting, and headache. After the initial symptoms, a period lasting from 2 to 24 hours occurs, during which an exposed individual seems free from any abnormalities. The patient then develops signs and symptoms of pulmonary edema. As edema progresses, general discomfort and dyspnea increase and frothy sputum develops. The patient may then demonstrate signs of hypovolemic or even cardiogenic shock. In general, if a person can rest and survive until the danger of the pulmonary edema is past, the patient has a higher recovery rate.

Removal of the patient to a fresh air environment and supportive airway and circulatory system management are generally all that is required. If the agent was released as a liquid, decontamination procedures are warranted. Note that the effects of an acute exposure to some of these agents may not immediately be seen but rather develop over a period of several hours. Exposed patients should be medically evaluated and, if necessary, kept for continued evaluation.

Chlorine. Chlorine is a common chemical used widely in industry, especially in the production of chlorinated inorganic and organic chemicals and in the manufacture of solvents and plastics. It is also used as a bleaching or cleaning agent and in water treatment facilities for purifying drinking water. Chlorine was the first chemical used in modern warfare when the Germans released 150 tons of it against the allied troops in 1915. Characteristics of chlorine include the following:

- A greenish-yellow gas or amber liquid (under pressure) with a pungent odor
- More than twice as heavy as air
- Highly volatile and nonpersistent
- A strong oxidizer and highly corrosive

The primary signs and symptoms from exposure to chlorine include eye and airway irritation, dyspnea, chest tightness, headache, vomiting, and delayed-onset pulmonary edema. In general, removal of the patient to a fresh air environment and oxygen and supportive airway and circulatory system management are all that is required. Note that the effects of an acute exposure to chlorine may not be seen immediately, but rather develop over a period of several hours. Exposed patients should be medically evaluated and, if necessary, kept for continued evaluation.

Anhydrous Ammonia. Anhydrous ammonia is used in both agriculture as a fertilizer and in industrial facilities as a refrigerant for cooling and freezing. It is commonly used in meat, poultry, and fish processing facilities; dairy and ice cream plants; cold storage warehouses; and other food processing facilities. Anhydrous ammonia is a colorless gas in lower concentrations. In higher concentrations it can form a white cloud. It is considered a volatile, nonpersistent agent. Eye and airway irritation, severe general pain, dyspnea, chest tightness, laryngeal edema, and pulmonary edema are expected signs and symptoms. Partial and full-thickness burns and/or frostbite may occur when in contact with the skin.

In general, removal of the patient to a fresh air environment and oxygen and supportive airway and circulatory system management are all that is required. Note that the effects of an acute exposure to ammonia may not be seen immediately, but rather develop over a period of several hours. Exposed patients should be medically evaluated and, if necessary, kept for continued evaluation.

Vesicants

Vesicants (also known as **blister agents**) are named after the most obvious injury they inflict on a person (Figure 66-7). Examples include mustard agents, lewisite, and a related chemical, phosgene oxime. These agents burn and blister the skin or any other part of the body with which they come into contact. Blisters are not the

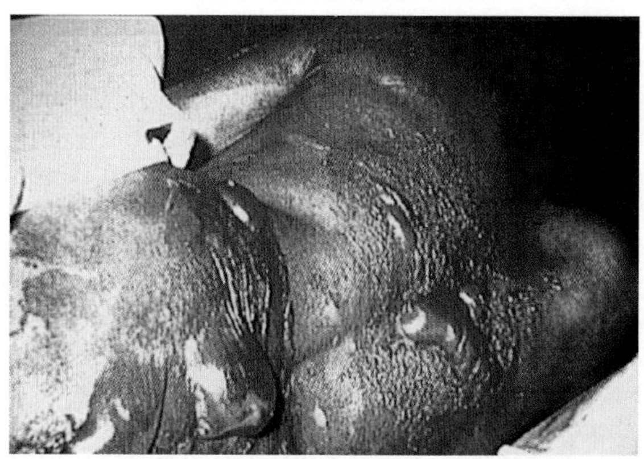

Figure 66-7 Blister formation from mustard agent exposure.

only risk that these agents pose. They severely damage the skin, eyes, lungs, gastrointestinal tract, and other internal organs. Blister agents are most commonly used on the battlefield to force enemy troops to use personal protective equipment during battle, thereby decreasing their effectiveness. These agents contaminate almost everything they contact.

Sulfur mustard is the most well known and used of the vesicants. Mustard produced the largest number of chemical casualties of World War I despite its late initial use. In its pure state, mustard is colorless and almost odorless (possibly an odor of mustard, garlic, or rotten onions). At room temperature, mustard is a liquid with a low volatility. These agents can be thickened with a polymer to create a persistent threat. At warmer temperatures, blister agents become a nonpersistent agent but have a higher concentration of vapor, increasing the respiratory threat. Under temperate conditions, mustard evaporates slowly and is primarily a liquid hazard, but its vapor hazard increases with increasing temperature. At 100°F or above, it is a definite vapor hazard. Mustard freezes at 57°F; because a solid is difficult to disperse, mustard is often mixed with substances with a lower freezing point.

Signs and symptoms can begin hours after exposure, but by then the damage has already be done. Erythema and blisters on skin; irritation, conjunctivitis, and corneal opacity and damage in the eyes; mild upper respiratory signs to marked airway damage; and gastrointestinal effects occur. No immediate pain is felt from exposure to mustards agents.

Mustard agent exposure has no antidote. Symptomatic management of lesions and supportive airway management are usually all that is required. Only a small portion of patients have long-term effects. Decontamination of these agents is critical.

Nerve Agents

The nerve agents are probably the most well-known type of chemical agent. They are the most toxic of the chemical agents, but are also the hardest to acquire or manufacture. Nerve agents are chemically related to organophosphate pesticides but are several times more deadly. The nerve agent group includes both G agents and V agents. The G agents were originally developed just before and during World War II by industry-rich Germany. These include tabun (GA), sarin (GB), soman (GD), and cyclohexyl methyl phosphonofluoridate (GF). The most familiar V agent is **VX,** which was developed in the United Kingdom. The only other known V agent is one developed by the former Soviet Union that has characteristics similar to VX. In their pure states nerve agents are a colorless liquid; when impure they tend to be a yellowish color. Some of the agents may have a fruity odor to them, but this is an unreliable sign. The G agents tend to be nonpersistent, volatile agents, whereas VX is a highly persistent, nonvolatile agent (it evaporates about as quickly as motor oil). The vapor hazard significantly increases when exposed to high temperatures or aerosolized.

The signs and symptoms for all nerve agents are similar. The only difference comes when discussing the onset, which varies greatly depending on several factors, including weather, geography, and whether the release was indoors or outdoors. The most important aspect to note at onset of symptoms is whether the individual was exposed to a vapor or liquid. A vapor exposure can lead to signs and symptoms in a few seconds to minutes, whereas symptoms of an exposure to a liquid agent may take several minutes to even hours. The specific signs and symptoms to note in a nerve agent event include muscle twitching, **miosis,** headache, rhinorrhea, salivation, and dyspnea in mild cases. A patient with a severe exposure may exhibit all of these signs and symptoms and develop severe difficulty breathing, generalized muscular twitching, weakness or paralysis, seizures, loss of bladder and bowel control, and loss of consciousness. The classic **SLUDGE-BBM** (***s***alivation, ***l***acrimation, ***u***rination, ***d***efecation, ***g***astrointestinal distress, ***e***mesis, ***b***radycardia, ***b***ronchoconstriction, and ***m***iosis) syndrome may be seen.

Nerve agents work by attaching to and deactivating a body enzyme known as *acetyl cholinesterase*. This enzyme controls the activity of the parasympathetic nervous system neurotransmitter acetylcholine. The deactivation of acetyl cholinesterase allows the parasympathetic nervous system to work in excess, which is what results in the symptoms listed previously.

Two specific antidotes are available for nerve agent exposure: atropine and pralidoxime chloride. Atropine works as an acetylcholine-blocking agent. Atropine takes the place of the acetylcholine in the organ receptor sites, corrects bradycardia, and dries secretions produced by overstimulation of the parasympathetic nervous system. Atropine does not correct respiratory muscle weakness, so the patient will likely need respiratory support. The second medication, pralidoxime chloride (2-PAM), works to remove the nerve agent from the enzyme, thereby returning normal function to acetyl cholinesterase. It also works to restore activity to the respiratory muscles. These two drugs are paired together in a kit called a **Mark 1 antidote kit** (Figure 66-8). The Mark 1 kit is a two-part autoinjector with 2 mg of atropine and 600 mg of 2-PAM. Valium (also in autoinjector form) also is used in combination with the Mark 1 kit. Consult medical direction for the appropriate dosing regimen. The success of 2-PAM depends on the aging process of the agent used. Aging is the time for the nerve agent/acetyl cholinesterase bond to mature. If the nerve agent/acetyl cholinesterase bond "ages," the acetyl cholinesterase enzyme is deactivated. Once the enzyme is deactivated, it must be regenerated over an extended period. The aging time varies by agent (soman, 2 minutes; sarin, 4 to 6 hours; VX, 1 hour). Decontamination of these patients is critical.

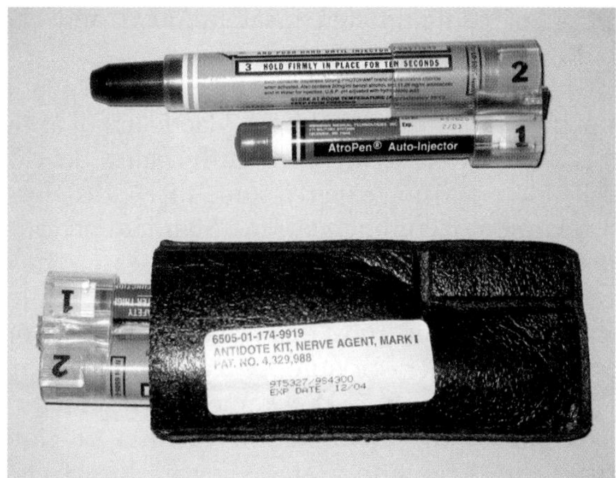

Figure 66-8 Mark 1 Antidote Kit for nerve agent exposure.

BOX 66-5 Biologic Agent Release Indicators

1. A large epidemic with greater case loads than expected, especially in a discrete population
2. More severe disease than expected for a given pathogen as well as unusual routes of exposure
3. Unusual disease for a given geographic area, found outside the normal transmission season, or impossible to transmit naturally in the absence of the normal vector for transmission
4. Multiple, simultaneous epidemics of different diseases
5. A zoonotic disease outbreak as well as a human outbreak (many of the potential threat agents are pathogenic to animals)
6. Unusual strains or variants or antimicrobial resistance patterns different from those circulating
7. Higher attack rates in those exposed in certain areas, such as inside a building if the agent was released indoors, or lower rates in those inside a sealed building if an aerosol was released outdoors
8. Intelligence that an adversary has access to a particular agent or agents
9. Claims by a terrorist of the release of a biologic agent
10. Direct evidence of the release of an agent with findings of equipment, munitions, or tampering.

Reprinted from Pavlin, J. A. (1999). *Epidemiology of bioterrorism.* Washington, DC: Walter Reed Army Institute of Research.

Riot Control Agents

Two forms of **2-chlorobenzalmalononitrile** (**CS** or **CN;** commonly known as *tear gas*) are listed together because the symptoms, delivery systems, decontamination, and treatment are the same for both. The primary difference is that CS is generally considered more potent. Both have relatively short action times, and the severity of symptoms decreases rapidly with time. CN and CS are both chemical irritants. They do not cause any permanent physical damage but irritate the mucous membranes (and to a much lesser, but still intense degree, the skin) on contact. Both have questionable effectiveness on intoxicated or emotionally disturbed persons because they only cause pain and have limited direct physiologic effects (compared with pepper spray, which causes an inflammatory response regardless of whether the subject can feel pain or not). CN and CS cause essentially the same symptoms, although CS is generally more severe. CN and CS in crystal form tend to cling to clothing, skin, and hair, and during large-scale deployments they often are visible on the patient. In smoke form they are usually not visible.

Removing as much clothing as practical is the single most effective decontamination action. In case of visible gross **contamination,** water is useful for removing large amounts of agent, but ultimately the remaining agent will not be removed until the water dries and the agent can blow away. Plain water or saline should be applied directly to the eyes, being careful to allow the water to run away from the eyes. In cases of pepper spray exposure, saline causes increased pain, so only plain water should be used for eye irrigation. Consider the use of Morgan therapeutic irrigation lenses (MorTan, Inc., Missoula, Mont.). For continued pain, evaluate the patient for the presence of corneal abrasions. Treat respiratory symptoms as necessary. Dyspnea or painful respiration (chest pain on breathing) is generally caused by deep inhalation of an agent. In otherwise healthy persons, it is not a danger to the patient. Screen the patient for underlying conditions such as asthma and other forms of chronic obstructive pulmonary disease that may be aggravated by a chemical agent.

Biologic Agents

[OBJECTIVE 9]

Covert attacks with biologic weapons require a different response from that of a chemical weapon. No signs of the attack may exist. **Biologic agents** have an incubation period lasting from days to weeks. The first clue that an attack has taken place may be ill patients weeks after the attack (Box 66-5) (Pavlin, 1999). No ground zero exists for response, and decontamination cannot take place. Medical personnel who work at hospitals, clinics, and physician offices are likely to be the first responders to this type of event.

Bioterrorism Agent Threat List

[OBJECTIVE 10]

Biologic agents can be bacteria, viruses, toxins, or rickettsia. Examples of bacterial agents include anthrax, plague, and tularemia. Examples of viral agents include smallpox, Ebola, Marburg, and Venezuelan equine encephalitis. Examples of toxins include botulinum toxin, ricin, and *Staphylococcus enterotoxin B*. Examples of rickettsia include epidemic typhus and Q fever. As weapons, pathogens each present unique risks and response challenges, making bioterrorism preparedness particularly difficult. The Centers for Disease Control and Prevention (CDC) have established a list of likely bioterrorism agents (CDC, 2000) (Table 66-1). This list includes three categories, A, B, and C. Category A pathogens are highly lethal agents that are easily dispersed or transmitted from person to person. In the early cold war era of the 1950s and 1960s, most of these organisms were successfully weaponized in the offensive biologic weapons programs of the United States and the former Soviet Union. Category B pathogens are also somewhat easy to deliver as a weapon, but result in much lower morbidity and mortality rates than category A pathogens. Category C pathogens are emerging diseases that could be harnessed for use by bioterrorists in the future.

Because of the number of possible agents, this chapter profiles the category A pathogens (see Table 66-1) (Rotz et al., 2000).

Anthrax

Anthrax is caused by the gram-positive, spore-forming bacterium ***Bacillus anthracis.*** Inhalational anthrax is the most lethal form of anthrax disease and results from the inhalation of spores. This results in a two-stage illness, including a prodromal and fulminant phase. The **prodromal** phase lasts from a few hours to a few days. It includes nonspecific, flulike symptoms, including fever, malaise, shortness of breath, nonproductive cough, and nausea. The **fulminant** stage includes the development of high-grade **bacteremia** characterized by fever, respiratory distress, profuse sweating, cyanosis, and shock. Patients with these symptoms usually die within several days. The most common form of the anthrax disease process is cutaneous anthrax (Figure 66-9). It is a local infection resulting from skin exposure to anthrax spores, which causes swelling that progresses to form an ulcer within several days. The ulcer develops into a depressed, painless lesion called an *eschar.* Cutaneous anthrax can occur naturally and is known as *wool sorter's disease.* It often is seen in patients who work with livestock and animal hides. A gastrointestinal form of the disease results from ingestion of *B. anthracis.* This may occur from consumption of contaminated meat products and can be difficult to diagnose.

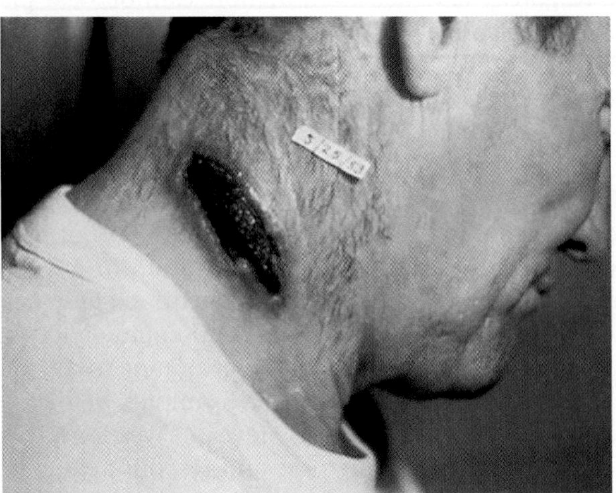

Figure 66-9 Cutaneous anthrax lesion on the neck.

Anthrax treatment recommendations include both treatment and postexposure prophylactic use of antibiotics. Because new data are constantly being developed, consult bioterrorism experts and the CDC for the latest treatment recommendations. Standard precautions are adequate for all forms of anthrax disease. The only risk to providers is direct contact with a cutaneous lesion or exposure to body substances during invasive procedures such as surgery or autopsy. Patient decontamination is warranted only in the immediate aftermath of a known release. Decontamination consists of clothing removal and soap and water shower; bleach is not necessary.

TABLE 66-1 Critical Biologic Agents for Public Health Preparedness

Biologic Agent	Disease
Category A	
Variola major	Smallpox
Bacillus anthracis	Anthrax
Yersinia pestis	Plague
Clostridium botulinum (botulinum toxins)	Botulism
Francisella tularensis	Tularemia
Filoviruses and arenaviruses (e.g., Ebola, Lassa fever)	Viral hemorrhagic fevers
Category B	
Coxiella burnetii	Q fever
Brucella spp.	Brucellosis
Burkholderia mallei	Glanders
Burkholderia pseudomallei	Melioidosis
Alphaviruses (VEE, EEE, WEE)	Encephalitis
Rickettsia prowazekii	Typhus fever
Toxins (e.g., ricin, staphylococcal enterotoxin B)	Toxic syndromes
Chlamydia psittaci	Psittacosis
Food safety threats (e.g., *Salmonella* spp., *Escherichia coli* O157:H7)	
Water safety threats (e.g., *Vibrio cholerae*, *Cryptosporidium parvum*)	
Category C	
Emerging threat agents (e.g., Nipah virus, hantavirus)	

VEE, Venezuelan equine encephalomyelitis; *EEE,* eastern equine encephalomyelitis; *WEE,* western equine encephalomyelitis.

Reprinted from Rotz, L., Khan, A., Lillibridge, S. R., Ostroff, M., & Hughes, J. M. (2000). *Public health assessment of potential biological terrorism agents.* Retreived August 9, 2008, from http://www.cdc.gov.

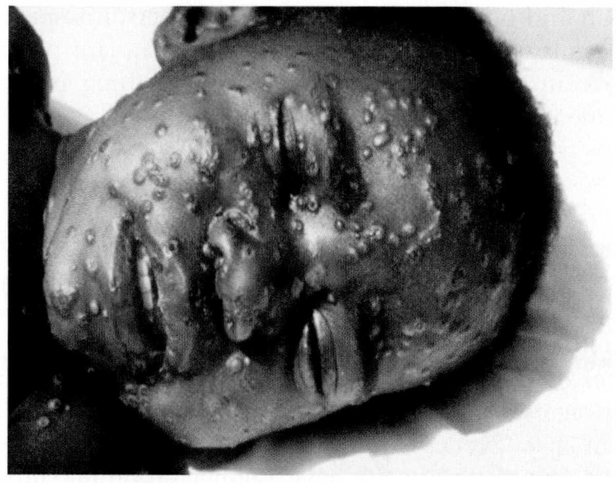

Figure 66-10 Child with smallpox.

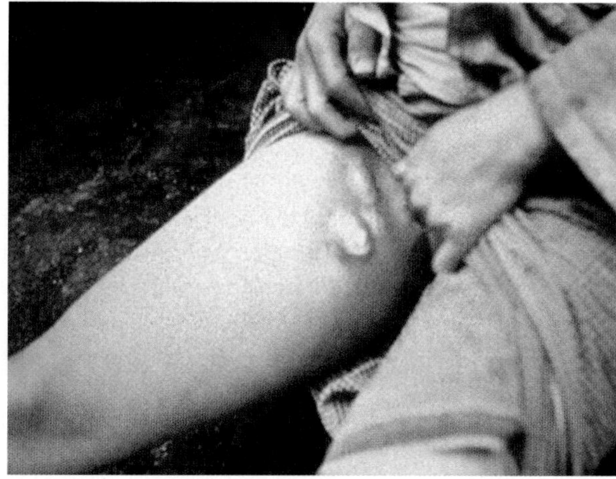

Figure 66-11 This patient with plague displays a swollen, ruptured inguinal lymph node, or bubo.

Smallpox

Smallpox is a disease caused by the Variola virus, a member of the Orthopox virus family. **Variola major** is the organism that causes classic smallpox epidemics. It is the virus most likely to be used as a weapon. The most similar patient presentation is the appearance of chickenpox. Smallpox lesions begin in the mouth and throat and then spread to the face and extremities (Figure 66-10). They concentrate centrifugally on the face, arms, and legs, with fewer lesions on the patient's trunk. In addition, the lesions appear on the palms of the hands and the soles of the feet. Across the body the lesions are uniform and in the same stage of development (vesicles, pustules, or scabs). In contrast, chickenpox concentrates centrally, not centrifugally, with large numbers of lesions on the patient's trunk and fewer lesions on the face and extremities. The patient should be kept in a negative-pressure room. Personnel and/or visitors must wear proper respiratory protection (e.g., N-95 mask), gown, and gloves for each patient contact. Any suspected cases must be immediately isolated until diagnosis is confirmed. Confirmed cases must remain isolated until all scabs separate, usually approximately 3 weeks.

Although an adequate supply of smallpox vaccine is available for everyone in the United States, no vaccination is recommended for the public unless it is in response to a confirmed outbreak. This is because of the serious risk of complications that accompanies the smallpox vaccine. Vaccination also may be effective in preventing some morbidity and significantly reducing mortality rate if given within 4 days of exposure.

Plague

Plague is a term often used as a general word to describe lethal outbreaks of infectious disease. However, plague is a specific disease resulting from the gram-negative bacillus *Yersinia pestis*. Three forms of plague disease exist: pneumonic, bubonic, and septicemic. Early symptoms for all forms of plague disease include fever, chills, myalgia, weakness, increased white blood cell count, and headaches.

Pneumonic plague is most severe form of the plague disease. Patients with pneumonic plague initially demonstrate dizziness, chest discomfort, and a productive cough with blood-tinged sputum. By the second day of the illness, the symptoms may worsen significantly and include tachypnea, chest pain, coughing, and sputum increase and may include dyspnea, hemoptysis, cardiopulmonary insufficiency, and circulatory collapse.

Bubonic plague is the most common form of plague disease. The bubonic form most commonly comes from the bite of an infected flea. Patients with bubonic plague have swollen, tender, and painful buboes (enlarged lymph nodes) (Figure 66-11). These symptoms typically occur within 24 hours of the onset of early symptoms and are generally located near the area of inoculation. Other possible symptoms include bladder distention, apathy, confusion, fright, agitation, oliguria, anuria, tachycardia, hypotension, and leukocytosis.

Septicemic plague is a systemic infection caused by direct inoculation of *Y. pestis* into the bloodstream or secondarily from untreated bubonic disease. Patients with septicemic plague initially have nausea, vomiting, and diarrhea. Skin lesions, gangrene, and necrosis often develop later in the disease process.

Rapid diagnosis is essential to reduce plague mortality. In the absence of appropriate antibiotic therapy, plague illness can rapidly progress and cause death within several days. Plague exposure is treated with antibiotics. As with anthrax, the CDC should be consulted for the latest treatment and postexposure prophylaxis recommendations. Infection control for bubonic and septicemic forms of plague disease consists of standard precautions. Pneumonic plague requires droplet isolation until at least 48 hours of appropriate antibiotic therapy. For all forms of plague disease, aerosol-generating surgical procedures should be avoided, including autopsy. If required, these procedures should be accomplished in a negative-pressure room. An N-95 respirator also is required for these procedures. Only standard cleaning of patient rooms and handling of linens are necessary.

Tularemia

Francisella tularensis is a hardy, highly infectious organism. Exposure to as few as 10 organisms can result in **tularemia,** also known as *rabbit fever* or *deer fly fever.* Inhalation of *F. tularensis* typically results in flulike symptoms after a 2- to 5-day incubation period. However, the onset of symptoms can occur within 1 day or as long as 14 days after exposure. The clinical presentation may include the rapid onset of fever, chills, myalgia, weakness, and headaches. In addition, these symptoms may progress to a nonproductive cough; sore throat; and inflammation of the bronchi, lungs, and lymph nodes.

Tularemia is treated with antibiotics. As with the other bioterrorism agents, consult the CDC for the latest treatment recommendations. Even though *F. tularensis* is highly infectious for individuals directly exposed to the organism, it is not spread from person to person. Standard precautions are adequate to protect healthcare workers and limit the risk of nosocomial infections.

Botulism

Clostridium botulinum is the only toxin listed as one of the six category A biologic agents by the CDC. Foodborne **botulism** is the most frequently occurring form of the disease. It results from ingesting foods that have been contaminated with *C. botulinum* and therefore contain the resulting toxin. Wound botulism occurs when *C. botulinum* infects the site of a wound, multiplies, and releases the toxin, causing illness. Infant or adult intestinal botulism also may occur. Three forms of the disease described occur naturally. Inhalational botulism does not occur naturally and is the most likely form expected from an aerosol release of botulinum toxin. The onset of botulism after exposure depends on the quantity and duration of the exposure. Initial symptoms include double or blurred vision and dryness of the mouth. The larger exposures may include progression of symptoms to include slurred speech, difficulty swallowing, and bilateral descending peripheral muscle weakness and paralysis. Severe disease may involve the respiratory muscles, leading to respiratory failure and death.

Treatment for botulism includes rapid administration of antitoxin and supportive care, including aggressive respiratory monitoring and support. The efficacy of the antitoxin therapy depends on how early it is initiated in the course of illness. Administration of antitoxin also involves either finding out what the specific serotype is or administering the trivalent antitoxin available through the CDC. Local hospitals do not have this on hand, so protocols and plans must be in place to address the issue of how to obtain it when it is needed. Therefore the local response must include well-trained providers with a high index of suspicion and a logistical system to deliver antitoxin rapidly where it is needed. Because botulinum is a toxin and not an infectious organism, person-to-person transmission does not occur and only standard precautions are needed. Exposed skin and clothing may be cleaned with soap and water.

Viral Hemorrhagic Fevers

Viral hemorrhagic fevers (VHFs) are caused by a number of viruses from the Arenavirus, Filovirus, Bunyavirus, and Flavivirus families. Included in these viral families are the organisms that cause diseases such as **Ebola, Marburg,** Rift Valley, and **Lassa fevers.** After a VHF aerosol release, an incubation period occurs ranging from 2 to 21 days depending on the pathogen used. Those exposed normally have a flulike prodromal illness of less than 1 week, including symptoms such as high fever, headache, malaise, myalgias, nausea, and bloody diarrhea. Severe cases may then show signs of bleeding from bodily orifices, under the skin, and in internal organs and progress to shock and multiorgan failure. Diagnosis is initially based on the clinical criteria and requires a high index of suspicion. Treatment options for VHFs are also limited and primarily consist of supportive care with close monitoring of blood pressure, maintenance of fluid balance and circulatory volume, and ventilatory support as needed. Although ribavirin may offer some benefit for certain kinds of VHFs, no approved antiviral drugs are available for treatment of these diseases. Given the inordinate risk posed by these organisms to healthcare workers, strict adherence to infection control precautions is essential. These recommendations include patient isolation in a negative-pressure room; strict hand hygiene; and use of double gloves, impermeable gown, face shield, eye protection, and leg and shoe coverings. In addition, an air-purifying respirator with a high-efficiency particulate air respiratory protection should be worn by anyone entering the patient room.

Radiologic Agents

Simple Radiologic Device

[OBJECTIVE 11]

A simple radiologic device could be a hidden radioactive source (usually a **gamma** source) placed in a heavily populated or congested area. It can consist of any material or combination of materials that spontaneously emit ionizing radiation. Potential sources include hospital radiation therapy (cobalt-60, cesium-137); nuclear power fuel rods (uranium-235, plutonium); and sources from universities, laboratories, and radiography (cobalt-60, cesium-137, iridium-192, radium-226). Patients exposed to electromagnetic radiation sources emitting gamma rays become irradiated. These patients are not contaminated and do not pose a secondary contamination risk. Conversely, exposure to particle radiation sources (**alpha** and **beta particles,** neutrons, protons, and positrons) in the form of dusts, liquids, or gases contaminates the patient and presents a secondary contamination risk unless properly handled.

Radiologic Dispersal Devices or Weapons

A radiologic dispersal device, sometimes called a **dirty bomb,** is designed to spread **radioactive** material contaminating patients, structures, and terrain. Unlike a nuclear weapon, it does not release radioactivity in a massive burst of energy. Radioactive contaminants can be delivered by a variety of means. A common device consists of a radioactive source and a conventional explosive. Potential sources for the radioactive component of these devices include all the sources listed above. The advantage of these devices is that nuclear technology is not required. Although a radiologic dispersal device may cause traumatic injuries as a result of the conventional explosion, their primary value is the psychological effect on patients and the need to carry out extensive structural decontamination procedures. Patients may be contaminated by the radiologic material and require decontamination.

In cases involving a dirty bomb, initial injuries will result from the blast effect of the conventional explosive. If patients accumulate a large enough dose through ingestion, inhalation, or exposure, radiation sickness may occur. With a simple radiologic device, the effects will be the delayed signs of radiation exposure. Radiation ionizes atoms, resulting in damage to the genetic material in the cells. Cells with high metabolic turnover rates such as those in the gastrointestinal tract and blood system are affected the most. Massive radiation exposures may result in extensive neurologic and gastrointestinal damage. Loss of bone marrow function also may occur with resulting immunocompromise and systemic infection. Soluble radioactive compounds may cause local symptoms as well. Products may act as carcinogens. Most symptoms from radioactive product exposure are delayed; treat other medical or trauma problems according to normal protocols. An accurate history of the exposure is essential to determine risk and proper treatment modalities. The dose of radiation determines the type and clinical course of exposure, as follows:

- 100 rads: Gastrointestinal symptoms (nausea, vomiting, abdominal cramps, diarrhea); symptom onset within hours.
- 600 rads: Severe gastrointestinal symptoms (necrotic gastroenteritis); may result in dehydration and death within a few days.
- Several thousand rads: Neurologic and cardiovascular symptoms (confusion, lethargy, ataxia, seizures, coma, cardiovascular collapse) within minutes to hours. Bone marrow depression, leukopenia, and infections usually follow severe exposures.

Acute radiation syndrome is a condition that occurs in the following four phases as the patient's illness progresses to either recovery or death:

- *Prodromal phase.* This initial phase of acute illness typically lasts 1 to 2 days and, depending on the dose, ranges from undetectable to generalized flulike symptoms, changes in skin sensation, and skin burns.
- *Latent phase.* A dormant period in which no symptoms occur, this phase may last from a few hours to weeks depending on the severity of the dose.
- *Manifest illness phase.* Severity of the exposure is revealed during this phase. Organs that have been affected and laboratory values demonstrate the level of damage.
- *Recovery or death.* The patient either recovers or dies. Both of the last two phases may be affected by rapid intervention and acute intensive care treatment.

Immediate rescue and lifesaving care are of primary importance, taking all reasonable precautions to avoid contact with the radioactive materials and their containers. The time responders spend in any potentially contaminated area should be guided by experts and contamination assessment findings.

For simple radiologic devices, most patients are away from the source of exposure and do not require decontamination. If a particulate source was used in the form of a dust or liquid, decontamination is required. Experts and contamination assessment techniques should guide the need for individual patient decontamination.

With dirty bombs, small numbers of patients with life-threatening injuries and particle or liquid exposure should have their clothing, jewelry, and shoes quickly removed and isolated. The patients should be treated and secured by using reverse isolation procedures such as transportation bags, plastic, or blankets. This helps prevent the spread of contamination during transport. Provide adequate ambulance ventilation (intake and exhaust fans of proper size). Use adequate personal protective equipment. Notify the emergency department that a potentially contaminated patient is en route and supply the staff with all available information concerning the identity and nature of the contaminant. In mass casualty cases, the number of contaminated patients will quickly overwhelm the available resources if field decontamination is not carried out. In these cases, follow standard field patient decontamination protocols.

Care for traumatic injuries and symptomatic treatment should be conducted in the field. For in-hospital therapy, chelating agents or pharmacologic blocking drugs (potassium iodine, diethylenetriamine pentaacetic acid, dimercaprol [British antilewisite], sodium bicarbonate, Prussian blue, calcium gluconate, ammonium chloride, barium sulfate, sodium alginate, d-penicillamine) may be useful if given before or immediately after exposure to radiation.

Assistance and advice on patient care concerns may be obtained from the Oak Ridge Radiation Emergency Assistance Center and Training Site 24 hours a day by calling 615-576-3131 or 615-481-1000, ext. 1502 or pager 241.

Nuclear Devices

The physical effects of a nuclear weapon detonation are blast, thermal radiation, and nuclear radiation (Figure 66-12). The effects depend on the size (yield) of the weapon, its physical design, and how the weapon is used (air, surface, or subsurface burst). An enhanced radiation weapon is designed to concentrate a much greater portion of the total energy release into neutrons and x-rays than a comparably sized standard nuclear weapon. Thus an enhanced radiation weapon produces less thermal radiation but much greater nuclear radiation. Significant prompt radiation occurs only within the area of severe blast damage for ground bursts. Radiation from a large enhanced radiation weapon exploded above the surface would cause radiation injuries beyond the blast-damaged area. Fallout and residual radiation is a hazard for survivors, rescuers, and medical response personnel.

The altitude at which a nuclear weapon is detonated determines the relative damage of blast, heat, and nuclear radiation.

Air Burst

An air burst is an explosion from the weapon being detonated in air at an altitude below 30 km but high enough that the fireball does not make contact with the ground. An air burst causes significant structural damage, skin burns, and eye injuries. A significant, initial radiation hazard and some neutron-induced activity may be present near ground zero. Fallout hazard is minimal with an air burst.

Surface Burst

A surface burst is detonated on or slightly above the earth surface, and the fireball touches the land or water surface. In the area affected by the blast, thermal radiation and initial nuclear radiation are less extensive than for an air burst of similar yield. Extensive damage and cratering will be present at ground zero. Radioactive fallout will be a hazard over a much larger downwind area than that affected by the blast and thermal radiation.

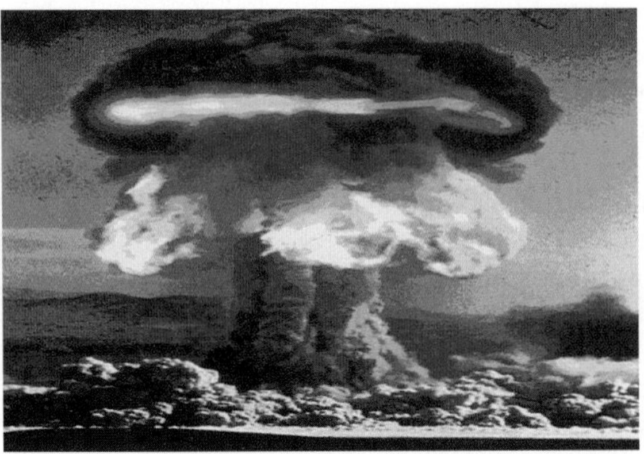

Figure 66-12 Nuclear explosion.

Subsurface Burst

Detonated beneath the surface of the land or water, a subsurface burst produces cratering. If the burst does not penetrate the surface, the only other hazard will be from ground and water shock. If the surface is penetrated by the blast, thermal, and initial radiation effects will occur. Local fallout also will be heavy.

High-Altitude Burst

A high-altitude burst above 30 km is designed to create significant ionization of the upper atmosphere, causing an intense electromagnetic pulse. This would affect equipment, instrumentation, and monitors, disrupting communications and patient care.

A nuclear detonation will result in the generation of four types of ionizing radiation: neutron, gamma, beta, and alpha. Neutrons and gamma rays characterize the initial burst, whereas the residual radiation is primarily alpha, beta, and gamma rays. There may also be neutron-induced radioactive material in a small area around ground zero. In most cases, blast and thermal effects will far outnumber radiation injuries. Nuclear detonation is accompanied by an electromagnetic pulse that will greatly affect operations by interfering with electronic medical equipment. This happens immediately after the blast and should not affect units arriving later.

Most injuries will be from the thermal and blast effects of the weapon. Massive radiation exposures may result in extensive neurologic and gastrointestinal damage. Loss of bone marrow function also may occur with resulting immunocompromise and systemic infection. Soluble radioactive compounds may cause local symptoms as well. Products also may act as carcinogens.

Explosive Agents

[OBJECTIVE 12]

Explosives and incendiaries have been the terrorist weapon of choice for many reasons. The components and instructions for bomb making are readily available. The effects of bombs are immediate and attention getting. Improvised explosive devices are relatively easy to make and hard to detect. They can range from small devices that can be concealed in a letter or package to a car or large truck bomb. A common terrorist tactic when using explosive devices is to plant secondary devices timed to explode after emergency personnel arrive at the scene. Always be alert for any unusual or suspicious objects at the emergency scene.

Four different injury classes are commonly seen from blast scenarios: primary, secondary, tertiary, and quaternary injuries.

Primary Blast Injury

[OBJECTIVE 13]

When detonated, explosive devices turn from a solid into a superheated gas in 1/10,000 of a second. These gases expand at a rate of 13,000 mph (mach 17.6). After the device explodes, waves of pressure are sent out from the seat of the blast called *blast waves*. These are the first to cause injury to patients by smashing and shattering anything in the way. The following four main target organs and organ systems are affected by this primary blast injury wave:

- Ears: specifically tympanic membrane rupture, leading to difficulties in communication. Patient may report ringing in their ears and be overly anxious.
- Lungs: hemothorax, affecting the patient's ability to breathe.
- Gastrointestinal system: as ruptured abdominal hollow organs that can lead to sepsis and hemorrhage.
- Central nervous system: caused by systemic air embolism.

Secondary Blast Injury

Secondary blast injuries are caused by shrapnel from the fragments of the device and from things that have been attached to the explosive device. This trauma is like any other penetrating trauma. The patient also may have bruising, bleeding, fractured extremities, and shock.

Tertiary Blast Injuries

Tertiary blast injuries are caused by the patient being thrown like a projectile. The injuries are similar to injuries seen from falls and motor vehicle accidents and treatment is the same. These patients also may have primary and secondary blast injuries.

Quaternary Blast Injuries

Quaternary blast injuries are all the other injuries caused by the incident. These can include burns, psychological injuries, and crush syndrome. Every incident involving explosive devices should be evaluated for the presence of radiation, chemical, or biologic agents.

Quinary Blast Injuries

Quinary blast injuries are those that occur as a result of additives to the explosive device and their associated health effects. These include radiation, chemicals, and microorganisms such as bacteria. With the increase in suicide bombings worldwide, biohazards have been added to this category. This occurs when human remains of the suicide bomber, such as shards of bone, become embedded in victims.

Incendiary devices are designed to burst into flames or start fires. The most popular incendiary device throughout history has been the Molotov cocktail. It is simply a glass bottle filled with gasoline or other flammable liquid. A fuel soaked rag is used to plug the bottle. The rag is ignited and the bottle thrown at the target. The bottle breaks on impact, igniting the fuel and spreading the fire. Incendiary devices cause typical burn injuries.

Case Scenario SUMMARY

1. *Define the National Response Plan.* The federal response to disasters is managed by the NRP, which describes the structure and processes that comprise a national approach to domestic incident management. It is designed to join the efforts and resources of federal, state, local, tribal, private sector, and nongovernmental organizations. The NRP includes planning assumptions, roles and responsibilities, concept of operations, incident management actions, and plan maintenance. It represents a concerted national effort to accomplish the following:
   - Prevent terrorist attacks within the United States
   - Reduce America's vulnerability to terrorism, major disasters, and other emergencies
   - Minimize the damage from attacks, major disasters, and other emergencies
   - Facilitate recovery from domestic incidents that occur

Continued

Case Scenario SUMMARY—continued

The NRP applies a functional approach that groups the capabilities of federal departments and agencies as well as the American Red Cross into ESFs, which provide the planning, support, resources, program implementation, and emergency services most likely to be needed during major incidents. The federal response to these incidents is typically provided through the full or partial activation of the ESF structure as necessary. The activation of this plan ensures that support agencies will be coordinated. This provides assistance from a national level and gains awareness for this event.

2. *What is a disaster medical assistance team?* DMATs are field-deployable hospital teams that include physicians, nurses, emergency medical technicians, and other medical and nonmedical support personnel. Specialty DMAT teams concentrate on areas such as burns, pediatrics, and mental health concerns. Hospitals may have similar teams that are smaller in nature but are available to help in such disasters.
3. *What is an incident command system?* The ICS is designed to focus the actions of all responders on safely and efficiently mitigating an incident. It is designed for use in all incidents, regardless of type or size. The use of ICS principles in small, routine incidents serves as practice to ensure that the system works when needed. It is organized in a modular format. It should be a top-down organizational structure that can be used for any incident. Modules are typically organized according to function, with five primary functional areas or sections. These five functional areas include command, operations, planning, logistics, and finance and administration. Each functional area is recognized in any implementation of the ICS; however, each area does not require independent staffing. In a small incident, one person may be responsible for several functions. As the incident expands, so does the ICS, with an individual in charge of each area.

   The ICS provides an organized, uniform format that ensures that all agencies, regardless of their place of origin, will work cohesively during a disaster. This system assigns one commander, with all others assigned to a subgroup of this command.
4. *What is the Federal Emergency Management Agency?* FEMA has field teams known as *urban search and rescue teams* that specialize in the location, rescue, and initial medical stabilization of victims trapped in confined spaces resulting from structural collapse and other incidents. They are considered multiple-hazard teams that may respond to a variety of disasters, including earthquakes, hurricanes, tornadoes, floods, terrorist attacks, and hazardous materials releases.
5. *Where should the police, FEMA, and DMAT report to in the ICS?* The operations section is responsible for managing all tactical operations at the incident. This section is coordinated by the operations section chief, who reports to the IC. Depending on the incident, fire control, police operations, public works, and EMS and hazardous materials team activities may all report to the operations section chief.
6. *Who is in charge of the construction equipment location and the Red Cross?* The logistics section is responsible for locating, organizing, and providing facilities, services, and materials needed for mitigation of the incident. This section is coordinated by the logistics section chief, who reports to the IC.
7. *Who is in charge of the media?* The media may need to report to logistics. Often a specific public relations person is identified and is the primary contact for the media.
8. *What is a unified command?* The unified command concept is used when a number of agencies have an overall responsibility to the incident. Senior representatives from each involved agency comprise the unified command group, which makes the decisions regarding the goals, objectives, and priorities for the response to the incident. The concept of unified command still requires a leader. The agency with the current incident focus usually takes the lead of the unified command group. In this scenario, a structure and planes have exploded. This will involve the fire department, confined rescue and tactical rescue personnel, FEMA, the Federal Bureau of Investigation, EMS, DMAT, Transportation Security Agency, police, hazardous materials, and government officials. The leaders of these of these organizations will participate in the unified command. The IC will be one of these individuals.
9. *What is a command post?* The establishment of a **command post** is an important benchmark. It is the location from which incident operations are directed. At small incidents, this may be the car of a senior officer. At larger incidents a specially designed mobile command post, command tent, or even a nearby structure may be used. Only one incident command post is used at an incident. It is usually marked with a green flag or light. In large or complex incidents, an emergency operations center may be established to support the IC.
10. *What is a consolidated response plan?* A plan is necessary when responding to any type of emergency. Each responding agency as well as the local, county, and state government will all have response plans. Coordination of these plans must be handled as a preplanning concern. These plans can help identify who will be responsible for each aspect of the incident. They also can assist with obtaining resources during the emergency.

    Disaster drills are typically held once every 1 to 2 years in communities so that responding personnel are familiar with the response plan. This adds structure and eliminates confusion.

Chapter Summary

- A response to a disaster tests every part of the EMS system. These situations mandate that the paramedic use skills usually practiced only in drills and exercises.
- The response to a natural disaster may force medical personnel to operate for extended periods in an austere environment.
- The response to technologic disasters may place the paramedic in an unsafe situation.
- The threat of WMD is always present.
- Responders must be able to recognize these events and respond appropriately.
- Responders should have a working knowledge of the different types of WMD expected to be used.

REFERENCES

Centers for Disease Control and Prevention. (2000). *Critical biological agents for public health preparedness.* Atlanta, GA: Centers for Disease Control and Prevention.

Pavlin, J. A. (1999). *Epidemiology of bioterrorism.* Washington, DC: Walter Reed Army Institute of Research.

Rotz, L., Khan, A., Lillibridge, S. R., Ostroff, M., & Hughes, J. M. (2000). *Public health assessment of potential biological terrorism agents.* Retrieved August 9, 2008, from http://www.cdc.gov.

Ryan, J., Mahoney, P. F., Greaves, I., Bowyer, G., et al. (Eds.). (2002). *Conflict and catastrophe medicine: A practical guide.* London: Springer-Verlag London Limited.

SUGGESTED RESOURCES

American Hospital Association. *Emergency readiness:* http://www.aha.org.

American Medical Association
Center for Public Health Preparedness and Disaster Response
515 N. State Street
Chicago, IL 60610
Phone: 800-621-8335
Website: http://www.ama-assn.org/go/DisasterPreparedness

Association for Professionals in Infection Control and Epidemiology. *Bioterrorism resources:* http://www.apic.org.

Briggs, S. M., Brinsfield, K. H., et al. (Eds.). (2003). *Advanced disaster medical response: Manual for providers.* Boston: Harvard Medical International Trauma & Disaster Institute.

Centers for Disease Control and Prevention. *Emergency preparedness and response:* http://www.bt.cdc.gov.

Currance, P. L., & Bronstein, A. C. (1995). *Hazardous materials for EMS.* St. Louis: Mosby–Year Book.

Currance, P. L., Clements, B., & Bronstein, A. C. (2005). *Emergency care for hazardous materials exposure* (3rd ed.). St. Louis: Mosby.

Currance, P. L. (2005). *Medical response to weapons of mass destruction.* St. Louis: Mosby.

Department of Homeland Security. *National domestic preparedness:* http://www.ojp.usdoj.gov.

MedlinePlus health topic on anthrax: http://www.nlm.nih.gov/medlineplus/anthrax.html.

MedlinePlus health topic on smallpox: http://www.nlm.nih.gov/medlineplus/smallpox.html.

Saint Louis University School of Public Health, Institute for Biosecurity: http://www.bioterrorism.slu.edu.

State of Wisconsin. *Hospital disaster plan:* http://www.dhfs.state.wi.us.

United States Army Medical Research Institute of Chemical Defense: http://chemdef.apgea.army.mil.

United States Army Medical Research Institute of Chemical Defense. Chemical Casualty Care Division: http://ccc.apgea.army.mil.

United States Army Medical Research Institute of Infectious Diseases. *Education and training:* http://www.usamriid.army.mil.

University of Alabama. *Bioterrorism and emerging infections education:* http://www.bioterrorism.uab.edu.

World Health Organization. *Epidemic and pandemic alert and response:* http://www.who.int/csr/en.

Chapter Quiz

1. In the past, the most common terrorist weapon has been _____.
  a. chemical weapons
  b. biologic weapons
  c. radiologic weapons
  d. explosives

2. A secondary device is ________.
  a. a type of detonator
  b. an additional device set up to harm emergency responders
  c. a type of high explosive that needs a primary detonator
  d. a second liquid that makes an incendiary device burn faster

3. A dirty bomb is an explosive device laced with a ________.
  a. fertilizer
  b. biologic agent
  c. chemical agent
  d. radioactive isotope

4. Primary blast injuries could include ________.
  a. eardrum damage
  b. lung damage
  c. gastrointestinal damage
  d. central nervous system damage
  e. all of the above

Chapter Quiz—continued

5. The four phases of illness associated with whole-body irradiation include all the following except a ________.
a. prodromal phase
b. symptom phase
c. latent phase
d. manifest illness phase
e. recovery phase or death

6. True or False: A dirty bomb would likely cause massive destruction and injuries.

7. All the following are bacterial weapons except ________.
a. anthrax
b. plague
c. smallpox
d. tularemia

8. True or False: Some biologic agent illnesses can be prevented by vaccination.

9. Which of the following diseases have potential for person-to-person transmission?
a. Inhalational anthrax and pneumonic plague
b. Pneumonic plague and botulism
c. Botulism and bubonic plague
d. Smallpox and pneumonic plague

10. Tabun, sarin, soman, and VX are examples of ________.
a. blood agents
b. nerve agents
c. vesicants or blister agents
d. pulmonary agents

11. Chemicals that produce burnlike injuries to the skin are known as ________.
a. blood agents
b. nerve agents
c. vesicants or blister agents
d. pulmonary agents

12. True or False: Exposure to mustard agent results in immediate blistering of unprotected skin.

13. Which is *not* an antidote for exposure to nerve agents?
a. Atropine
b. Diazepam
c. Epinephrine
d. 2-PAM

14. What is the one position of the ICS that will always be filled at every incident?
a. Staging
b. Operations
c. IC
d. Planning

15. Which one of the concepts below is not part of the ICS standard operating procedure?
a. Span of control
b. Integrated communications
c. Consolidated response plan
d. use of 10 codes

16. An ICS should be implemented ________.
a. only when federal agencies are involved
b. at all incidents regardless of the size
c. only when patients are involved
d. only when the incident involves fire departments
e. only when directed to do so by the Federal Bureau of Investigation

17. The ICS functional area responsible for obtaining resources needed for incident management is ________.
a. operations
b. finance
c. safety
d. logistics
e. planning

18. At a hazardous materials or WMD incident, EMS responders primarily work under the ________,
a. operations section
b. planning section
c. finance and administration section
d. logistics section

19. What is the first priority when responding to a manmade or natural disaster?
a. Patient assessment
b. Chemical evaluation
c. Ensuring responder safety
d. Notification of receiving hospital

20. A WMD may consist of ________.
a. biologic agents
b. chemical agents
c. explosives
d. radioactivity
e. all the above

Terminology

Alpha particle A positively charged particle emitted by certain radioactive materials.

Anthrax An acute bacterial infection caused by inhalation, contact, or ingestion of *Bacillus anthracis* organisms. Three forms of anthrax disease may occur depending on the route of exposure. Inhalational anthrax disease occurs after the inhalation of anthrax spores. Cutaneous anthrax disease is the most common form and occurs after the exposure of compromised skin to anthrax spores. Gastrointestinal anthrax disease occurs after the ingestion of live *B. anthracis* in contaminated meat.

Bacillus anthracis Gram-positive, spore-forming bacteria that cause anthrax disease in human beings and animals.

Bacteremia The presence of bacteria in the blood; fever, chills, tachycardia, and tachypnea are common manifestations of bacteremia.

Beta particle A negatively charged particle emitted by certain radioactive materials.

Biologic agent A disease-causing pathogen or a toxin that may be used as a weapon to cause disease or injury to people.

Blister agent A chemical used as a weapon designed specifically to injure the body tissue internally and externally of those exposed to its vapors or liquid; the method of injury is to cause painful skin blisters or tissue destruction of the exposed surface area (e.g., mustard, lewisite).

Blood agents Chemicals absorbed into the body through the action of breathing, skin absorption, or ingestion (e.g., hydrogen cyanide, cyanogen chloride).

Botulism A severe neurologic illness caused by a potent toxin produced by the *Clostridium botulinum* organism; the three forms are foodborne, wound, and intestinal (also called *infant*) botulism.

Bubonic Relating to an inflamed, enlarged lymph gland.

Chloracetophenone Tear gas; commercially known as Mace.

Choking agent An industrial chemical used as a weapon to kill those who inhale the vapors or gases; the method of injury is asphyxiation resulting from lung damage from hydrochloric acid burns (e.g., chlorine, phosgene); also known as a *pulmonary agent*.

Clostridium botulinum Bacteria that produce a powerful toxin that causes botulism disease in human beings, waterfowl, and cattle.

Command post The location from which incident operations are directed.

Contamination The deposition or absorption of chemical, biologic, or radiologic materials onto personnel or other materials.

Cyanogen chloride A highly toxic blood agent.

Dirty bomb A conventional explosive device used as a radiologic agent dispersal device.

Disaster Medical Assistance Team (DMAT) Field-deployable hospital teams that include physicians, nurses, emergency medical technicians, and other medical and nonmedical support personnel.

Disaster Mortuary Operations Teams Teams composed of forensic and mortuary professionals trained to deal with human remains after disaster situations.

Ebola A viral hemorrhagic fever illness caused by the Ebola virus (Filovirus family); seen mostly in Africa; transmitted by person-to-person contact with body fluids of infected individuals; no specific treatment is available, and it often is fatal within several days.

Explosive Any chemical compound, mixture, or device, the primary or common purpose of which is to function by detonation or rapid combustion (i.e., with substantial instantaneous release of gas and heat); found in liquid or solid forms (e.g., dynamite, TNT, black powder, fireworks, ammunition).

Francisella tularensis A hardy, slow-growing, highly infectious, aerobic organism; human infection may result in tularemia, also known as *rabbit fever* or *deer fly fever.*

Fulminant Sudden, intense occurrence.

Gamma A type of electromagnetic radiation.

Hospital Incident Command System An emergency management system that uses a logical management structure, defined responsibilities, clear reporting channels, and a common nomenclature to help unify hospitals with other emergency responders.

Hydrogen cyanide A highly toxic blood agent.

Incendiary device A device designed to ignite a fire.

Incident commander (IC) The person responsible for the overall management of an emergency scene.

International medical surgical response teams Specialty surgical teams that can respond both in the United States and internationally.

Lassa fever A viral hemorrhagic fever illness caused by the Lassa virus (Arenavirus family).

Marburg A viral hemorrhagic fever illness caused by the Marburg virus (Filovirus family).

Mark 1 antidote kit Self-injected nerve agent antidote kit consisting of atropine and 2-PAM.

Miosis Constricted pupils.

National Disaster Medical System A systemic response that includes field units, coordination of patient transportation, and provision of hospital beds. The field component is composed of many volunteer teams of medical professionals.

National Medical Response Team Quick response specialty teams trained and equipped to provide mass casualty decontamination and patient care after

Terminology—continued

the release of a chemical, biologic, or radiologic agent.

National Veterinary Response Team (NVRT) Teams designed to provide animal care and assistance during disasters.

Plague An acute infectious disease caused by anaerobic, gram-negative bacteria *Yersinia pestis;* transmitted naturally from rodents to human beings through flea bites; three common syndromes are bubonic (most likely form of the disease to be seen from naturally occurring infections), pneumonic (most likely form of the disease to result from an act of terrorism), and septicemic plague.

Prodromal An early symptom of a disease.

Radioactive The ability to emit ionizing radioactive energy.

Secondary device An additional explosive or other type of device specifically designed to harm personnel responding to the emergency.

SLUDGE-BBM Mnemonic for ***s***alivation, ***l***acrimation, ***u***rination, ***d***efecation, ***g***astrointestinal pain, ***e***mesis, ***b***radycardia, ***b***ronchoconstriction, and ***m***iosis.

Smallpox A disease caused by variola viruses, which are members of the Orthopoxvirus family; eradicated in the 1970s but still remains a threat as a bioterrorism agent.

Sulfur mustard The most well known and commonly used vesicant.

Surge capacity The ability to expand care based on a sudden mass casualty incident developed in the emergency management plan.

Tularemia A disease resulting from infection of *Francisella tularensis;* normally transmitted through handling infected small mammals such as rabbits or rodents or through the bites of ticks, deerflies, or mosquitoes that have fed on infected animals; also known as *rabbit fever* or *deer fly fever.*

Variola major A member of the Orthopoxvirus family that causes the most common form of smallpox; the most likely form of the organism to be used as a weapon.

Vesicants Agents named from the most obvious injury they inflict on a person; will burn and blister the skin or any other part of the body they touch; also known as *blister agents* or *mustard agents*.

Viral hemorrhagic fevers (VHFs) A group of viral diseases of diverse etiology (arenaviruses, filoviruses, bunyaviruses, and flaviviruses) having many similar characteristics, including increased capillary permeability, leukopenia, and thrombocytopenia, resulting in a severe multisystem syndrome.

Yersinia pestis The anaerobic, gram-negative bacteria that cause plague disease in human beings and rodents.

APPENDIX A

Quiz Answers

CHAPTER 35

1. An ectopic pregnancy occurs outside the uterus, most commonly in the fallopian tube. Ectopic pregnancies cause bleeding and pain as they grow and can eventually rupture through the wall of the fallopian tube, causing life-threatening bleeding. Ectopic pregnancies are diagnosed in the first trimester of pregnancy, sometimes before a woman even knows she is pregnant. They may appear with vaginal bleeding, abdominal pain, or both.

2. Seizures in pregnancy should initially be managed the same as for the nonpregnant patient. This includes management of the airway, including rescue position, airway maneuvers, airway devices as necessary, and supplemental oxygen. If protocols allow, consider IV access, administration of benzodiazepines, and intubation if indicated. In the pregnant patient, however, any seizure in the second half of pregnancy should be assumed to be eclampsia until proved otherwise. Eclampsia is a condition unique to pregnancy that can lead to strokes and death if not rapidly controlled. The seizures of eclampsia do not respond well to benzodiazepines, and magnesium sulfate, 4 to 6 g IV, is the drug of choice.

3. Placenta previa and abruptio placentae are the two most common causes of vaginal bleeding in the third trimester. Placenta previa occurs when the placenta implants over the cervical opening. It can lead to painless bright red blood from the vagina. Abruptio placentae is separation of a part of the placenta away from the wall of the uterus. It classically presents as darker vaginal bleeding accompanied by cramping abdominal pain.

4. 500 mL of blood loss is considered normal after a vaginal delivery. Excessive bleeding can be controlled with uterine massage or by having the mother breastfeed her infant. Both maneuvers cause the uterus to contract, thereby slowing bleeding. As for any patient with active hemorrhage, IV access and volume replacement, initially with normal saline or lactated Ringer's solution, is critical.

5. Stage I is from the onset of cervical dilation until the cervix is completely dilated. It is accompanied by contractions that steadily increase in frequency and duration. Stage II is from the time the cervix is fully dilated until expulsion of the fetus from the birth canal. During this stage the mother usually feels a strong urge to push. Stage III is from the delivery of the infant until delivery of the placenta.

6. The contents of an obstetric kit should include gown, gloves, mask, and protective eyewear for the delivery attendant. The kit should also include clean towels, blankets, a bulb syringe, two plastic umbilical cord clamps, gauze sponges, one pair of scissors, and a container for the placenta.

7. In the left lateral recumbent position, the mother is placed on her left side, with pillows or blankets to support the hips, back, and abdomen as needed. This position decreases pressure from the uterus on the inferior vena cava and thus increases venous return to the heart.

8. For a breech presentation, the hips and legs are often born spontaneously. As the hips appear, gently grasp the infant over the bony part of the pelvis to help guide the body out. Then rotate the torso so that the shoulders are oriented anteriorly to posteriorly. Guide the infant's body upward to allow the posterior shoulder to deliver, then downward to deliver the anterior shoulder. If the head does not deliver shortly, follow steps 1 to 6 as listed in the section on breech presentation to assist the delivery.

9. Cervical spine precautions in a pregnant patient should be placed for the same indications as in the nonpregnant patient. In a patient at more than 20 weeks' gestation who requires cervical spine immobilization, avoid supine hypotensive syndrome by immobilizing the patient on a backboard, then tilting the backboard 30 degrees to the left with blankets or pillows used to elevate the right side of the backboard.

CHAPTER 36

1. **b.** In secondary apnea, a lack of oxygen persists. The newborn takes several gasping respirations. The skin is cyanotic, bradycardia ensues, and blood pressure falls. Gasping ventilations become weaker and then stop (secondary apnea).

2. **c.** Heart rate and ventilatory effort are the most important assessment parameters during resuscitation of the newly born.

3. **c.** Because central and peripheral pulses in the neck and extremities often are difficult to feel in newborns, heart rate should be assessed by auscultating the apical pulse with a stethoscope or palpating the base of the umbilical cord. The umbilical pulse is readily accessible in the newly born and permits assessment of heart rate without interruption of ventilation for auscultation.

4. **d.** The assisted ventilation rate should be 40 to 60 breaths/min and 30 breaths/min when chest compressions are also being delivered.

5. **b.** An Apgar score of 8 is assigned based on the following: some flexion of the extremities (1 point), regular respirations (2 points), blue extremities/pink body (1 point), heart rate greater than 100 beats/min (2 points), and vigorous crying on stimulation (2 points).

6. **d.** *Newly born,* describes the time from the first minute to first hours of life. A neonate (also called a newborn infant) is from this time to 1 month. An infant is from 1 month to 1 year of age.

7. **c.** The history and findings are most consistent with increased intracranial pressure.

8. **b.** Choanal atresia is a narrowing or blockage of one or both nares. A fistula is an abnormal passage, and meningocele is a type of spina bifida.

CHAPTER 37

1. **d.** The pediatric chain of survival represents a sequential series of events to assess, support, or restore effective ventilation and circulation to the child in respiratory or cardiopulmonary arrest. The sequence consists of five important steps: (1) prevention of illness or injury, (2) early cardiopulmonary resuscitation, (3) early EMS activation, (4) rapid advanced life support, and (5) post-cardiac arrest care.

2.

	Croup	Epiglottitis	Bacterial Tracheitis
Age	6 months to 3 years	2 to 7 years	Any age
Cause	Viral	Bacterial	Bacterial
Seasonal preference	Late fall, early winter	None	None
Onset	Gradual	Sudden	Gradual
Fever	Low	High	High
Appearance	Nontoxic	Toxic	Toxic
Posture	No preference	Upright, leaning forward, drooling	Upright
Sore throat	No	Yes	Minimal
Cry	Bark, stridor	Muffled	Bark, stridor

3. In the pediatric patient, dysrhythmias are divided into four broad categories on the basis of heart rate: (1) normal for age, (2) slower than normal for age (bradycardia), (3) faster than normal for age (tachycardia), or (4) absent/pulseless (cardiac arrest).

4. The spleen is the most frequently injured abdominal organ during blunt trauma. The liver is the second most commonly injured solid organ in the pediatric patient with blunt abdominal trauma but the most common cause of lethal hemorrhage.

5. Falls are the single most common cause of injury in children.

6. **a.** If an infant or child is symptomatic because of bradycardia, initial treatment is directed at assessment of the airway and breathing rather than administration of epinephrine, atropine, or other drugs. This is because problems with adequate oxygenation and ventilation are more common in children than are cardiac causes of bradycardia.

7. **c.** Hypovolemia and sepsis are the most common causes of shock in children.

8. *Appearance:* unresponsive to verbal stimuli, limp; *breathing:* increased work of breathing evident; *circulation:* pale.

9. **d.** Pneumonia, asthma, and bronchiolitis are conditions that affect the lower airway. Croup, epiglottitis, and bacterial tracheitis are conditions that affect the upper airway.

10. "Normal" values for a 3-year-old child are as follows:
    - **a.** Ventilatory rate: 24 to 40 breaths/min
    - **b.** Heart rate: 90 to 150 beats/min
    - **c.** Blood pressure: more than 70 mm Hg

CHAPTER 38

1. **b.** Chest pain and shortness of breath account for 25% of EMS responses for elderly people.

2. False. Elderly people's lungs do not have an increased ability for oxygen to cross the membrane into the bloodstream.

3. True. Elderly people who exercise regularly are able to maintain cardiac function much better than their sedentary counterparts.

4. **d.** Risk factors for heart disease in the elderly include diabetes, known coronary disease, and increasing age.

5. **d.** Unintentional injury is the leading cause of nonfatal illness in the elderly population.

6. **c.** As we age, our brains lose volume.

7. **a.** Beta-blockers are generally not well tolerated in patients with chronic obstructive pulmonary disease.

8. **a.** The most serious signs of digoxin toxicity are conduction disturbances and cardiac dysrhythmias.

9. **d.** Metabolic disorder is the most likely cause of delirium.

10. **c.** Poor short-term memory is typical of dementia.

11. **c.** Trauma patients older than 85 years have nine times the mortality rate of patients aged 29 to 65 years.

12. **a.** Decreased lean muscle mass contributes to changes in drug distribution with age.

13. **d.** An elderly patient with head trauma and no apparent neurologic deficits may still have significant intracranial hemorrhage.

14. **a.** Increased vascular resistance leads to hypertension.

CHAPTER 39

1. **d.** The underlying issue with all domestic violence relationships is power and control.

2. **a.** Interpersonal violence is the leading cause of injuries to women between the ages of 15 and 44 years of age.

3. **b.** The abuser commonly appears charming, concerned, and solicitous of the EMS crew.

4. **d.** The cycle of abuse begins with verbal attacks.

5. **c.** Your first consideration is scene safety.

6. **a.** You should consider asking the patient, when alone, if domestic violence is a problem.

7. **c.** The mechanism of injury does not correlate with the injuries observed.

8. **d.** Retinal hemorrhage is the ocular finding associated with shaken baby syndrome.

9. **b.** Elder abuse may be difficult to assess in the prehospital setting because of normal physiologic processes that affect the geriatric population.

10. **c.** Your first priority after your initial conversation is to preserve the crime scene as much as possible while waiting for law enforcement to arrive.

11. **d.** While taking the history from a victim of sexual assault, you should remain as nonjudgmental as possible.

12. **c.** When an EMS crew is dispatched to a crime scene, personal safety must be the first priority.

13. **a.** When considering legal considerations of any case that involves the prehospital environment, the first priority is confidentiality.

CHAPTER 40

1. True. When assessing a patient with a speech impairment, be sure to allow adequate time for the patient to respond to questions.

2. Causes of visual impairment include cataracts; glaucoma; macular problems that result in visual disturbances; degeneration of the eyeball, optic nerve, or nerve pathways; disease (such as diabetes or hypertension); eye or brain injury; infection (such as cytomegalovirus, herpes simplex virus, or bacterial ulcers); and vitamin A deficiency in children living in developing countries.

3. **b.** Conductive deafness is defined as faulty transportation of sound from the outer to the inner ear.

4. Treatment for an obese patient includes obtaining a thorough medical history, using appropriate-size diagnostic devices (such as a large blood pressure cuff), requesting additional staff to assist with moving the patient for transport, being sensitive to patients who are self-conscious about their weight, and maintaining professionalism.

5. True. The presence of a medical identification bracelet or necklace may indicate a special challenge.

6. **a.** The head is placed in a neutral position when performing airway maneuvers on a patient with spina bifida because an Arnold-Chiari malformation may be present.

7. False. You should still explain procedures to a person with a mental illness. Adjust assessment and treatment strategies based on the level of understanding of the patient. Allow extra time to obtain a history and explain procedures whenever possible.

8. Patients with spina bifida are prone to latex allergies. Because of repeated exposure to products containing latex (such as catheters, gloves), children become sensitive to the latex and develop life-threatening allergic reactions. These allergies continue into adulthood.

9. Characteristics of Down syndrome include rounded and small skull, flat occiput, enlarged anterior fontanel; upward slant to eyes with short, sparse eyelashes; flat nasal bridge; protruding tongue; mottled skin; hypotonia; short and broad hands with stubby fingers; shortened rib cage; protruding abdomen; short stature; and reduced birth weight.

10. A vascular access device may be present in a patient requiring repeated blood testing, frequent intravenous medications, or large quantities or concentrations of fluids.

11. **c.** Patients who cannot eat by mouth for whatever reason may be fed through a gastrostomy tube.

12. **c.** Prehospital care for patients with emotional impairments is primarily supportive.

13. Arthritis is the inflammation of a joint.

14. False. It is an inherited metabolic disease of the lungs and digestive system that manifests in childhood.

15. Signs and symptoms of spinal cord involvement in a patient with multiple sclerosis include tingling, numbness, or feeling of constriction in any part of the body; extremities that feel heavy and become weak; and spasticity.

16. **a.** The most common form of muscular dystrophy is Duchenne muscular dystrophy.

17. **a.** A patient with poliomyelitis may require advanced airway support to ensure adequate ventilation.

18. True. A patient with a previous head injury may have cognitive deficits of language, communication, information processing, memory, and perceptual skills.

19. **c.** Myasthenia gravis causes muscles to become weak and tire easily.

20. **b.** False. Not all people identify with their ethnic cultural background.

21. Personal protection should be used on every emergency response.

CHAPTER 41

1. According to statistics, an estimated 760,000 people are homeless in the United States on any given night.

2. True. At least half of the homeless population has a coexisting substance abuse problem.

3. Codependency is defined by the exhibition of too much and often inappropriate caring behavior.

4. True. A codependent person believes he or she is the only one qualified enough to care for a particular individual.

5. Allowing an individual to continue with a persistent problem, often times interfering with that person getting the help they need, is known as enabling behavior.

6. False. Once resettled in the United States, immigrants frequently retain aspects of the culture and civilization they left behind.

7. The most common barrier to providing prehospital care with new residents to the United States is the language barrier.

8. False. The ability to pay for services is not the chief criteria for rendering care in EMS.

CHAPTER 42

1. Types of patients who receive home care include the following:
   - Patients who have mobility problems
   - Patients who have a terminal illness
   - Patients who have a developmental delay
   - Patients who have a congenital condition, such as congenital heart disease
   - Patients recuperating from surgery or an acute illness
   - Transplant candidates
   - Chronically ill infants, children, and adults
   - Maternal/child care
   - Patients who require wound care, enteral nutrition, respiratory therapy, physical therapy, chronic pain management, or home chemotherapy
   - Psychosocial support of the home care family

2. CPAP is the delivery of a steady, gentle flow of air through a soft mask worn over the nose (nasal CPAP) or over the mouth and nose (mask CPAP). BiPAP is a form of noninvasive, mechanical ventilation in which two (bi) levels of positive pressure are delivered: one during inspiration (to keep the airway open as the patient inhales) and the other (lower) pressure during expiration to reduce the work of exhalation.

3. **c.** Listen to breath sounds and then ventilate the patient with a bag-mask device.

4. **c.** Left side with head down.

5. Although many types of vascular access devices exist, they can be classified into one of these four general categories: dialysis shunts, central venous catheters, implanted ports, and peripherally inserted central catheters.

6. ***D***isplaced tube (right mainstem or esophageal intubation) or ***D***isconnection of the tube or ventilator circuit; reassess tube position, ventilator connections

   Obstructed tube (blood or secretions are obstructing air flow); suction

   Pneumothorax (tension); needle thoracostomy

   Equipment problem/failure (empty oxygen source, inadvertent change in ventilator settings, low battery); check equipment and oxygen source

7. False. Placement of an orogastric or nasogastric tube should be checked after insertion, before giving fluids and medications, and again after giving fluids and medications.

CHAPTER 43

1. **c.** Trauma. Trauma is a leading cause of death, second to heart disease, cancer, stroke, and chronic lower respiratory diseases.

2. The paramedic plays a significant role in injury prevention, interfacility transport, and emergency department care.

3. **a.** Level I. Level I trauma centers have requirements for research, patient care, education, and teaching programs.

4. **c.** When transport by ground would cause a significant delay. Transporting 45 minutes by ground versus 5 minutes by air to the facility is not in the patient's best interest.

5. **c.** Four times. As you double the speed you increase the energy fourfold because energy is the square of the velocity.

6. **b.** Predicting injuries. Kinematics is the process of predicting injury patterns based on certain mechanisms.

7. **d.** Down and under. In down and under impact, if the leg impacts at or slightly above the knee, the femur is the site of impact. If the femur hits the dashboard, the likely primary injuries include fractured femur.

8. **d.** New Hampshire.

9. **d.** Laying the bike down. This protective maneuver separates the rider from the motorcycle, allowing the rider to slide away from the object. The rider can sustain injuries, but they are generally less severe than those that can occur from hitting an object while still on the motorcycle.

10. True. An adult turns away from the threat but a child tends to face the threat; therefore the child's injuries most often are frontal in nature.

CHAPTER 44

1. **a.** Tachycardia, hypotension, and narrowed pulse pressure are signs of internal hemorrhage.

2. **a.** Arterial bleeding presents with bright red blood that sprays in a pulsing manner.

3. **c.** Direct pressure is the first step in controlling external hemorrhage.

4. **d.** If the patient has internal bleeding, transport to the closest medical facility will benefit him the most.

5. The difference between controlled and uncontrolled bleeding.

6. Signs and symptoms of internal bleeding include the following:
   - Anxiety, restlessness, combativeness, or altered mental status
   - Weakness, faintness, or dizziness
   - Rapid, shallow breathing (with no other respiratory problems present)
   - Rapid, weak pulse
   - Pale, cool, clammy skin
   - Narrowing pulse pressure
   - Excessive thirst
   - Pain, tenderness, swelling, or discoloration of suspected site of injury
   - Bleeding from the mouth, rectum, vagina, or other body opening
   - Vomiting bright red blood or dark coffee ground–colored blood
   - Coughing up blood
   - Sudden, severe headache
   - Dark, tarry stools (melena) or bloody stools (hematochezia)
   - Tender, rigid, and/or distended abdomen

7. Orthostatic vital signs (also called the *tilt test* or *postural vital signs*) are serial measurements of the patient's pulse and blood pressure with the patient recumbent and then standing. Orthostatic vital signs have been used for many years to assess for possible volume depletion in patients reporting dizziness, lightheadedness, nausea, vomiting, diarrhea, or gastrointestinal bleeding.

CHAPTER 45

1. **c.** Evaluate for underlying life-threatening trauma.

2. Apply a gloved hand to the injury and apply direct pressure. Do not wait to apply pressure to an arterial hemorrhage, even for dressing supplies. By applying pressure immediately you can initiate the clotting process and decrease the amount of blood the patient loses.

3. Compartment syndrome.

4. **b.** Secondary. Terrorists commonly add material to their explosive devices to increase the amount of material/shrapnel that is blasted out of the device. Therefore you would likely see an increase in the injuries common to the secondary effects of the blast.

5. **a.** Removal of a tourniquet. The common mechanism for crush syndrome is crushing force but it can also occur a result of any prolonged hypoxia of tissue, particularly with associated tissue damage from trauma. Tourniquets create both circumstances, and their removal can result in crush syndrome.

6. **b.** Venous.

7. **c.** Sterile, adherent dressings.

8. The large vessels of the neck, in addition to profuse bleeding, may be capable of aspirating air, resulting in emboli. The use of occlusive dressings may prevent this.

9. Their bites are often punctures with less tearing or crushing, as with a dog bite. Puncture wounds are difficult to clean and can penetrate deep into underlying tissue, spreading bacteria.

10. **c.** Diabetes. Diabetic patients are prone to peripheral vascular disease and diabetic neuropathy. Both conditions increase the risk of infection and necrosis from even minor injuries to the extremities, especially the feet.

CHAPTER 46

1. **b.** Epidermis. The layers of the skin from outermost to deepest are epidermis, dermis, subcutaneous.

2. **b.** Thermal. Thermal injuries account for 80% of all burn injuries treated in the United States and Canada. Causes include flame, scald, and contact with hot objects. When combined, chemical, electrical, and radiation burns account for just over 8% of all injuries.

3. False. Burn deaths are relatively rare. The most common cause of death in burn-related trauma is sepsis/infection. However, in large burns, underresuscitation could certainly prove detrimental to outcome.

4. **d.** Zone of coagulation. Extension of burn injury because of improper resuscitation is an important cause of increased morbidity in the burn patient. The innermost zone of injury is where the majority of

the skin damage occurs. This is an area of necrotic tissue lacking blood supply and nerve sensation.

5. **c.** Third degree. The common nomenclature for a full-thickness burn, that is, one involving the entire depth of the dermis, or deeper, is *third degree* burn.

6. False. Because partial-thickness burns do not involve the deeper structures of the dermis, healing without surgery is almost always possible. The cells responsible for skin regeneration come from the deep dermal structures.

7. **c.** 40%. Using the Rule of Nines for adults, the following percentages of body surface area are calculated:
   - Entire left leg: 18%
   - Half of the right arm: 4.5%
   - Anterior trunk: 18%

8. **b.** 32%. Using the pediatric rule of nines, the following body surface area calculations are made:
   - Entire head: 18%
   - Entire leg: 14%

   Recall that the pediatric patient has a disproportionate body surface area compared with an adult.

9. **d.** Lactated Ringer's solution. All relevant research regarding burns thus far points at a balanced salt solution, such as lactated Ringer's solution, as the best choice in the early resuscitation of burns. Normal saline (0.9% sodium chloride solution) may also be used.

10. False. If signs of inhalation injury are noted, and the paramedic is trained to do so, emergent airway control should be obtained. Swelling will continue to worsen and may do so in a very short period. When this happens complete obliteration of normal airway anatomy occurs, making late intubation dangerous, difficult, and potentially impossible.

CHAPTER 47

1. The areas assessed when using the Glasgow Coma Scale are eye opening, motor response, and verbal response.

2. True. A patient who has a traumatic brain injury has a cervical spine injury until proven otherwise.

3. **b.** Dilation of the pupil on the left side. If the oculomotor nerve is compressed, the patient will have dilation of the pupil on the same side as the injury.

4. **a.** Increased intracranial pressure. Increases in intracranial pressure cause characteristic changes in vital signs called Cushing's triad. The triad includes hypertension (often with a widening pulse pressure), bradycardia, and an irregular breathing pattern.

5. True. Permanent scarring always occurs with an alkaline burn of the cornea and sometimes permanent vision loss.

6. **d.** Basilar skull fracture. In patients with a skull fracture, cerebrospinal fluid often is draining from the nose or ear.

7. **a.** Altered mental status, unequal pupils, decreased heart rate, increased blood pressure. As pressure is exerted on brain tissue, the patient will have an altered level of responsiveness, increased blood pressure, bradycardia, and dilation of the pupil on the same side as the injury.

8. False. An injury to the head may or may not result in an injury to the brain.

9. False. Whether to remove a helmet is a controversial subject. Several factors such as fit, spinal immobilization, and airway and breathing need to be considered.

10. **d.** Epidural hematoma. Most epidural hematomas involve arterial bleeding.

CHAPTER 48

1. **a.** Your first action when dealing with a trauma patient is to stabilize the head and neck manually while assessing airway and breathing.

2. **c.** T4.

3. **b.** The spinous process.

4. **c.** Axis.

5. **a.** Has an odontoid process that allows the head to pivot in any direction.

6. **c.** You should straighten the head and neck because it maximizes the vertebral foramen space, giving the spine room to swell. Placing a patient in a neutral position should be performed unless resistance is met because this also allows for a better airway.

7. **b.** Between L1 and L2.

8. **a.** Areas of skin innervated by a single spinal nerve.

9. **c.** Sensation of sharp and soft.

10. **d.** Perform a full spine assessment.

11. **b.** False.

12. **a.** Continue to test motor and sensory skills in all extremities; if they are normal, clear the spine.

13. **d.** After completing the physical examination and managing any distracting injuries.

14. **d.** All the other patients have distracting injuries, significant mechanism of injury, or are unreliable.

15. **b.** A hanging.

16. **c.** Secondary cord injuries.

CHAPTER 49

1. Severe respiratory distress, unilaterally diminished or absent breath sounds, and jugular venous distension.

2. Hypotension, muffled heart tones, and jugular venous distention, which may be found in the setting of acute pericardial tamponade.

3. Sudden deceleration.

4. Flail chest results when three or more adjacent ribs are fractured at two points, allowing a freely moving segment of the chest wall to move in paradoxic motion.

5. A crunching sound heard upon auscultation of the heart, which may be present with tracheobronchial injuries.

6. An open pneumothorax, which is associated with a defect in the chest wall. Air can sometimes be heard flowing in and out of the defect, prompting the term "sucking chest wound."

7. An excessive drop in systolic blood pressure during the inspiratory phase of the normal respiratory cycle, which is associated with the presence of cardiac tamponade.

8. Traumatic asphyxia is a syndrome characterized by a deep purple color of the skin of the head and neck, bilateral subconjunctival hemorrhages, petechiae, and facial edema.

9. Cover the wound with an occlusive dressing of petrolatum gauze taped to the skin on only three sides.

10. False.

CHAPTER 50

1. True. The main cause of morbidity and mortality in abdominal trauma is hemorrhage.

2. True. The two main goals of prehospital care for patients with abdominal trauma are to control hemorrhage and transport the patient rapidly to an appropriate receiving facility.

3. True. Important host factors that may worsen hemorrhage in abdominal trauma include alcohol and medications such as warfarin (Coumadin).

4. True. The superior border of the abdomen is the diaphragm.

5. True. The kidneys, as well as parts of the duodenum, pancreas, and colon, are located retroperitoneally.

6. True. Injuries are described as open if the abdominal contents are exposed to the external environment.

7. True. Abdominal injuries may be subtle, so a high index of suspicion is important when assessing patients with abdominal trauma.

8. True. If the contents of hollow organs spill into the abdominal cavity, peritonitis may result.

9. True. In a car crash the internal organs may continue to move forward after the car has stopped and may be squeezed between the anterior abdominal wall and the spinal column. This is an example of compression force.

10. True. In a car crash the aortic arch may be sheared off as it continues forward while the descending aorta is fixed and stationary. This is an example of shear, or deceleration, force.

11. True. A pedestrian struck by a moving car may likely be injured in three phases. First the car's bumper strikes the patient, then the patient is thrown onto the hood, and the patient finally hits the ground. As a result knee, head, and abdominal injuries often occur.

12. True. Flying objects striking the body because of a nearby explosion are considered secondary blast injuries and are similar to other penetrating injuries.

13. True. The two major factors determining the severity of penetrating abdominal injuries are the region of the abdomen involved and the amount of energy making contact with the body.

14. False. A gunshot wound to the right upper quadrant of the abdomen that exits the right back can reliably be predicted to have injured the liver with little risk of injuring other intraabdominal structures.

15. True. For gunshot wounds the maximal amount of energy that could possibly be applied to the body is the kinetic energy of the projectile, described as mass multiplied by half of the velocity squared.

16. True. Critical findings in the assessment of the victim of abdominal trauma include altered mental status, airway compromise, and shock.

17. True. If critical findings are noted on the initial assessment, the patient should be transported without delay.

18. True. The four parts of the abdominal trauma assessment are described as inspection, auscultation, palpation, and percussion.

19. True. Things to look for during the inspection phase of the abdominal assessment include bruising, bleeding, distension, eviscerations, and the presence of impaled objects.

20. False. The goal of the complete abdominal assessment is to diagnose which specific organ(s) have been injured as a result of abdominal trauma.

21. True. The only effective therapy for most abdominal injuries is surgical intervention. Thus rapid transport to a facility capable of pro-

viding this is the main prehospital treatment for most patients with abdominal trauma.

22. True. While the patient is being transported treatment for shock with intravenous fluids often is indicated.

23. True. PASG may have a role in controlling abdominal hemorrhage and stabilizing pelvic fracture. Local protocol should guide its use.

24. True. Hollow organ injuries result in morbidity and mortality from two causes: hemorrhage and contamination.

25. True. The spleen is the most commonly injured solid organ.

26. True. Improperly worn lap and/or shoulder belts increase the risk of vascular injuries.

27. True. It requires a lot of force to fracture the pelvis. Therefore these injuries often are associated with injuries to the intraabdominal contents and vascular structures as well.

28. True. All penetrating abdominal injuries are critical findings and require rapid transportation to an appropriate receiving facility.

29. False. Impaled objects should be removed and the wound covered to prevent contamination.

30. True. In abdominal evisceration the protruding contents should be covered with a moistened sterile dressing and the patient immediately transported to the hospital.

31. False. The major cause of death in diaphragmatic rupture is severe damage to the diaphragm muscle, impeding respiration and causing herniation and protrusion of the abdominal contents into the thorax.

32. True. Striking the handlebars in a bicycle crash may cause injury to the pancreas as this retroperitoneal structure is compressed against the spinal column.

33. True. Trauma in pregnancy can lead to several problems for both the mother and the baby, including placental abruption and premature labor.

34. True. Women in the later stages of pregnancy should be transported on their left side to avoid having the gravid uterus compress the vena cava.

35. False. Pregnant women should not wear their seat belts because this increases the risk of uterine rupture or placental abruption if they are involved in a car crash.

36. True. Injuries to the genitourinary system often occur in association with abdominal trauma.

CHAPTER 51

1. d. The signs and symptoms of compartment syndrome can be subtle. One of the most identifiable symptoms is pain that is out of proportion to the injury and may be unresponsive to typical analgesic therapy.

2. a. A fracture of the radius or ulna could result in blood loss of 250 to 500 mL.

3. c. Check distal pulses before and after splinting an extremity. If distal pulses are no longer present after you have applied the splint, the splint may have been applied too tightly.

4. a. Traction splints are a specialized splint designed for midshaft closed femur fractures.

5. a. An injury in which the patient lands on his outstretched arm is likely to result in a Colles fracture.

6. True. In some cases, you may want to consider administering pain medication before immobilizing the patient to make the procedure more tolerable for the patient.

7. d. Follow the ABCs.

8. a. First reevaluate the splint and bandage to determine whether it is limiting circulation.

9. c. Evaluating a painful, swollen, deformed extremity may be difficult in a patient with arthritis. It can mimic fractures and dislocations, and it can hide fractures and dislocations. Your physical assessment will reveal joints that are swollen, painful, and deformed and have a limited range of motion. Patients with arthritis, regardless of the cause, live with this limited function and pain daily and it may be hard to identify a new injury in the field.

10. b. Sprains are injuries that occur when ligaments are stretched beyond their normal range of motion, sometimes resulting in tearing of the ligament.

CHAPTER 52

1. c. Lightning has struck mountain gullies, the middle of flagpoles, and even the bottom of the space shuttle gantry and other tall objects.

2. b. Conduction occurs when an object comes in direct contact with another object and heat is transferred. This is the case when a warm body comes in contact with a cool park bench.

3. b. Many harmless snakes have similar color combinations, but true coral snakes (with the exception of rare albino specimens) always have contiguous red and yellow bands. This has generated a helpful memory aid: "red on yellow, kill a fellow; red on black, venom lack."

4. False. Those susceptible to exertional heatstroke include all age groups. Common to this type of heatstroke are athletes and military personnel who often have little choice as to when exercise and activity take place.

5. a. The most common medication taken for the prevention of acute mountain sickness is acetazolamide (Diamox). It increases the amount of alkali excreted in the blood in the urine, making the blood more acidic.

6. c. Decompression sickness, decompression illness, or "the bends" is caused by the formation of nitrogen bubbles in the bloodstream and tissues of the body.

7. c. Methods to prevent cold emergencies include the following:
- Avoid long periods of exposure
- Intake plenty of clear fluids
- Intake adequate amounts of carbohydrates, proteins, and nutrients
- Cover exposed body surfaces
- Layer clothing
  - Clothing should be polypropylene or other wicking fabric
  - The outer layer of clothing should be waterproof and breathable
  - Avoid use of cotton layers, which will increase heat loss when wet
- Keep clothing and body dry if possible
- Wear comfortable and loose clothing
- Add heat from an external source
- Increase heat production of the body through exercise
- Get plenty of sleep and rest to allow the body to replenish energy supplies

8. d. The hallmark of black widow bites is widespread, sustained muscle spasms with an absence of dramatic local tissue injury. Severe abdominal pain and rigidity may be present and has been mistaken for an "acute abdomen" (a surgical emergency such as appendicitis or perforated bowel). The worst pain is generally present for 8 to 12 hours and then subsides, but symptoms may remain severe for several days.

9. c. Despite long periods of submersion some patients will recover if the water is cold enough. Similar to hypothermia treatment, patients submerged in cold water are not dead until they are warm and dead.

10. a. Hypothermia is a result of core temperatures dropping below 35°C (95°F).

CHAPTER 53

1. d. Tractors and machines.

2. d. The overturn not being immediately discovered.

3. c. Crush injury syndrome.

4. c. Rapid extrication if entrapment has been less than 1 hour.

5. b. Intravenous fluid.

6. c. Power take-off shaft.

7. d. A substance that prevents, repels, or destroys the growth of an unwanted host.

8. b. Organophosphate chemicals.

9. False. Emergency responders must always follow confined space standards when entering any farm confined space.

10. a. Silo fillers disease.

11. c. Two weeks after the silo is filled.

12. b. Hydrogen sulfide.

CHAPTER 54

1. False. A few states do recognize some type of wilderness EMS certification.

2. b. The mnemonic INDIAN is used to assess if a patient's spine can be clinically cleared in the field. The patient must be assessed for ***i***ntoxication, ***n***eurological deficit, ***d***istracting ***i***njury, ***a***ltered level of consciousness/mental status, and ***n***eck and back pain or tenderness. If none of these conditions are present, the patient has negative examination findings. Arm pain is not one of the conditions that would result in a positive examination finding.

3. b. A WEMS system is a formally structured organization, integrated into or part of the standard EMS system, and configured to provide wilderness medical care to a discrete region or activity.

4. a, c, d. In both wilderness EMS and disaster EMS settings, scope of care may be expanded to address the fact that transfer to comprehensive care may be delayed. Expanded scope of care in wilderness settings may include medications (antibiotics, steroidal medications, etc.) and interventions (reduction of dislocations, suturing, etc.) that can temporize or reverse a condition that might otherwise be detrimental to a patient if managed by traditional EMS practices. Field appendectomy is not part of the expanded scope of care.

5. True. Although wilderness EMS providers may rarely have access to ambulances, ambulance-based gear, and online medical direction while at the scene of injury or illness, they usually have increased access to other resources, such as helicopter services (air medical and rescue, hospital and military based), rescue gear, specialists in wilderness rescue, volunteer help, and extended care equipment, when compared with traditional EMS providers.

6. False. In the United States, rescues and wilderness EMS medical care are usually volunteer or provided by the government and no charge is applied to those rescued. This partly stems from the philosophical convictions of those providing the rescue, such as the policy of the MRA that no charge be levied by affiliate organizations. Another reason is that governmental bodies, such as the National Park Service and state providers, are obligated to protect the safety of participants in their regions and thus medical care and by extension rescue often are considered an obligation of the state (although some authorities do point out that no specific mandated "duty to rescue" exists on the part of state or national parks).

7. **a, b, d.** Although many wilderness EMS services are volunteer based, and EMS services and funding in many park services can be tight, the NDMS/FEMA system represents one of the most comprehensive and well-funded disaster/austere medical care systems in the world.

8. **a, b, d.** For the purposes of this text, wilderness medicine is considered to be medical management in situations where care and prevention are limited by environmental considerations, prolonged extrication, or resource availability.

CHAPTER 55

1. **c.** This patient would be a high priority.
2. **b.** False.
3. **a.** True.
4. **a.** True.
5. **c.** Pattern recognition.
6. **d.** When responding to a chest pain call, the equipment that should be brought in with you to the patient should include stretcher, airway bag, drug box, and cardiac monitor.
7. **a.** Stretcher, airway bag, trauma bag, backboard, spinal immobilization supplies.
8. **b.** You suspect congestive heart failure.
9. **d.** You suspect pneumothorax.
10. **c.** You should immediately assess the airway.

CHAPTER 56

1. **b.** They do not promote paramedic critical thinking.
2. **c.** They provide a standardized approach to patient care.
3. **e.** Reflection on actions.
4. ***R***ead the patient, ***r***ead the scene, ***r***eact, ***r***eevaluate, ***r***evise management plan, and ***r***eview performance.
5. **a.** Application of principle.
6. The paramedic's knowledge of anatomy, physiology, and pathophysiology.
7. **a.** Consider alternative treatments and protocols to respond to the current patient condition.
8. Develop and use a mental checklist. Practice assessment and treatment skills to the near-instinct level. Plan for the worst case possible.
9. **c.** Sick patient with vital signs that do not present a classic clinical condition.
10. **d.** Situational awareness.

CHAPTER 57

1. False. There is no national standard for critical care ground transport.
2. True. The Centers for Medicare and Medicaid Services policy specifically states that critical care ground transport is transportation provided between facilities for critically ill or injured persons.
3. True. Critical care ground transport units should be equipped comparable to mobile intensive care units.
4. True. The best available information credits Igor Sikorsky with the invention of military helicopters.
5. **b.** Available information notes that the first documented rescue of a patient took place in the jungles of Burma in 1944.
6. True. Henry's law is associated with decompression sickness and is related to the solubility of gases in liquids in equilibrium because the amount of gas dissolved in a liquid is proportional to the gas pressure.
7. Three things that cause stress in transport are decreased humidity, fatigue, and noise.
8. **d.** An isolated extremity fracture is unlikely to meet the criteria for air medical transport because the patient is usually stable. Transport of this type of patient may unnecessarily put the flight crew and patient at risk.
9. True. According to a majority of activation criteria, airway compromise meets the physiologic criteria for air medical transport. Local protocols should be kept in mind when making the decision.
10. False. Prolonged extrication typically meets the mechanism of injury criteria for air medical transport.
11. True. Limb paralysis typically meets the *anatomic criteria* for the activation of an air medical helicopter because of the possible loss of limb or use as an outcome.
12. **b.** Concrete is considered the best surface for a landing zone because it is likely to be the most level and debris-free surface.
13. **c.** Most flight services require a 100 ×100-ft area to land a medical helicopter. You should know the expectations of the flight services in your area to provide a safe location for the helicopter to land.

CHAPTER 58

1. EMS deployment and system status management can be defined as the art and science of matching the production capacity of an ambulance system to the changing patterns of demand placed on that system. It involves strategies and tactics used to continuously manage the resources available to anticipate and prepare for the next call.

2. Strategies for ambulance deployment may include (1) station-based or static deployment, (2) full deployment, and (3) combination of station and full deployment.

3. UhU is an indicator of productivity.

4. (a) For periods of predicted demand, resources are moved closer to where calls are known to have occurred. (b) Less time is required to travel less distance. (c) When crews are fully deployed and already in their units the chute time is reduced, improving overall response time.

5. By matching supply of available crews with call demand or requests for service, fewer crews are required during periods of low demand and more crews can be made available at peak demand periods. Matching supply with demand reduces cost and can improve response time and even the workload among crews. If deployment is well managed and expectations are realistic, these goals can be achieved without undue negative impact on employee satisfaction.

6. • Required response times
   • Level-of-care requirements
   • Population density
   • Geographic density
   • Call-demand patterns
   • Call acuity (severity)
   • Road systems
   • Location of healthcare facilities

7. Because EMS is a service industry, 55% to 80% of the cost is in personnel.

8. Offload delay is the most common reason for increased time on task.

9. Temporal demand is the measurement of call demand by hour of the day.

10. The basic UhU-T ratio is determined by dividing the number of transports by the system's net unit hours available for coverage.

CHAPTER 59

1. **b.** The difference between cover and concealment relates to the degree to which you are protected from bullets.

2. **b.** A brown paper bag. A plastic bag may destroy evidence.

3. **d.** Your assessment for dangerous situations should begin several blocks from the scene, looking for evidence of possible danger.

4. **a.** Approach the vehicle from the passenger side, which provides protection from traffic and is usually the opposite approach the driver would expect from law enforcement personnel.

5. Fingerprints, footprints, blood and body fluids, hair, carpet fibers, clothing fibers, dropped personal effects of an aggressor, weapons.

6. You should retreat and seek cover to protect against the projectiles and the possibility of further crowd violence. Consider taking the patient with you if doing so does not increase the danger to you and your partner.

7. You should use unconventional pathways to approach the residence. In addition, you should avoid positioning yourself between the ambulance lights and the residence, listens for signs of danger before entry, and do not stand in front of the door.

8. **a.** True. Body armor is soft and made from a series of fibers woven tightly together to form a vest. It offers protection from handgun bullets, most knives, and blunt trauma. Body armor does not protect against high-velocity bullets (e.g., rifles) or thin or dual-edged weapons (e.g., ice pick), and protection is reduced when wet.

9. Only record the facts about the scene of a crime. You must record them accurately because they will be used in court. Record any remarks made by the patient or bystanders in quotation marks. Avoid opinions and keep the documentation objective.

10. Shouting or increasingly loud voices, pushing or shoving, hostilities toward anyone on scene, rapid increase in crowd size, and inability of law enforcement officials to control the crowd.

CHAPTER 60

1. 9-1-1/emergency call receiving; incident address verification; call triage and call processing; identification of scene hazards; telephone treatment (prearrival instructions); responder case assignment/unit alerting; incident communications and coordination; response time measurement; unit status tracking; critical staff notifications; posting and unit deployment; scheduling interfacility and nonemergency transports.

2. Automatic number identification/automatic location identification.

3. **b.** False. 12 hours per year.

4. **b.** False.

5. Telephone aid is an ad-libbed instruction, relying solely on the dispatcher's prior experience. It is much less effective than protocols because this type of instruction is not scripted and not formally approved for use.

6. Address verification.

7. Emergency medical dispatch protocols, training, certification, prearrival instructions, and quality improvement.

8. **a.** True.

9. Timely, objective case evaluation feedback.

10. CAD, or computer-aided dispatch.

CHAPTER 61

1. **b.** Type II ambulances are typically the most affordable to purchase and operate.

2. **a.** When responding to a call, lights and sirens should be used in a life-threatening emergency.

3. **d.** Stopping distances in an ambulance are longer than in a car. There should be 4 seconds worth of space between the ambulance and the vehicle it is following.

4. **b.** The recommended size for a helicopter landing zone is 100 × 100 ft.

5. **a.** While responding to a call with lights and sirens the ambulance approaches an intersection with a red light. The driver should come to a complete stop, check for other vehicles, then proceed.

6. **a.** True. A bariatric ambulance is designed to transport morbidly obese patients.

7. **b.** You should have the light replaced. The ambulance should be in good working order.

8. **b.** A two-person crew is called to transport a patient who weighs 500 lb. The crew should call for a lift assist.

9. **a.** True. Responding with other emergency vehicles can increase the risk of being involved in a collision at intersections.

10. **a.** The transport vehicle should be cleaned at the beginning of each shift, after each call, and at the end of each shift.

CHAPTER 62

1. Three to seven, with five being optimum.

2. Multiple-patient incidents involve two to 25 persons, and multiple-casualty incidents involve 26 to 99 persons.

3. The basic elements of an incident command system are command finance, logistics, operations, and planning and safety.

4. Unified and singular.

5. The command post should be located in a stationary location that affords a quiet, safe workspace.

6. Situation found, actions taken, resources needed, confirmation of command.

7. Communication to the incident commander should be concise and limited to essential transmissions. Unnecessary traffic can distract the incident commander.

8. START.

9. Immediate, delayed minor, and dead/dying.

10. The safety officer is responsible for preventing unsafe actions from occurring during emergency incidents.

CHAPTER 63

1. Rescue is a patient-driven event.

2. The three levels of skill for responders to a technical rescue incident are awareness, operations, and technician.

3. The priorities for safety in any rescue are personal safety, safety for the rescue team, safety of bystanders and other involved persons, and safety of the rescue subject.

4. When EMS personnel are the first at the rescue site, they need to size-up the scene for any risks to rescuers first and report them to incoming responders.

5. Types of personal protective equipment include protection from blood-borne pathogens, helmets, eye protection, hearing protection, foot protection, and protective clothing.

6. The type III personal flotation device is preferred for most rescue work.

7. **d.** Airbags are also known as supplemental restraint systems.

8. **d.** These cylinder-like containers can contain pressurized gas at a pressure of 4000 psi.

9. A vehicle's battery may not be under the hood within the engine compartment. Potential alternate battery locations include inside the front wheel well, under the front or rear seat, and inside the trunk.

10. **d.** If the rescuer cuts the negative battery cable, he or she should cut the same cable a second time to remove a minimum 2-inch section.

11. **d.** Scanning, similar to a patient assessment, is a brief and systematic look around the interior of the vehicle to determine the location and status of all airbags within the vehicle.

12. **c.** The airbag inflation zone distances for front driver, front passenger, and side-impact airbags are 10 inches, 18 inches, and 5 inches.

13. **b.** The concern about accidentally cutting into a stored gas inflator unit for an undeployed side impact roof airbag can be alleviated if

rescue teams strip away the roof pillar trim before cutting a roof pillar.

14. True. Hybrid gasoline/electric vehicles contain two electrical systems: the standard 12-volt system and a high-voltage system.

15. **d.** At a hybrid vehicle crash incident, once the gear selector lever has been moved, the inside rescuer must attempt to turn the ignition to the OFF position.

16. **c.** All vehicle crash scene hazards fall into one of three general categories: environmental hazards, scene hazards, and hazards presented by the vehicle itself.

17. **a.** Placing the emergency vehicle at an angle to approaching traffic is referred to as *blocking.*

18. **c.** The area of highest risk for EMS personnel at a crash scene is closest to the crashed vehicles and typically where the patients are located. This primary danger zone is commonly referred to as the *hot zone.*

19. True. Electricity can leave an energized wire and travel invisibly through the ground. When this happens at a crash scene, the ground becomes energized with what is referred to as *ground gradient.*

20. True. Real-world experiences demonstrate that there really is such a thing as a typical vehicle crash. They typically occur on a dry, level road surface and more than likely at an intersection.

21. **a.** To better understand what happens at an extrication scene and promote improved training for vehicle rescue, all tasks that take place can be organized into four categories. These groupings are known collectively as the phases of rescue.

22. Potential hazards in moving water include hydraulics, strainers, dams, hydroelectric or irrigation intakes, and foot or extremity pins.

23. Never underestimate the power of moving water; do not enter moving water without highly specialized training and equipment; the priorities at the scene are always self rescue first, the rescue and security of fellow rescuers second, and the victims last; and all rescuers must wear a personal flotation device even if using shore-based rescue techniques.

24. The basic water rescue model is talk, reach, throw, and row.

25. Atmospheric problems are most often the danger in confined space situations.

26. Lock out is the placing of a locking mechanism on an energy-isolating device to ensure that the device and the equipment being controlled cannot be operated until the lock-out mechanism is removed. Tag out is the placing of a tag-out mechanism on an energy-isolating device that indicates that the energy-isolating device and the equipment being controlled may not be operated until the tag-out mechanism is removed.

27. Two common medical issues in trench collapse are asphyxia and crush syndrome.

28. Three personal skills needed in high-angle rescue are belaying, rappelling, and ascending.

29. Immobilization on rigid spine boards for longer periods can result in tissue interface pressure, or pressure points. Over time, sufficient pressure at these points can result in pressure necrosis, or bed sores.

30. Anchors are the means of securing the ropes and other elements in the high-angle system.

31. Ground safety concerns for EMS personnel working around helicopters include the following:
    - Keep well clear of helicopter rotors
    - Always get the approval of a flight crew member before approaching a starting or operating helicopter
    - Only approach and depart as directed, in a slightly crouched position and in full view of a crew member
    - Keep seat belt and shoulder harness fastened until instructed by the pilot to unbuckle
    - Wear eye protection when working around helicopters
    - Aircraft must be loaded by qualified personnel only
    - No smoking within 100 feet of an aircraft
    - Do not throw objects to or from an aircraft

CHAPTER 64

1. **b.** Because responders performing this function will possibly be exposed to hazardous substances and will be required to wear PPE, the operations level training is the appropriate answer.

2. **d.** The first priority in any response is ensuring response crew safety.

3. False. The NFPA 704 system is designed to warn emergency responders of the presence of hazardous materials and the possible severity of the hazard. However, it does not identify specific chemicals that may be present.

4. **a.** Simple asphyxiants displace oxygen. Chemical asphyxiants interfere with the body's ability to use oxygen.

5. **c.** The six hazardous materials recognition clues include occupancy and location, container shape, markings and colors, placards and labels, shipping papers, and senses. The Materials Safety Data Sheet is an industrial reference document that can be accessed once the hazardous material has been identified.

6. **b.** The hot and warm zones will be contaminated. The cold zone is a safe area free of contamination. The command post should always be located in the cold zone.

7. **a.** The safest position at a hazardous materials scene is away from the route of material movement. That would be upwind and uphill.

8. **c.** Although all of these reasons are true, the *most* important reason to set up control zones is the safety of the public and emergency responders.

9. **d.** Level A protective ensembles provide the highest degree of both respiratory and skin protection. This will require the use of a self-contained breathing apparatus and a vapor-tight total encapsulating suit.

10. **b.** Both level A and level B use the same type of respiratory protection, a self-contained breathing apparatus. The difference is in the degree of skin protection. Level A is designed for vapor protection and level B is designed for splash or particulate protection.

11. True. The use of PPE creates both physical and physiologic stress. Heat stress is one of the major concerns. Overprotection and underprotection should be avoided.

12. **c.** The dose/response relation is based on the fact that the larger the amount taken into the body, the greater the toxicologic response.

13. **a.** Emergency decontamination operations, usually having patients walk through a water spray, may not result in complete decontamination. Many variables exist, including the type of agent, time spent in the spray, and whether clothing was removed.

14. True. If patients are not decontaminated before transport, the contamination will be spread to the ambulance, transport crew, and hospital. Contaminated patients should be decontaminated before transport. The only exception would be small numbers of patients with radiologic contamination, life-threatening trauma, and hospital resources that are able to handle the situation.

15. False. NFPA level I provides adequate training to operate in the cold zone of a hazardous materials incident. NFPA level II is adequate training to operate in the warm zone.

16. **b.** The top section of the NFPA 704 symbol is red and represents fire danger.

17. False. The sense of smell is not considered adequate warning for the presence of hazardous materials. By the time you smell a chemical you are being exposed. In addition, many chemicals cause olfactory fatigue and deaden the sense of smell.

18. True. Air has a vapor density of 1, so any chemical with a vapor density of greater than 1 will be heavier than air.

19. **a.** The lowest level that a gas will burn is the LEL.

20. **c.** Vapor pressure is the physical property that indicates how quickly a liquid will evaporate. The higher the vapor pressure, the faster the evaporation.

21. **b.** The specific gravity of water is 1, so any chemical with a specific gravity of more than 1 will sink in water. Water solubility must also be assessed. If the chemical is water soluble it will mix with water no matter what the specific gravity is.

22. **b.** Most hazardous materials exposures involve inhalation.

23. **c.** Patient decontamination takes place in the warm zone.

CHAPTER 65

1. **d.** Field medicine, tactical skills, and personal fitness.

2. **c.** Cover and concealment. *Cover* is defined as protection from enemy fire. *Concealment* is defined as protection from enemy observation. Cover depends on the weapons system deployed against it. In this scenario, sheet rock or studs may provide some cover.

3. **c.** Critically important; a TEMS medic must qualify to the same physical and psychological standards of the respective SWAT team.

4. **c.** Assessment. A TEMS medic should have years of experience with thousands of field patients.

5. **a.** 90%.

6. **b.** Exsanguination from external hemorrhage.

7. **c.** Fire superiority.

8. **c.** Control exsanguinating hemorrhage from an external bleed with a tourniquet and extricate from the line of fire. SCAB is a mnemonic used for the order of priority for tactical medicine: ***s***cene safety, ***c***irculation, ***a***irway, and ***b***reathing. This differs from the traditional ABCs.

9. **b.** Tourniquets, tactical battle dressings, airways, chest seals, 3.25-inch 14-gauge needles, trauma shears.

10. **b.** The law enforcement agency and the agency that employs the medics.

CHAPTER 66

1. **d.** To date, more than 90% of terrorist attacks have involved the use of explosives.

2. **b.** Many terrorists use an additional explosive device set to explode after the arrival of emergency responders.

3. **d.** The use of a radioactive substance combined with a conventional explosive is commonly known as a "dirty bomb" or a radiation dispersal device.

4. **e.** The primary blast injury is caused by the atmospheric overpressure created by the explosion. This overpressure can cause injuries to all the listed systems.

5. **b.** The four phases of illness associated with whole-body irradiation include the prodromal phase, the latent phase, the manifest illness phase, and the recovery phase or death.

6. False. The immediate destruction and injuries will be limited to the size of the conventional explosive. The purpose of a dirty bomb is to disperse radioactive contamination. The immediate damage will be far less than that of a nuclear detonation.

7. **c.** Smallpox is a virus. All the others listed are bacteria.

8. True. Anthrax and smallpox are examples of biologic agent illnesses that can be prevented by vaccination.

9. **d.** Smallpox and pneumonic plague can be spread person to person. Inhalational anthrax, botulism, and bubonic plague have no potential for person-to-person transmission.

10. **b.** Tabun, sarin, soman, and VX are members of the nerve agent class of chemical weapons.

11. **c.** Chemicals that produce blisters and burnlike injuries to the skin are known as *vesicants* or *blister agents.* Mustard agent and lewisite are members of the vesicant class of chemical weapons.

12. **b.** False. The blisters associated with exposure to mustard agent have a delayed onset. Although the injury occurs almost immediately, the symptoms (including the blisters) may take hours to appear.

13. **c.** The common antidote therapy for nerve agent exposure includes atropine, pralidoxime chloride, and diazepam. Epinephrine is not indicated.

14. **c.** The incident command system should be modular and a top-down structure. Only the positions needed should be filled. If the incident command system is implemented, there will always be an incident commander.

15. **d.** Communication should always be in plain English. A "10 code" may mean different things to different agencies, creating confusion.

16. **b.** The incident command system will be needed at major incidents. Its use at small incidents will ensure that it is familiar and practiced.

17. **d.** The logistics section is responsible for obtaining resources needed for incident management.

18. **a.** The most obvious use of EMS resources at a hazardous materials or WMD incident is the care of patients. This is carried out under the operations section.

19. **c.** Ensuring responder safety should be the top priority of any response.

20. **e.** A WMD could be composed of chemical, biologic, radiologic, or explosive agents.

APPENDIX B

Compilation of Drug Profiles

Abciximab (ReoPro)

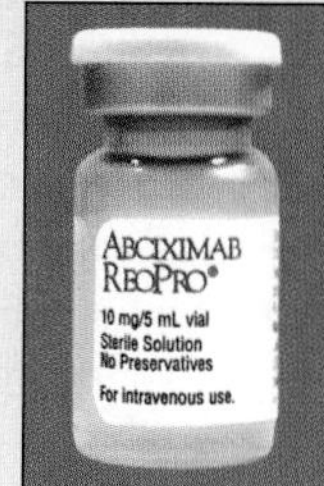

Classification: GP IIb/IIIa inhibitor
Action: Prevents the aggregation of platelets by inhibiting the integrin GP IIb/IIIa receptor.
Indications: UA/NSTEMI patients undergoing planned or emergent PCI.
Adverse Effects: Bleeding from the GI tract, internal bleeding, intracranial hemorrhage, hypotension, stroke, anaphylactic shock.
Contraindications: Bleeding from any source, severe uncontrolled hypertension, surgery or trauma within the previous 6 weeks, stroke within the previous 30 days, renal failure, thrombocytopenia, intracranial mass.
Dosage:
UA/NSTEMI with Planned PCI within 24 Hours:
- 0.25 mg/kg IV, IO (10 to 60 minutes prior to procedure), then 0.125 mcg/kg/min IV, IO infusion for 12 to 24 hours.

Percutaneous Coronary Intervention Only:
- 0.25 mg/kg IV, IO, then 10 mcg/min IV, IO infusion.

Special Considerations: Pregnancy class C

Activated Charcoal

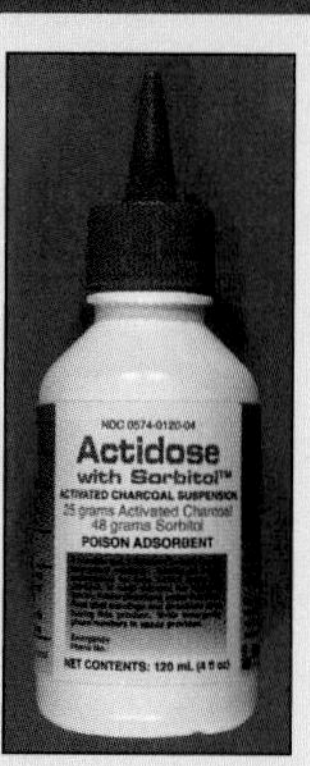

Classification: Antidote, adsorbent
Action: When certain chemicals and toxins are in proximity to the activated charcoal, the chemical will attach to the surface of the charcoal and become trapped.
Indications: Toxic ingestion
Adverse Effects: Nausea/vomiting, constipation, or diarrhea. If aspirated into the lungs, charcoal can induce a potentially fatal form of pneumonitis.
Contraindications: Ingestion of acids, alkalis, ethanol, methanol, cyanide, ferrous sulfate or other iron salts, lithium; coma; GI obstruction.
Dosage:
- **Adult:** 50 to 100 g/dose.
- **Pediatric:** 1 to 2 g/kg.

Special Considerations: Pregnancy class C

Adenosine (Adenocard)

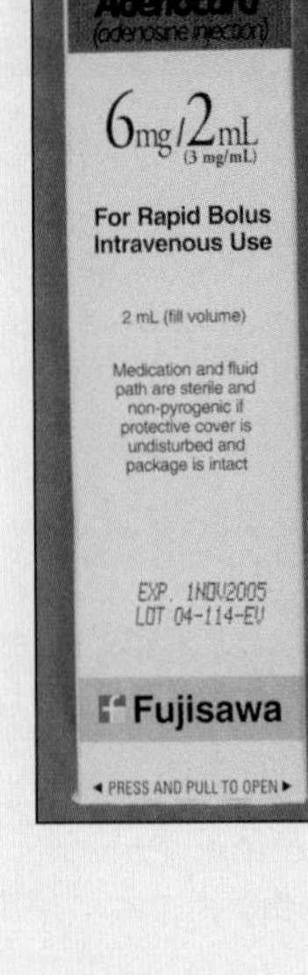

Classification: Antiarrhythmic

Action: Slows the conduction of electrical impulses at the AV node.

Indications: Stable reentry SVT. Does not convert AF, atrial flutter, or VT.

Adverse Effects: Common adverse reactions are generally mild and short-lived: sense of impending doom, complaints of flushing, chest pressure, throat tightness, numbness. Patients will have a brief episode of asystole after administration.

Contraindications: Sick sinus syndrome, second- or third-degree heart block, or poison-/drug-induced tachycardia.

Dosage: Note: Adenosine should be delivered only by rapid IV bolus with a peripheral IV or directly into a vein, in a location as close to the heart as possible, preferably in the antecubital fossa. Administration of adenosine must be immediately followed by a saline flush, and then the extremity should be elevated.

- **Adult:** Initial dose 6 mg rapid IV, IO (over a 1- to 3-second period) immediately followed by a 20-mL rapid saline flush. If the first dose does not eliminate the rhythm in 1 to 2 minutes, 12 mg rapid IV, IO, repeat a second time if required.
- **Pediatric:**
  - **Children >50 kg:** Same as adult dosing.
  - **Children <50 kg:** Initial dose 0.1 mg/kg IV, IO (max dose: 6 mg) immediately followed by a $\geq$5-mL rapid saline flush; may repeat at 0.2 mg/kg (max dose: 12 mg).

Special Considerations:

- Use with caution in patients with preexisting bronchospasm and those with a history of AF.
- Elderly patients with no history of PSVT should be carefully evaluated for dehydration and rapid sinus tachycardia requiring volume fluid replacement rather than simply treated with adenosine.
- Pregnancy class C

Albumin

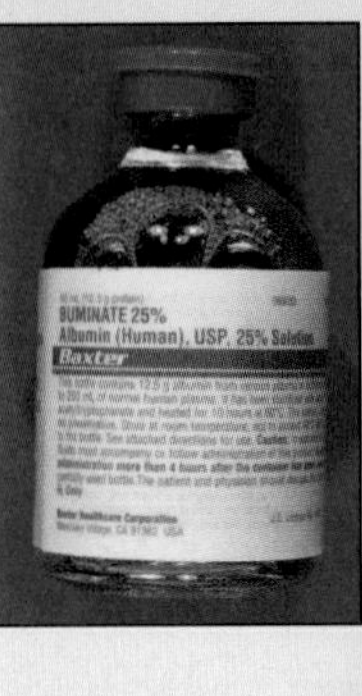

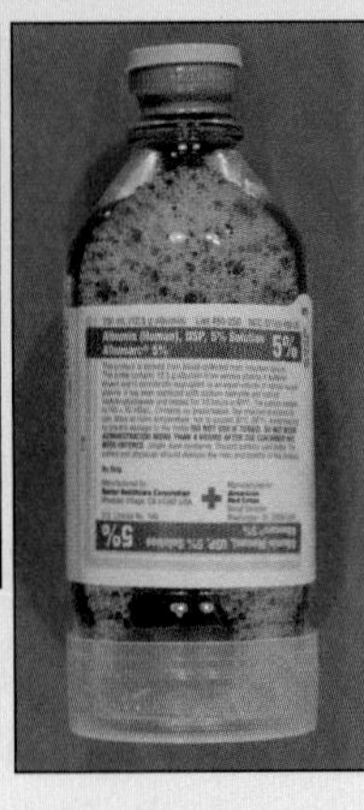

Classification: Volume expander, colloid

Action: Increases oncotic pressure in intravascular space.

Indications: Expand intravascular volume.

Adverse Effects: Allergic reaction in some patients; an excessive volume of fluid can result in CHF and pulmonary edema in susceptible patients.

Contraindications: Severe anemia or cardiac failure in the presence of normal or increased intravascular volume, solution appears turbid or after 4 hours since opening the container, known sensitivity.

Dosage: Two preparations: 500 mL of a 5% solution and 100 mL of a 25% solution.

- **Adult:**
  - **5% albumin:** 500 to 1000 mL IV, IO.
  - **25% albumin:** 50 to 200 mL IV, IO.
- **Pediatric:**
  - **5% albumin:** 12 to 20 mL/kg IV; the initial dose may be repeated in 15 to 30 minutes if the clinical response is inadequate.
  - **25% albumin:** 2.5 to 5 mL/kg IV, IO.
  - Alternatively, one may administer based on grams of albumin at 0.5 to 1 g/kg/dose IV, IO. May repeat as needed (max dose: 6 g/kg/day).

Special Considerations:

- Patients with a history of CHF, cardiac disease, hypertension, and pulmonary edema should be given 5% albumin, or the 25% albumin should be diluted. Because 25% of albumin increases intravascular volume greater than the volume administered, slowly administer 25% albumin in normovolemic patients to prevent complications such as pulmonary edema.
- Pregnancy class C

Albuterol (Proventil, Ventolin)

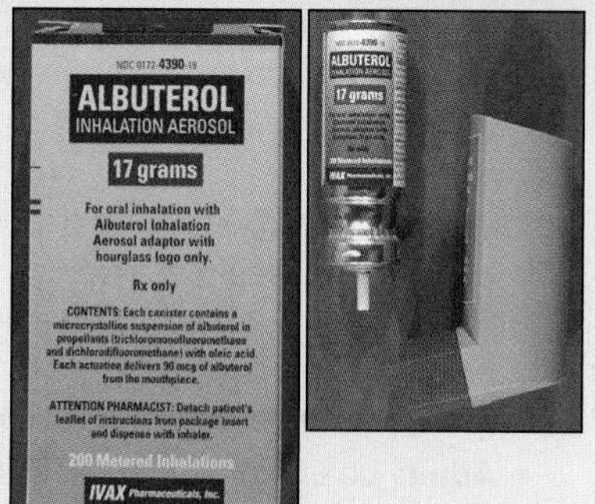

Classification: Bronchodilator, beta agonist
Action: Binds and stimulates $beta_2$ receptors, resulting in relaxation of bronchial smooth muscle.
Indications: Asthma, bronchitis with bronchospasm, and COPD.
Adverse Effects: Hyperglycemia, hypokalemia, palpitations, sinus tachycardia, anxiety, tremor, nausea/vomiting, throat irritation, dry mouth, hypertension, dyspepsia, insomnia, headache, epistaxis, paradoxical bronchospasm.
Contraindications: Angioedema, sensitivity to albuterol or levalbuterol. Use with caution in lactating patients, cardiovascular disorders, cardiac arrhythmias.
Dosage:
Acute Bronchospasm:

- **Adult:**
  - **MDI:** 4 to 8 puffs every 1 to 4 hours may be required.
  - **Nebulizer:** 2.5 to 5 mg every 20 minutes for a maximum of three doses. After the initial three doses, escalate the dose or start a continuous nebulization at 10 to 15 mg/hr.
- **Pediatric:**
  - **MDI:**
    - **4 years and older:** 2 inhalations every 4 to 6 hours; however, in some patients, 1 inhalation every 4 hours is sufficient. More frequent administration or more inhalations are not recommended.
    - **Younger than 4 years:** Administer by nebulization.
  - **Nebulizer:**
    - **Older than 12 years:** The dose for a continuous nebulization is 0.5 mg/kg/hr.
    - **Younger than 12 years:** 0.15 mg/kg every 20 minutes for a maximum of three doses. Alternatively, continuous nebulization at 0.5 mg/kg/hr can be delivered to children younger than 12 years.

Asthma in Pregnancy:

- **MDI:** Two inhalations every 4 hours. In acute exacerbation, start with 2 to 4 puffs every 20 minutes.
- **Nebulizer:** 2.5 mg (0.5 mL) by 0.5% nebulization solution. Place 0.5 mL of the albuterol solution in 2.5 mL of sterile normal saline. Flow is regulated to deliver the therapy over a 5- to 20-minute period. In refractory cases, some physicians order 10 mg nebulized over a 60-minute period.

Special Considerations: Pregnancy class C

Albuterol/Ipratropium (Combivent)

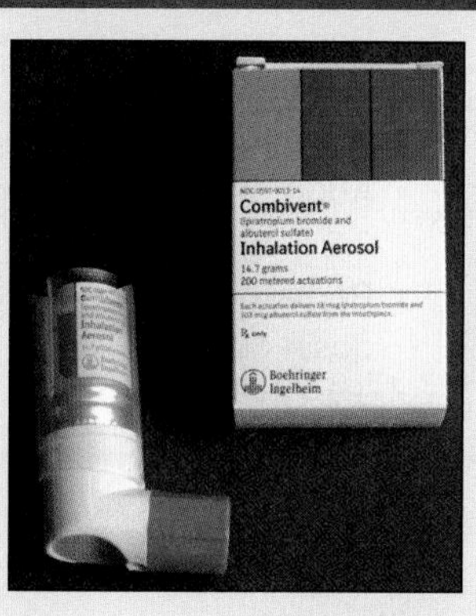

Classification: Combination bronchodilator
Action: Binds and stimulates $beta_2$ receptors, resulting in relaxation of bronchial smooth muscle, and antagonizes the acetylcholine receptor, producing bronchodilation.
Indications: Second-line treatment (if bronchodilator is ineffective) in COPD or severe acute asthma exacerbations during medical transport.
Adverse Effects: Headache, cough, nausea, arrhythmias, paradoxical acute bronchospasm.
Contraindications: Allergy to soybeans or peanuts; known sensitivity to atropine, albuterol, or their respective derivatives. Used with caution in patients with asthma, hypertension, angina, cardiac arrhythmias, tachycardia, cardiovascular disease, congenital long QT syndrome, closed-angle glaucoma.
Dosage:

- **Adult:** 2 puffs inhaled every 6 hours by MDI, with a maximum daily dose of 12 puffs/day.
- **Pediatric:** Not recommended for pediatric patients.

Special Considerations: Pregnancy class C

Aminophylline

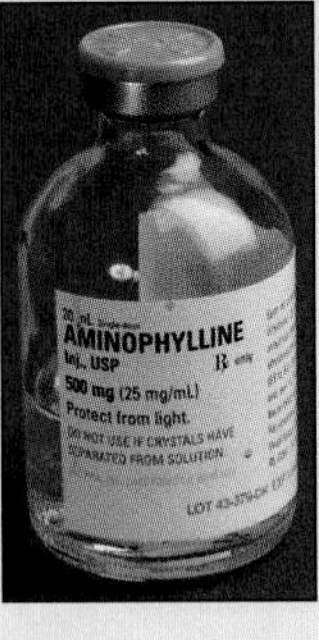

Classification: Bronchodilator

Action: Relaxes the smooth muscle of the bronchial airways and pulmonary blood vessels. May also have antiinflammatory properties.

Indications: Bronchospasm

Adverse Effects: Seizures, cardiac arrest, arrhythmias, nausea/vomiting, abdominal pain or cramping, headache, tachycardia, palpitations, anxiety, ventricular arrhythmias.

Contraindications: Known sensitivity. Use with caution in liver disease, kidney disease, seizures, cardiac arrhythmias.

Dosage: A loading dose is first administered, followed by an infusion.

- **Adult:** Load with 5 mg/kg IV, IO slowly over a 20- to 30-minute period, followed by an infusion. An infusion rate of 0.4 mg/kg/hr is effective for a nonsmoker, but a patient who smokes can require a high infusion rate at 0.8 mg/kg/hr IV, IO. When treating patients with CHF, reduce the dose to 0.2 mg/kg/hr.
- **Pediatric:** Load with 5 mg/kg slow IV, IO over a 20-minute period.
  - **Older than 12 years:** 0.4 mg/kg/hr IV, IO.
  - **10 to 12 years:** 0.7 mg/kg/hr IV, IO.
  - **1 to 9 years:** 0.8 to 1 mg/kg/hr IV, IO.
  - **6 months to 1 year:** 0.6 to 0.7 mg/kg/hr IV, IO.
  - **6 to 24 weeks:** 0.5 mg/kg/hr IV, IO.

Special Considerations: Pregnancy class C

Amiodarone (Cordarone)

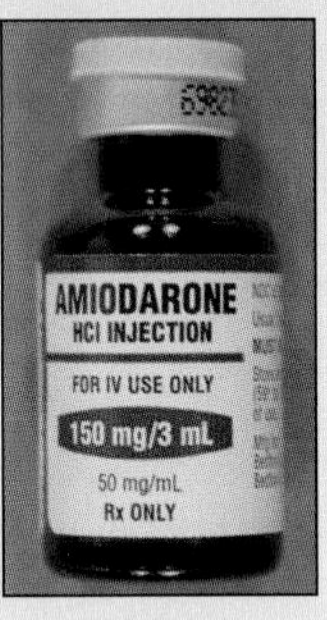

Classification: Antiarrhythmic, class III

Action: Acts directly on the myocardium to delay repolarization and increase the duration of the action potential.

Indications: Ventricular arrhythmias; second-line agent for atrial arrhythmias.

Adverse Effects: Burning at the IV site, hypotension, bradycardia.

Contraindications: Sick sinus syndrome, second- and third-degree heart block, cardiogenic shock, when episodes of bradycardia have caused syncope, sensitivity to benzyl alcohol and iodine.

Dosage:

Ventricular Fibrillation and Pulseless Ventricular Tachycardia:

- **Adult:** 300 mg IV/IO. May be followed by one dose of 150 mg in 3 to 5 minutes. After conversion, follow with a 1-mg/min infusion for 6 hours, then a 0.5-mg/min maintenance infusion over 18 hours.
- **Pediatric:** 5 mg/kg (max dose: 300 mg); may repeat 5 mg/kg IV, IO up to 15 mg/kg.

Relatively Stable Patients with Arrhythmias such as Premature Ventricular Contractions or Wide Complex Tachycardias with a Strong Pulse:

- **Adult:** 150 mg in 100 mL D_5W IV, IO over a 10-minute period; may repeat in 10 minutes up to a maximum dose of 2.2 g over 24 hours.
- **Pediatric:** 5 mg/kg very slow IV, IO (over 20 to 60 minutes); may repeat in 5-mg/kg doses up to 15 mg/kg (max dose: 300 mg).

Special Considerations: Pregnancy class D

Angiotensin-Converting Enzyme (ACE) Inhibitors: Captopril (Capoten), Enalapril (Vasotec), Lisinopril (Prinivil, Zestril), Ramipril (Altace)

Classification: Angiotensin-converting enzyme (ACE) inhibitors
Action: Blocks the enzyme responsible for the production of angiotensin II, resulting in a decrease in blood pressure.
Indications: Congestive heart failure, hypertension, post–myocardial infarction.
Adverse Effects: Headache, dizziness, fatigue, depression, chest pain, hypotension, palpitations, cough, dyspnea, upper respiratory infection, nausea/vomiting, rash, pruritus, angioedema, hypotension, renal failure.
Contraindications: Angioedema related to previous treatment with an ACE inhibitor, known sensitivity. Use with caution in aortic stenosis, bilateral renal artery stenosis, hypertrophic obstructive cardiomyopathy, pericardial tamponade, elevated serum potassium levels, acute kidney failure.
Dosage:

- **Adult:** Medication is administered orally. Dosage is individualized.
- **Pediatric:** Medication is administered orally. Dosage is individualized.

Special Considerations: Pregnancy class D

Aspirin, ASA

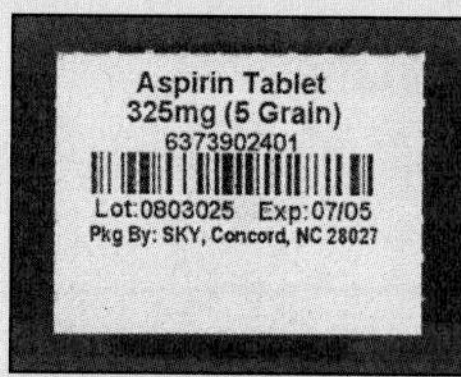

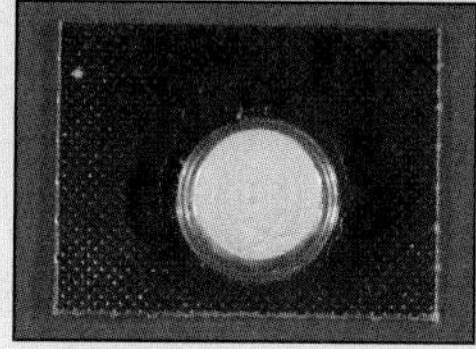

Classification: Antiplatelet agent, nonnarcotic analgesic, antipyretic
Action: Prevents the formation of a chemical known as thromboxane A_2, which causes platelets to clump together, or aggregate, and form plugs that cause obstruction or constriction of small coronary arteries.
Indications: Fever, inflammation, angina, acute MI, and patients complaining of pain, pressure, squeezing, or crushing in the chest that may be cardiac in origin.
Adverse Effects: Anaphylaxis, angioedema, bronchospasm, bleeding, stomach irritation, nausea/vomiting.
Contraindications: GI bleeding, active ulcer disease, hemorrhagic stroke, bleeding disorders, children with chickenpox or flulike symptoms, known sensitivity.
Dosage: Note: "Baby aspirin" 81 mg, standard adult aspirin dose 325 mg.

Myocardial Infarction:

- **Adult:** 160 to 325 mg PO (alternatively, four 81-mg baby aspirin are often given), 300-mg rectal suppository.
- **Pediatric:** 3 to 5 mg/kg/day to 5 to 10 mg/kg/day given as a single dose.

Pain or Fever:

- **Adult:** 325 to 650 mg PO (1 to 2 adult tablets) every 4 to 6 hours.
- **Pediatric:** 60 to 90 mg/kg/day in divided doses every 4 to 6 hours.

Special Considerations: Pregnancy class C except the last 3 months of pregnancy, when aspirin is considered pregnancy class D.

Atenolol (Tenormin)

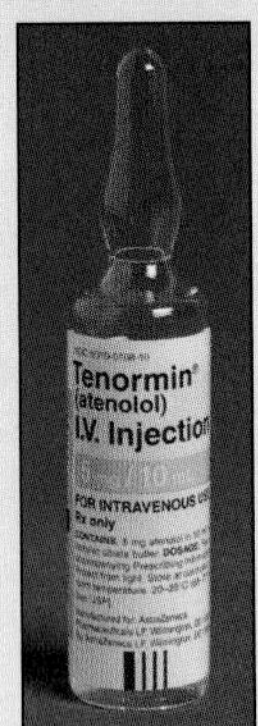

Classification: Beta adrenergic antagonist, antianginal, antihypertensive, class II antiarrhythmic

Action: Inhibits the strength of the heart's contractions and heart rate, resulting in a decrease in cardiac oxygen consumption. Also saturates the beta receptors and inhibits dilation of bronchial smooth muscle ($beta_2$ receptor).

Indications: ACS, hypertension, SVT, atrial flutter, AF.

Adverse Effects: Bradycardia, bronchospasm, hypotension.

Contraindications: Cardiogenic shock, AV block, bradycardia, known sensitivity. Use with caution in hypotension, chronic lung disease (asthma and COPD).

Dosage: ACS:

- **Adult:** 5 mg IV, IO over a 5-minute period; repeat in 5 minutes.
- **Pediatric:** Not recommended for pediatric patients.

Special Considerations: Pregnancy class D

Atracurium (Tracrium)

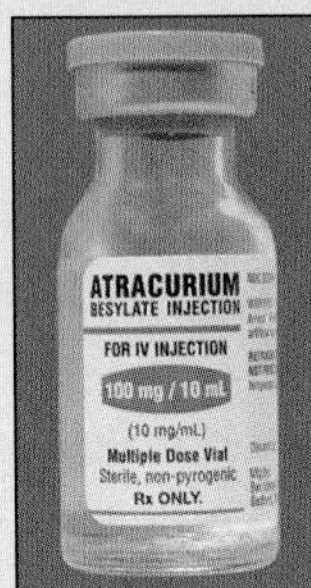

Classification: Nondepolarizing neuromuscular blocker

Action: Antagonizes acetylcholine receptors at the motor end plate, producing muscle paralysis.

Indications: Neuromuscular blockade to facilitate ET intubation.

Adverse Effects: Flushing, edema, urticaria, pruritus, bronchospasm and/or wheezing, alterations in heart rate, decrease in blood pressure.

Contraindications: Cardiac disease, electrolyte abnormalities, dehydration, known sensitivity.

Dosage:

- **Adult:** 0.4 to 0.5 mg/kg IV, IO; repeat with 0.08 mg/kg to 0.10 mg/kg every 20 to 45 minutes as needed for prolonged paralysis.
- **Pediatric:**
  - **Older than 2 years:** Same as adult dosing.
  - **Younger than 2 years:** 0.3 to 0.4 mg/kg IV, IO.

Special Considerations:

- Do not give by IM injection.
- Pregnancy class C

Atropine Sulfate

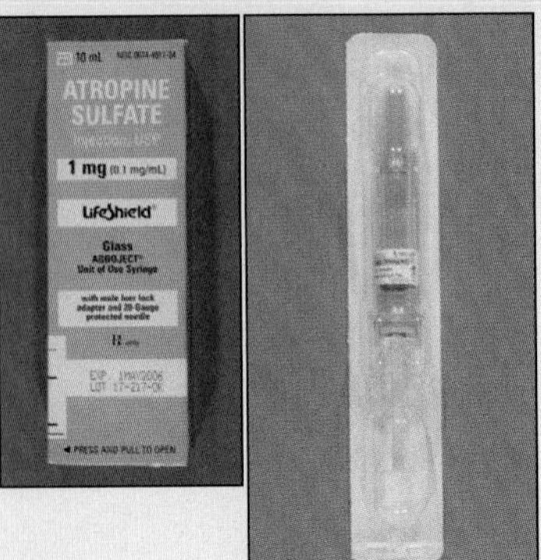

Classification: Anticholinergic (antimuscarinic)

Action: Competes reversibly with acetylcholine at the site of the muscarinic receptor. Receptors affected, in order from the most sensitive to the least sensitive, include salivary, bronchial, sweat glands, eye, heart, and GI tract.

Indications: Symptomatic bradycardia, asystole or PEA, nerve agent exposure, organophosphate poisoning.

Adverse Effects: Decreased secretions resulting in dry mouth and hot skin temperature, intense facial flushing, blurred vision or dilation of the pupils with subsequent photophobia, tachycardia, restlessness. Atropine may cause paradoxical bradycardia if the dose administered is too low or if the drug is administered too slowly.

Contraindications: Acute MI; myasthenia gravis; GI obstruction; closed-angle glaucoma; known sensitivity to atropine, belladonna alkaloids, or sulfites. Will not be effective for infranodal (type II) AV block and new third-degree block with wide QRS complex.

Continued

Atropine Sulfate—continued

Dosage:

Symptomatic Bradycardia:

- **Adult:** 0.5 mg IV, IO every 3 to 5 minutes to a maximum dose of 3 mg.
- **Adolescent:** 0.02 mg/kg (minimum 0.1 mg/dose; maximum 1 mg/dose) IV, IO up to a total dose of 2 mg.
- **Pediatric:** 0.02 mg/kg (minimum 0.1 mg/dose; maximum 0.5 mg/dose) IV, IO, to a total dose of 1 mg.

Asystole/Pulseless Electrical Activity:

- 1 mg IV, IO every 3 to 5 minutes, to a maximum dose of 3 mg. May be administered via ET tube at 2 to 2.5 mg diluted in 5 to 10 mL of water or normal saline.

Nerve Agent or Organophosphate Poisoning:

- **Adult:** 2 to 4 mg IV, IM; repeat if needed every 20 to 30 minutes until symptoms dissipate. In severe cases, the initial dose can be as large as 2 to 6 mg administered IV. Repeat doses of 2 to 6 mg can be administered IV, IM every 5 to 60 minutes.
- **Pediatric:** 0.05 mg/kg IV, IM every 10 to 30 minutes as needed until symptoms dissipate.
- **Infants <15 lb:** 0.05 mg/kg IV, IM every 5 to 20 minutes as needed until symptoms dissipate.

Special Considerations:

- Half-life 2.5 hours.
- Pregnancy class C; possibly unsafe in lactating mothers.

Butorphanol (Stadol)

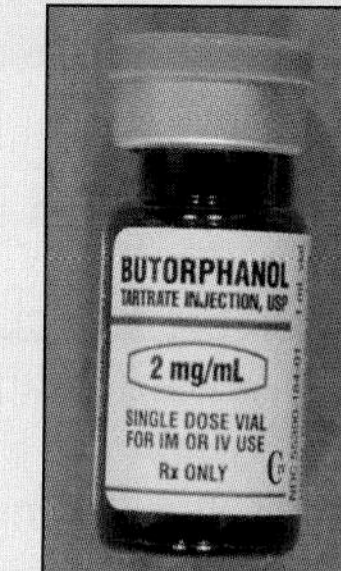

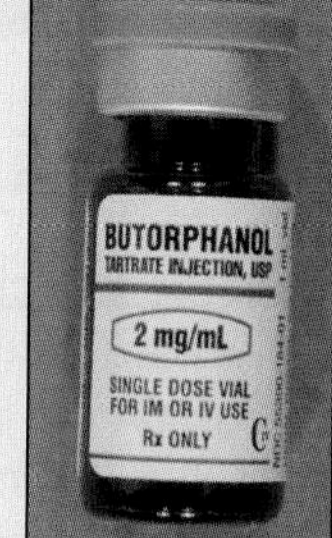

Classification: Opioid agonist-antagonist; schedule C-IV controlled substance
Action: Produces analgesia by binding to the opioid receptor.
Indications: Moderate to severe pain.
Adverse Effects: Drowsiness, dizziness, confusion, respiratory depression, nausea/vomiting, bradycardia, hypotension.
Contraindications: Patients with active substance abuse, sensitivity to opiate agonists. Use with caution in kidney, liver, or pulmonary problems.
Dosage:

- **Adult:** 0.5 to 2 mg IV, IO every 3 to 4 hours.
- **Pediatric:** Not recommended for pediatric patients.

Special Considerations: Pregnancy class C

Calcium Gluconate

Classification: Electrolyte solution
Action: Counteracts the toxicity of hyperkalemia by stabilizing the membranes of the cardiac cells, reducing the likelihood of fibrillation.
Indications: Hyperkalemia, hypocalcemia, hypermagnesemia.
Adverse Effects: Soft tissue necrosis, hypotension, bradycardia (if administered too rapidly).
Contraindications: VF, digitalis toxicity, hypercalcemia.
Dosage: Supplied as 10% solution; therefore each milliliter contains 100 mg of calcium gluconate.

- **Adult:** 500 to 1000 mg IV, IO administered slowly at a rate of approximately 1 to 1.5 mL/min maximum dose 3 g IV, IO.
- **Pediatric:** 60 to 100 mg/kg IV, IO slowly over a 5- to 10-minute period; maximum dose 3 g IV, IO.

Special Considerations:

- Do not administer by IM or Sub-Q routes, which causes significant tissue necrosis.
- Pregnancy class C

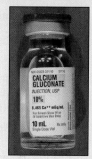

Carbamazepine (Tegretol)

Classification: Anticonvulsant

Action: Decreases the spread of the seizure.

Indications: Partial and generalized tonic-clonic seizures.

Adverse Effects: Dizziness, drowsiness, ataxia, nausea/vomiting, blurred vision, confusion, headache, transient diplopia, visual hallucinations, life-threatening rashes.

Contraindications: AV block, bundle branch block, agranulocytosis, bone marrow suppression, MAOI therapy, hypersensitivity to carbamazepine or tricyclic antidepressants. Use with caution in petit mal, atonic, or myoclonic seizures; liver disease, patients with blood dyscrasia caused by drug therapies or blood disorders, patients with a history of cardiac disease, or patients with a history of alcoholism.

Dosage:

- **Adult:** 200 mg PO every 12 hours.
- **Pediatric:**
  - **6 to 11 years:** 100 mg PO twice daily.
  - **Younger than 6 years:** 10 to 20 mg/kg/day PO 2 or 3 times per day.

Special Considerations: Pregnancy class D

Clopidogrel (Plavix)

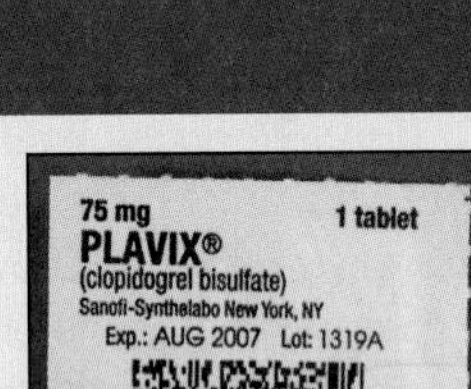

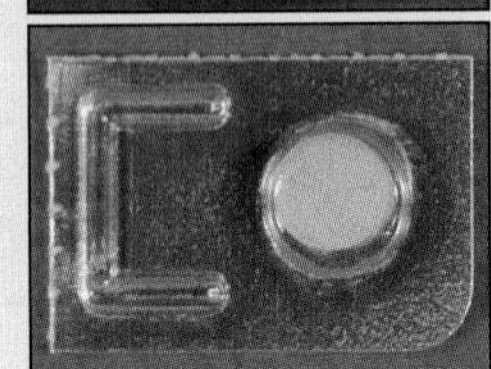

Classification: Antiplatelet

Action: Blocks platelet aggregation by antagonizing the GP IIb/IIIa receptors.

Indications: ACS, chronic coronary and vascular disease, ischemic stroke.

Adverse Effects: Nausea, abdominal pain, and hemorrhage.

Contraindications: History of intracranial hemorrhage, GI bleed or trauma, known sensitivity.

Dosage:

Unstable Angina Pectoris or Non–Q-Wave Acute Myocardial Infarction:

- **Adult:** Single loading dose of 300 mg PO followed by a daily dose of 75 mg PO.
- **Pediatric:** Not recommended for pediatric patients.

Special Considerations: Pregnancy class B

Dexamethasone (Decadron)

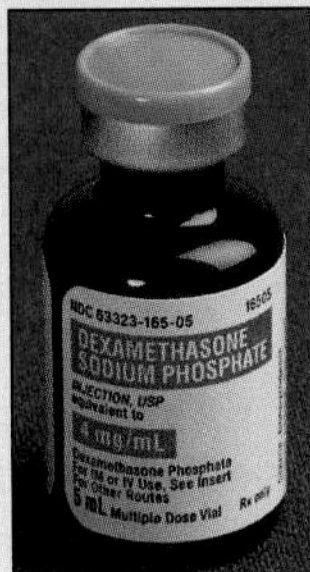

Classification: Corticosteroid

Action: Reduces inflammation and immune responses.

Indications: Various inflammatory conditions, adrenal insufficiency, nonresponsive forms of shock.

Adverse Effects: Nausea/vomiting, edema, hypertension, hyperglycemia, immunosuppression.

Contraindications: Fungal infections, known sensitivity.

Dosage:

- **Adult:** 1 to 6 mg/kg IV to a maximum dose of 40 mg.
- **Pediatric:** 0.03 to 0.3 mg/kg IV, IO divided into doses every 6 hours.

Special Considerations: Pregnancy class C

Dextrose (Dextrose 50%, Dextrose 25%, Dextrose 10%)

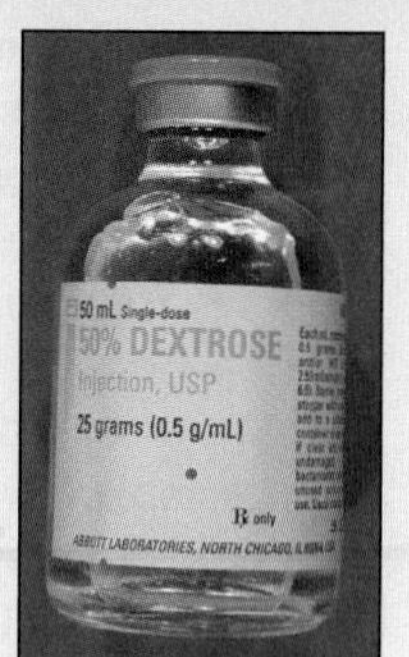

Classification: Antihypoglycemic
Action: Increases blood glucose concentrations.
Indications: Hypoglycemia
Adverse Effects: Hyperglycemia, warmth, burning from IV infusion. Concentrated solutions may cause pain and thrombosis of the peripheral veins.
Contraindications: Intracranial and intraspinal hemorrhage, delirium tremens, solution is not clear, seals are not intact.
Dosage:
Hyperkalemia:
- **Adult:** 25 g dextrose 50% IV, IO.
- **Pediatric:** 0.5 to 1 g/kg IV, IO.

Hypoglycemia:
- **Adult:** 10 to 25 g of dextrose 50% IV (20 to 50 mL of dextrose solution).
- **Pediatric:**
  - **Older than 2 years:** 2 mL/kg of dextrose 50%.
  - **Younger than 2 years:** 2 to 4 mL/kg of dextrose 10%.

Special Considerations: Pregnancy class C

Diazepam (Valium)

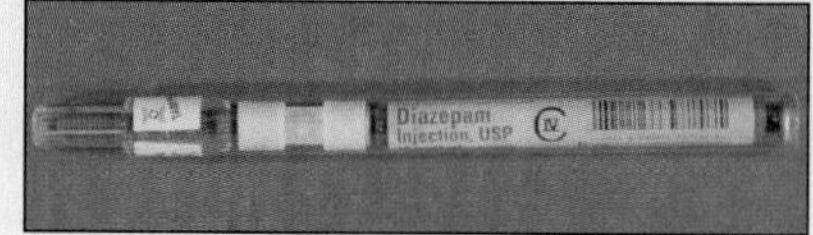

Classification: Benzodiazepine; schedule C-IV
Action: Binds to the benzodiazepine receptor and enhances the effects of GABA. Benzodiazepines act at the level of the limbic, thalamic, and hypothalamic regions of the CNS and can produce any level of CNS depression required (including sedation, skeletal muscle relaxation, and anticonvulsant activity).
Indications: Anxiety, skeletal muscle relaxation, alcohol withdrawal, seizures.
Adverse Effects: Respiratory depression, drowsiness, fatigue, headache, pain at the injection site, confusion, nausea, hypotension, oversedation.
Contraindications: Children younger than 6 months, acute-angle glaucoma, CNS depression, alcohol intoxication, known sensitivity.
Dosage:
Anxiety:
- **Adult:**
  - **Moderate:** 2 to 5 mg slow IV, IM.
  - **Severe:** 5 to 10 mg slow IV, IM (administer no faster than 5 mg/min).
  - **Low:** Low dosages are often required for elderly or debilitated patients.
- **Pediatric:** 0.04 to 0.3 mg/kg/dose IV, IM every 4 hours to a maximum dose of 0.6 mg/kg.

Delirium Tremens from Acute Alcohol Withdrawal:
- **Adult:** 10 mg IV

Seizure:
- **Adult:** 5 to 10 mg slow IV, IO every 10 to 15 minutes; maximum total dose 30 mg.
- **Pediatric:**
  - **IV, IO:**
    - **5 years and older:** 1 mg over a 3-minute period every 2 to 5 minutes to a maximum total dose of 10 mg.
    - **Older than 30 days to younger than 5 years:** 0.2 to 0.5 mg over a 3-minute period; may repeat every 2 to 5 minutes to a maximum total dose of 5 mg.
    - **Neonate:** 0.1 to 0.3 mg/kg/dose given over a 3- to 5-minute period; may repeat every 15 to 30 minutes to a maximum total dose of 2 mg. (Not a first line agent due to sodium benzoic acid in the injection.)

Continued

Diazepam (Valium)—continued

- **Rectal administration:** If vascular access is not obtained, diazepam may be administered rectally to children.
  - **12 years and older:** 0.2 mg/kg.
  - **6 to 11 years:** 0.3 mg/kg.
  - **2 to 5 years:** 0.5 mg/kg.
  - **Younger than 2 years:** Not recommended.

Special Considerations:

- Make sure that IV, IO lines are well secured. Extravasation of diazepam causes tissue necrosis.
- Diazepam is insoluble in water and must be dissolved in propylene glycol. This produces a viscous solution; give slowly to prevent pain on injection.
- Pregnancy class D

Digoxin (Lanoxin)

Classification: Cardiac glycoside

Action: Inhibits sodium-potassium-adenosine triphosphatase membrane pump, resulting in an increase in calcium inside the heart muscle cell, which causes an increase in the force of contraction of the heart.

Indications: CHF, to control the ventricular rate in chronic AF and atrial flutter, narrow-complex PSVT.

Adverse Effects: Headache, weakness, GI disturbances, arrhythmias, nausea/vomiting, diarrhea, vision disturbances.

Contraindications: Digitalis allergy, VT and VF, heart block, sick sinus syndrome, tachycardia without heart failure, pulse lower than 50 to 60 beats/min, MI, ischemic heart disease, patients with preexcitation AF or atrial flutter (i.e., a delta wave, characteristic of Wolff-Parkinson-White syndrome, visible during normal sinus rhythm).

Dosage: Dosage is individualized.

Special Considerations:

- Low levels of serum potassium can lead to digoxin toxicity and bradycardia. Conditions such as administration of steroids or diuretics or vomiting and diarrhea can produce low levels of potassium and subsequent digoxin toxicity.
- Pregnancy class C

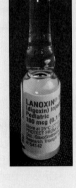

Diltiazem (Cardizem)

Classification: Calcium channel blocker, class IV antiarrhythmic

Action: Blocks calcium from moving into the heart muscle cell, which prolongs the conduction of electrical impulses through the AV node.

Indications: Stable narrow-QRS tachycardia caused by reentry, stable narrow-QRS tachycardia caused by automaticity, to control the ventricular rate in patients with AFib or atrial flutter (NOTE: Should *not* be given to patients with Afib or atrial flutter associated with known preexcitation [e.g., WPW syndrome]).

Adverse Effects: Flushing; headache; bradycardia; hypotension; heart block; myocardial depression; severe AV block; and, at high doses, cardiac arrest.

Contraindications: Hypotension, heart block, heart failure.

Dosage:

- **Adult:** Optimum dose is 0.25 mg/kg IV, IO over a 2-minute period; 20 mg is a reasonable dose for the average adult patient. A second, higher dose of 0.35 mg/kg IV, IO (25 mg is a typical second dose) may be administered over a 2-minute period if rate control is not obtained with the lower dose. For continued reduction in heart rate, a continuous infusion can be started at a dose range of 5 to 15 mg/hr.
- **Pediatric:** Not recommended for pediatric patients.

Special Considerations:

- Use with extreme caution in patients who are taking beta blockers because these two drug classes potentiate each other's effects and toxicities.
- Patients with a history of heart failure and heart block are at a higher risk for toxicity.
- Pregnancy class C

Diphenhydramine Hydrochloride (Benadryl)

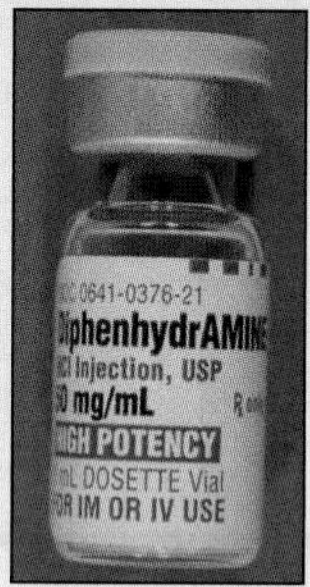

Classification: Antihistamine
Action: Binds and blocks H_1 histamine receptors.
Indications: Anaphylactic reactions, dystonic reactions
Adverse Effects: Drowsiness, dizziness, headache, excitable state (children), wheezing, thickening of bronchial secretions, chest tightness, palpitations, hypotension, blurred vision, dry mouth, nausea/vomiting, diarrhea.
Contraindications: Acute asthma, which thickens secretions; patients with cardiac histories; known sensitivity.
Dosage:

- **Adult:** 25 to 50 mg IV, IO, IM.
- **Pediatric:** 2 to 12 years: 1 to 1.25 mg/kg IV, IO, IM.

Special Considerations: Pregnancy class B

Dobutamine (Dobutrex)

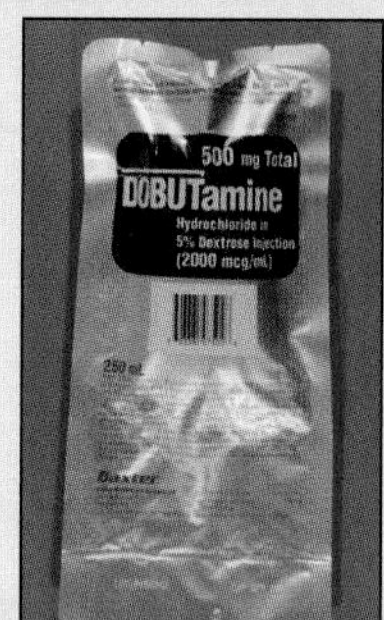

Classification: Adrenergic agent
Action: Acts primarily as an agonist at $beta_1$ adrenergic receptors with minor $beta_2$ and $alpha_1$ effects. Consequently, dobutamine increases myocardial contractility and stroke volume with minor chronotropic effects, resulting in increased cardiac output.
Indications: CHF, cardiogenic shock.
Adverse Effects: Tachycardia, PVCs, hypertension, hypotension, palpitations, arrhythmias.
Contraindications: Suspected or known poisoning/drug-induced shock, systolic blood pressure <100 mm Hg with signs of shock, idiopathic hypertrophic subaortic stenosis, known sensitivity (including sulfites). Use with caution in hypertension, recent MI, arrhythmias, hypovolemia.
Dosage:

- **Adult:** 2 to 20 mcg/kg/min IV, IO. At doses >20 mcg/kg/min, increases of heart rate of >10% may induce or exacerbate myocardial ischemia.
- **Pediatric:** Same as adult dosing.

Special Considerations:

- Half-life 2 minutes
- Pregnancy class C

Dolasetron (Anzemet)

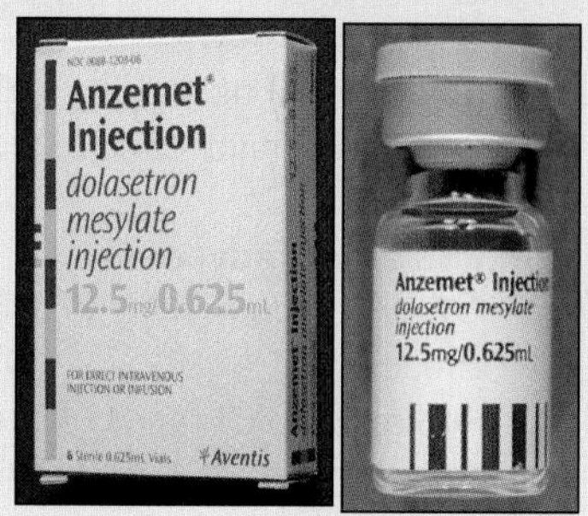

Classification: Antiemetic
Action: Prevents/reduces nausea/vomiting by binding and blocking a receptor for the brain chemical serotonin.
Indications: Prevent and treat nausea/vomiting.
Adverse Effects: Headache, fatigue, diarrhea, dizziness, abdominal pain, hypotension, hypertension, ECG changes (prolonged PR and QT intervals, widened QRS), bradycardia, tachycardia, syncope.
Contraindications: Known sensitivity. Use with caution in hypokalemia, hypomagnesemia, cardiac arrhythmias.
Dosage:

- **Adult:** 12.5 mg IV, IO.
- **Pediatric:** 2 to 16 years: 0.35 mg/kg IV, IO (max dose: 12.5 mg).

Special Considerations: Pregnancy class B

Dopamine (Intropin)

Classification: Adrenergic agonist, inotrope, vasopressor

Action: Stimulates alpha and beta adrenergic receptors. At moderate doses (2-10 mcg/kg/min), dopamine stimulates $beta_1$ receptors, resulting in inotropy and increased cardiac output while maintaining dopaminergic-induced vasodilatory effects. At high doses (>10 mcg/kg/min), alpha adrenergic agonism predominates, and increased peripheral vascular resistance and vasoconstriction result.

Indications: Hypotension and decreased cardiac output associated with cardiogenic shock and septic shock, hypotension after return of spontaneous circulation following cardiac arrest, symptomatic bradycardia unresponsive to atropine.

Adverse Effects: Tachycardia, arrhythmias, skin and soft tissue necrosis, severe hypertension from excessive vasoconstriction, angina, dyspnea, headache, nausea/vomiting.

Contraindications: Pheochromocytoma, VF, VT, or other ventricular arrhythmias, known sensitivity (including sulfites). Correct any hypovolemia with volume fluid replacement before administering dopamine.

Dosage:

- **Adult:** 2 to 20 mcg/kg/min IV, IO infusion. Starting dose 5 mcg/kg/min; may gradually increase the infusion by 5 to 10 mcg/kg/min to desired effect. Cardiac dose is usually 5 to 10 mcg/kg/min; vasopressor dose is usually 10 to 20 mcg/kg/min. Little benefit is gained beyond 20 mcg/kg/min.
- **Pediatric:** Same as adult dosing

Special Considerations:

Half-life 2 minutes

Pregnancy class C

Epinephrine

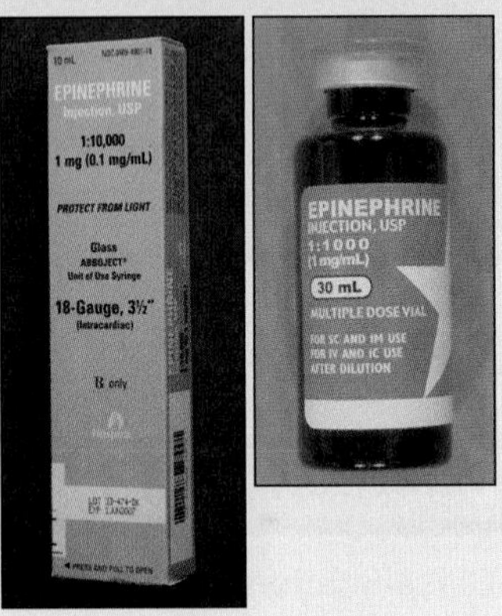

Classification: Adrenergic agent, inotrope

Action: Binds strongly with both alpha and beta receptors, producing increased blood pressure, increased heart rate, bronchodilation.

Indications: Bronchospasm, allergic and anaphylactic reactions, cardiac arrest.

Adverse Effects: Anxiety, headache, cardiac arrhythmias, hypertension, nervousness, tremors, chest pain, nausea/vomiting.

Contraindications: Arrhythmias other than pulseless VT/VF, asystole, PEA; cardiovascular disease; hypertension; cerebrovascular disease; shock secondary to causes other than anaphylactic shock; closed-angle glaucoma; diabetes; pregnant women in active labor; known sensitivity to epinephrine or sulfites.

Dosage:

Cardiac Arrest:

- **Adult:** Initial dose 1 mg (1:10,000 solution) IV, IO; may repeat every 3 to 5 minutes.
- **Pediatric:** Initial dose 0.01 mg/kg (1:10,000 solution) IV, IO; repeat every 3 to 5 minutes as needed (max dose: 1 mg).

Symptomatic Bradycardia:

- **Adult:** 1 mcg/min (1:10,000 solution) as a continuous IV infusion; usual dosage range: 2 to 10 mcg/min IV; titrate to effect.
- **Pediatric:** 0.01 mg/kg (1:10,000 solution) IV, IO; may repeat every 3 to 5 minutes (max dose: 1 mg). If giving epinephrine by ET tube, administer 0.1 mg/kg.

Asthma Attacks and Certain Allergic Reactions:

- **Adult:** 0.3 to 0.5 mg (1:1000 solution) IM or Sub-Q; may repeat every 10 to 15 minutes (max dose: 1 mg).
- **Pediatric:** 0.01 mg/kg (1:1000 solution) IM or Sub-Q (max dose: 0.5 mg).

Continued

Epinephrine—continued

Anaphylactic Shock:

- **Adult:** 0.1 mg (1 : 10,000 solution) IV slowly over 5 minutes, or IV infusion of 1 to 4 mcg/min, titrated to effect.
- **Pediatric:** Continuous IV infusion rate of 0.1 to 1 mcg/kg/min (1 : 10,000 solution); titrate to response.

Special Considerations:

- Half-life 1 minute
- Pregnancy class C

Epinephrine Autoinjectors (EpiPen, EpiPen Jr)

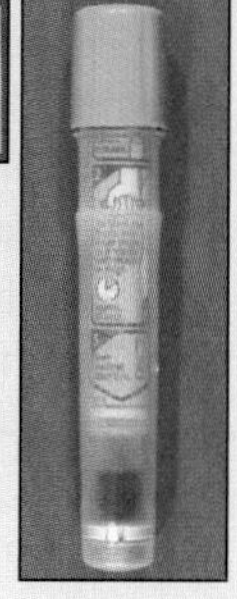

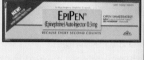

Classification: Adrenergic agonist, inotrope

Action: Binds strongly with both alpha and beta receptors, producing increased blood pressure, increased heart rate, bronchodilation.

Indications: Anaphylactic shock, certain allergic reactions, asthma attacks.

Adverse Effects: Headaches, nervousness, tremors, arrhythmias, hypertension, chest pain, nausea/vomiting.

Contraindications: Arrhythmias other than VF, asystole, PEA; cardiovascular disease; hypertension; cerebrovascular disease; shock secondary to causes other than anaphylactic shock; closed-angle glaucoma; diabetes; pregnant women in active labor; known sensitivity to epinephrine or sulfites.

Dosage:

- **Adult:** An EpiPen contains 0.3 mg epinephrine to be administered IM into the anterolateral thigh.
- **Pediatric:** For children weighing <30 kg, an EpiPen Jr delivers 0.15 mg IM.

Special Considerations:

- Half-life 1 minute
- Pregnancy class C

Eptifibatide (Integrilin)

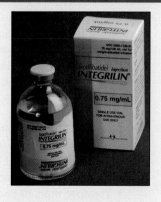

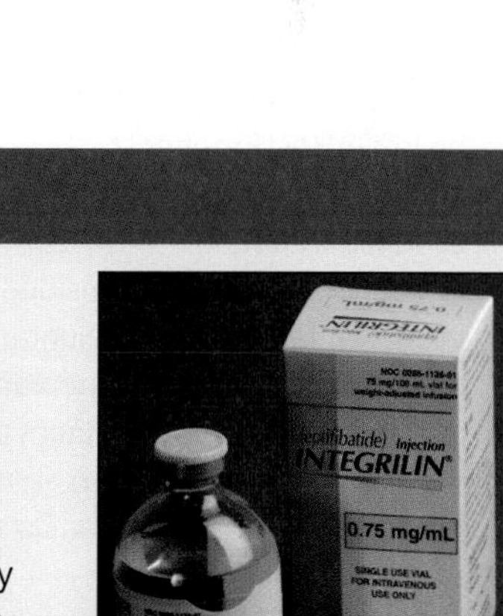

Classification: GP IIb/IIIa inhibitor

Action: Prevents the aggregation of platelets by binding to the GP IIb/IIIa receptor.

Indications: UA/NSTEMI—to manage medically and for those undergoing percutaneous coronary intervention.

Adverse Effects: Bleeding from the GI tract, internal bleeding, intracranial hemorrhage, hypotension, stroke, anaphylactic shock.

Contraindications: Bleeding from any source, severe uncontrolled hypertension, surgery or trauma within the previous 6 weeks, stroke within the previous 30 days, renal failure, thrombocytopenia.

Dosage:

- **Adult:** Loading dose: 180 mcg/kg IV, IO (max dose: 22.6 mg) over 1 to 2 minutes, then 2 mcg/kg/min IV, IO infusion (max dose: 15 mg/hr).
- **Pediatric:** No current dosing recommendations exist for pediatric patients.

Special Considerations:

- Half-life approximately 90 to 120 minutes
- Pregnancy class B

Esmolol (Brevibloc)

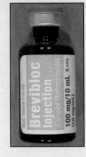

Classification: Beta adrenergic antagonist, class II antiarrhythmic

Action: Inhibits the strength of the heart's contractions, as well as heart rate, resulting in a decrease in cardiac oxygen consumption.

Indications: ACS, MI, acute hypertension, supraventricular tachyarrhythmias, thyrotoxicosis.

Adverse Effects: Hypotension, sinus bradycardia, AV block, cardiac arrest, nausea/vomiting, hypoglycemia, injection site reaction.

Contraindications: Acute bronchospasm, COPD, second- or third-degree heart block, bradycardia, cardiogenic shock, pulmonary edema, sick sinus syndrome, known sensitivity. Use with caution in patients with pheochromocytoma, Prinzmetal's angina, cerebrovascular disease, stroke, poorly controlled diabetes mellitus, hyperthyroidism, thyrotoxicosis, renal disease.

Dosage:

- **Adult:** 500 mcg/kg (0.5 mg/kg) IV, IO over a 1-minute period, followed by a 50 mcg/kg/min (0.05 mg/kg) infusion over a 4-minute period (maximum total: 200 mcg/kg). If patient response is inadequate, administer a second bolus 500 mcg/kg (0.5 mg/kg) over a 1-minute period, and then increase infusion to 100 mcg/kg/min. Maximum infusion rate: 300 mcg/kg/min.
- **Pediatric:** 500 mcg/kg (0.5 mg/kg) IV, IO over a 1-minute period, followed by an infusion at 25 to 200 mcg/kg/min.

Special Considerations:

- Half-life 5 to 9 minutes
- Any adverse effects caused by administration of esmolol are brief because of the drug's short half-life.
- Resolution of effects usually within 10 to 20 minutes.
- Pregnancy class C

Etomidate (Amidate)

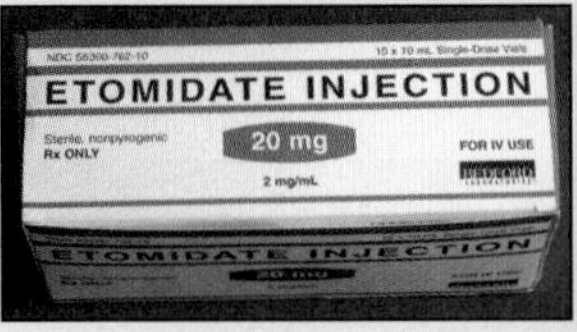

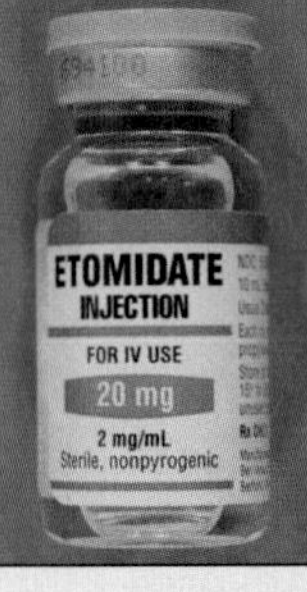

Classification: Hypnotic, anesthesia induction agent

Action: Although the exact mechanism is unknown, etomidate appears to have GABA-like effects.

Indications: Induction for rapid sequence intubation and pharmacologic-assisted intubation, induction of anesthesia.

Adverse Effects: Hypotension, respiratory depression, pain at the site of injection, temporary involuntary muscle movements, frequent nausea/vomiting on emergence, adrenal insufficiency, hyperventilation, hypoventilation, apnea of short duration, hiccups, laryngospasm, snoring, tachypnea, hypertension, cardiac arrhythmias.

Contraindications: Known sensitivity. Use in pregnancy only if the potential benefits justify the potential risk to the fetus. Do not use during labor and avoid in nursing mothers.

Dosage:

- **Adult:** 0.2 to 0.6 slow mg/kg IV, IO (over 30 to 60 seconds). A typical adult intubating dose of etomidate is 20 mg slow IV. Consider less (e.g., 10 mg) in the elderly or patients with cardiac conditions.
- **Pediatrics:**
  - **Older than 10 years:** Same as adult dosing.
  - **Younger than 10 years:** Safety has not been established.

Special Considerations:

- Etomidate is used to prepare a patient for orotracheal intubation. Both personnel and equipment must be present to manage the patient's airway before administration.
- Pregnancy class C

Felbamate (Felbatol)

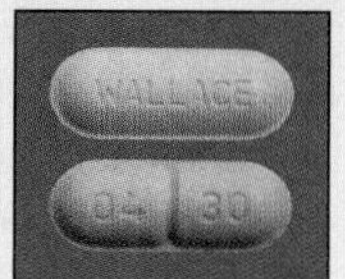

Classification: Anticonvulsant

Action: Although the mechanism of action is not known, it is believed that it antagonizes the effects of glycine, increases the seizure threshold in absence seizures, and prevents the spread of generalized tonic-clonic and partial seizures.

Indications: Partial seizures with and without generalization in epileptic adults; partial and generalized seizures associated with Lennox-Gastaut syndrome in children.

Adverse Effects: Nausea/vomiting, suicidal ideation and behavior, depression, insomnia, dyspepsia, upper respiratory tract infection, fatigue, headache, constipation, diarrhea, rhinitis, anxiety, aplastic anemia, photosensitivity.

Contraindications: Blood dyscrasias, hepatic disease, known sensitivity to carbomates.

Dosage: Should be individualized based on condition.

Special Considerations: Pregnancy class C

Fentanyl Citrate (Sublimaze)

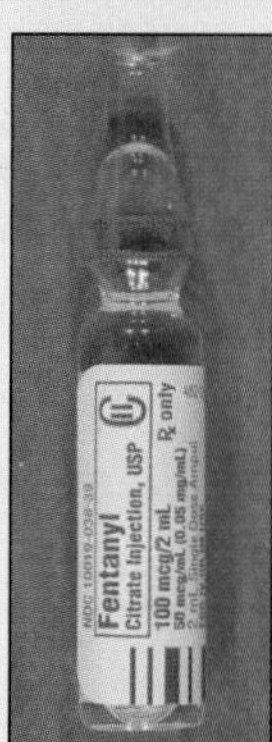

Classification: Narcotic analgesic; schedule C-II

Action: Binds to opiate receptors, producing analgesia and euphoria.

Indications: Pain

Adverse Effects: Respiratory depression, apnea, hypotension, nausea/vomiting, dizziness, sedation, euphoria, sinus bradycardia, sinus tachycardia, palpitations, hypertension, diaphoresis, syncope, pain at injection site.

Contraindications: Known sensitivity. Use with caution in traumatic brain injury, respiratory depression.

Dosage: Note: Dosage should be individualized.

- **Adult:** 50 to 100 mcg/dose (0.05 to 0.1 mg) IM or slow IV, IO (administered over 1 to 2 minutes).
- **Pediatric:** 1 to 2 mcg/kg IM or slow IV, IO (administered over 1 to 2 minutes).

Special Considerations: Pregnancy class B

Fibrinolytics: Tissue Plasminogen Activator (tPA), Streptokinase (Streptase, Kabikinase), Reteplase (Retavase), Tenecteplase (TNKase)

Classification: Fibrinolytic agent

Action: Alters plasmin in the body, which then breaks down fibrinogen and fibrin clots and reestablishes blood flow.

Indications: ST segment elevation (≥1 mm in two or more contiguous leads), new or presumed-new left bundle branch block.

Adverse Effects: Bleeding, intracranial hemorrhage, stroke, cardiac arrhythmias, hypotension, bruising.

Contraindications: ST segment depression, cardiogenic shock, recent (within 10 days) major surgery, cerebrovascular disease, recent (within 10 days) GI bleeding, recent trauma, hypertension (systolic blood pressure ≥180 mm Hg or diastolic blood pressure ≥110 mm Hg), high likelihood of left heart thrombus, acute pericarditis, subacute bacterial endocarditis, severe renal or liver failure with bleeding complications, significant liver dysfunction, diabetic hemorrhagic retinopathy, septic thrombophlebitis, advanced age (older than 75 years), patients taking warfarin (Coumadin).

Dosage: Dosing per medical direction.

Special Considerations: Pregnancy class C

Flumazenil (Romazicon)

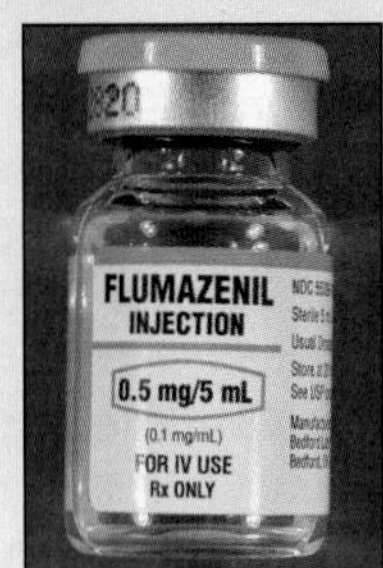

Classification: Benzodiazepine receptor antagonist, antidote

Action: Competes with benzodiazepines for binding at the benzodiazepine receptor, reverses the sedative effects of benzodiazepines.

Indication: Benzodiazepine oversedation

Adverse Effects: Resedation, seizures, dizziness, pain at injection site, nausea/vomiting, diaphoresis, headache, visual impairment.

Contraindications: Cyclic antidepressant overdose; life-threatening conditions that require treatment with benzodiazepines, such as status epilepticus and intracranial hypertension; known sensitivity to flumazenil or benzodiazepines. Use with caution where there is the possibility of unrecognized benzodiazepine dependence and in patients who have a history of substance abuse or who are known substance abusers.

Dosage:

- **Adult:** Initial dose is 0.2 mg IV, IO over a 15-second period. If the desired effect is not observed after 45 seconds, administer a second 0.2-mg dose, again over a 15-second period. Doses can be repeated a total of four times until a total dose of 1 mg has been administered.
- **Pediatric:** Children older than 1 year, 0.01 mg/kg IV, IO given over a 15-second period. May repeat in 45 seconds and then every minute to a maximum cumulative dose of 0.05 mg/kg or 1 mg, whichever is the lower dose.

Special Considerations:

- Monitor for signs of hypoventilation and hypoxia for approximately 2 hours.
- If the half-life of the benzodiazepine is longer than flumazenil, an additional dose may be needed.
- May precipitate withdrawal symptoms in patients dependent on benzodiazepines.
- Flumazenil has not been shown to benefit patients who have overdosed on multiple drugs.
- Pregnancy class C

Fosphenytoin (Cerebyx)

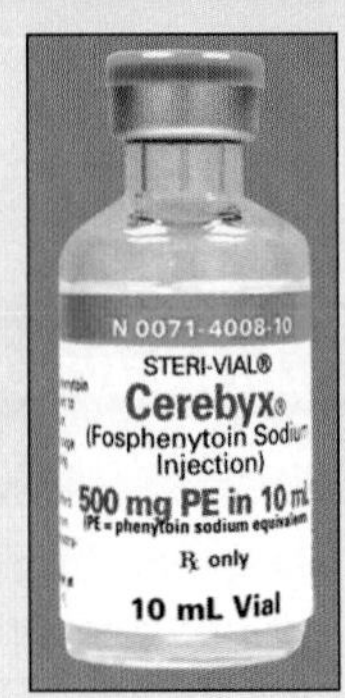

Classification: Anticonvulsant

Action: Alters the movement of sodium and calcium into nervous tissue and prevents the spread of seizure activity.

Indications: Partial and generalized seizures, status epilepticus, seizure prophylaxis.

Dosage: The dose and concentration of fosphenytoin is expressed in PE to simplify the conversion between phenytoin and fosphenytoin.

- **Adult:** The usual loading dose of fosphenytoin is 15 to 20 mg PE/kg IV, not to exceed 150 mg PE/min IV rate.
- **Pediatric:** The usual loading dose of fosphenytoin is 15 to 20 mg PE/kg IV, not to exceed 3 mg PE/kg/min (max dose: 150 mg PE/min) IV rate.

Adverse Effects: Phenytoin can cause several adverse effects often related to drug dose, including sedation, nystagmus, tremors, ataxia, dysarthria, gingival hypertrophy, hirsutism, and facial coarsening. Too-rapid administration can cause hypotension.

Contraindications:

- Bradycardia, bundle branch blocks, agranulocytosis, Adams-Stokes syndrome, hydantoin hypersensitivity
- Pregnancy class D
- Compatible with breast-feeding

Furosemide (Lasix)

Classification: Loop diuretic

Action: Inhibits the absorption of the sodium and chloride ions and water in the loop of Henle, as well as the convoluted tubule of the nephron. This results in decreased absorption of water and increased production of urine.

Indications: Pulmonary edema, CHF, hypertensive emergency.

Adverse Effects: Vertigo, dizziness, weakness, orthostatic hypotension, hypokalemia, thrombophlebitis. Patients with anuria, severe renal failure, untreated hepatic coma, increasing azotemia, and electrolyte depletion can develop life-threatening consequences.

Contraindications: Known sensitivity to sulfonamides or furosemide.

Dosage:

Congestive Heart Failure and Pulmonary Edema:

- **Adult:** The initial dose is 0.5 to 1 mg/kg IV push, given at a rate no faster than 20 mg/min.
- **Pediatric:** 1 mg/kg IV, IO or IM. If the response is not satisfactory, an additional dose of 2 mg/kg may be administered no sooner than 2 hours after the first dose.

Hypertensive Emergency:

- **Adult:** 40 to 80 mg IV, IO.
- **Pediatric:** 1 mg/kg IV or IM.

Special Considerations:

- Onset of action for IV, IO administration occurs within 5 minutes and will peak within 30 minutes.
- Furosemide is a diuretic, so the patient will likely have urinary urgency. Be prepared to help the patient void.
- Pregnancy class C

Gabapentin (Neurontin)

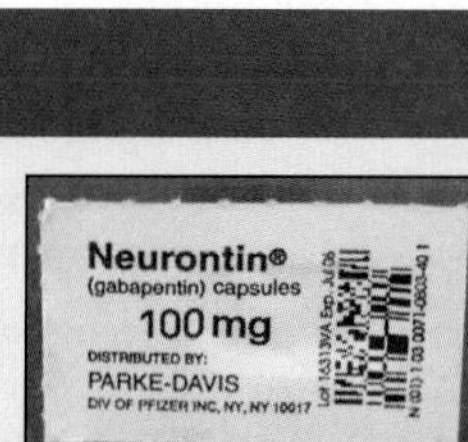

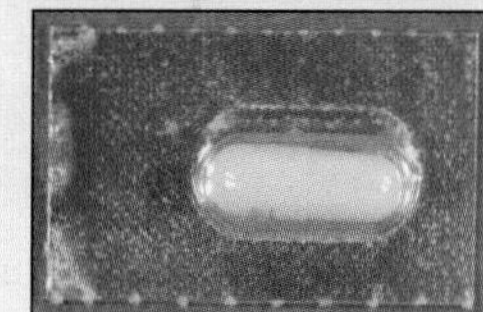

Classification: Anticonvulsant

Action: The exact mechanism of action has not been determined.

Indications: Seizures, neuropathic pain syndromes.

Adverse Effects: Dizziness, ataxia, sleepiness, gait disturbances, upset stomach.

Contraindications: Known sensitivity. Use with caution in elderly patients, renal impairment.

Dosage:

- **Adult:** 300 to 1800 mg PO daily.
- **Pediatric:**
  - **5 to 12 years:** 25 to 35 mg/kg/day PO divided in three divided doses daily.
  - **3 to 4 years:** 40 mg/kg/day PO divided in three divided doses daily.

Special Considerations: Pregnancy class C

Glucagon (GlucaGen)

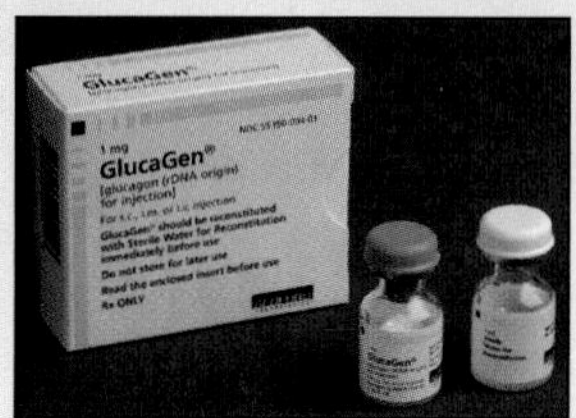

Classification: Hormone

Action: Converts glycogen to glucose.

Indication: Hypoglycemia, beta blocker overdose.

Adverse Effects: Nausea/vomiting, rebound hyperglycemia, hypotension, sinus tachycardia.

Contraindications: Pheochromocytoma, insulinoma, known sensitivity.

Continued

Glucagon—continued

Dosage:

Hypoglycemia:

- **Adult:** 1 mg IM, IV, IO, Sub-Q.
- **Pediatric:** (<20 kg) 0.5 mg IM, IV, IO, Sub-Q.

Beta blocker overdose:

- **Adult:** 2 to 5 mg IV, IO over a 1-minute period, followed by a second dose of 10 mg IV if the symptoms of bradycardia and hypotension recur. (Note that this dose is much higher than the dose required to treat hypoglycemia.)
- **Pediatric:** For patients weighing <20 kg, the dose is 0.5 mg.

Special Considerations: Pregnancy class B

Haloperidol (Haldol)

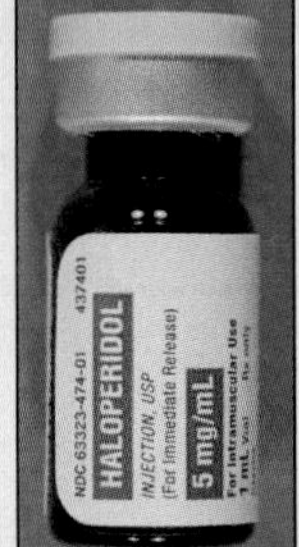

Classification: Antipsychotic agent
Action: Selectively blocks postsynaptic dopamine receptors.
Indications: Psychotic disorders, agitation.
Adverse Effects: Extrapyramidal symptoms, drowsiness, tardive dyskinesia, hypotension, hypertension, VT, sinus tachycardia, QT prolongation, torsades de pointes.
Contraindications: Depressed mental status, Parkinson's disease.
Dosage:

- **Adult:**
  - **Mild agitation:** 0.5 to 2 mg PO or IM.
  - **Moderate agitation:** 5 to 10 mg PO or IM.
  - **Severe agitation:** 10 mg PO or IM.
- **Pediatric:** Not recommended for pediatric patients.

Special Considerations: Pregnancy class C

Heparin (Unfractionated Heparin)

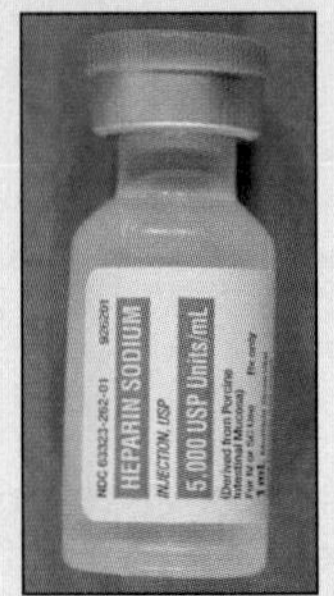

Classification: Anticoagulant
Action: Acts on antithrombin III to reduce the ability of the blood to form clots, thus preventing clot deposition in the coronary arteries.
Indications: ACS, acute pulmonary embolism, deep venous thrombosis.
Adverse Effects: Bleeding, thrombocytopenia, allergic reactions.
Contraindications: Predisposition to bleeding, aortic aneurysm, peptic ulceration; known sensitivity or history of heparin-induced thrombocytopenia, severe thrombocytopenia, sulfite sensitivity.
Dosage:

Cardiac Indications:

- **Adult:** 60 U/kg IV (max 4000 units), followed by 12 U/kg/hr (max 1000 units). Once in the hospital, additional dosing is determined based on laboratory blood tests.
- **Pediatric:** 75 U/kg followed by 20 U/kg/hr.

Pulmonary Embolism and Deep Vein Thrombosis:

- **Adult:** 80 U/kg IV, followed by 18 U/kg/hr.
- **Pediatric:** 75 U/kg IV followed by 20 U/kg/hr.

Special Considerations:

- Half-life approximately 90 minutes
- Pregnancy class C

Hetastarch (Hespan)

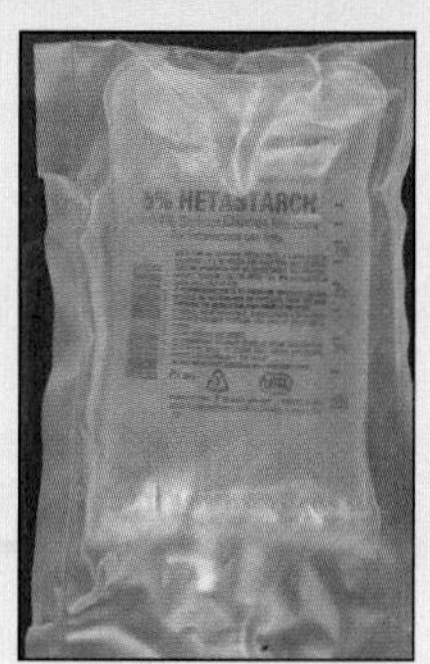

Classification: Volume expander, colloid

Action: Causes water to move from interstitial spaces, thereby increasing the oncotic pressure within the intravascular space.

Indications: Hypovolemia when volume must be increased only in the intravascular compartment.

Adverse Effects: Anaphylactic reactions, CHF, pulmonary edema, cardiac arrhythmias, cardiac arrest, severe hypotension, pruritus, edema, platelet dysfunction, bleeding complications, dilution of the serum proteins responsible for the formation of blood clots, nausea/vomiting.

Contraindications: Bleeding disorders, intracranial bleeding, CHF, pulmonary edema, renal failure, thrombocytopenia or other coagulopathy (e.g., hemophilia), known sensitivity to hetastarch or corn.

Dosage: Note: The dosage of hetastarch required is determined by the clinical situation and the severity of the hypovolemia.

- **Adult:** 500 to 1000 mL IV, IO; more than 1500 mL of hetastarch typically is not administered because of concerns that larger doses can interfere with platelet function and promote bleeding.
- **Pediatric:** 10 mL/kg per dose IV; the total daily dosage should not exceed 20 mL/kg.

Special Considerations: Pregnancy class C

HMG Coenzyme A Statins: Atorvastatin (Lipitor), Fluvastatin (Lescol), Lovastatin (Mevacor), Pravastatin (Pravachol), Rosuvastatin (Crestor), Simvastatin (Zocor)

Classification: HMG coenzyme A statins

Action: Reduces the level of circulating total cholesterol, LDL-cholestrol, and serum triglycerides; reduces the incidence of reinfarction, recurrent angina, rehospitalization, and stroke when initiated within a few days after onset of ACS.

Indications: Acute coronary syndromes/acute myocardial infarction prophylaxis, hypercholesterolemia, hyperlipoproteinemia, hypertriglyceridemia, stroke prophylaxis.

Adverse Effects: Constipation, flatulence, dyspepsia, abdominal pain, infection, headache, flu-like symptoms, back pain, allergic reaction, asthenia, diarrhea, sinusitis, pharyngitis, rash, arthralgia, nausea/vomiting, myopathy, myasthenia, renal failure, rhabdomyolysis, chest pain, bronchitits, rhinitis, insomnia.

Contraindications: Active hepatic disease, pregnancy, breast-feeding, rhabdomyolysis

Dosage:

- **Adult:** Medication is administered orally. Dosage is individualized.
- **Pediatric:** Safe use has not been established.

Special Considerations: Pregnancy class X

Hydralazine (Apresoline)

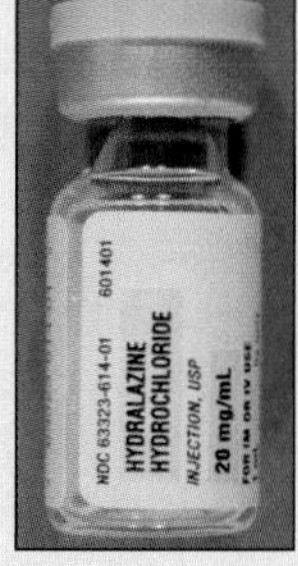

Classification: Antihypertensive agent, vasodilator

Action: Directly dilates the peripheral blood vessels.

Indications: Hypertension associated with preeclampsia and eclampsia, hypertensive crisis.

Adverse Effects: Headache, angina, flushing, palpitations, reflex tachycardia, anorexia, nausea/vomiting, diarrhea, hypotension, syncope, peripheral vasodilation, peripheral edema, fluid retention, paresthesias.

Contraindications: Patients taking diazoxide or MAOIs, coronary artery disease, stroke, angina, dissecting aortic aneurysm, mitral valve and rheumatic heart diseases.

Dosage:

Preeclampsia and Eclampsia:

- **Adult:** 5 to 10 mg IV, IO. Repeat every 20 to 30 minutes until systolic blood pressure of 90 to 105 mm Hg is attained.

Acute Hypertension Not Associated with Preeclampsia:

- **Adult:** 10 to 20 mg IV, IO, or IM.
- **Pediatric:**
  - **1 month to 12 years:** 0.1 to 0.6 mg/kg IV, IO, or IM (max: 20 mg/dose).

Special Considerations: Pregnancy class C

Hydrocortisone Sodium Succinate (Cortef, Solu-Cortef)

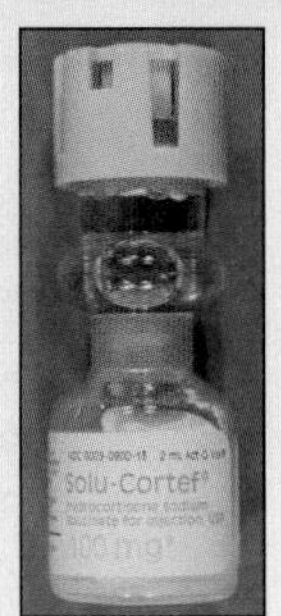

Classification: Corticosteroid

Action: Reduces inflammation by multiple mechanisms. As a steroid, it replaces the steroids that are lacking in adrenal insufficiency.

Indications: Adrenal insufficiency, allergic reactions, anaphylaxis, asthma, COPD.

Adverse Effects: Leukocytosis, hyperglycemia, increased infection, decreased wound healing, increased rate of death from sepsis.

Contraindications: Cushing's syndrome, known sensitivity to benzyl alcohol. Use with caution in diabetes, hypertension, CHF, known systemic fungal infection, renal disease, idiopathic thrombocytopenia, psychosis, seizure disorder, GI disease, glaucoma.

Dosage:

Anaphylactic Shock:
- **Adult:** 100 to 500 mg IV, IO, or IM.
- **Pediatric:** 2 to 4 mg/kg/day IV, IO, or IM (max: 500 mg).

Adrenal Insufficiency:
- **Adult:** 100 to 500 mg IV, IO, or IM.
- **Pediatric:** 1 to 2 mg/kg IV, IO, or IM.

Asthma and Chronic Obstructive Pulmonary Disease:
- **Adult:** 100 to 500 mg IV, IO, IM.
- **Pediatric:** 1 mg/kg IV, IO. The dose may be reduced for infants and children, but it is governed more by the severity of the condition and response of the patient than by age or body weight. Dose should not be less than 25 mg daily.

Special Considerations: Pregnancy class C

Hypertonic Saline (3% Saline)

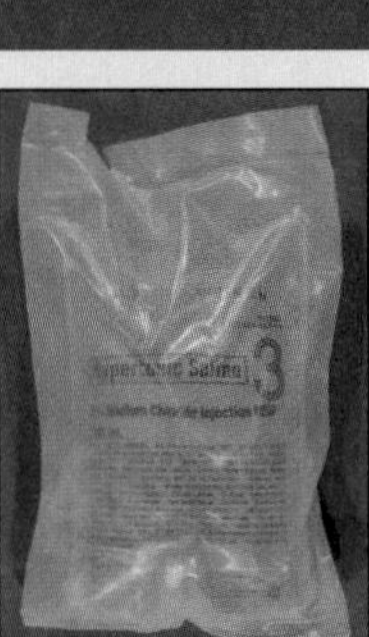

Classification: Volume expander, electrolyte solution

Action: The hyperonic nature of this fluid pulls extravascular fluid into the vascular space. Hypertonic saline may therefore be used as a volume expander in cases of hypovolemia or to reduce the edema of the swollen brain. Three percent saline has an electrolyte concentration of 514 mEq/L sodium.

Indications: Reduction of increased intracranial pressure resulting from traumatic brain injury, hypovolemic shock.

Adverse Effects: Increased rate of bleeding, alteration of blood clotting ability, osmotic demyelination syndrome.

Contraindications: Pulmonary congestion, pulmonary edema, known sensitivity. Hypertonic saline should not be administered by the IO route.

Dosage: Note: Hypertonic saline is available in several concentrations from 3% to 5%.
- **Adult:** 250-mL bag of hypertonic saline infused IV slowly over a 1-hour period.
- **Pediatric:** 6.5 to 10 mL/kg infused slowly IV over a 2-hour period.

Special Considerations:
- Hypertonic saline can cause damage to the vein in which it is administered.
- Pregnancy class C

Insulin, Regular (Humulin R, Novolin R)

Classification: Hormone
Action: Binds to a receptor on the membrane of cells and facilitates the transport of glucose into cells.
Indications: Hyperglycemia, insulin-dependent diabetes mellitus, hyperkalemia.
Adverse Effects: Hypoglycemia, tachycardia, palpitations, diaphoresis, anxiety, confusion, blurred vision, weakness, depression, seizures, coma, insulin shock, hypokalemia.
Contraindications: Hypoglycemia, known sensitivity.
Dosage:
Diabetic Ketoacidosis:

- **Adult:** 0.1 U/kg IV, IO, or Sub-Q. Because of poor perfusion of the peripheral tissues, Sub-Q administration is much less effective than the IV, IO route. IV, IO insulin has a very short half-life; therefore IV, IO insulin without an infusion is not that effective. The rate for an insulin infusion is 0.05 to 0.1 U/kg/hr IV, IO. When dosing insulin, use a U-100 insulin syringe to measure and deliver the insulin. The time from administration to action, as well as the duration of action, varies greatly among different individuals, as well as at different times in the same individual.

Hyperkalemia:

- **Adult:** 10 U IV, IO of regular insulin (Insulin R), coadministered with 50 mL of $D_{50}W$ over 5 minutes.
- **Pediatric:** 0.1 U/kg Insulin R IV, IO.

Special Considerations:

- Only regular insulin can be given IV, IO.
- Pregnancy class B

Ipratropium Bromide (Atrovent)

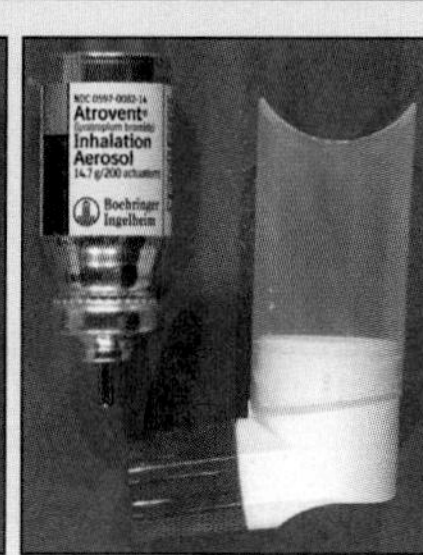

Classification: Bronchodilator, anticholinergic
Action: Antagonizes the acetylcholine receptor on bronchial smooth muscle, producing bronchodilation.
Indications: Asthma, bronchospasm associated with COPD.
Adverse Effects: Paradoxical acute bronchospasm, cough, throat irritation, headache, dizziness, dry mouth, palpitations.
Contraindications: Closed-angle glaucoma, bladder neck obstruction, prostatic hypertrophy, known sensitivity including peanuts or soybeans and atropine or atropine derivatives.
Dosage:
Nebulization:

- **Adult:** 0.5 mg every 6 to 8 hours.
- **Pediatric:** 5 to 14 years: 0.25 to 0.5 mg every 20 minutes for 3 doses as needed.

Metered-Dose Inhaler:

- **Adult:** 4 inhalations every 10 minutes, with no more than 24 inhalations per day or closer than 4 hours apart.
- **Pediatric:**
  - **Older than 12 years:** 2 to 3 puffs inhaled every 6 to 8 hours. Maximum of 12 puffs/day.
  - **5 to 12 years:** 1 to 2 puffs inhaled every 6 to 8 hours. Maximum of 8 puffs/day.

Special Considerations:

- Ipratropium bromide is not typically used as a sole medication in the treatment of acute exacerbation of asthma. Ipratropium bromide is commonly administered after a beta agonist.
- Care should be taken to not allow the aerosol spray (especially in the MDI) to come into contact with the eyes. This can cause temporary blurring of vision that resolves without intervention within 4 hours.
- Pregnancy class B

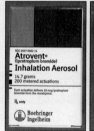

Ketamine (Ketalar)

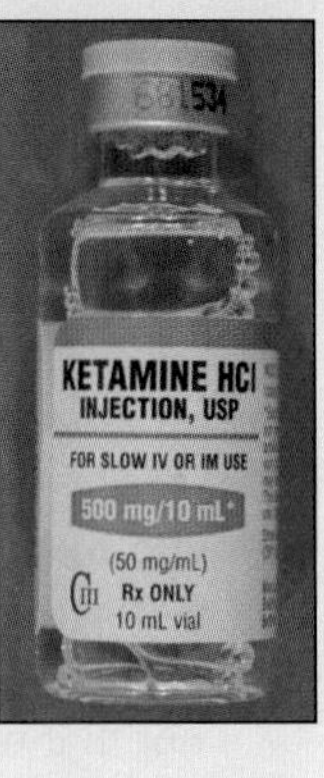

Classification: General anesthetic

Action: Produces a state of anesthesia while maintaining airway reflexes, heart rate, and blood pressure.

Indications: Pain and as anesthesia for procedures of short duration.

Adverse Effects: Emergence phenomena, hypertension and sinus tachycardia, hypotension and sinus bradycardia, other cardiac arrhythmias (rare), respiratory depression, apnea, laryngospasms and other forms of airway obstruction (rare), tonic and clonic movements, vomiting.

Contraindications: Patients in whom a significant elevation in blood pressure would be hazardous (hypertension, stroke, head trauma, increased intracranial mass or bleeding, MI). Use with caution in patients with increased ICP or increased intraocular pressure (glaucoma) and patients with hypovolemia, dehydration, or cardiac disease (especially angina and CHF).

Dosage: Administer slowly over a period of 60 seconds.

IV, IO:

- **Adult:** 1 to 4.5 mg/kg IV/IO. 1 to 2 mg/kg produces anesthesia typically within 30 seconds that typically lasts 5 to 10 minutes.
- **Pediatric:** 0.5 to 2 mg IV, IO over a 1-minute period.

IM:

- **Adult:** 6.5 to 13 mg/kg IM. 10 mg/kg IM is capable of producing anesthesia within 3 to 4 minutes with an effect typically lasting 12 to 25 minutes. In adults, concomitant administration of 5 to 15 mg of diazepam reduces the incidence of emergence phenomena.
- **Pediatric:** 3 to 7 mg IM.

Special Considerations: Pregnancy class C

Ketorolac (Toradol)

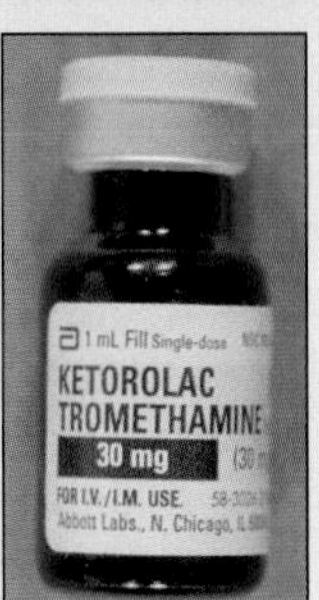

Classification: NSAID

Action: Inhibits the production of prostaglandins in inflamed tissue, which decreases the responsiveness of pain receptors.

Indications: Moderately severe acute pain.

Adverse Effects: Headache, drowsiness, dizziness, abdominal pain, dyspepsia, nausea/vomiting, diarrhea.

Contraindications: Patients with a history of peptic ulcer disease or GI bleed, patients with renal insufficiency, hypovolemic patients, pregnancy (third trimester), nursing mothers, allergy to aspirin or other NSAIDs, stroke or suspected stroke or head trauma, need for major surgery in the immediate or near future (i.e., within 7 days).

Dosage: Note: The following dosage regimen applies to single-dose administration only. IV, IO administration should occur over a period of at least 15 seconds.

- **Adult:**
  - **Younger than 65 years:** 30 mg IV, IO or 60 mg IM.
  - **Older than 65 years:** 15 mg IV, IO or 30 mg IM.
- **Pediatric:** 0.5 mg/kg IV, IO to a maximum dose of 15 mg, or 1 mg/kg IM to a maximum dose of 30 mg.

Special Considerations: Pregnancy class C; class D in third trimester

Labetalol (Normodyne, Trandate)

Classification: Beta adrenergic antagonist, antianginal, antihypertensive

Action: Binds with both the $beta_1$ and $beta_2$ receptors and $alpha_1$ receptors in vascular smooth muscle. Inhibits the strength of the heart's contractions, as well as heart rate. This results in a decrease in cardiac oxygen consumption.

Indications: ACS, SVT, severe hypertension.

Adverse Effects: Usually mild and transient; hypotensive symptoms, nausea/vomiting, bronchospasm, arrhythmia, bradycardia, AV block.

Contraindications: Hypotension, cardiogenic shock, acute pulmonary edema, heart failure, severe bradycardia, sick sinus syndrome, second- or third-degree heart block, asthma or acute bronchospasm, cocaine-induced ACS, known sensitivity. Use caution in pheochromocytoma, cerebrovascular disease or stroke, poorly controlled diabetes, with hepatic disease. Use with caution at lowest effective dose in chronic lung disease.

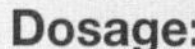

Dosage:

Cardiac Indications: Note: Monitor blood pressure and heart rate closely during administration.

Adult: 10 mg IV, IO over a 1- to 2-minute period. May repeat every 10 minutes to a maximum dose of 150 mg or give initial bolus and then follow with infusion at 2 to 8 mg/min.

Pediatric: 0.4 to 1 mg/kg/hr to a maximum dosage of 3 mg/kg/hr.

Severe Hypertension:

- **Adult:** Initial dose is 20 mg IV, IO slow infusion over a 2-minute period. After the initial dose, blood pressure should be checked every 5 minutes. Repeat doses can be given at 10-minute intervals. The second dose should be 40 mg IV, IO, and subsequent doses should be 80 mg IV, IO, to a maximum total dose of 300 mg. The effect on blood pressure typically will occur within 5 minutes from the time of administration. Alternatively, may be administered via IV infusion at 2 mg/min to a total maximum dose of 300 mg.
- **Pediatric:** 0.4 to 1 mg/kg/hr IV, IO infusion with a maximum dose of 3 mg/kg/hr.

Special Considerations: Pregnancy class C

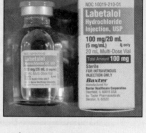

Lamotrigine (Lamictal)

Classification: Anticonvulsant, antimanic agent

Action: The exact mechanism of action has not been determined. Studies suggest lamotrigine stabilizes neuronal membranes by acting at voltage-sensitive sodium channels, thereby decreasing presynaptic release of glutamate and aspartate, resulting in decreased seizure activity.

Indications: Seizures, bipolar disorders.

Adverse Effects: Headache, dizziness, nausea/vomiting, ataxia, diplopia.

Contraindications: Known sensitivity.

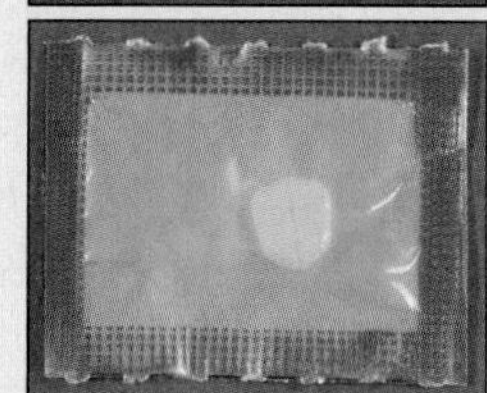

Dosage:

- **Adult:** Medication is administered orally. Dosage is individualized.
- **Pediatric:** Medication is administered orally. Dosage is individualized.

Special Considerations: Pregnancy class C

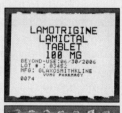

Lidocaine (Xylocaine)

Classification: Antiarrhythmic, class IB

Action: Blocks sodium channels, increasing the recovery period after repolarization; suppresses automaticity in the His-Purkinje system and depolarization in the ventricles.

Indications: Ventricular arrhythmias, when amiodarone is not available: cardiac arrest from VF/VT, stable monomorphic VT with preserved ventricular function, stable polymorphic VT with normal baseline QT interval and preserved left ventricular function (when ischemia and electrolyte imbalance are treated), stable polymorphic VT with baseline QT-prolongation suggestive of torsades de pointes.

Adverse Effects: Toxicity (signs may include anxiety, apprehension, euphoria, nervousness, disorientation, dizziness, blurred vision, facial paresthesias, tremors, hearing disturbances, slurred speech, seizures, sinus bradycardia), seizures without warning, cardiac arrhythmias, hypotension, cardiac arrest), pain at injection site.

Contraindications: AV block; bleeding; thrombocytopenia; known sensitivity to lidocaine, sulfite, or paraben. Use with caution in bradycardia, hypovolemia, cardiogenic shock, Adams-Stokes syndrome, Wolff-Parkinson-White syndrome.

Dosage:

Pulseless Ventricular Tachycardia and Ventricular Fibrillation:

- **Adult IV, IO:** 1 to 1.5 mg/kg IV, IO; may repeat at half the original dose (0.5-0.75 mg/kg) every 5 to 10 minutes to a maximum dose of 3 mg/kg. If a maintenance infusion is warranted, the rate is 1 to 4 mg/min.
- **Adult ET tube:** 2 to 10 mg/kg ET tube, diluted in 10 mL normal saline or sterile distilled water.
- **Pediatric IV, IO:** 1 mg/kg IV, IO (maximum 100 mg). If a maintenance infusion is warranted, the rate is 20 to 50 mcg/kg/min.
- **Pediatric ET tube:** 2 to 3 mg/kg ET tube, followed by a 5-mL flush of normal saline.

Perfusing Ventricular Rhythms:

- **Adult:** 0.5 to 0.75 mg/kg IV, IO (up to 1-1.5 mg/kg may be used). Repeat 0.5 to 0.75 mg/kg every 5 to 10 minutes to a maximum total dose of 3 mg/kg. A maintenance infusion of 1 to 4 mg/min (30-50 mcg/kg/min) is acceptable.
- **Pediatric:** 1 mg/kg IV, IO. May repeat every 5 to 10 minutes to a maximum dose of 3 mg/kg. Maintenance infusion rate is 20 to 50 mcg/kg/min.

Special Considerations:

- Half-life approximately 90 minutes
- Pregnancy class B

Lorazepam (Ativan)

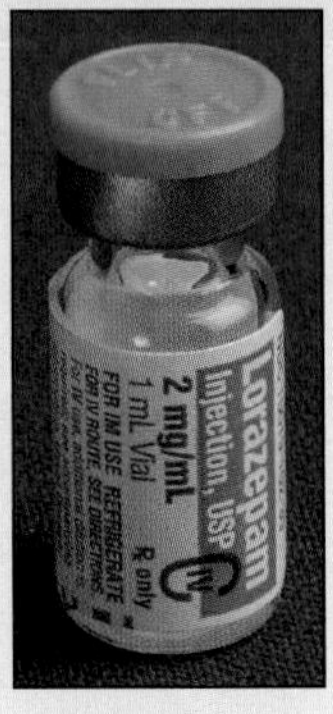

Classification: Benzodiazepine; schedule C-IV

Action: Binds to the benzodiazepine receptor and enhances the effects of the brain chemical GABA, an inhibitory transmitter, and may result in a state of sedation, hypnosis, skeletal muscle relaxation, anticonvulsant activity, coma.

Indications: Preprocedure sedation induction, anxiety, status epilepticus.

Adverse Effects: Headache, drowsiness, ataxia, dizziness, amnesia, depression, dysarthria, euphoria, syncope, fatigue, tremor, vertigo, respiratory depression, paradoxical CNS stimulation.

Contraindications: Known sensitivity to lorazepam, benzodiazepines, polyethylene glycol, propylene glycol, or benzyl alcohol; COPD; sleep apnea (except while being mechanically ventilated); shock; coma; acute closed-angle glaucoma.

Dosage: Note: IV, IO lorazepam needs to be administered slowly.

Analgesia and Sedation:

- **Adult:** 2 mg or 0.44 mg/kg IV, IO, whichever is smaller. This dose will provide adequate sedation in most patients and should not be exceeded in patients older than 50 years.
- **Pediatric:** 0.05 mg/kg IV, IO. Each dose should not exceed 2 mg IV, IO.

Continued

Lorazepam (Ativan)—continued

Seizures:

- **Adult:** 4 mg IV, IO given over 2 to 5 minutes; may repeat in 10 to 15 minutes (max total dose: 8 mg in a 12-hour period).
- **Pediatric:**
  - **Adolescents:** 0.07 mg/kg slow IV, IO given over 2 to 5 minutes (max single dose: 4 mg). May repeat in 10 to 15 minutes (max dose: 8 mg in a 12-hour period).
  - **Children and infants:** 0.1 mg/kg slow IV, IO given over 2 to 5 minutes (max single dose: 4 mg). May repeat at half the original dose in 10 to 15 minutes if seizure activity resumes.
  - **Neonates:** 0.05 mg/kg slow IV, IO given over 2 to 5 minutes. May repeat in 10 to 15 minutes.

Special Considerations:

- Be prepared to support the patient's airway and ventilation.
- Pregnancy class D

Magnesium Sulfate

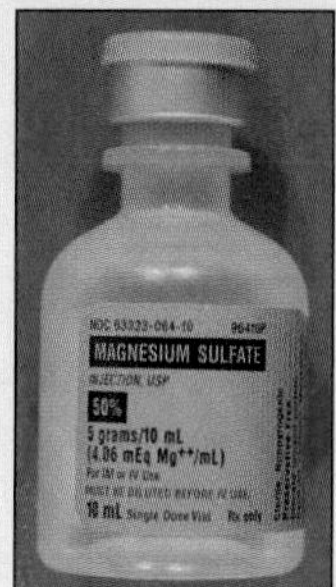

Classification: Electrolyte, tocolytic, mineral

Action: Required for normal physiologic functioning. Magnesium is a cofactor in neurochemical transmission and muscular excitability. Magnesium sulfate controls seizures by blocking peripheral neuromuscular transmission. Magnesium is also a peripheral vasodilator and an inhibitor of platelet function.

Indications: Torsades de pointes, cardiac arrhythmias associated with hypomagnesemia, eclampsia and seizure prophylaxis in preeclampsia, status asthmaticus.

Adverse Effects: Magnesium toxicity (signs include flushing, diaphoresis, hypotension, muscle paralysis, weakness, hypothermia, and cardiac, CNS, or respiratory depression).

Contraindications: AV block, GI obstruction. Use with caution in renal impairment.

Dosage:

Ventricular Fibrillation/Pulseless Ventricular Tachycardia with Torsades De Pointes or Hypomagnesemia:

- **Adult:** 1 to 2 g in 10 mL D_5W IV, IO administered over 5 to 10 minutes.
- **Pediatric:** 25 to 50 mg/kg IV, IO over 10 to 20 minutes; may administer faster for torsades de pointes (max single dose: 2 g).

Torsades De Pointes with a Pulse or Cardiac Arrhythmias with Hypomagnesemia:

- **Adult:** 1 to 2 g in 50 to 100 mL D_5W IV, IO administered over 5 to 60 minutes. Follow with 0.5 to 1 g/hr IV, IO titrated to control torsades de pointes.
- **Pediatric:** 25 to 50 mg/kg IV, IO over 10 to 20 minutes (max single dose: 2 g).

Eclampsia and Seizure Prophylaxis in Preeclampsia:

- **Adult:** 4 to 6 g IV, IO over 20 to 30 minutes, followed by an infusion of 1 to 2 g/hr.

Status Asthmaticus:

- **Adult:** 1.2 to 2 g slow IV, IO (over 20 minutes).
- **Pediatric:** 25 to 50 mg/kg (diluted in D_5W) slow IV, IO (over 10 to 20 minutes).

Special Considerations: Pregnancy class A

Mannitol (Osmitrol)

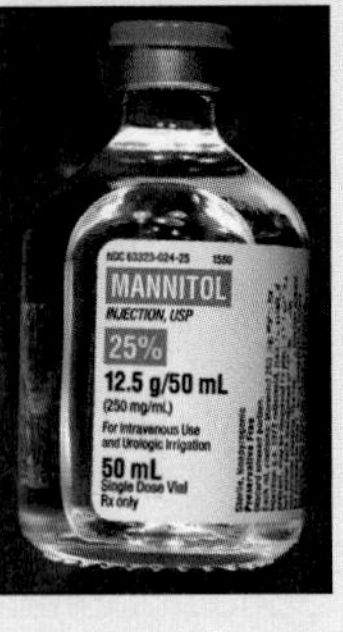

Classification: Osmotic diuretic

Action: Facilitates the flow of fluid out of tissues (including the brain) and into interstitial fluid and blood, thereby dehydrating the brain and reducing swelling. Reabsorption by the kidney is minimal, consequently increasing urine output.

Indications: Increased ICP.

Adverse Effects: Pulmonary edema, headache, blurred vision, dizziness, seizures, hypovolemia, nausea/vomiting, diarrhea, electrolyte imbalances, hypotension, hypertension, sinus tachycardia, PVCs, angina, phlebitis.

Contraindications: Active intracranial bleeding, CHF, pulmonary edema, severe dehydration. Use with caution in hypovolemia, renal failure.

Dosage:

- **Adult:** 0.5 to 2 g/kg IV, IO followed by 0.25 to 1 g/kg administered every 4 hours.
- **Pediatric:** 0.25 to 1 g/kg IV, IO followed by 0.25-0.5 g/kg every 4 hours.

Special Considerations:

- Mannitol should not be given in the same IV, IO line as blood.
- Pregnancy class C

Meperidine (Demerol)

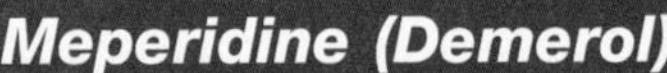

Classification: Narcotic analgesic, schedule C-II

Action: Binds to opiate receptors, producing analgesia and euphoria.

Indications: Moderate to severe pain.

Adverse Effects: Respiratory depression, nausea/vomiting, sinus bradycardia, sinus tachycardia, palpitations, hypertension, hypotension, orthostatic hypotension, diaphoresis, syncope, shock, cardiac arrest.

Contraindications: Patients who have taken a MAOI in the past 2 weeks, patients who are using other CNS depressants or alcohol, known sensitivity. Use with caution in patients with chronic respiratory conditions (asthma or COPD), pregnant or nursing women, atrial flutter.

Dosage: If given IV, IO, administer slowly.

- **Adult:** 50 to 150 mg IV, IO, IM, or Sub-Q. Elderly: 50 mg IV, IO, IM, or Sub-Q.
- **Pediatric:** 1 to 2 mg/kg IV, IO, IM, or Sub-Q.

Special Considerations:

- In adults, half-life approximately 4 hours, but its active metabolites may last 30 hours.
- Pregnancy class C; class D near term.

Methylprednisolone Sodium Succinate (Solu-Medrol)

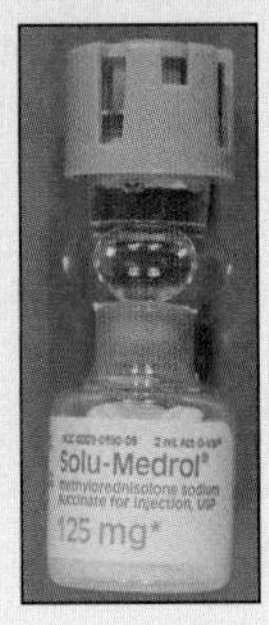

Classification: Corticosteroid

Action: Reduces inflammation by multiple mechanisms.

Indications: Anaphylaxis, asthma, COPD.

Adverse Effects: Depression, euphoria, headache, restlessness, hypertension, bradycardia, nausea/vomiting, swelling, diarrhea, weakness, fluid retention, paresthesias.

Contraindications: Cushing's syndrome, fungal infection, measles, varicella, known sensitivity (including sulfites). Use with caution in active infections, renal disease, penetrating spinal cord injury, hypertension, seizures, CHF.

Dosage:

Asthma and Chronic Obstructive Pulmonary Disease:

- **Adult:** 40 to 80 mg IV.
- **Pediatric:** 1 mg/kg (up to 60 mg) IV, IO per day in two divided doses.

Continued

Methylprednisolone Sodium Succinate (Solu-Medrol)—continued

Anaphylactic Shock:

- **Adult:** 1 to 2 mg/kg/dose, then 0.5 to 1 mg/kg every 6 hours.
- **Pediatric:** Same as adult dosing.

Blunt Spinal Cord Injury:

- **Adult:** 30 mg/kg IV, IO over a period of 1 hour, then as an infusion to run for the remaining 23 hours at a dose of 5.4 mg/kg/hr.
- **Pediatric:** Same as adult dosing.

Special Considerations:

- May mask signs and symptoms of infection.
- Pregnancy class C

Metoprolol (Lopressor, Toprol XL)

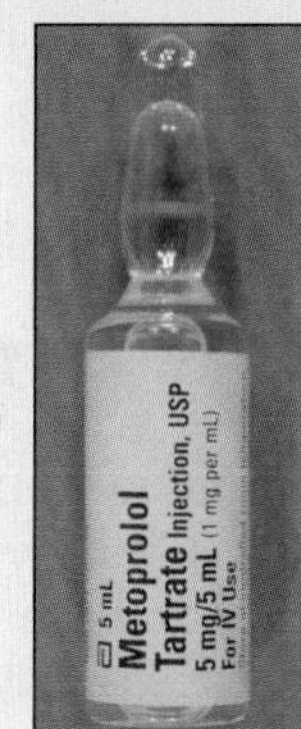
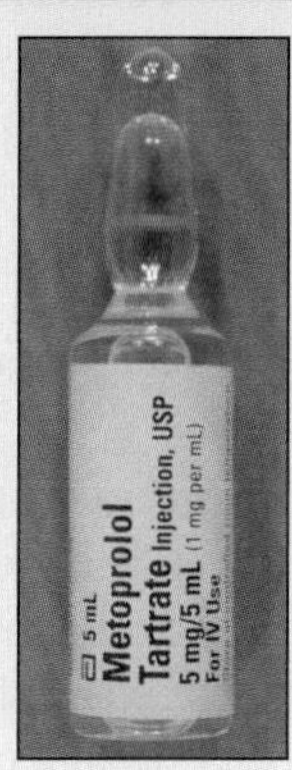

Classification: Beta adrenergic antagonist, antianginal, antihypertensive, class II antiarrhythmic

Action: Inhibits the strength of the heart's contractions as well as heart rate. This results in a decrease in cardiac oxygen consumption. Also saturates the beta receptors and inhibits dilation of bronchial smooth muscle (beta$_2$ receptor).

Indications: ACS, hypertension, SVT, atrial flutter, AF, thyrotoxicosis.

Adverse Effects: Tiredness, dizziness, diarrhea, heart block, bradycardia, bronchospasm, drop in blood pressure.

Contraindications: Cardiogenic shock, AV block, bradycardia, known sensitivity. Use with caution in hypotension, chronic lung disease (asthma and COPD).

Dosage:

Cardiac Indications:

- **Adult:** 5 mg slow IV, IO over a 5-minute period; repeat at 5-minute intervals up to a total of three infusions totaling 15 mg IV, IO.
- **Pediatric:** Not recommended for pediatric patients; no studies available.

Special Considerations:

- Blood pressure, heart rate, and ECG should be monitored carefully.
- Use with caution in patients with asthma.
- Pregnancy class C

Midazolam (Versed)

Classification: Benzodiazepine, schedule C-IV

Action: Binds to the benzodiazepine receptor and enhances the effects of the brain chemical (neurotransmitter) GABA. Benzodiazepines act at the level of the limbic, thalamic, and hypothalamic regions of the CNS to produce short-acting CNS depression (including sedation, skeletal muscle relaxation, and anticonvulsant activity).

Indications: Sedation, anxiety, skeletal muscle relaxation.

Adverse Effects: Respiratory depression, respiratory arrest, hypotension, nausea/vomiting, headache, hiccups, cardiac arrest.

Contraindications: Acute-angle glaucoma, pregnancy, known sensitivity.

Dosage:

Sedation:

Note: The dose of midazolam needs to be individualized. Every dose should be administered slowly over a period of 2 minutes. Allow 2 minutes to evaluate the clinical effect of the dose given.

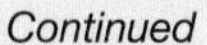

Continued

Midazolam (Versed)—continued

- **Adult:**
  - **Adult (healthy and younger than 60 years):** *Some patients require as little as 1 mg IV, IO. No more than 2.5 mg should be given over a 2-minute interval.* If additional sedation is required, continue to administer small increments over 2-minute periods (max dose: 5 mg). If the patient also has received a narcotic, he or she will typically require 30% less midazolam than the same patient not given the narcotic.
  - **Adult (60 years and older and debilitated or chronically ill patients):** This group of patients has a higher risk of hypoventilation, airway obstruction, and apnea. The peak clinical effect can take longer in these patients; therefore dose increments should be smaller, and the rate of injection should be slower. *Some patients require a dose as small as 1 mg IV, IO, and no more than 1.5 mg should be given over a 2-minute period.* If additional sedation is required, additional midazolam should be given at a rate of no more than 1 mg over a 2-minute period (max dose: 3.5 mg). If the patient also has received a narcotic, he or she will typically require 50% less midazolam than the same patient not given the narcotic.
  - **Adult—continuous infusion:** Continuous infusions can be required for prolonged transport of intubated, critically ill, and injured patients. After an initial bolus dose, the adult patient will require a maintenance infusion dose of 0.02 to 0.1 mg/kg/hr (1-7 mg/hr).
- **Pediatric (weight-based):** Pediatric patients typically require higher doses of midazolam than do adults on the basis of weight (in mg/kg). Younger pediatric patients (younger than 6 years) require higher doses (in mg/kg) than older pediatric patients. Midazolam takes approximately 3 minutes to reach peak effect; therefore wait at least 2 minutes to determine effectiveness of drug and need for additional dosing.
  - **12 to 16 years:** Same as adult dosing. Some patients in this age group require a higher dose than that used in adults, but rarely does a patient require more than 10 mg.
  - **6 to 12 years:** 0.025 to 0.05 mg/kg IV, IO up to a total dose of 0.4 mg/kg. Exceeding 10 mg as total dose usually is not necessary.
  - **6 months to 5 years:** 0.05 to 0.1 mg/kg IV, IO up to a total dose of 0.6 mg/kg. Exceeding 6 mg as total dose usually is not necessary.
- **Younger than 6 months:** Dosing recommendations for this age group is unclear. Because this age group is especially vulnerable to airway obstruction and hypoventilation, use small increments with frequent clinical evaluation. Dose: 0.05 to 0.1 mg/kg IV, IO.

Special Considerations:

- Patients receiving midazolam require frequent monitoring of vital signs and pulse oximetry. Be prepared to support patient's airway and ventilation.
- Pregnancy class D

Milrinone (Primacor)

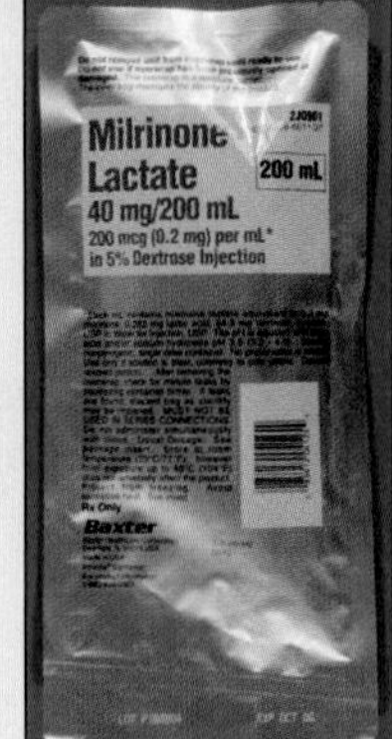

Classification: Inotrope

Action: Milrinone is a positive inotrope and vasodilator with minimal chronotropic effect. Milrinone inhibits an enzyme, cAMP phosphodiesterase, which results in an increase in the concentration of calcium inside the cardiac cell. The result is improvement in diastolic function and myocardial contractility.

Indications: Cardiogenic shock, CHF.

Adverse Effects: Cardiac arrhythmias, nausea/vomiting, hypotension.

Contraindications: Valvular heart disease, known sensitivity.

Dosage:

- **Adult:** 50 mcg/kg IV, IO over a period of 10 minutes, followed by an infusion of 0.375 to 0.5 mcg/kg/min (max dose: 0.75 mcg/kg/min).
- **Pediatric:** Same as adult dosing.

Special Considerations: Pregnancy class C

Morphine Sulfate

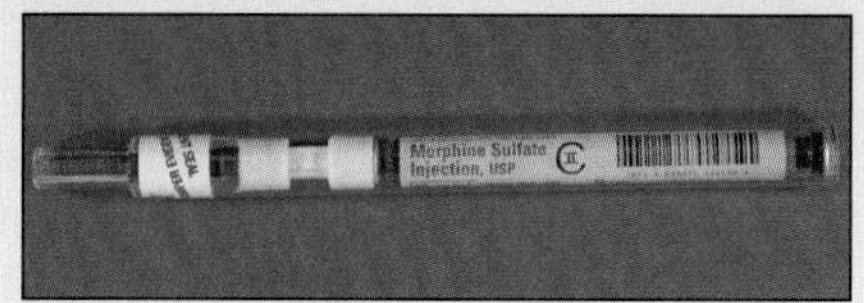

Classification: Opiate agonist, schedule C-II

Action: Binds with opioid receptors. Morphine is capable of inducing hypotension by depression of the vasomotor centers of the brain, as well as release of the chemical histamine. In the management of angina, morphine reduces stimulation of the sympathetic nervous system caused by pain and anxiety. Reduction of sympathetic stimulation reduces heart rate, cardiac work, and myocardial oxygen consumption.

Indications: Moderate to severe pain, including chest pain associated with ACS, CHF, pulmonary edema.

Adverse Effects: Respiratory depression, hypotension, nausea/vomiting, dizziness, lightheadedness, sedation, diaphoresis, euphoria, dysphoria, worsening of bradycardia and heart block in some patients with acute inferior wall MI, seizures, cardiac arrest, anaphylactoid reactions.

Contraindications: Respiratory depression, shock, known sensitivity. Use with caution in hypotension, acute bronchial asthma, respiratory insufficiency, head trauma.

Dosage:

Pain:

- **Adult:** 2.5 to 15 mg IV, IO, IM, or Sub-Q administered slowly over a period of several minutes. The dose is the same whether administered IV, IO, IM, or Sub-Q.
- **Pediatric:**
  - **6 months to 12 years:** 0.05 to 0.2 mg/kg IV, IO, IM, or Sub-Q.
  - **Younger than 6 months:** 0.03 to 0.05 mg/kg IV, IO, IM, or Sub-Q.

Chest Pain Associated with Acute Coronary Syndromes, Congestive Heart Failure, and Pulmonary Edema:
Administer small doses and reevaluate the patient. Large doses may lead to respiratory depression and worsen the patient's hypoxia.

- **Adult:** 2 to 4 mg slow IV, IO over a 1- to 5-minute period with increments of 2 to 8 mg repeated every 5 to 15 minutes until patient relieved of chest pain.
- **Pediatric:** 0.1 to 0.2 mg/kg/dose IV, IO.

Special Considerations:

- Monitor vital signs and pulse oximetry closely. Be prepared to support patient's airway and ventilations.
- Overdose should be treated with naloxone.
- Pregnancy class C

Nalbuphine (Nubain)

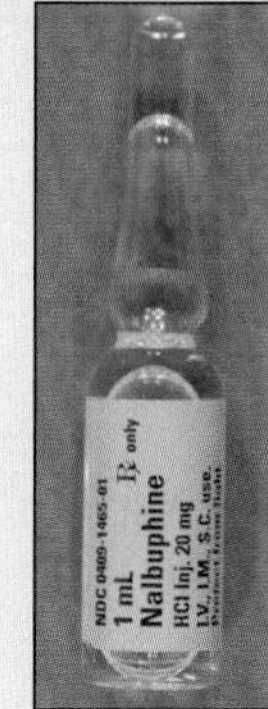

Classification: Synthetic opioid agonist-antagonist

Action: Produces analgesia by binding to the opioid receptor.

Indications: Moderate to severe pain.

Adverse Effects: Drowsiness, diaphoresis, headache, nausea/vomiting, dry mouth, respiratory depression, hypotension, bradycardia.

Contraindications: Known sensitivity.

Dosage:

- **Adult:** 10 mg IV, IO, IM, or Sub-Q.
- **Pediatric:** Not recommended for pediatric patients.

Special Considerations: Pregnancy class B

Naloxone (Narcan)

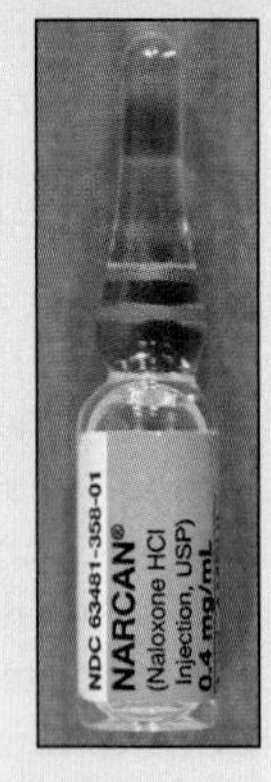

Classification: Opioid antagonist

Action: Binds the opioid receptor and blocks the effect of narcotics.

Indications: Narcotic overdoses, reversal of narcotics used for procedure-related anesthesia.

Adverse Effects: Nausea/vomiting, restlessness, diaphoresis, tachycardia, hypertension, tremulousness, seizures, cardiac arrest, narcotic withdrawal. Patients who have gone from a state of somnolence from a narcotic overdose to wide awake may become combative.

Contraindications: Known sensitivity to naloxone, nalmefene, or naltrexone. Use with caution in patients with supraventricular arrhythmias or other cardiac disease, head trauma, brain tumor.

Dosage:

- **Adult:** 0.4 to 2 mg IV, IO, ET, IM, or Sub-Q. Alternatively, administer 2 mg intranasally. Higher doses (10-20 mg) may be required for overdoses of synthetic narcotics. A repeat dose of one-third to two-thirds the original dose is often necessary.
- **Pediatric:**
  - **5 years or older or weight >20 kg:** 2 mg IV, IO, ET, IM, or Sub-Q.
  - **Younger than 5 years or weight <20 kg:** 0.1 mg/kg IV, IO, ET, IM, or Sub-Q; may repeat every 2 to 3 minutes.

Special Considerations: Pregnancy class C

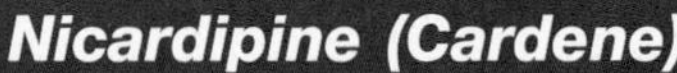

Nicardipine (Cardene)

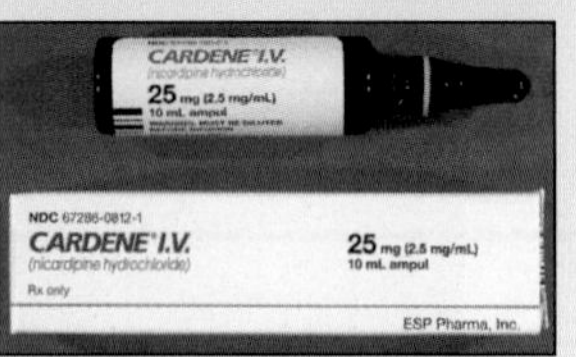

Classification: Calcium channel blocker

Action: Blocks calcium movement into the smooth muscle of the blood vessel walls, causing vasodilation.

Indications: Hypertension

Adverse Effects: Edema, headaches, flushing, sinus tachycardia, hypotension.

Contraindications: Aortic stenosis, hypotension, known sensitivity. Use with caution in heart failure, cardiac conduction abnormalities, cerebral vascular disease, depressed AV node conduction.

Dosage:

- **Adult:** 5 mg/hr IV, IO; may increase by 2.5 mg/hr every 5 to 15 minutes (max dose: 15 mg/hr). Once the patient has achieved the desired blood pressure, decrease infusion to a maintenance dose of 3 mg/hr.
- **Pediatric:** 0.5 to 1 mcg/kg/min IV, IO infusion.

Special Considerations: Pregnancy class C

Nitroglycerin (Nitrolingual, NitroQuick, NitroStat Nitro-Dur)

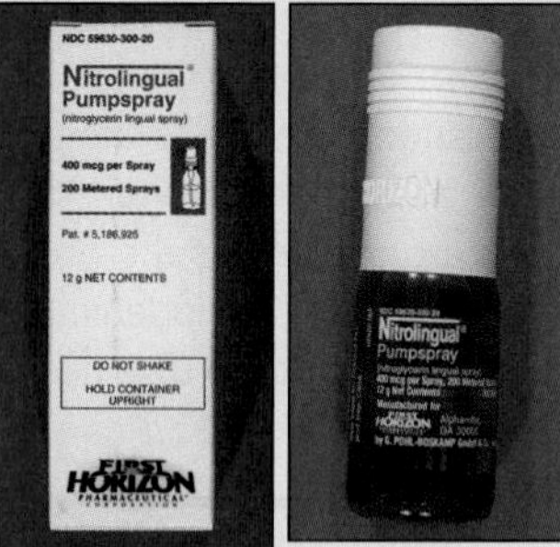

Classification: Antianginal agent

Action: Relaxes vascular smooth muscle, thereby dilating peripheral arteries and veins. This causes pooling of venous blood and decreased venous return to the heart, which decreases preload. Nitroglycerin also reduces left ventricular systolic wall tension, which decreases afterload.

Indications: Angina, ongoing ischemic chest discomfort, hypertension, myocardial ischemia associated with cocaine intoxication.

Adverse Effects: Headache, hypotension, bradycardia, lightheadedness, flushing, cardiovascular collapse, methemoglobinemia.

Contraindications: Hypotension, severe bradycardia or tachycardia, increased ICP, intracranial bleeding, patients taking any medications for erectile dysfunction (such as sildenafil [Viagra], tadalafil [Cialis], or vardenafil [Levitra]), known sensitivity to nitrates. Use with caution in anemia, closed-angle glaucoma, hypotension, postural hypotension, uncorrected hypovolemia.

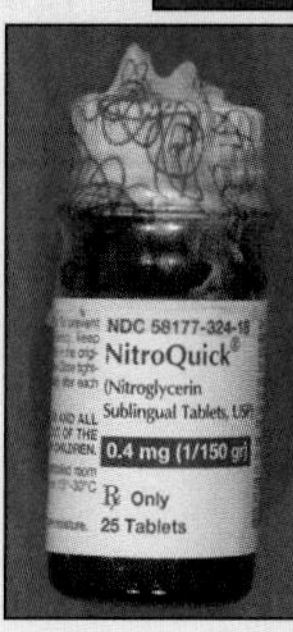

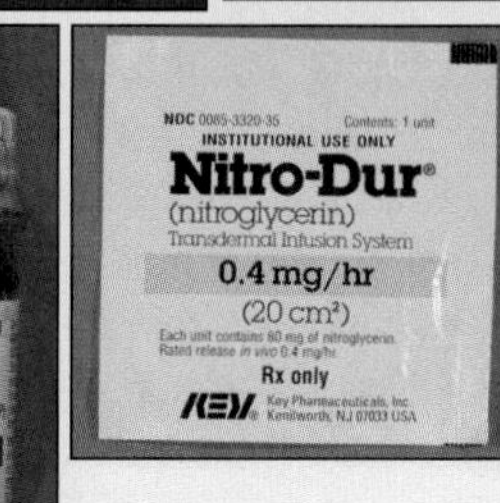

Dosage:

- **Adult:**
  - **Sublingual tablets:** 1 tablet (0.3-0.4 mg) at 5-minute intervals to a maximum of 3 doses.
  - **Translingual spray:** 1 (0.4 mg) spray at 5-minute intervals to a maximum of 3 sprays.
  - **Ointment:** 2% topical (Nitro-Bid ointment): Apply 1 to 2 inches of paste over the chest wall, cover with transparent wrap, and secure with tape.
  - **IV:**
    - **Bolus:** 12.5 to 25 mcg
    - **Infusion:** 5 mcg/min; may increase rate by 5 to 10 mcg/min every 5 to 10 minutes as needed. End points of dose titration for nitroglycerin include a drop in the blood pressure of 10%, relief of chest pain, and return of ST-segment to normal on a 12-lead ECG.
- **Pediatric IV infusion:** The initial pediatric infusion is 0.25 to 0.5 mcg/kg/min IV, IO titrated by 0.5 to 1 mcg/kg/min. Usual required dose is 1 to 3 mcg/kg/min to a maximum dose of 5 mcg/kg/min.

Special Considerations:

- Administration of nitroglycerin to a patient with right ventricular MI can result in hypotension.
- Pregnancy class C

Nitrous Oxide

Classification: Inorganic gas, inhaled anesthetic

Action: Exact mechanism is not known.

Indications: Mild to severe pain.

Adverse Effects: Delirium, hypoxia, respiratory depression, nausea/vomiting.

Contraindications: Use with caution in head trauma, increased ICP, pneumothorax, bowel obstruction, patients with COPD who require a hypoxic respiratory drive.

Dosage: Inhaled: 20% to 50% concentration mixed with oxygen.

Special Considerations:

- Ensure the safety of healthcare professionals. Only use with a scavenger gas system to ensure that unused gas is collected, or scavenged, and that providers are not exposed to significant levels of the agent.
- Pregnancy class not noted

Norepinephrine (Levophed)

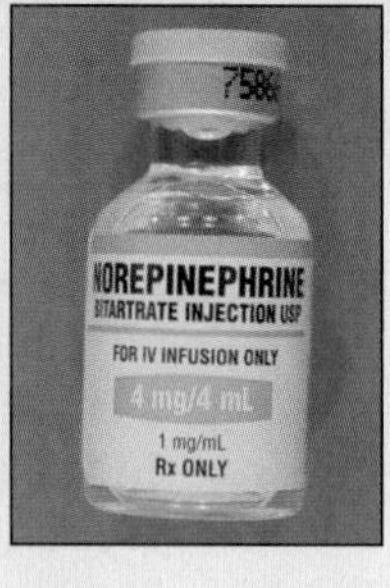

Classification: Adrenergic agonist, inotrope, vasopressor

Action: Norepinephrine is an $alpha_1$, $alpha_2$, and $beta_1$ agonist. Alpha-mediated peripheral vasoconstriction is the predominant clinical result of administration, resulting in increasing blood pressure and coronary blood flow. Beta adrenergic action produces inotropic stimulation of the heart and dilates the coronary arteries.

Indications: Cardiogenic shock, septic shock, severe hypotension.

Adverse Effects: Dizziness, anxiety, cardiac arrhythmias, dyspnea, exacerbation of asthma.

Contraindications: Patients taking MAOIs, known sensitivity. Use with caution in hypovolemia.

Dosage:

- **Adult:** Add 4 mg to 250 mL of D_5W or D_5NS, but not normal saline alone. 0.5 to 1 mcg/min as IV, IO, titrated to maintain blood pressure >80 mm Hg. Refractory shock may require doses as high as 30 mcg/min.
- **Pediatric:** 0.05 to 2 mcg/kg/min IV, IO infusion, to a maximum dose of 2 mcg/kg/min.

Special Considerations:

- Do not administer in same IV line as alkaline solutions.
- Half-life 1 minute
- Pregnancy class C

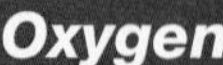

Oxygen

Classification: Elemental gas

Action: Facilitates cellular energy metabolism

Indications: Hypoxia, ischemic chest pain, respiratory distress, suspected carbon monoxide poisoning, traumatic injuries, shock, cardiac arrest.

Adverse Effects: High concentrations can cause decreased level of consciousness and respiratory depression in patients with chronic carbon dioxide retention or chronic lung disease.

Contraindications: Known paraquat poisoning.

Dosage:

Low-Concentration Oxygen:

- A dose of 1 to 4 L/min by a nasal cannula is appropriate.

High-Concentration Oxygen:

- A dose of 10 to 15 L/min via nonrebreather mask is appropriate.

Special Considerations: Pregnancy class A

Pancuronium (Pavulon)

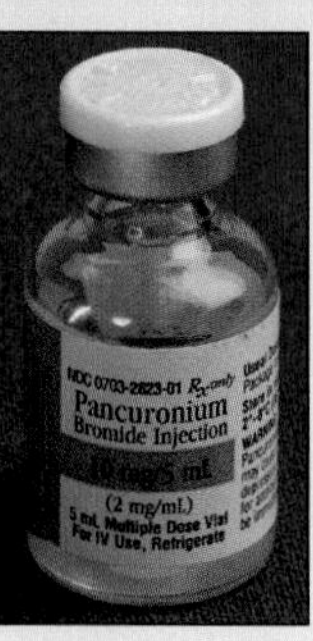

Classification: Nondepolarizing neuromuscular blocker

Action: Antagonizes acetylcholine at the motor end plate, producing skeletal muscle paralysis.

Indications: To induce neuromuscular blockade for the facilitation of ET intubation.

Adverse Effects: Muscle paralysis, apnea, dyspnea, respiratory depression, cutaneous flushing, sinus tachycardia.

Contraindications: Known sensitivity to bromides. Use with caution in heart disease, renal disease.

Dosage:

- **Adult:** 0.04 to 0.1 mg/kg IV, IO; repeat dosing is 0.01 mg/kg every 25 to 60 minutes.
- **Pediatric:** Same as adult dosing.

Special Considerations: Pregnancy class C

Phenobarbital (Luminal)

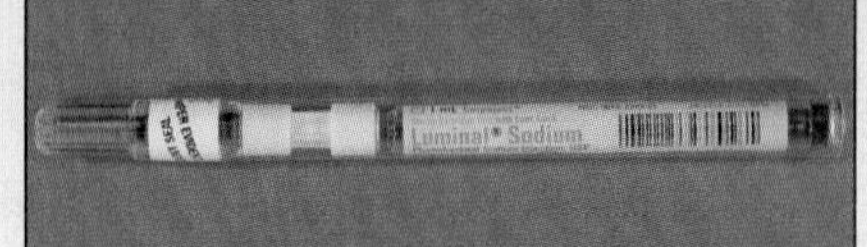

Classification: Anticonvulsant, barbiturate, schedule C-IV

Action: Depresses seizure activity in the cortex, thalamus, and limbic system; increases threshold for electrical stimulation of motor cortex; produces state of sedation.

Indications: Seizures

Adverse Effects: Depression, agitation, respiratory depression, accelerated metabolism of several other medications.

Contraindications: Liver dysfunction, porphyria, agranulocytosis, known sensitivity to barbiturates. Use with caution with respiratory dysfunction.

Dosage:

- **Adult:** 15 to 18 mg/kg IV, IO; infuse at a rate not faster than 60 mg/min.
- **Pediatric:** 15 to 20 mg/kg IV, IO; infuse at a rate not faster than 2 mg/kg/min.

Special Considerations:

- Be prepared to manage the patient's airway.
- Pregnancy class D

Phentolamine (Regitine)

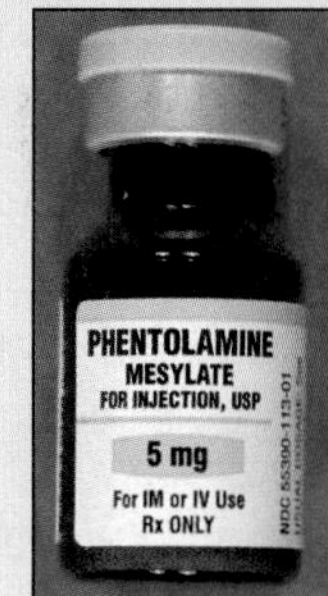

Classification: Alpha antagonist, antihypertensive

Action: Blocks alpha adrenergic receptors, causing vasodilation.

Indications: Hypertensive emergencies and hypertension caused by pheochromocytoma, cocaine-induced vasospasm of the coronary arteries.

Adverse Effects: Sinus tachycardia, angina, dizziness, orthostatic hypotension, prolonged hypotensive episodes, nausea/vomiting, diarrhea, weakness, flushing, nasal congestion.

Contraindications: Known sensitivity. Use with caution in acute MI, angina, coronary insufficiency, evidence suggestive of coronary artery disease, peptic ulcer disease.

Dosage:

Hypertensive Crisis:

- **Adult:** 5 to 15 mg IV, IO or IM.
- **Pediatric:** Not recommended for pediatric patients.

Cocaine-Induced Vasospasm:

- **Adult:** 5 mg IV, IO or IM.
- **Pediatric:** Not recommended for pediatric patients.

Special Considerations: Pregnancy class C

Phenylephrine (Neo-Synephrine)

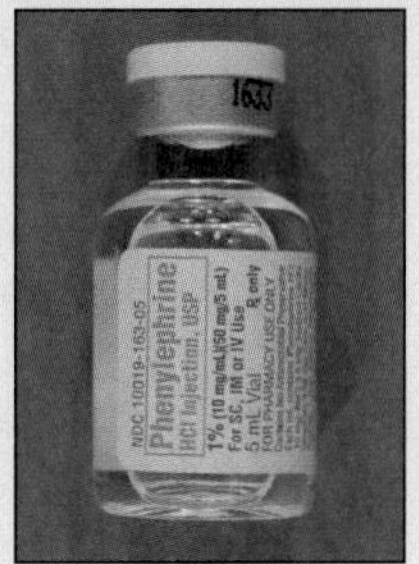

Classification: Adrenergic agonist

Action: Stimulates the alpha receptors, causing vasoconstriction, which results in increased blood pressure.

Indications: Neurogenic shock, spinal shock, cases of shock in which the patient's heart rate does not need to be increased, drug-induced hypotension.

Adverse Effects: Hypertension, VT, headache, excitability, tremor, MI, exacerbation of asthma, cardiac arrhythmias, reflex bradycardia, soft tissue necrosis.

Contraindications: Acute MI, angina, cardiac arrhythmias, severe hypertension, coronary artery disease, pheochromocytoma, narrow-angle glaucoma, cardiomyopathy, MAOI therapy, known sensitivity to phenylephrine or sulfites.

Continued

Phenylephrine (Neo-Synephrine)—continued

Dosage:

- **Adult:** 100 to 180 mcg/min IV, IO. Once the blood pressure has been stabilized, the dose can be reduced to 40 to 60 mcg/min.
- **Pediatric (2 to 12 years):** 5 to 20 mcg/kg IV, IO followed by 0.1 to 0.5 mcg/kg/min IV, IO (max dose: 3 mcg/kg/min IV, IO).

Special Considerations: Pregnancy class C

Phenytoin (Dilantin)

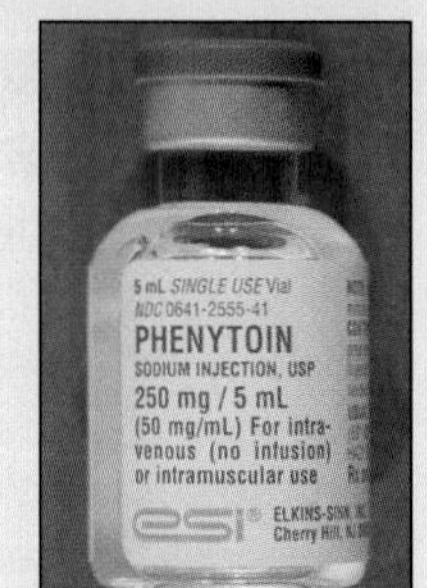

Classification: Anticonvulsant

Action: Depresses seizures by affecting the movement of sodium and calcium into neural tissue.

Indications: Generalized tonic-clonic seizures.

Adverse Effects: Nausea/vomiting, depression of cardiac conduction, sedation, nystagmus, tremors, ataxia, dysarthria, gingival hypertrophy, hirsutism, facial coarsening, hypotension.

Contraindications: Sinus bradycardia, sinoatrial block, second- and third-degree heart block, Adams-Stokes syndrome, known sensitivity to hydantoins.

Dosage:

- **Adult:** 15 to 20 mg/kg IV, IO should be administered slowly at a rate not exceeding 50 mg/min (this requires approximately 20 minutes in a 70-kg patient).
- **Pediatric:** 15 to 20 mg/kg IV, IO, administered at a rate of 1 to 3 mg/kg/min.

Special Considerations:

- Continuously monitor the ECG and blood pressure during administration.
- Pregnancy class D

Potassium Chloride

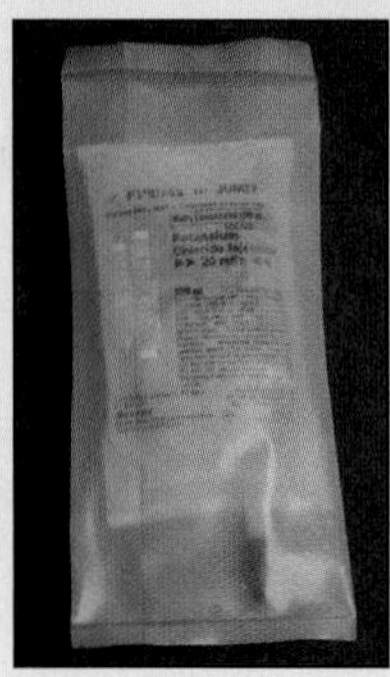

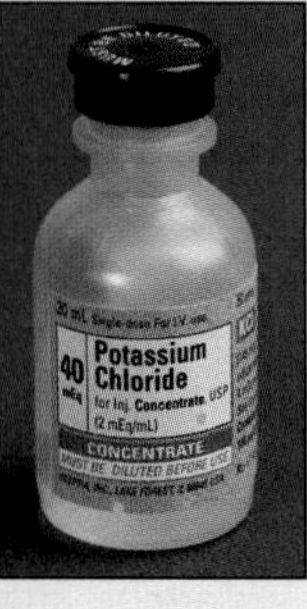

Classification: Electrolyte replacement

Action: Replaces potassium. Slight alterations in extracellular potassium levels can cause serious alterations in both cardiac and nervous function.

Indications: Hypokalemia

Adverse Effects: Hyperkalemia; AV block; cardiac arrest; GI bleeding, obstruction, or perforation; tissue necrosis if the infusion infiltrates into the soft tissues.

Contraindications: Use with caution in patients with cardiac arrhythmias, renal failure, muscle cramps, severe tissue trauma.

Dosage:

- **Adult:** Dosage must be individualized according to patient serum potassium concentration.
- **Pediatric:** Dosage must be individualized according to patient serum potassium concentration.

Special Considerations: Pregnancy class C

Pralidoxime (2-PAM)

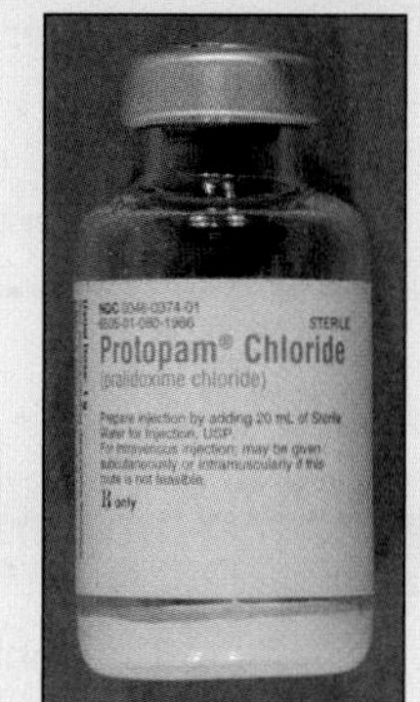

Classification: Cholinergic agonist, antidote

Action: Reactivates cholinesterase.

Indications: Toxicity from nerve agents (organophosphates) having cholinesterase activity.

Adverse Effects: Dizziness, blurred vision, hypertension, diplopia, hyperventilation, laryngospasm, nausea/vomiting, sinus tachycardia.

Contraindications: Myasthenia gravis, renal failure, inability to control the airway.

Dosage:

- **Adult:** 1 to 2 g (dilute in 100 mL normal saline) over a 15- to 30-minute period. If this is not practical or if pulmonary edema is present, the dose should be given slowly (≥5 min) by IV as a 5% solution in water.
- **Autoinjector:** Pralidoxime is also available as an autoinjector that delivers 600 mg IM. Repeat doses can be given every 15 minutes to a total of three doses (1800 mg). Pralidoxime autoinjector is not recommended for pediatric patients.
- **Pediatric:** 20 to 50 mg/kg IV, IO over a 10-minute period.

Special Considerations: Pregnancy class C

Prednisone

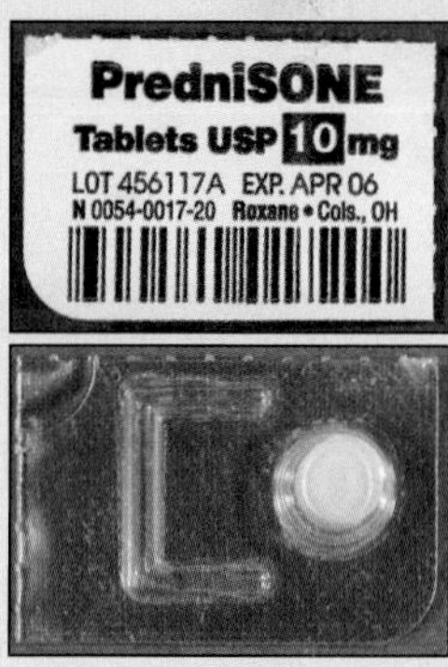

Classification: Corticosteroid

Action: Reduces inflammation

Indications: Inflammatory conditions, such as asthma with bronchospasm.

Adverse Effects: Many adverse effects of steroid use are not related to short-term use but typically are seen with long-term use and during withdrawal.

Contraindications: Cushing's syndrome, fungal infections, measles, varicella, known sensitivity.

Dosage:

- **Adult:** Dosage must be individualized.
- **Pediatric:** Dosage must be individualized.

Procainamide (Pronestyl)

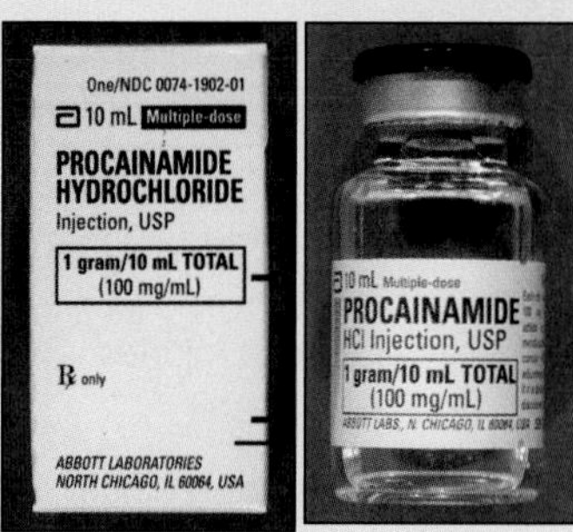

Classification: Antiarrhythmic, class IA

Action: Blocks influx of sodium through membrane pores, consequently suppresses atrial and ventricular arrhythmias by slowing conduction in myocardial tissue.

Indications: Alternative to amiodarone for stable monomorphic VT with normal QT interval and preserved ventricular function, reentry SVT if uncontrolled by adenosine and vagal maneuvers if blood pressure stable, AF with rapid rate in Wolff-Parkinson-White syndrome.

Adverse Effects: Asystole, VF, flushing, hypotension, PR prolongation, QRS widening, QT prolongation.

Contraindications: AV block, QT prolongation, torsades de pointes. Use with caution in hypotension, heart failure.

Dosage:

- **Adult:** 20 mg/min slow IV, IO (max total dose: 17 mg/kg until one of the following occurs: arrhythmia resolves, hypotension, QRS widens by >50% of original width, total dose of 17 mg/kg).

Continued

Procainamide (Pronestyl)—continued

- **Maintenance:** Infusion (after resuscitation from cardiac arrest): mix 1 g in 250 mL solution (4 mg/mL), infuse at 1 to 4 mg/min.
- **Pediatric:** 15 mg/kg slow IV, IO over 30 to 60 minutes.

Special Considerations: Pregnancy class C

Promethazine (Phenergan)

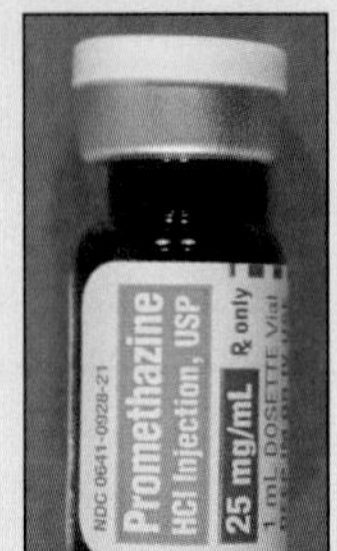

Classification: Antiemetic, antihistamine

Action: Decreases nausea and vomiting by antagonizing H_1 receptors.

Indications: Nausea/vomiting

Adverse Effects: Paradoxic excitation in children and elderly patients.

Contraindications: Altered level of consciousness, jaundice, bone marrow suppression, known sensitivity. Use with caution in seizure disorder.

Dosage:

- **Adult:** 12.5 to 25 mg IV, IO or IM.
- **Pediatric:**
  - **2 years and older:** 0.25 to 1 mg/kg IV, IO, IM (maximum rate of IV, IO administration is 25 mg/min).

Special Considerations: Pregnancy class C

Propofol (Diprivan)

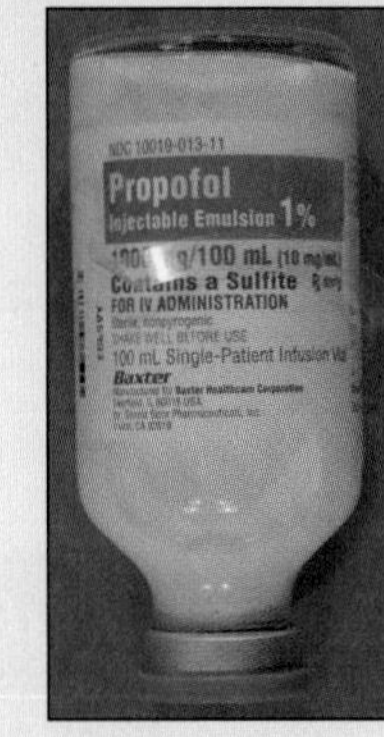

Classification: Anesthetic

Action: Produces rapid and brief state of general anesthesia.

Indications: Anesthesia induction.

Adverse Effects: Apnea, cardiac arrhythmias, asystole, hypotension, hypertension, pain at injection site.

Contraindications: Hypovolemia, known sensitivity (including soybean oil, eggs).

Dosage: A general induction dose used to produce a state of unconsciousness rapidly is 1.5 to 3 mg/kg IV, IO.

Patient Group	Dose	Rate of Administration (10 mg/mL)
Healthy adults younger than 55 years	2 to 2.5 mg/kg IV, IO	40 mg every 10 seconds
Elderly or debilitated patients	1 to 1.5 mg/kg IV, IO	20 mg every 10 seconds
Cardiac patients	0.5 to 1.5 mg/kg IV, IO	20 mg every 10 seconds
Patients with head injuries	1 to 2 mg/kg IV, IO	20 mg every 10 seconds
Pediatric (3-16 years)	2.5 to 3.5 mg/kg IV, IO	20 mg every 10 seconds

After the induction bolus, the patient must be given intermittent boluses or a maintenance infusion. For an average adult, an intermittent dose is 20 to 50 mg as needed. Alternatively, a propofol infusion may be ordered. Maintenance of anesthesia with a propofol infusion can be achieved by following the following protocols:

- **Adult patients:** 25 to 75 mcg/kg/min IV, IO
- **Elderly, debilitated, or head-injured patients:** Use approximately 80% of the normal adult dose.
- **Pediatric:** 125 to 300 mcg/kg/min IV, IO.

Continued

Propofol (Diprivan)—continued

Special Considerations:

Propofol should be administered only by personnel trained and equipped to manage the patient's airway and provide mechanical ventilation. In elderly and debilitated patients, avoid rapid administration to prevent hypotension, apnea, airway obstruction, and/or oxygen desaturation. Continue to monitor the patient's oxygenation and vital signs and try to limit use of propofol to patients who are intubated. Propofol should not be administered through the same IV catheter as blood or plasma. Pain can occur at the site of injection, which can be minimized by use of larger veins, slower rates of administration, and administration of 1 mL 1% lidocaine before propofol administration.

Propofol is listed as a pregnancy class B; however, propofol should be avoided in pregnant women because it crosses the placenta and can cause neonatal depression.

Propranolol (Inderal)

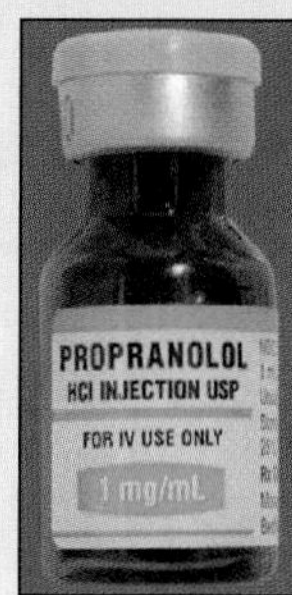

Courtesy Gold Standard.

Classification: Beta adrenergic antagonist, antianginal, antihypertensive, antiarrhythmic class II

Action: Nonselective beta antagonist that binds with both the $beta_1$ and $beta_2$ receptors. Propranolol inhibits the strength of the heart's contractions, as well as heart rate. This results in a decrease in cardiac oxygen consumption.

Indications: Angina; narrow-complex tachycardias that originate from either a *reentry mechanism* (reentry SVT) or an *automatic focus* (junctional, ectopic, or multifocal tachycardia) uncontrolled by vagal maneuvers and adenosine in patients with preserved ventricular function; AF and atrial flutter in patients with preserved ventricular function; hypertension; migraine headaches.

Adverse Effects: Bradycardia, AV block, bronchospasm, hypotension.

Contraindications: Cardiogenic shock, heart failure, AV block, bradycardia, pulmonary edema, sick sinus syndrome, known sensitivity. Use with caution in chronic lung disease (asthma and COPD).

Dosage:

- **Adult:** 1 to 3 mg IV, IO at a rate of 1 mg/min; may repeat the dose 2 minutes later.
- **Pediatric:** 0.01 to 0.1 mg/kg slow IV, IO over a 10-minute period.

Special Considerations:

- Monitor blood pressure and heart rate closely during administration.
- Pregnancy class C

Racemic Epinephrine/Racepinephrine (microNefrin, S_2)

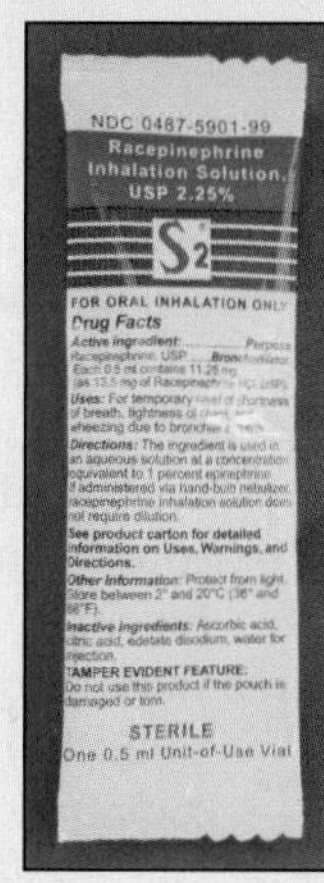

Classification: Bronchodilator, adrenergic agent

Action: Stimulates both alpha and beta receptors, causing vasoconstriction, reduced mucosal edema, and bronchodilation.

Indications: Bronchial asthma, croup.

Adverse Effects: Anxiety, dizziness, headache, tremor, palpitations, tachycardia, cardiac arrhythmias, hypertension, nausea/vomiting.

Contraindications: Glaucoma, elderly, cardiac disease, hypertension, thyroid disease, diabetes, known sensitivity to sulfites.

Dosage:

- **Adult:** Add 0.5 mL to nebulizer; for hand-bulb nebulizer, administer 1 to 3 inhalations; for jet nebulizer, add 3 mL of diluent, swirl the nebulizer and administer for 15 minutes.
- **Pediatric:**
  - **Older than 4 years:** Same as adult dosing.
  - **Younger than 4 years:** Safe and effective use has not been demonstrated.

Special Considerations:

- Monitor blood pressure, heart rate, and cardiac rhythm for changes.
- Onset of action is 1 to 5 minutes.
- Pregnancy class C

Rocuronium (Zemuron)

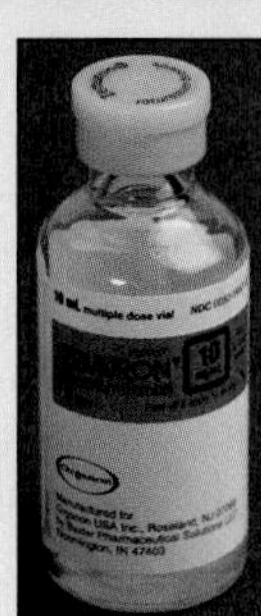

Classification: Neuromuscular blocker, nondepolarizing
Action: Antagonizes acetylcholine at the motor end plate, producing skeletal muscle paralysis.
Indications: To induce neuromuscular blockade for the facilitation of ET intubation.
Adverse Effects: Muscle paralysis, apnea, dyspnea, respiratory depression, sinus tachycardia, urticaria.
Contraindications: Known sensitivity to bromides. Use with caution in heart disease, liver disease.
Dosage:

- **Adult:** 0.6 to 1.2 mg/kg IV, IO.
- **Pediatric (older than 3 months):** 0.6 mg/kg IV, IO.

Special Considerations:

- Onset of action is 2 to 8 minutes.
- Duration of action is 31 minutes.
- Pregnancy class B

Scopolamine (Transderm Scop)

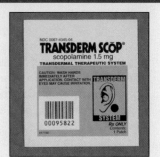

Classification: Neurologic antivertigo, antimuscarinic
Action: Antagonizes acetylcholine at muscarinic receptors.
Indications: Motion sickness
Adverse Effects: Dry mouth, drowsiness, dilated pupils and blurred vision, hallucinations, confusion.
Contraindications: Glaucoma, cardiac arrhythmias, coronary artery disease, known sensitivity.
Dosage:
Adult and children older than 12 years: 1 disc applied to skin behind ear.
Special Considerations:

- Half-life 8 hours
- Pregnancy class C

Sodium Bicarbonate

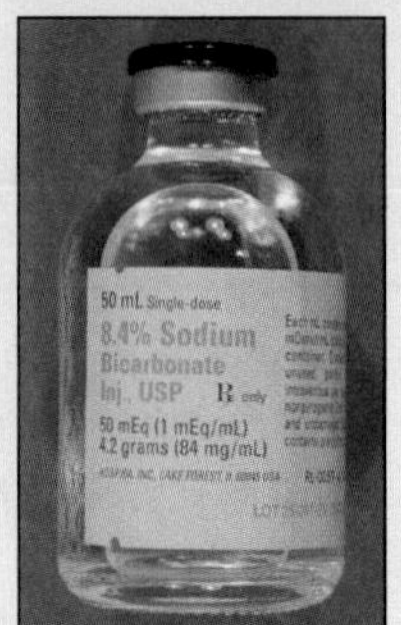

Classification: Electrolyte replacement
Action: Counteracts existing acidosis.
Indications: Acidosis, drug intoxications (e.g., barbiturates, salicylates, methyl alcohol).
Adverse Effects: Metabolic alkalosis, hypernatremia, injection site reaction, sodium and fluid retention, peripheral edema.
Contraindications: Metabolic alkalosis.
Dosage:
Metabolic Acidosis during Cardiac Arrest:

- **Adult:** 1 mEq/kg slow IV, IO; may repeat at 0.5 mEq/kg in 10 minutes.
- **Pediatric:** Same as adult dosing.

Metabolic Acidosis Not Associated with Cardiac Arrest:

- **Adult:** Dosage should be individualized.
- **Pediatric:** Dosage should be individualized.

Special Considerations:

- Do not administer into an IV, IO line in which another medication is being given.
- Because of the high concentration of sodium within each ampule of sodium bicarbonate, use with caution in patients with CHF and renal disease.
- Pregnancy class C

Sodium Nitroprusside (Nipride, Nitropress)

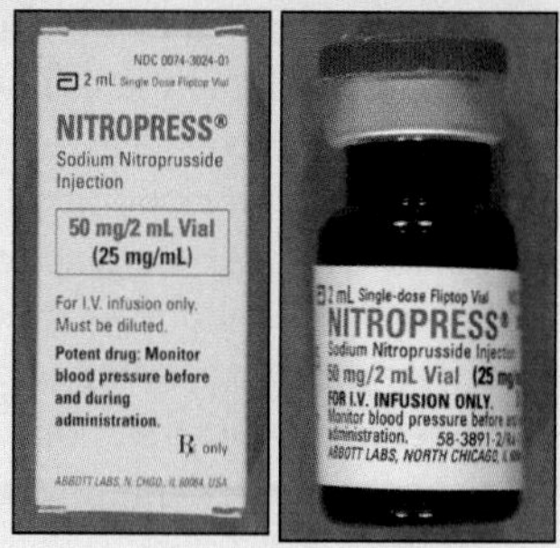

Classification: Antihypertensive agent
Action: Causes direct relaxation of both arteries and veins.
Indications: Hypertensive emergencies.
Adverse Effects: Cyanide or thiocyanate toxicity, nausea/vomiting, dizziness, headache, restlessness, abdominal pain, methemoglobinemia.
Contraindications: Hypotension, increased ICP, cerebrovascular disease, coronary artery disease, hepatic disease, renal disease, pulmonary disease.
Dosage:

- **Adult:** 0.3 to 10 mcg/kg/min IV, IO. Titrate to desired blood pressure.
- **Pediatric:** Same as adult dosing.

Special Considerations:

- Nitroprusside will break down when exposed to ultraviolet light. Therefore the infusion should be shielded from light by wrapping the bag with aluminum foil.
- Pregnancy class C

Succinylcholine (Anectine)

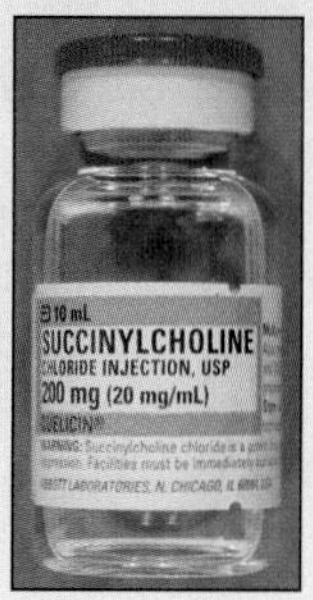

Classification: Neuromuscular blocker, depolarizing
Action: Competes with the acetylcholine receptor of the motor end plate on the muscle cell, resulting in muscle paralysis.
Indications: To induce neuromuscular blockade for the facilitation of ET intubation.
Adverse Effects: Anaphylactoid reactions, respiratory depression, apnea, bronchospasm, cardiac arrhythmias, malignant hyperthermia, hypertension, hypotension, muscle fasciculation, postprocedure muscle pain, hypersalivation, rash.
Contraindications: Malignant hyperthermia, burns, trauma. Use with caution in children, cardiac disease, hepatic disease, renal disease, peptic ulcer disease, cholinesterase-inhibitor toxicity, pseudocholinesterase deficiency, digitalis toxicity, glaucoma, hyperkalemia, hypothermia, rhabdomyolysis, myasthenia gravis.
Dosage:

- **Adult:**
  - **IV:** 0.6 mg/kg IV, IO (range 0.3-1.1 mg/kg).
  - **IM:** 3 to 4 mg/kg (max dose: 150 mg).
- **Pediatric:**
  - **IV:**
    - **Adolescents and older children:** 1 mg/kg IV, IO.
    - **Small children and infants:** 2 mg/kg IV, IO.
  - **IM:** 3 to 4 mg/kg (max dose: 150 mg).

Special Considerations:

- IV administration results in neuromuscular blockade in 0.5 to 1 minute. IM administration results in neuromuscular blockade in 2 to 3 minutes.
- IV administration in infants and children can potentially result in profound bradycardia and, in some cases, asystole. The incidence of bradycardia is greater after the second dose. The occurrence of bradycardia can be reduced with the pretreatment of atropine.
- Succinylcholine can have a significantly prolonged effect in the setting of poisoning with nerve gas agents and organophosphate pesticides.
- Pregnancy class C

Terbutaline (Brethine)

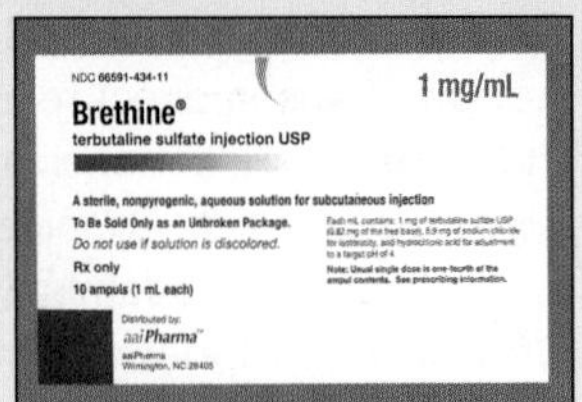

Classification: Adrenergic agonist

Action: Stimulates the $beta_2$ receptor, producing relaxation of bronchial smooth muscle and bronchodilation.

Indications: Prevention and reversal of bronchospasm.

Adverse Effects: Cardiac arrhythmias, arrhythmia exacerbation, angina, anxiety, headache, tremor, palpitations, dizziness.

Contraindications: Known sensitivity to sympathomimetics. Use with caution in hypertension, cardiac disease, cardiac arrhythmias, diabetes, elderly, MAOI therapy, pheochromocytoma, thyrotoxicosis, seizure disorder.

Dosage:

- **Adult:** 0.25 mg Sub-Q every 20 minutes for 3 doses. The usual site for the Sub-Q injection is the lateral deltoid.
- **Pediatric:** 0.01 mg/kg Sub-Q every 20 minutes for 3 doses.

Special Considerations: Pregnancy class B

Thiamine (Vitamin B_1)

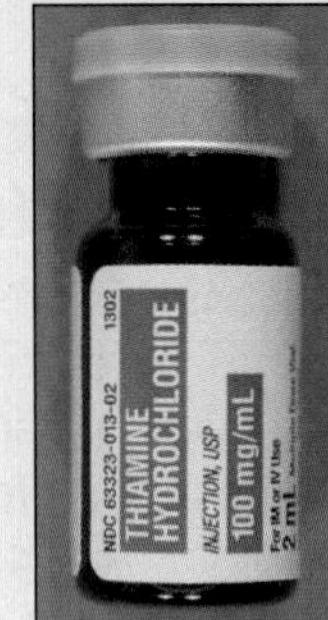

Classification: Vitamin B_1

Action: Thiamine combines with adenosine triphosphate to produce thiamine diphosphate, which acts as a coenzyme in carbohydrate metabolism.

Indication: Wernicke-Korsakoff syndrome, beriberi, nutritional supplementation.

Adverse Effects: Itching, rash, pain at injection site.

Contraindications: Known sensitivity.

Dosage:

Wernicke-Korsakoff Syndrome:

- **Adult:** 100 mg IV, IO.
- **Pediatric:** Not recommended for pediatric patients.

Special Considerations: Pregnancy class A

Tirofiban (Aggrastat)

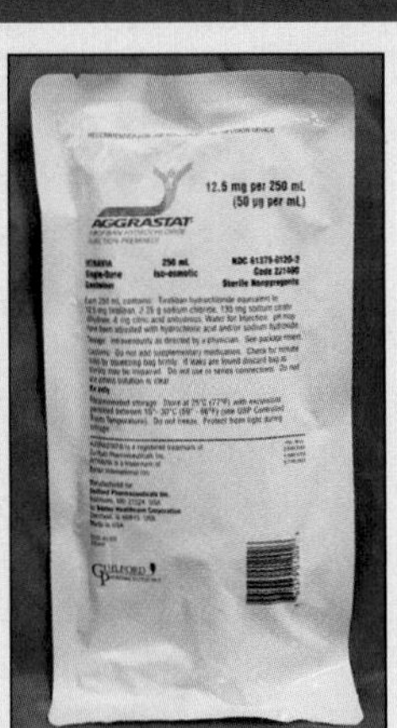

Classification: GP IIb/IIIa inhibitor

Action: Prevents the aggregation of platelets by binding to the GP IIb/IIIa receptor.

Indications: UA/NSTEMI—to manage medically and for those undergoing PCI.

Adverse Effects: Bleeding from the GI tract, internal bleeding, intracranial hemorrhage, hypotension, stroke, anaphylactic shock.

Contraindications: Bleeding from any source, severe uncontrolled hypertension, surgery or trauma within the previous 6 weeks, stroke within the previous 30 days, renal failure, thrombocytopenia.

Dosage: 0.4 mcg/kg/min IV, IO for 30 minutes, then 0.1 mcg/kg/min IV, IO infusion for 48 to 96 hours.

Special Considerations:

- Half-life approximately 2 hours
- Pregnancy class B

Valproic Acid (Depakote)

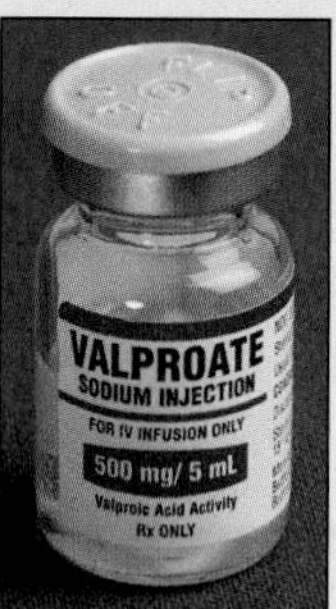

Classification: Anticonvulsant, antimanic

Action: Although the exact mechanism of action is unknown, it is suggested that valproic acid increases brain concentrations of GABA.

Indications: Seizures, mood disorders.

Adverse Effects: Tremor, transient hair loss, weight gain, weight loss.

Contraindications: Liver disease.

Dosage: Dosing is individualized.

Special Considerations:

- Although generally well tolerated, valproic acid does require regular monitoring of blood levels to ensure maintenance of therapeutic levels while minimizing adverse drug reactions.
- Pregnancy class D

Vasopressin

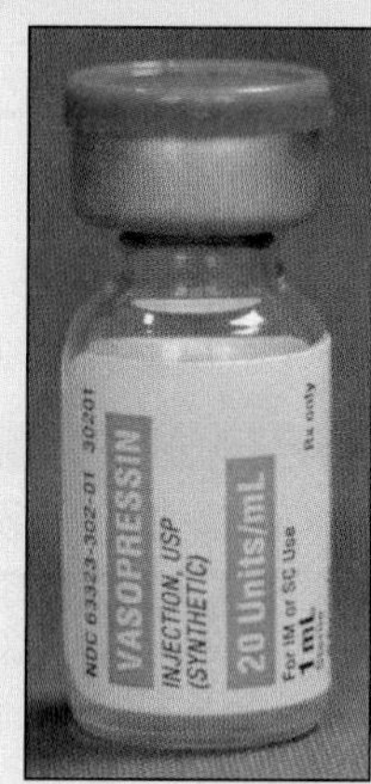

Classification: Nonadrenergic vasoconstrictor

Action: Vasopressin causes vasoconstriction independent of adrenergic receptors or neural innervation.

Indications: Adult shock-refractory VF or pulseless VT, asystole, PEA, vasodilatory shock.

Adverse Effects: Cardiac ischemia, angina

Contraindications: Responsive patients with cardiac disease

Dosage:

- **Adult:** 40 U IV/IO may replace either the first or second dose of epinephrine.
- May be given ET but the optimal dose is not known.

Special Considerations: Pregnancy class C

Vecuronium (Norcuron)

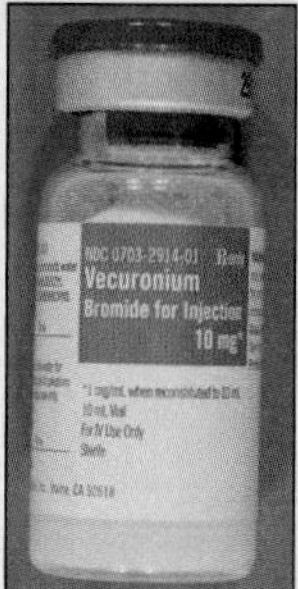

Classification: Neuromuscular blocker, nondepolarizing

Action: Antagonizes acetylcholine at the motor end plate, producing skeletal muscle paralysis.

Indications: To induce neuromuscular blockade for the facilitation of ET intubation.

Adverse Effects: Muscle paralysis, apnea, dyspnea, respiratory depression, sinus tachycardia, urticaria.

Contraindications: Known sensitivity to bromides. Use with caution in heart disease, liver disease.

Dosage:

- **Adult:** 0.08-0.1 mg/kg IV, IO.
- **Pediatric:** Dosage is individualized.

Special Considerations: Pregnancy class C

Verapamil (Isoptin)

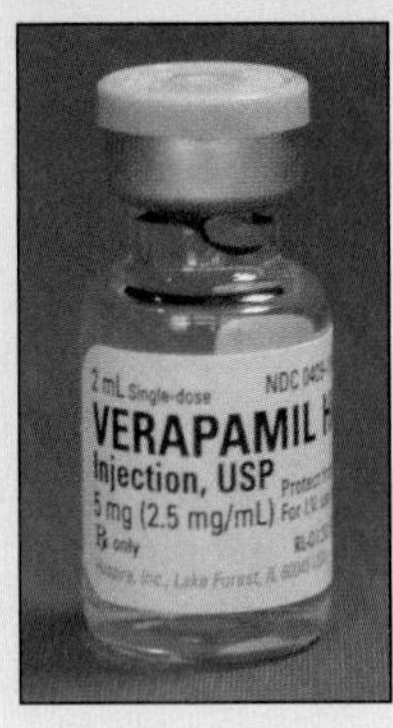

Classification: Calcium-channel blocker; class IV antiarrhythmic

Action: Blocks calcium from moving into the heart muscle cell, which prolongs the conduction of electrical impulses through the AV node. Also dilates arteries.

Indications: Atrial fibrillation, hypertension, PSVT, PSVT prophylaxis.

Adverse Effects: Sinus bradycardia; first-, second-, or third-degree AV block; congestive heart failure; reflex sinus tachycardia; transient asystole; AV block; hypotension.

Contraindications: Second- or third- degree AV block (except in patients with a functioning artificial pacemaker; hypotension (systolic pressure <90 mm Hg) or cardiogenic shock; sick sinus syndrome (except in patients with a functioning artificial pacemaker); Wolff-Parkinson-White syndrome; Lown-Ganong-Levine syndrome; severe left ventricular dysfunction; known sensitivity to verapamil or any component of the formulation; atrial flutter or fibrillation and an accessory bypass tract (WPW, Lown-Ganong-Levine syndrome); in infants <1 yr.

Dosage:

- **Adult:** 2.5 to 5 mg IV, IO over 2 minutes (3 minutes in elderly patients). May repeat at 5 to 10 mg every 15-30 minutes to a maximum dose of 30 mg.
- **Pediatric:**
  - **Children 1-16 yrs:** 0.1 mg/kg IV, IO (maximum 5 mg/dose) over 2 minutes. May repeat in 30 minutes to a maximum dose of 10 mg.
  - **Infants <1 year:** Not recommended.

Special Considerations: Pregnancy class C

Warfarin (Coumadin)

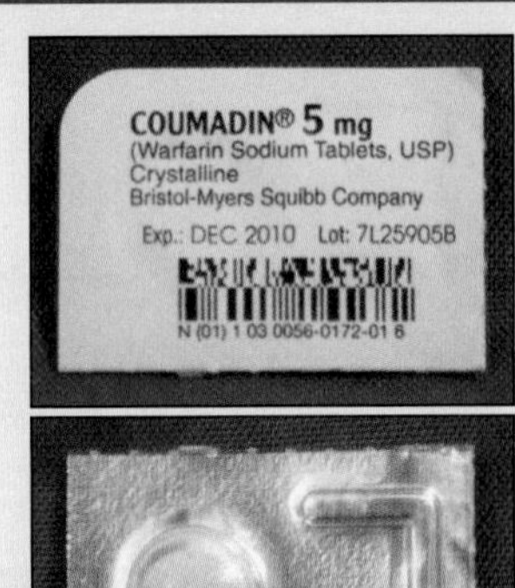

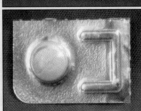

Classification: Anticoagulant

Action: Inhibit the synthesis of vitamin K dependent clotting factors.

Indications: Treatment and/or prophylaxis of thrombosis related to acute coronary syndromes, stroke, deep venous thrombosis, pulmonary embolism, atrial fibrillation, cardiac valve replacement.

Adverse Effects: Bleeding, angina, edema, rash, abdominal cramps, gastrointestinal bleeding, vomiting, hematuria, retroperitoneal hematoma, anaphylactoid reactions, skin necrosis.

Contraindications: Bleeding tendencies, recent or potential surgery of the eye or CNS, major regional lumbar block anesthesia or surgery resulting in large, open surfaces, patient who has a history of falls or is a significant fall risk, unsupervised senile or psychotic patient, eclampsia/preeclampsia, threatened abortion, pregnancy.

Dosage: Dosage is individualized.

Special Considerations: Pregnancy class X

Glossary

800 MHz A type of radio signal in the ultra-high-frequency range that allows splitting a frequency into individual talk groups used as communication links with other system users.

9-1-1/E9-1-1 A set of three numbers that automatically sends the call to the emergency dispatch center. E9-1-1 is enhanced 9-1-1, which gives the dispatcher the ability to determine the caller's location by routing the call through several CAD systems.

Abandonment Terminating care when it is still needed and desired by the patient and without ensuring that appropriate care continues to be provided by another qualified healthcare professional.

Abbreviation A shorter way of writing something.

Abdominal compartment syndrome Syndrome caused by diffuse intestinal edema, a result of fluid accumulation in the bowel wall. It may be caused by overresuscitation with crystalloids and results in shock and renal failure.

Abdominal evisceration An injury in which a severe laceration or incision of the abdomen breaches through all layers of muscle to allow abdominal contents, most often the intestines, to protrude above the surface of the skin.

Aberrant Abnormal.

Abortion The ending of a pregnancy for any reason before 20 weeks' gestation; the lay term miscarriage is referred to as a *spontaneous abortion.*

Abruptio placentae Separation of the placenta from the uterine wall after the twentieth week of gestation.

Abscess A collection of pus.

Absence seizure A generalized seizure characterized by a blank stare and an alteration of consciousness.

Absolute refractory period Corresponds with the onset of the QRS complex to approximately the peak of the T wave; cardiac cells cannot be stimulated to conduct an electrical impulse, no matter how strong the stimulus.

Absorption Movement of small organic molecules, electrolytes, vitamins, and water across the digestive tract and into the circulatory system. Also the movement of a drug from the site of input into the circulation.

Abuse Use of a substance for other than its approved, accepted purpose or in a greater amount than prescribed.

Acalculus cholecystitis Inflammation of the gallbladder in the absence of gallstones.

Acceptance A grief stage in which the individual has come to terms with the reality of his or her (or a loved one's) imminent death.

Accessory muscles Muscles of the neck, chest, and abdomen that become active during labored breathing.

Accessory pathway An extra bundle of working myocardial tissue that forms a connection between the atria and ventricles outside the normal conduction system.

Accreditation Recognition given to an EMD center by an independent auditing agency for achieving a consistently high level of performance based on industry best practice standards.

Acetylation A mechanism in which a drug is processed by enzymes.

Acetylcholinesterase A body chemical that stops the action of acetylcholine (a neurotransmitter involved in the stimulation of nerves).

Acid Fluid produced in the stomach; breaks down the food material within the stomach into chyme.

Acid-base balance Delicate balance between the body's acidity and alkalinity.

Acidic pH less than 7.0.

Acids Materials that have a pH value less than 7.0 (e.g., hydrochloric acid, sulfuric acid).

Acquired immunity Specific immunity directed at a particular pathogen that develops after the body has been exposed to it once (e.g., immunity to chickenpox after first exposure).

Acquired immunodeficiency syndrome (AIDS) An acquired immunodeficiency disease that can develop after infection with HIV.

Acrocyanosis Cyanosis of the extremities.

Action potential A five-phase cycle that reflects the difference in the concentration of charged particles across the cell membrane at any given time.

Activated charcoal An adsorbent made from charred wood that effectively binds many poisons in the stomach; most effective when administered within 1 hour of intake.

Activation phase In phases of immunity, the stage at which a single lymphocyte activates many other lymphocytes and significantly expands the scope of immune response in a process known as amplification.

Active immunity Induced immunity in which the body can continue to mount specific immune response when exposed to the agent (e.g., vaccination).

Active listening Listening to the words that the patient is saying as well as paying attention to the significance of those words to the patient.

Active range of motion The degree of movement at a joint as determined by the patient's own voluntary movements.

Active transport A process used to move substances against the concentration gradient or toward the side that has a higher concentration; requires the use of energy by the cell but is faster than diffusion.

Acute arterial occlusion A sudden blockage of arterial blood flow that occurs because of a thrombus, embolus, tumor, direct trauma to an artery, or an unknown cause.

Acute care Short-term medical treatment usually provided in a hospital for patients who have an illness or injury or who are recovering from surgery.

Acute coronary syndrome (ACS) A term used to refer to patients presenting with ischemic chest discomfort. Acute coronary syndromes consist of three major syndromes: unstable angina, non–ST-segment elevation myocardial infarction, and ST-segment elevation myocardial infarction.

Acute exposure An exposure that occurs over a short timeframe (less than 24 hours); usually occurs at a spill or release.

Acute renal failure (ARF) When the kidneys suddenly stop functioning, either partially or completely, but eventually recover full or nearly full functioning over time.

Acute respiratory distress syndrome (ARDS) Collection of fluid in the alveoli of the lung, usually as a result of trauma or serious illness.

Addiction The involvement in a repetitive behavior (gambling, substance abuse, etc.). In physical addiction the individual has become dependent on an external substance and develops physical withdrawal symptoms if the substance is unavailable.

Additive effect The combined effect of two drugs given at the same time that have similar effects.

Adenosine triphosphate (ATP) Formed from metabolism of nutrients in the cell; serves as an energy source throughout the body.

Adipocyte A fat cell; a connective tissue cell that has differentiated and become specialized in the synthesis (manufacture) and storage of fat.

Adipose (fat) connective tissue Tissue that stores lipids; acts as an insulator and protector of the organs of the body.

Administrative law A branch of law that deals with rules, regulations, orders, and decisions created by governmental agencies.

Adrenergic Having the characteristics of the sympathetic division of the autonomic nervous system.

Adrenocortical steroids Hormones released by the adrenal cortex essential for life; assist in the regulation of blood glucose levels, promote peripheral use of lipids, stimulate the kidneys to reabsorb sodium, and have antiinflammatory effects.

Adsorb To gather or stick to a surface in a condensed layer.

Adult respiratory distress syndrome (ARDS) A life-threatening condition that causes lung swelling and fluid buildup in the air sacs.

Advance directive A document in which a competent person gives instructions to be followed regarding his or her healthcare in the event the person later becomes incapacitated and unable to make or communicate those decisions to others.

Advanced emergency medical technician (AEMT) An EMS professional who provides basic and limited advanced skills to patients who access the EMS system.

Adverse effect (reaction) An unintentional, undesirable, and often unpredictable effect of a drug used at therapeutic doses to prevent, diagnose, or treat disease.

Advocate A person who assists another person in carrying out desired wishes; a paramedic should function as a patient's advocate in all aspects of prehospital care.

Aerosol A collection of particles dispersed in a gas.

Affect Description of the patient's visible emotional state.

Afferent division Nerve fibers that send impulses from the periphery to the central nervous system.

Affinity The intensity or strength of the attraction between a drug and its receptor.

Afterload Pressure or resistance against which the ventricles must pump to eject blood.

Ageism Stereotypical and often negative bias against older adults.

Agonal respirations Slow, shallow, irregular respirations resulting from anoxic brain injury.

Agonist A drug that causes a physiologic response in the receptor to which it binds.

Agonist-antagonist A drug that blocks a receptor. It may provide a partial agonist activity, but it also prevents an agonist from exerting its full effects.

Agoraphobia Consistent anxiety and avoidance of places and situations where escape during a panic attack would be difficult or embarrassing.

Air emboli Bubble of air that has entered the vasculature. Emboli can result in damage similar to a clot in the vasculature, typically resulting in brain injury or pulmonary emboli when neck vessels are damaged.

Air embolism Introduction of air into venous circulation, which can ultimately enter the right ventricle, closing off circulation to the pulmonary artery and leading to death.

Air trapping A respiratory pattern associated with an obstruction in the pulmonary tree; the breathing rate increases to overcome resistance in getting air out, the respiratory effort becomes more shallow, the volume of trapped air increases, and the lungs inflate.

Airbag identification The various shapes, sizes, colors, and styles of visual identification labels indicating that an airbag is present.

Airbags Inflatable nylon bags designed to supplement the protection of occupants during crashes; one of the most common new technology items confronting responders at crash scenes; also known as *supplemental restraint systems.*

Air-reactive materials Materials that react with atmospheric moisture and rapidly decompose.

Alarm reaction The body's autonomic, sympathetic nervous system response to stimuli designed to prepare the individual to fight or flee.

Alcoholic ketoacidosis (AKA) Condition found in patients who chronically abuse alcohol accompanied by vomiting, a build-up of ketones in the blood, and little or no food intake.

Alcoholism Addiction and dependence on ethanol; often develops over many years.

Aldosterone A hormone responsible for the reabsorption of sodium and water from the kidney tubules.

Alkali A substance with a pH above 7.0; also known as a *base* or *caustic.*

Alkaline pH greater than 7.0.

Alkaloids A group of plant-based substances containing nitrogen and found in nature.

Allergen A substance that can provoke an allergic reaction.

Allergic reaction An abnormal immune response, mediated by immunoglobulin E antibodies, to an allergen that should not cause such a response and to which the patient has already been exposed; usually involves excessive release of immune agents, especially histamines.

All-hazards emergency preparedness A cross-cutting approach in which all forms of emergencies, including manmade and natural disasters, epidemics, and physical or biologic terrorism, are managed from a common template that uses consistent language and structure.

Allografting Transplanting organs or tissues from genetically nonidentical members of the same species.

All-terrain vehicle (ATV) Any of a number of models of small open motorized vehicles designed for off-road and wilderness use; three-wheeled (all-terrain cycles) and four-wheeled (quads) versions are most often used for personnel insertion; six- and eight-wheeled models exist for specialized applications.

Alpha particle A positively charged particle emitted by certain radioactive materials.

Altered mental status Disruption of a person's emotional and intellectual functioning.

Altitude illness A syndrome associated with the relatively low partial pressure of oxygen in the atmosphere at altitudes encountered during mountain climbing or travel in unpressurized aircraft.

Alveolar air volume In contrast to dead air space, alveolar volume is the amount of air that does reach the alveoli for gas exchange (approximately 350 mL in the adult male). It is the difference between tidal volume and dead-space volume.

Alveoli Functional units of the respiratory system; area in the lungs where the majority of gas exchange takes place; singular form is *alveolus.*

Alzheimer's disease Progressive dementia seen mostly in the elderly and marked by decline of memory and cognitive function.

Amniotic sac (bag of waters) The fluid-filled protective sac that surrounds the fetus inside the uterus.

Amplitude Height (voltage) of a waveform on the ECG.

Ampule A sealed sterile container that holds a single dose of liquid or powdered medication.

Amygdala Almond-shaped structure at the end of each hippocampus that attaches emotional significance to incoming stimuli; has a large role in the fear response; plural form is *amygdale.*

Amylase Enzyme in pancreatic juice.

Amyotrophic lateral sclerosis (ALS) Autoimmune disorder affecting the motor roots of the spinal nerves, causing progressive muscle weakness and eventually paralysis.

Anal canal Area between the rectum and the anus.

Analgesia A state in which pain is controlled or not perceived.

Anaphylactic reaction An unusual or exaggerated allergic reaction to a foreign substance.

Anaphylactoid reaction Reaction that clinically mimics an allergic reaction but is not mediated by immunoglobulin E antibodies, so it is not a true allergic reaction.

Anaphylaxis Life-threatening allergic reaction.

Anasarca Massive generalized body edema.

Anatomic plane The relation of internal body structures to the surface of the body; imaginary straight line divisions of the body.

Anatomic position The position of a person standing erect with his or her feet and palms facing the examiner.

Anatomy Study of the body's structure and organization.

Anchor point A single secure connection for an anchor.

Anchors The means of securing the ropes and other elements of the high-angle system.

Anemia Deficiency in red blood cells or hemoglobin; most common form is iron-deficiency anemia.

Anesthesia A process in which pain is prevented during a procedure.

Aneurysm Localized dilation or bulging of a blood vessel wall or wall of a heart chamber.

Anger A stage in the grieving process in which the individual is upset by the stated future loss of life.

Angina pectoris Chest discomfort or other related symptoms of sudden onset that may occur because the increased oxygen demand of the heart temporarily exceeds the blood supply.

Anginal equivalents Symptoms of myocardial ischemia other than chest pain or discomfort.

Angioedema Swelling of the tissues, including the dermal layer; often found in and around the mouth, tongue, and lips.

Angle of Louis An angulation of the sternum that indicates the point where the second rib joins the sternum; also called the *manubriosternal junction.*

Anhedonia Lack of enjoyment in activities one used to find pleasurable.

Anion A negatively charged ion.

Anorexia nervosa Eating disorder characterized by a preoccupation that one is obese; drastic, intentional weight loss; and bizarre attitudes and rituals associated with food and exercise.

Anoxia A total lack of oxygen availability to the tissues.

Antagonist A drug that does not cause a physiologic response when it binds with a receptor.

Antegrade amnesia The inability to remember short-term memory information after an event during which the head was struck.

Antepartum The period before childbirth.

Anterior The front, or ventral, surface.

Anterior cord syndrome Collection of symptoms seen after the compression, death, or transection of the anterior portion of the spinal cord.

Anthrax An acute bacterial infection caused by inhalation, contact, or ingestion of *Bacillus anthracis* organisms. Three forms of anthrax disease may occur depending on the route of exposure. Inhalational anthrax disease occurs after the inhalation of anthrax spores. Cutaneous anthrax disease is the most common form and occurs after the exposure of compromised skin to anthrax spores. Gastrointestinal anthrax disease occurs after the ingestion of live *B. anthracis* in contaminated meat.

Antiarrhythmic Medications used to correct irregular heartbeats and slow hearts that beat too fast.

Antibacterial Medication that kills or limits bacteria.

Antibiotic In common medical terms, a drug that kills bacteria.

Antibody Agents produced by B lymphocytes that bind to antigens, thus killing or controlling them and slowing or stopping an infection; also called *immunoglobulin.*

Antidiuretic hormone (ADH) A hormone released in response to detected loss of body water; prevents further loss of water through the urinary tract by promoting the reabsorption of water into the blood.

Antidote A substance that can reverse the adverse effects of a poison.

Antifungal Agent that kills fungi.

Antigen A marker on a cell that identifies the cell as "self" or "not self"; antigens are used by antibodies to identify cells that should be attacked as not self.

Antihistamine Medication that reduces the effects of histamine.

Antiinflammatory mediators Protein entities, often produced in the liver, that act as modulators of the immune response to the proinflammatory response to injury; also called *cytokines.*

Antipyretic medication A medication that reduces or eliminates a fever.

Antisepsis Prevention of sepsis by preventing or inhibiting the growth of causative microorganisms; in the field, the process used to cleanse local skin areas before needle puncture with products that are alcohol or iodine based.

Antivenin A substance that can reverse the adverse effects of a venom by binding to it and inactivating it.

Antiviral An agent that kills or impedes a virus.

Antonym A root word, prefix, or suffix that has the *opposite* meaning of another word.

Anucleated Cells of the body that do not have a central nucleus, such as those in cardiac muscle.

Anus The end of the anal canal.

Anxiety The sometimes vague feeling of apprehension, uneasiness, dread, or worry that often occurs without a specific source or cause identified. It is also a normal response to a perceived threat.

Aorta Delivers blood from the left ventricle of the heart to the body.

Aortic valve Semilunar valve on the left of the heart; separates the left ventricle from the aorta.

Apex Tip.

Apex of the heart Lower portion of the heart, tip of the ventricles (approximately the level of the fifth left intercostal space); points leftward, downward, and forward.

Apgar score A scoring system applied to an infant after delivery; key components include appearance, pulse, grimace, activity, and respiration.

Aphasia Loss of speech.

Apnea Respiratory arrest.

Apnea monitor A technologic aid used to warn of cessation of breathing in a premature infant; also may warn of bradycardia and tachycardia.

Apocrine glands Sweat glands that open into hair follicles, including in and around the genitalia, axillae, and anus; secrete an organic substance (which is odorless until acted upon by surface bacteria) into the hair follicles.
Appendicitis Inflammation of the appendix.
Appendicular region Area that includes the extremities (e.g., arms, pelvis, and legs).
Appendicular skeleton Consists of all the bones not within the axial skeleton: upper and lower extremities, the girdles, and their attachments.
Appendix Accessory structure of the cecum.
Application of principles The step at which the paramedic applies critical thinking in a clinical sense and arrives at a field impression or a working diagnosis.
Aqueous humor Fluid that fills the anterior chamber of the eye; maintains intraocular pressure.
Arachnoid mater Second layer of the meninges.
Arachnoid membrane Weblike middle layer of the meninges.
Areolar connective tissue A loose tissue found in most organs of the body; consists of weblike collagen, reticulum, and elastin fibers.
Arnold-Chiari malformation A complication of spina bifida in which the brainstem and cerebellum extend down through the foramen magnum into the cervical portion of the vertebrae.
Arrector pili Smooth muscle that surrounds each follicle; responsible for "goose bumps," which pull the hair upwards.
Arrhythmia Term often used interchangeably with dysrhythmia; any disturbance or abnormality in a normal rhythmic pattern; any cardiac rhythm other than a sinus rhythm.
Arterial puncture Accidental puncture into an artery instead of a vein.
Arterioles Small arterial vessels; supply oxygenated blood to the capillaries.
Arteriosclerosis A chronic disease of the arterial system characterized by abnormal thickening and hardening of the vessel walls.
Arthritis Inflammation of a joint that results in pain, stiffness, swelling, and redness.
Artifact Distortion of an ECG tracing by electrical activity that is noncardiac in origin (e.g., electrical interference, poor electrical conduction, patient movement).
Artificial anchors The use of specially designed hardware to create anchors where good natural anchors do not exist.
Arytenoid cartilages Six paired cartilages stacked on top of each other in the larynx.
Ascending colon Part of the large intestine.
Ascites Marked abdominal swelling from a buildup of fluid in the peritoneal cavity.
Asepsis Sterile; free from germs, infection, and any form of life.
Asphyxiants Chemicals that impair the body's ability to either get or use oxygen.
Aspiration Inhalation of foreign contents into the lungs.
Aspiration pneumonitis Inflammation of the bronchi and alveoli caused by inhaled foreign objects, usually acids such as stomach acid.
Assault A threat of imminent bodily harm to another person by someone with the obvious ability to carry out the threat.
Assay A test of a substance to determine its components.
Assessment-based management Taking the information you obtain from your assessment and using it to treat the patient.
Asthma A reversible obstructive airway disease characterized by chronic inflammation, hyperreactive airways, and episodes of bronchospasm.
Asynchronous pacemaker Fixed-rate pacemaker that continuously discharges at a preset rate regardless of the patient's intrinsic activity.
Asystole A total absence of ventricular electrical activity.
Ataxia Inability to control voluntary muscle movements; unsteady movements and staggering gait.
Atelectasis An abnormal condition characterized by the collapse of alveoli, preventing the respiratory exchange of carbon dioxide and oxygen in a part of the lungs.
Atherosclerosis A form of arteriosclerosis in which the thickening and hardening of the vessel walls are caused by a buildup of fatty deposits in the inner lining of large and middle-sized muscular arteries (from *athero*, meaning gruel or paste, and *sclerosis*, meaning hardness).
Atlas First cervical vertebra.
Atopic A genetic disposition to an allergic reaction that is different from developing an allergy after one or more exposures to a drug or substance.
Atresia Absence of a normal opening.
Atria Two receiving chambers of the heart; singular form is *atrium.*
Atrial kick Remaining 20% to 30% of blood forced into the right ventricle during atrial contraction.
Atrioventricular junction The atrioventricular node and the nonbranching portion of the bundle of His.
Atrioventricular node A group of cells that conduct an electrical impulse through the heart; located in the floor of the right atrium immediately behind the tricuspid valve and near the opening of the coronary sinus.
Atrioventricular sequential pacemaker Type of dual-chamber pacemaker that stimulates first the atrium, then the ventricle, mimicking normal cardiac physiology.
Atrioventricular valve Valve located between each atrium and ventricle; the tricuspid separates the right

atrium from the right ventricle, and the mitral (bicuspid) separates the left atrium from the left ventricle.

Atrophy Decrease in cell size that negatively affects function.

Attenuated vaccine A vaccine prepared from a live virus or bacteria that has been physically or chemically weakened to produce an immune response without causing the severe effects of the disease.

Attributes Qualities or characteristics of a person.

Auditory ossicles Three small bones (malleus, incus, and stapes) that articulate with each other to transmit sounds waves to the cochlea.

Augmented limb lead Leads aVR, aVL, and aVF; these leads record the difference in electrical potential at one location relative to zero potential rather than relative to the electrical potential of another extremity, as in the bipolar leads.

Aura Sensory disturbances caused by a partial seizure; may precede a generalized seizure.

Auricle Outer ear; also called the *pinna.*

Auscultation The process of listening to body noises with a stethoscope.

Authority having jurisdiction The local agency having legal authority for the type of rescue and the location at which it occurs.

Autoantibodies Antibodies produced by B cells that mistakenly attack and destroy "self" cells belonging to the patient; autoantibodies are the pathophysiologic agent of most autoimmune disorders.

Autografting Transplanting organs or tissues within the same person.

Autoignition point The temperature at which a material ignites and burns without an ignition source.

Autologous skin grafting The transplantation of skin of one patient from its original location to that of a wound on the same patient, such as a burn. Autologous means "derived from the same individual."

Automatic location identification Telephone technology used to identify the location of a caller immediately.

Automatic number identification Telephone technology that provides immediate identification of the caller's 10-digit telephone number.

Automaticity Ability of cardiac pacemaker cells to initiate an electrical impulse spontaneously without being stimulated from another source (such as a nerve).

Autonomic dysreflexia Massive sympathetic stimulation unbalanced by the parasympathetic nervous system because of spinal cord injury, usually at or above T6.

Autonomic dysreflexia syndrome A condition characterized by hypertension superior to an SCI site caused by overstimulation of the sympathetic nervous system.

Autonomic nervous system Division of the peripheral nervous system that regulates many involuntary processes.

AVPU Mnemonic for *a*wake, *v*erbal, *p*ain, *u*nresponsive; used to evaluate a patient's mental status.

Axial compression (loading) The application of a force of energy along the axis of the spine, often resulting in compression fractures of the vertebrae.

Axial loading Application of excessive pressure or weight along the vertical axis of the spine.

Axial region Area that includes the head, neck, thorax, and abdomen.

Axial skeleton Part of the skeleton composed of the skull, hyoid bone, vertebral column, and thoracic cage.

Axis Imaginary line joining the positive and negative electrodes of a lead; also the second cervical vertebra.

Axon Branching extensions of the neuron where impulses exit the cell.

Azotemia The increase in nitrogen-containing waste products in the blood secondary to renal failure.

B lymphocytes Cells present in the lymphatic system that mediate humoral immunity (also known as *B cells*).

B pillar The structural roof support member on a vehicle located at the rear edge of the front door; also referred to as the *B post.*

Babinski's sign An abnormal finding indicated by the presence of great toe extension with the fanning of all other toes on stimulation of the sole of the foot when it is stroked with a semi-sharp object from the heel to the ball of the foot.

Bacillus anthracis A gram-positive, spore-forming bacterium that causes anthrax disease in human beings and animals.

Bacteremia The presence of bacteria in the blood. This condition could progress to septic shock. Fever, chills, tachycardia, and tachypnea are common manifestations of bacteremia.

Bacteria Prokaryotic microorganisms capable of infecting and injuring patients; however, some bacteria, as part of the normal flora, assist in the processes of the human body.

Bacterial tracheitis A potentially serious bacterial infection of the trachea.

Band A range of radio frequencies.

Bargaining A stage of the grieving process. The individual may attempt to "cut a deal" with a higher power to accomplish a specific goal or task.

Bariatric ambulance Ambulance designed to transport morbidly obese patients.

Barotrauma An injury resulting from rapid or extreme changes in pressure.

Barrier device A thin film of material placed on the patient's face used to prevent direct contact with the patient's mouth during positive-pressure ventilation.

Base of the heart Top of the heart; located at approximately the level of the second intercostal space.

Baseline Straight line recorded on ECG graph paper when no electrical activity is detected.

Bases Materials with a pH value greater than 7.0; also known as *caustic*.

Basilar skull fracture Loss of integrity to the bony structures of the base of the skull.

Basophils Type of granulocyte (white blood cell or leukocyte) that releases histamine.

Battery Touching or contact with another person without that person's consent.

Battle's sign Significant bruising around the mastoid process (behind the ears).

Beck's triad Classic signs of cardiac tamponade that include jugular venous distention, hypotension, and muffled heart sounds.

Behavior The conduct and activity of a person that is observable by others.

Behavioral emergency Actions or ideations by the patient that are harmful or potentially harmful to the patient or others.

Belay A safety technique used to safeguard personnel exposed to the risk of falling; the belayer is the person responsible for operation of the belay.

Bell's palsy An inflammation of the facial nerve (cranial nerve VII) that is thought to be caused by herpes simplex virus.

Benchmarking Comparison of operating policies, procedures, protocols, and performance with those of other agencies in an effort to improve results.

Benzodiazepine Any of a group of minor tranquilizers with a common molecular structure and similar pharmacologic activity, including antianxiety, sedative, hypnotic, amnestic, anticonvulsant, and muscle-relaxing effects.

Beriberi Disease caused by a deficiency of thiamine and characterized by neurologic symptoms, cardiovascular abnormalities, and edema.

Beta particle A negatively charged particle emitted by certain radioactive materials.

Bevel The slanted tip at the end of the needle.

Bicuspid valve Left atrioventricular valve in the heart; also called the *mitral valve*.

Bile salts Manufactured in the liver; composed of electrolytes and iron recovered from red blood cells when they die.

Bilevel positive airway pressure (BiPAP) A form of noninvasive, mechanical ventilation in which two (bi) levels of positive-pressure ventilation; one during inspiration (to keep the airway open as the patient inhales) and the other (lower) pressure during expiration to reduce the work of exhalation.

Bilevel positive airway pressure (BiPAP) device Breathing device that can be set at one pressure for inhaling and a different pressure for exhaling.

Bioassay A test that determines the effects of a substance on an organism and compares the result with some agreed standard.

Bioavailability The speed with which and how much of a drug reaches its intended site of action.

Bioburden Accumulation of bacteria in a wound; does not necessarily imply an infection is present.

Biologic agent A disease-causing pathogen or a toxin that may be used as a weapon to cause disease or injury to people.

Biot respirations Irregular respirations varying in rate and depth and interrupted by periods of apnea; associated with increased intracranial pressure, brain damage at the level of the medulla, and respiratory compromise from drug poisoning.

Biphasic Waveform that is partly positive and partly negative.

Bipolar disorder An illness of extremes of mood, alternating between periods of depression and episodes of mania (type I) or hypomania (type II).

Bipolar limb lead ECG lead consisting of a positive and negative electrode; a pacing lead with two electrical poles that are external from the pulse generator; the negative pole is located at the extreme distal tip of the pacing lead, and the positive pole is located several millimeters proximal to the negative electrode. The stimulating pulse is delivered through the negative electrode.

Birth canal Part of the female reproductive tract through which the fetus is delivered; includes the lower part of the uterus, the cervix, and the vagina.

Blast lung syndrome Injuries to the body from an explosion, characterized by anatomic and physiologic changes from the force generated by the blast wave hitting the body's surface and affecting primarily gas-containing structures (lungs, gastrointestinal tract, and ears).

Bleeding Escape of blood from a blood vessel.

Blister agent A chemical used as a weapon designed specifically to injure the body tissue internally and externally of those exposed to its vapors or liquid; the method of injury is to cause painful skin blisters or tissue destruction of the exposed surface area (e.g., mustard, lewisite).

Blocked premature atrial complex Premature atrial contraction not followed by a QRS complex.

Blocking A position that places the emergency vehicle at an angle to the approaching traffic, across several lanes of traffic if necessary; this position begins to shield the work area and protects the crash scene from some of the approaching traffic.

Blood Liquid connective tissue; allows transport of nutrients, oxygen, and waste products.

Blood agents Chemicals absorbed into the body through the action of breathing, skin absorption, or ingestion (e.g., hydrogen cyanide, cyanogen chloride).

Blood alcohol content Milligrams of ethanol per deciliter of blood divided by 100; a fairly standard measure of how intoxicated a person is.

Blood-brain barrier A layer of tightly adhered cells that protects the brain and spinal cord from exposure to medications, toxins, and infectious particles.

Blood pressure Force exerted by the blood against the walls of the arteries as the ventricles of the heart contract and relax.

Bloody show Passage of the protective blood and mucus plug from the cervix; often is an early sign of labor.

Body mass index A calculation strongly associated with subcutaneous and total body fat and with skinfold thickness measurements.

Body surface area (BSA) Area of the body covered by skin; measured in square meters.

Boiling liquid expanding vapor explosion An explosion that can occur when a vessel containing a pressurized liquid ruptures.

Boiling point The temperature at which the vapor pressure of the material being heated equals atmospheric pressure (760 mm Hg); water boils to steam at 100°C (212°F).

Bone Hard connective tissue; consists of living cells and a matrix made of minerals.

Borborygmi Hyperactivity of bowel sounds.

Borderline personality disorder Cluster B disorder marked by unstable emotions, relationships, and attitudes.

Botulism A severe neurologic illness caused by a potent toxin produced by *Clostridium botulinum* organisms; the three forms are food borne, wound, and infant (also called intestinal) botulism.

Bowel sounds The noises made by the intestinal smooth muscles as they squeeze fluids and food products through the digestive tract.

Bowman's capsule Located in the renal corpuscle.

Boyle's law Gas law that demonstrates that as pressure increases, volume decreases; explains the pain that can occur in flight in the teeth and ears and barotrauma in the gastrointestinal tract.

Bradycardia Heart rate slower than 60 beats/min (from *brady*, meaning "slow").

Bradykinesia Abnormal slowness of muscular movement.

Bradypnea A respiratory rate that is persistently slower than normal for age; in adults, a rate slower than 12 breaths/min.

Brain injury A traumatic insult to the brain capable of producing physical, intellectual, emotional, social, and vocational changes.

Brainstem Part of the brain that connects it to the spinal cord; responsible for many of the autonomic functions the body requires to survive (also called *vegetative functions*).

Brake bar rack A descending device consisting of a U-shaped metal bar to which several metal bars are attached that create friction on the rope. Some racks are limited to use in personal rappelling, whereas others also may be used for lowering rescue loads.

Braxton-Hicks contractions (false labor) Benign and painless contractions that usually occur after the third month of pregnancy.

Breach of duty Violation by the defendant of the standard of care applicable to the circumstances.

Breech presentation Presentation of the buttocks or feet of the fetus as the first part of the infant's body to enter the birth canal.

Bronchioles Smallest of the air passages.

Bronchiolitis An acute, infectious, inflammatory disease of the upper and lower respiratory tracts that results in obstruction of the small airways.

Bronchitis Inflammation of the lower airways, usually with mucus production. Often chronic and related to tobacco abuse.

Bronchopulmonary dysplasia (BPD) Respiratory condition in infants usually arising from preterm birth.

Bronchospasm Wheezing.

Brown-Séquard syndrome Group of symptoms that develop after the herniation or transection of half of the spinal cord manifested with unilateral damage.

Bruit The blowing or swishing sound created by the turbulence within a blood vessel.

Bubonic Relating to an inflamed, enlarged lymph gland.

Buccal An administration route in which medication is placed in the mouth between the gum and the mucous membrane of the cheek and absorbed into the bloodstream.

Buffer systems Compensatory mechanisms that act together to control pH.

Bulbourethral glands Pair of small glands that manufacture a mucous-type secretion that unites with the prostate fluid and spermatozoa to form sperm.

Bulimia nervosa Eating disorder consisting of a pattern of eating large amounts of food in one sitting (binging) and then forcing oneself to regurgitate (purging), with associated guilt and depression.

Bulk containers Large containers and tanks used to transport large quantities of hazardous materials.

Bulla A localized, fluid-filled lesion usually greater than 0.5 cm.

Bundle branch block (BBB) Abnormal conduction of an electrical impulse through either the right or left bundle branches.

Bundle of His Fibers located in the upper portion of the interventricular septum that conduct an electrical impulse through the heart.

Burnout Exhaustion to the point of not being able to perform one's job effectively.

Bursitis Chronic or acute inflammation of the small synovial sacs known as bursa.

Burst Three or more sequential ectopic beats; also referred to as a *salvo* or *run*.

Cadaveric transplantation Transplantation of organs from an already deceased person to a living person.

Calibration Regulation of an ECG machine's stylus sensitivity so that a 1-mV electrical signal will produce a deflection measuring exactly 10 mm.

Call processing time The elapsed time from the moment a call is received by the communications center to the time the responding unit is alerted.

Cancer A group of diseases that allow unrestrained growth of cells in one or more of the body organs or tissues.

Capacitance vessels Venules that have the capability of holding large amounts of volume.

Capillaries Tiny vessels that connect arterioles to venules; deliver blood to each cell in the body.

Capillary leak Loss of intravascular fluid (plasma, water) from a loss of capillary integrity or an opening of gap junctions between the cells of the capillaries. May be caused by thermal injury to capillaries or the intense inflammatory reaction to burn injury, infection, or physical trauma.

Caplet A tablet with an oblong shape and a film-coated covering.

Capnograph A device that provides a numerical reading of exhaled CO_2 concentrations and a waveform (tracing).

Capnography Continuous analysis and recording of CO_2 concentrations in respiratory gases.

Capnometer A device used to measure the concentration of CO_2 at the end of exhalation.

Capnometry A numeric reading of exhaled CO_2 concentrations without a continuous written record or waveform.

Capsid Layer of protein enveloping the genome of a virion; composed of structural units called the capsomeres.

Capsule A membranous shell surrounding certain microorganisms, such as the pneumococcus bacterium; also a small gelatin shell in which a powdered or granulated form of medication is placed.

Capture Ability of a pacing stimulus to depolarize successfully the cardiac chamber being paced; with one-to-one capture, each pacing stimulus results in depolarization of the appropriate chamber.

Carbamate A pesticide that inhibits acetylcholinesterase.

Carbon dioxide narcosis Condition mostly seen in patients with chronic obstructive pulmonary disease, in whom carbon dioxide is excessively retained, causing mental status changes and decreased respirations.

Carboys Glass or plastic bottles commonly used to transport corrosive products.

Carbuncle A series of abscesses in the subcutaneous tissues that drain through hair follicles.

Cardiac arrest Absence of cardiac mechanical activity confirmed by the absence of a detectable pulse, unresponsiveness, and apnea or agonal, gasping respirations.

Cardiac cycle Period from the beginning of one heartbeat to the beginning of the next; normally consisting of PQRST waves, complexes, and intervals.

Cardiac output Amount of blood pumped into the aorta each minute by the heart.

Cardiac rupture An acute traumatic perforation of the ventricles or atria.

Cardiac sphincter Circular muscle that controls the movement of material into the stomach.

Cardiogenic shock A condition in which heart muscle function is severely impaired, leading to decreased cardiac output and inadequate tissue perfusion.

Cardiomyopathy A disease of the heart muscle.

Cardiovascular disorders A collection of diseases and conditions that involve the heart (cardio) and blood vessels (vascular).

Carina Area in the bronchial tree that separates into the right and left mainstem bronchi.

Carotid bruit The noise made when blood in the carotid arteries passes over plaque buildups.

Carpal tunnel syndrome A medical condition in which the median nerve is compressed at the wrist (within the carpal tunnel), resulting in pain and numbness of the hand.

Carpopedal spasm Cramping of the extremities secondary to hyperventilation-induced hypocalcemia.

Cartilage Connective tissue composed of chondrocytes; exact makeup depends on the location and function in the body.

Cartilaginous joint Unites two bones with hyaline cartilage or fibrocartilage.

Case law Interpretations of constitutional, statutory, or administrative law made by the courts; also known as *common law* or *judge-made law*.

Catabolic Refers to the metabolic breakdown of proteins, lipids, and carbohydrates by the body to produce energy.

Catabolism Process of breaking down complex substances into more simple ones.

Catalepsy Abnormal state characterized by a trancelike level of consciousness and postural rigidity; occurs in hypnosis and in certain organic and psychological disorders such as schizophrenia, epilepsy, and hysteria.

Cataract A partial or complete opacity on or in the lens or lens capsule of the eye, especially one impairing vision or causing blindness.

Catatonia A state of psychologically induced immobility with muscular rigidity, at times interrupted by agitation.

Catatonic schizophrenia A form of schizophrenia characterized by alternating periods of extreme withdrawal and extreme excitement. During the withdrawal stage stupor, waxy flexibility, muscular rigidity, mutism, blocking, negativism, and catalepsy may be seen; during the period of excitement, purposeless and impulsive activity may range from mild agitation to violence. See *Catatonia.*

Cathartics Substances that decrease the time a poison spends in the gastrointestinal tract by increasing bowel motility.

Catheter shear/catheter fragment embolism Breaking off the tip of the intravenous catheter inside the vein, which then travels through the venous system; it can lodge in pulmonary circulation as a pulmonary embolism.

Cation A positively charged ion.

Cauda equina Peripheral nerve bundles descending through the spinal column distal to the conus medullaris. Cauda equina are not spinal nerves.

Cauda equina syndrome A group of symptoms associated with the compression of the peripheral nerves still within the spinal canal below the level of the first lumbar vertebra, characterized by lumbar back pain, motor and sensory deficits, and bowel or bladder incontinence.

Caudal A position toward the distal end of the body; usually inferior.

Causation In a negligence case, the negligence of the defendant must have caused or created the harm sustained by the plaintiff; also referred to as *proximate cause.*

Caustic A substance with a pH above 7.0; also known as a *base* or *alkali.*

Cecum First segment of the large intestine; the appendix is its accessory structure.

Cell body Portion of the neuron containing the organelles, where essential cellular functions are performed.

Cell-mediated immunity Form of acquired immunity; results from activation of T lymphocytes that were previously sensitized to a specific antigen.

Cellular swelling Swelling of cellular tissues, usually from injury.

Cellulitis An inflammation of the skin.

Cementum A layer of tough tissue that anchors the root of a tooth to the periodontal membrane/ligament.

Central cord syndrome Collection of symptoms seen after the death of the central portion of the spinal cord.

Central nervous system (CNS) The brain and spinal cord.

Central neurogenic hyperventilation Similar to Kussmaul respirations; characterized as deep, rapid breathing; associated with increased intracranial pressure.

Central retinal artery occlusion (CRAO) A condition in which the blood supply to the retina is blocked because of a clot or embolus in the central retinal artery or one of its branches.

Central vein A major vein of the chest, neck, or abdomen.

Central venous catheter A catheter through a vein to end in the superior vena cava or right atrium of the heart for medication or fluid administration.

Centrioles Paired, rodlike structures that exist in a specialized area of the cytoplasm known as the centrosome.

Centrosome Specialized area of the cytoplasm; plays an important role in the process of cell division.

Cephalic A position toward the head; usually superior.

Cerebellum Area of the brain involved in fine and gross coordination; responsible for interpretation of actual movement and correction of any movements that interfere with coordination and the body's position.

Cerebral contusion A brain injury in which brain tissue is bruised in a local area but does not puncture the pia mater.

Cerebral palsy Neuromuscular condition in which the patient has difficulty controlling the voluntary muscles because of damage to a portion of the brain.

Cerebral perfusion pressure (CPP) Pressure inside the cerebral arteries and an indicator of brain perfusion; calculated by subtracting intracranial pressure from mean arterial pressure (CPP = MAP – ICP).

Cerebrospinal fluid (CSF) Fluid that bathes, protects, and nourishes the central nervous system.

Cerebrovascular accident (CVA) Blockage or hemorrhage of the blood vessels in the brain, usually causing focal neurologic deficits; also known as a *stroke.*

Cerebrum Largest part of the brain, divided into right and left hemispheres.

Certification An external verification of the competencies that an individual has achieved and typically involves an examination process; in healthcare these processes are typically designed to verify that an individual has achieved minimal competency to ensure safe and effective patient care.

Certified Flight Paramedic (FP-C) A certification obtained by paramedics on successful completion of the Flight Paramedic Examination.

Certified Flight Registered Nurse (CFRN) A nurse who has completed education, training, and certification beyond a registered nurse with a focus on air medical transport of potentially critically ill or injured patients.

Cerumen Earwax.

Ceruminous glands Glands lining the external auditory canal; produce cerumen or earwax.

Cervical spondylosis Degeneration of two or more cervical vertebrae, usually resulting in a narrowing of the space between the vertebrae.

Cervical vertebrae First seven vertebrae in descending order from the base of the skull.

Cervix Inferior portion of the uterus.

Chalazion A small bump on the eyelid caused by a blocked oil gland.

Charles' law Law stating that oxygen cylinders can have variations in pressure readings in different ambient temperatures.

Chelating agent A substance that can bind metals; used as an antidote to many heavy metal poisonings.

Chemical Abstracts Services (CAS) number Unique identification number of chemicals, much like a person's Social Security number.

Chemical asphyxiants Chemicals that prevent the transportation of oxygen to the cells or the use of oxygen at the cellular level.

Chemical name A precise description of a drug's chemical composition and molecular structure.

Chemical restraints Agents such as sedatives that can suppress a patient's neurologic and/or motor capabilities and reduce the threat to the paramedic; also known as *pharmacologic restraints.*

Cheyne-Stokes respirations A pattern of gradually increasing rate and depth of breathing that tapers to slower and shallower breathing with a period of apnea before the cycle repeats itself; often described as a crescendo-decrescendo pattern or periodic breathing.

Chief complaint The reason the patient has sought medical attention.

Child maltreatment An all-encompassing term for all types of child abuse and neglect, including physical abuse, emotional abuse, sexual abuse, and neglect.

Chloracetophenone Tear gas; commercially known as *Mace.*

Choanal atresia Narrowing or blockage of one or both nares by membranous or bony tissue.

Choking agent An industrial chemical used as a weapon to kill those who inhale the vapors or gases; the method of injury is asphyxiation resulting from lung damage from hydrochloric acid burns (e.g., chlorine, phosgene); also known as a pulmonary agent.

Cholangitis Inflammation of the bile duct.

Cholecystitis Inflammation of the gallbladder.

Choledocholithiasis The presence of gallstones in the common bile duct.

Cholelithiasis The presence of stones in the gallbladder.

Cholinergic Having the characteristics of the parasympathetic division of the autonomic nervous system.

Cholinesterase inhibitor A chemical that blocks the action of acetylcholinesterase; thus the neurotransmitter acetylcholine is allowed to send its signals continuously to innervate nerve endings.

Chordae tendineae Fibrous bands of tissue in the valves that attach to each part or cusp of the valve.

Chorioamnionitis Infection of the amniotic sac and its contents.

Choroid Vascular layer of the eyeball.

Choroid plexus Group of specialized cells in the ventricles of the brain; filters blood through cerebral capillaries to create the cerebrospinal fluid.

Chromatin Material within a cell nucleus from which the chromosomes are formed.

Chromosomes Any of the threadlike structures in the nucleus of a cell that function in the transmission of genetic information; each consists of a double strand of DNA attached to proteins called histones.

Chronic Long, drawn out; applied to a disease that is not acute.

Chronic exposure An exposure to low concentrations over a long period.

Chronic obstructive pulmonary disease (COPD) A progressive and irreversible condition characterized by diminished inspiratory and expiratory capacity of the lungs.

Chronic renal failure The gradual, long-term deterioration of kidney function.

Chronology The arrangement of events in time.

Chronotropism A change in heart rate.

Chute time The time required to get a unit en route to a call from dispatch.

Chyme Semifluid mass of partly digested food expelled by the stomach into the duodenum.

Ciliary body Consists of muscles that change the shape of the lens in the eye; includes a network of capillaries that produce aqueous humor.

Circadian A daily rhythmic activity cycle based on 24-hour intervals or events that occur at approximately 24-hour intervals, such as certain physiologic occurrences.

Circadian rhythm The 24-hour cycle that relates to work and rest time.

Circumflex artery Division of the left coronary artery.

Circumoral paresthesia A feeling of tingling around the lips and mouth caused by hyperventilation.

Circumstantial thinking Adding detours and extra details to conversations but eventually returning to the main topic.

Cirrhosis A chronic degenerative disease of the liver.

Civil law A branch of law that deals with torts (civil wrongs) committed by one individual, organization, or group against another.

Clarification Using a phrase or question in an attempt to clarify any ambiguous statements or words.

Classic heat stroke Heat stroke caused by environmental exposure that results in core hyperthermia greater than 40°C (104°F).

Clean To wash with soap and water.

Cleft lip Incomplete closure of the upper lip.

Cleft palate Incomplete closure of the hard and/or soft palate of the mouth.

Clinical performance indicator A definable, measurable, skilled task completed by the dispatcher that has a significant impact on the delivery of patient care.

Clitoris Small, erectile structure superior to the entrance to the vagina.

Closed-ended questions A form of interview question that limits a patient's response to simple, brief words or phrases (e.g., "yes or no," "sharp or dull").

Closed fracture Fracture of the bone tissue that has not broken the skin tissue.

Clostridium botulinum A bacterium that produces a powerful toxin that causes botulism disease in human beings, waterfowl, and cattle.

Cluster A personality disorders Odd and eccentric type of personality disorders, including paranoid, schizoid, and schizotypal; characterized by social isolation and odd thought processes.

Cluster B personality disorders Emotional and dramatic type of personality disorders, including histrionic, borderline, antisocial, and narcissistic; characterized by impulsive, unpredictable behavior, and manipulation of others.

Cluster C personality disorders Anxious and fearful type of personality disorders, including avoidant, dependent, and compulsive; marked by anxiety, shyness, and avoidance of conflict.

Cluster headache A migraine-like condition characterized by attacks of intense unilateral pain. The pain occurs most often over the eye and forehead and is accompanied by flushing and watering of the eyes and nose. The attacks occur in groups, with a duration of several hours.

CNS-PAD An acronym for ***c***entral ***n***ervous ***s***ystem padding: ***p***ia mater, ***a***rachnid mater, ***d***ura mater.

Coagulation Formation of blood clots with the associated increase in blood viscosity.

Coagulation cascade A set of interactions of the circulating clotting factors.

Coagulation necrosis Dead or dying tissue that forms a scar or eschar.

Cocaine hydrochloride Fine, white powdered form of cocaine, a powerful central nervous system stimulant; typically snorted intranasally.

Coccyx (coccygeal vertebrae) Terminal end of the spinal column; a tail-like bone composed of three to five vertebra. No nerve roots travel through the coccyx.

Cochlea Bony structure in the inner ear resembling a tiny snail shell.

Code of ethics A guide for interactions between members of a specific profession (such as physicians) and the public.

Codependence A psychological concept defined as exhibiting too much and often inappropriate caring behavior.

Cognition Operation of the mind by which one becomes aware of objects of thought or perception; includes all aspects of perceiving, thinking, and remembering.

Cognitive disability An impairment that affects an individual's awareness and memory as well as his or her ability to learn, process information, communicate, and make decisions.

Cognitive phase In the phases of immune response, the stage at which a foreign antigen is recognized to be present.

Cold diuresis The occurrence of increased urine production on exposure to cold.

Cold protective response The mechanism associated with cold water in which individuals can survive extended periods of submersion.

Cold zone A safe area isolated from the area of contamination; also called the *support zone*. This zone has safe and easy access. It contains the command post and staging areas for personnel, vehicles, and equipment. EMS personnel are stationed in the cold zone.

Collagen A fibrous protein that provides elasticity and strength to skin and the body's connective tissue.

Collapsed lung See *Pneumothorax*.

Colostomy Incision in the colon for the purpose of making a temporary or permanent opening between the bowel and the abdominal wall.

Combination deployment Using a mix of geographic coverage and demand posts to best serve the community given the number of ambulances available at any one time.

Combining form A word root followed by a vowel.

Combining vowel A vowel that is added to a word root before a suffix.

Comfort care Medical care intended to provide relief from pain and discomfort, such as the control of pain with medications.

Command post The location from which incident operations are directed.

Comminuted skull fracture Breakage of a bone or bones of the skull into multiple fragments.

Communicable period The period after infection during which the diease may be transmitted to another host.

Communication The exchange of thoughts, messages, and information.

Compartment syndrome (CS) A condition in which compartment pressures increase in an injured extremity to the point that capillary circulation is stopped; often only correctable through surgical opening of the compartment.

Compensatory pause Pause for which the normal beat after a premature complex occurs when expected; also called a *complete pause*.

Complete abortion Passage of all fetal tissue before 20 weeks of gestation.

Complex Several waveforms.

Complex partial seizure A seizure affecting only one part of the brain that does alter consciousness.

Compliance The resistance of the patient's lung tissue to ventilation.

Compound presentation Presentation of an extremity beside the major presenting fetal part.

Compound skull fracture Open skull fracture.

Compound word Word that contains more than one root.

Computer-aided dispatch (CAD) A computer-aided system that automates dispatching by enhanced data collection, rapid recall of information, dispatch mapping, as well as unit tracking and the ability to track and dispatch resources.

Concealment To hide or put out of site; provides no ballistic protection.

Concept formation The initial formation of an overall concept of care for a particular patient begins when the paramedic arrives on location of the incident.

Conception The act or process of fertilization; beginning of pregnancy.

Concurrent medical direction Consultation with a physician or other advanced healthcare professional by telephone, radio, or other electronic means, permitting the physician and paramedic to decide together on the best course of action in the delivery of patient care.

Concussion A brain injury with a transient impairment of consciousness followed by a rapid recovery to baseline neurologic activity.

Conducting arteries Large arteries of the body (e.g., aorta and the pulmonary trunk); have more elastic tissue and less smooth muscle; stretch under great pressures and then quickly return back to their original shapes.

Conduction system A system of pathways in the heart composed of specialized electrical (pacemaker) cells.

Conductive hearing loss Type of deafness that occurs where there is a problem with the transfer of sound from the outer to the inner ear.

Conductivity Ability of a cardiac cell to receive an electrical stimulus and conduct that impulse to an adjacent cardiac cell.

Confidentiality Protection of patient information in any form and the disclosure of that information only as needed for patient care or as otherwise permitted by law.

Confined space By Occupational Safety and Health Administration (OSHA) definition, a space large enough and configured so that an employee can enter and perform assigned work but has limited or restricted means for entry or exit (e.g., tanks, vessels, silos, storage bins, hoppers, vaults, and pits are spaces that may have limited means of entry); not designed for continuous employee occupancy.

Confrontation Focusing on a particular point made during the interview.

Congenital Present at or before birth.

Conjunctiva Thin, transparent mucous membrane that covers the inner surface of the eyelids and the outer surface of the sclera.

Conjunctivitis Inflammation of the conjunctiva.

Connective tissue Most abundant type of tissue in the body; composed of cells that are separated by a matrix.

Conscious sedation A medication or combination of medications that allows a patient to undergo what could be an unpleasant experience by producing an altered level of consciousness but not complete anesthesia. The goal is for the patient to breathe spontaneously and maintain his or her own airway.

Consensus formula Formula used to calculate the volume of fluid needed to properly resuscitate a burn patient. The formula is 2 to 4 mL/kg/% total body surface area burned. This is the formula currently regarded by the American Burn Association as the standard of care in adult burn patients. Several other, similar formulas exist that also may be used.

Consent Permission.

Constricted affect Emotion shown in degrees less than expected.

Contamination The deposition or absorption of chemical, biologic, or radiologic materials onto personnel or other materials.

Contamination reduction zone See *Warm zone.*

Continuing education (CE) Lifelong learning.

Continuous positive airway pressure (CPAP) The delivery of slight positive pressure throughout the respiratory cycle to prevent airway collapse, reduce the work of breathing, and improve alveolar ventilation.

Continuous positive airway pressure (CPAP) device Breathing device that allows delivery of slight positive pressure to prevent airway collapse and improve oxygenation and ventilation in spontaneously breathing patients.

Continuous quality improvement (CQI) Programs designed to improve the level of care; commonly driven by quality assurance.

Contractility Ability of cardiac cells to shorten, causing cardiac muscle contraction in response to an electrical stimulus.

Contraction Rhythmic tightening of the muscular uterine wall that occurs during normal labor and leads to expulsion of the fetus and placenta from the uterus.

Contraction interval The time from the beginning of one contraction to the beginning of the next contraction.

Contraction time The time from the beginning to the end of a single uterine contraction.

Contraindication Use of a drug for a condition when it is not advisable.

Contrecoup injury An injury at another site, usually opposite the point of impact.

Contributory negligence An injured plaintiff's failure to exercise due care that, along with the defendant's negligence, contributed to the injury.

Conus medullaris Terminal end of the spinal cord.

Conus medullaris syndrome Complications resulting from injury to the conus medullaris.

Conventional silo A vertical structure used to store ensiled plant material in a aerobic environment.

Cor pulmonale Right-sided heart failure caused by pulmonary disease.

Core body temperature The measured body temperature within the core of the body; generally measured with an esophageal probe; normal is 98.6° F.

Cornea Avascular, transparent structure that permits light through to the interior of the eye.

Coronary artery disease Disease of the arteries that supply the heart muscle with blood.

Coronary heart disease Disease of the coronary arteries and their resulting complications, such as angina pectoris or acute myocardial infarction.

Coronary sinus Venous drain for the coronary circulation into the right atrium.

Corrosive A substance able to corrode tissue or metal (e.g., acids and bases).

Corticosteroids See *Adrenocortical steroids.*

Cosmesis Of or referring to the improvement of physical appearance.

Costal angle The angle formed by the margins of the ribs at the sternum.

Costochondritis Inflammation of the cartilage in the anterior chest that causes chest pain.

Coughing A protective mechanism usually induced by mucosal irritation; the forceful, spastic expiration experienced during coughing aids in the clearance of the bronchi and bronchioles.

Coup contrecoup An injury most often associated with a blow to the skull in which the force of the impact is transmitted through the skull bones to the opposite side of the head, where the bruise, fracture, or other sign of injury appears.

Coup injury An injury directly below the point of impact.

Couplet Two consecutive premature complexes.

Cover A type of concealment that hides the body and offers ballistic protection.

Crack cocaine Solid, brownish-white crystal form of cocaine, a powerful central nervous system stimulant; typically smoked.

Crackles (rales) As the name implies, when fluid accumulates in the smaller airway passages, air passing through the fluid creates a moist crackling or popping sound heard on inspiration.

Cranial nerve Twelve pairs of nerves that exit the brain and innervate the head and face; some also are part of the visceral portion of the peripheral nervous system.

Cranium The vaultlike portion of the skull, behind and above the face.

Creatinine End product of creatine metabolism; released during anaerobic metabolism. Elevated levels of creatinine are common in advanced stages of renal failure.

Creatine kinase An enzyme in skeletal and cardiac muscles that is released into circulation as a result of tissue damage. Can be used as a laboratory indicator of muscle damage.

Credentialing A local process by which an individual is permitted by a specific entity (e.g., medical director) to practice in a specific setting (e.g., EMS agency).

Crepitation A crackling sound indicative of bone ends grinding together.

Crepitus The grating, crackling, or popping sounds and sensations experienced under skin and joints.

Cricoid cartilage Most inferior cartilage of the larynx; only complete ring in the larynx.

Cricothyroid membrane A fibrous membrane located between the cricoid and thyroid cartilages.

Cricothyrotomy An emergency procedure performed to allow rapid entrance to the airway (by the cricothyroid membrane) for temporary oxygenation and ventilation.

Crime scene A location where any part of a criminal act has occurred or where evidence relating to a crime may be found.

Criminal law A branch of law in which the federal, state, or local government prosecutes individuals on behalf of society for violating laws designed to safeguard society.

Cross tolerance Decreasing responsiveness to the effects of a drug in a drug classification (such as narcotics) and the likelihood of development of decreased responsiveness to another drug in that classification.

Crossmatch The process by which blood compatibility is determined by mixing blood samples from the donor and recipient.

Croup A viral infection of the upper airway; respiratory distress caused by narrowing below the glottis and characterized by hoarseness, inspiratory stridor, and a barking cough.

Crown The visible part of a tooth.

Crowning The appearance of the first part of the infant at the vaginal opening during delivery.

Crush points Formed when two objects are moving toward each other or when one object is moving toward a stationary object and the gap between the two is decreasing.

Crush syndrome Renal failure and shock after crush injuries.

Crust A collection of cellular debris or dried blood; often called a *scab.*

Cryogenic Pertaining to extremely low temperatures.

CSM ***C***irculation, ***s***ensation, and ***m***ovement.

Cullen's sign Yellow-blue ecchymosis surrounding the umbilicus.

Cultural beliefs Values and perspectives common to a racial, religious, or social group of people.

Cultural imposition The tendency to impose your beliefs, values, and patterns of behavior on an individual from another culture.

Cumulative action Increased intensity of drug action evident after administration of several doses.

Current Flow of electrical charge from one point to another.

Current health status Focus on the environmental and personal habits of the patient that may influence the patient's general state of health.

Cushing syndrome Disorder caused by the overproduction of corticosteroids; characterized by a "moon face," obesity, fat accumulation on the upper back, increased facial hair, acne, diabetes, and hypertension.

Cushing's triad Characteristic pattern of vital signs during rising intracranial pressure, presenting as rising hypertension, bradycardia, and abnormal respirations.

Customs A practice or set of practices followed by a group of people.

Cyanogen chloride A highly toxic blood agent.

Cyanosis A bluish coloration of the skin as a result of hypoxemia, or deoxygenation of hemoglobin.

Cyclohexyl methyl phosphonofluoridate G nerve agent. The G agents tend to be nonpersistent, volatile agents.

Cyclothymia A less-severe form of bipolar disorder marked by more frequently alternating periods of a dysphoric mood that does not meet the criteria for depression and hypomania.

Cylinders Nonbulk containers that normally contain liquefied gases, nonliquified gases, or mixtures under pressure; cylinders also may contain liquids or solids.

Cyst A walled cavity that contains fluid or purulent material.

Cystic fibrosis (CF) Genetic disease marked by hypersecretion of glands, including mucus glands in the lungs.

Cystic medial degeneration A connective tissue disease in which the elastic tissue and smooth muscle fibers of the middle arterial layer degenerate.

Cystitis Infection isolated in the bladder.

Cytokines Protein molecules produced by white blood cells that act as chemical messengers between cells; released in response to injury.

Cytoplasm Fluid-like material in which the organelles are suspended; lies between the plasma membrane and the nucleus.

Cytoplasmic membrane Encloses the cytoplasm and its organelles; forms the outer border of the cell.

Cytosol Liquid medium of the cytoplasm.

Dalton's law (law of partial pressure) Law relating to the partial pressure of oxygen during transport; defines that it is more difficult for oxygen to transfer from air to blood at lower pressures.

Damages Compensable harm or other losses incurred by an injured party (plaintiff) because of the negligence of the defendant.

Data interpretation The step that uses all the data gathered in the concept formation stage with the paramedic's knowledge of anatomy, physiology, and pathophysiology to continue the decision-making process.

Daughter cells Two cells that result from mitosis.

Dead air space Not all the air inspired during a breath participates in gas exchange and can be further classified as anatomic or physiologic dead space. In the average adult male this equates to approximately 150 mL. Anatomic dead space includes airway passages such as the trachea and bronchi, which are incapable of participating in gas exchange. Alveoli that have the potential to participate in gas exchange but do not because of disease or obstruction, as in chronic obstructive pulmonary disease (COPD) or atelectasis, are referred to as physiologic dead space.

Deafness A complete or partial inability to hear.

Debridement Removal of foreign material or dead tissue from a wound (pronounced *da brēd'*).

Decannulation Removal of a tracheostomy tube.

Decompensated shock A clinical state of tissue perfusion that is inadequate to meet the body's metabolic demands; accompanied by hypotension; also called *progressive* or *late shock*.

Decompression sickness An illness occurring during or after a diving ascent that results when nitrogen in compressed air converts back from solution to gas, forming bubbles in tissues and blood.

Decontamination The process of removing dangerous substances from the patient; may involve removing substances from the skin (external decontamination) and/or removing substances from the gastrointestinal tract (internal decontamination).

Deep fascia Fibrous, nonelastic connective tissue that forms the boundaries of muscle compartments.

Deep partial-thickness burn A burn in which the mid- or deeper dermis is injured. Results in injury to the deeper hair follicle, glandular, nerve, and blood vessel structures.

Deep venous thrombosis (DVT) A blood clot that forms in the deep venous system of the pelvis or legs; may progress to a pulmonary embolism.

Defamation The publication of false information about a person that tends to blacken the person's character or injure his or her reputation.

Defendant The person or institution being sued; also called the *respondent*.

Defibrillation Therapeutic use of electric current to terminate lethal cardiac dysrhythmias.

Degenerative joint disease See *Osteoarthritis*.

Dehydration A state in which the body has an excessive water loss from the tissues.

Delayed reaction A delay between exposure and onset of action.

Delirium Short-term and temporary mental confusion and fluctuating level of consciousness, often caused by intoxication from various substances, hypoglycemia, or acute psychiatric episodes.

Delirium tremens (DT) The most severe form of ethanol withdrawal, including hallucinations, delusions, confusion, and seizures.

Delta wave Slurring of the beginning portion of the QRS complex caused by preexcitation.

Delusion False perception and interpretation of situations and events that a person believes to be true no matter how convincing evidence is to the contrary.

Delusions of reference A belief that ordinary events have a special, often dangerous, meaning to the self.

Demand pacemaker Synchronous pacemaker that discharges only when the patient's heart rate drops below the preset rate for the pacemaker.

Dementia Long-term decline in mental faculties such as memory, concentration, and judgment; often seen with degenerative neurologic disorders such as Alzheimer's disease.

Dendrite Branchlike projections from a neuron that receive impulses or sensory information.

Denial A common defense mechanism that presents with feelings of disbelief, such as "no, that can't be right" when a life-threatening or terminal diagnosis is received; one of the stages of the grief response.

Denominator The number or mathematic expression below the line in a fraction; the denominator is the sum of the parts.

Dentin A hard but porous tissue found under the enamel and cementum of a tooth.

Deoxyribonucleic acid (DNA) Specialized structure within the cell that carries genetic material for reproduction.

Depersonalization A sudden sense of the loss of one's identity.

Deployment Matching production capacity of an ambulance system to the changing patterns of call demand.

Depolarization Movement of ions across a cell membrane, causing the inside of the cell to become more positive; an electrical event expected to result in contraction.

Depressed skull fracture A fracture of the skull with inward displacement of bone fragments.

Depression Sorrow and lack of interest in the things that previously produced pleasure.

Derealization A sudden feeling that one's surroundings are not real, as if one is watching a movie or television, not reality.

Dermatomes Areas of the body innervated by specific sensory spinal nerves; also a device used to remove healthy skin from somewhere on the body of the burn patient for the purpose of transplanting (grafting) at another site, such as an excised burn wound or other open wound.

Dermis Located below the epidermis and consists mainly of connective tissue containing both collagen and elastin fibers; contains specialized nervous tissue that provides sensory information, pain, pressure, touch, and temperature, to the central nervous system; also contains hair follicles, sweat and sebaceous glands, and a large network of blood vessels.

Descending colon Part of the large intestine.

Desired action The intended beneficial effect of a drug.

Developmental disabilities Disabilities that involve some degree of impaired adaptation in learning, social adjustment, or maturation.

Diabetes insipidus (DI) Disorder caused by insufficient production of ADH in the posterior pituitary gland, causing a larger than normal increase in the secretion of free water in the urine and poor absorption of water into the bloodstream.

Diabetic ketoacidosis (DKA) Condition found in diabetic patients caused by the lack or absence of insulin, leading to an increase of ketone bodies and acidosis in the blood.

Dialysis The process of diffusing blood across a semipermeable membrane to remove substances that the kidney would normally eliminate.

Dialysis shunt Shunt composed of two plastic tubes (one inserted into an artery, the other into a vein) that stick out of the skin to allow easy access and attachment to a dialysis machine for filtering waste products from the blood.

Diapedesis Migration of phagocytes through the endothelial wall of the vasculature into surrounding tissues.

Diaphragm Muscle that separates the thoracic cavity from the abdominal cavity.

Diaphragmatic hernia Protrusion of the abdominal contents into the chest cavity through an opening in the diaphragm.

Diaphysis Shaft of the bone where marrow is found that forms red and white blood cells.

Diastole Phase of the cardiac cycle in which the atria and ventricles relax between contractions and blood enters these chambers; when the term is used without reference to a specific chamber of the heart, the term implies ventricular diastole.

Diastolic blood pressure The pressure exerted against the walls of the large arteries during ventricular relaxation.

Diencephalon Portion of the brain between the brainstem and cerebrum; contains the thalamus and hypothalamus and the temperature regulatory centers for the body.

Differential diagnosis The list of problems that could produce the patient's chief complaint.

Differentiation Process of cell maturation; the cell becomes specialized for a specific purpose, such as a cardiac cell versus a bone cell.

Diffuse axonal injury (DAI) A type of brain injury caused by shearing forces that occur between different parts of the brain as a result of rotational acceleration.

Diffusion Spreading out of molecules from an area of higher concentration to an area of lower concentration.

Digestion Chemical breakdown of food material into smaller fragments that can be absorbed into the circulatory system.

Digestive tract Series of muscular tubes designed to move food and liquid.

Digoxin A medication derived from digitalis that acts by increasing the force of myocardial contraction and the refractory period and decreasing the conduction rate of the atrioventricular node; used to treat heart failure, most supraventricular tachycardias, and cardiogenic shock.

Dilation Spontaneous opening of the cervix that occurs as part of labor.

Diplomacy Tact and skill in dealing with people.

Direct (closed-ended) questions Questions that can be answered with short responses such as "yes" or "no."

Direct communication Method of intercellular communication in which one cell communicates with the cell adjacent to it by using minerals and ions.

Dirty bomb A conventional explosive device used as a radiologic agent dispersal device.

Disaster An incident involving 100 or more persons.

Disaster Medical Assistance Team (DMAT) Field-deployable hospital teams that include physicians, nurses, emergency medical technicians, and other medical and nonmedical support personnel.

Disaster Mortuary Operations Teams Teams composed of forensic and mortuary professionals trained to deal with human remains after disaster situations.

Discrimination Treatment or consideration based on class or category rather than individual merit.

Disease period The interval between the first appearance of symptoms and resolution.

Disinfect To clean with an agent that should kill many of, or most, surface organisms.

Disinfection Process of cleaning the ambulance, the cot, and equipment; disinfectant substances are toxic to body tissues.

Disorganized schizophrenia A subtype of schizophrenia characterized by an earlier age of onset, usually at puberty, and a more severe disintegration of personality than occurs in other forms of the disease; symptoms include incoherence, loose associations, gross disorganization or behavior, and flat or inappropriate affect.

Dispatch A central location that receives information and collects, disseminates, and transmits the information to the proper resources.

Dispatch factors Training and education of communications personnel, rapid call taking, call prioritization (selecting the most appropriate resources to respond), managing out-of-chute times (getting crews on the road quickly), and providing crews with route selection assistance.

Dispatch life support The provision of clinically approved, scripted instructions by telephone by a trained and certified emergency medical dispatcher.

Disseminated intravascular coagulation (DIC) A complex, systemic, thrombohemorrhagic disorder involving the generation of intravascular fibrin and the consumption of procoagulants and platelets.

Dissociatives Substances that cause feelings of detachment (dissociation) from one's surroundings and self; includes PCP, ketamine, and dextromethorphan.

Distal A position farthest away from the attachment of a limb to the trunk.

Distracting injury An injury that occupies the patient's attention and focus. The injury causes significant enough pain that the patient may not feel pain from other injuries, particularly spine injuries.

Distraction A self-defense measure that creates diversion in a person's attention.

Distress Stress that is perceived as negative; it may be seen as physical or mental pain or suffering.

Distributing arteries Blood vessels that have well-defined adventitia layers and larger amounts of smooth muscle; capable of altering blood flow.

Distribution The movement of drugs from the bloodstream to target organs.

Distributive shock Inadequate tissue perfusion as a result of fluid shifts between body compartments. Burn shock is a distributive shock in which plasma and water are lost from the vascular tree into the surrounding tissues. This shock also is seen in the setting of sepsis, in which a similar fluid redistribution occurs.

Diuretic An agent that promotes the excretion of urine.

Diversity Differences of any kind such as race, class, religion, gender, sexual preference, personal habitat, and physical ability.

Diverticulitis Inflammation of a diverticulum, especially of the small pockets in the wall of the colon that fill with stagnant fecal material and become inflamed.

Diverticulosis A condition of the colon in which outpouches develop.

Documentation Written information to support actions that lead to conclusive information; written evidence.

Donor skin site A site on the body from which healthy skin is removed for the purpose of grafting a burn or other open wound.

Do not resuscitate (DNR) orders Orders limiting cardiopulmonary resuscitation or advanced life support treatment in the case of a cardiac arrest. These orders may be individualized in that they may allow for differing levels of interventions. When individualized, they usually grant or deny permission for chest compressions, intubation or ventilation, and life-saving medications.

Dorsal Referring to the back of the body; posterior.

Dosage The amount of medication that can be safely given for the average person for a specified condition. Also the administration of a therapeutic agent in prescribed amounts.

Dose The exact amount of medication to be given or taken at one time.

Down syndrome A genetic syndrome characterized by varying degrees of mental retardation and multiple physical defects.

Downregulation The process by which a cell decreases the number of receptors exposed to a given substance to reduce its sensitivity to that substance.

Dromotropism The speed of conduction through the atrioventricular junction.

Drop (or drip) factor The number of drops per milliliter that an intravenous administration set delivers.

Drowning The process of experiencing respiratory impairment from immersion or submersion in a liquid.

Drug Any substance (other than a food or device) intended for use in the diagnosis, cure, relief, treatment, or prevention of disease or intended to affect the structure or function of the body of human beings or animals.

Drug allergy The reaction to a medication with an adverse outcome.

Drug antagonism The interaction between two drugs in which one partially or completely inhibits the effects of the other.

Drug dependence A physical need or adaptation to the drug without the psychological need to take the drug.

Drug interaction The manner in which one drug and a second drug (or food) act on each other.

Drug overdose Internalization of more than the safe amount of a medication or drug; often associated with illegal drugs when a user administers too great an amount of substance; may be used to commit suicide.

Drug-food interaction Changes in a drug's effects caused by food or beverages ingested during the same period.

Dual-chamber pacemaker Pacemaker that stimulates the atrium and ventricle.

Dual-stage airbags An airbag with two inflation charges inside; only one of the two charges may deploy during the initial crash, causing the bag to inflate; the second charge of the dual-stage airbag may remain.

Ductus arteriosus Blood vessel that connects the pulmonary trunk to the aorta in a fetus.

Ductus deferens Also known as *vas deferens;* tubes that extend from the end of the epididymis and through the seminal vesicles.

Ductus venosus Fetal blood vessel that conects the umbilical vein and the inferior vena cava.

Due process The constitutional guarantee that laws and legal proceedings must be fair regarding an individual's legal rights.

Due regard Principle used when driving an emergency vehicle of ensuring that all other vehicles and citizens in the area see and grant the emergency vehicle the right of way.

Duodenum First part of the small intestine; has important accessory structures that help digest various types of nutrients.

Duplex A radio system that allows transmitting and receiving at the same time through two different frequencies.

Dura mater Toughest layer of the meninges; top layer.

Durable power of attorney for healthcare A type of advanced directive that allows an individual to appoint someone to make healthcare decisions for him or her if the person's ability to make these decisions or communicate wishes is lost.

Duty to act A legal obligation (created by statute, contract, or voluntarily) to provide services.

Dysarthria An articulation disorder in which the patient is not able to produce speech sounds.

Dyspareunia Pain during sexual intercourse.

Dyspepsia Epigastric discomfort often occurring after meals.

Dysphagia Difficulty swallowing.

Dysphoric mood (dysphoria) An unpleasant emotional state characterized by sadness, irritability, or depression.

Dysplasia Abnormal cell growth; cells take on an abnormal size, shape, and organization as a result of ongoing irritation or inflammation.

Dyspnea An uncomfortable awareness of one's breathing that may be associated with a change in the breathing rate, effort, or pattern.

Dysrhythmia An abnormal heart rhythm.

Dysthymia A constant, chronic, low-grade form of depression.

Dystonia Impairment of muscle tone, particularly involuntary muscle contractions of the face, neck, and tongue; often caused by a reaction to certain antipsychotic medications.

Ebola A viral hemorrhagic fever illness caused by the Ebola virus (Filovirus family); seen mostly in Africa; transmitted by person-to-person contact with body fluids of infected individuals; no specific treatment is available, and it often is fatal within several days.

Ecchymosis Collection of blood within the skin that appears blue-black, eventually fading to a greenish-brown and yellow. Commonly called a *bruise*.

Eclampsia A life-threatening condition of pregnancy and the postpartum period characterized by hypertension, edema, and seizures.

Economic abuse Preventing others from having or keeping a job; forcing control of another's paycheck; restricting access or forcing conditions on others to receive an allowance; stealing money; not allowing others to know about or have access to economic assets.

Ecstasy (MDMA) A synthetic, hallucinogenic stimulant drug similar to both methamphetamine and mescaline.

Ectopic Impulse(s) originating from a source other than the sinoatrial node.

Ectopic pregnancy A pregnancy that implants outside the uterus, usually in the fallopian tube.

Eczema A disorder of the skin characterized by inflammation, itching, blisters, and scales.

Edema A collection of water in the interstitial space.

Effector The muscle, gland, or organ on which the autonomic nervous system exerts an effect; target organ.

Effector phase In phases of immunity, the stage at which the infection is eradicated.

Efferent division Nerve fibers that send impulses from the central nervous system to the periphery.

Efficacy The ability of a drug to produce a physiologic response after attaching to a receptor.

Efflux Flowing out of.

Ejection fraction Fraction (expressed as a percentage) of blood ejected from the ventricle of the heart with each contraction. Generally at least 60% of the blood entering the ventricle should be forced to the lungs or systemic circulation.

Elasticity Ability of muscle to rebound toward its original length after contraction.

Electrical alternans A beat-to-beat change in waveform amplitude on the ECG.

Electrodes Adhesive pads that contain a conductive gel and are applied at specific locations on the patient's chest wall and extremities and connected by cables to an ECG machine.

Electrolytes Elements or compounds that break into charged particles (ions) when melted or dissolved in water or another solvent.

Elevated mood (euphoria) Exaggerated sense of happiness and joy; a feeling of being on top of the world.

Elimination The process of removing a drug from the body.

Elixir A clear, oral solution that contains the drug, water, and some alcohol.

Emancipated minor A self-supporting minor. This status often depends on the minor receiving an actual court order of emancipation.

Embryo The developing egg from fertilization until approximately 8 weeks of pregnancy.

Emergency decontamination The process of decontaminating people exposed to and potentially contaminated with hazardous materials by rapidly removing most of the contamination to reduce exposure and save lives, with secondary regard for completeness of decontamination.

Emergency medical dispatching (EMD) The science and skills associated with the tasks of an emergency medical dispatcher.

Emergency medical responder (EMR) An EMS professional who provides initial basic life-support care to patients who access the EMS system; formerly called *first responder*.

Emergency Medical Treatment and Active Labor Act (EMTALA) A federal law that requires a hospital to provide a medical screening examination to anyone who comes to that hospital and to provide stabilizing treatment to anyone with an emergency medical condition without considering the patient's ability to pay.

Emergency operations center A gathering point for strategic policymakers during an emergency incident.

Emergency service function (ESF) A grouping of government and certain private sector capabilities into an organizational structure to provide the support, resources, program implementation, and services most likely to be needed to save lives, protect property and the environment, restore essential services and critical infrastructure, and help victims and communities return to normal, when feasible, after domestic incidents.

Emesis Vomiting.

Emotional/mental impairment Impaired intellectual functioning (such as mental retardation), which results in an inability to cope with normal responsibilities of life.

Empathy Identification with and understanding of another's situation, feelings, and motives.

Emphysema Lung disease in which destruction of the alveoli creates dyspnea; often associated with tobacco abuse.

Empyema A collection of pus in the pleural cavity.

EMS Emergency medical services.

EMS system A network of resources that provides emergency care and transportation to victims of sudden illness or injury.

Emulsification The breakdown of fats on the skin surface by alkaloids, creating a soapy substance; penetrates deeply.

Emulsion A water and oil mixture containing medication.

Enabling behavior Behavior that allows another individual to continue to stay ill.

Enamel Hard, white outer surface of a tooth.

Encephalitis Inflammation and usually infection of brain tissue.

Encephalopathy A condition of disturbances of consciousness and possible progression to coma.

Endocardium Innermost layer of the heart that lines the inside of the myocardium and covers the heart valves.

Endocrine communication Method of intercellular communication in which one cell communicates with target cells throughout the body by using hormones.

Endocrine gland Where hormones are manufactured.

Endogenous Produced within the organism.

Endolymph Fluid that fills the labyrinth.

Endometriosis Growth of endometrial tissue outside the uterus, often causing pain.

Endometritis Infection of the endometrium.

Endometrium Innermost tissue lining of the uterus that is shed during menstruation.

Endoplasmic reticulum (ER) Chain of canals or sacs that wind through the cytoplasm.

Endorphins Neurotransmitters that function in the transmission of signals within the nervous system.

Endothelial cells A thin layer of flat epithelial cells that lines serous cavities, lymph vessels, and blood vessels.

Endotoxin A substance contained in the cell wall of gram-negative bacteria, generally released during the destruction of the bacteria by either the host organism's defense mechanisms or by treatment with medications.

Endotracheal (ET) Within or through the trachea.

Endotracheal intubation An advanced airway procedure in which a tube is placed directly into the trachea.

End-stage renal disease (ESRD) When the kidneys function at 10% to 15% of normal and dialysis or transplantation is the only option for the patient's survival.

Enlargement Implies the presence of dilation or hypertrophy or both.

Enteral A drug given for its systemic effects that passes through the digestive tract.

Enteric-coated tablets Tablets that have a special coating so they break down in the intestines instead of the stomach.

Enteral drug One that is given and passed through any portion of the digestive tract.

Entrapment A state of being pinned or entrapped.

Envenomation The process of injecting venom into a wound; venomous animals include snakes, insects, and marine creatures.

Environmental emergency A medical condition caused or exacerbated by weather, terrain, atmospheric pressure, or other local environmental factors.

Environmental hazards Hazards related to the weather and time of day, including extremes of heat, cold, wetness, dryness, and darkness, that increase risks to crews and patients.

Enzyme A large molecule (protein) that performs a biochemical reaction in the cell.

Eosinophils Type of granulocyte (white blood cell, or leukocyte) involved in immune response to parasites as well as in allergic responses.

Epicardium Also known as the *visceral pericardium;* the external layer of the heart wall that covers the heart muscle.

Epidemiologist Medical professional who studies the causes, distribution, and control of disease in populations.

Epidemiology The study of the causes, patterns, prevalence, and control of disease in groups of people.

Epidermis The outermost layer of the skin; made of tightly packed epithelial cells.

Epididymis Convoluted series of tubes located in the posterior portion of the scrotum; final maturation of sperm occurs here.

Epidural hematoma A collection of blood between the skull and dura mater.

Epidural space Potential area above the dura mater; contains arterial vessels.

Epiglottitis An inflammation of the epiglottis.

Epilepsy Group of neurologic disorders characterized by recurrent seizures, often of unknown cause.

Epiphyseal plate Found in children who are still generating bone growth; also known as the *growth plate.*

Epiphysis Either end of the bone where bone growth occurs during the developmental years.

Epistaxis Bloody nose.

Epithelial tissue Covers most of the internal and external surfaces of the body.

Epithelialization Migration of basal cells across a wound and the growth of skin over a wound.

Eponym A word that derives its name from the specific person (or place or thing) for whom (or which) it is named.

Erosion A partial focal loss of epidermis. This lesion is depressed, moist, and does not bleed; usually heals without scarring.

Erythema multiforme An internal (immunologic) reaction in the skin characterized by a variety of lesions.

Erythrocytes Red blood cells.

Erythropoiesis The development and differentiation of red blood cells; typically occurs in the bone marrow.

Erythropoietin A hormone that stimulates peripheral stem cells in the bone marrow to produce red blood cells.

Escape Term used when the sinus node slows or fails to initiate depolarization and a lower pacemaker site spontaneously produces electrical impulses, assuming responsibility for pacing the heart.

Eschar A thick wound covering that consists of necrotic or otherwise devitalized tissue or cellular components. In a burn wound, this is the burned tissue or skin of the wound.

Esophageal atresia (EA) A condition in which the section of the esophagus from the mouth and the section of the esophagus from the stomach end as a blind pouch without connecting to each other.

Esophagitis Inflammation of the esophagus.

Esophagoduodenoscopy Medical procedure in which an endoscope is used to look at the esophagus, stomach, and duodenum.

Esophagus Tube surrounded by smooth muscle that propels material into the stomach.

Essential hypertension High blood pressure for which no cause is identifiable; also called *primary hypertension*.

Estimated date of confinement The due date of the fetus.

Estrogen A female hormone produced mainly by the ovaries from puberty to menopause that is responsible for the development of secondary sexual characteristics and cyclic changes in the thickness of the uterine lining during the first half of the menstrual cycle.

Ethanol (ETOH) Colorless, odorless alcohol found in alcoholic beverages such as beer, wine, and liquor.

Ethics Societal principles of conduct that people or groups of people adopt as guidelines for personal behavior.

Ethnocentrism Viewing your life as the most desirable, acceptable, or best and acting a manner conveying superiority to another culture's way of life.

Eukaryotes One of the two major classes of cells found in higher life forms (more complex in structure).

Eustachian tube A small tube connecting the middle ear to the posterior nasopharynx; allows the ear to adjust to atmospheric pressure.

Eustress Stress that occurs from events, people, or influences that are perceived as good or positive. Eustress can increase productivity and performance.

Euthymic mood A normal, baseline emotional state.

Evaluation of treatment A reassessment of the patient overall and specifically the body system(s) affected by that treatment to answer two critical questions: Did the treatment work as intended? What is the clinical condition of the patient after the treatment?

Evasive tactic A self-defense measure in which the moves and actions of an aggressor are anticipated and unconventional pathways are used during retreat for personal safety.

Excision In reference to burn surgery, this is the sharp, surgical removal of burned tissue that will never regain function. Excision is carried out before skin grafting.

Excitability Ability to respond to a stimulus.

Excited delirium Acute and sudden agitation, paranoia, aggression, hyperthermia, dramatically increased strength, and decreased sensitivity to pain related to long-term use of stimulant drugs; often ends in sudden death.

Excoriation A linear erosion created by scratching. It is a hollowed out area that is sometimes crusted.

Excretion Removal of waste products from the body.

Exertional heat stroke A condition primarily affecting younger, active persons characterized by rapid onset (developing in hours) and frequently associated with high core temperatures.

Exhaled CO_2 detector A capnometer that provides a noninvasive estimate of alveolar ventilation, the concentration of exhaled CO_2 from the lungs, and arterial carbon dioxide content; also called an *end-tidal CO_2 detector.*

Exhaustion The last stage of the stress response and the body's inability to respond appropriately to subsequent stressors.

Exhaustion stage Occurs when the body's resistance to a stressor (decreased reaction to the stress, tolerance) and the ability to adapt fail; the ability to respond appropriately to other stressors may then fail; the immune system can be affected, and the individual may be at risk physically or emotionally.

Exogenous Produced outside the organism.

Exotoxin Proteins released during the growth phase of the bacteria that may cause systemic effects.

Expiratory reserve volume Amount of gas that can be forcefully expired at the end of a normal expiration.

Explanation Sharing objective information related to a message.

Explosive Any chemical compound, mixture, or device, the primary or common purpose of which is to function by detonation or rapid combustion (i.e., with substantial instantaneous release of gas and heat); found in liquid or solid forms (e.g., dynamite, TNT, black powder, fireworks, ammunition).

Exposure When blood or body fluids come in contact with eyes, mucous membranes, nonintact skin, or through a needlestick; it also can occur through inhalation and ingestion.

Expressed consent Permission given by a patient or his or her responsible decision maker either verbally or through some physical expression of consent.

Exsanguinate Near complete loss of blood; not conducive with life.

Exsanguination Bleeding to death.

Extensibility Ability to continue to contract over a range of lengths.

Extension posturing (decerebrate) Occurs as a result of an injury to the brainstem; presents as the patient's arms at the side with wrists turned outward.
External anal sphincter Muscle under voluntary control that allows a controlled bowel movement.
External auditory canal Tube from the external ear to the middle ear; lined with hair and ceruminous glands.
External bleeding Observable blood loss.
External ear Includes the auricle and external auditory canal.
External respiration The exchange of gases between the alveoli of the lungs and the blood cells traveling through the pulmonary capillaries.
External urinary sphincter Ring of smooth muscle in the urethra under voluntary control.
Extracellular Outside the cell or cytoplasmic membrane.
Extracellular fluid (ECF) The fluid found outside of the cells.
Extubation Removal of an endotracheal tube from the trachea.
Exudate Drainage from a vesicle or pustule.
Eyebrows Protect the eyes by providing shade and preventing foreign material (sweat, dust, etc.) from entering the eyes from above.
Eyelids Protect the eyes from foreign objects.
Facilitated diffusion Movement of substances across a membrane by binding to a helper protein integrated into the cell wall and highly selective about the chemicals allowed to cross the membrane.
Facilitated transport The transport of substances through a protein channel carrier with no energy input.
Facilitation Encouraging the patient to provide more information.
Factitious disorder Condition in which patients intentionally produce signs and symptoms of illness to assume the sick role.
Fainting (syncope) A brief loss of consciousness caused by a temporary decrease in blood flow to the brain.
Fallopian tube Paired structures extending from each side of the uterus to each ovary; they provide a way for the egg to reach the uterus.
False imprisonment Confinement or restraint of a person against his or her will or without appropriate legal justification.
False motion Abnormal movement of a bone or joint typically associated with a fracture or dislocation.
Fascia Anatomically, the tough connective tissue covering of the muscles of the body. Fascia contains the muscles within a compartment.
Fascicle Small bundle of nerve fibers.
Fasciotomy A surgical incision into the muscle fascia to relieve intracompartmental pressures; the emergency treatment for compartment syndrome.
Fear Physical and emotional reaction to a real or perceived threat.
Febrile seizure Seizure caused by too rapid of a rise in body temperature; rarely seen after age 2 years.
Fecalith A hard impacted mass of feces in the colon.
Feces Undigested food material that has been processed in the colon.
Federal Communication Commission (FCC) An independent U.S. government agency, directly responsible to Congress, established by the Communications Act of 1934; it regulates interstate and international communications by radio, television, wire, satellite, and cable. The FCC's jurisdiction covers the 50 states, the District of Columbia, and U.S. possessions.
Fetus The term used for an infant from approximately 8 weeks of pregnancy until birth.
Fibrin A threadlike protein formed during the clotting process that crisscrosses the wound opening and forms a matrix that traps blood cells and platelets, thereby creating a clot. Fibrin is formed by the action of thrombin and fibrinogen.
Fibrinolysis The breakdown of fibrin, the main component of blood clots.
Fibrinolytic agent Clot-busting drug; used in very early treatment of acute myocardial infarction, stroke, deep vein thrombosis, pulmonary embolism, and peripheral arterial occlusion.
Fibroblasts A cell that gives rise to connective tissue.
Fibrous connective tissue Composed of bundles of strong, white collagenous fibers (protein) in parallel rows; tendons and ligaments are composed of this type of tissue; relatively strong and inelastic.
Fibrous joints Two bones united by fibrous tissue that have little or no movement.
Fibrous tunic Layer of the eye that contains the sclera and the cornea.
Fick principle Describes the components needed for the oxygenation of the body's cells.
Finance officer The person responsible for providing a cost analysis of an incident.
Fine ventricular fibrillation Ventricular fibrillation with fibrillatory waves less than 3 mm in height.
FiO_2 Fraction of inspired oxygen.
"First on the Scene" program An educational program that teaches people what to do and what not to do when they come upon an injury emergency.
First-degree burn Superficial burn involving only the epidermis, such as a minor sunburn.
First-pass effect The breakdown of a drug in the liver and walls of the intestines before it reaches the systemic circulation.
First responder unit The closest trained persons and vehicle assigned to respond to a call; often the closest available fire department vehicle.
Fissure A vertical loss of epidermis and dermis with sharply defined walls (sometimes called a *crack*).

Fistula An abnormal tunnel that has formed from within the body to the skin.

Fixed positioning Establishing a single location in a central point to station an emergency vehicle, such as a fire station.

Fixed-rate pacemaker Asynchronous pacemaker that continuously discharges at a preset rate regardless of the patient's heart rate.

Fixed-station deployment Deployment method of using only geographically based stations.

Fixed-wing aircraft Airplanes used for longer distance medical flights; they can travel higher and faster than rotor-wing aircraft.

Flail segment A free-floating section of the chest wall that results when two or more adjacent ribs are fractured in two or more places or when the sternum is detached.

Flammable The capacity of a substance to ignite.

Flammable gases Any compressed gas that meets requirements for lower flammability limit, flammability limit range, flame projection, or flame propagation as specified in CFR Title 49, Sec. 173.300(b) (e.g., acetylene, butane, hydrogen, propane).

Flammable range The concentration of fuel and air between the lower flammable limit or lower explosive limit and the upper flammable limit or upper explosive limit; the mixture of fuel and air in the flammable range supports combustion.

Flammable solid A solid material other than an explosive that is liable to cause fires through friction or retained heat from manufacturing or processing or that can be ignited readily; when ignited, it burns so vigorously and persistently that it creates a serious transportation hazard (e.g., phosphorus, lithium, magnesium, titanium, calcium resinate).

Flash electrical burn A burn resulting from indirect contact with an electrical explosion.

Flashpoint The minimal temperature at which a substance evaporates fast enough to form an ignitable mixture with air near the surface of the substance.

Flat affect A complete or near-complete lack of emotion.

Flat bones Specialized bones that protect vital anatomic structures (e.g., ribs and bones of the skull).

Flexible deployment See *System status management.*

Flexion posturing (decorticate) Occurs from an injury to the cerebrum; presents as a bending of the arms at the elbow, the patient's arms pulled upwards to the chest, and the hands turned downward at the wrists.

Flight of ideas Moving quickly from topic to topic during conversation but without any connection or transition.

Flow rate The number of drops per minute an intravenous administration set will deliver.

Fluctuance A wavelike motion felt between two fingertips when palpating a fluid-filled structure such as a subcutaneous abscess.

Fluctuant nodule A movable and compressible mass; typically a pocket of pus or fluid within the dermis.

Focal atrial tachycardia Atrial tachycardia that begins in a small area (focus) within the heart.

Focal deficit Alteration or lack of strength or sensation in the body caused by a neurologic problem.

Focal injury An injury limited to a particular area of the brain.

Follicle Small, tubelike structure in which hair grows; contains a small cluster of cells known as the hair papilla.

Follicles Vesicles within the cortex of the ovary.

Folliculitis Inflammation of the follicle; localized to hair follicles and is more common in immunocompromised patients; are usually multiple and measure 5 mm or less in diameter; erythematous, pruritic, and frequently have a central pustule on top of a raised lesion, often with a central hair.

Fontanelles Membranous spaces at the juncture of an infant's cranial bones that later ossify.

Foramen Open passage.

Foramen magnum Opening in the floor of the cranium where the spinal cord exits the skull.

Foramen ovale The opening in the interatrial septum in a fetal heart.

Foreign body Any object or substance found in a organ or tissue where it does not belong under normal circumstances.

Form of thought Ability to compose thoughts in a logical manner.

Formed elements Located in the bloodstream; erythrocytes, leukocytes, and thrombocytes, or platelets.

Formulary A book that contains a list of medicinal substances with their formulas, uses, and methods of preparation.

Fractile response time Method used to determine the time at which 90% of all requests for service receive a response; considered a more definitive measure of performance than averages.

Francisella tularensis A hardy, slow-growing, highly infectious, aerobic organism; human infection may result in tularemia, also known as *rabbit fever* or *deer fly fever.*

Free nerve endings Most common type of dermal nerve ending; responsible for sensing pain, temperature, and pressure.

Free radical A molecule containing an extra electron, which allows it to form potentially harmful bonds with other molecules.

Frontal lobe Section of cerebrum important in voluntary motor function and the emotions of aggression, motivation, and mood.

Frontal plane Imaginary straight line that divides the body into anterior (ventral) and posterior (dorsal) sections.
Frostbite A condition in which the skin and underlying tissue freeze.
Frostnip Reversible freezing of superficial skin layer marked by numbness and whiteness of the skin.
Fully deployed Assigning ambulances to a street corner post.
Fulminant Sudden, intense occurrence.
Functional reserve capacity At the end of a normal expiration, the volume of air remaining in the lungs.
Fundus Superior aspect of the uterus.
Fungi Plantlike organisms that do not contain chlorophyll; the two classes of fungi are yeasts and molds.
Furuncles Inflammatory nodules that involve the hair follicle (e.g., boils).
Gag reflex A normal neural reflex elicited by touching the soft palate or posterior pharynx; the responses are symmetric elevation of the palate, retraction of the tongue, and contraction of the pharyngeal muscles.
Gagging A reflex caused by irritation of the posterior pharynx that can result in vomiting.
Gamma A type of electromagnetic radiation.
Gamma-hydroxybutyrate (GHB) A drug structurally related to the neurotransmitter gamma-aminobutyric acid, usually dissolved in liquid, that causes profound central nervous system depression.
Gamma rays A type of electromagnetic radiation that can travel great distances; can be stopped by heavy shielding, such as lead.
Gamow bag Portable hyperbaric chamber that can help with altitude sickness emergencies.
Ganglion The junction between the preganglionic and postganglionic nerves.
Gangrenous necrosis Tissue death over a large area.
Gases Substances inhaled and absorbed through the respiratory tract.
Gasoline and electric hybrid vehicle Vehicle designed to produce low emissions by combining a smaller than normal internal combustion gasoline engine with a special electric motor to power the vehicle.
Gasping Inhaling and exhaling with quick, difficult breaths.
Gastric The route used when a tube is placed into the digestive tract, such as a nasogastric, orogastric, or gastrostomy tube.
Gastric distention Swelling of the abdomen caused by an influx of air or fluid.
Gastric lavage A method of internal decontamination that involves emptying the stomach contents through an orogastric or nasogastric tube.
Gastritis Inflammation of the stomach.
Gastroenteritis Inflammation of the stomach and the intestines.
Gastrostomy tube A tube placed in a person's stomach that allows continuous feeding for an extended time.
Gay-Lussac's law A gas law sometimes combined with Charles' law that deals with the relation between pressure and temperature; in an oxygen cylinder, as the ambient temperature decreases, so does the pressure reading.
Gel cap Soft gelatin shell filled with liquid medication.
Gene The biologic unit of inheritance, consisting of a particular nucleotide sequence within a DNA molecule that occupies a precise locus on a chromosome and codes for a specific polypeptide chain.
Generalized anxiety disorder Condition characterized by excessive worries about everyday life.
Generalized seizure Excessive electrical activity in both hemispheres of the brain at the same time.
Generic name The name proposed by the first manufacturer when a drug is submitted to the FDA for approval; often an abbreviated form of the drug's chemical name, structure, or formula.
Geospatial demand analysis Understanding the different locations of demand within a community.
Germ theory Controversial theory developed in the 1600s in which microorganisms were first identified as the possible cause of some disease processes.
Germinativum Basal layer of the epidermis where the epidermal cells are formed.
Gestation or gestational age The number of completed weeks of pregnancy from the last menstrual period.
Glasgow Coma Scale (GCS) Neurologic assessment of a patient's best verbal response, eye opening, and motor function.
Glaucoma Increased intraocular pressure caused by a disruption in the normal production and drainage of aqueous humor; causes often are unknown.
Global positioning system (GPS) A satellite-based geographic locating system often placed on an ambulance to track its exact location.
Glomerulus Network of capillaries in the renal corpuscle.
Glottis The true vocal cords and the space between them.
Gluconeogenesis Creation of new glucose in the body by using noncarbohydrate sources such as fats and proteins.
Glycogenolysis Breakdown of glycogen to glucose in the liver.
Glycolysis Process by which glucose and other sugars are broken down to yield lactic acid (anaerobic glycolysis) or pyruvic acid (aerobic glycolysis). The breakdown releases energy in the form of adenosine triphosphate.

Glycoside A compound that yields a sugar and one or more other products when its parts are separated.

Golgi apparatus Substance that concentrates and packages material for secretion out of the cell.

Gomphoses Joint in which a peg fits into a socket.

Gout A metabolic disease in which uric acid crystals are deposited onto the cartilaginous surfaces of a joint, resulting in pain, swelling, and inflammation.

Graft Connection by a surgeon of a piece of the patient's saphenous vein to an artery and vein; in lieu of using the patient's own blood vessel, a cow's artery or a synthetic graft may be used.

Graham's law Law stating that gases move from a higher pressure or concentration to an area of lower pressure or concentration; takes into consideration the effect of simple diffusion at a cellular level.

Gram-negative bacteria Bacteria that do not retain the crystal violet stain used in Gram's stain and that take the color of the red counterstain.

Gram-positive bacteria Bacteria that retain the crystal violet stain used in Gram's stain.

Grandiose delusions Dramatically inflated perceptions of one's own worth, power, or knowledge.

Granulocyte A form of leukocyte that attacks foreign material in the wound.

Gravida Number of pregnancies.

Gravidity The number of times a patient has been pregnant.

Great vessels Large vessels that carry blood to and from the heart; superior and inferior venae cavae, pulmonary veins, aorta, and pulmonary trunk.

Greenstick fracture The incomplete fracturing of an immature bone.

Grey-Turner's sign Bruising along the flanks that may indicate pancreatitis or intraabdominal hemorrhage.

Ground effect The cushion of air created by downdraft when a helicopter is in a low hover. Ground effect benefits the helicopter flight because it increases lift capacity, meaning less power is required for the helicopter to hover. When the helicopter has ground effect, it is said to be in ground effect. If a helicopter does not have ground effect, it is said to be operating out of ground effect.

Ground electrode Third ECG electrode (the first and second are the positive and negative electrodes), which minimizes electrical activity from other sources.

Grunting A short, low-pitched sound heard at the end of exhalation that represents an attempt to generate positive end-expiratory pressure by exhaling against a closed glottis, prolonging the period of oxygen and carbon dioxide exchange across the alveolar-capillary membrane; a compensatory mechanism to help maintain patency of small airways and prevent atelectasis.

Guarding The contraction of abdominal muscles in the anticipation of a painful stimulus.

Guidelines For emergency medical dispatchers, an unstructured, subjective, unscripted method of telephone assessment and treatment; a less-effective process than protocols.

Guillain-Barré syndrome Autoimmune neurologic disorder marked by weakness and paresthesia that usually travel up the legs.

Gum Plant residue used for medicinal or recreational purposes.

Gurgling Abnormal respiratory sound associated with collection of liquid or semisolid material in the patient's upper airway.

Gurney Stretcher or cot used to transport patients.

Gustation Sense of taste.

Hair papilla Small cluster of cells within a follicle; growth of hair starts in this cluster of cells, which is hidden in the follicle.

Half Duplex A radio system that use two frequencies: one to transmit and one to receive; however, like a simplex system, only one person can transmit at a time.

Half-life The time required to eliminate half of a substance from the body.

Hallucination False sensory perceptions originating inside the brain.

Hallucinogen Substance that causes hallucinations and intense distortions and perceptions of reality; includes LSD, psilocybin mushrooms, peyote, and mescaline.

Hamman's sign A crunching sound occasionally heard on auscultation of the heart when air is in the mediastinum.

Hangman's fracture A fracture of the axis, the second cervical vertebra. This may occur with or without axis dislocation.

Hazard Communication Standard (HAZCOM) Occupational Safety and Health Administration standard regarding worker protection when handling chemicals.

Hazardous materials A substance (solid, liquid, or gas) capable of posing an unreasonable risk to health, safety, environment, or property.

Hazardous Waste Operations and Emergency Response (HAZWOPER) Occupational Safety and Health Administration and Environmental Protection Agency regulations regarding worker safety when responding to hazardous materials emergencies.

Head bobbing Indicator of increased work of breathing in infants; the head falls forward with exhalation and comes up with expansion of the chest on inhalation.

Head injury A traumatic insult to the head that may result in injury to the soft tissue or bony structures of the head and/or brain injury.

Headache A pain in the head from any cause.

Health A state of complete physical, mental, and social well-being, not merely the absence of disease or infirmity.

Health Insurance Portability and Accountability Act (HIPAA) Rules governing the protection of a patient's identifiable information.

Healthcare professional An individual who has special skills and knowledge in medicine and adheres to the standards of conduct and performance of that medical profession.

Healthcare A business associated with the provision of medical care to individuals.

Heart disease A broad term referring to conditions affecting the heart.

Heart failure A condition in which the heart is unable to pump enough blood to meet the metabolic needs of the body.

Heartbeat Organized mechanical action of the heart.

Heat emergencies Conditions in which the body's thermoregulation mechanisms begin to fail in response to ambient heat, causing illness.

Hematemesis Vomiting of bright red blood.

Hematochezia Bright red blood in the stool.

Hematocrit A measure of the relative percentage of blood cells (mainly erythrocytes) in a given volume of whole blood; also called *volume of packed red cells* or *packed cell volume.*

Hematoma Collection of blood beneath the skin or within a body compartment.

Hematuria Blood found in the urine.

Hemiparesis Muscle weakness of one half of the body.

Hemiplegia Paralysis of one side of the body.

Hemoglobin A protein found on red blood cells that is rich in iron.

Hemolytic anemia Anemia that results from the destruction of red blood cells.

Hemopoietic tissue Connective tissue found in the marrow cavities of bones (mainly long bones).

Hemoptysis The coughing up of blood.

Hemorrhage Heavy bleeding.

Hemorrhagic anemia Anemia caused by hemorrhage.

Hemorrhagic stroke Rupture of a blood vessel in the brain causing decreased perfusion and potentially leading to rising intracranial pressure.

Hemorrhoids Swollen, distended veins in the anorectal area.

Hemostasis Stopping a hemorrhage.

Hemothorax Blood within the thoracic cavity, a potentially life-threatening injury.

Henry's law Law associated with decompression sickness that deals with the solubility of gases in liquids at equilibrium.

Hepatic artery The artery that supplies the liver with blood and nutrients from the circulatory system.

Hepatic duct Connects the gallbladder to the liver; secretes bile into the gallbladder.

Hepatitis Inflammation of the liver.

Hering-Breuer reflex A reflex that limits inspiration to prevent overinflation of the lungs in a conscious, spontaneously breathing person; also called the *inhibito-inspiratory reflex.*

Hernia Protrusion of any organ through an abdominal opening in the muscle wall of the cavity that surrounds it.

Herniated disc A condition in which an intervertebral disc weakens and protrudes out of position, often affecting adjacent nerve roots.

Herniation Protrusion of the brain through an abnormal opening, often the foramen magnum.

Heroin (diacetylmorphine) The most popular, powerful, and addictive member of the opioids.

Herpes simplex A skin eruption caused by the herpes simplex virus, divided into two types; HSV-1 causes oral infection and HSV-2 causes genital infections.

Herpes zoster A skin eruption that follows a particular nerve distribution (dermatome); caused by the varicella zoster virus in persons who have had varicella sometime in their lives (also called *shingles*).

Hiatus A gap or a cleft.

Hiccup (hiccoughing) Intermittent spasm of the diaphragm resulting in sudden inspiration with spastic closure of the glottis; usually annoying and serves no known physiologic purpose.

High angle An environment in which the load is predominantly supported by the rope rescue system.

High voltage Greater than 1000 V.

High-altitude cerebral edema The most severe high-altitude illness, characterized by increased intracranial pressure.

High-altitude pulmonary edema A high-altitude illness characterized by increased pulmonary artery pressure and edema, leading to cough and fluid in the lungs (pulmonary edema).

High-angle terrain (vertical terrain) A steep environment such as a cliff or building side where hands must be used for balance when ascending.

Hilum Point of entry for bronchial vessels, bronchi, and nerves in each lung.

Hilus Indentation through which the renal artery, vein, lymphatic vessels, and nerves enter and leave the kidney.

Hippocampi Structures within the limbic system that filter incoming information, determine what stimuli is important, and commit the experiences to memory.

His-Purkinje system Portion of the conduction system consisting of the bundle of His, bundle branches, and Purkinje fibers.

Histamine A substance released by mast cells that promotes inflammation.

History of present illness A narrative detail of the symptoms the patient is experiencing.

Hollow organ An organ (a part of the body or group of tissues that performs a specific function) that contains a channel or cavity within it, such as the large and small intestines.

Homan's sign Pain and tenderness in the calf muscle on dorsiflexion of the foot.

Home care The provision of health services by formal and informal caregivers in the home to promote, restore, and maintain a person's maximal level of comfort, function, and health, including care toward a dignified death.

Homeostasis A state of equilibrium in the body with respect to functions and composition of fluids and tissues.

Homeotherm Organism with a stable independent body temperature; an organism whose stable body temperature is generally independent of the surrounding environment.

Homonyms Terms that sound alike but are spelled differently and have different meanings.

Honeymoon phase A period of remorse by the abuser characterized by the abuser's denial and apologies.

Hordeolum A common acute infection of the glands of the eyelids.

Hormones Chemicals within the body that reach every cell through the circulatory system.

Hospice A care program that provides for the dying and their special needs.

Hospital Incident Command System An emergency management system that uses a logical management structure, defined responsibilities, clear reporting channels, and a common nomenclature to help unify hospitals with other emergency responders.

Hospital off-load time The time necessary for a crew to become available once they arrive at a hospital.

Hot load Loading a patient into a helicopter while the rotors are spinning.

Hot zone The primary danger zone around a crash scene that typically extends approximately 50 feet in all directions from the wreckage.

Hover The condition in which a helicopter remains fairly stationary over a given point, moving neither vertically nor horizontally.

Hub The plastic piece that houses a needle and fits onto a syringe.

Human immunodeficiency virus (HIV) The virus that can cause AIDS.

Human leukocyte antigen Leukocyte antigen that transplant surgeons attempt to match to prevent incompatibility.

Humoral immunity Immunity from antibodies in the blood.

Humoral Pertaining to elements in the blood or other body fluids.

Huntington's disease Programmed cell death of certain neurons in the brain, leading to behavioral abnormalities, movement disorders, and a decline in cognitive function.

Hydration Process of taking in fluids with the normal daily output.

Hydraulic A water hazard caused when water moves over a uniform obstruction to flow.

Hydraulic injection injuries High-pressure fluid that leaks from hydraulic hoses and is injected into the body.

Hydrocarbon A member of a large class of chemicals belonging to the petroleum derivative family; they have a variety of uses, such as solvents, oils, reagents, and fuels; the psychoactive ingredient in many abused inhalants.

Hydrocele Collection of fluid in the scrotum or along the spermatic cord.

Hydrocephalus An excessive amount of cerebrospinal fluid.

Hydrogen cyanide A highly toxic blood agent.

Hydrogen ion concentration Concentration of hydrogen ions in a given solution, such as water or blood; used to calculate the pH of a substance.

Hydrogen sulfide A hazardous gas produced by the decomposition of organic material prevalent when manure is stored in a liquid form for an extended period.

Hydrophilic Attracts water molecules.

Hydrophobic Repels water molecules.

Hydrostatic pressure Pressure exerted by a fluid from its weight.

Hydroxylysine An amino acid found in collagen.

Hymen Thin of layer of tissue that may cover the vaginal orifice in women who have not had sexual intercourse.

Hypercalcemia A state in which the body has an abnormally high level of calcium.

Hypercapnia An increased amount of carbon dioxide in the blood; may be a result of hypoventilation.

Hypercarbia An excess of CO_2 in the blood.

Hyperdynamic Excessively forceful or energetic. Term is used to describe shock states in which the heart is pumping aggressively to make up for fluid losses, such as in burn or septic shock.

Hyperextension Extension beyond a joint's normal range of motion.

Hyperflexion Flexion beyond a joint's normal range of motion.

Hyperkalemia A state in which the body has an abnormally elevated potassium level.

Hypermagnesemia A state in which the body has an abnormally elevated concentration of magnesium in the blood.

Hypermetabolic A state or condition of the body characterized by excessive production and utilization of energy molecules such as protein.

Hyperopia Farsightedness; difficulty seeing objects close to the person.

Hyperosmolar hyperglycemic nonketotic coma (HHNC) Condition caused by a relative insulin insufficiency that leads to extremely high blood sugar levels while still allowing for normal glucose metabolism and an absence of ketone bodies.

Hyperplasia Abnormal cell division that increases the number of a specific type of cell.

Hyperpnea Increased respiratory rate or deeper than normal breathing; also called *hyperventilation.*

Hyperresonant A high-pitched sound.

Hypersensitivity disorder A disorder in which the immune system responds inappropriately and excessively to an antigen (in this response, known as allergens).

Hypersensitivity pneumonitis Inflammation in and around the tiny air sacs (alveoli) and smallest airways (bronchioles) of the lung caused by an allergic reaction to inhaled organic dusts or, less commonly, chemicals; also called *extrinsic allergic alveolitis, allergic interstitial pneumonitis,* or *organic dust pneumoconiosis.*

Hypersensitivity reaction An immune response that is excessive beyond the bounds of normalcy to a point that it leads to damage (as with endotoxins) or is potentially damaging to the individual.

Hypersensitivity An altered reactivity to a medication that occurs after prior sensitization; response is independent of the dose.

Hypertension Elevated blood pressure.

Hypertensive emergencies Situations that require rapid (within 1 hour) lowering of blood pressure to prevent or limit organ damage.

Hypertensive urgencies Significant elevations in blood pressure with nonspecific symptoms that should be corrected within 24 hours.

Hyperthermia A core body temperature greater than 98.6°F.

Hypertonic In a membrane, the side with the higher concentration in an imbalance in the ionic concentration from one side to the other.

Hypertrophic scar Scar that forms with excessive amounts of scar tissue. The scar remains contained by the wound boundaries but may be slightly raised and can impair function.

Hypertrophy Enlargement or increase in the size of a cell(s) or tissue.

Hyperventilation Blowing off too much carbon dioxide.

Hyphema Blood in the anterior chamber of the eye.

Hypocalcemia A state in which the body has an abnormally low calcium level.

Hypocarbia An inadequate amount of carbon dioxide in the blood.

Hypokalemia A state in which the level of potassium in the serum falls below 3.5 mEq/L.

Hypomagnesemia A state in which the body has an abnormally low serum concentration of magnesium.

Hypomania An episode of a lesser form of mania that may transition into mania or alternate with depression.

Hypoperfusion The inadequate circulation of blood through an organ or a part of the body; shock.

Hypotension Low blood pressure significant enough to cause inadequate perfusion.

Hypothalamus Interface between the brain and the endocrine system; provides control for many autonomic functions.

Hypothermia A core body temperature below 95°F (35°C).

Hypotonic In a membrane, the side with the lower concentration when an imbalance exists in the ionic concentration from one side to the other.

Hypoventilation Occurs when the volume of air that enters the alveoli and takes part in gas exchange is not adequate for the body's metabolic needs.

Hypovolemic shock Inadequate tissue perfusion caused by inadequate vascular volume.

Hypoxemia An abnormal deficiency in the concentration of oxygen in arterial blood.

Hypoxia Inadequate oxygenation of the cells.

Iatrogenic drug response An unintentional disease or drug effect produced by a physician's prescribed therapy; *iatros* means "physician," and *-genic* is a word root meaning "produce."

Icterus Jaundice.

Idiosyncrasy The unexpected and usually individual (genetic) adverse response to a drug.

Ileostomy Surgical creation of a passage through the abdominal wall into the ileum.

Ileum Last segment of the small intestine; area of decreased absorption where chyme is prepared for entry into the large intestine.

Ileus Decreased peristaltic movement of the colon.

Immediately dangerous to life or health concentrations (IDLHs) Maximal environmental air concentration of a substance from which a person could escape within 30 minutes without symptoms of impairment or irreversible health effects.

Immersion Covering of the face and airway in water or other fluid.

Immunity Protection from legal liability in accordance with applicable laws; also the body's ability to resist a particular disease.

Immunodeficiency Deficit in the immune system and its response to infection or injury.

Immunoglobulin See *Antibody.*

Impetigo A highly contagious infection caused by staphylococcal or streptococcal bacteria. A superficial vesicopustular skin infection that primarily occurs on exposed areas of the face and extremities from scratching infected lesions; usually begins at a traumatized region of the skin, where a combination of vesicles and pustules develops; the pustules rupture and crust, leaving a characteristic thick, golden or honeylike appearance.

Implied consent The presumption that a patient who is ill or injured and unable to give consent for any reason would agree to the delivery of emergency health care necessitated by his or her condition.

Incarcerated hernia Hernia of intestine that cannot be returned or reduced by manipulation; it may or may not become strangulated.

Incendiary device A device designed to ignite a fire.

Incidence The rate at which a certain event occurs, such as the number of new cases of a specific disease occurring during a certain period in a population at risk.

Incidence rate The rate of contraction of a disease versus how many are currently sick with the disease.

Incident commander The person responsible for the overall management of an emergency scene.

Incident scene hazards Hazards directly related to the specific incident scene, including control of crowds, traffic, the danger of downed electrical wires, the presence of hazardous materials, and the location of an emergency.

Incomplete abortion An abortion in which the uterus retains part of the products of the pregnancy.

Incomplete cord transection A partial cutting (severing) of the spinal cord in which some cord function remains distal to the injury site.

Incontinence Inability to control excretory functions; usually refers to the involuntary passage of urinary or fecal matter.

Incubation period The time between exposure to a disease pathogen and the appearance of the first signs or symptoms.

Incus The anvil-shaped bone located between the malleus and stapes in the middle ear.

Index of suspicion The expectation that certain injuries or patterns of injuries have resulted to a body part, organ, or system based on the mechanism of injury and the force of impact to the patient.

Indication The appropriate use of a drug when treating a disease or condition.

Indicative change ECG changes seen in leads looking directly at the wall of the heart in an infarction.

Induration Hardened mass within the tissue typically associated with inflammation.

Infarction Death of tissue because of an inadequate blood supply.

Inferior Toward the feet; below a point of reference in the anatomic position.

Inferior vena cava Vessels that return venous blood from the lower part of the body to the right atrium.

Infiltration Complication of intravenous therapy when the catheter tip is outside the vein and the intravenous solution is dispersed into the surrounding tissues.

Inflammation A tissue reaction in an injury, infection, or insult.

Influx Flowing into.

Ingestion Process of bringing food into the digestive tract.

Inhalants Substances such as aerosols, fuels, paints, and other chemicals that produce fumes at room temperature; they are breathed in, producing a high.

Inhalation A route in which the medication is aerosolized and delivered directly to the lung tissue.

Injury Intentional or unintentional damage to a person resulting from acute exposure to thermal, mechanical, electrical, or chemical energy or from the absence of such essentials as heat or oxygen.

Injury risk A real or potential hazardous situation that puts individuals at risk for sustaining an injury.

Injury surveillance An ongoing systematic collection, analysis, and interpretation of injury data essential to the planning, implementation, and evaluation of public health practice, closely integrated with the timely dissemination of the data to those who need to know.

Inner ear Holds the sensory organs for hearing and balance.

Inotropic Relating to the force of cardiac contraction.

Inotropism A change in myocardial contractility.

Inspiratory reserve volume Amount of gas that can be forcefully inspired in addition to a normal breath's tidal volume.

Integrity Doing the right thing even when no one is looking.

Integumentary system The largest organ system in the body, consisting of the skin and accessory structures (e.g., hair, nails, glands).

Intense affect Heated and passionate emotional responses.

Intentional injury Injuries and deaths self-inflicted or perpetrated by another person, usually involving some type of violence.

Intentional tort A wrong in which the defendant meant to cause the harmful action.

Interatrial septum Septum dividing the atria in the heart.

Intercalated discs The cell-to-cell connection with gap junctions between cardiac muscle cells.

Interference The ability of one drug to limit the physiologic function of another drug.

Intermittent claudication Pain, cramping, muscle tightness, fatigue, or weakness of the legs when walking or during exercise.

Internal anal sphincter Muscle under autonomic control; has stretch receptors that provide the sensation of the need to defecate.

Internal bleeding Escape of blood from blood vessels into tissues and spaces within the body.

Internal respiration The exchange of gases between blood cells and tissues.

Internal urinary sphincter Ring of smooth muscle in the urethra that is under autonomic control.

International medical surgical response teams Specialty surgical teams that can respond both in the United States and internationally.

Interoperability Describes a radio system that can use the components of several different systems; it can use specialized equipment to connect several different radio systems and components together and have them communicate with each other.

Interpretation Stating the conclusions you have drawn from the information.

Interstitial compartment Area consisting of fluid outside cells and outside the circulatory system.

Interstitium Extravascular and extracellular milieu; also known as the *third space*.

Interval Waveform and a segment; in pacing, the period, measured in milliseconds, between any two designated cardiac events.

Interventricular septum Septum dividing the ventricles in the heart.

Intimal In reference to blood vessels, the innermost lining of an artery; composed of a single layer of cells.

Intimate partner violence and abuse (IPVA) Formerly called *domestic violence,* this is a learned pattern of assaultive and controlling behavior, including physical, sexual, and psychological attacks as well as economic control, which adults or adolescents use against their intimate partners to gain power and control.

Intimate space The area within 1.5 feet of a person.

Intoxication Being under the effect of a toxin or drug; common terminology (nonmedical) refers to intoxication as being under the effect of alcohol or illegal drugs.

Intracardiac The injection of a drug directly into the heart.

Intracellular Inside of the cell or cytoplasmic membrane.

Intracellular fluid (ICF) Fluid found within cells.

Intracerebral hematoma Bleeding within the brain tissue itself.

Intracerebral hemorrhage Bleeding within the brain tissue, often from smaller blood vessels.

Intracranial pressure (ICP) Pressure inside the brain cavity; should be very low, usually less than 15 mm Hg.

Intradermal Route of the injection of medication between the dermal layers of skin.

Intralingual Direct injection into the underside of the tongue with a small volume of medication.

Intramuscular (IM) An injection of medication directly into the muscle.

Intranasal The route that offers direct delivery of medications into the nasal passages and sinuses.

Intraosseous An administration route used in emergency situations when peripheral venous access is not established; a needle is passed through the cortex of the bone and the medication is infused into the capillary network within the bone matrix.

Intraosseous infusion The process of infusing medications, fluids, and blood products into the bone marrow cavity for subsequent delivery to the venous circulation.

Intraperitoneal Abdominopelvic organs surrounded by the peritoneum.

Intrathecal The direct deposition of medication into the spinal canal.

Intravascular compartment Area consisting of fluid outside cells but inside the circulatory system; the majority of intravascular fluid is plasma, which is the fluid component of blood.

Intravenous (IV) Administration route offering instantaneous and nearly complete absorption through peripheral or central venous access.

Intravenous (IV) bolus The delivery of a drug directly into an infusion port on the administration set using a syringe.

Intravenous cannulation Placement of a catheter into a vein to gain access to the body's venous circulation.

Intravenous therapy Administration of a fluid into a vein.

Intrinsic rate Rate at which a pacemaker of the heart normally generates impulses.

Intussusception Invagination of a part of the colon into another part of the colon; also referred to as *telescoping*.

Invasion of privacy Disclosure or publication of personal or private facts about a person to a person or persons not authorized to receive such information.

Invasive wound infection An infection involving the deeper tissues of a wound that may be destructive to blood vessels and other structures of the skin and soft tissues.

Investigational drug A drug not yet approved by the Food and Drug Administration.

Involuntary consent The rendering of care to a person under specific legal authority, even if the patient does not consent to the care.

Ion Electrically charged particle.

Ionizing radiation Particles or pure energy that produces changes in matter by creating ion pairs.

Iris Colored part of the eye; ring of smooth muscle that surrounds the pupil; controls the size (diameter) of the pupil.

Irregular bones Unique bones with specialized functions not easily classified into the other types of bone (e.g., vertebrae).

Ischemia Decreased supply of oxygenated blood to a body part or organ.

Ischemic phase Vascular response to shock when precapillary and postcapillary sphincters constrict, halting blood to distal tissues.

Ischemic stroke Lack of perfusion to an area of brain tissue; caused by a blood clot, air, amniotic fluid, or a foreign body.

Islets of Langerhans Groups of cells located in the pancreas that produce insulin, glucagon, somatostatin, and pancreatic polypeptide.

Isoelectric line Absence of electrical activity; observed on the ECG as a straight line.

Isografting Transplanting tissue from a genetically identical person (i.e., identical twin).

Isolation The seclusion of individuals with an illness to prevent transmission to others.

Isotonic A balance in the ionic concentration from one side of the membrane to the other.

Jacking the dash Making cuts into the front pillar and A pillar and lifting the dash, instrument panel, steering wheel, column, and even the pedals off a trapped driver or front seat passenger.

Jejunum Second part of the small intestine; major site of nutrient absorption.

Joint dislocation Disruption of articulating bones from their normal location.

Joints Point where two or more bones make contact to allow movement and provide mechanical support.

J-point Point where the QRS complex and ST segment meet.

Jugular venous distension (JVD) The presence of visually enlarged external jugular neck veins.

Jump kit A hard- or soft-sided bag used by paramedics to carry supplies and medications to the patient's side.

Junctional bradycardia A rhythm that begins in the atrioventricular junction with a rate of less than 40 beats/min.

Jurisprudence The theory and philosophy of law.

Kehr's sign Acute left shoulder pain caused by the presence of blood or other irritants in the peritoneal cavity.

Keloid An excessive accumulation of scar tissue that extends beyond the original wound margins.

Keratinized Accumulation of the protein keratin within the cytoplasm of skin cells. These cells comprise the epidermis of the skin. These dead cells function as the first defense against invaders and minor trauma.

Keratinocytes Epidermal cells.

Keratitis Inflammation and swelling of the cornea.

Kernicterus Excessive fetal bilirubin; associated with hemolytic disease.

Ketonemia The presence of ketones in the blood.

Kinetic energy M [mass] × $^1/_2$ V [velocity]^2; also called the *energy of motion.*

Knee bags Airbags mounted low on the instrument panel designed to deploy against the driver's and front seat passenger's knees in a frontal collision.

Korotkoff sounds The noise made by blood under pressure tumbling through the arteries.

Kussmaul respirations An abnormal respiratory pattern characterized by deep, gasping respirations that may be slow or rapid.

Kwashiorkor A form of malnutrition caused by inadequate protein intake compared with the total needed or required calorie intake.

Kyphosis Abnormally increased convexity in the curvature of the thoracic spine as viewed from the side; also called *hunchback.*

Labeling The application of a derogatory term to a patient on the basis of an event, habit, or personality trait that may not be accurate about the underlying condition.

Labia majora Rounded folds of external adipose tissue of the external female genitalia.

Labia minora Thinner, pinkish folds of skin that extend anteriorly to form the prepuce of the external female genitalia.

Labile Affect that changes frequently and rapidly.

Labor The process by which the fetus and placenta are expelled from the uterus. Usually divided into three stages, starting with the first contraction and ending with delivery of the placenta.

Labyrinth Series of bony tunnels inside the inner ear.

Labyrinthitis An inflammation of the structures in the inner ear.

Lacrimal ducts Small openings at the medial edge of the eye; drain holes for water from the surface of the eye.

Lacrimal fluid Watery, slightly alkaline secretion that consists of tears and saline that moisten the conjunctiva.

Lacrimal gland One of a pair of glands situated superior and lateral to the eye bulb; secretes lacrimal fluid.

Lacrimation Tearing of the eyes.

Lactic acid Byproduct of anaerobic metabolism.

Landing zone An area used to land a helicopter that is 100 feet × 100 feet and free of overhead wires.

Large intestine Organ where a large amount of water and electrolytes is absorbed and where undigested food is concentrated into feces.

Laryngoscope An instrument used to examine the interior of the larynx; during endotracheal intubation the device is used to visualize the glottic opening.

Laryngotracheobronchitis Croup.

Larynx Lies between the pharynx and the lungs; outer case of nine cartilages that protect and support the vocal cords.

Lassa fever A viral hemorrhagic fever illness caused by the Lassa virus (Arenavirus family).

Latent period Period during and after infection in which the disease is no longer transmissable.

Lateral A position away from the midline of the body.

Lateral recumbent Lying on either the right or left side.

Lead Electrical connection attached to the body to record electrical activity.

Left A position toward the left side of the body.

Left coronary artery Vessel that supplies oxygenated blood to the left side of the heart muscle.

Legally blind Less than 20/200 vision in at least one eye or a extremely limited field of vision (such as 20 degrees at its widest point).

Lens Transparent, biconvex elastic disc suspended by ligaments.

Leptomeningitis Inflammation of the inner brain coverings.

Lesions A wound, injury, or pathologic change in body tissue; any visible, local abnormality of the tissues of the skin, such as a wound, sore, rash, or boil.

Lethal concentration 50% (LC50) The air concentration of a substance that kills 50% of the exposed animal population; also commonly noted as LCt50; this denotes the concentration and the length of exposure time that results in 50% fatality in the exposed animal population.

Lethal dose 50% (LD50) The oral or dermal exposure dose that kills 50% of the exposed animal population in 2 weeks.

Leukocytes White blood cells.

Leukocytosis An increase in the number of white blood cells in the blood; typically results from infection, hemorrhage, fever, inflammation, or other factors.

Leukopenia A decrease in the total number of white blood cells in the blood.

Liability The legal responsibility of a party for the consequences of his or her acts or omissions.

Libel False statements about a person made in writing that blacken the person's character or injure his or her reputation.

Lice Wingless insects that live in human hair.

Licensure Permission granted to an individual by a governmental authority, such as a state, to perform certain restricted activities.

Life-threatening conditions A problem to the circulatory, respiratory, or nervous system that will kill a patient within minutes if not properly managed.

Ligaments Fibrous connective tissue that connects bones to bones, forming joint capsules.

Limbic system The part of the brain involved in mood, emotions, and the sensation of pain and pleasure.

Linear laceration Laceration that generally has smooth margins, although not as precise as those of an incision.

Linear skull fracture A line crack in the skull.

Lipid accumulation Accumulation of lipids in cells, usually as a result of the failure or inadequate performance of the enzyme that metabolizes fats.

Lipid peroxidation Process of cellular membrane destruction from exposure of the membrane to oxygen free radicals.

Lipophilic Substances that tend to seek out and bind to fatty substances.

Liquefaction necrosis Dead or dying tissue in which the necrotic material becomes softened and liquefied.

Liver Largest internal organ in the body; serves as a major detoxifier in the body.

Living will A type of advanced directive with written and signed specific instructions to healthcare providers about the individual's wishes regarding what types of healthcare measures or treatments should be undertaken to prolong life.

Loaded airbag An airbag that has not deployed during the initial crash.

Local damage Damage present at the point of chemical contact.

Local effect The effects of a drug at the site where the drug is applied or in the surrounding tissues.

Lock out, tag out An industrial workplace safety term describing actions taken to shut off power to a device, appliance, machine, or vehicle and to ensure that power remains off until work is completed.

Logistics officer The person responsible for assembling supplies used during an incident.

Long bones Bones that are longer than they are wide, have attachments for muscles to allow movement, and are found in limbs (e.g., the femur).

Looseness of associations (LOA) Going off track during conversation to varying degrees.

Low-angle terrain An environment in flat or mildly sloping areas in which rescuers primarily support themselves with their feet on the terrain surface.

Low vision Level of visual impairment in which an individual is unable to read a newspaper at the usual viewing distance even if wearing glasses or contact lenses. It is not limited to distance vision and can be a severe visual impairment.

Low voltage Less than 1000 V.

Lower airway Portion of the respiratory tract below the glottis.

Lower airway inhalation injury Injury to the anatomic portion of the respiratory tree below the level of the glottis. Generally caused by the inhalation of the toxic byproducts of combustion.

Lower flammable limit The minimal concentration of fuel in the air that will ignite; below this point too much oxygen and not enough fuel are present to burn (too lean); also called the *lower explosive limit.*

Ludwig's angina A bacterial infection of the floor of the mouth resulting from an infection in the root of the teeth, an abscessed tooth, or an injury to the mouth.

Lumbar vertebrae Vertebrae of the lower back that do not attach to any ribs and are superior to the pelvis.

Lumen An opening in the bevel of a needle.

Lungs Organs that allow the mechanical movement of air to and from the respiratory membrane.

Lymph Fluid that flows through the lymphatic ducts and aids in immune response and debris removal.

Lymph nodes Filter out foreign materials and collect infection-fighting cells that kill pathogens.

Lymphadenopathy Swelling of lymph nodes.

Lymphatic system The network of vessels, ducts, nodes, valves, and organs involved in protecting and maintaining the internal fluid environment of the body; part of the circulatory system.

Lymphatic vessels Unidirectional tubes that carry fluid or lymph within the lymphatic system.

Lymphedema Edema that follows when lymphatic pathways are blocked and fluid accumulates in the interstitial space.

Lymphocyte A form of leukocyte.

Lyse To destroy a cell.

Lysergic acid diethylamide (LSD) A powerful synthetic hallucinogen, often called *acid* and found on small squares of blotter paper.

Lysosomes Membrane-walled structures that contain enzymes.

Macrophages A monocyte that has matured and localized in one particular type of tissue; active in the immune system by activating agents that kill pathogens, absorbing foreign materials, and slowing infections and infectious agents.

Macule A flat, circumscribed, discolored lesion (e.g., freckle) measuring less that 1 cm.

Mainstem bronchi Each of two main breathing tubes that lead from the trachea into the lungs. There is one right mainstem bronchus and one left mainstem bronchus.

Malaise General feeling of illness without any specific symptoms.

Malfeasance Performing a wrongful act.

Malignant Highly dangerous or virulent; often used to describe a deadly form of cancer or a spreading of cancer.

Malignant hypertension Severe hypertension with signs of acute and progressive damage to end organs such as the heart, brain, and kidneys.

Malingering Faking illness for a tangible gain (missing work, avoiding incarceration, etc.).

Malleus Hammer-shaped bone located at the front of the middle ear; receives vibrations from the tympanic membrane.

Malocclusion The condition in which the teeth of the upper and lower jaws do not line up.

Mammary glands Female organs of milk production; located within the breast tissue.

Mania An excessively intense enthusiasm, interest, or desire; a craze.

Manure gas A name used for several different gases formed by decomposition of manure (methane, carbon dioxide, ammonia, hydrogen sulfide, and hydrogen disulfide); in certain concentrations all are toxic to animals and human beings.

Marasmus A form of nutritional deficiency from an overall lack of calories that results in wasting.

Marburg A viral hemorrhagic fever illness caused by the Marburg virus (Filovirus family).

Margination Process of phagocytes adhering to capillary and venule walls in the early phases of inflammation.

Marijuana Dried mixture of shredded leaves, stems, and seeds of the hemp plant that are usually smoked and contain many psychoactive compounds, most notably tetrahydrocannabinol (THC).

Mark 1 antidote kit Self-injected nerve agent antidote kit consisting of atropine and 2-pralidoxime (2-PAM).

Mast cells Connective tissue cell that contains histamine; important in initiating the inflammatory response.

Material safety data sheet (MSDS) A document that contains information about the specific identity of a hazardous chemical; information includes exact name and synonyms, health effects, first aid, chemical and physical properties, and emergency telephone numbers.

Matrix Nonliving material that separates cells in the connective tissue.

Mechanical processing Physical manipulation and breakdown of food.

Mechanism of action The manner in which a drug works to produce its intended effect.

Mechanism of injury The way an injury occurs on the body.

Meconium A dark green substance that represents the infant's first bowel movement.

Medial A position toward the midline of the body.

Median lethal dose The dose that kills 50% of the drug-tested population.

Mediastinitis Infection of the mediastinum; a serious medical condition.

Mediastinoscopy Surgical procedure of looking into the mediastinum with an endoscope.

Mediastinum Area that includes the trachea, esophagus, thymus gland, heart, and great vessels.

Medical asepsis Medically clean, not sterile; the goal in prehospital care because complete asepsis is not always possible.

Medical direction Physician oversight of paramedic practice; also called *medical control*.

Medical director A physician responsible for the oversight of the EMS system and the actions of the paramedics; also known as a *physician advisor*.

Medical ethics A field of study that evaluates the decisions, conduct, policies, and social concerns of medical activities.

Medical practice act Legislation that governs the practice of medicine; may prescribe how and to what extent a physician may delegate authority to a paramedic to perform medical acts; varies from state to state.

Medical terminology Greek- and Latin-based words (typically) that function as a common language for the medical community.

Medically clean Disinfected.

Medulla Most inferior part of the brainstem; responsible for some vegetative functions.

Medulla oblongata Lowest portion of brain tissue and the interface between the brain and the spinal cord; responsible for maintenance of basic life functions such as heart rate and respirations.

Meissner corpuscle Encapsulated nerve endings in the superficial dermis responsible for sensing vibrations and light touch.

Melancholy An episode of dysphoric mood with disruptions of homeostasis, including alterations in appetite, activities, and sleep patterns; also called *major* or *severe depression.*

Melena Foul-smelling, dark, and tarry stools stained with blood pigments or with digested blood, often indicating gastrointestinal bleeding.

Melting point The temperature at which a solid changes to a liquid (e.g., ice melting to water at 0°C (32°F).

Membrane potential Difference in electrical charge across the cell membrane.

Menarche The onset of the menstrual cycle.

Meninges Covering of the brain and spinal cord; layers include the dura mater, arachnoid, and pia mater.

Meningitis Irritation of the connective tissue covering the central nervous system, often from infection or hemorrhage.

Meningocele A type of spina bifida in which the spinal cord develops normally but a saclike cyst that contains the meninges and cerebrospinal fluid protrudes from an opening in the spine, usually in the lumbosacral area.

Meningomyelocele The severest form of spina bifida in which the meninges, cerebrospinal fluid, and a portion of the spinal cord protrude from an opening in the spine and are encased in a sac covered by a thin membrane; also called *myelomeningocele.*

Menopause Cessation of menstruation in the human female.

Menstruation Cyclical shedding of endometrial lining.

Mental illness Any form of psychiatric disorder.

Mental retardation Developmental disability characterized by a lower than normal IQ.

Merocrine glands Sweat glands that open directly to the surface of the body; produce a fluid (mainly water) when the temperature rises that allows the body to dispel large amounts of heat through the evaporation process.

Mesentery Layers of connective tissue found in the peritoneal cavity.

Metabolism Sum of all physical and chemical changes that occur within an organism.

Metabolites The smaller molecules from the breakdown that occurs during metabolism.

Metaplasia The transformation of one type of mature differentiated cell into another type of mature differentiated cell.

Metastatic Spread of cancerous cells to a distant site.

Metered-dose inhaler (MDI) A handheld device that disperses a measured dose of medication in the form of a fine spray directly into the airway.

Methamphetamine A powerful, highly addictive central nervous system stimulant found in either a white powder form or a clear crystal form ("crystal meth").

Methemoglobinemia The oxidation of hemoglobin from the ferrous iron to the ferric iron state.

Methicillin-resistant Staphylococcus aureus Any of several bacterial strains of *S. aureus* resistant to methicillin (a penicillin) and related drugs; typically acquired in the hospital.

Micturition Urination.

Midbrain Lies below the diencephalon and above the pons; works with the pons to route information from higher within the brain to the spinal cord and vice versa.

Middle ear Air-filled chamber within the temporal bone; contains the auditory ossicles.

Migraine headache A recurring vascular headache characterized by unilateral onset, severe pain, sensitivity to light, and autonomic disturbances during the acute phase, which may last for hours or days.

Milliampere (mA) Unit of measure of electrical current needed to elicit depolarization of the myocardium.

Millivolt (mV) Difference in electrical charge between two points in a circuit.

Minor In most states, a person younger than 18 years.

Minute volume Amount of gas moved in and out of the respiratory tract per minute. Tidal volume multiplied by ventilatory rate equals minute volume. The minute volume is the true measurement of a patient's ventilatory status and is vital in assessing pulmonary function. It ascertains the ventilatory rate and the depth of each inhalation.

Miosis Pinpoint pupils.

Miscarriage (spontaneous abortion) Loss of the products of conception before the fetus can survive on its own.

Misfeasance Performing a legal act in a harmful manner.

Mitochondria Power plant of the cell and body; site of aerobic oxidation.

Mitosis Process of division and multiplication in which one cell divides into two cells.

Mitral valve Left atrioventricular valve in the heart; also called the *bicuspid valve.*

Mittelschmerz Pain occurring at time of ovulation.

Mixed episode A period of manic-like energy and agitation coupled with the pessimism and dysphoria of severe depression.

Mobile data computer A device used in an ambulance or first responder vehicle to retrieve and send call information; has its own memory storage and processing capability.

Mobile data terminal A device used like a mobile data computer but without its own memory storage and processing capability.

Mobile radio A radio installed in an emergency vehicle; usually transmits by higher wattage than a portable radio.

Modern deployment Deployment that considers workload and how available resources can achieve a balance among coverage, response times, and crew satisfaction.

Mold A multicellular type of fungus that grows hyphae.

Monoblasts Immature monocytes.

Monocytes Type of white blood cell (leukocyte) designed to consume foreign material and fight pathogens; generally become macrophages within a few days after release into the bloodstream.

Monomorphic Having the same shape.

Mons pubis A hair-covered fat pad overlying the symphysis pubis.

Mood The dominant and sustained emotional state of a patient; the emotional lens through which a patient views the world.

Morals Values that help a person define right (what a person ought to do) versus wrong (what a person ought not to do).

Morbid obesity Having a body mass index of 40 or more; equates to approximately 100 lb more than ideal weight.

Morbidity Nonfatal injury rates; state of being diseased; propensity to cause disease or illness.

Mortality Death rate.

Mortality rate The number of patients who have died from a disease in a given period.

Motor cortex Area of brain tissue on the frontal lobe that controls voluntary movements.

Mucosa Layer of cells lining body cavities or organs (e.g., the lining of the mouth and digestive tract); generally implies a moist surface.

Multiformed atrial rhythm Cardiac dysrhythmia that occurs because of impulses originating from various sites, including the sinoatrial node, the atria, and/or the atrioventricular junction; requires at least three different P waves seen in the same lead for proper diagnosis.

Multipara A woman who has given birth multiple times.

Multiple-casualty incident An incident involving 26 to 99 persons.

Multiple organ dysfunction syndrome Altered organ function in an acutely ill person in whom homeostasis cannot be maintained without intervention.

Multiple-patient incident An incident involving two to 25 persons.

Multiple sclerosis (MS) Autoimmune disorder in which the immune system attacks the myelin sheath surrounding neurons, causing widespread motor problems and pain.

Multiplex A system that allows the crew to transmit voice and data at the same time, enabling the crew to call in a patient report while transmitting an ECG strip to the hospital.

Murphy's sign An inspiratory pause when the right upper quadrant is palpated.

Muscle tissue Contractile tissue that is the basis of movement.

Muscular dystrophy (MD) Hereditary condition causing malformation of muscle tissue and leading to malformation of the musculoskeletal system and physical disability.

Mutate To change in an unusual way.

Mutism A condition in which a person will not speak.

Myasthenia gravis Autoimmune disorder affecting acetylcholine receptors throughout the body, causing widespread muscle weakness.

Mycoses Diseases caused by fungi.

Mydriasis Dilation of the pupils.

Myelomeningocele Developmental anomaly of the central nervous system in which a hernial sac containing a portion of the spinal cord, the meninges, and cerebrospinal fluid protrudes through a congenital cleft in the vertebral column; occurs in approximately two of every 1000 live births, is readily apparent, and is easily diagnosed at birth.

Myocardial cells Working cells of the myocardium that contain contractile filaments and form the muscular layer of the atrial walls and the thicker muscular layer of the ventricular walls.

Myocardial depressant factor An inflammatory mediator (cytokine) produced as a result of significant burn injury; known to affect the contractile function of the cardiac ventricles.

Myocardial infarction (MI) Necrosis of some mass of the heart muscle caused by an inadequate blood supply.

Myocarditis Inflammation of the middle and thickest layer of the heart, the myocardium.

Myocardium Middle and thickest layer of the heart; contains the cardiac muscle fibers that cause contraction of the heart as well as the conduction system and blood supply.

Myoglobin A protein within muscle that functions as an oxygen carrier. When released in large quantities into the bloodstream, these proteins block the small vessels of the kidneys.

Myoglobinuria Presence of myoglobin in the urine; almost always a result of a pathologic (disease) state such as widespread muscle injury.

Myometrium Muscular region of the uterus.
Myopia Nearsightedness; difficulty seeing objects at a distance.
Myositis A rare muscle disease in which the body's immune system is activated, resulting in inflammation and pain of muscle tissue.
Myotomes Areas of the body controlled by specific motor spinal nerves.
Myxedema Severe form of hypothyroidism characterized by hypothermia and unresponsiveness.
N-95 particulate mask (medical) A facial mask worn over the nose and mouth that removes particulates from the inspired and expired air.
Nasal flaring Widening of the nostrils on inhalation; an attempt to increase the size of the airway and increase the amount of available oxygen.
Nasal polyps Small, saclike growths consisting of inflamed nasal mucosa.
Nasogastric (NG) The administration route used when a nasogastric tube is in place; bypasses the voluntary swallowing reflex.
Nasogastric tube A tube placed by way of the nose into the stomach.
Nasolacrimal duct Opening at the medial corner of the eye that drains excess fluid into the nasal cavity.
Natal Connected with birth.
National Disaster Medical System An organized response to an event that includes field units, coordination of patient transportation, and provision of hospital beds. The field component is composed of many volunteer teams of medical professionals.
National Fire Protection Association (NFPA) International voluntary membership organization that promotes improved fire protection and prevention and establishes safeguards against loss of life and property by fire; writes and publishes national voluntary consensus standards.
National Flight Paramedics Association (NFPA) Association established in 1984 to differentiate the critical care paramedic from the flight paramedic; has developed a position statement recommending the training considered necessary to perform the duties of a flight paramedic.
National Highway Traffic Safety Administration (NHTSA) An agency within the U.S. Department of Transportation that was first given the authority to develop EMS systems, including the development of curriculum.
National Medical Response Team Quick response specialty teams trained and equipped to provide mass casualty decontamination and patient care after the release of a chemical, biologic, or radiologic agent.
National Registry of EMTs (NREMT) A national organization developed to ensure that graduates of EMS training programs have met minimal standards by measuring competency through a uniform testing process.
National Standard Curriculum (NSC) Document providing information or course planning and structure, objectives, and detailed lesson plans. It also suggests hours of instruction for the EMT-A.
Natural immunity Nonspecific immunity that mounts a generalized response to any foreign material or pathogen (e.g., inflammation).
Natural killer cells Specialized lymphocytes capable of killing infected or malignant cells.
Nebulizer A machine that turns liquid medication into fine droplets in aerosol or mist form.
Necrosis Death of an area of tissue.
Necrotizing Causing the death (necrosis) of tissue.
Negative battery cable An electrical power cable that allows the vehicle's electrical system to be grounded or neutral as an electrical circuit.
Negative pressure Pressure that acts as a vacuum, pulling more fluid from the vascular space at a faster rate than before, further depleting the intravascular volume; also known as *inhibition pressure*.
Neglect Failure of a parent or other person with responsibility for the child to provide needed food, clothing, shelter, medical care, or supervision such that the child's health, safety, and well-being are threatened with harm
Negligence The failure to act as a reasonably prudent and careful person would under similar circumstances.
Negligence per se Conduct that may be declared and treated as negligent without having to prove what would be reasonable and prudent under similar circumstances, usually because the conduct violates a law or regulation.
Nematocyst The stinging cells many marine creatures use to envenomate and immobilize prey.
Neonatal abstinence syndrome Withdrawal symptoms that occur in newborns born to opioid-addicted mothers.
Neonate An infant from birth to 1 month of age also called a newborn infant.
Neoplasm Cancerous growth; a tumor that may be malignant or benign.
Neovascularization New blood vessel growth to support healing tissue.
Nephron Functional unit of the kidney.
Nephrotoxic Chemicals, medications, or other substances that can be toxic to the kidneys.
Nerve Neurons and blood vessels wrapped together with connective tissue; the body's information highways.
Nervous tissue Tissue that can conduct electrical impulses.
Neural tube defects Congenital anomalies that involve incomplete development of the brain, spinal cord, and/or their protective coverings.
Neuralgia Pain caused by chronic nerve damage.
Neuroeffector junction Interface between a neuron and its target tissue.
Neurogenic shock Shock with hypotension caused by a sudden loss of control over the sympathetic

nervous system. Loss can be caused by a variety of mechanisms from traumatic injury to disease and infection.

Neuroglia Supporting cells of nervous tissue; functions include nourishment, protection, and insulation.

Neurons Conducting cells of nervous tissue; composed of a cell body, dendrites, and axon.

Neuropeptide A protein that may interact with a receptor after circulation through the blood.

Neuroses Mental diseases related to upbringing and personality in which the person remains "in touch" with reality.

Neurotransmitters A chemical released from one nerve that crosses the synaptic cleft to reach a receptor.

Neutralizing agent A substance that counteracts the effects of acids or bases; brings the pH of a solution back to 7.0.

Neutron radiation Penetrating radiation that can result in whole-body irradiation.

Neutrophils A form of granulocyte that is short lived but often first to arrive at the site of injury; capable of phagocytosis.

Newborn asphyxia The inability of a newborn to begin and continue breathing at birth.

Newly born An infant in the first minutes to hours after birth.

Nodule An elevated, solid lesion in the deep skin or subcutaneous tissues.

Noncardiogenic pulmonary edema (NCPE) Fluid collection in the alveoli of the lung that does not result from heart failure.

Nonfeasance Failure to perform a required act or duty.

Nonproprietary name Generic name.

Nonsteroidal antiinflammatory drug (NSAID) Medications used primarily to treat inflammation, mild to moderate pain, and fever.

Nonverbal cues Expressions, motions, gestures, and body language that may be used to communicate other than with words.

Normal flora Nonthreatening bacteria found naturally in the human body that, in some cases, are necessary for normal function.

Nuclear envelope The outer boundary between the nucleus and the rest of the cell to the endoplasmic reticulum for protein synthesis.

Nuclear membrane Membrane in the cell that surrounds the nucleus.

Nucleoplasm Protoplasm of the nucleus as contrasted with that of the cell.

Nucleus Area within a cell where the genetic material is stored.

Nullipara A woman who has not borne a child.

Numerator The number or mathematic expression written above the line in a fraction; the numerator is a portion of the denominator.

Nystagmus Involuntary rapid movement of the eyes in the horizontal, vertical, or rotary planes of the eyeball.

Obesity An excessively high amount of body fat or adipose tissue in relation to lean body mass.

Objective information Verifiable findings, such as information seen, felt, or heard by the paramedic.

Obsessive-compulsive disorder (OCD) An anxiety disorder marked by frequent, intrusive, unwanted, and bothersome thoughts (obsessions) and repetitive rituals (compulsions).

Obstructed lane +1 Blocking with an emergency vehicle to stop the flow of traffic in the lane in which the damaged vehicle is positioned plus one additional lane or the shoulder of the roadway.

Occipital lobe Most rearward portion of the cerebrum; mainly responsible for processing the sense of sight.

Occupational Safety and Health Administration (OSHA) A unit of the U.S. Department of Labor that establishes protective standards, enforces those standards, and reaches out to employers and employees through technical assistance and consultation programs.

Official name A drug's name as listed in the *United States Pharmacopoeia.*

Offline medical direction Prospective and retrospective medical direction (e.g., protocols and standard operating procedures).

Oils In medicine, substances extracted from flowers, leaves, stems, roots, seeds, or bark for use as therapeutic treatments.

Olfactory Sense of smell.

Olfactory fatigue Desensitization of the sense of smell.

Olfactory tissue Located within the nasopharynx; contains receptors that enable the ability of smell (olfaction).

Omphalocele Protrusion of abdominal organs into the umbilical cord.

Oncotic pressure The net effect of opposing osmotic pressures in the capillary beds.

Online medical direction Direct voice communication by a medical director (or designee) to a prehospital professional while he or she is attending to the patient; also called *direct medical direction.*

Oocyte The female gamete; product of the female reproductive system.

Oogenesis Egg production.

Open-ended questions A form of interview question that allows patients to respond in narrative form so that they may feel free to answer in their own way and provide details and information that they believe to be important.

Open fracture Fracture of the bone tissue that breaks the skin and may or may not still be exposed.

Open pneumothorax Injury to the thoracic cavity in which the cavity is breached, allowing air into the space between the lung and the chest wall.

Operations Carries out the tactical objectives of the incident commander.

Ophthalmic Route of administration in which medications are applied to the eye, such as antibiotic eye drops.

Ophthalmoscope An instrument used to examine the inner parts of the eye; consists of an adjustable light and multiple magnification lenses.

Opioids Powerful pain-relieving drugs derived from the seed pods of the poppy plant or drugs that are similar in molecular structure.

Oral A route of administration in which the medication is placed in the mouth and swallowed; the drug is absorbed through the gastrointestinal tract.

Oral cavity First part of the gastrointestinal tract; includes salivary glands, teeth, and tongue.

Organ A structure composed of two or more kinds of tissues organized to perform a more complex function than any one tissue alone can.

Organ of Corti Organ of hearing located in the cochlea.

Organ systems The coordination of several organs working together.

Organelles Structures within the cell that perform specialized functions.

Organic An etiology of an illness that stems from a biologic cause, such as a stroke or electrolyte imbalance.

Organism An entity composed of cells and capable of carrying on life functions.

Organophosphate A pesticide that inhibits acetylcholinesterase.

Orogastric (OG) tube A tube placed by way of the mouth into the stomach.

Oropharynx Starts at the uvula; back of the oral cavity that extends down to the epiglottis.

Orphan drugs Products developed for the diagnosis and/or treatment of rare diseases or conditions, such as sickle cell anemia and cystic fibrosis.

Orthopnea Dyspnea relieved by a change in position (either sitting upright or standing).

Orthostatic vital signs Serial measurements of the patient's pulse and blood pressure taken with the patient recumbent, sitting, and standing. Results are used to assess possible volume depletion; also called the *tilt test* or *postural vital signs*.

Osmolarity The number, or concentration, of solute per liter of water.

Osmosis The passive movement of water from a higher to a lower concentration.

Osmotic gradient The difference in the concentration from one side of a membrane to the other in the presence of an imbalance in the ionic concentration.

Osmotic pressure The pressure exerted by the concentration of the solutes in a given space.

Osteoarthritis A disorder in which the cartilaginous covering of the joint surface starts to wear away, resulting in pain and inflammation of a joint; also known as *degenerative joint disease*.

Osteomyelitis An infection of bone.

Osteoporosis Reduction in the amount of bone mass, which leads to fractures after minimal trauma.

Ostomy Hole; usually refers to a surgically made hole in some part of the body (e.g., tracheostomy, gastrostomy, colostomy).

Otic Route of administration in which medications are applied to the ear, such as antibiotic drops.

Otitis externa A condition manifested by redness and irritation of the external auditory canal; also called *swimmer's ear*.

Otosclerosis Abnormal growth of bone that prevents structures in the ear from working properly; thought to be a hereditary disease.

Otoscope An instrument used to examine the inner ear; consists of a light source and magnifying lens; the tip is covered with a disposable cone.

Oval window A membranous structure that separates the middle ear from the inner ear.

Ovarian follicle The ovum and its surrounding cells.

Ovarian medulla Inner portion of the ovary.

Ovarian torsion Twisting of an ovary on its axis such that the venous flow to the ovary is interrupted.

Ovaries Site of egg production in females.

Overdose The accidental or intentional ingestion of an excess of a substance with the potential for toxicity.

Over-the-counter (OTC) Drugs that can be purchased without a prescription.

Overweight State of increased body weight in relation to height.

Ovulation Mid-cycle release of an ovum during the menstrual cycle.

Ovum (oocyte) Human egg that, when fertilized, implants in the lining of the uterus and results in pregnancy.

Oxidation A normal chemical process in the body caused by the release of oxygen atoms created during normal cell metabolism.

Oxidation ability The ability of a substance to readily release oxygen to stimulate combustion.

Oxygen-limiting silo A vertical structure used to store ensiled plant material in an anaerobic environment.

Oxyhemoglobin Hemoglobin that has oxygen molecules bound to it.

P wave First wave in the cardiac cycle; represents atrial depolarization and the spread of the electrical impulse throughout the right and left atria.

Pacemaker Artificial pulse generator that delivers an electrical current to the heart to stimulate depolarization.

Pacemaker cells Specialized cells of the heart's electrical conduction system capable of spontaneously generating and conducting electrical impulses.

Packaging Placing the injured or ill patient in a litter and securing him or her for evacuation.

Painful stimulus Any stimulus that causes discomfort to the patient, triggering some sort of response.

Palliative care Provision of comfort measures (physical, social, psychological, and spiritual) to terminally ill patients.

Pallor Pale, washed-out coloration of skin. Often a result of extreme anemia or chronic illness. A patient with pallor can be referred to as pallid.

Palpation The process of applying pressure against the body with the intent of gathering information.

Palpitations An unpleasant awareness of one's heartbeat.

Pancreatitis Inflammation of the pancreas.

Pandemic A disease that affects the majority of the population of a single region or that is epidemic at the same time in many different regions.

Panic attack A sudden, paralyzing anxiety reaction characterized by an overwhelming sense of fear, anxiety, and impending doom, often with physical symptoms such as chest pain and difficulty breathing.

Papillary dermis Section of the dermis composed of loose connective tissue that contains vasculature that feeds the epidermis.

Papillary muscles Muscles attached to the chordae tendineae of the heart valves and the ventricular muscle of the heart.

Papule An elevated, solid lesion usually less than 0.5 centimeters in diameter; may arise from the epidermis, dermis, or both.

Para The number of pregnancies carried to 20 weeks or more.

Paracrine communication Method of intercellular communication in which cells communicate with cells in close proximity through the release of paracrine factors, or cytokines.

Paradoxic motion (of a segment of the chest wall) Part of the chest moves in an opposite direction from the rest during respiration.

Paranoid delusions False perceptions of persecution and the feeling that one is being hunted or conspired against; this is the most common type of delusion.

Paranoid schizophrenia A form of schizophrenia characterized by persistent preoccupation with illogical, absurd, and changeable delusions, usually of a persecutory, grandiose, or jealous nature, accompanied by related hallucinations.

Paraphimosis Tight, constricting band caused by the foreskin when it is retracted behind the glans penis.

Paraplegia Paralysis of the lower extemities. The injury can be either complete (a complete loss of muscle control and sensation below the injury site) or incomplete (a partial loss of muscle control or sensation below the injury site).

Parasites An organism that lives within or on another organism (the host) but does not contribute to the host's survival.

Parasympathetic division A division of the autonomic nervous system; responsible for the relaxed state of the body known as "feed and breed."

Parasympathetic nervous system The subdivision of the autonomic nervous system usually involved in activating vegetative functions, such as digestion, defecation, and urination.

Parasympatholytics Drugs that block or inhibit the function of the parasympathetic receptors.

Parasympathomimetics Drugs that mimic the parasympathetic division of the autonomic nervous system.

Parenteral Administration route used for systemic effects and given by a route other than the digestive tract.

Paresthesia Abnormal sensation described as numbness, tingling, or pins and needles.

Parietal lobe Section of the cerebrum responsible for the integration of most sensory information from the body.

Parietal pleura Lining of the pleural cavity attached tightly to the interior of the chest cage.

Parity The number of pregnancies that have resulted in birth.

Parkinson's disease Progressive movement disorder caused by dysfunction in the cerebellum; rigidity, tremor, bradykinesia, and postural instability are characteristic.

Parkmedic A National Park Service ranger who has undergone additional wilderness medical training and who operates in certain parks under the medical direction of emergency physicians from University of Southern California–Fresno; scope of practice lies between a traditional EMT-Intermediate and EMT-Paramedic, with additional wilderness medical training.

Paroxysmal atrial tachycardia Atrial tachycardia that starts or ends suddenly.

Paroxysmal nocturnal dyspnea (PND) A sudden onset of difficulty breathing that awakens the patient from sleep.

Paroxysmal supraventricular tachycardia (PSVT) A regular, narrow QRS tachycardia that starts or ends suddenly.

Partial agonist A drug that when bound to a receptor may elicit a physiologic response, but it is less than that of an agonist; may also may block the response of a competing agonist.

Partial pressure The pressure exerted by an individual gas in a mixture.

Partial seizure A seizure confined to one area of the brain.

Partial-thickness burn Burns that involve any layer of the dermis. The depth of these burns varies and depends on location, so they are further subcategorized as superficial partial-thickness or deep partial-thickness burns. Also called *second-degree burns*.

Partially sighted Level of vision in persons who have some type of visual problem and may need assistance.

Passive immunity Induced immunity that only lasts as long as the injected immune agents are alive and active (e.g., immunoglobulin injection).

Passive range of motion Degree of movement at a joint determined when the examiner causes the movement with the patient at rest.

Passive transport The ability of a substance to traverse a barrier without any energy input; generally occurs from a higher to a lower concentration.

Past medical history A summary of all past health-related events.

Patch A flat, circumscribed, discolored lesion measuring greater than 1 cm.

Pathologic fracture Fractures that occur as a result of an underlying disease process that weakens the mechanical properties of the bone.

Pathophysiology Functional changes that accompany a particular syndrome or disease.

Patients with terminal illness Patients with advanced stage of illness or disease with an unfavorable prognosis and no known cure.

Pattern recognition Gathering patient information, relating it to the healthcare professional's knowledge of pathophysiology and the signs and symptoms of illnesses and injuries, and determining whether the patient's presentation fits a particular pattern.

Pattern response Anticipating the equipment and emergency care interventions needed on the basis of the patient's history and physical examination findings.

Patterned injuries Those that leave a distinctive mark, indicating that an object was used in the assault (e.g., cigarette burns, electrical cord whipping, human bites, glove injuries, attempted strangulation, and slaps).

Peak expiratory flow The greatest rate of airflow that can be achieved during forced expiration beginning with the lungs fully inflated.

Peak flow meter A device used to assess the severity of respiratory distress.

Pediculosis Human infestation with lice.

Pelvic inflammatory disease (PID) An infection of a woman's reproductive organs, usually from a bacterial infection, that spreads from the vagina to the upper parts of the reproductive tract.

Penetrating trauma Any mechanism of injury that causes a cut or piercing of skin.

Penis Male sex organ with three columns of erectile tissue; transfers sperm during copulation.

Percussion A diagnostic technique that uses tapping on the body to differentiate air, solids, and fluids.

Performance-based response system A contractual agreement between the EMS provider and the government authority to provide ambulance response to a particular municipality or region with time requirements for each response and total responses on a monthly basis.

Perfusion Circulation of blood through an organ or a part of the body.

Pericardial cavity The potential space between the two layers of the pericardium.

Pericardial effusion An increase in the volume and/or character of pericardial fluid that surrounds the heart.

Pericardial tamponade Life-threatening injury in which blood collects within the pericardium until the increasing pressure prevents the heart from filling with blood, causing death.

Pericardiocentesis A procedure in which a needle is inserted into the pericardial space and the excess fluid is drawn out (aspirated) through the needle.

Pericarditis Inflammation of the double-walled sac (pericardium) that encloses the heart.

Pericardium Two-layer serous membrane lining the pericardial cavity.

Perinatal From the twenty-eighth week of gestation through the first 7 days after delivery.

Perineal body See *Perineum*.

Perineum The tissue between the mother's vaginal and rectal openings; may be torn during delivery.

Periodontal membrane/ligament Ligamentous attachment between the root of a tooth and the socket of the bone within which it sits.

Periosteum Fibrous connective tissue rich in nerve endings that envelops bone.

Peripheral nervous system All the nerves outside the central nervous system.

Peripheral vein A vein outside the chest or abdomen, such as the veins of the upper and lower extremities.

Peripherally inserted central catheter (PICC) line A thin tube inserted into a peripheral vein (usually the arm) and threaded into the superior vena cava to allow fluid or medication administration.

Peristalsis The wavelike contraction of the smooth muscle of the gastrointestinal tract.

Peritoneal cavity The space between the parietal and visceral peritoneum; also called the *peritoneal space*.

Peritoneum Double-layered serous membrane that lines the abdominal cavity and covers the organs located in the abdominopelvic cavity.

Peritonitis Inflammation of the peritoneum, typically caused by infection or in response to contact with blood or digestive fluids.

Peritonsillar abscess (PTA) An infection of tissue between the tonsil and pharynx, usually the result of a significant infection in the tonsils.

Permeability Ability of a membrane channel to allow passage of electrolytes once it is open.

Permissible exposure limit Allowable air concentration of a substance in the workplace as established by the Occupational Safety and Health Administration; these values are legally enforceable.

Permit-required confined space A confined space with one or more of the following characteristics: (1) contains or has a potential to contain a hazardous atmosphere; (2) contains a material with the potential for engulfing an entrant; (3) has an internal configuration such that an entrant could be trapped or asphyxiated by inwardly converging walls or by a floor that slopes downward and tapers to a smaller cross-section; or (4) contains any other recognized serious safety or health hazard.

Personal protective equipment (PPE) Equipment used to protect personnel; includes items such as gloves, eyewear, masks, respirators, and gowns.

Personal space The area around an individual that the person perceives as an extension of himself or herself. In the United States, personal distance is 1.5 to 4 feet.

Personality disorders Patterns of interacting with others and the world that are rigid and harmful, causing social and occupational problems.

Pertinent negative In a patient assessment, the signs and symptoms found not to be present that support a working diagnosis.

Pertinent positive In a patient assessment, the signs and symptoms found to be present that support a working diagnosis.

Pesticide A chemical material used to control a pest (insect, weed, etc.).

Petechiae A tiny pinpoint rash on the upper area of the neck and the face; may indicate near strangulation or suffocation; caused by an occlusion of venous return from the head while arterial pressure remains normal; may be present in mothers after childbirth.

pH A numeric assignment used to define the hydrogen ion concentration of a given chemical. The lower the pH, the higher the hydrogen ion concentration and the more acidic the solution.

Phagocyte Cells that are part of the body's immune system that play a predominant role in the destruction of invading microorganisms.

Phagocytosis Ingestion and digestion of foreign materials by phagocytes (cells, such as macrophages, designed to perform this function).

Pharmaceutics The science of preparing and dispensing drugs.

Pharmacogenetics The study of inherited differences (variation) in drug metabolism and response.

Pharmacokinetics The process by which a drug is absorbed, distributed, metabolized, and eliminated by the body.

Pharmacologic restraints Agents such as sedatives that can suppress a patient's neurologic and/or motor capabilities so that the threat to the paramedic is reduced; also known as *chemical restraints*.

Pharmacology The study of drugs, including their actions and effects on the host.

Pharmacopoeia A book describing drugs, chemicals, and medicinal preparations in a country or specific geographic area, including a description of the drug, its formula, and dosage.

Phases of rescue The training and organizational concept that groups all the activities that take place at a typical vehicle crash with entrapment into four categories, with each known as a phase of rescue.

Phlebitis Inflammation of a vein.

Phobia An intense fear of a particular object or situation.

Phosphate A salt of phosphoric acid that is important in the maintenance of the acid-base balance of the blood.

Phospholipid bilayer A double layer composed of three types of lipid molecules that comprise the plasma membrane.

Photoreceptor cells Rods and cones contained in the sensory part of the retina; they relay impulses to the optic nerve.

Photosensitivity A condition in which the patient's eyes are sensitive or feel pain when exposed to bright light.

Physical abuse Inflicting a nonaccidental physical injury on another person such as punching, kicking, hitting, or biting.

Physical disabilities Disabilities that involve limitation of mobility.

Physical restraints Straps, splints, and other devices that prevent movement of all or part of the patient's body.

Physician advisor A physician responsible for the oversight of the EMS system and the actions of the paramedics; also known as a *medical director*.

Physiology Study of how the body functions.

Pia mater Last meningeal layer; adheres to the central nervous system.

Pierre Robin sequence A congenital anomaly characterized by a very small lower jaw (micrognathia), a tongue that tends to fall back and downward (glossoptosis), and cleft palate.

Pill Dried powder forms of medication in the form of a small pellet; the term "pill" has been replaced with tablet and capsule.

Pinch points A machinery entanglement hazard formed when two machine parts move together and at least one of the parts moves in a circle.

Pinocytosis Absorption or ingestion of nutrients, debris, and fluids by a cell.

Placards Diamond-shaped signs placed on the sides and ends of bulk transport containers (e.g., truck, tank car, freight container) that carry hazardous materials.

Placenta (afterbirth) The organ inside the uterus that exchanges nutrition and waste between mother and fetus.

Placenta previa Placement of the placenta such that it partially or completely covers the cervix.

Placental abruption (abruptio placenta) Separation of part of the placenta away from the wall of the uterus.

Placental barrier Many layers of cells that form between maternal and fetal circulation that protect the fetus from toxins.

Plague An acute infectious disease caused by the anaerobic, gram-negative bacterium *Yersinia pestis;* transmitted naturally from rodents to human beings through flea bites; three common syndromes are bubonic (most likely form of the disease to be seen from naturally occurring infections), pneumonic (most likely form of the disease to result from an act of terrorism), and septicemic plague.

Plaintiff The person who initiates a lawsuit by filing a complaint; also known as a *claimant, petitioner,* or *applicant.*

Planning Supplies past, present, and future information about the incident.

Plaque An elevated, solid lesion usually greater than 0.5 cm in diameter that lacks any deep component.

Plasma Pale, yellow material in the blood; made of approximately 92% water and 8% dissolved molecules.

Plasma level profile The measurement of blood level of a medication versus the dosage administered.

Plasma membrane The outer covering of a cell that contains the cellular cytoplasm; also known as the *cell membrane.*

Platelets One of three formed elements in the blood; also called *thrombocytes.*

Pleura Serous membrane that lines the pleural cavity.

Pleural cavities Areas that contain the lungs.

Pleural effusion Collection of fluid in the pleural space, usually fluid that has seeped through the lung or chest wall tissue.

Pleural friction rub Noise made when the visceral and parietal pleura rub together.

Pleurisy Painful rubbing of the pleural lining.

Plural Amount that refers to more than one person, place, or thing.

Pluripotent Cell line that has the ability to differentiate into multiple different cell lines based on the right physiologic stimulus.

Pneumomediastinum Air entrapped within the mediastinum; a serious medical condition.

Pneumonia An inflammation and infection of the lower airway and lungs caused by a viral, bacterial, parasitic, or fungal organism.

Pneumonia Infection of the lungs.

Pneumothorax A collection of air in the pleural space, usually from either a hole in the lung or a hole in the chest wall.

Pocket mask A clear, semirigid mask designed for mouth-to-mask ventilation of a nonbreathing adult, child, or infant.

Poikilothermic An organism whose temperature matches the ambient temperature.

Point of maximum impulse (PMI) The apical impulse; the site where the heartbeat is most strongly felt.

Poison Any substance that can harm the human body; also known as a *toxin.*

Poisoning Exposure to a substance that is harmful in any dosage.

Poisonous Describes gases, liquids, or other substances of such nature that exposure to a very small amount is dangerous to life or is a hazard to health; also known as *toxic* (e.g., cyanide, arsenic, phosgene, aniline, methyl bromide, insecticides, pesticides).

Polarized state Period after repolarization of a myocardial cell (also called the *resting state*) when the outside of the cell is positive and the interior of the cell is negative.

Poliomyelitis Viral infection that tends to attack the motor roots of the spinal nerves, often leading to physical disability and even paralysis of the diaphragm.

Polydipsia Excessive thirst.

Polymorphic Varying in shape.

Polyphagia Excessive eating.

Polypharmacy The concurrent use of several medications.

Polyuria Excessive urination.

Pons Area of the brainstem that contains the sleep and respiratory centers for the body, which along with the medulla control breathing.

Portable radio Also referred to as a *walkie-talkie.* These radios are carried by emergency personnel and have a lower wattage output than the mobile or base unit. To use these portable radios with a higher watt output, the units can be connected through a repeater system to increase their output, which increases range.

Portal hypertension Increased venous pressure in the portal circulation.

Portal vein A vein composed of a group of vessels that originate from the digestive system.

Positive battery cable Also known as the *hot cable,* this electrical power cable allows a vehicle's electrical system to carry the current or electrical energy from the battery to the electrically powered appliances throughout the vehicle.

Positive end-expiratory pressure (PEEP) The amount of pressure above atmospheric pressure present in the airway at the end of the expiratory cycle. When forcing air into the lungs (positive-pressure ventilation), airway pressure is maintained above atmospheric pressure at the end of exhalation by means of a mechanical device, such as a PEEP valve.
Positive-pressure ventilation Forcing air into the lungs.
Postconcussion syndrome Symptoms of a concussion that persist for weeks to 1 year after an initial injury to the head.
Posterior The back, or dorsal, surface.
Postganglionic neuron The nerve that travels from the ganglia to the desired organ or tissue.
Postictal State that begins at the termination of seizure activity in the brain and ends with the patient returning to a level of normal behavior.
Postnatal The period immediately following the birth of a child and lasting for approximately 6 weeks.
Postpartum Pertaining to the mother after delivery.
Posttraumatic stress disorder (PTSD) An anxiety disorder that occurs after a traumatic, often life-threatening event.
Posture A patient's overall attitude and frame of mind.
Potassium The main intracellular ion (electrolyte), with the chemical designation K^+.
Potential difference Difference in electrical charge between two points in a circuit; expressed in volts or millivolts.
Potentiating To augment or increase the action of.
Potentiation A prolongation or increase in the effect of a drug by another drug.
Pounds per square inch (psi) The amount of pressure on an area that is 1 inch square.
Poverty of speech A disorder of thought form characterized by very little spontaneous, voluntary speech and short answers to questions.
Powder Medication ground into a fine substance.
Power take-off Element that connects a tractor to an implement; also called a *driveshaft*.
Prearrival instructions Clinically approved instructions provided by telephone by a trained and certified emergency medical dispatcher.
Precapillary sphincters Smooth muscle located at the entrances to the capillaries; responsive to local tissue needs.
Preeclampsia A complication of pregnancy that includes hypertension, swelling of the extremities and, in its most severe form, seizures (see *Eclampsia*).
Preexcitation Term used to describe rhythms that originate from above the ventricles but in which the impulse travels by a pathway other than the atrioventricular node and bundle of His; thus the supraventricular impulse excites the ventricles earlier than normal.
Prefix A sequence of letters that comes before the word root and often describes a variation of the norm.
Preganglionic neuron The nerve that extends from the spinal cord (central nervous system) to the ganglion.
Prehospital care report (PCR) The report written by the paramedic after the call has been completed. The report becomes part of the patient's permanent medical record.
Preload Force exerted by the blood on the walls of the ventricles at the end of diastole.
Premature birth Delivery between the twentieth and thirty-seventh weeks of pregnancy.
Premature complex Early beat occurring before the next expected beat; can be atrial, junctional, or ventricular.
Premature or preterm infant Infant born before 37 completed weeks of gestation.
Prenatal Preceding birth.
Preoccupation A topic or theme that consistently recurs in a person's thought process and conversations.
Prepuce A fold formed by the union of the labia minora over the clitoris.
Presbycusis Age-related hearing loss.
Presbyopia Loss of function of the lens to adjust to close reading; usual onset in middle age.
Presenting part The first part of the infant to appear at the vaginal opening, usually the head.
Pressured speech Rapid, loud, and intense speech that often results from racing thoughts and is frequently seen during manic episodes.
Preterm birth Birth before 37 weeks of gestation.
Preterm delivery Delivery between the twentieth and thirty-seventh weeks of pregnancy.
Prevalence rate The fraction of the population that currently has a certain disease.
Priapism A prolonged and painful erection.
Primary apnea The newly born's initial response to hypoxemia consisting of initial tachypnea, then apnea, bradycardia, and a slight increase in blood pressure; if stimulated, responds with resumption of breathing.
Primary blast injury Injuries caused by an explosive's pressure wave.
Primary cord injury A spinal cord injury caused by a direct traumatic blow.
Primary hypertension High blood pressure for which no cause is identifiable; also called *essential hypertension*.
Primary injury prevention Keeping an injury from occurring.
Primary skin lesion A lesion that has not been altered by scratching, rubbing, scrubbing, or other types of trauma.
Primary triage The initial sorting of patients to determine which are most injured and in need of immediate care.

Primary tumor A collection of cells that grow out of control, far in excess of normal rates. A primary tumor is a tumor that develops in one tissue only (e.g., a liver primary tumor originates in the liver).

Primigravida A woman who is pregnant for the first time.

Primipara A woman who has given birth to her first child.

Primum non nocere Latin for "first, do no harm."

Prions Infectious agents composed of only proteins.

Prodromal An early symptom of a disease.

Prodrome A symptom indicating the onset of a disease.

Prodrug A substance that is inactive when it is given and is converted to an active form within the body.

Profession A group of similar jobs or fields of interest that involve a responsibility to serve the public and require mastery of specific knowledge and specialized skills.

Professional A person who has special knowledge and skills and conforms to high standards of conduct and performance.

Professional malpractice A type of tort case addressing whether a professional person failed to act as a reasonably prudent and careful person with similar training would act under similar circumstances.

Professionalism Following the standards of conduct and performance for a profession.

Progesterone A female hormone secreted after ovulation has occurred that causes changes in the lining of the uterus necessary for successful implantation of a fertilized egg.

Prokaryotes One of the kingdoms of cells; simpler in structure and found in lower life forms such as bacteria.

Proliferative phase Portion of the menstrual cycle in which the endometrial lining grows under the influence of estrogen.

Prone Position in which the patient is lying on his or her stomach (face down).

Proprioception Ability to sense the orientation, location, and movement of the body's parts relative to other body parts.

Prospective medical direction Physician participation in the development of EMS protocols and procedures, and participation in the education and testing of EMS professionals; a type of offline medical direction.

Prostaglandins A class of fatty acids that has many of the properties of hormones.

Prostate Glandular tissue that produces prostatic fluid and muscular portion that contracts during ejaculation to prevent urine flow; dorsal to the symphysis pubis and the base of the urinary bladder.

Protein Any one of a number of large molecules composed of amino acids that form the structural components of cells or carry out biochemical functions.

Protocols A set of treatment guidelines written for the paramedic to follow. A written form of medical direction.

Protoxin A substance converted to a toxin through a biochemical process in the body; would be harmless if they were not converted (e.g., methanol and ethylene glycol).

Proximal A position nearer to the attachment of a limb to the trunk.

Pruritus Itching of the skin.

Psoriasis A common chronic skin disorder characterized by erythematous papules and plaques with a silver scale.

Psychological abuse The verbal or psychological misuse of another person, including threatening, name calling, ignoring, shaming unfairly, shouting, and cursing; mind games are another form of psychological abuse.

Psychomotor Pertaining to motor effects of cerebral or psychic activity.

Psychomotor agitation Excessive motor activity that is usually nonproductive and tedious, resulting from inner tensions (pacing, fidgeting, hand wringing, etc.)

Psychoses A group of mental disorders in which the individual loses contact with reality; psychosis is thought to be related to complex biochemical disease that disorders brain function. Examples include schizophrenia, bipolar disease (also known as *manic-depressive illness*), and organic brain disease.

Psychosis An abnormal state of widespread brain dysfunction characterized by bizarre thought content, typically delusions and hallucinations.

Psychosocial development The social and psychological changes human beings undergo as they grow and age.

Psychosocial factors Life events that affect a person's emotional state, such as marriage, divorce, or death of a loved one.

Public health The discipline that studies the overall health of populations and intervenes on behalf of those populations rather than on behalf of individuals.

Public Safety Answering Point (PSAP) A dispatch center set up to receive and dispatch 9-1-1 calls.

Pull-in point Machinery entanglement hazard created when an operator attempts to remove material being pulled into a machine.

Pulmonary abscess A collection of pus within the lung itself.

Pulmonary arteries Left and right pulmonary arteries supplying the lungs.

Pulmonary bleb Cavity in the lung much like a balloon; may rupture to create a pneumothorax.

Pulmonary circulation Blood from the right ventricle is pumped directly to the lungs for oxygenation through the pulmonary trunk; blood becomes oxygenated and is then delivered through the pulmonary arteries for the left atrium.

Pulmonary edema A buildup of fluid in the lungs, usually a complication of left ventricular fibrillation.

Pulmonary embolism Movement of a clot into the pulmonary circulation.

Pulmonary embolus A blood clot that has lodged in the pulmonary artery, causing shortness of breath and hypoxia.

Pulmonary trunk Vessels that deliver blood from the right ventricle of the heart to the lungs for oxygenation.

Pulmonary veins Vessels that return blood to the left atrium of the heart.

Pulmonic valve Right semilunar valve; separates the right ventricle and the pulmonary trunk.

Pulp Center of a tooth that contains nerves, blood vessels, and connective tissue.

Pulse deficit A difference between the apical pulse and the peripheral pulse rates.

Pulse generator Power source that houses the battery and controls for regulating a pacemaker.

Pulse oximetry A noninvasive method of measuring the percentage of oxygen-bound hemoglobin.

Pulse pressure The difference between the systolic and diastolic blood pressures.

Pulseless electrical activity (PEA) Organized electrical activity observed on a cardiac monitor (other than ventricular tachycardia) without the patient having a palpable pulse.

Pulsus alternans A beat-to-beat difference in the strength of a pulse (also called *mechanical alternans*).

Pulsus paradoxus A fall in systolic blood pressure of more than 10 mm Hg during inspiration (also called *paradoxic pulse*).

Pupil Central opening in the iris.

Purkinje fibers Fibers found in both ventricles that conduct an electrical impulse through the heart.

Purpura Reddish-purple nonblanchable discolorations greater than 0.5 cm in diameter; large purpura are called ecchymoses.

Pustule A lesion that contains purulent material.

Pyelonephritis Infection of the kidney.

Pyrogens Substances, such as endotoxins from certain bacteria, that stimulate the body to produce a fever.

Pyrophorics Substances that form self-ignitable flammable vapors when in contact with air.

QRS complex Several waveforms (Q wave, R wave, and S wave) that represent the spread of an electrical impulse through the ventricles (ventricular depolarization).

Quadriplegia Paralysis affecting all four extremities.

Quality assurance Programs designed to achieve a desired level of care.

Quality improvement Programs designed to improve the level of care; commonly driven by quality assurance.

Quality improvement unit (QIU) Trained and certified quality specialists who have the knowledge and skills to measure dispatcher performance against established standards accurately and consistently.

Quarantine The seclusion of groups of exposed but asymptomatic individuals for monitoring.

Quick response unit A type of responder with paramedic-level skills but no transport capability.

R wave On an EGG, the first positive deflection in the QRS complex, representing ventricular depolarization.

Raccoon eyes Bruising around the orbits of the eyes.

Racing thoughts The subjective feeling that one's thoughts are moving so fast that one cannot keep up; often seen during manic episodes.

Radio frequency Channel that allows communication from one specific user to another. For simple communication, both users must be on the same frequency or channel.

Radioactive The ability to emit ionizing radioactive energy.

Radioactive substances Any material or combination of materials that spontaneously emit ionizing radiation and have a specific activity greater than 0.002 mcCi/g (e.g., plutonium, cobalt, uranium 235, radioactive waste).

Radioactivity The spontaneous disintegration of unstable nuclei accompanied by the emission of nuclear radiation.

Range of motion The full and natural range of a joint's movement.

Rapid medical assessment A quick head-to-toe assessment of a medical patient who is unresponsive or has an altered mental status.

Rapid sequence intubation (RSI) The use of medications to sedate and paralyze a patient to achieve endotracheal intubation rapidly.

Rapid trauma assessment A quick head-to-toe assessment of a trauma patient with a significant mechanism of injury.

Rattles (rhonchi) Attributable to inflammation and mucus or fluid in the larger airway passages; descriptive of airway congestion heard on inspiration. Rhonchi are commonly associated with bronchitis or pneumonia.

Red blood cell count The number of red blood cells per liter of blood.

Rebound tenderness Discomfort experienced by the patient that occurs when the pressure from palpation is released.

Receptor A molecule, such as a protein, found inside or on the surface of a cell that binds to a specific substance (such as hormones, antigens, drugs, or neurotransmitters) and causes a specific physiologic effect in the cell.

Reciprocal change Mirror image ECG changes seen in the wall of the heart opposite the location of an infarction.

Reciprocity The ability for an EMS professional to use his or her certification or license to be able to practice in a different state.

Recompression A method used to treat divers with certain diving disorders, such as decompression sickness.

Rectal The drug administration route for suppositories; the drug is placed into the rectum (colon) and is absorbed into the venous circulation.

Rectum End of the sigmoid colon; feces are further compacted into waste here.

Reentry Spread of an impulse through tissue already stimulated by that same impulse.

Referred pain Pain felt at a site distant to the organ of origin.

Reflection Echoing the patient's message using your own words.

Reflection on actions A final step that may involve a personal reflection or a run critique; in certain instances this may be done formally, but in most instances it is accomplished informally.

Refractoriness Period of recovery that cells need after being discharged before they are able to respond to a stimulus.

Refresher education The process of refreshing information and skills previously learned.

Registration The process of entering an individual's name and essential information into a record as a means of verifying initial certification and monitoring recertification.

Regurgitation Backward flow of blood through a valve during ventricular contraction of the heart.

Rejection In terms of organ transplantation, the process by which the body uses its immune system to identify a transplanted organ and kill it; the medical management of posttransplant patients is largely directed at preventing rejection.

Relative refractory period Corresponds with the downslope of the T wave; cardiac cells can be stimulated to depolarize if the stimulus is strong enough.

Relief medic Emergency medical technician who has obtained additional training and certification in disaster and relief medical operations.

Rem Roentgen equivalent man.

Renal calculi Kidney stones formed by substances such as calcium, uric acid, or cystine.

Renal corpuscle Large terminal end of the nephron.

Renal insufficiency A decrease in renal function to approximately 25% of normal.

Renal pyramids Number of divisions in the kidney.

Repeater A system that receives transmissions from a low-wattage radio and rebroadcasts the signal at a higher wattage to the dispatch center.

Reperfusion phenomenon Series of events that result from the reperfusion of tissue damaged in a crush injury or tissue that is profoundly hypoxic; can lead to crush syndrome (rhabdomyolysis).

Repolarization Movement of ions across a cell membrane in which the inside of the cell is restored to its negative charge.

Res ipsa loquitur Latin phrase meaning "the thing speaks for itself." In negligence cases, this doctrine can be imposed when the plaintiff cannot prove all four components of negligence, but the injury itself would not have occurred without negligence (e.g., a sponge left in a patient after surgery).

Rescue The act of delivery from danger or entrapment.

Residual volume After a maximal forced exhalation, the amount of air remaining in the lungs and airway passages not able to be expelled.

Resistance The amount of weight moved or lifted during isotonic exercise. Also the ability of the body to defend itself against disease-causing microorganisms.

Resistance stage The stage of the stress response in which the specific stimulus no longer elicits an alarm reaction.

Respiration The exchange of gases between a living organism and its environment.

Respiratory arrest Absence of breathing.

Respiratory distress Increased work of breathing (ventilatory effort).

Respiratory failure A clinical condition in which there is inadequate blood oxygenation and/or ventilation to meet the metabolic demands of the body tissues.

Respiratory membrane Where gas exchange takes place; oxygen is picked up in the bloodstream and carbon dioxide is eliminated through the lungs.

Respiratory syncytial virus A virus linked to bronchiolitis in infants and children.

Respiratory tract Passages to move air to and from the exchange surfaces.

Respondeat superior Latin phrase meaning "let the master answer." Under this legal doctrine, an employer is liable for the acts of employees within their scope of employment.

Response area The geographic area assigned to an emergency vehicle for responding to the sick and injured.

Response assignment plan An approved, consistent plan for responding to each call type.

Response mode A type of response, either with or without lights and sirens use.

Response time The time from when the call is received until the paramedics arrive at the scene.

Restraint Any mechanism that physically restricts an individual's freedom of movement, physical activity, or normal access to his or her body.

Restraint asphyxia Suffocation of a patient stemming from an inability to expand the chest cavity during inspiration because of restraint and immobilization.

Reticular activating system Group of specialized neurons in the brainstem; involved in sleep and wake cycles; maintains consciousness.

Reticular cells The cells forming the reticular fibers of connective tissue; those forming the framework of lymph nodes, bone marrow, and spleen are part of the reticuloendothelial system and under appropriate stimulation may differentiate into macrophages.

Reticular dermis Section of the dermis composed of larger and denser collagen fibers; provides most of the skin's elasticity and strength. This layer contains most of the skin structures located within the dermis.

Reticular formation A cloud of neurons in the brainstem and midbrain responsible for maintaining consciousness.

Retina Outer pigmented area and inner sensory layer that responds to light.

Retinal detachment A condition in which the retina is lifted or pulled from its normal position, resulting in a loss of vision.

Retractions Use of accessory muscles of respiration to assist in ventilation during times of distress; sinking in of the soft tissues above the sternum or clavicle or between or below the ribs during inhalation.

Retreat Leaving the scene when danger is observed or when violence or indicators of violence are displayed; requires immediate and decisive action.

Retrograde Moving backward or moving in the opposite direction to that which is considered normal.

Retrograde amnesia The inability to remember events or recall memories from before an event in which the head was struck.

Retroperitoneal Abdominopelvic organs found behind the peritoneum.

Retrospective medical direction Physician review of prehospital care reports and participation in the quality improvement process; a type of offline medical direction.

Reuptake Absorption of neurotransmitters from the synapse into the presynaptic neuron to be reused or destroyed.

Review of systems A review of symptoms for each organ system.

Rhabdomyolysis Complex series of events that occur in patients with severe muscle injury (e.g., crush injuries); destruction of the muscle tissues results in a release of cellular material and acidosis that can lead to acute renal failure.

Rheumatoid arthritis (RA) A painful, disabling disease in which the body's immune system attacks the joints.

Rhinitis Inflammation of the mucous membranes of the nose, usually accompanied by swelling of the mucosa and a nasal discharge.

Rhinorrhea Persistent discharge of fluid (such as blood or cerebrospinal fluid) from the nose.

Rhonchi Rattling or rumbling in the lungs.

Ribonucleic acid (RNA) Specialized structures within the cell that carry genetic material for reproduction.

Ribosome Substance in organelle where new protein is synthesized; forms the framework for the genetic blueprint.

Right A position toward the right side of the body.

Right block or left block Terms describing a responding vehicle arriving on scene and turning at a right or left angle. In this block position, the emergency vehicle acts as a physical barrier between the crash scene work area and approaching traffic.

Right coronary artery Blood vessel that provides oxygenated blood to the right side of the heart muscle.

Risk factors Traits and lifestyle habits that may increase a person's chance of developing a disease.

Risus sardonicus Distorted grinning expression caused by involuntary contraction of the facial muscles.

Roentgens Denote ionizing radiation passing through air.

Rolling the dash Rescue tasks involving strategic cuts to the firewall structure followed by pushing, spreading, or even pulling equipment to move the dash, firewall, steering wheel, column, and pedals away from front seat occupants.

Rollover protective structure A structure mounted on a tractor designed to support the weight of the tractor if an overturn occurs; if a tractor has this structure and the operator wears a seat belt, the operator will stay in the safety zone if the tractor overturns.

Root word In medical terminology, the part of the word that gives the primary meaning.

Rotor-wing aircraft Helicopter that can be used for hospital-to-hospital and scene-to-hospital transports; usually travels a shorter distance and is used in the prehospital setting for certain types of transport.

Routes of administration Various methods of giving drugs, including oral, enteral, parenteral, and inhalational.

Rovsing's sign Pain in the right lower quadrant elicited by palpation of the abdomen in the left lower quadrant.

S1 The sound of the tricuspid and mitral valves closing.

S2 The sound of the closing of the pulmonary and aortic valves.

Sacrum (sacral vertebrae) A heavy, large bone at the base of the spinal cord between the lumbar vertebrae and the coccyx. Roughly triangular in shape, it comprises the back of the pelvis and is made of the five sacral vertebrae fused together.

Safety officer The person responsible for ensuring that no unsafe acts occur during the emergency incident.

Sagittal plane Imaginary straight line that runs vertically through the middle of the body, creating right and left halves.

Saliva Mucus that lubricates material like food that is placed in it; enzymes begin the digestive process of starchy material.

Salivary glands Located in the oral cavity; produce saliva.

Saponification A form of necrosis in which fatty acids combine with certain electrolytes to form soaps.

Sarin A nerve agent.

Saturation of peripheral oxygen The percentage of hemoglobin saturated with oxygen (SpO_2).

Scabies A contagious skin disease of the epidermis marked by itching and small raised red spots caused by the itch mite *(Sarcoptes scabiei).*

Scale Thick stratum corneum that results from hyperproliferation or increased cohesion of keratinocytes (can include eczema or psoriasis).

Scar A collection of new connective tissue; may be hypertrophic or atrophic and implies dermoepidermal damage.

Schizophrenia A group of disorders characterized by psychotic symptoms, thought disorder, and negative symptoms (social isolation and withdrawal); types include paranoid, disorganized, and catatonic.

Sciatica Pain in the lumbar back and leg caused by irritation and impingement of the sciatic nerve, usually from a herniated disc.

Sclera Firm, opaque, white outer layer of the eye; helps maintain the shape of the eye.

Scope of practice A predefined set of skills, interventions, or other activities that the paramedic is legally authorized to perform when necessary; usually set by state law or regulation and local medical direction.

Scrotum Loose layer of connective tissue that support the testes.

Sebaceous glands Found in the dermis; secrete oil (sebum) in the shaft of the hair follicle and the skin.

Sebum Oil secreted by the sebaceous glands in the shaft of the hair follicle and the skin; prevents excessive drying of the skin and hair; also protects from some forms of bacteria.

Second messenger A molecule that relays signals from a receptor on the surface of a cell to target molecules in the cell's nucleus or internal fluid where a physiologic action is to take place; also called a *biochemical messenger.*

Secondary apnea When asphyxia is prolonged, a period of deep, gasping respirations with a simultaneous fall in blood pressure and heart rate; gasping becomes weaker and slower and then ceases.

Secondary blast injury Injuries caused by shrapnel from the fragments of an explosive device and from things that have been attached to it.

Secondary contamination The risk of another person or healthcare provider becoming contaminated with a hazardous material by contact with a contaminated victim.

Secondary cord injury A spinal cord injury that develops over time after a traumatic injury to the spinal column or the blood vessels that supply the spinal cord with blood. Generally caused by ischemia, swelling, or compression.

Secondary device An explosive, chemical, or biologic device hidden at the scene of an emergency and set to detonate or release its agent after emergency response personnel are on scene.

Secondary hypertension High blood pressure that has an identifiable cause, such as medications or an underlying disease or condition.

Secondary injury prevention Preventing further injury from an event that has already occurred.

Secondary skin lesion Any lesion that has been altered by scratching, scrubbing, or other types of trauma.

Secondary triage Conducted after the primary search; determines the order of treatment and transport of the remaining patients.

Secondary tumor A tumor that has spread from its original location (e.g., lung tumor that spreads to brain); also called *metastasis.*

Secretion Release of water, acids, enzymes, and buffers that aid in the breakdown and digestion of food in the digestive tract.

Secretory phase Portion of the menstrual cycle in which the corpus luteum secretes progesterone to maintain the endometrial lining in case of fertilization.

Sedative-hypnotics Prescription central nervous system depressant drugs that cause powerful relaxation and euphoria when abused; typically barbiturates and benzodiazepines.

Segment Line between waveforms; named by the waveform that precedes and follows it.

Seizure A temporary alteration in behavior or consciousness caused by abnormal electrical activity of one or more groups of neurons in the brain.

Self-injury An unhealthy coping mechanism involving intentionally injuring one's own body, often through cutting or burning oneself to relieve emotional tension; also known as *self-mutilation.*

Sellick maneuver Technique used to compress the cricoid cartilage against the cervical vertebrae, causing occlusion of the esophagus, thereby reducing the risk of aspiration; cricoid pressure.

Semicircular canals Three bony fluid-filled loops in the internal ear; involved in balance of the body.

Semilunar (SL) valves Valves shaped like half moons that separate the ventricles from the aorta and pulmonary artery.

Seminal fluid Liquid produced in the seminal vesicles.

Seminal vesicles Ducts that produce seminal fluids.

Sensing Ability of a pacemaker to recognize and respond to intrinsic electrical activity.

Sensorineural hearing loss A type of deafness that occurs when the tiny hair cells in the cochlea are damaged or destroyed. In addition, damage to the auditory nerve prevents sounds from being transmitted from the cochlea to the brain.

Sensory cortex Area of brain tissue on the frontal lobe responsible for receiving sensory information from different parts of the body.

Sepsis Pathologic state, usually accompanied by fever, resulting from the presence of microorganisms or their poisonous products in the bloodstream; commonly called *blood poisoning*.

Septic abortion An abortion associated with intrauterine infection.

Septic arthritis Invasion of microorganisms into a joint space, causing infection of the joint.

Septic shock Sepsis with hypotension, despite adequate fluid resuscitation, along with the presence of perfusion abnormalities that may include lactic acidosis, decreased urine output, and a sudden change in mental status.

Septicemia A serious medical condition characterized by vasodilation that leads to hypotension, tissue hypoxia, and eventually shock; usually caused by gram-negative bacteria; diagnosed by blood tests called cultures.

Septum Tough piece of tissue that divides the left and right halves of the heart.

Serious apnea Cessation of breathing for longer than 20 seconds or any duration if accompanied by cyanosis and sinus bradycardia.

Serosanguineous discharge Blood and fluid discharged from the body.

Serous membrane Membrane that lines the thoracic, abdominal, and pelvic cavities; composed of the parietal membrane, which adheres to the cavity wall, and the visceral membrane, which adheres to the organ.

Serum base deficit Implies that the blood buffer, bicarbonate, is being used to combat a metabolic acidosis. Metabolic acidosis occurs in the setting of numerous shock states, such as burn shock. This number is reported on a standard blood gas assay and is detected in an arterial or venous blood sample.

Serum lactate Measure in the blood; a byproduct of anaerobic metabolism. As such, it is a good measure of end organ and cellular perfusion in shock states. Elevated serum lactate levels, or lactic acidemia, implies that cells, tissues, or organs are not receiving adequate oxygen to carry out their metabolic activities.

Sesamoid bones Specialized bones found within tendons where they cross a joint; designed to protect the joint (e.g., the patella [kneecap]).

Severe sepsis Sepsis associated with organ dysfunction, shock, or hypotension.

Sexual abuse Child sexual abuse includes a range of behaviors such as oral, anal, or genital penile penetration; anal or genital digital or other penetration; genital contact with no intrusion; fondling of a child's breasts or buttocks; indecent exposure; inadequate or inappropriate supervision of a child's voluntary sexual activities; and use of a child in prostitution, pornography, Internet crimes, or other sexually exploitative activities.

Sexual assault Sexually explicit conduct used as an expression of interpersonal violence against another individual; nonconsenting sexual acts achieved through power and control.

Shaft The length of a needle; the needle shaft connects to the hub. Also called the *cannula*.

Shear points Hazardous machinery locations created when the edges of two objects are moved toward or next to one another closely enough to cut a relatively soft material.

Shingles Infection of a nerve, often by the herpes zoster virus, causing severe pain and a rash along a unilateral dermatome.

Shock Inadequate systemic perfusion that results from the failure of the cardiovascular system to deliver sufficient oxygen and nutrients to sustain vital organ function.

Short bones Specialized bones of the skeleton designed for compactness and strength, often with limited movement (e.g., bones of the wrist [carpals])

Short haul The transport of one or more people externally suspended below a helicopter.

Shoulder dystocia Impaction of a newborn's anterior shoulder underneath the mother's pubic bone, slowing or preventing delivery.

Shunt Insertion of catheters into an artery and a vein from outside the body. Most shunts are located on the forearm. When not in use to dialize a patient, the catheters are connected to each other with clear tubing, allowing the continuous flow of blood from artery to vein, then covered with self-adhering roller gauze for protection.

Side effect An effect of a drug other than the one for which it was given; may or may not be harmful.

Side impact airbags Deployable airbags located inside any or all vehicle doors, front and rear outboard seatbacks, as well as along all or a portion of the roof line.

Sighing Involuntary and periodic slow, deep breath followed by a prolonged expiratory phase. Occurring approximately once per minute, the act of sighing is thought to open atelectatic (collapsed) alveoli.

Sigmoid colon Part of the large intestine.

Signs and symptoms Signs are a medical or trauma condition of the patient that can be seen, heard, smelled, measured, or felt during an examination. Symptoms are conditions described by the patient, such as shortness of breath, or pieces of information bystanders tell you about the patient's chief complaint.

Silo gas The gases produced from the fermentation of plant material inside a silo.

Simple asphyxiants Inert gases and vapors that displace oxygen in inspired air (e.g., carbon dioxide, nitrogen).

Simple partial seizure A seizure affecting only one part of the brain without an alteration in consciousness.

Simple pneumothorax Injury to the thoracic cavity in which a lung is ruptured, allowing air into the space between the chest wall and the lungs.

Simplex A system that allows only one-at-a-time communication. The transmission cannot be interrupted; both operators use the same frequency.

Singular command Command type involving one agency.

Sinoatrial node Pacemaker site of the heart; where impulse formation begins in the heart.

Sinus block (barosinusitis) A condition of acute or chronic inflammation of one or more of the paranasal sinuses; produced by a negative pressure difference between the air in the sinuses and the surrounding atmospheric air.

Sinus rhythm A normal heart rhythm.

Sinuses Cavities within the bones of the skull that connect to the nasal cavity.

Situational awareness The state of being aware of everything occurring in the surrounding environment and the relative importance of all these events.

Size-up The art of assessing conditions that exist or can potentially exist at an incident scene.

Skeletal muscles Muscles that affect movement of the skeleton, usually by voluntary contractions.

Skin grafting Transplantation of skin, either from the same person or from a cadaver, to the site of a wound, such as a burn.

Skin turgor The elasticity of the skin; good skin turgor returns the skin's natural shape within 2 seconds.

Slander False statements spoken about a person that blacken the person's character or injure his or her reputation.

Slipped capital femoral epiphysis A disease in which a posterior displacement of the growth plate of the femur occurs (the epiphysis).

SLUDGEM Mnemonic for ***s***alivation, ***l***acrimation, ***u***rination, ***d***efecation, ***g***astrointestinal pain, ***e***mesis, and ***m***iosis.

Smallpox A disease caused by variola viruses, which are members of the Orthopoxvirus family; eradicated in the 1970s but still remains a threat as a bioterrorism agent.

Sneezing Occurs from nasal irritation and allows clearance of the nose.

Sniffing position Neck flexion at the fifth and sixth cervical vertebrae, with the head extended at the first and second cervical vertebrae. This position aligns the axes of the mouth, pharynx, and trachea, opening the airway and increasing airflow.

Snoring Noisy breathing through the mouth and nose during sleep; caused by air passing through a narrowed upper airway.

Social distance The acceptable distance between strangers used for impersonal business transactions. In the United States, social distance is 4 to 12 feet.

Sodium bicarbonate Neutralizes hydrochloric acid from the stomach.

Solid organ An organ (a part of the body or group of tissues that performs a specific function) without any channel or cavity within it; examples include the kidneys, pancreas, liver, and spleen.

Solubility Pertaining to the ease with which a drug can dissolve.

Solution A medication dissolved in a liquid, often water.

Soman A G nerve agent. The G agents tend to be nonpersistent, volatile agents.

Somatic Portion of the peripheral nervous system that carries impulses to and from the skin and musculature; responsible for voluntary muscle control.

Somatic delusions False perceptions of the appearance or functioning of one's own body.

Somatic nervous system Division of the peripheral nervous system whose motor nerves control movement of voluntary muscles.

Somatic pain Pain that arises from either the cutaneous tissues of the body's surface or deep tissues of the body, such as musculoskeletal tissue or the parietal peritoneum.

Somatoform disorders A group of disorders characterized by the manifestation of psychological problems as physical symptoms; this includes conversion disorder, hypochondriasis, somatization disorder, and body dysmorphic disorder.

Sore throat Any inflammation of the larynx, pharynx, or tonsils.

Space blanket A blanket resembling aluminum foil used to help the patient maintain body temperature.

Space-occupying lesion A mass, such as a tumor or blood collection, within a contained body space, such as the skull.

Spacer A hollow plastic tube that attaches to the metered-dose inhaler on one end and has a mouthpiece on the other; sometimes called a *holding chamber*.

Span of control The amount of resources that one person can effectively manage.

Special needs Conditions with the potential to interfere with usual growth and development;

may involve physical disabilities, developmental disabilities, chronic illnesses, and forms of technologic support.

Specialty center A hospital that has met criteria to offer special care as a burn center, level I trauma center, stroke center, or pediatric center.

Specific gravity The ratio of a liquid's weight compared with an equal volume of water (which has a constant value of 1); materials with a specific gravity of less than 1.0 float on water and materials with a specific gravity greater than 1.0 sink.

Sperm Mucus-type secretion made of prostatic fluid and spermatozoa.

Spermatic cord Nerves, blood vessels, and smooth muscle that surround the vas (ductus) deferens.

Spermatocele Benign accumulation of sperm at the epididymis presenting as a firm mass.

Spermatogenesis Spermatozoa formation.

Spermatozoa Product of the male reproductive system.

Sphincters Smooth muscles that regulate flow through the capillary beds.

Spina bifida (SB) A neural tube defect that affects the back portion of the vertebrae, which fail to close, usually in the area of the lower back; meninges, the spinal cord, or both may protrude through this opening.

Spina bifida occulta Mildest form of spina bifida in which the spinal cord is intact but one or more vertebrae fail to close in the lumbosacral area.

Spinal cord Long stalk of nerve tissue that is the interface between the brain and the body; extends from the foramen magnum to the lumbar spine and contains the main reflex centers of the body.

Spinal cord injury (SCI) An injury to the spinal cord that results from trauma; usually a permanent injury.

Spinal cord injury without radiological abnormality A spinal cord injury not detected on a standard radiograph.

Spinal nerves Paired nerves that originate from the spinal cord and exit the spine on either side between vertebrae; each has a sensory root and a motor root.

Spinal shock Shock with hypotension caused by an injury to the spinal cord.

Spirit A medication that contains volatile aromatic substances.

Split-thickness skin graft A skin graft in which only a fraction of the thickness of the natural dermis is taken.

Spontaneous abortion See *Miscarriage.*

Spontaneous bacterial peritonitis (SBP) Infection of cirrhotic fluid in the abdominal cavity.

Spontaneous pneumothorax Pneumothorax occurring without trauma, usually by rupture of a pulmonary bleb.

Sprain An injury to a ligament that results when the ligament is overstretched, leading to tearing or complete disruption of the ligament.

Stagnant phase Vascular response in shock when precapillary sphincters open, allowing the capillary beds to engorge with fluid; follows the ischemic phase.

Stair chair A collapsible, portable chair with handles on the front and back used to carry patients in sitting position down stairs.

Standard of care Conduct exercising the degree of care, skill, and judgment that would be expected under like or similar circumstances by a similarly trained, reasonable paramedic in the same scenario.

Standard operating procedures (SOPs) An organized set of guidelines distributed across the organization.

Standing orders Written instructions that authorize EMS personnel to perform certain medical interventions before establishing direct communication with a physician.

Standard precautions Infection control practices in healthcare designed to be observed with every patient and procedure and prevent the exposure to bloodborne pathogens.

Stapes The stirrup-shaped bone that links the middle ear to the inner ear; connects to the malleus and incus.

Status asthmaticus Condition of severe asthma that is minimally responsive to therapy; a serious condition.

Status epilepticus Any prolonged series of similar seizures without return to full consciousness between them.

Statute A law passed by a legislature.

Statute of limitations A law that sets the time limits within which parties must take action to enforce their rights.

Statutory law Statutes and ordinances enacted by Congress, state legislatures, and city councils.

Steady state An evenly distributed concentration of a drug in the plasma.

Stellate laceration A laceration with jagged margins.

Stem cells Formative cells whose daughter cells may give rise to other cell types.

Stenosis Abnormal constriction or narrowing of a structure.

Stereotyping The attribution of some trait or characteristic to one person on the basis of the interviewer's preconceived notions about a general class of people of similar characteristics.

Sterile Free of any living organism.

Sterilization Process that makes an object free of all forms of life (e.g., bacteria) by using extreme heat or certain chemicals.

Sterilize To kill all microorganisms.

Stimuli Anything that excites or incites an organism or part to function, become active, or respond.

Stomach Organ located at the inferior end of the esophagus; large storage vessel surrounded by multiple layers of smooth muscle; cells within it produce acid.

Stored energy Any energy (mechanical, electrical, hydraulic, compressed air, etc.) that has the potential of being released either intentionally or inadvertently, causing further injury or problems.

Strain An injury to a muscle that results when the muscle is overstretched, leading to tearing of the individual muscle fibers.

Strainer A water hazard formed by an object or structure in the current that allows water to flow but that strains out large objects, such as boats and people.

Strangulation Compression of the vessels that carry blood, leading to ischemia.

Stratum corneum Outer layer of the epidermis where skin cells are shed.

Stress Mental, emotional, or physical pressure, strain, or tension resulting from stimuli.

Stressor A stimulus that produces stress.

Stricture A specific form of narrowing, usually from scar tissue formation.

Stridor A harsh, high-pitched sound heard on inspiration associated with upper airway obstruction; often described as a high-pitched crowing or "seal-bark" sound.

Stroke volume Amount of blood ejected by either ventricle during one contraction; can be calculated as cardiac output divided by heart rate.

Struck-by A situation in which a responder, working in or near moving traffic, is struck, injured, or killed by traffic passing the incident scene.

Stye An external hordeolum.

Stylet A relatively stiff but flexible metal rod covered by plastic and inserted into an endotracheal tube; used for maintaining the shape of the relatively pliant tube and "steering" it into position.

Subarachnoid hemorrhage Bleeding from the arteries between the arachnoid membrane and the pia mater that occurs suddenly and often is fatal.

Subcutaneous (Sub-Q) Injection of medication in a liquid form underneath the skin into the subcutaneous tissue.

Subcutaneous emphysema Air entrapped beneath the skin, typically caused by rupture of a structure containing air; feels like crackling when palpated.

Subcutaneous tissue Thick layer of connective tissue found between the layers of the skin; composed of adipose tissue and areolar tissue; insulates, protects, and stores energy (in the form of fat).

Subdural hematoma A collection of blood in the subdural space, which is between the dura mater and arachnoid layer of the meninges.

Subdural space Area below the dura mater; contains large venous vessels, drains, and a small amount of serous fluid.

Subjective information Information told to the paramedic.

Sublingual Medication placed under the tongue.

Sucking chest wound Open thoracic injury characterized by air being pulled into and pushed out of the wound during respiration.

Sudden cardiac death (SCD) An unexpected death from a cardiac cause that either occurs immediately or within 1 hour of the onset of symptoms.

Suffix Added to the end of a root word to change the meaning; usually identifies the condition of the root word.

Suicide The act of ending one's own life.

Sulfur mustard The most well known and commonly used of the vesicants.

Summarization Briefly reviewing the interview and your conclusions.

Summation The combined effects of two or more drugs equaling the sum of each of their effects.

Superficial burn A burn with a pink appearance that does not exhibit blister formation; painful both with and without tactile stimulation (e.g., sunburn); also known as a *first-degree burn.*

Superficial fascia Connective tissue that contains the subcutaneous fat cells.

Superficial partial-thickness burn Burns involving the more superficial dermis. These burns have a moist, pink appearance, and when lightly touched, are painful and sensate. Blood vessels, hair shafts, nerves, and glands may be injured, but not to the extent that regeneration cannot take place.

Superior Situated above or higher than a point of reference in the anatomic position; top.

Superior vena cava Vessel that returns venous blood from the upper part of the body to the right atrium of the heart.

Supernormal period Period during the cardiac cycle when a weaker than normal stimulus can cause cardiac cells to depolarize; extends from the end of phase 3 to the beginning of phase 4 of the cardiac action potential.

Supine Position in which the patient is lying on his or her back (face up).

Supine hypotensive syndrome A fall in the pregnant patient's blood pressure when she is placed supine; caused by the developing fetus and uterus pressing against the inferior vena cava.

Suppository Medications combined to make them a solid at room temperature; when placed in a body opening such as the rectum, vagina, or urethra, they dissolve because of the increase in body temperature and are absorbed through the surrounding mucosa.

Supraglottic Any airway structure above the vocal cords (e.g., the epiglottis).

Suprasternal notch A depression easily felt at the base of the anterior aspect of the neck, just above the angle of Louis.

Supraventricular Originating from a site above the bifurcation of the bundle of His, such as the sinoatrial node, atria, or atrioventricular junction.

Supraventricular dysrhythmias Rhythms that begin in the sinoatrial node, atrial tissue, or the atrioventricular junction.

Surfactant Specialized cells within each alveolus that keep it from collapsing when little or no air is inside.

Surge capacity The ability to expand care based on a sudden mass casualty incident; developed in the emergency management plan.

Susceptibility Vulnerability or weakness; the opposite of resistance.

Suspension Medication suspended in a liquid, such as an oral antibiotic.

Sutures Seams between flat bones.

Sweat glands Odor-forming glands in the body; two types are merocrine and apocrine.

Swimmer's ear See *Otitis externa.*

Sympathetic division of the autonomic nervous system Division of the autonomic nervous system that, when stimulated, provides a fight-or-flight response, including increased heart rate, pupil dilation, bronchodilation, and the shunting of blood to the muscles.

Sympathetic nervous system Division of the autonomic nervous system that prepares the body for stress or the classic fight-or-flight response.

Sympatholytics Drugs that block or inhibit adrenergic receptors.

Sympathomimetics Drugs that mimic the sympathetic division of the autonomic nervous system.

Sympathy Sharing the patient's feelings or emotional state in relation to an illness.

Symphysis Cartilaginous joint; unites two bones by means of fibrocartilage.

Synapse Microscopic space at the neuroeffector junction that neurotransmitters cross to stimulate target tissues.

Synaptic communication Method of intercellular communication in which neural cells communicate to adjacent neural cells by using neurotransmitters.

Synaptic junction The open space in which neurotransmitters traverse to reach a receptor.

Synchondroses Cartilaginous joint; unites the bones by means of hyaline cartilage.

Synchronized intermittent mandatory ventilation (SIMV) A ventilator setting that generally allows the patient to inspire at will and to the depth that he or she desires.

Syncope A transient loss of consciousness and inability to maintain postural tone, typically resulting in a ground-level fall; also know as *passing out* or *fainting.*

Syndesmosis Joint in which the bones are united by fibrous, connective tissue forming an intraosseous membrane or ligament.

Synergism The interaction of drugs such that the total effect is greater than the sum of the individual effects.

Synonym A root word, prefix, or suffix that has the same or almost the same meaning as another word, prefix, or suffix.

Synovial fluid Fluid located within the joint capsules of synovial joints; provides lubrication and cushioning during manipulation of the joint.

Synovial joint Freely movable; enclosed by a capsule and synovial membrane.

Synovium Soft tissue that lines the noncartilaginous surfaces of a joint.

Synthetic drugs Drugs chemically developed in a laboratory; also called *manufactured drugs.*

Syrup A medication dissolved in water with sugar or a sugar substitute to disguise taste.

System At least two kinds of organs organized to perform a more complex task than can a single organ.

System Status Management The dynamic process of staffing, stationing, and moving ambulances based on projected call volumes; also called *flexible deployment.*

Systemic damage Damage remote to the site of exposure or absorption.

Systemic effect Drug action throughout the body.

Systemic inflammatory response syndrome A response to infection manifested by a change in two or more of the following: temperature, heart rate, respiratory rate, and white blood cell count.

Systole Contraction of the heart (usually referring to ventricular contraction) during which blood is propelled into the pulmonary artery and aorta; when the term is used without reference to a specific chamber of the heart, the term implies ventricular systole.

Systolic blood pressure The pressure exerted against the walls of the large arteries at the peak of ventricular contraction.

T lymphocytes Cells present in the lymphatic system that mediate cell-mediated immunity (also known as *T cells*).

Tablets Medications that have been pressed into a small form that is easy to swallow. They are a specific shape, color, and may have engraving for identification.

Tachycardia A heart rate grater than 100 beats/min.

Tachyphylaxis The rapidly decreasing response to a drug or physiologically active agent after administration of a few doses; rapid cross-tolerance.

Tachypnea An increased respiratory rate, usually greater than 30 breaths/min.

Tactical EMS EMS personnel specially trained and equipped to provide prehospital emergency care in tactical environments.

Tactical patient care Patient care activities that occur inside the scene perimeter or hot zone.

Tangential thinking A progression of thoughts related to each other but that become less and less related to the original topic.

Tardive dyskinesia A neurologic syndrome caused by the long-term or high-dose use of dopamine agonists, usually antipsychotic medications; characterized by repetitive, involuntary, and purposeless movements such as grimacing, rapid movements of the face, lip smacking, and eye blinking. Symptoms may last for a significant period after removal of the offending agent.

Teachable moment The time just after an injury has occurred when the patient and observers remain acutely aware of what has happened and may be more receptive to learning how the event or illness could have been prevented.

Teamwork The ability to work with others to achieve a common goal.

Teeth Provide mastication of food products in preparation for entry into the stomach.

Telematic A system set up as mayday call reporting, such as On-Star and Tele-aid. This system can send information from an automobile that has been involved in an accident directly to an emergency dispatch center with the exact location and the amount of damage that may have occurred.

Telephone aid Ad-libbed instructions most often used in emergency dispatch centers by dispatchers who have had previous training as paramedics, EMTs, or cardiopulmonary resuscitation providers; strictly relies on the dispatcher's experience and prior knowledge of a particular situation or medical condition and is considered an ineffective form of telephone treatment.

Telson Venom-containing portion of a scorpion's abdomen that is capable of venomous injection into human beings.

Temporal demand Measurement of call demand by hour of the day.

Temporal lobe Cerebrum beneath the temporal bone; area where processing of hearing and language occurs.

Temporal modeling Predicting the times when calls occur.

Tendonitis Inflammation of a tendon, often caused by overuse.

Tendons Tough, fibrous bands of connective tissue that connect muscle to muscle and muscle to bones.

Tension-building phase Period when tension in the relationship is high and heightened anger, blaming, and arguing may occur between the victim and the abuser.

Tension pneumothorax Life-threatening injury in which air enters the space between the lungs and the chest wall but cannot exit. With each breath, the pressure increases until it prevents ventilation and causes death.

Teratogen A drug or agent that is harmful to the development of an embryo or fetus.

Term gestation A gestation equal to or longer than 37 weeks.

Terminal drop A theory that holds that mental and physical functioning decline drastically only in the few years immediately preceding death.

Terminal illness Advanced stage of illness or disease with an unfavorable prognosis and no known cure.

Tertiary blast injury Injuries caused by the patient being thrown like a projectile.

Testes Male reproductive organs suspended within the scrotum.

Testicular torsion Twisting of the spermatic cord inside the scrotum that cuts off the blood supply to the testis.

Testosterone Male hormone secreted within the testes.

Tetany Repeated, prolonged contraction of muscles, especially of the face and limbs.

Tetraplegia Paralysis to all four extremities as a result of a spinal cord injury high in the spine. The injury can either be complete (a complete loss of muscle control and sensation below the injury site) or incomplete (a partial loss of muscle control or sensation below the injury site).

Thalamus Structure located within the limbic system that is the switchboard of the brain, through which almost all signals travel on their way in or out of the brain.

Therapeutic abortion Planned surgical or medical evacuation of the uterus.

Therapeutic dose The dose required to produce a beneficial effect in 50% of the drug-tested population; also called *effective dose*.

Therapeutic index The ratio between the amount of drug required to produce to produce a therapeutic dose and a lethal dose of the same drug. A narrow therapeutic index is dangerous because the possibility of underdosing or overdosing is higher.

Therapeutic threshold The level of a drug that elicits a beneficial physiologic response.

Thermogenesis The process of heat generation.

Thermolysis A chemical process by which heat is dissipated from the body; sometimes results in chemical decomposition.

Thermoreceptor A sensory receptor that responds to heat and cold.

Third space Extravascular and extracellular milieu; also known as the *interstitium*.

Thirst mechanism Sensation activated by cells in the hypothalamus when cells called osmoreceptors detect an imbalance in body water; as the body is replenished by drinking fluid, the osmoreceptors sense a return to baseline and turn off this mechanism.

Thoracic vertebrae A group of 12 vertebrae in the middle of the spinal column that connect to ribs.

Thought blocking A symptom of thought disorder in which a patient is speaking and then stops mid-sentence, unable to remember what he or she was saying and unable to continue.

Thought content The dominant themes and ideas of a patient; may include delusions, hallucinations, and preoccupations.

Threatened abortion Vaginal bleeding or uterine cramping during the first half of pregnancy without cervical dilation.

Threshold limit value The airborne concentrations of a substance; represents conditions under which nearly all workers are believed to be repeatedly exposed day after day without adverse effects.

Thrombocytes One of three formed elements in the blood; also known as *platelets*.

Thrombocytopenia A lower than normal number of platelets circulating in the blood.

Thromboembolism Movement of a clot within the vascular system.

Thrombophlebitis Development of a clot in a vein in which inflammation is present.

Thromboplastin Blood coagulation factor.

Thrombus Blood clot.

Thrush A fungal infection of the mouth.

Thyroid storm Severe form of hyperthyroidism characterized by tachypnea, tachycardia, shock, hyperthermia, and delirium.

Thyrotoxicosis A condition in which the thyroid gland produces excess thyroid hormone; also called *hyperthyroidism* or *Graves' disease*.

Tidal volume The volume of air moved into or out of the lungs during a normal breath; can be indirectly evaluated by observing the rise and fall of the patient's chest and abdomen.

Time on task The average time a unit is committed to manage an incident.

Tincture A medicine consisting of an extract in an alcohol solution (e.g., tincture of iodine, tincture of mercurochrome).

Tinea capitis Located on the head and scalp; appears as a round, scaly area where no hair is growing; diffuse scaling.

Tinea corporis Located on the body; appears annular (e.g. ringworm).

Tinea cruris Located on the groin and genitalia; appears as a sharply demarcated area with elevated scaling, geographic borders.

Tinea manuum Located on the hands; appears as dry, diffuse scaling, usually on the palm.

Tinea pedis Located on the feet; appears as maceration between the toes, scaling on soles or sides of the foot, sometimes vesicles and/or pustules.

Tinea unguium Located on or under fingernails or toenails; appears as dark debris under the nails.

Tinea versicolor Located on the trunk; appears as pink, tan, or white patches with fine, desquamating scale.

Tinnitus A ringing, roaring sound or hissing in the ears that is usually caused by certain medicines or exposure to loud noise.

Tissue A group of cells that are similar in structure and function.

Tocolytic A medication used to slow uterine contractions.

Tolerance Decreasing responsiveness to the effects of a drug; increasingly larger doses are necessary to achieve the effect originally obtained by a smaller dose.

Tongue Muscular organ that provides for the sensation of taste; also directs food material toward the esophagus.

Tonic-clonic seizure Form of generalized seizure with a tonic phase (muscle rigidity) and a clonic phase (muscle tremors).

Topical Medication administered by applying it directly to the skin or mucous membrane.

Tort A wrong committed on the person or property of another.

Total body surface area burned (TBSAB) Used to describe the amount of the body injured by a burn and expressed as a percentage of the entire body surface area.

Total body water (TBW) The total amount of fluid in the body at any given time.

Totally blind Description of someone who has no vision and uses nonvisual media or reads Braille.

Toxic organic dust syndrome A flulike illness caused by the inhalation of grain dust, with symptoms including fever, chest tightness, cough, and muscle aches; inhalation may occur in an agricultural setting or from covering a floor with straw.

Toxicology The study of poisons.

Toxidrome A classification system of toxic syndromes by signs and symptoms.

Toxin A poisonous substance of plant or animal origin.

TP segment Interval on the ECG between two successive PQRST complexes during which electrical activity of the heart is absent; begins with the end of the T wave through the onset of the following P wave and represents the period from the end of ventricular repolarization to the onset of atrial depolarization.

Trachea Air passage that connects the larynx to the lungs.

Tracheal stoma A surgical opening in the anterior neck that extends from the skin surface into the trachea, opening the trachea to the atmosphere.

Tracheitis Inflammation of the mucous membranes of the trachea.

Tracheostomy A surgically created hole in the anterior trachea for breathing.

Tracheoesophageal fistula (TEF) An abnormal opening between the trachea and the esophagus.

Trade name The name given a chemical compound by the company that makes it; also called the *brand name* or *proprietary name*.

Transcellular compartment Compartment classified as extracellular but distinct because it is formed from the transport activities of cells; cerebrospinal fluid, bladder urine, the aqueous humor, and the synovial fluid of the joints are considered transcellular.

Transdermal Through the skin.

Transection A complete cutting (severing) across the spinal cord.

Transient ischemic attack (TIA) Neurologic dysfunction caused by a temporary blockage in blood flow; by definition the symptoms resolve within 24 hours but usually within 1 or 2 hours.

Transient synovitis A nonspecific inflammation of a joint, usually the hip, that affects the synovium and synovial fluid in children.

Transverse colon Part of the large intestine.

Transverse plane Imaginary straight line that divides the body into top (superior) and bottom (inferior) sections; also known as the *horizontal plane.*

Traumatic asphyxia Life-threatening injury in which the thorax is severely crushed, preventing ventilation; typically results in death.

Traumatic iritis An inflammation of the iris caused by blunt trauma to the eye.

Triage Classifying patients based on the severity of illness or injury.

Tricuspid valve Right atrioventricular valve of the heart.

Trigeminal neuralgia Irritation of the seventh cranial nerve (trigeminal nerve), causing episodes of severe, stabbing pain in the face.

Trip audit The review of a prehospital care report written by a paramedic to a peer or a third party.

Tripod position Position used to maintain an open airway that involves sitting upright and leaning forward with the neck slightly extended, chin projected, and mouth open and supported by the arms.

Trismus Spasm of the muscles used for chewing, resulting in limited movement of the mouth because of pain.

Trunking system A system that uses multiple repeaters (five or more) so that the computer can search for an open channel to transmit by.

Tube trailers Trailers that carry multiple cylinders of pressurized gases.

Tuberculosis (TB) A highly contagious bacterial infection known for causing pneumonia and infecting other parts of the body.

Tularemia A disease resulting from infection of *Francisella tularensis;* normally transmitted through handling infected small mammals such as rabbits or rodents or through the bites of ticks, deerflies, or mosquitoes that have fed on infected animals; also known as *rabbit fever* or *deer fly fever.*

Tumor, benign An abnormal growth of cells that is not malignant (i.e., is not known for spreading and growing aggressively).

Tumor, malignant An abnormal growth of cells that is known for being aggressive and spreading to other parts of the body.

Tumor necrosis factor-alpha An inflammatory cytokine released in response to a variety of physical trauma, including burns. In burn injuries, massive quantities are produced by the liver; has been implicated as the causative agent in myocardial depression seen in burns.

Tumor, primary A tumor in the location where it originates (e.g., a primary lung tumor is in the lung).

Tumor, secondary A tumor that has spread from its original location (e.g., lung tumor that spreads to the brain); also called *metastasis.*

Tunica adventitia Outermost layer of the blood vessel; made of mainly elastic connective tissue; allows the vessel to expand to great pressure or volume.

Tunica intima Innermost layer of the blood vessel; composed of a single layer of epithelial cells; provides almost no resistance to blood flow.

Tunica media Middle layer of the blood vessel; mainly composed of smooth muscle; functions to alter the diameter of the lumen of the vessel and is under autonomic control, which enables the body to adjust blood flow quickly to meet immediate needs.

Tunics Layers of an elastic tissue and smooth muscle in the blood vessels.

Tunnel vision Focusing on or considering only one aspect of a situation without first taking into account all possibilities.

Turbinates Large folds found in the nasal cavity; highly vascular area in the nose that warms and humidifies inhaled air.

Turgor Normal tension of a cell or tissue.

Tympanic membrane A thin, translucent, pearly gray oval disk that protects the middle and conducts sound vibrations; eardrum.

Type and crossmatch Mixing a sample of a recipient's and donor's blood to evaluate for incompatibility.

Type I ambulance Regular truck cab and frame with a modular ambulance box mounted on the back.

Type II ambulance Van-style ambulance.

Type III ambulance A van chassis with a modified modular back.

Type IV (quaternary) blast injuries All other miscellaneous injuries caused by an explosive device.

Ulcer A full-thickness crater that involves the dermis and epidermis, with loss of the surface epithelium; this lesion is depressed and may bleed; it usually heals with scarring.

Umbilical An administration route that may be used on a newborn infant; because the umbilical cord was the primary source of nutrient and waste exchange, it provides an immediate source of drug exchange.

Umbilical cord The cord, containing two arteries and a vein, that connects the fetus to the placenta.

Umbilical cord prolapse Appearance of the umbilical cord in front of the presenting part, usually with compression of the cord and interruption of blood supply to the fetus.

Umbilical vein route Route of administration that achieves access through the one umbilical vein set between the two umbilical arteries.

Unethical Conduct that does not conform to moral standards of social or professional behavior.

Unified command Command type involving multiple agencies.

Unintentional injury Injuries and deaths not self-inflicted or perpetrated by another person (accidents).

Unintentional tort A wrong that the defendant did not mean to commit; a case in which a bad outcome occurred because of the failure to exercise reasonable care.

Unipolar lead Lead that consists of a single positive electrode and a reference point; a pacing lead with a single electrical pole at the distal tip of the pacing lead (negative pole) through which the stimulating pulse is delivered. In a permanent pacemaker with a unipolar lead, the positive pole is the pulse generator case.

Unit hour utilization (UhU) A measure of ambulance service productivity and staff workload.

United Nations (UN) number The four-digit number assigned to chemicals during transit by the U.S. Department of Transportation; the *2008 Emergency Guidebook* lists useful information about these chemicals.

Upper airway Portion of the respiratory tract above the glottis.

Upper flammable limit The concentration of fuel in the air above which the vapors cannot be ignited; above this point too much fuel and not enough oxygen are present to burn (too rich); also called the *upper explosive limit.*

Upper respiratory tract infection (URI) Viral syndrome causing nasal congestion, coughing, fever, and runny nose.

Upregulation The process by which a cell increases the number of receptors exposed to a given substance to improve its sensitivity to that substance.

Upstream A term describing the approaching traffic side of the damaged vehicles and the crash scene.

Uremia A term used to describe the signs and symptoms that accompany chronic renal failure.

Uremic frost Dried crystals of urea excreted through the skin that appear to be a frosting on the patient's body.

Ureter A thin-walled pair of tubes that drain urine from each kidney to the bladder.

Urethra Passageway for both urine and male reproductive fluids; opening at the end of the bladder.

Urethral meatus Opening of the urethra between the clitoris and vagina.

Urinary bladder A muscular sac responsible for storing urine before it is eliminated from the body.

Urinary retention The inability to empty the bladder or completely empty the bladder when urinating.

Urinary system Eliminates dissolved organic waste products by urine production and elimination.

Urticaria Also known as *hives;* a skin condition in uhich a wheal on the skin forms from edema; often caused by a reaction to a drug or through contact with substances (skin contact or even inhaled), causing hypersensitivity in the patient.

Uterine cavity Innermost region of the uterus.

Uterine prolapse Protrusion of part or all of the uterus out of the vagina.

Uterine tubes Tubular structures that extend from each side of the superior end of the body of the uterus to the lateral pelvic wall; they pick up the egg released by the ovary and transport it to the uterus; also known as *fallopian tubes.*

Uterus Muscular organ approximately the size of a pear; grows with the developing fetus.

Uvula Fleshy tissue resembling a grape that hangs down from the soft palate.

Vagina Female organ of copulation, the lower part of the birth canal, extending from the uterus to the outside of the body; extends from the cervix to the outside of the body.

Vaginal orifice Opening of the vagina.

Vaginitis An inflammation of the vaginal tissues.

Vallecula The depression or pocket between the base of the tongue and the epiglottis.

Vancomycin-resistant *Enterococcus* Bacteria resistant to vancomycin (a potent antibiotic); commonly acquired by patients in the hospital or patients who have indwelling catheters.

Vapor density The weight of a volume of pure gas compared with the weight of an equal volume of pure dry air (which has a constant value of 1); materials with a vapor density less than 1.0 are lighter than air and rise when released; materials with a vapor density greater than 1.0 are heavier than air and sink when released.

Vapor pressure The pressure exerted by a vapor against the sides of a closed container; a measure of volatility—high vapor pressure means it is a volatile substance.

Varicella An acute contagious vesicular skin eruption caused by the varicella zoster virus (chickenpox).

Varices Distended veins.

Varicocele Dilation of the venous plexus and internal spermatic vein, presenting as a lump in the scrotum.

Variola major A member of the *orthopoxvirus* family that causes the most common form of smallpox; the most likely form of the organism to be used as a weapon.

Vas deferens Tubes that extend from the end of the epididymis and through the seminal vesicles; also known as the *ductus deferens.*

Vascular access device Type of intravenous device used to deliver fluids, medications, blood, or nutritional therapy; usually inserted in patients who require long-term intravenous therapy.

Vascular headaches Headaches that involve changes in the diameter or size and chemistry of blood vessels that supply the brain.

Vascular resistance Amount of opposition that the blood vessels give to the flow of blood.

Vascular tunic Layer of the eye that contains most of the vasculature of the eye.

Vector A mode of transmission of a disease, typically from an insect or animal.

Vegetative functions Autonomic functions the body requires to survive.

Vehicle hazards Hazards directly related to the vehicle itself, including undeployed airbags; fuel system concerns; electrical system and battery electricity; stability of the vehicle; sharp glass and metal; leaking hot antifreeze; and engine oil, transmission oil, or antifreeze spills. Even the contents inside a vehicle's trunk or cargo area are typical vehicle hazards that can be encountered.

Vehicle stabilization Immediate action taken to prevent any unwanted movement of a crash-damaged vehicle.

Vena cava One of two large veins returning blood from the peripheral circulation to the right atrium of the heart.

Venipuncture Piercing of a vein.

Venom The poison injected by venomous animals such as snakes, insects, and marine creatures.

Venous return Amount of blood flowing into the right atrium each minute from the systemic circulation.

Ventilation The mechanical process of moving air into and out of the lungs.

Ventral Referring to the front of the body; anterior.

Ventricles Either of the two lower chambers in the heart.

Ventricular fibrillation Disorganized electrical activity of the ventricular conduction system of the heart, resulting in inefficient contractile force. This is the main cause of sudden cardiac death in electrical injuries.

Venules Small venous vessels that return blood to the capillaries.

Verbal apraxia Speech disorder in which the person has difficulty saying what he or she wants to say in a correct and consistent manner.

Verbal stimulus Any noise that elicits some sort of response from the patient.

Vertebrae Specialized bones comprising the spinal column.

Vertebral foramen Open space in the middle of vertebra.

Vertigo An out-of-control spinning sensation not relieved by lying down that may get worse when the eyes are closed.

Very high frequency A type of radio signal used to make two-way radio contact between the communications center and the responders. Now considered old technology compared with more contemporary 800-MHz radio systems.

Vesicants Agents named from the most obvious injury they inflict on a person; will burn and blister the skin or any other part of the body they touch; also known as *blister agents* or *mustard agents.*

Vesicles The "shipping containers" of the cell. They are simple in structure, consisting of a single membrane filled with liquid; they transport a wide variety of substances both inside and outside the cell.

Vestibule Space or cavity that serves as the entrance to the inner ear.

Veterinary medical assistance team Teams designed to provide animal care and assistance during disasters.

Vials Glass containers with rubber stoppers at the top.

Viral hemorrhagic fevers A group of viral diseases of diverse etiology (arenaviruses, filoviruses, bunyaviruses, and flaviviruses) having many similar characteristics, including increased capillary permeability, leukopenia, and thrombocytopenia, resulting in a severe multisystem syndrome.

Viral shedding Release of viruses from an infected host through some vector (e.g., sneezing, coughing, bleeding).

Virions Small particles of viruses.

Virulence A term to refer to the relative pathogenicity or the relative ability to do damage to the host of an infectious agent.

Virus Microorganism that invades cells and uses their machinery to live and replicate; cannot survive without a host, does not have a cell wall of its own, and consists of a strand of DNA or RNA surrounded by a capsid.

Visceral Portion of the peripheral nervous system that processes motor and sensory information from the internal organs; includes the autonomic nervous system.

Visceral pain Deep pain that arises from internal areas of the body that are enclosed within a cavity.

Visceral pleura Lining of the pleural cavity that adheres tightly to the lung surface.

Viscosity The thickness of a liquid; a high-viscosity liquid does not flow easily (e.g., oils and tar); a low-viscosity liquid flows easily (e.g., gasoline) and poses a greater risk for aspiration and consequent pulmonary damage.

Visual acuity card A standardized board used to test vision.

Vitreous chamber The most posterior chamber of the eyeball.

Vitreous humor Thick, jellylike substance that fills the vitreous chamber of the eyeball.

Voice over Internet protocol Telephone technology that gives Internet users the ability to make voice telephone calls.

Volatility A measure of how quickly a material passes into the vapor or gas state; the greater the volatility, the greater its rate of evaporation.

Volkmann contracture A deformity of the hand, fingers, and wrist caused by injury to the muscles of the forearm; also known as *ischemic contracture.*

Voltage Difference in electrical charge between two points.

Volume of packed red cells A measure of the relative percentage of blood cells (mainly erythrocytes) in a given volume of whole blood; also called *hematocrit* or *packed cell volume.*

Voluntary guarding Conscious contraction of the abdominal muscles in an attempt to prevent painful palpation.

Volvulus Intestinal obstruction caused by a knotting and twisting of the bowel.

Vomiting Forceful ejection of stomach contents through the mouth.

Vowel The letters *a*, *e*, *i*, *o*, *u*, and sometimes *y.*

Vulva The region of the external genital organs of the female, including the labia majora, labia minora, mons publis, clitoris, and vagina.

Vulvovaginitis Inflammation of the external female genitalia and vagina.

VX Most toxic of the nerve agent class of military warfare agents.

Warm zone Area surrounding the hot zone that functions as a safety buffer area, decontamination area, and as an access and egress point to and from the hot zone; also called the *contamination reduction zone.*

Warts Benign lesions caused by the papillomavirus.

Washout phase Vascular response in shock when postcapillary sphincters open, allowing fluid in the capillary beds to be pushed into systemic circulation; follows the stagnant phase.

Water solubility The degree to which a material or its vapors are soluble in water.

Water-reactive materials Materials that violently decompose and/or burn vigorously when they come in contact with moisture.

Waveform Movement away from the baseline in either a positive or negative direction.

Wernicke-Korsakoff syndrome Neurologic disorder caused by a thiamine deficiency; most often seen in chronic alcoholics; characterized by ataxia, nystagmus, weakness, and mental derangement in the early stages. In later stages, the condition is much more likely to become permanent and is characterized by amnesia, disorientation, delirium, and hallucinations.

Wheal A firm, rounded, flat-topped elevation of skin that is evanescent and pruritic (itches); also known as a *hive.*

Wheeze A musical, whistling sound heard on inspiration and/or expiration resulting from constriction or obstruction of the pharynx, trachea, or bronchi. Wheezing is commonly associated with asthma.

Wilderness command physician A physician who has received additional training by a Wilderness Emergency Medical Services Institute–endorsed course in wilderness medical care and medical direction of wilderness EMS providers and operations.

Wilderness emergency medical technician An emergency medical technician who has obtained EMT certification by Department of Transportation criteria and has completed additional modules in wilderness care; sometimes abbreviated as WEMT, W-EMT, or EMT-W.

Wilderness EMS An individual or group that preplans to administer care in an austere environment and then is called on to perform these duties when needed.

Wilderness EMS system A formally structured organization integrated into or part of the standard EMS system and configured to provide wilderness medical care to a discrete region.

Wilderness first aid A level of certification indicating a provider has been trained in traditional first aid with added training in wilderness care and first aid administration in austere environments.

Wilderness first responder A first responder who has obtained certification by Department of Transportation criteria and has completed additional modules in wilderness care.

Wilderness medicine Medical management in situations where care and prevention are limited by environmental considerations, prolonged extrication, or resource availability.

Window phase The period after infection during which the antigen is present but no antibody is detectable.

Withdrawal Physical and/or psychological signs and symptoms that result from discontinuing regular administration of a drug; effects are usually the opposite of the effects of the drug itself because the body has changed itself to maintain homeostasis.

Wolff-Parkinson-White syndrome Type of preexcitation syndrome characterized by a slurred upstroke of the QRS complex (delta wave) and wide QRS.

Word root The foundation of a word; establishes the basic meaning of a word.

Word salad The most severe form of looseness of associations in which the topic shifts so rapidly that it interrupts the flow of sentences themselves, producing a jumble of words.

Workload management Planning resources and support services around demand.

Wrap point A machinery entanglement hazard formed when any machine component rotates.

Xenografting Transplanting tissue from a member of a different species (e.g., porcine heart valves harvested from pigs).

Years of potential life lost (YPLL) A method that assumes that, on average, most people will live a productive life until the age of 65 years.

Yeast A unicellular type of fungus that reproduces by budding.

Yersinia pestis The anaerobic, gram-negative bacterium that causes plague disease in human beings and rodents.

Zone of coagulation In a full-thickness burn wound, the central area of the burn devoid of blood flow. This tissue is not salvageable and becomes visibly necrotic days after the injury.

Zone of stasis or ischemia Outside the zone of coagulation, where blood supply is tenuous. The capillaries may be damaged but oxygenated blood can still pass through them to perfuse the surrounding tissues.

Illustration Credits

Chapter 35

Figures 35-1, 35-2. Lowdermilk, D. L., & Perry, S. E. (2004). *Maternity and women's health care* (8th ed.). St. Louis: Mosby.

Figures 35-3, 35-6, 35-7, 35-8, 35-9, 35-10, 35-13. McSwain, N. E. (2003). *The basic EMT: Comprehensive prehospital care* (2nd ed.). St. Louis: Mosby.

Figures 35-4, 35-12. Chapleau, W. (2007). *Emergency first responder: Making the difference.* St. Louis: Mosby.

Figure 35-5. Seidel, H., Ball, J., Dains, J., Benedict, G. W. (2006). *Mosby's guide to physical examination* (6th ed.). St. Louis: Mosby.

Figure 35-11. Roberts, J., & Hedges, J. (2003). *Clinical procedures in emergency medicine* (4th ed.). Philadelphia: Saunders.

Figure 35-14. Shade, B., Collins, T., Wertz, E., Jones, S. A., & Rothenberg, M. A. (2007). *Mosby's EMT-Intermediate textbook for the 1999 National Standard Curriculum* (3rd ed.). St. Louis: Mosby/JEMS.

Figure 35-15. Chapleau, W., & Pons, P. (2007). *Emergency medical technician: Making the difference.* St. Louis: Mosby/JEMS.

Chapter 36

Figures 36-1, A and B; 36-12. Thibodeau, G. A., & Patton, K. T. (2004). *Structure and function of the body* (12th ed.). St. Louis: Mosby.

Figure 36-2. Thibodeau, G., & Patton, K. (2005). *The human body in health and disease* (4th ed.). St. Louis: Mosby.

Figures 36-3, A and B; 36-5; 36-7, A; 36-9, A and B; 36-19; 36-20. Zitelli, B., & Davis, H. (2002). *Atlas of pediatric physical diagnosis* (4th ed.). St. Louis: Mosby.

Figure 36-4, A, B, and C. Zitelli, B., & Davis, H. (2002). *Atlas of pediatric physical diagnosis* (4th ed.). St. Louis: Mosby. Courtesy Christine Williams.

Figures 36-6, B; 36-7, B. Chaudhry, B., & Harvey, D. (2001). *Mosby's color atlas and text of pediatrics and child health* (4th ed.). Oxford: Mosby Ltd.

Figure 36-8, A and B. Cummings, C. W., Haughey, B. H., Thomas, J. R., Harker, L. A., Robbins, K. T., Schuller, D. E., et al. (2005). *Cummings otolaryngology, head and neck surgery* (4th ed.). St. Louis: Mosby.

Figures 36-10; 36-11; 36-13, A and B. Aehlert, B. (2007). *Mosby's comprehensive pediatric emergency care* (Rev. ed.). St. Louis: Mosby.

Figure 36-17, A and B. Henry, M., & Stapleton, E. (2007). *EMT prehospital care* (3rd ed.). St. Louis: Mosby/JEMS.

Figures 36-14, 36-15. Chapleau, W., & Pons, P. (2007). *Emergency medical technician: making the difference.* St. Louis: Mosby/JEMS.

Chapter 37

Figures 37-1; 37-7, A; 37-8; 37-14; 37-15; 37-16. Aehlert, B. (2007). *Mosby's comprehensive pediatric emergency care* (Rev. ed.). St. Louis: Mosby.

Figure 37-2, 37-10, 37-12, 37-17, 37-22, 37-23. Zitelli, B., & Davis, H. (2002). *Atlas of pediatric physical diagnosis* (4th ed.). St. Louis: Mosby.

Figure 37-3, 37-21. Hockenberry, M., & Wilson, D. (2007). *Wong's nursing care of infants and children* (8th ed.). St. Louis: Mosby.

Figure 37-4, 37-11. Seidel, H., Ball, J., Dains, J., et al. (2002). *Mosby's guide to physical examination* (5th ed.). St. Louis: Mosby.

Figures 37-5, 37-6. National Association of Emergency Medical Technicians. (2007). *PHTLS prehospital trauma life support* (6th ed.). St. Louis: Mosby.

Figures 37-7, B and C; 37-9, B. EMSC Slide Set. (1996). Courtesy the Emergency Medical Services for Children Program, administered by the U.S. Department of Health and Human Services Health Resources and Services Administration, Maternal and Child Health Bureau.

Figure 37-9, A. Dieckman, R. A., Fiser, D. H., & Selbst, S. M. (1996). *Illustrated textbook of pediatric emergency & critical care procedures.* St. Louis: Mosby–Year Book.

Figure 37-13. Aehlert, B. (2004). *ECGs Made easy study cards* (2nd ed.). St. Louis: Mosby.

Figures 37-18, 37-19, 37-20, 37-24. Shade, B., Collins, T., Wertz, E., et al. (2002). *Mosby's EMT-Intermediate textbook for the 1999 National Standard Curriculum* (2nd ed.). St. Louis: Mosby/JEMS.

Figure 37-21. Wong-Baker FACES Pain Scale.

Figures 37-25, 37-26. Cohen, J., & Powderly, W. G. (2004). *Infectious diseases* (2nd ed.). St. Louis: Mosby.

Chapter 39

Figures 39-1, 39-5. Courtesy Duluth Domestic Abuse Intervention Project, MN.

Figures 39-2, 39-3, 39-4, 39-9. Polsky, S. S., & Markowitz, J. *Color atlas of domestic violence.* St. Louis: Mosby.

Figures 39-6, 39-7, A and B. Zitelli, B., & Davis, H. (2002). *Atlas of pediatric diagnosis* (4th ed.). St. Louis: Mosby.

Figure 39-7, C. Courtesy Kent Hymel.

Figures 39-8, 39-10. Girardin, B. W., Faugno, D. K., Seneski, P. C., et al. (1998). *Color atlas of sexual assault.* St. Louis: Mosby.

Chapter 40

Figures 40-1, 40-4. EMSC slide set (CD-ROM), 1996. Courtesy Emergency Medical Services for Children Program, administered y the U.S. Department of Health and Human Services Health Resources and Services Administration, Maternal and Child Health Bureau.

Figure 40-3. Courtesy PMT/Permark Corporation, New York.

Figure 40-5. Chaudhry, B., & Harvey, D. (2001). *Mosby's color atlas and text of pediatrics and child health* (4th ed.). Oxford: Mosby Ltd.

Figures 40-6, 40-7, 40-8. Zitelli, B., & Davis, H. (2002). *Atlas of pediatric physical diagnosis* (4th ed.). St. Louis: Mosby.

Chapter 41

Figures 41-1, 41-2. Copyright 2007 Jupiter Images Corporation.

Chapter 42

Figure 42-1. Sorrentino, S., & Gorek, B. (2007). *Mosby's textbook for long-term care nursing assistants* (5th ed.). St. Louis: Mosby.

Figures 42-2, 42-4. Birchenall, J., & Straight, E. (2003). *Mosby's textbook for the home care aide* (2nd ed.). St. Louis: Mosby.

Figures 42-3, 42-6, 42-8, 42-14. Courtesy Nellcor Puritan Bennett, Pleasanton, CA.

Figures 42-5, 42-20, 42-21, 42-25. Hockenberry, M. J., & Wilson, D. (2003). *Wong's nursing care of infants and children* (7th ed.). St. Louis: Mosby.

Figure 42-7. Roberts, J., & Hedges, J. (2003). *Clinical procedures in emergency medicine* (4th ed.). Philadelphia: Saunders.

Figure 42-9. Newport HT51 ventilator courtesy Newport Medical Instruments, Inc., Costa Mesa, CA.

Figure 42-10. Esprit critical care ventilator courtesy of Respironics, Inc., Murrysville, PA.

Figure 42-11. Image of SmartMonitor 2 provided by Children's Medical Ventures, a subsidiary of Respironics, Inc., Murrysville, PA.

Figures 42-13, 42-26. Henry, M., & Stapleton, E. (2007). *EMT prehospital care* (3rd ed.). St. Louis: Mosby/JEMS.

Figures 42-15, 42-17. Dieckman, R. A., Fiser, D. H., & Selbst, S. M. (1996). *Illustrated textbook of pediatric emergency & critical care procedures.* St. Louis: Mosby–Year Book.

Figure 42-16. McSwain, N. E. (2003). *The basic EMT: Comprehensive prehospital care* (2nd ed.). St. Louis: Mosby.

Figure 42-22. Courtesy Cook Incorporated, Bloomington, IN.

Figures 42-23, 42-24, 42-28, 42-29, 42-31, 42-32. deWit, S. (2005). *Fundamental concepts and skills for nursing* (2nd ed.). Philadelphia: Saunders.

Figure 42-27. Chaudhry, B., & Harvey, D. (2001). *Mosby's color atlas and text of pediatrics and child health* (4th ed.). Oxford: Mosby Ltd.

Figure 42-30. Leahy, J. M., & Kizilay, P. E. (1998). *Foundation of nursing: A nursing process approach.* Philadelphia: W. B. Saunders.

Chapter 43

Figures 43-1, 43-3, 43-4, 43-7, 43-8, 43-9, 43-11, 43-15, 43-23, 43-24, 43-26, 43-27, 43-30. National Association of Medical Technicians. (2007). *PHTLS prehospital trauma life support* (6th ed.). St. Louis: Mosby.

Figures 43-2, 43-6, 43-10, 43-13, 43-14, 43-17, 43-20, 43-25, 43-28, 43-29, 43-31. McSwain, N. E. (2003). *The basic EMT: Comprehensive prehospital care* (2nd ed.). St. Louis: Mosby.

Figure 43-16. National Association of Emergency Medical Technicians. (2007). *PHTLS prehospital trauma life support* (6th ed.). St. Louis: Mosby.

Figures 43-18, 43-19. Drake, R., Vogl, W., & Mitchell, A. (2005). *Gray's anatomy for students.* New York: Churchill Livingstone.

Figure 43-21. Currance, P. (2005). *Medical response to weapons of mass destruction.* St. Louis: Mosby.

Chapter 45

Figure 45-1. Courtesy Associated Bag Company, 400 West Boden Street, Milwaukee, WI 53207.

Figures 45-4, 45-5. Drake, R., Vogl, W., & Mitchell, A. (2005). *Gray's anatomy for students.* New York: Churchill Livingstone.

Figure 45-6. Trott, A. (2005). *Wounds and lacerations: Emergency care and closure* (3rd ed.). St. Louis: Mosby.

Figures 45-7, 45-10, 45-13, 45-15, 45-16, 45-18, 45-20. Heuther, S., & McCance, K. (2004). *Understanding pathophysiology* (3rd ed.). St. Louis: Mosby.

Figures 45-8, 45-21, 45-23. Courtesy Department of Dermatology, School of Medicine, University of Utah.

Figure 45-9. Goldman, M. P., Fitzpatrick, R. E. (1998). *Cutaneous laser surgery: the art and science of selective photothermolysis* (2nd ed.). St. Louis: Mosby.

Figures 45-11, 45-12, 45-14, 45-17, 45-19. Henry, M., & Stapleton, E. (2007). *EMT prehospital care* (3rd ed.). St. Louis, Mosby.

Figure 45-22. Habif, T. B. (1996). *Clinical dermatology: A color guide to diagnosis and therapy* (3rd ed.). St. Louis: Mosby.

Figure 45-24. Modified from Stern, P. J. (1999). Fractures of the metacarpals and phalanges. In D. P. Green (Ed.), *Green's operative hand surgery* (4th ed.). New York: Churchill Livingstone.

Figures 45-25, 45-27, Marx, J., Hockberger, R., & Walls, R. (2006). *Rosen's emergency medicine: Concepts and clinical practice* (6th ed., Vol. 1). St. Louis: Mosby.

Figure 45-26. Crenshaw, A. H. (Ed.) (1992). *Campbell's operative orthopedics* (8th ed.). St. Louis: Mosby.

Figure 45-28. Green, D. P. (Ed.) (1993). *Operative hand surgery* (3rd ed.). New York: Churchill Livingstone.

Chapter 46

Figure 46-1. Chapleau, W., & Pons, P. (2007). *Emergency medical technician: Making the difference.* St. Louis: Mosby/JEMS.

Figures 46-2, 46-9. National Association of Emergency Medical Technicians. (2007). *PHTLS prehospital trauma life support* (6th ed.). St. Louis: Mosby.

Figure 46-7. Marx, J., Hockberger, R., & Walls, R. (2006). *Rosen's emergency medicine: Concepts and clinical practice* (6th ed.). St. Louis: Mosby.

Chapter 47

Figures 47-1, 47-2, 47-3, 47-4, 47-6, 47-7, 47-8, 47-11, 47-14, 47-15, 47-19, 47-20, 47-21, 47-24, 47-25, 47-26. Drake, R., Vogl, W., & Mitchell, A. (2005). *Gray's anatomy for students.* New York: Churchill Livingstone.

Figure 47-5. Marx, J., Hockberger, R., & Walls, R. (2006). *Rosen's emergency medicine: Concepts and clinical practice* (6th ed., Vol. 2). St. Louis: Mosby.

Figure 47-9. Zitelli, B., & Davis, H. (2002). *Atlas of pediatric physical diagnosis* (4th ed.). St. Louis: Mosby.

Figure 47-10. Cummings, C. W., Haughey, B. H., Thomas, J. R., et al. (2005). *Cummings otolaryngology, head and neck surgery* (4th ed.). St. Louis: Mosby.

Figures 47-12, 47-13, 47-27, 47-28. Herlihy, B. (2007). *The human body in health and illness* (3rd ed.). Philadelphia: Saunders.

Figures 47-16, 47-18, 47-30. Seidel, H., Ball, J., Dains, J., et al. (2002). *Mosby's guide to physical examination* (5th ed.). St. Louis: Mosby.

Figures 47-22, 47-23, 47-29. Gould, B. E. (2006). *Pathophysiology for the health professions* (3rd ed.). Philadelphia: Saunders.

Skill 47-2. National Association of Emergency Medical Technicians. (2007). *PHTLS prehospital trauma life support* (6th ed.). St. Louis: Mosby.

Chapter 48

Figures 48-2, 48-3, 48-4, 48-5, 48-7, 48-8. Drake, R., Vogl, W., & Mitchell, A. (2005). *Gray's anatomy for students.* New York: Churchill Livingstone.

Figure 48-6. Thibodeau, G., & Patton, K. (2005). *The human body in health and disease* (4th ed.). St. Louis: Mosby.

Figure 48-17, A. Henry, M., & Stapleton, E. (2007). *EMT prehospital care* (3rd ed.). St. Louis: Mosby/JEMS.

Figure 48-17, B and C. Stoy, W., Platt, T., & Lejeune, D. (2007). *Mosby's EMT-Basic textbook* (2nd ed.). St. Louis: Mosby/JEMS.

Figure 48-17, A. National Association of Emergency Medical Technicians. (2007). *PHTLS prehospital trauma life support* (6th ed.). St. Louis: Mosby.

Skill 48-4. Chapleau, W., Pons, P. (2007). *Emergency medical technician: Making the difference.* St. Louis: Mosby.

Chapter 49

Figure 49-1. Green, N., & Swiontkowski, M. (2003). *Skeletal trauma in children* (3rd ed.). Philadelphia: Saunders.

Figures 49-2, 49-4, 49-7, 49-8, 49-10. Marx, J., Hockberger, R., & Walls, R. (2006). *Rosen's emergency medicine: Concepts and clinical practice* (6th ed.). St. Louis: Mosby.

Figure 49-3. Ferrera, P., Colucciello, S. A., Marx, J., et al. (2001). *Trauma management: An emergency medicine approach.* St. Louis: Mosby.

Figure 49-5. National Association of Emergency Medical Technicians. (2007). *PHTLS prehospital trauma life support* (6th ed.). St. Louis: Mosby.

Figure 49-6. Auerbach, P. (2007). *Wilderness medicine* (5th ed.). St. Louis: Mosby.

Figure 49-11. Modified from Townsend, C. M., Beauchamp, D., Evers, M., et al. (2004). *Sabiston textbook of surgery: The biological basis of modern surgical practice* (17th ed.). Philadelphia: Saunders.

Chapter 50

Figures 50-1, 50-3. Drake, R., Vogl, W., & Mitchell, A. (2005). *Gray's anatomy for students.* New York: Churchill Livingstone.

Figure 50-2. Modified from Drake, R., Vogl, W., & Mitchell, A. (2005). *Gray's anatomy for students.* New York: Churchill Livingstone.

Figure 50-4. Grieg, J. D. (1996). *Color atlas of surgical diagnosis* (2nd ed.). London: Mosby/Wolfe.

Figure 50-5. Jarvis, C. (2004). *Physical examination and health assessment* (4th ed.). Philadelphia: Saunders.

Chapter 51

Figures 51-4, 51-5, 51-6. Drake, R., Vogl, W., & Mitchell, A. (2005). *Gray's anatomy for students.* New York: Churchill Livingstone.

Figure 51-7. Leonard, P. (2005). *Building a medical vocabulary* (6th ed.). Philadelphia: Saunders.

Figure 51-8. Barkin, R., & Rosen, P. (2004). *Emergency pediatrics: A guide to ambulatory care* (6th ed.). St. Louis: Mosby.

Figure 51-9. Canale, S. T. (1998). *Operative orthopedics* (9th ed.). St. Louis: Mosby.

Figures 51-12, 51-17, 51-19, 51-22. Chapleau, W., & Pons, P. (2007). *Emergency medical technician: Making the difference.* St. Louis: Mosby/JEMS.

Figures 51-18, 51-20. Mettler, F. (2004). *Essentials of radiology* (2nd ed.). Philadelphia: Saunders.

Figure 51-23; Skill 51-1. Shade, B., Collins, T., Wertz, E., Jones, S. A., Rothenberg, M. A. (2007). *Mosby's EMT-Intermediate textbook for the 1999 National Standard Curriculum* (3rd ed.). St. Louis: Mosby/JEMS.

Chapter 52

Figures 52-1, 52-2. Courtesy National Weather Service, Pueblo, CO.

Figure 52-3. Auerbach, P. (2007). *Wilderness medicine* (5th ed.). St. Louis: Mosby.

Box 52-17. Courtesy Divers Alert Network, Durham, NC.

Chapter 53

Figures 53-1, 53-4, 53-5, 53-6, 53-9, 53-10. Courtesy David Oliver, Emergency Services Rescue Training, Inc.

Figure 53-2. Copyright 2007 Jupiter Images Corporation.

Figures 53-3, 53-7, 53-8, 53-14, 53-15, 53-16, 53-17, 53-18, 53-19. Courtesy Pennsylvania State University, State College, PA.

Chapter 54

Figure 54-1. Vines, T., & Hudson, S. (2005). *High angle rescue techniques* (3rd ed.), St. Louis: Mosby.

Figure 54-2. National Association of Emergency Medical Technicians. (2007). *PHTLS prehospital trauma life support* (6th ed.). St. Louis: Mosby.

Chapter 57

Figure 57-4. Courtesy Datascope Corporation, Montvale, NJ.

Figure 57-5. Lewis, S. M., Heitkemper, M. M., Dirksen, S. R. (2000). *Medical-surgical nursing: Assessment and management of clinical problems (5th ed.).* St. Louis, Mosby.

Figure 57-6. Courtesy Robert Vroman.

Figures 57-7, 57-8. Chapleau, W., & Pons, P. (2007). *Emergency medical technician: Making the difference.* St. Louis: Mosby/JEMS.

Chapter 60

Figure 60-1. Chapleau, W., & Pons, P. (2007). *Emergency medical technician: Making the difference.* St. Louis: Mosby/JEMS.

Figure 60-2. Henry, M., & Stapleton, E. (2007). *EMT prehospital care* (3rd ed.). St. Louis: Mosby/JEMS.

Chapter 61

Figures 61-1, 61-2, 61-4, 61-5. Henry, M., & Stapleton, E. (2007). *EMT prehospital care* (3rd ed.). St. Louis: Mosby/JEMS.

Figure 61-6. McSwain, N. E. (2003). *The basic EMT: Comprehensive prehospital care* (2nd ed.). St. Louis: Mosby.

Chapter 62

Figures 62-1, 62-2, 62-3. U.S. Department of Homeland Security: *FEMA 511: National Incident Management System,* draft, August 2007.

Figures 62-4, 62-5. Henry, M., & Stapleton, E. (2007). *EMT prehospital care* (3rd ed.). St. Louis: Mosby/JEMS.

Chapter 63

Figure 63-1. Courtesy Todd Hoffman.

Figure 63-3. Moore, R. E. (2003). *Vehicle rescue and extrication* (2nd ed.). St. Louis: Mosby.

Figures 63-4 63-5, 63-6, 63-7, 63-8, 63-9, 63-10, 63-11, 63-12, 63-13, 63-14, 63-15, 63-16, 63-17, 63-18, 63-19. Courtesy Ron Moore.

Figure 63-22. Centers for Disease Control and Prevention, National Institute for Occupational Safety and Health: *Electronic Library of Construction Occupational Safety and Health.* Available at: www.cdc.gov/eLCOSH.

Figure 63-23. U.S. Department of Labor, Occupational Safety and Health Administration. (1999). *OSHA technical manual, section V, chapter 2: Excavations: hazard recognition in trenching and shoring.*

Figures 63-24, 63-25, 63-27, 63-28, 63-29, 63-30, 63-31, 63-32, 63-33. Vines, T., & Hudson, S. (2005). *High angle rescue techniques* (3rd ed.). St. Louis: Mosby.

Figure 63-26. Courtesy Skedco, Inc., Tualatin, OR.

Chapter 64

Figures 64-1, 64-2, 64-3, 64-4, 64-5, 64-6, 64-7, 64-8, 64-9, 64-10, 64-11, 64-12, 64-14, 64-16, 64-17, 64-18, 64-19, 64-20, 64-21, 64-22, 64-23, 64-24, 64-28, 64-29, 64-30, 64-31, 64-32, 64-34, 64-35, 64-36, 64-37. Currance, P., & Bronstein, A. C. (1999). *Hazardous materials for EMS: Practices and procedures.* St. Louis: Mosby. Photographs courtesy Phil Currance.

Figures 64-13, 64-15, 64-25, 64-27. Modified from Currance, P., & Bronstein, A. C. (1999). *Hazardous materials for EMS: Practices and procedures.* St. Louis: Mosby.

Figure 64-26. Chapleau, W., & Pons, P. (2007). *Emergency medical technician: Making the difference.* St. Louis: Mosby/JEMS.

Chapter 65

Figures 65-2, 65-6, 65-7, 65-8. Courtesy North American Rescue Products, Inc., Greer, SC.

Chapter 66

Figures 66-1, 66-2. Courtesy Phil Currance.

Figure 66-3. Currance, P. (2005). *Medical response to weapons of mass destruction.* St. Louis: Mosby/JEMS.

Figures 66-4, 66-6. Courtesy Phil Currance.

Figures 66-7, 66-13. Courtesy Medical Management of Chemical Casualties.

Figure 66-8. Courtesy Lana Blackwell.

Figures 66-9, 66-10, 66-11. Courtesy Centers for Disease Control and Prevention, Public Health Image Library.

Figure 66-12. Courtesy National Audiovisual Center, Department of Commerce, Springfield, VA.

Index

Page numbers followed by f, t, or b indicate figures, tables, or boxed material, respectively. Numbers in **boldface** indicate volume number.

J

M

O

Q

R

S

X

Y